a LANGE medical book

AF767044

ENDOCRINE SURGERY: Clinical Diagnosis and Management

Edited by

Alexander Shifrin, MD, FACS, FACE, ECNU, FEBS (Endocrine Surgery), FISS
Surgical Director of Endocrinology
Statesir Cancer Center
Atlantic Health, CentraState Medical Center
Freehold, New Jersey

Thomas J. Fahey, III, MD, FACS
Johnson and Johnson Professor
Vice-Chair, Department of Surgery
Chief, Endocrine Surgery
Director, Endocrine Oncology Program
The New York Presbyterian Hospital-Weill Cornell Medical Center
New York, New York

Mc Graw Hill

Endocrine Surgery: Clinical Diagnosis and Management

1 2 3 4 5 6 7 8 9 DSS 29 28 27 26 25 24

ISBN 978-1-26465714-8
MHID 1-264-65714-5

Notice

Medicine is an ever-changing science. As new research and clinical experience broaden our knowledge, changes in treatment and drug therapy are required. The authors and the publisher of this work have checked with sources believed to be reliable in their efforts to provide information that is complete and generally in accord with the standards accepted at the time of publication. However, in view of the possibility of human error or changes in medical sciences, neither the authors nor the publisher nor any other party who has been involved in the preparation or publication of this work warrants that the information contained herein is in every respect accurate or complete, and they disclaim all responsibility for any errors or omissions or for the results obtained from use of the information contained in this work. Readers are encouraged to confirm the information contained herein with other sources.

This book was set in Minion Pro by KnowledgeWorks Global Ltd.
The editors were Sydney Keen Vitale and Kim J. Davis.
The production supervisor was Catherine Saggese.
Project management was provided by Revathi Viswanathan of KnowledgeWorks Global Ltd.

This book is printed on acid-free paper.

Library of Congress Cataloging-in-Publication Data

Names: Shifrin, Alexander, editor. | Fahey, Thomas J., III, editor.
Title: Endocrine surgery : clinical diagnosis and management / edited by Alexander Shifrin, Thomas J Fahey, III.
Other titles: Endocrine surgery (Shifrin)
Description: New York : McGraw Hill, [2025] | Includes bibliographical references and index. | Summary: "This book provides a concise introduction to clinical diagnosis and management for endocrine diseases of the thyroid, parathyroid, adrenal glands, and pancreas"—Provided by publisher.
Identifiers: LCCN 2023049815 (print) | LCCN 2023049816 (ebook) | ISBN 9781264657148 (paperback ; alk. paper) | ISBN 9781264657476 (ebook)
Subjects: MESH: Endocrine Surgical Procedures | Endocrine System Diseases—surgery | Endocrine Glands—surgery
Classification: LCC RD599 (print) | LCC RD599 (ebook) | NLM WK 148 | DDC 617.4/4—dc23/eng/20240228
LC record available at https://lccn.loc.gov/2023049815
LC ebook record available at https://lccn.loc.gov/2023049816

To everyone involved in the surgical and medical care of patients with endocrine gland diseases; to all endocrine surgeons, head and neck surgeons, otolaryngology surgeons, surgical oncologists, general surgeons, endocrinologists, medical oncologists, and other health-care providers devoting their lives to cure patients with endocrine diseases.

To our families, our loved ones, and our children, supporting us and patiently waiting for us to complete this book.

To our teachers, who taught us the science of medicine and surgery.

To all of the patients we had the pleasure of caring for, we learned from them and presented some of their cases in this book.

Contents

PART C. PARATHYROID

PART D. ADRENALS

PART H. FAMILIAL ENDOCRINE SYNDROMES

PART I. ENDOCRINE EMERGENCIES

Contributors

Amr H. Abdelhamid, MBBCH, MMSc
Division of Thyroid and Parathyroid Endocrine Surgery
Department of Otolaryngology—Head and Neck Surgery
Massachusetts Eye and Ear Infirmary
Harvard Medical School
Boston, Massachusetts

Dev Abraham, MD, MRCP (UK)
Professor
Division of Endocrinology, Metabolism and Diabetes
University of Utah School of Medicine and Huntsman Cancer Institute
Salt Lake City, Utah

Arthur G. Affleck III, MD
Department of General Surgery
Oregon Health Sciences University General Surgery Residency
Portland, Oregon

Ahmed Ahmed, MD
Division of Endocrine and Metabolic Disorders
Department of Internal Medicine
Eastern Virginia Medical School
Norfolk, Virginia

Tobias Åkerström, MD, PhD
Department of Surgical Sciences
Uppsala University
Uppsala, Sweden

John D. Allendorf, MD
Chair, Department of Surgery
Chief, Endocrine Surgery
NYU Grossman Long Island School of Medicine
Mineola, New York

Wilson M. Alobuia, MD, MS
General Surgery Resident
Department of Surgery
Stanford University School of Medicine
Stanford, California

Defne Altan, AB
Department of Surgery
Massachusetts General Hospital
Boston, Massachusetts

Peter Angelos, MD, PhD
Department of Surgery
MacLean Center for Clinical Medical Ethics
University of Chicago
Chicago, Illinois

Megan K. Applewhite, MD
Faculty, Endocrine Surgery
Albany Medical Center
Albany, New York

Aljehani Ashwaq, MD
University of Lorraine
Department of Surgery (CVMC)
Unit of Endocrine, Thyroid and Metabolic Surgery, and INSERM
CHRU Nancy—Hospital Brabois Adultes
Nancy, France
Department of Surgery
Imam Mohammad Ibn Saud Islamic University (IMSIU) College of Medicine
Riyadh, Saudi Arabia

Sara Abou Azar, MD
Endocrine Surgery Fellow
University of Chicago Medicine
Chicago, Illinois

Marisa A. Bartz-Kurycki, MD, MS
Medical College of Wisconsin
Milwaukee, Wisconsin

Andrew J. Bauer, MD
Director, The Thyroid Center
Division of Endocrinology and Diabetes
Children's Hospital of Philadelphia
Professor of Pediatrics
Department of Pediatrics
Perelman School of Medicine
University of Pennsylvania
Philadelphia, Pennsylvania

Kamal Bhusal, MD, FACE
Associated Professor of Clinical Medicine
Program Director of Fellowship in Endocrinology, Diabetes and Metabolism
Division of Endocrinology, Diabetes & Metabolism
Department of Internal Medicine
LSU Health Sciences Center Shreveport
Shreveport, Louisiana

Maria Luisa Brandi, MD, PhD
F.I.R.M.O. Italian Foundation for the Research on Bone Diseases
Florence, Italy

James D. Brierley, BSc, MB, FRCP, FRCR, FRCP(C)
Princess Margaret Cancer Centre
University Health Network
Department of Radiation Oncology
University of Toronto
Toronto, Ontario, Canada

David Butrón-Hernández, MD
Assistant Professor of Radiology and Interventional Radiology
Department of Radiology
Salvador Zubirán National Institute for Medical Sciences and Nutrition
Mexico City, Mexico

Virginia Cappagli, MD, PhD
Department of Clinical and Experimental Medicine
Endocrine Unit
University of Pisa
Pisa, Italy

Denise Carneiro-Pla, MD, FACS
Professor of Surgery
Division of Oncologic and Endocrine Surgery
Department of Surgery
Medical University of South Carolina
Charleston, South Carolina

David Carty, FRCP (UK), PhD
Department of Diabetes and Endocrinology
Glasgow Royal Infirmary
School of Cardiovascular and Metabolic Health
University of Glasgow
Glasgow, Scotland, United Kingdom

Sally E. Carty, MD
Department of Surgery
Division of Endocrine Surgery
University of Pittsburgh
Pittsburgh, Pennsylvania

Jennifer T. Castle, MD
Department of Surgery
University of Kentucky College of Medicine
Lexington, Kentucky

John A. Chabot, MD
David V. Habif Professor of Surgery
Associate Director, HICCC for Clinical Affairs
Director, The Pancreas Center; Chief, GI & Endocrine Surgery
Columbia University
New York, New York

Herbert Chen, MD
Department of Surgery
University of Alabama at Birmingham
Birmingham, Alabama

Alexander S. Chiu, MD
Endocrine Surgery Fellow
Department of Surgery, Division of Endocrine Surgery
University of Wisconsin School of Medicine and Public Health
Madison, Wisconsin

Paladino Nunzia Cinzia, MD, PhD
Division of General, Endocrine and Metabolic Surgery
Department of endocrinology
Aix-Marseille University
Marseille, France

Uriel Clemente, MD
Department of Surgical Oncology
Section of Surgical Endocrinology
University of Texas MD Anderson Cancer Center
Houston, Texas

Gemma Currie, MRCP (UK), PhD
Department of Diabetes and Endocrinology
Glasgow Royal Infirmary
School of Cardiovascular and Metabolic Health
University of Glasgow
Glasgow, Scotland, United Kingdom

Despoina Daskalaki, MD
Abdominal Transplant Institute
Tufts Medical Center
Boston, Massachusetts

Taïeb David, MD, PhD
Division of Medical Imaging
Department of Nuclear Medicine
Aix-Marseille University
Marseille, France

Stephanie Davis, MD
Endocrine Surgery Fellow
University of California, San Francisco
San Francisco, California

Georgiana A. Dobri, MD
Departments of Neurosurgery and Endocrinology
New York Presbyterian Hospital/Weill Cornell Medical Center
New York, New York

Gerard M. Doherty, MD
Moseley Professor of Surgery
Harvard Medical School
Boston, Massachusetts

Amanda R. Doubleday, DO, MBA
Clinical Assistant Professor
Department of Surgery, Division of Endocrine Surgery
University of Wisconsin School of Medicine and Public Health
Madison, Wisconsin

Frederick Thurston Drake, MD, MPH
Associate Professor of Surgery
Department of Surgery
Boston University School of Medicine
Boston Medical Center
Boston, Massachusetts

William Drake, FRCP, DM
Barts Health NHS Trust
London, United Kingdom

Henning Dralle, MD
Department of General, Visceral and Transplantation Surgery
Section of Endocrine Surgery
University of Duisburg-Essen
Essen, Germany

Quan-Yang Duh, MD
Chief, Section of Endocrine Surgery and Professor
Department of Surgery
University of California, San Francisco
San Francisco, California

Rossella Elisei, MD
Department of Clinical and Experimental Medicine
Endocrine Unit
University of Pisa
Pisa, Italy

Douglas B. Evans, MD
Donald C. Ausman Family Foundation Professor of Surgery and Chair
Department of Surgery
Medical College of Wisconsin
Milwaukee, Wisconsin

Oliver J. Fackelmayer, MD, FACS
Division of General, Endocrine & Metabolic Surgery
Department of Surgery
University of Kentucky
Lexington, Kentucky

Thomas J. Fahey, III, MD, FACS
Johnson and Johnson Professor
Vice-Chair, Department of Surgery
Chief, Endocrine Surgery
Director, Endocrine Oncology Program
The New York Presbyterian Hospital-Weill Cornell Medical Center
New York, New York

Anna Z. Fashandi, MD
Norman W. Thompson Endocrine Surgery Fellow
Department of Surgery
Division of Endocrine Surgery
Michigan Medicine
Ann Arbor, Michigan

Alahmed Feras, MD
University of Lorraine
Department of Surgery (CVMC)
Unit of Endocrine, Thyroid and Metabolic Surgery, and INSERM
CHRU Nancy–Hospital Brabois Adultes
Nancy, France
Surgery Department
Division of General Surgery
Security Forces Hospital
Riyadh, Saudi Arabia

Gustavo Fernandez-Ranvier, MD, PhD
Division of Metabolic, Endocrine and Minimally Invasive Surgery
Department of Surgery
Mount Sinai Hospital
Icahn School of Medicine at Mount Sinai
New York, New York

Deshka S. Foster, MD
Department of Surgery
Stanford University School of Medicine
Palo Alto, California

Sebag Frédéric, MD
Division of General, Endocrine and Metabolic Surgery
Department of endocrinology
Aix-Marseille University
Marseille, France

Rajshri M. Gartland, MD, MPH
Department of Surgery
Massachusetts General Hospital
Boston, Massachusetts

Paul G. Gauger, MD
William J. Fry Professor of Surgery
Professor of Learning Health Sciences
Department of Surgery
Division of Endocrine Surgery
Michigan Medicine
Ann Arbor, Michigan

Courtney E. Gibson, MD, FACS
Division of Surgical Oncology
Department of Surgery
Yale Medical School/Yale-New Haven Hospital (YNHH)
New Haven, Connecticut

Oliver Gimm, MD, FEBS (Endocrine)
Head, Division of Surgery, Orthopedics and Oncology
Department of Surgery and Department of Biomedical and Clinical Sciences
Linköping University
Linköping, Sweden

Francesca Giusti, MD, PhD
Department of Experimental and Clinical Biomedical Sciences
University of Florence
Florence, Italy

David Goldenberg, MD
Department of Otolaryngology—Head and Neck Surgery
Penn State Health
Milton S. Hershey Medical Center
Hershey, Pennsylvania

Jessica E. Gosnell, MD
Department of Surgery
Section of Endocrine Surgery
University of California, San Francisco
San Francisco, California

Kathryn Graham, MB ChB, BSc (Hons), MRCP, PhD, FRCR
Consultant in Clinical Oncology
Beatson West of Scotland Cancer Centre
NHS Greater Glasgow & Clyde
Glasgow, Scotland, United Kingdom

Paul H. Graham, MD
Associate Professor
Department of Surgical Oncology
University of Texas MD Anderson Cancer Center
Houston, Texas

Robert Grant, MD
Surgical Oncology Program
National Cancer Institute
National Institutes of Health
Bethesda, Maryland

Claire E. Graves, MD
Assistant Professor
Section of Endocrine Surgery
Department of Surgery
University of California, Davis
Sacramento, California

Avital Harari, MD, MBA, MSc
Section of Endocrine Surgery
University of California, Los Angeles
Los Angeles, California

Per Hellman, MD, PhD
Department of Surgical Sciences
Uppsala University
Uppsala, Sweden

Fraser Henderson, Jr., MD
Department of Neurosurgery
New York Presbyterian Hospital/Weill Cornell Medical Center
New York, New York

Miguel F. Herrera, PhD
Program Director, Endocrine Surgery
Department of Surgery
Salvador Zubirán National Institute for Medical Sciences and Nutrition
Mexico City, Mexico

Richard A. Hodin, MD
Department of Surgery
Massachusetts General Hospital
Boston, Massachusetts

James R. Howe, MD
University of Iowa Hospital and Clinics
Department of Surgery
Iowa City, Iowa

Bernice Huang, MD
Fellow, Surgical Endocrinology
Department of Surgical Oncology
University of Texas MD Anderson Cancer Center
Houston, Texas

William B. Inabnet, III, MD, MHA, FACS
Department of Surgery
University of Kentucky College of Medicine
Lexington, Kentucky

Mahsa Javid, MB, BChr, MA, DPhil, FRCS, FRCSC
Assistant Professor of Surgery
Division of Oncologic and Endocrine Surgery
Department of Surgery
Medical University of South Carolina
Charleston, South Carolina

Crystal D. C. Kamilaris, MD
Section on Endocrinology and Genetics & Endocrinology Inter-institute Training Program
Eunice Kennedy Shriver National Institute of Child Health & Human Development
National Institutes of Health
Bethesda, Maryland

Ken Kazahaya, MD, MBA
Associate Director
Division of Pediatric Otolaryngology
Children's Hospital of Philadelphia
Co-Lead Surgeon, The Thyroid Center
Children's Hospital of Philadelphia
Associate Professor of Clinical Otorhinolaryngology—Head and Neck Surgery
The University of Pennsylvania
Philadelphia, Pennsylvania

Allison Keane, MD
Department of Otolaryngology—Head and Neck Surgery
Penn State Health
Milton S. Hershey Medical Center
Hershey, Pennsylvania

Electron Kebebew, MD, FACS
Professor of Surgery
Chief, Division of General Surgery
Stanford Medicine Harry A. Oberhelman, Jr. and Mark L. Welton Professor
Department of Surgery
Stanford University School of Medicine
Stanford, California

Tahsin M. Khan, MD
Surgical Oncology Program
National Cancer Institute
National Institutes of Health
Bethesda, Maryland

Jina Kim, MD
Assistant Professor of Medical Education
Inova Health System/University of Virginia
Fairfax, Virginia

Christine E. Kolwitz, DO
Department of Surgery
Division of Abdominal Organ Transplantation and Hepatobiliary Surgery
Oregon Health & Science University
Portland, Oregon

Ananya V. Kondapalli, MD
Department of Medicine
Division of Endocrinology
Columbia University Irving Medical Center
New York, New York

Matthew A. Krell, MD
Department of Surgery
New York University Grossman Long Island School of Medicine
Mineola, New York

Amanda M. Laird, MD, FACS
Rutgers Robert Wood Johnson Medical School
Rutgers Cancer Institute of New Jersey
New Brunswick, New Jersey

Terry C. Lairmore, MD, FACS
Professor of Clinical Surgery
Donnie and Gail Juneau Endowed Chair in Surgical Oncology
Director Division of Surgical Oncology
Department of Surgery
LSU Health Shreveport
Shreveport, Louisiana

Brunaud Laurent, MD
University of Lorraine
Department of Surgery (CVMC)
Unit of Endocrine, Thyroid and Metabolic Surgery, and INSERM
CHRU Nancy–Hospital Brabois Adultes
Nancy, France

Anderson Lee, BA
Medical Student
University of Toledo College of Medicine and Life Sciences
Toledo, Ohio

James A. Lee, MD
Professor of Surgery
Chief of Endocrine Surgery
Columbia University Medical Center
New York, New York

Alice C. Levine, MD
Division of Endocrinology, Diabetes, and Bone Metabolism
Department of Medicine
Icahn School of Medicine at Mount Sinai Hospital
New York, New York

Steven K. Libutti, MD, FACS
Rutgers Robert Wood Johnson Medical School
Rutgers Cancer Institute of New Jersey
New Brunswick, New Jersey

Whitney Liddy, MD
Department of Otolaryngology—Head and Neck Surgery
Feinberg School of Medicine
Northwestern University
Chicago, Illinois

David Lieb, MD, FACE, FACP
Division of Endocrine and Metabolic Disorders
Department of Internal Medicine
Eastern Virginia Medical School
Norfolk, Virginia

Benjamin Lieberman, DO
Research Fellow
Mount Sinai Hospital
Icahn School of Medicine at Mount Sinai
New York, New York

Dimitrios A. Linos, MD, PhD
Professor of Surgery
National & Kapodistrian University of Athens Medical School
Marousi, Greece
Lecturer in Surgery, Harvard Medical School
Boston, Massachusetts

Rachel Liou, MD
Assistant Professor of Surgery
Division of GI & Endocrine Surgery
Department of Surgery
Columbia University Medical Center
New York City, New York

Loredana Lorusso, MD, PhD
Department of Clinical and Experimental Medicine
Endocrine Unit
University of Pisa
Pisa, Italy

Jelena Lukovic, MD, FRCPC, MPH
Princess Margaret Cancer Centre
University Health Network
Department of Radiation Oncology
University of Toronto
Toronto, Ontario, Canada

Nicole Lunardi, MD
General Surgery Resident
Department of Surgery
University of Texas Southwestern Medical Center
Dallas, Texas

Andreas Machens, MD
Department of Visceral, Vascular and Endocrine Surgery
Martin Luther University Halle-Wittenberg
Halle (Saale), Germany

Sharon T. Mackin, MRCP (UK), MD
Department of Diabetes and Endocrinology
Glasgow Royal Infirmary
School of Cardiovascular and Metabolic Health
University of Glasgow
Glasgow, Scotland, United Kingdom

Richard C. Maduka, MD
Yale School of Medicine
Department of Surgery
New Haven, Connecticut

Ujjal Mallick, MBBS, MS, FRCPE (Hon), FRCP (Hon), FRCR
Chief Investigator "IoN" and "HiLo" Thyroid Cancer Trials
Consultant Clinical Oncologist (Hon)
Northern Centre for Cancer Care
Freeman Hospital
Newcastle upon Tyne NHS Hospitals Foundation Trust
London, United Kingdom

Alexander Manzella, MD
Rutgers Robert Wood Johnson Medical School
New Brunswick, New Jersey

Francesca Marini, PhD
Department of Experimental and Clinical Biomedical Sciences
University of Florence
F.I.R.M.O. Italian Foundation for the Research on Bone Diseases
Florence, Italy

Aarti Mathur, MD, PhD
Department of Surgery
Johns Hopkins Hospital
Baltimore, Maryland

Matthew Matson, MRCP, FRCR
Barts Health NHS Trust
London, United Kingdom

Jessica E. Maxwell, MD, MBA
University of Texas MD Anderson Cancer Center
Department of Surgical Oncology
Houston, Texas

Peter J. Mazzaglia, MD, FACS
Department of Surgery
Rhode Island Hospital
The Warren Alpert Medical School of Brown University
Providence, Rhode Island

Christopher R. McHenry, MD
Vice Chairman of Surgery and Director of the Division of General Surgery
MetroHealth Medical Center
Professor of Surgery
Case Western Reserve University School of Medicine
Cleveland, Ohio

Robert McIntyre, Jr., MD
Cynthia H. and John H. Schultz Chair in Surgery
Division Chief, GI Trauma and Endocrine Surgery
Vice Chair Finance
Department of Surgery
University of Colorado
Associate Chief Medical Officer for Perioperative Services
University of Colorado Hospital
Aurora, Colorado

Travis J. McKenzie, MD
Mayo Clinic
Rochester, Minnesota

Gopal Menon, MBBS, MD, MPH
Surgical Oncology Fellow
Roswell Park Cancer Institute
Buffalo, New York

Barbra S. Miller, MD
Professor of Surgery
Co-Director, OSU Comprehensive Adrenal Program
Division Director of Clinical Operations
Division of Surgical Oncology
Department of Surgery
The James Cancer Hospital and Solove Research Institute
Wexner Medical Center
The Ohio State University
Columbus, Ohio

Alessandra L. Moore, MD
2021-2022 Harvard Combined Endocrine Surgery Fellow
Brigham and Women's and Massachusetts General Hospital
Boston, Massachusetts
Assistant Professor of Surgery
University of Rochester Medical Center
Rochester, New York

Matthew A. Nehs, MD
Department of Surgery
Brigham and Women's Hospital
Boston, Massachusetts

Patrick N. Nguyen, MD
PGY-4 Resident, General Surgery
Albany Medical Center
Albany, New York

Naris Nilubol, MD
Endocrine Surgery section, Surgical Oncology Program
National Cancer Institute, National Institutes of Health
Bethesda, Maryland

Jeffrey A. Norton, MD
Department of Surgery
Stanford University School of Medicine
Palo Alto, California

Jennifer B. Ogilvie, MD, FACS
Section of Endocrine Surgery
Division of Surgical Oncology
Department of Surgery
Yale University School of Medicine
New Haven, Connecticut

Sarah C. Oltmann, MD, FACS
Associate Professor of Surgery
Dedman Family Scholar in Clinical Care
Department of Surgery
University of Texas Southwestern Medical Center
Dallas, Texas

Roy Oommen, MD
Assistant Professor of Surgery
Columbia University Medical Center
Section of Thoracic Surgery
Price Center for Comprehensive Chest Care
New York-Presbyterian Hospital
New York, New York

Radwa Osman, MD
Division of Endocrine and Metabolic Disorders
Department of Internal Medicine
Eastern Virginia Medical School
Norfolk, Virginia

Nicci Owusu-Brackett, MD
Fellow, Complex General Surgical Oncology
Division of Surgical Oncology
Department of Surgery
The James Cancer Hospital and Solove Research Institute
Wexner Medical Center
The Ohio State University
Columbus, Ohio

Pia Pace-Asciak, MASc, MD, FRCSC
Department of Otolaryngology—Head and Neck Surgery
University of Toronto
Toronto, Ontario, Canada

Janice L. Pasieka, MD, FRCSC, FACS
Clinical Professor of Surgery and Oncology
Department of Surgery, Section of General Surgery
Divisions of Endocrine Surgery and Surgical Oncology
Cumming School of Medicine
University of Calgary
Calgary, Alberta, Canada

Jesse D. Pasternak, MD, MPH, FRCSC, FACS
Section Head, Endocrine Surgery and Oncology
Division of General Surgery, Sprott Department of Surgery—University Health Network
Department of Surgical Oncology, Princess Margaret Cancer Centre
Director, Endocrine Surgery Fellowship Program
Assistant Professor of Surgery, University of Toronto
UHN–Toronto General Hospital
Toronto, Ontario, Canada

Kepal N. Patel, MD
NYU Langone Health
New York, New York

Natalia S. Pellegata, PhD
Department of Biology and Biotechnology "L. Spallanzani"
University of Pavia
Pavia, Italy

Terrance Peng, MPH
Keck School of Medicine
University of Southern California
Los Angeles, California

Rafael Humberto Pérez-Soto, MD
Assistant Professor, Endocrine Surgery
Department of Surgery
Salvador Zubirán National Institute for Medical Sciences and Nutrition
Mexico City, Mexico

Nancy D. Perrier, MD
Department of Surgical Oncology
Section of Surgical Endocrinology
University of Texas MD Anderson Cancer Center
Houston, Texas

Rodney F. Pommier, MD, FACS
Professor of Surgery
Division of Surgical Oncology
Oregon Health & Science University School of Medicine
Portland, Oregon

Rajam Raghunathan, MD, CM, PhD
Department of General Surgery
University of Ottawa
Ottawa, Ontario, Canada

Kimberly M. Ramonell, MD
Department of Surgery
Division of Endocrine Surgery
University of Pittsburgh
Pittsburgh, Pennsylvania

Gregory W. Randolph, MD, FACS, FACE, FEBS (Endocrine)
Professor of Otolaryngology—Head and Neck Surgery
Claire and John Bertucci Endowed Chair in Thyroid Surgical Oncology, Harvard Medical School
Chief of Division of Thyroid and Parathyroid Endocrine Surgery
Department of Otolaryngology—Head and Neck Surgery
Massachusetts Eye and Ear Infirmary
Harvard Medical School
Boston, Massachusetts

Nick Reed, MBBS, MRCP (UK), FRCR, FRCP (Glas)
Professor in Clinical Oncology
Beatson West of Scotland Cancer Centre
NHS Greater Glasgow & Clyde
Glasgow, Scotland, United Kingdom

Rosyli F. Reveron-Thornton, MD
Department of Surgery
Stanford University School of Medicine
Palo Alto, California

Sanziana A. Roman, MD
Professor of Surgery
University of California, San Francisco
San Francisco, California

Gustavo Romero-Velez, MD
Clinical Associate
Endocrine and Metabolism Institute
Cleveland Clinic
Cleveland, Ohio

Jennifer E. Rosen, MD, FACS
Division of Endocrine Surgery
Department of Surgery
MedStar Georgetown University and Washington Hospital Center
Washington, DC

Aaron Schulman, MD
Assistant Professor of Medicine
Division of Endocrinology, Diabetes and Metabolism
Weill Cornell Medicine
New York, New York

Theodore H. Schwartz, MD
Department of Neurosurgery
New York Presbyterian Hospital/Weill Cornell Medical Center
New York, New York

Elliot Scott, MD
Endocrine Surgery Fellow
Department of Surgery
Mount Sinai Hospital
Icahn School of Medicine at Mount Sinai
New York, New York

Nimesh Shah, BSc (Hons), PGDip Med Ed, FRCR
Barts Health NHS Trust
London, United Kingdom

Ashok R. Shaha, MD
Professor of Surgery
Head and Neck Service, Department of Surgery
Memorial Sloan Kettering Cancer Center
New York, New York

Alexander Shifrin, MD, FACS, FACE, ECNU, FEBS (Endocrine Surgery), FISS
Surgical Director of Endocrinology
Statesir Cancer Center
Atlantic Health, CentraState Medical Center
Freehold, New Jersey

Shonni J. Silverberg, MD
Department of Medicine
Division of Endocrinology
Columbia University Irving Medical Center
New York, New York

William F. Simonds, MD
Senior Clinical Investigator
Metabolic Diseases Branch
National Institute of Diabetes and Digestive and Kidney Diseases
Bethesda, Maryland

Allan Siperstein, MD
Chair Endocrine Surgery
Endocrine and Metabolism Institute
Cleveland Clinic
Cleveland, Ohio

Rebecca S. Sippel, MD
Vice Chair of Academic Affairs and Professional Development
Chief, Division of Endocrine Surgery
Department of Surgery, Division of Endocrine Surgery
University of Wisconsin School of Medicine and Public Health
Madison, Wisconsin

Maheshwaran Sivarajah, MD, MSc
Department of Surgery
University Hospitals Portage Medical Centre
Case Western Reserve University
Ravenna, Ohio

Catherine M. Skefos, MA, MS, CGC
Clinical Cancer Genetics
University of Texas MD Anderson Cancer Center
Houston, Texas

Vivian Sobel, MD
Assistant Professor of Medicine
Division of Endocrinology, Diabetes and Metabolism
Weill Cornell Medicine
New York, New York

Justin M. Soffer, MD
Department of Surgery
Vanderbilt University Medical Center
Nashville, Tennessee

Carmen C. Solórzano, MD, FACS
Professor and Chair, Department of Surgery
John L. Sawyers Chair in Surgical Sciences
Director, Vanderbilt Endocrine Surgery
Vanderbilt University Medical Center
Nashville, Tennessee

Joshua Sonett, MD
Professor of Surgery
Columbia University Medical Center
Section of Thoracic Surgery
Price Center for Comprehensive Chest Care
New York-Presbyterian Hospital
New York, New York

Julie A. Sosa, MD, MA
Leon Goldman, MD Distinguished Professor of Surgery and Chair
Department of Surgery
Professor, Department of Medicine
Affiliated Faculty
Philip R. Lee Institute for Health Policy Studies
University of California, San Francisco
San Francisco, California

Taylor C. St. Amour, MD
Resident Physician
Department of General Surgery
Vanderbilt University Medical Center
Nashville, Tennessee

Constantine A. Stratakis, MD, D(Med)Sc, PhD
Section on Endocrinology and Genetics & Endocrinology Inter-institute Training Program
Eunice Kennedy Shriver National Institute of Child Health & Human Development
National Institutes of Health
Bethesda, Maryland
Human Genetics & Precision Medicine
Institute for Molecular Biology & Biotechnology
Foundation for Research & Technology Hellas
Heraklion, Greece
ELPEN Pharmaceuticals, Inc.
Athens, Greece

Vivian E. Strong, MD
Memorial Sloan-Kettering Cancer Center
New York, New York

Chad K. Sudoko, MD
Resident Physician
Department of Otorhinolaryngology—Head and Neck Surgery
Hospital of the University of Pennsylvania
Philadelphia, Pennsylvania

Iwao Sugitani, MD, PhD
Graduate School Professor and Chairman
Department of Endocrine Surgery
Nippon Medical School Graduate School of Medicine
Tokyo, Japan

Vishnu Sundaresh, MD, MSCI
Associate Professor
Division of Endocrinology, Metabolism and Diabetes
University of Utah School of Medicine
Salt Lake City, Utah

Martha E. Teke, MD
Surgical Oncology Program
National Cancer Institute
National Institutes of Health
Bethesda, Maryland

Angela E. Thelen, MD
General Surgery Resident
MetroHealth Medical Center
Cleveland, Ohio

Jennifer F. Tseng, MD, MPH
Surgeon-in-Chief, Boston Medical Center
James Utley Professor and Chair
Department of Surgery
Boston University School of Medicine
Boston, Massachusetts

Effie Tsomos, MD
Division of Endocrinology, Diabetes, and Bone Metabolism
Department of Medicine
Icahn School of Medicine at Mount Sinai (South Nassau)
Mount Sinai South Nassau
Oceanside, New York

Ralph P. Tufano, MD, MBA, FACS
Division of Otolaryngology—Head and Neck Surgery
Johns Hopkins University
Baltimore, Maryland

Rhea Udyavar, MD
Department of Surgery
Johns Hopkins Hospital
Baltimore, Maryland

Hunter J. Underwood, MD
Assistant Professor of Surgery
Division of Endocrine Surgery
University of Michigan
Ann Arbor, Michigan

Danica M. Vodopivec, MD
Endocrine Neoplasia and Hormonal Disorders
University of Texas MD Anderson Cancer Center
Houston, Texas

Marcella Donovan Walker, MD, MS
Department of Medicine
Division of Endocrinology
Columbia University Irving Medical Center
New York, New York

Martin K. Walz, MD, PhD
Department of Surgery and Center of Minimally Invasive Surgery
Evang. Kliniken Essen-Mitte
Essen, Germany

Tracy S. Wang, MD, MPH, FACS
Medical College of Wisconsin
Milwaukee, Wisconsin

Michael A. Weintraub, MD
Department of Endocrinology
New York Presbyterian Hospital/Weill Cornell Medical Center
New York, New York

Lauren Williams, MD
Department of Surgery
Division of Otolaryngology—Head and Neck Surgery
Yale School of Medicine
New Haven, Connecticut

Alison P. Woods, MD, MHS
Post-Doctoral Research Fellow
Department of Surgery
Boston University School of Medicine
Boston Medical Center
Boston, Massachusetts
Department of Surgery
Johns Hopkins University School of Medicine
Baltimore, Maryland

Sean Wrenn, MD
Department of Surgery
Rush University Medical Center
Chicago, Illinois

Thomas Szabo Yamashita, MD
Mayo Clinic
Rochester, Minnesota

Rajini K. Yatavelli, MD
Assistant Professor
Division of Endocrinology, Diabetes & Metabolism
Department of Internal Medicine
LSU Health Sciences Center Shreveport
Shreveport, Louisiana

Caitlin T. Yeo, MD, FRCSC
Clinical Lecturer of Surgery and Oncology
Department of Surgery
Section of General Surgery
Divisions of Endocrine Surgery and Surgical Oncology
Cumming School of Medicine
University of Calgary
Calgary, Alberta, Canada

Rasa Zarnegar, MD
Professor of Surgery
New York Presbyterian–Weill Cornell Medicine
New York, New York

Martha A. Zeiger, MD
Surgical Oncology Program
National Cancer Institute
National Institutes of Health
Bethesda, Maryland

Hui Zheng, MD
Division of Endocrine Surgery
Department of Surgery
MedStar Georgetown University and Washington Hospital Center
Washington, DC

Polina V. Zmijewski, MD, MA
Department of Surgery
University of Alabama at Birmingham
Birmingham, Alabama

Preface

"To study the phenomena of disease without books is to sail an uncharted sea, while to study books without patients is not to go to sea at all."

—William Osler

Endocrine surgery developed as a separate subspecialty of general surgery several decades ago. Endocrine surgery fellowships grew from about 10 in the world in the 1990s to more than 40 currently, with 22 to 25 within the United States. In addition to endocrine surgical fellowships, other disciplines—ENT/head and neck surgeons and surgical oncologists among them—have also created special training programs dedicated to caring for patients with endocrine surgical diseases of the thyroid, parathyroid, and adrenal glands and intestines and pancreas. Medical endocrinologists are now often closely associated with endocrine surgeons in the same practice setting to form single specialty groups. Major universities in the country have established endocrine surgery divisions and conduct weekly endocrine surgery tumor boards. Standard of care approach to the treatment of endocrine surgical disease has resulted in the development of the Collaborative Endocrine Surgery Quality Improvement Program (CESQIP), designated by the American Board of Surgery as a primary nationally validated, risk-adjusted, outcomes-based program quality reporting system for all endocrine surgeons in the United States and all over the world, similar to NSQIP for general surgeons. Starting in the United States, CESQIP has now spread to other countries and continents, including Canada, Mexico, Europe, and Asia. Based on the CESQIP data, endocrine surgery reporting volume for the last 5 years has increased by 31% in the United States for thyroid, parathyroid, and adrenal procedures; in 2014, there were 1380 procedures reported in CESQIP; in 2015, 1753 procedures; in 2016, 1951 procedures; in 2017, 1995 procedures; and in 2018, 2011 procedures.

The American Association of Endocrine Surgeons (AAES) counted about 300 members a decade ago and is now approaching almost 1000. In addition, other societies such as the European Society of Endocrine Surgeons (ESES), the International Association of Endocrine Surgeons (IAES), the Asian Association of Endocrine Surgeons (AAES), and other societies have grown over the past two decades, making the community of endocrine surgeons one of the fastest growing surgical subspecialties. The European Division of Endocrine Surgery (DES) established an Endocrine Surgery Board Examination and determined the curriculum for the Endocrine Surgery Board Examination and the Neck Endocrine Surgery Examination.

This book is a ready source of information related to endocrine surgical diseases managed by endocrine surgeons, head and neck surgeons, surgical oncologists, and ENT surgeons. It includes endocrine surgical disorders of the thyroid, parathyroid, and adrenal glands, as well as neuroendocrine tumors of the intestines and pancreas. In addition, familial endocrine syndromes, including the multiple endocrine neoplasia syndromes, are covered. Epidemiology, pathophysiology, and pathology are discussed to the extent that they contribute to the book's ultimate purpose, which is patient care guidance. It emphasizes quick recall of major diagnostic features and brief descriptions of the disease process, followed by approaches for definitive diagnosis and treatment. All treatment options are based on the current national and international guidelines. Emphasis is given to the multidisciplinary approach to all endocrine surgical conditions, which has been increasingly recognized as the standard of care. This book will help practitioners understand the best care options for endocrine surgical patients and point out how to utilize the multidisciplinary expertise available at their institutions. The book includes current references to the journal literature for the reader who wishes to pursue a specific area.

We hope that this book will be the primary source and reference for daily practice, be utilized in preparation for Endocrine Surgery examinations, and elevate the level of expertise in Endocrine Surgery by augmenting the standard of training for current and future endocrine surgeons.

Alexander Shifrin, MD
Thomas J. Fahey, III, MD

Acknowledgments

The creation of this textbook, covering the entire scope of endocrine surgery, was dependent on a team effort, which was possible only with the support and enthusiasm of the many individuals who contributed to this book, our colleagues who trusted us and dedicated their time and effort to make it happen, without whom this book would have never come to life!

Special thanks to Senior McGraw Hill Editors Jason Malley, who started to work with us, and then Sydney Keen Vitale and Kim Davis, who helped us to complete this project and believed in us, and for their hard work and dedication.

Finally, we would like to thank the entire staff at McGraw Hill, who were very supportive from the first idea of this manuscript and maintained their enthusiasm until the end.

Multidisciplinary Approach to Endocrine Surgical Patients

1

Alexander Shifrin, MD, FACS
Thomas J. Fahey, III, MD, FACS

INTRODUCTION

In the modern era, the comprehensive approach to patient care involves a group of experts experienced in different aspects of patient's specific conditions. This is probably especially true for endocrine surgical patients given the significant medical implications of many endocrine surgical problems. Complex problems may be best addressed by a multidisciplinary group—both in the diagnostic and pretreatment phase, as well as in post-surgical phase for patients who require surgery. Involvement of an endocrinologist is desirable prior to surgery, especially for complex endocrine problems where there are multiple treatment options. The input of radiology and pathology is crucial during all stages of patient care, and review of radiographic and pathologic images at multidisciplinary conferences can be both enlightening and educational.

Multidisciplinary communication can be divided into three distinct stages: preoperative evaluation, intraoperative management based on preoperative plan and intraoperative findings, and postoperative care.[1-4]

ASPECTS OF THE MULTIDISCIPLINARY APPROACH TO PREOPERATIVE CARE

Preoperative Evaluation

The preoperative evaluation can be divided into two phases—the diagnostic phase and presurgical phase. The most important aspect of the diagnostic phase is to ensure that the proper diagnosis has been made and that the appropriate operation has been planned. An errant diagnosis can lead to an unnecessary operation, or inadequate (incomplete) procedure, which exposes the patient to risks without the potential benefits normally expected from the surgery. Examples of potential diagnostic pitfalls are listed in Table 1–1.

The presurgical phase involves evaluation of comorbidities and coordination of care with cardiology, pulmonology, and anesthesia prior to the day of surgery. Managing a patient with multiple comorbidities or a potentially difficult airway should be discussed with the anesthesia team prior to surgery—and preferably with an anesthesiologist who is familiar with endocrine surgical problems.[5] Communication with the anesthesia team is particularly important to allow for proper preparation for patients with compressive or substernal goiters, thyroid tumors with local invasion, and pheochromocytomas or large adrenal tumors. For patients with a history of cervical spine disease undergoing neck surgery, it is important to consider whether an evaluation by a spine surgeon is necessary prior to positioning for a neck operation.

Special Considerations

A. Patients With Thyroid Nodules and Thyroid Cancer

While traditionally thought of as a forum for discussion of adjuvant postoperative treatment for thyroid cancer, the multidisciplinary endocrine conference or tumor board can be particularly useful for deciding the best management strategy for patients with complicated and/or recurrent thyroid cancers. Per American Thyroid Association (ATA) guidelines, the basic goals of initial therapy for patients with differentiated thyroid carcinoma (DTC) are to improve overall and disease-specific survival, reduce the risk of persistent and recurrent disease and associated morbidity, and permit accurate disease staging and risk stratification, while minimizing treatment-related morbidity and unnecessary therapy.[2-7] As the therapeutic options for advanced thyroid cancers evolve, neoadjuvant treatment is one example of a situation where preoperative discussion at a multidisciplinary conference will prove to be very helpful. At the other end of the spectrum, determination of whether a papillary microcarcinoma is a candidate for active surveillance

Table 1–1. Diagnostic pitfalls in endocrine surgery.

Expected Diagnosis	Potential Diagnostic Pitfall	Modification to the Surgical Plan
Primary hyperparathyroidism	Familial hypocalciuric hypercalcemia MEN 1 syndrome MEN 2A syndrome Parathyroid carcinoma Jaw-Tumor syndrome	No surgery There is a high possibility of parathyroid hyperplasia. To include thyroidectomy. Be prepared for parathyroid tumor debulking, possible thyroid lobectomy if invasion into the thyroid lobe detected intraoperatively.
Primary hyperparathyroidism	Not identifying a thyroid nodule preoperatively	Thyroid nodule biopsy should be performed prior to a parathyroidectomy, if indicated. The patient might need simultaneous thyroid surgery in addition to a parathyroidectomy.
Unilateral, less than 4 cm, thyroid nodule with cancer	Extrathyroidal extension or gross lymph node metastasis might be found during the surgery	Make sure that the patient is consented not only for a thyroid lobectomy, but total thyroidectomy with possible central neck lymph node dissection is also included into the consent.
Patient presents for a thyroidectomy, no preoperative calcium level is checked	Missed diagnosis of concurrent primary hyperparathyroidism	If concurrent primary hyperparathyroidism is diagnosed, parathyroidectomy should be added to the consent.
Thyroid nodule with cancer	Lymph node mapping to evaluate for lateral neck spread is not performed.	Modify the procedure to include a modified radical neck dissection if lateral neck metastases are detected.
Non-functioning adrenal nodule	Mild autonomous cortisol excess	Surgery is needed for mild autonomous cortisol secretion. Perioperative steroid administration may be required to treat postoperative hypotension.
Cushing syndrome	Adrenocortical carcinoma	Be ready to convert to an open adrenalectomy.
Primary aldosteronism due to unilateral adenoma	Idiopathic primary hyperaldosteronism	No surgery is required due to the presence of bilateral adrenal hyperplasia.

or an ablative treatment (radiofrequency or ethanol ablation) may require input from radiology and the treating endocrinologist, in addition to the treating surgeon.[8,9] In addition, for routine thyroid cancer cases, preoperative discussion regarding the extent of the surgery should include evaluation of thyroid function and communication with the patient's endocrinologist and primary care provider to decide whether a hemithyroidectomy or total thyroidectomy is recommended—with input from the patient, of course.[10]

B. Patients With Hyperthyroidism

The utilization of antithyroid medication, duration of treatment, and the timing of surgery in patients with hyperthyroidism—and particularly those with Graves' disease—should be discussed with a multidisciplinary team that includes the endocrinologist and nuclear medicine physician at a minimum, and for patients with ophthalmopathy an ophthalmologist as well. As the treatment paradigms for Graves' disease are slowly shifting, a multidisciplinary approach has become more important. The pros and cons of extended medical therapy, RAI, or surgery should be reviewed and discussed with the patient.[11,12]

C. Patients With Hyperparathyroidism

The timing of referral for patients with primary hyperparathyroidism (PHPT) is easy for a patient with a classic presentation such as nephrolithiasis, hypercalcemia, and elevated parathyroid hormone levels. However, many patients with hyperparathyroidism do not present with classic signs and symptoms and these patients warrant a multidisciplinary discussion that should include the primary care physician, endocrinologist, and endocrine surgeon at a minimum. Many physicians delay referral of patients with biochemical evidence of PHPT if they do not meet criteria for surgery or if imaging studies do not identify a classic adenoma.

Since up to 40% of patients who do not meet criteria may develop complications over their lifetime, referral should still be considered.[13] In addition, the failure of imaging studies to identify an enlarged parathyroid gland should not preclude surgery as the culprit gland or glands will be identified at surgery in the vast majority of cases.[14,15] For patients with secondary and tertiary HPT, discussion with the referring nephrologist should include the extent of parathyroidectomy—specifically whether a subtotal parathyroidectomy or total with autotransplantation would be preferable.

D. Patients With Adrenal Tumors

The utility of a multidisciplinary approach in patients with adrenal tumors depends on the type of functional excess. For patients with hyperaldosteronism, the critical discussion is centered on the diagnostic phase of preoperative evaluation—and specifically whether the patient has unilateral or bilateral disease. For young patients (<40 years) with a clearly defined adenoma on one side whether adrenal venous sampling is advised is largely dependent on the assessment of the contralateral gland, and thus the input of radiology is critical.

For patients with a pheochromocytoma the diagnosis and localization is typically not subtle, but the presurgical phase of preoperative planning is critical. Multidisciplinary input from endocrinology or hypertension into the antihypertensive regimen is highly desirable as alpha blockade is initiated. Communication with the anesthesia team is essential so that appropriate planning for the intraoperative phase is completed prior to the day of surgery. Recent guidelines published for patients with pheochromocytoma and paraganglioma recommend that these patients should be evaluated and treated by a multidisciplinary team at an appropriate center of expertise given the complexity in biochemical diagnosis, localization performance and interpretation of genetic testing, preoperative preparation, surgical treatment and follow-up.[16,17] Finally, for large adrenal tumors with suspected malignancy, consultation with additional surgical teams such as vascular, cardiac (for a tumor with intracaval extension), or hepatobiliary should be completed prior to surgery.

E. Patients With Pancreatic or Gastrointestinal Neuroendocrine Tumors (NETs)

While most pancreatic NETs (pNETs) are sporadic and about 65% to 85% are non-functioning, pNETs can be associated with genetic syndromes such as multiple endocrine neoplasia type 1 (MEN1), von Hippel-Lindau disease (VHL), neurofibromatosis 1 (NF1), or tuberous sclerosis complex and can be the source of hormone excess. Though functioning pNETs now account for less than 20% of cases, the diagnosis and treatment of patients with functioning PNETs—and in particular insulinomas or gastrinomas—can be complex and requires a multidisciplinary approach between the surgeon, gastroenterologist (frequently an interventional gastroenterologist), radiologist, pathologist, and at times an oncologist.[18]

F. Pediatric Patients

Pediatric patients comprise a special population of patients with endocrine surgical problems due to the unique aspects of care of endocrine tumors or diseases and increased incidence of inherited diseases in this age group. The guidelines for management of children with DTC strongly recommend that these patients should be cared for by teams of physicians experienced in the management of DTC in children. Interdisciplinary decisions regarding optimal therapy in this age group will help to reduce the possibility that treatment and long-term follow-up will be either overly aggressive or inadequate.[19] In addition, it is recommended that pediatric thyroid surgery should be performed in a hospital with the full spectrum of pediatric specialty care, including pediatric endocrinology, genetic medicine, radiology (ultrasound and anatomic imaging), nuclear medicine, anesthesia and intensive care expertise, as well as a high-volume thyroid surgeon. Thyroid surgery performed under these guidelines is associated with lower complications rates, decreased hospital stay, and lower cost.[19]

ASPECTS OF THE MULTIDISCIPLINARY APPROACH TO INTRAOPERATIVE CARE

Communication with the anesthesia team is the lynchpin of the multidisciplinary approach to intraoperative care. An anesthesia team that is familiar with endocrine surgical problems is optimal and is particularly important in caring for patients with pheochromocytoma, adrenal tumors with invasion of adjacent organs or major blood vessels, substernal goiter, or thyroid carcinomas with invasion of adjacent structures. Intraoperative consultation with other specialists, including pathology, radiology, or endocrinology may be desirable based on intraoperative findings.

ASPECTS OF THE MULTIDISCIPLINARY APPROACH TO POSTOPERATIVE CARE

Patients with benign endocrine surgical diseases can often return to the care of their endocrinologist and primary care physician without continued multidisciplinary input. However, management of postoperative patients with endocrine cancer is best served through a multidisciplinary approach including presentation at a multidisciplinary tumor board. For differentiated thyroid cancers the merits of adjuvant RAI are best discussed and coordinated through a multidisciplinary conference.[20] For more advanced cancers, discussion of treatment options should include an oncologist with expertise in the use of the expanding numbers of tyrosine kinase inhibitors, which may be the first line of treatment. Studies of thyroid cancer patients have demonstrated that most patients with thyroid cancer appreciate and are clearly in favor of using a multidisciplinary approach to their disease, as well as desire to have their opinion integrated into the management of their disease.[2] However, most health-care professionals feel that it is neither desirable nor practical to include patients in multidisciplinary conferences.[3]

The recent study by Volkan Kisioglu investigated the effect of making surgical decisions in a council through a multidisciplinary approach after clinical, ultrasonographic, and pathological evaluation of nodules on the accuracy of the decisions. The multidisciplinary approach was shown to be superior to the non-multidisciplinary approach in the detection of malignancy.[7]

BUILDING A MULTIDISCIPLINARY PROGRAM

Building a multidisciplinary program (MDP) takes a substantial amount of time and effort. However, there are significant clinical and financial benefits of an MDP to patients, the health-care providers, and ultimately to health-care systems. Many hospitals implement tumor boards that function as a multidisciplinary conference with attendance of a variety of specialty providers who discuss their own patient cases and then relay that information back to the patient.

The first step in building an MDP is to create a business plan that would be presented to hospital administration with a vision of the MDP, market share analysis, a detailed description of the MDP, upfront costs, anticipated financial revenue, and ideas for marketing and outreach.

The next step is to secure participation from the different subspeciality physicians and providers involved in the multidisciplinary care of the specific disease category or service line.

Once the physicians are on board, the support of hospital administration is critical to the success of the program for simple things like identifying a conference room with appropriate technology to more resource-intense factors like hiring a nurse navigator to coordinate the program efforts and organize the multidisciplinary conferences. A nurse navigator is defined by the Academy of Oncology Nurse & Patient Navigators as "a medical professional whose clinical expertise and training guides patients and their caregivers to make informed decisions, collaborating with a multidisciplinary team to allow for timely cancer screening, diagnosis, treatment, and increased supportive care across the cancer continuum."[21,22] In addition to organizing the efforts of the physicians on the multidisciplinary team, a nurse navigator can facilitate communication of team decisions to patients and is critical in educating patients and locating and providing necessary resources to optimize patient care.[23-27]

Finally, in addition to the proven benefits to patient care, an MDP benefits the hospital through the attraction of new patients to the system that ultimately receive a higher level of care.

REFERENCES

1. Carty S, Doherty G, Inabnet W, et al. American Thyroid Association statement on the essential elements of interdisciplinary communication of perioperative information for patients undergoing thyroid cancer surgery. *Thyroid.* 2012;22(4):395-399.
2. Díez J, Galofré J. Thyroid cancer patients' view of clinician professionalism and multidisciplinary approach to their management. *J Multidiscip Healthc.* 2021;14:1053-1061.
3. Taylor C, Ramirez AJ. Multidisciplinary team members' views about MDT working: results from a survey commissioned by the National Cancer Action Team. National Cancer Action Team; 2009. Available from: http://www.ncin.org.uk/view.aspx?rid=137. Accessed April 30, 2021.
4. Pillay B, Wootten AC, Crowe H, et al. The impact of multidisciplinary team meetings on patient assessment, management and outcomes in oncology settings: a systematic review of the literature. *Cancer Treat Rev.* 2016;42:56-72.
5. Patel K, Yip L, Lubitz C, et al. Executive Summary of the American Association of Endocrine Surgeons guidelines for the definitive surgical management of thyroid disease in adults. *Annals of Surgery.* 2020;271(3):399-410.
6. Haugen B, Alexander E, Bible K, et al. 2015 American Thyroid Association Management guidelines for adult patients with thyroid nodules and differentiated thyroid cancer: the American Thyroid Association Guidelines task force on thyroid nodules and differentiated thyroid cancer. *Thyroid.* 2016;26(1):1-133.
7. Kisioglu SV, Atacan H, Cakir E, et al. Efficacy of multidisciplinary approach in thyroid nodules: analysis of factors used for predicting malignancy. *Endocrine Abstracts.* 2021;73:AEP640.
8. Sugitani I, Ito Y, Takeuchi D, et al. Indications and strategy for active surveillance of adult low-risk papillary thyroid microcarcinoma: consensus statements from the Japan Association of Endocrine Surgery task force on management for papillary thyroid microcarcinoma. *Thyroid.* 2021;31(2):183-192.
9. Haser G, Tuttle RM, Su H, et al. Active surveillance for papillary thyroid microcarcinoma: new challenges and opportunities for the health care system. *Endocr Pract.* 2016;22(5):602-611.
10. Russell M, Kamani D, Randolph G. Modern surgery for advanced thyroid cancer: a tailored approach. *Gland Surg.* 2020;9(Suppl 2):S105-S119.
11. Ross DS, Burch HB, Cooper DS, et al. 2016 American Thyroid Association guidelines for diagnosis and management of hyperthyroidism and other causes of thyrotoxicosis. *Thyroid.* 2016;26(10):1343-1421. Erratum in: *Thyroid.* 2017;27(11):1462.
12. Scappaticcio L, Longo M, Maiorino M, et al. Abnormal liver blood tests in patients with hyperthyroidism: systematic review and meta-analysis. *Thyroid.* 2021;31(6):884-894.
13. Bilezikian JP. Primary Hyperparathyroidism. *J Clin Endocrinol Metab.* 2018;103(11):3993-4004.
14. Bilezikian J, Brandi M, Eastell R, et al. Guidelines for the management of asymptomatic primary hyperparathyroidism: summary statement from the Fourth International Workshop. *J Clin Endocrinol Metab.* 2014;99(10):3561-3569.
15. Wilhelm SM, Wang TS, Ruan DT, et al. The American Association of Endocrine Surgeons guidelines for definitive management of primary hyperparathyroidism. *JAMA Surg.* 2016;151(10):959-968.
16. Zeiger MA, Thompson GB, Duh QY, et al. American Association of Clinical Endocrinologists and American Association of Endocrine Surgeons Medical guidelines for the management of adrenal incidentalomas: executive summary of recommendations. *Endocr Pract.* 2009;15(5):450-453.
17. Lenders JW, Duh QY, Eisenhofer G, et al. Pheochromocytoma and paraganglioma: an endocrine society clinical practice guideline. *J Clin Endocrinol Metab.* 2014;99(6):1915-1942.
18. Souche R, Hobeika C, Hain E, Gaujoux S. Surgical management of neuroendocrine tumours of the pancreas. *J Clin Med.* 2020;9(9):2993.
19. Francis G, Waguespack S, Bauer A, et al. Management guidelines for children with thyroid nodules and differentiated thyroid cancer: the American Thyroid Association Guidelines task force on pediatric thyroid cancer. *Thyroid.* 2015;25(7):716-759.
20. Moore MD, Postma E, Gray KD, et al. Less is more: the impact of multidisciplinary thyroid conference on the treatment of well-differentiated thyroid carcinoma. *World J Surg.* 2018;42:343-349.

21. Hedman C, Djärv T, Strang P, Lundgren CI. Determinants of long-term quality of life in patients with differentiated thyroid carcinoma: a population-based cohort study in Sweden. *Acta Oncol.* 2016;55(3):365-369.
22. Miaskowski C. Outcome measures to evaluate the effectiveness of pain management in older adults with cancer. *Oncol Nurs Forum.* 2010;37(suppl):27-32.
23. Academy of Oncology Nurse & Patient Navigators. Helpful Definitions. www.aonnonline.org/about/helpful-definitions/. Accessed August 31, 2015.
24. Psooy BJ, Schreuer D, Borgaonkar J, Caines JS. Patient navigation: improving timeliness in the diagnosis of breast abnormalities. *Can Assoc Radiol J.* 2004;55:145-150.
25. Gilbert JE, Green E, Lankshear S, et al. Nurses as patient navigators in cancer diagnosis: review, consultation and model design. *Eur J Cancer Care (Engl).* 2011;20:228-236.
26. Seek A, Hogle WP. Modeling a better way: navigating the healthcare system for patients with lung cancer. *Clin J Oncol Nurs.* 2007;11:81-85.
27. Meguid C, Ryan C, Edil B, et al. Establishing a framework for building multidisciplinary programs. *J Multidiscip Healthc.* 2015;8:519-526.

2 Ethical Considerations in Endocrine Surgery

Patrick N. Nguyen, MD
Peter Angelos, MD, PhD
Megan K. Applewhite, MD

INTRODUCTION

Endocrine surgeons, like all surgeons, play a central role in patient care from the preoperative work-up to complex intraoperative decision-making and extending into the post-operative care of their patients. In each of these phases of care, there arise ethical considerations that range from small and nuanced word choice during the informed consent discussion to more significant decisions in the operating room and postoperatively when there may be unexpected findings or outcomes. Here, we will further elucidate the role of ethics and endocrine surgery as viewed through the lens of the patient care continuum from initial clinic visit to postoperative follow-up.

INFORMED CONSENT

Informed consent is often discussed from a medicolegal point of view. While a signed and witnessed surgical consent form must be present at surgical time-out, informed consent is more than a sheet of paper with signatures. It is a conversation that should encompass the preoperative, intraoperative, and postoperative periods.

The conversation should begin with disclosure. The surgeon must disclose the patient's diagnosis, the implications of the diagnosis, treatment options, alternatives, and their potential consequences. As the conversation progresses, the surgeon should first determine the patient's decision-making capacity. The patient must be able to understand their diagnosis and its implications, the treatment options, and their consequences, and then communicate a voluntary and independent decision regarding their treatment plan.[1] If the patient does not have decision-making capacity, the surgeon should turn toward the surrogate decision-maker, who may be the patient's medical power of attorney, spouse, next of kin, etc. Regardless of the identity of the medical decision-maker, informed consent remains a shared decision-making process during which the surgeon helps the patient (or their surrogate) understand their condition and then weigh the risks of complications against the benefits of surgery to make an informed decision.[2]

Patients vary in both their medical literacy and their wish to know the technical aspects and risks of surgery. Because trust and patient autonomy is a central tenet in every surgeon-patient relationship, patients undergoing surgery should be able to acquire and communicate a reasonable understanding of the surgery and its risks. However, some studies indicate that as many as one-third of surgical patients might not have an adequate understanding of the operation that they are having performed on them.[3] Furthermore, some patients might avoid discussing complications because they believe the procedure is unavoidable or because they want to avoid fear of the complications.[4] The art and essence of informed consent is discussing the risks of complications with the patients, and then assisting them with weighing these risks against the benefits of the procedure. Educational aids such as brochures, drawings, models, or videos may help the surgeon better describe the proposed surgery and its associated risks.[5]

The success of the conversation is contingent on both the surgeon and the patient. The verbiage and demeanor of the surgeon should be sensitive to the reactions, concerns, and responses of the patient. Informed consent is thus a dialogue between the surgeon and their patient that culminates in a relationship of trust.

RISKS, BENEFITS, & ALTERNATIVES

A discussion of risks, benefits, and alternative modalities of therapy lies at the core of informed consent and the preoperative conversation. A coarse-grained view of endocrine surgery shows the same risks and complications as with any other surgical procedure: surgical site infection, bleeding requiring transfusions and/or repeat operations, and locoregional injury. The specific nature of these complications reveals themselves in a finer view. For instance, neck operations on the thyroid and parathyroid glands carry the risk of hypocalcemia, a postoperative neck hematoma which would require reoperation in the case of airway compromise, or an intraoperative recurrent laryngeal nerve (RLN) injury that may lead to hoarseness or tracheostomy placement in the worst cases. Adrenalectomies carry the risk of postoperative adrenal insufficiency and crisis as well as risk of visceral injuries. The surgeon should discuss the statistical risk of these complications, as well as the signs and symptoms that the patient should recognize postoperatively.

Since surgery carries risks that can be avoided by not having surgery, the surgeon should discuss alternatives to surgery with the patient. However, the benefits and risks of these alternatives should be weighed against those of surgery. Consider the case of an indeterminate thyroid nodule. A viable alternative to surgery for many low-risk thyroid cancers would actually be no surgery or "active surveillance." Evolving alternatives also include alcohol ablation or radiofrequency ablation. Although these modalities avoid the complications of surgery, the risk of cancer progression (in "active surveillance") or non-oncologic margins (ablation) are higher. These discussions should account for patient factors and goals of care. For instance, a 99-year-old gentleman with advanced heart failure and previous total thyroidectomy with lateral neck dissection for thyroid cancer is likely not a good re-operative surgical candidate for a new lesion within the previous area of resection. The surgeon need not know all of the specifics of nonoperative alternatives, but the surgeon should know enough to help the patient weigh the pros and cons of surgery against the nonsurgical alternatives.

SETTING REALISTIC EXPECTATIONS

Beyond describing rates and consequences of RLN injury and permanent hypoparathyroidism, the endocrine surgeon must educate the patient on the more common postoperative outcomes, such as anticipated neck swelling and throat soreness from the endotracheal tube after thyroidectomy and transient hypocalcemia following parathyroidectomy. For many patients, an understanding of the experiences of other patients in similar circumstances provides reassurance preoperatively while also preparing them to identify and acclimate to the changes they may encounter in the postoperative setting.

In discussing expectations, the surgeon should tailor the conversation not just to the operation proposed, but to the patient's identity. In a study assessing quality of life in survivors of thyroid cancer, the experience of survivorship differs based on gender, age, and medical literacy.[6] It also identified a discrepancy between patient-reported adverse outcomes and those cited in the peer-reviewed surgical literature. While the incidence of RLN injury after thyroidectomy is cited at 1% to 5% in the surgical literature, the North American Thyroid Cancer Survivorship Study (NATCSS), a survey of more than 1100 thyroid cancer survivors, found the prevalence of patient-reported voice change following thyroidectomy at 54.9%. Similar trends toward higher rates of patient-reported adverse outcomes following surgery are observed for weight gain, hypoglycemia, and side effects from surgery, all reported at rates more than 10-fold above what might be expected from peer-reviewed surgical studies. Certainly, retrospective quality of life surveys may be subject to selection bias, but the perspective of these survivors is valuable and can help shape the preoperative conversation.

For cancers with a higher burden of disease, discussions about expectations will necessarily be different than for those with disease contained to the thyroid. For a patient with papillary carcinoma with lateral neck disease, or a follicular cancer with more distant metastases, while a worse prognosis is expected, and this ought to be communicated, it is critical that the surgeon avoids the "hanging of crepe." This strategy consists of describing the grimmest picture of potential outcomes to prepare patients for the worst-case scenario. If the worst-case scenario does occur, the expectations had been set, and the patients and their families had been prepared. If the worst-case scenario does not pan out, the surgeon is regarded in a better light.[7] Although "crepe hanging" can prepare patients and their families for the worst possible scenario, there are several disadvantages to this approach. Firstly, it inflicts an intense emotional distress upon the patient and their families that is potentially unnecessary. The associated perception of inevitable doom can affect the behaviors of other members of the patient's care team as well, leading to potentially nonstandard levels of care. Furthermore, it is disingenuous of the surgeon to suggest the worst possible outcome when they know the patient will likely do better than that. What the family loses in worry and anxiety, the surgeon gains in praise and laud if/when operation and subsequent therapy is successful, which could be seen as manipulative. Ultimately, it is better to accurately prognosticate patients based on their presentation and available data, then faithfully relaying their prognosis to them in a controlled, professional manner.

SURGICAL INNOVATION & TECHNOLOGY

Modern surgical innovation proceeds with the adoption of new technologies and new techniques. For instance, there has been interest in robot-assisted approaches to thyroidectomies and parathyroidectomies. Transoral surgery is yet another approach for neck endocrine gland surgeries. In theory, these alternative approaches to endocrine surgery may provide a more minimally invasive approach. In reality, the specific advantages these approaches afford are difficult to study because the prevalence of complications is already low. Surgeons should be cautious when advocating for one approach over the other if objective evidence is sparse or unconvincing; however, it is important to recognize that innovation is critical to evolution of surgical techniques. Without early adopters of technology and innovative approaches, the field risks not moving forward and improving. For this reason, early adopters ought to be encouraged to push techniques and technology to work for patients in novel ways as long as safety to the patient is always kept in the forefront. For mid and late adopters of innovation, addition to understanding emerging data, surgeon awareness of their own skillset, and comfort with innovation is critical, and becomes important when deciding whether to adapt new techniques into one's own practice.

PATIENT FACTORS IN THE SURGEON-PATIENT RELATIONSHIP

Due to the nature of the endocrine glands, endocrine surgery requires that the patient upholds certain responsibilities to increase the chances of a successful postoperative outcome. For instance, adherence to hormone replacement and surveillance visits and lab draws are essential to favorable long-term outcomes in both benign and oncologic endocrine disease.[8]

Globalization and an increasingly accessible Internet have made a wealth of information available to patients with a few touches of the fingertips. While this generates opportunities to become more medically literate, this also creates opportunities for medical misinformation or even disinformation. Yet another layer of complexity is that patients may feel more empowered to make their own choices based on what they have read. Though occasionally difficult, the surgeon should help the patient filter correct information from incorrect information. Ideally, this should be part of the preoperative discussion focused on the risks and benefits of surgery and alternatives to surgery. Having a readily available list of reliable and evidence-based websites to share with patients can help guide them in their educational process when they have questions that arise outside the office setting.

GENETIC COUNSELING

Endocrine pathologies are sometimes entangled in genetic syndromes, most frequently discussed for trainees is the multiple endocrine neoplasia syndromes. However, endocrine cancers, such as thyroid cancer, may be a part of a more subtle cancer syndrome with genetic disorders, such as Cowden syndrome, Familial Non-Medulary Thyroid Cancer, Li-Fraumeni, Lynch syndrome, and others. Although the prevalence of these syndromes is rare overall, the family history remains a critical component of the surgeon interview with a patient. If suspicion of a genetic syndrome is high, genetic testing should be discussed with the patient. Although genetic testing may not help the patient any more than providing a unifying diagnosis, patients must understand that their relatives may be similarly affected by the same genetic syndrome.

INTRAOPERATIVE DECISION-MAKING & UNEXPECTED INTRAOPERATIVE FINDINGS

Intraoperative decision-making frequently arises during endocrine surgeries. For instance, in a four-gland exploration for hyperparathyroidism, the surgeon must decide whether or not a thyroid lobectomy is indicated when all locations for an ectopic parathyroid gland have been exhausted. In surgeries for thyroid cancer, the surgeon may have to do a central neck dissection if grossly abnormal nodes are encountered. In unexpected situations, the surgeon must make an evidence-based or experience-based decision that the patient may not have explicitly consented to. The surgical consent form may cover the unexpected finding and associated management. In the case, the surgeon would certainly wish to engage the surrogate decision-maker if possible, and would proceed to keep the patient safe and make decisions in their best interest to minimize harm and maximize benefit of the operation with the circumstances as they are.

DISCLOSURE OF ERRORS & COMPLICATIONS

Errors and complications are not always avoidable. However, errors and complications are distinct entities. Errors are made, and complications occur. An error is a deviation from the ideal maneuver or decision. On the other hand, a complication is the postoperative sequelae of an error. An error does not always result in a complication. Certainly, complications should be disclosed to the patient. The central question is thus: Do all errors need to be disclosed to the patient, even when they do not result in a complication? Patients have a right to know their medical history, but if all imperfections of the operation were disclosed to the patient, then the list would be detailed and lengthy in many cases, given variation in anatomy, unexpected findings, and varied levels of proficiency in cases where trainees are participating. A focus-group study of patients and physicians examined both perspectives of disclosure.[9] In general, patients felt that physicians should disclose the following: (1) an explicit statement that an error occurred, (2) a basic description of what the error was, why it happened, and how it will be prevented from happening again, and (3) an apology. The physician group generally agreed that harmful errors should be disclosed, but many were reluctant to formally apologize due to concerns of legal liability. We would argue that honesty and clarity in discussing intraoperative and postoperative complications is extremely important to respect the autonomy of the patient, and to maintain patient trust in the surgeon-patient relationship. Interestingly, the study suggested that physicians were adversely affected by complications as well and frequently do not feel there is adequate support when complications happen. This represents an opportunity for the surgical community to encourage discussion between peers when complications occur, as this can offer much-needed support that stabilizes or improves the well-being of the surgeon, who frequently feels the negative impact of serious patient complications in a significant way.

REFERENCES

1. Informed Consent. American Medical Association.
2. Bernat JL, Peterson LM. Patient-centered informed consent in surgical practice. *Arch Surg*. 2006;141(1):86-92.
3. Pugliese OT, Solari JL, Ferreres AR. The extent of surgical patients' understanding. *World J Surg*. 2014;38(7):1605-1609.
4. McNair AGK, MacKichan F, Donovan JL, et al. What surgeons tell patients and what patients want to know before major cancer surgery: a qualitative study. *BMC Cancer*. 2016;16:258.
5. Bollschweiler E, Apitzsch J, Obliers R, et al. Improving informed consent of surgical patients using a multimedia-based program? Results of a prospective randomized multicenter study of patients before cholecystectomy. *Annals of Surgery*. 2008;248(2):205-211.
6. Aschebrook-Kilfoy B, James B, Nagar S, et al. Risk factors for decreased quality of life in thyroid cancer survivors: initial findings from the North American thyroid cancer survivorship study. *Thyroid*. 2015;25(12):1313-1321.
7. Siegler M. Pascal's wager and the hanging of crepe. *N Engl J Med*. 1975;293(17):853-857.
8. Dhillon VK, Russell JO, Al Khadem MG, Tufano RP. Preoperative information for thyroid surgery. *Gland Surg*. 2017;6(5):482-487.
9. Gallagher TH, Waterman AD, Ebers AG, Fraser VJ, Levinson W. Patients' and physicians' attitudes regarding the disclosure of medical errors. *JAMA*. 2003;289(8):1001-1007.

3 Genetic Basis & Clinical Management of Familial Thyroid Cancer

Hunter J. Underwood, MD
Kepal N. Patel, MD

GENERAL CONSIDERATIONS

The overwhelming majority of non-medullary thyroid cancer (NMTC) is attributable to sporadic somatic mutations. NMTC diagnosed in the setting of thyroid cancer present in 2 to 3 first-degree relatives with the absence of known environmental risk factors is defined as familial non-medullary thyroid cancer (FNMTC).[1] Current literature suggests that FNMTC represents 3% to 9% of new thyroid cancer diagnoses with 5% representing syndromic forms with well-established driver mutations. The non-syndromic forms are defined as non-syndromic familial non-medullary thyroid cancer (NFNMTC), whereas those with established genotype/phenotype correlation are described as syndromic familial non-medullary thyroid cancer (SFNMTC). The most common syndromes associated with SFNMTC include familial adenomatous polyposis (FAP), PTEN-Hamartoma tumor (Cowden) syndrome, Carney complex, Werner syndrome, and DICER syndrome.

In contrast, medullary thyroid cancer (MTC) is associated with germline *RET* proto-oncogene mutation in 25% of cases. Although *RET* mutations can occur sporadically, germline *RET* mutations are associated with multiple endocrine neoplasia (MEN) syndromes 2A and 2B. Among MEN syndromes, MEN2A is most common and includes the variants of classical MEN2A, MEN2A with cutaneous lichen amyloidosis, MEN2A with Hirschsprung disease, and familial MTC. MEN2B is the least common variant subtype of MEN; however, it is associated with high-risk MTC that occurs early in infancy. As the penetration of MTC within these syndromes is 100%, early identification and genetic testing are critical to offer prophylactic thyroidectomy and screen for other associated conditions at the appropriate time.

A thorough understanding of the phenotypical presentations of syndromes associated with SFNMTC and MTC is critical for diagnosis which allows for surveillance of other associated malignancies and genetic testing of index patients' family members if indicated. In this chapter, we aim to summarize both the genetic and molecular bases of these syndromes, as well as their clinical implications.

NONSYNDROMIC FAMILIAL NON-MEDULLARY THYROID CANCER

NFNMTC is defined as the presence of follicular cell thyroid carcinoma affecting 2 to 3 first-degree relatives without a known familial syndrome or known exposure to environmental risk factors. Although all histologic subtypes of NMTC have been described in this entity, papillary thyroid cancer (PTC) represents the overwhelming majority of cases. The genetic basis for NFNMTC is currently not well-defined and is thought to be a polygenic process without a clear driver mutation; thus, germline genetic testing is not possible. Interestingly, common somatic mutations seen in PTC (eg, *BRAF*, *RAS*) are not present as germline mutations in NFNMTC kindreds. Although culpable germline mutations for NFNMTC have not been identified, several susceptibility genes have been reported including *HAP2, SRGAP1, FOXE1, TITF-1/NKX2.1,* and *MAP2K5.*

Multiple studies have demonstrated NFNMTC presents at an earlier age; however, there is conflicting literature regarding the aggressiveness of NFNMTC compared to sporadic NMTC. Given this controversy, a meta-analysis was conducted by Wang et al. which included 12 studies with 12,741 patients with NFNMTC and sporadic NMTC.[2] They found that NFNMTC had increased rates of recurrence, decreased disease-free survival, high risk of multifocality, extrathyroidal extension, and lymph node metastasis when compared to sporadic cases. While there is no evidence to suggest prophylactic thyroidectomy is warranted for NFNMTC patients, total thyroidectomy (as opposed to hemithyroidectomy) should be considered for the initial surgical approach given higher rates of multifocality and recurrence.

Given the concordant data regarding earlier age of presentation about NFNMTC kindreds, thyroid cancer screening should be performed in those with appropriate family history. Screening should include both physical and ultrasound exam of the thyroid gland and lymph node basins. A recent prospective study investigating screening protocols for patients with NFNMTC found that the prevalence of thyroid cancer detected by screening in at-risk individuals with two first-degree relatives was the same as the general population (4.6% vs 4.5%, respectively).[3] However, among at-risk patients with three or more first-degree relatives, the prevalence of thyroid cancer detected by screening was 22.7%. Despite the controversy regarding the definition of NFNMTC, this suggests that active screening should only be performed in individuals with three or more first-degree relatives affected. Currently, there is no consensus regarding when screening should occur; however, the American Association of Endocrine Surgeons (AAES) recent guidelines suggest screening 5 years prior to the youngest adult family member being diagnosed.[4]

SYNDROMIC FAMILIAL NON-MEDULLARY THYROID CANCER

Familial Adenomatous Polyposis & Gardner Syndrome

Familial adenomatous polyposis (FAP) and Gardner syndrome are both caused by germline mutation of the adenomatous polyposis coli (APC) tumor suppressor gene located on chromosome 5q21. While FAP is largely defined by intestinal polyps, the variant known as Gardner syndrome is also associated with extraintestinal tumors such as osteomas of the skull, fibromas, and epithelial cysts. Both syndromes have autosomal dominant inheritance and are associated with an increased risk of thyroid cancer. As with the general population, PTC is the most common cancer type among FAP/Gardner patients; however, 20% to 40% of these tumors have a distinct variant on histopathology designated the cribriform-morular variant. Thus, the diagnosis of FAP/Gardners should be strongly considered in any patient with cribriform-morular variant of PTC seen unexpectedly on final pathology after thyroidectomy.

A recent meta-analysis of 9821 patients with FAP demonstrated a pooled prevalence of thyroid cancer, benign structural thyroid disease, and functional thyroid disease of 2.6%, 48.8%, and 6.9%, respectively.[5] Of significance, in 34% of the study population the diagnosis of thyroid cancer preceded the diagnosis of FAP. Although the rate of PTC is significantly higher in FAP patients than in the general population, the role of thyroid cancer screening in FAP patients remains controversial. Current guidelines from the American College of Gastroenterology suggest yearly ultrasound screening starting in adolescence.[6] A recent prospective study of 267 patients with FAP undergoing thyroid cancer screening with ultrasound showed that on initial sonogram 63.3% had normal appearing thyroid glands without nodularity, 27.7% had the presence of low-risk nodules, and 9.0% with high-risk nodules.[7] The patients were observed for a mean of 4.8 years and underwent an average of three ultrasounds. None of the patients with normal thyroid glands on initial ultrasound developed thyroid cancer or new nodules. Among those with nodules on initial ultrasound, a total of six patients (2.3%) developed thyroid cancer with five patients being from the low-risk group and one patient being from the high-risk group. This suggests that the surveillance strategy and frequency of imaging can be tailored to the individual patient based on the coexisting presence of structural thyroid disease on initial exam.

Cowden (PTEN-Hamartoma Tumor) Syndrome

Cowden syndrome is an autosomal dominant disease characterized by the presence of multiple benign hamartomas and mucocutaneous lesions with an increased risk of developing breast, thyroid, and uterine malignancy. Germline mutations in the tumor suppressor gene PTEN are associated with approximately 80% of cases; however, alterations in SDHB-D, PIK3CA, AKT1, and KLLN promoter methylation may also play a role. Given the lack of concrete genotype-phenotype correlation, the diagnosis of Cowden syndrome is currently based on clinical criteria as opposed to strictly being based on the detection of associated mutations.[8]

Previous studies have demonstrated that the lifetime risk of developing thyroid cancer in the setting of Cowden syndrome is 35% with a younger age of incidence. As a result, the National Comprehensive Cancer Network (NCCN) recommends annual screening via thyroid ultrasound annually starting at 18 years for patients with Cowden syndrome. A recent retrospective study from the Mayo Clinic investigated the incidence and progression of thyroid cancer in patients with Cowden syndrome from 1979 to 2017 with an average follow-up of 10 years. Of the 47 patients identified, 23 (48.9%) underwent total thyroidectomy during the study period.[9] The majority of the patients who underwent surgery initially presented for surgical consultation due to the presence of multinodular goiter. Only nine patients (19.1%) had thyroid cancer detected on final pathology with the majority being classical PTC or follicular-variant of PTC and had similar clinical behavior as with sporadic PTC. Of these patients, seven were diagnosed with Cowden syndrome after thyroidectomy, which redemonstrates the importance of maintaining a high index of suspicion for genetic syndromes after thyroid cancer diagnosis in younger patients or those with significant family history. Although there is no current data to support prophylactic thyroidectomy, it can be considered in those with Cowden syndrome with severe developmental delay due to the impracticality of screening. This, however, must be balanced with the simultaneous impracticality of lifelong thyroid hormone.

Carney Complex

Carney complex displays autosomal-dominant inheritance and is associated with cardiac and soft-tissue myxomas, cutaneous changes, schwannomas, and tumors of the adrenal, pituitary, and thyroid glands. The molecular pathogenesis of Carney complex is most often due to an inactivating germline mutation of *PRKAR1A* tumor-suppressor gene which is present in 70% of patients with the syndrome. Less commonly, Carney complex is caused by a variety of genetic changes on chromosome 2 at locus 2p16. Regardless of molecular etiology, the phenotype remains the same. Thyroid cancer or structural thyroid disease is noted in 5% of patients with Carney complex; thus, screening and prophylactic thyroidectomy are not currently recommended.

Werner Syndrome

Werner syndrome, also known as "adult progeria," is an autosomal recessive disease caused by multiple mutations of WRN on chromosome 8p11-21. The diagnosis of Werner syndrome is often made in the second decade of life when rapid aging begins to occur after puberty. Premature aging is associated with skin changes, cataracts, atherosclerosis, osteoporosis, and a high occurrence of neoplasms. In a large case series, 16% of 189 patients with Werner syndrome developed thyroid cancer at a median age of 40 years.[10] Follicular thyroid carcinoma is the most common histologic subtype among patients with Werner syndrome. Due to the rarity of the syndrome, no defined screening guidelines exist and the role of prophylactic thyroidectomy has not been established.

DICER1 Syndrome

DICER1 syndrome is characterized by autosomal dominant loss of function mutation in the *DICER1* protein, which aids in cleaving RNA precursors to functional miRNA. Phenotypically, DICER1 syndrome is associated with pleuropulmonary blastoma (PBB), Sertoli-Leydig ovarian tumors, pineoblastoma, and multinodular goiter. The penetrance of any of these phenotypes is estimated at 15%. Treatment of PPB with alkylating chemotherapy was thought to drive the risk of thyroid cancer; however, newer data suggest an increased risk of thyroid cancer in DICER1 patients who are not treated with systemic chemotherapy.[11] No guidelines for screening currently exist; however, AAES guidelines suggest screening with ultrasound at 5 years after completion of chemotherapy for PBB or 10 years of age, whichever occurs first.

HEREDITARY MEDULLARY THYROID CANCER

Multiple Endocrine Neoplasia 2

Although the majority of MTC is sporadic, 25% of index cases are associated with germline mutation of the RET proto-oncogene located on chromosome 10. RET is expressed in all cells that arise from the neural crest, branchial arches, and the urogenital system. As parafollicular C-cells within the thyroid gland arise from the neural crest, a majority of MTC harbor RET mutations. The autosomal dominant inheritance of RET mutations is the molecular hallmark of multiple endocrine neoplasia syndrome, type 2, and its variants. The penetration of MTC within those with MEN2 approaches 100% throughout a lifetime; however, the specific codon mutated within the gene helps guide screening protocols for other associated malignancies and/or the age at which prophylactic thyroidectomy is recommended. MEN2A has four described variants, which include classical MEN2A, MEN2A with cutaneous lichen amyloidosis (CLA), MEN2A with Hirschsprung disease (HD), and familial MTC. MEN2B, however, only has one defined phenotype. The American Thyroid Association (ATA) guidelines have categorized common RET mutations seen in MEN2 into moderate risk, high risk, and highest risk based on the phenotypical aggressiveness of MTC observed.[12]

Classical MEN2A

Classical MEN2A represents the majority (95%) of MEN2 cases and is associated with germline RET mutations occurring in codons 609, 611, 618, or 620 of exon 10 or codon 634 of exon 11. Nearly all patients with classical MEN2A develop MTC; however, the penetrance of pheochromocytoma and hyperparathyroidism varies depending on the specific codon mutation. RET codon 634 mutations are associated with the highest incidence of pheochromocytoma. A Japanese series of 493 registered MEN2 patients displayed penetrance of pheochromocytoma of 25% by 30 years of age, 52% by 50 years of age, and 88% by 77 years of age. Pheochromocytoma in MEN2A patients tends to be benign, bilateral, and multicentric. In one study, 52% of patients with MEN2A who underwent unilateral adrenalectomy for isolated pheochromocytoma developed a contralateral tumor within 10 years of resection.[13] Hyperparathyroidism penetrance typically varies from 2% to 12%, with the exception of codon 634 mutations, which has displayed penetrance of up to 30%.[14] The presentation of primary hyperparathyroidism is often mild biochemical profile disease; however, there are reports of both single and multigland disease. Historically, the timing of prophylactic thyroidectomy in MEN2A patients was based on calcitonin levels; however, current management focuses on ATA risk category based on patient-specific mutations. Those with moderate risk RET mutations should have calcitonin monitored annually and total thyroidectomy with prophylactic central neck dissection when levels begin to rise. Those with high-risk RET mutations should undergo total thyroidectomy and prophylactic central neck dissection by 5 years of age or earlier if calcitonin levels begin to increase.

MEN2A With Cutaneous Lichen Amyloidosis

MEN2A with CLA can occur from germline inheritance or sporadically and is characterized by hyperpigmented lesions that most often occur overlying the scapulae bilaterally. These lesions are associated with intense pruritus that improves with sun exposure and worsens with stress. CLA often presents at a young age prior to the development of MTC; thus, detection of these lesions in adolescence should prompt genetic testing. MEN2A with CLA is only associated with codon 634 and 804 mutations of the RET proto-oncogene. Among patients with codon 634 mutation, CLA phenotype is present in up to 34%.[15]

MEN2A With Hirschsprung Disease

Germline RET mutations are seen in 50% of patients with hereditary HD and 15% to 20% of patients with sporadic HD. MEN2A with HD is associated with point mutations of exon 10 of the RET gene with codon 620 mutation being the most prevalent.[16] HD occurs in approximately 7% of patients with MEN2A, whereas MEN2A occurs in 2% to 5% of patients who clinically have HD. The clinical phenotype seen with MEN2 syndromes is associated with "gain of function" mutations of the RET proto-oncogene, whereas RET mutations in HD are associated with "loss of function." The paradox of HD and MEN2A existing simultaneously is hypothesized to be due to constitutive activation of RET that is sufficient to trigger neoplastic change in certain cell types (eg, C cells), yet insufficient to create trophic response in precursor neurons.

Familial Medullary Thyroid Cancer

Familial medullary thyroid cancer (FMTC) is characterized by kindreds with germline RET mutation and hereditary MTC without associated pheochromocytoma or hyperparathyroidism.[17] The most common mutations seen in FMTC involve extracellular cysteine codons in RET exon 10.

Multiple Endocrine Neoplasia 2B

MEN2B is characterized by aggressive MTC that presents early in infancy. Of note, 75% of novel MEN2B cases are due to sporadic RET mutations, whereas 25% arise from germline mutations inherited in autosomal dominant manner.[18] The vast majority (95%) have RET mutations within codon M918T. The penetrance of pheochromocytoma within this genotype is approximately 50%. MEN2B is also classically associated with ophthalmologic abnormalities, marfanoid body habitus, and ganglioneuromatosis. The diagnosis of MEN2B is often made after MTC is clinically evident and too advanced to be cured. As patients with MEN2B are in the highest ATA risk category, prophylactic thyroidectomy is recommended within the first year of life with surgery being offered as soon as deemed appropriate by a multidisciplinary team. Pheochromocytoma screening is recommended annually starting at 11 years of age.

REFERENCES

1. Capezzone M, Robenshtok E, Cantara S, Castagna MG. Familial non-medullary thyroid cancer: a critical review. *J Endocrinol Invest.* 2021;44(5):943-950.
2. Wang X, Cheng W, Li J, et al. Familial nonmedullary thyroid carcinoma is a more aggressive disease: a systematic review and meta-analysis. *Eur J Endocrinol.* 2015;172(6):253-262.
3. Klubo-Gwiezdzinska J, Yang L, Merkel R, et al. Results of screening in familial non-medullary thyroid cancer. *Thyroid.* 2017;27(8):1017-1024.
4. Patel KN, Yip L, Lubitz CC, et al. The American Association of Endocrine Surgeons guidelines for the definitive surgical management of thyroid disease in adults. *Annal Surg.* 2020; *271*(3):e21-e93.
5. Chenbhanich J, Atsawarungruangkit A, Korpaisarn S, Phupitakphol T, Osataphan S, Phowthongkum P. Prevalence of thyroid diseases in familial adenomatous polyposis: a systematic review and meta-analysis. *Fam Cancer.* 2019;18(1):53-62.
6. Lamartina L, Grani G, Durante C, Filetti S, Cooper DS. Screening for differentiated thyroid cancer in selected populations. *Lancet Diabetes Endocrinol.* 2020;8(1):81-88.
7. Monachese M, Mankaney G, Lopez R, et al. Outcome of thyroid ultrasound screening in FAP patients with a normal baseline exam. *Fam Cancer.* 2019;18(1):75-82.
8. Pilarski R, Burt R, Kohlman W, Pho L, Shannon, KM, Swisher E. Cowden syndrome and the PTEN hamartoma tumor syndrome: systematic review and revised diagnostic criteria. *J Natl Cancer Inst.* 2013;105(21):1607-1616.
9. Yamashita TS, Baky FJ, McKenzie TJ, et al. Occurrence and natural history of thyroid cancer in patients with Cowden syndrome. *Eur Thyroid J.* 2020;9(5):243-246.
10. Lauper JM, Krause A, Vaughan TL, Monnat RJ Jr. Spectrum and risk of neoplasia in Werner syndrome: a systematic review. *PLoS One*, 2013;8(4):e59709.
11. Rutter MM, Jha P, Schultz K. et al. DICER1 mutations and differentiated thyroid carcinoma: evidence of a direct association. *J Clin Endocrinol.* 2016;101(1):1-5.
12. Wells SA Jr, Asa SL, Dralle H, et al. Revised American Thyroid Association guidelines for the management of medullary thyroid carcinoma: the American Thyroid Association Guidelines Task Force on medullary thyroid carcinoma. *Thyroid.* 2015;25(6):567-610.

13. Lairmore TC, Ball DW, Baylin SB, Wells SA Jr. Management of pheochromocytomas in patients with multiple endocrine neoplasia type 2 syndromes. *Ann Surg*. 1993; 217(6):595.
14. Imai T, Uchino S, Okamoto T, et al. High penetrance of pheochromocytoma in multiple endocrine neoplasia 2 caused by germline RET codon 634 mutation in Japanese patients. *Eur J Endocrinol*. 2013;168(5):683-687.
15. Verga U, Fugazzola L, Cambiaghi S, et al. Frequent association between MEN 2A and cutaneous lichen amyloidosis. *Clin Endocrinol*. 2003;59(2):156-161.
16. Attié T, Pelet A, Edery P, et al. Diversity of RET proto-oncogene mutations in familial and sporadic Hirschsprung disease. *Hum Mol Genet*. 1995;4(8):1381-1386.
17. Wells SA Jr, Pacini F, Robinson BG, Santoro M. Multiple endocrine neoplasia type 2 and familial medullary thyroid carcinoma: an update. *J Clin Endocrinol Metabol*. 2013;98(8):3149-3164.
18. Eng C, Clayton D, Schuffenecker I, et al. The relationship between specific RET proto-oncogene mutations and disease phenotype in multiple endocrine neoplasia type 2: International RET Mutation Consortium analysis. *JAMA*. 1996;276(19):1575-1579.

Quality Measures in Endocrine Surgery

4

Jennifer E. Rosen, MD, FACS
Hui Zheng, MD

BRIEF HISTORY OF QUALITY IMPROVEMENT IN SURGERY

Every hospital should follow every patient it treats, long enough to determine whether or not the treatment has been successful, and then to inquire, 'if not, why not' with a view to preventing similar failure in future.

—Dr Ernest Codman

Although we take it for granted today, quality improvement in medicine was a controversial idea in the early 20th century. Dr Ernest Codman, an orthopedic surgeon in Boston, Massachusetts, first advocated for a system where hospitals would not only track but also publish their "end results" from surgical interventions.[1] Dr Codman was ahead of his time, not only for recognizing the practical need for quality improvement but also for the educational value. Unfortunately, his revolutionary idea at the time fell on uninterested ears in the medical community.[2] Therefore, he took his "end result" idea to establish his own hospital, which he aptly named the "End Result Hospital."[3] From the Codman Hospital, he published annual reports and sent them to leading hospitals across the United States, urging them to follow his suit. Dr Codman's insistence on transparency in surgical outcomes inspired contemporary visionaries such as Dr Franklin Martin and eventually led to the founding of the American College of Surgeons (ACS) in 1913.[4]

The ACS initiated the Hospital Standardization Program in 1917 to accredit hospitals in the United States based on a set of "minimum standards."[5] Out of 692 reviewed hospitals with more than 100 beds, only 89 passed the muster initially, highlighting the overdue need for quality control at the time. As hospitals, medical, and surgical specialties grew both in numbers and complexity, the ACS joined forces with the American College of Physicians, the American Hospital Association, and the American Medical Association to establish the Joint Commission on Accreditation of Hospitals in 1951.[4] Later, quality improvement in medicine expanded its scope to include not only the end results of care but also the efficiency and cost-effectiveness, among others outlined in Dr Avedis Donabedian's paper from 1966.[6]

Due to a high mortality rate and surgical complications among the Veterans Administration (VA) hospitals in 1985, the US Federal Government issued a mandate to improve surgical outcomes in the VA system. The National VA Surgical Risk Study was conducted recognizing the challenge of comparing patients with differing risk factors and disease severities.[7] This hallmark study established the parameters of risk adjustment that were subsequently incorporated into the VA National Surgical Quality Improvement Program (VA-NSQIP). The program proved to be a resounding success, reducing 30-day postoperative morbidity and mortality by 27% and 45%, respectively, in the ensuing decade within the VA hospital system.[8] The ACS, as a champion organization for quality improvement in surgery, took notice and tested the program in a small number of civilian hospitals. In 2004, the ACS rolled out its own version of the VA-NSQIP (ACS NSQIP) nationwide, which now encompasses more than 700 participating hospitals.[9]

AMERICAN ASSOCIATION OF ENDOCRINE SURGEONS & CESQIP

Endocrine surgery is a relatively young subspecialty of surgery. A flurry of ground-breaking discoveries and inventions related to the treatment of endocrine diseases from 1950 to 1960 has made endocrine surgery more nuanced. In the same meeting where the International Association of Endocrine Surgeons (IAES) was founded, the American Association of Endocrine Surgeons (AAES) was established in 1979 by five surgeons, namely, Dr Orlo Clark, Dr Norman Thompson, Dr Anthony Edis, Dr Edwin Kaplan, and Dr Jack Monchik.[10] They held their very first meeting the next year at Ann Arbor, Michigan, with approximately 90 attendants.

The organization grew rapidly in the next few decades. While endocrine surgery fellowships were created in the 1980s, a defined curriculum was not developed until 2004, the first match in 2006, and an accreditation process in 2013.[11]

The Collaborative Endocrine Surgery Quality Improvement Program (CESQIP) was created by the AAES in 2012.[12] It is a voluntary collaboration to collect data for quality improvement as well as collaborative learning. There are 14 published studies in the English-language literature at the time of this writing that used data from the CESQIP database to evaluate quality outcomes in endocrine surgery. The development and utilization of CESQIP are in their infancy but hold great promise for advancing the field of quality outcomes in endocrine surgery and for patients who undergo endocrine surgery procedures.

ENDOCRINE OPERATIONS: WHAT AFFECTS PATIENT OUTCOME?

Thyroidectomy, parathyroidectomy, and adrenalectomy are within the scope of practice for endocrine surgeons, although not exclusively. Traditionally performed by general surgeons as well as otolaryngologists, the growing complexity and sophistication of treatments for thyroid and parathyroid conditions led to the formation of the subspecialty of endocrine surgery in the 1970s and culminated in the foundation of the AAES in 1978.[13] Many aspects of an endocrine surgeon's scope of practice continue to be shared with various other surgical subspecialties such as urology, minimally invasive surgery, surgical oncology, and otorhinolaryngology.

Thyroid and parathyroid operations comprise more than 90% of endocrine surgeons' practice. More than 100,000 thyroidectomies and 18,000 parathyroidectomies are performed every year in the United States. Many of them are performed by general surgeons and those without subspecialty training, however. More importantly, 75% of thyroidectomies are performed by low-volume thyroid surgeons, commonly defined as fewer than 30 to 35 procedures per year.[14] This has significant implications because studies have demonstrated that high-volume surgeons and hospitals produce superior outcomes concerning complication rates, length of stay, and cost.[15] It has also been laid bare that the obstacles to access high-volume surgeons fall disproportionally on racial minorities and socioeconomically disadvantaged patients.[16] This highlights the need for greater organization of the subspecialty and concentration of cases to improve the quality of care patients receive.

Adrenal resections are another operation performed by endocrine surgeons, although at a much lower volume than thyroid or parathyroid procedures. Adrenal surgery has a low mortality rate, but the complication rate of adrenal operations is significantly higher than that of thyroid and parathyroid operations, ranging from 8% to 19%. More than two-thirds of adrenalectomies are performed by general surgeons and related subspecialists including endocrine surgery and surgical oncology.[17] The lesson that has been repeatedly demonstrated across surgical specialties is that operative volume in the procedure of interest supersedes the training discipline a surgeon receives.[18] This is likely to drive a trend toward superspecialization of surgical specialties. However, the balance between expert care and accessibility remains difficult. It may be of interest for health-care insurance companies to incentivize and perhaps even cover the cost of traveling to improve access and reduce cost, so long as outcomes are reliably demonstrated to be linked to subspecialty expertise.

Neuroendocrine tumors (NETs) are a heterogenous entity of neoplasms that can arise from many parts of the body. Their incidence is approximately 5.86 per 100,000 people per year.[19] NETs most commonly arise from the gastrointestinal tract (62%-67%) followed by the lung (22%-27%). Their low prevalence qualifies for orphan disease status. Because of the heterogenous origin of NETs, multiple surgical disciplines including surgical oncologists, colorectal surgeons, and thoracic surgeons can be involved in addition to endocrine surgeons. This decentralized patient base poses a challenge to studying this uncommon neoplasm in terms of oncologic outcomes. We will discuss the challenges rare endocrine neoplasms pose for surgeons in another subsection.

WHAT OUTCOMES MATTER IN ENDOCRINE SURGERY?

When talking about outcomes in surgery, it is important to consider what you are trying to measure and for whom it matters. There are patient-reported outcomes: quality of life, financial toxicity, voice handicap index ratings, etc. There are objective measures of morbidity- and mortality-related outcomes: postoperative readmission most often for hypocalcemia, reoperation for hematoma, and recurrent laryngeal nerve injury. There are more disease-specific measures of outcomes: cure rate in primary hyperparathyroidism, postoperative length of stay after surgery for secondary hyperparathyroidism, postoperative thyroglobulin level in early-stage thyroid cancer as a proxy for complete resection, resolution of primary aldosteronism after adrenalectomy, etc.

Quality metrics are currently popular to use as proxies for quality care. Measurement of quality metrics in endocrine surgery can be difficult depending on the metric. Surgeons are now being asked for quality metrics that will be linked to bonus or incentive pay. Process measures such as completion of medical records are attractive metrics because they have a high incidence and therefore can be compared over time. However, measurable metrics are not necessarily good proxies for quality care. Surgeons should choose a metric that they can improve with institutional help, not just because they are already doing the work necessary or because they can be measured. Hypocalcemia, for example, is a poor-quality metric because it has a low incidence and is often managed as an outpatient issue and thus is not easily tracked. Most importantly, hypocalcemia after endocrine surgery is a poor proxy for quality care because it is not necessarily just due to surgeon-specific factors; for example, it can be due to a complicated case mix or patient noncompliance. In summary, the ideal quality metric would be reliable, measurable, have a high incidence, serve as a good proxy for what is considered quality care, and ideally be related to improved patient outcomes.

ENDOCRINE SURGERY OUTCOMES IN CHILDREN

Endocrine disorders in the pediatric population are relatively rare. Thyroid nodules are prevalent in 0.2% to 1.8% of the pediatric population, and the incidence of primary hyperparathyroidism (PHPT) is 2 to 5 per 100,000 children.[20] Adrenocortical tumors in the pediatric population are extremely rare, with a reported worldwide incidence of 0.3 cases per million children per year. We will therefore focus on thyroid and parathyroid diseases in children.

Thyroid nodules in children are more likely to be malignant than their adult counterparts. In children, similar to the adult population, the incidence of thyroid cancer has been increasing over the last four decades, albeit at a less dramatic pace.[21]

Again, there is an overlap in the number of surgical specialties involved in the care of thyroid and parathyroid diseases in the pediatric population. Due to their general interests in pathologies arising from organs within head and neck, otolaryngologists are often involved in the care of thyroid disorders and parathyroid conditions as well. Pediatric surgeons, being a general surgical discipline for children, usually do not accrue high volumes of thyroid or parathyroid cases.[22]

In fact, the majority of the pediatric thyroid and parathyroid operations are not performed by high-volume endocrine surgeons, akin to the patterns seen in adults. Only 18% of pediatric thyroid and parathyroid surgeries are attributed to surgeons who perform at least 30 cases per year on patients of all ages. While the rates of complications in thyroid and parathyroid operations are low, both general and endocrine-specific complications occur more frequently in the pediatric population compared to adults. Moreover, the superior outcome produced by high-volume endocrine surgeons has been demonstrated in pediatric populations as well.

Thyroid cancer in children differs from adults in significant ways. Pediatric thyroid cancer often presents with larger tumors and more extensive disease with metastasis to cervical lymph nodes and distant organs. Despite this, children with thyroid cancer often have a good prognosis. The use of radioactive iodine (RAI) should be judicious due to an increased risk of secondary malignancies and mortality later in life. The long latent period between RAI therapy and manifestation of risk poses a unique challenge to optimizing treatment strategy for thyroid cancer in the pediatric patient population. The data on the efficacy of this hazardous treatment modality is scarce.[23] A more centralized and collective approach should be adopted to study a disease that is uncommon and yet has profound impact on young lives for decades to come.

DISPARITY IN ENDOCRINE SURGERY

A growing body of literature on outcome disparity in endocrine surgery is painting a perplexing picture revealing an uncomfortable truth: not all patients receive equivalent treatment or have equivalent outcomes for the same disorders. We know that surgical volume and surgeon's experience are important factors in the outcome of patients undergoing endocrine surgery. Although not discriminatory at face value, studies using epidemiological data have demonstrated that Black and Hispanic patients are more likely to be operated on by low-volume surgeons and in low-volume hospitals.[24] There are many potential causes for these disparities. Insurance coverage, health-care access, geographical variation, familial background, genetic predisposition, and comorbidities may all play a role. It has been well demonstrated that Black and Hispanic patients are more likely to have a longer length of stay, higher cost of care, and higher rates of postoperative complications and mortality. The issue of access is highlighted even more in the case of parathyroid operations. A single institution study found that African Americans were likely to undergo surgery for PHPT later than their Caucasian counterparts after diagnosis.[25]

The disparity extends beyond the perioperative period. Thyroid cancer is the most common endocrine cancer and its incidence has been increasing in the last few decades. While the nature of the increase in thyroid cancer incidence is controversial, epidemiologic studies have consistently demonstrated that racial minorities, Black patients in particular, experienced lower survival rates than Caucasians.[26] However, this is complicated by the finding that Black patients often presented with less extensive disease.[27] One possibility is that Black patients were at greater risk of undertreatment for their disease after surgery.[16] Another factor is that this patient population may have more comorbidities that predispose them to higher mortality. This point is evidenced by the lack of significant difference in thyroid cancer-specific survival between White and Black patients.[28] There is a lack of data on genetic differences between Black patients and others to determine whether thyroid cancer behaves differently among these groups. Environmental exposures have also been implicated in explaining these differences but it is difficult to prove causality as well as to determine the degree of impact and on what aspect of the disease.[29]

Disparity also extends beyond the surgical outcome, physical health, and survival rate. Quality of life has been placed under the spotlight in recent years as the paradigm has shifted to value-based thinking and the importance of patient-reported outcomes. Overall, racial minorities tend to report worse quality of life after undergoing endocrine surgery. While patients with thyroid cancer overall report slightly lower quality of life, the deterioration is amplified in racial minorities. Specifically, Hispanic and Asian populations reported greater worries about mortality after being diagnosed with thyroid cancer. This is attributed in some part to overestimation of recurrence and mortality risk, highlighting the challenge of communicating prognosis to patients.[30] Functionally, Black patients reportedly experienced worse voice outcome after thyroid and parathyroid operations.[31] While surgical treatment has been shown to improve the quality of life in most patients with PHPT and functional adrenal tumors, it is unclear whether disparities exist in the degree of improvement.[32] In the future, it would be of great interest to study all aspects of disparities in care, including members of the LGBTQIA community who are under-represented in quality-of-life studies.

RARE & ORPHAN ENDOCRINE DISEASES

Rare disease is defined as a condition that affects fewer than 200,000 people in the United States. The Orphan Drug Act of 1983 was enacted to promote research and development of treatments for rare diseases. Rare disease treatments were often deemed unprofitable due to the small market, and the Act was intended to work by offering generous tax incentives and strategic regulatory laxity. There are approximately 7000 known rare conditions affecting 10% of the US population. The list is growing as we learn more from the human genome and discover subvariants of common diseases.[33]

Outlooks for rare endocrine and neuroendocrine malignancies are often grave, complicated, and lack substantial data for decision-making. While there are many rare endocrine disorders, most are treated medically and are nonsurgical. It may be a surprise to some that PHPT is included in this list. "Benign" endocrine conditions such as PHPT have excellent outcomes after surgery. On the other hand, other rare disorders such as adrenocortical carcinoma, NETs outside of the digestive tract, parathyroid carcinoma, subtypes of primary thyroid lymphoma, and endocrine malignancies in children have an incidence of less than 1 per million. They are also more aggressive in nature with patients often presenting with extensive or advanced disease. Because of their rarity, these endocrine diseases are not well understood. The treatment for rare endocrine diseases is largely based on expert opinions which in turn are often based on low-quality evidence such as case reports and case series.[19]

The collective damage of the rare diseases on individual patients is considerable. Patients and physicians need to advocate for greater resources devoted toward studying and treating these rare diseases. This collective will has proven formidable, as demonstrated by the passing of the Orphan Drug Act of 1983. We must now pool the most crucial and scarcest resource, the patients themselves, to make further strides. As we move toward personalized medicine, the future may be a world where we encounter more uncommon variants of common diseases. Therefore, we must strategize a new gold standard beyond the unachievable double-blinded randomized clinical trial for patients with rare diseases to adapt to a likely new reality.

CHALLENGES IN MEASURING OUTCOMES IN ENDOCRINE SURGERY

We would be remiss without addressing the challenges in measuring outcomes in endocrine surgery. National-level data require data entry that requires a data registrar or entrant, which can be expensive. One must define who the outcome matters to: The patient? The physician? The hospital system? The insurance company? The cost of health care as a whole to society? While automation and use of the electronic medical record can facilitate or ease the collection of data, not all outcomes are coded and entered in language that can be easily accessed for measurement and tracking. The infrastructure of patient sharing data is available but currently not organized. The ubiquity of the internet and use of telemedicine are perfect for this purpose. The world's renowned experts can be one click away; and conversely, the clinicians can have access to patients and colleagues all over the world. Of course, the legal groundwork for care that crosses state lines and the equitable financial structure for telemedicine remains uncertain. There is much work to be done in measuring outcomes that matter in endocrine surgery, and great promise to improve diagnosis, treatment, and survival in patients with endocrine disease.

REFERENCES

1. Codman EA. The classic: the registry of bone sarcomas as an example of the end-result idea in hospital organization. 1924. *Clin Orthop*. 2009;467(11):2766-2770.
2. Wright JR Jr. The American College of Surgeons, Minimum Standards for Hospitals, and the Provision of High-Quality Laboratory Services. *Arch Pathol Lab Med*. 2017; 141(5):704-717.
3. Mueller K. Commentary: Ernest Codman and the impact of quality improvement in neurosurgery: a century since the idea of the "end result." *Neurosurgery*. 2019;84(2):E116-E119.
4. Coale JG, Redman RR. A history of the Joint Commission on accreditation of hospitals.
5. Hines K, Mouchtouris N, Knightly JJ, Harrop J. A brief history of quality improvement in health care and spinal surgery. *Glob Spine J*. 2020;10(1_suppl):5S-9S.
6. Donabedian A. Evaluating the quality of medical care. 1966. *Milbank Q*. 2005;83(4):691-729.

7. Khuri SF, Daley J, Henderson W, et al. The Department of Veterans Affairs' NSQIP: the first national, validated, outcome-based, risk-adjusted, and peer-controlled program for the measurement and enhancement of the quality of surgical care. National VA Surgical Quality Improvement Program. *Ann Surg*. 1998;228(4):491-507.
8. Khuri SF, Daley J, Henderson WG. The comparative assessment and improvement of quality of surgical care in the Department of Veterans Affairs. *Arch Surg*. 2002;137(1):20-27.
9. Hall BL, Hamilton BH, Richards K, Bilimoria KY, Cohen ME, Ko CY. Does surgical quality improve in the American College of Surgeons National Surgical Quality Improvement Program: an evaluation of all participating hospitals. *Ann Surg*. 2009;250(3):363-376.
10. Thompson NW. The founding of the American Association of Endocrine Surgeons: the time was right. *Surgery*. 2011;150(6):1303-1307.
11. Chen HA, Krishnamurthy VD, Siperstein A, Carty S, Chen H. Four decades of the American Association of Endocrine Surgeons (AAES): past, present, and future. *Surgery*. 2020;167(1):1-3.
12. Collaborative Endocrine Surgery Quality Improvement Program (CESQIP. Accessed January 13, 2024. https://cesqip.org/
13. Thompson NW. The evolution of endocrine surgery as a subspecialty of general surgery: fragmentation or enhancement? *Arch Surg*. 1996;131(5):465-471.
14. Smith JA, Watkinson JC, Shaha A. Who should perform thyroid surgery? United Kingdom (UK) and United States (US) perspectives with recommendations. *Eur Arch Otorhinolaryngol*. 2012;269(1):1-4.
15. Meltzer C, Klau M, Gurushanthaiah D, et al. Surgeon volume in parathyroid surgery-surgical efficiency, outcomes, and utilization. *JAMA Otolaryngol–Head Neck Surg*. 2017; 143(8):843-847.
16. Shah SA, Adam MA, Thomas SM, et al. Racial disparities in differentiated thyroid cancer: have we bridged the gap? *Thyroid*. 2017;27(6):762-772.
17. Lindeman B, Hashimoto DA, Bababekov YJ, et al. Fifteen years of adrenalectomies: impact of specialty training and operative volume. *Surgery*. 2018;163(1):150-156.
18. Park HS, Roman SA, Sosa JA. Outcomes from 3144 adrenalectomies in the United States: which matters more, surgeon volume or specialty? *Arch Surg*. 2009;144(11):1060-1067.
19. Oronsky B, Ma PC, Morgensztern D, Carter CA. Nothing but NET: a review of neuroendocrine tumors and carcinomas. *Neoplasia N Y N*. 2017;19(12):991-1002.
20. Tuggle CT, Roman SA, Wang TS, et al. Pediatric endocrine surgery: who is operating on our children? *Surgery*. 2008;144(6):869-877.
21. Stack BC, Twining C, Rastatter J, et al. Consensus statement by the American Association of Clinical Endocrinology (AACE) and the American Head and Neck Society Endocrine Surgery Section (AHNS-ES) on pediatric benign and malignant thyroid surgery. *Head Neck*. 2021;43(4):1027-1042.
22. Kundel A, Thompson GB, Richards ML, et al. Pediatric endocrine surgery: a 20-year experience at the Mayo Clinic. *J Clin Endocrinol Metab*. 2014;99(2):399-406.
23. Prasad PK, Mahajan P, Hawkins DS, Mostoufi-Moab S, Venkatramani R. Management of pediatric differentiated thyroid cancer: an overview for the pediatric oncologist. *Pediatr Blood Cancer*. 2020;67(6):e28141.
24. Noureldine SI, Abbas A, Tufano RP, et al. The impact of surgical volume on racial disparity in thyroid and parathyroid surgery. *Ann Surg Oncol*. 2014;21(8):2733-2739.
25. Mallick R, Xie R, Kirklin JK, Chen H, Balentine CJ. Race and gender disparities in access to parathyroidectomy: a need to change processes for diagnosis and referral to surgeons. *Ann Surg Oncol*. 2021;28(1):476-483.
26. Harari A, Li N, Yeh MW. Racial and socioeconomic disparities in presentation and outcomes of well-differentiated thyroid cancer. *J Clin Endocrinol Metab*. 2014;99(1):133-141.
27. Zheng H, Lai V, Lu J, et al. Comparing the rate and extent of malignancy in surgically excised thyroid nodules across race and ethnicity. *Am J Surg*. Published online September 29, 2021:S0002-9610(21)00544-4.
28. Tang J, Kong D, Cui Q, et al. Racial disparities of differentiated thyroid carcinoma: clinical behavior, treatments, and long-term outcomes. *World J Surg Oncol*. 2018;16(1):45.
29. Crepeau P, Zhang Z, Udyavar R, et al. Socioeconomic disparity in the association between fine particulate matter exposure and papillary thyroid cancer. *Environ Health Glob Access Sci Source*. 2023;22(1):20.
30. Chen DW, Reyes-Gastelum D, Wallner LP, et al. Disparities in risk perception of thyroid cancer recurrence and death. *Cancer*. 2020;126(7):1512-1521.
31. Radowsky JS, Helou LB, Howard RS, Solomon NP, Stojadinovic A. Racial disparities in voice outcomes after thyroid and parathyroid surgery. *Surgery*. 2013;153(1):103-110.
32. Ejlsmark-Svensson H, Sikjaer T, Webb SM, Rejnmark L, Rolighed L. Health-related quality of life improves 1 year after parathyroidectomy in primary hyperparathyroidism: a prospective cohort study. *Clin Endocrinol (Oxf)*. 2019;90(1): 184-191.
33. Commissioner of the Orphan Drug Act—Relevant Excerpts. *FDA*. Published online April 24, 2019. Accessed September 7, 2021. https://www.fda.gov/industry/designating-orphan-product-drugs-and-biological-products/orphan-drug-act-relevant-excerpts

Thyroid Physiology

5

Marisa A. Bartz-Kurycki, MD, MS
Tracy S. Wang, MD, MPH

EMBRYOLOGY

The thyroid gland originates from the endoderm of the foregut. Thickening of the endodermal epithelium of the foregut occurs at day 16 or 17. The thyroid anlage buds anteriorly and migrates caudad with myocardial cells via the thyroglossal duct. During this migration, the thyroid anlage fuses with the ventral aspect of the fourth pharyngeal pouch. The steps are completed around embryonic day 60 resulting in a bilobed gland. By the seventh embryonic week, the thyroglossal duct undergoes involution leaving behind a dimple between the middle and posterior two-thirds of the tongue called the foramen cecum.[1] At the caudal aspect of the thyroglossal duct, cells differentiate into thyroid tissue, which develops into the pyramidal lobe of the thyroid gland. Parafollicular cells (also referred to as C cells) are derived from the neural crest and are incorporated into the thyroid gland when the lobes come in contact with the ultimobranchial glands. During embryologic weeks 12 to 14, the cells undergo differentiation with the development of follicles and colloid.

ANATOMY

The thyroid gland is a bilobed solid organ joined by the isthmus. It is one of the largest endocrine organs, weighing 15 to 20 g. Anatomically, the thyroid gland lies anterior to the trachea. The two lobes of the thyroid gland extend lateral to the trachea and esophagus, medial to the carotid sheath, and deep to the sternohyoid, sternothyroid, and sternocleidomastoid muscles. The superior pole of the thyroid tends to be well-defined while the inferior lobe is somewhat poorly defined. In approximately 30% of people, a pyramidal lobe will be evident as a fingerlike projection extending cephalad from the isthmus. Posteriorly, the fascial layer surrounding the thyroid gland coalesces to form the suspensory ligament to the trachea and cricoid cartilage, known as the ligament of Berry.

Blood Supply

The arterial blood supply is derived from multiple sources. The superior thyroid artery arises from the external carotid artery and enters the gland at the apex of the superior pole. The inferior thyroid artery arises from the subclavian artery via the thyrocervical trunk. Generally, the inferior thyroid artery enters at the posterior aspect of the thyroid gland near the ligament of Berry. Rarely, a *thyroidea ima* artery may be present, which arises from the innominate artery or the aorta to supply the gland inferiorly.

Venous drainage occurs via the superior, middle, and inferior thyroid veins. The superior and middle thyroid veins drain into the internal jugular vein. Two to three inferior thyroid veins may be present and typically drain into the innominate and brachiocephalic veins.

Lymphatic System

Lymphatic drainage for the thyroid gland is typically to the cervical nodal basins. The majority of nodal metastases for thyroid cancers will be found in the central nodal basins (level VI). The central compartment is bordered by the carotid artery laterally, the midline medially, the hyoid bone superiorly, and the plane of the innominate artery inferiorly. Cancers at the superior pole may spread directly to the lateral neck compartments (levels II-IV), as opposed to the central compartment first, which is more typical for initial nodal metastases.

Laryngeal Nerves

The superior laryngeal nerve arises from the vagus nerve near the base of the skull and travels along the internal carotid artery toward the superior pole of the thyroid. The internal branch provides sensory function to the larynx. The external branch of the superior laryngeal artery nerve supplies motor function to the cricothyroid muscle.

Injury to this branch of the superior laryngeal nerve results in poor projection of the voice and inability to modulate pitch.

The recurrent laryngeal nerve also arises from the vagus nerve. However, its path varies based on laterality. On the right side, the recurrent laryngeal nerve originates from the vagus nerve at the level of the subclavian artery and travels posterior to the subclavian artery. It ascends lateral to the trachea in the tracheoesophageal groove. Typically, the recurrent laryngeal nerve is found in close proximity to the inferior thyroid artery in the tracheoesophageal groove. Rarely, a nonrecurrent laryngeal nerve is present—almost exclusively on the right—and generally arises from the vagus and travels medially to the larynx without looping into the superior mediastinum. Typically, patients with this anatomy also have an aberrant right subclavian artery.

The anatomy of the left recurrent laryngeal nerve tends to be less variable. It arises from the vagus at the level of the aortic arch, travels inferior and medial to the ligamentum arteriosum, and ascends cephalad via the tracheoesophageal groove. A nonrecurrent left laryngeal nerve is also possible, though much less common than a nonrecurrent right laryngeal nerve.

The recurrent laryngeal nerve provides motor, sensory, and autonomic innervation to the intrinsic muscles of the larynx. Injury to one of the recurrent laryngeal nerves will lead to ipsilateral paralysis of the vocal cord, which is manifested by a hoarse or raspy voice. Bilateral injury to the recurrent laryngeal nerves results in a complete loss of voice and/or airway obstruction if the cords are paralyzed in a medialized position. If the vocal cords are damaged in an abducted position, the airway may not be obstructed; however, the patient will be predisposed to upper respiratory infections related to aspiration and an ineffective cough.

HISTOLOGY

The thyroid gland is comprised of spherical units called follicles. Follicles are lined by follicular cells which surround a lumen filled with colloid. A rich network of capillaries surrounds follicles. Follicular cells are essential to thyroid hormone production and secretion. The other prominent non-stromal cell type within the thyroid gland is the parafollicular cell (or C cell). Parafollicular cells are responsible for the production of calcitonin.

IODINE & THE SYNTHESIS OF THYROID HORMONES

Two primary functions of the thyroid gland are the production of thyroid hormones and calcitonin, which helps to regulate calcium. Iodine is necessary for thyroid hormone production. At least 100 μg of dietary iodine is needed each day to synthesize adequate amounts of thyroid hormone. The thyroid gland stores the majority (90%) of the iodide in the body in the form of colloid.

Iodine deficiency is common in certain parts of the world with mountainous terrain or where glaciers were formerly located. For example, cities around the Alpine valleys, Pyrenees, Himalayan, and Andes mountains, and the states bordering the Great Lakes have a higher incidence of endemic goiter. Iodine deficiency can lead to compensatory enlargement of the gland mediated by thyroid-stimulating hormone (TSH) causing goiter. Hypothyroidism, cretinism, and possibly follicular thyroid carcinoma can also arise in the setting of iodine deficiency. Endemic goiter and cretinism are the most common endocrine disorders worldwide. If iodine deficiency occurs during pregnancy, it can lead to irreparable damage to the fetus' developing central nervous system and varying degrees of mental disability (cretinism).[2]

Iodine Metabolism

Iodine is absorbed from the gastrointestinal tract in the inorganic form of iodide. Iodide is transported from the extracellular fluid by an active, sodium-dependent process mediated by the sodium-iodide symporter (NIS) at the basal membrane of follicular cells. *NIS* gene transcription is stimulated by TSH. TSH also prolongs the half-life of NIS protein. Conversely, high intracellular concentrations of iodide negatively feedback on the NIS which results in reduced uptake and organification of iodide. Mutations in the *NIS* gene may result in iodide transport defects that lead to congenital hypothyroidism. In addition, there is research that suggests "cold" nodules on radioiodine uptake (RAIU) scans are due to alterations in NIS expression within neoplastic thyroid cells.

Oxidation & Organification of Iodine

Oxidation of iodide occurs at the follicular lumen by thyroid peroxidase (TPO), which results in iodination of tyrosine molecules on thyroglobulin. This step in thyroid hormone production is also stimulated by TSH. *DUOX1* and *DUOX2* genes transcribe the calcium, NADPH-dependent oxidases which generate the hydrogen peroxide necessary for TPO-mediated iodination of thyroglobulin.

Iodothyronine Synthesis

Monoiodotyrosine (MIT) and diiodotyrosine (DIT) are the products of organification, which is also catalyzed by the enzyme, TPO. The coupling of two DIT molecules mediated by TPO generates thyroxine (T4). Coupling of one MIT and one DIT results in triiodothyronine (T3). Thyroglobulin is essential to this process with each molecule of thyroglobulin containing three to four molecules of T4 (Figure 5–1).

Storage & Secretion of Thyroid Hormone

Thyroid hormone is stored bound to thyroglobulin in the form of colloid in the follicular lumen. In euthyroid patients,

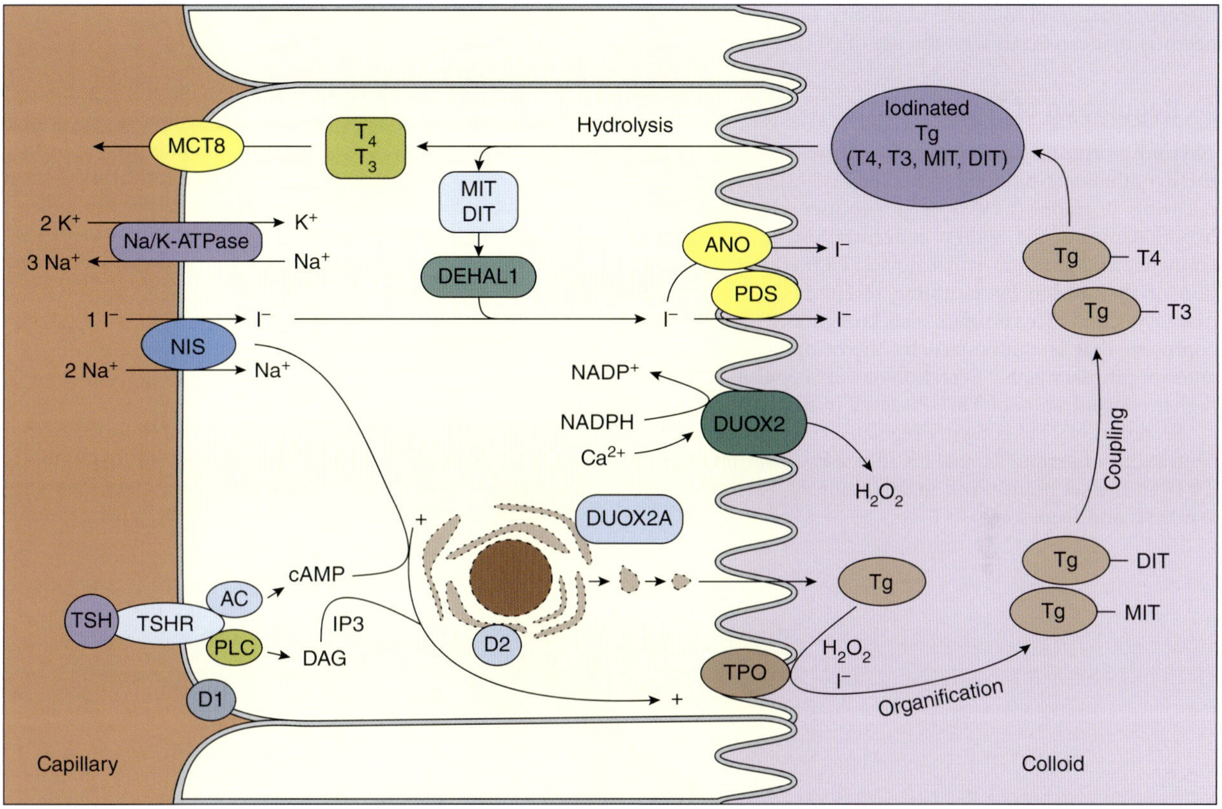

Figure 5–1. Cellular synthesis, storage, and secretion of thyroid hormones. Iodine is actively transported into the cell via sodium-iodide symporter (NIS). Iodide undergoes oxidation and organification with thyroglobulin (Tg) via thyroid peroxidase (TPO). Coupling of diiodotyrosine (DIT) and monoiodotyrosine (MIT) generates thyroxine (T4) and triiodothyronine (T3), which are stored in colloid. Secretion of thyroid hormones occurs via endocytosis and hydrolysis with transport from the cell via MCT8. Excess MITs and DITs are recycled within thyroid follicular cells. (Reproduced with permission from Salvatore D. Cohen R, Kopp PA, et al. Thyroid Pathophysiology and Diagnostic Evaluation. In: Melmed S, Polonsky KS, Larsen PR, Kronenberg HM, eds. *Williams Textbook of Endocrinology.* 13th ed. Philadelphia, PA: Elsevier;2016:334.)

there is enough thyroid hormone stored to last approximately 2 weeks. One benefit of this type of storage is that it helps to protect against the depletion of circulating thyroid hormone. However, thyrotoxicosis can arise in patients with subacute or painless thyroiditis from this reservoir.

Secretion of thyroid hormone is mediated by TSH. Colloid and thyroglobulin are endocytosed from the follicular lumen. Thyroglobulin is cleaved into T3 and T4 within lysosomes. T3 and T4 are transported from follicular cells via MCT 8 transporter at the basal lateral membrane. Iodotyrosine deiodinase is an NADPH-dependent enzyme that releases iodine from MITs and DITs, which is ultimately recycled and reused for thyroid hormone synthesis.

Thyroid hormone is primarily secreted as T4 and is converted in peripheral tissues to the active form, T3. High concentrations of iodide inhibit release of T4. Lithium also inhibits the release of thyroid hormone, though the mechanism by which it happens is not completely known. Antithyroid medications affect levels of T3 and T4 by different mechanisms. Methimazole (MMI) inhibits the function of TPO thereby reducing synthesis of T4 within the thyroid gland. Propylthiouracil (PTU) both reduces the synthesis of T4 and inhibits the peripheral conversion of D1-mediated conversion of T4 to T3 and is used to reduce levels of circulating T3 in patients with Graves' disease. Common adverse effects of antithyroid medications include rash, gastrointestinal irritation, and agranulocytosis. MMI is typically first-line therapy because of the rare possibility of fulminant liver necrosis that can occur with the use of PTU.

Regulation of Thyroid Hormone

Thyroid hormone synthesis and release is regulated by the hypothalamic-pituitary axis (Figure 5–2). Thyrotropin-releasing hormone (TRH) is a peptide released by the hypothalamus at the highest concentrations in the median eminence and paraventricular nuclei. TRH stimulates secretion of thyrotropin by activating receptors in the anterior pituitary gland. Thyrotropin, also known as TSH, is a glycoprotein that is synthesized by thyrotrophic cells of the anterior pituitary gland. Secretion of TSH is pulsatile, with a higher concentration of TSH observed in the evening.

Secretion of TSH is tightly regulated in response to concentrations of serum T4 and T3. Increases in serum T3 and T4 from the set point result in inhibition of TSH and TRH synthesis and secretion.

LABORATORY ASSESSMENT

Thyroid Function

When patients present with signs and symptoms suggestive of thyroid pathology, laboratory assessment is used to further confirm a diagnosis. The first step in biochemical assessment is typically ordering TSH. Thyrotropin levels are an indirect reflection of thyroid hormone supply. Abnormalities in TSH levels must be confirmed with levels of thyroid hormone (usually T4).

Indirect Assessment

A. TSH

Immunometric assays have made it possible to determine the normal range of serum TSH, which is 0.4 to 4.2 mU/L. The assays use TSH antibodies, which are quantified with chemiluminescence using a different labeled TSH epitope.

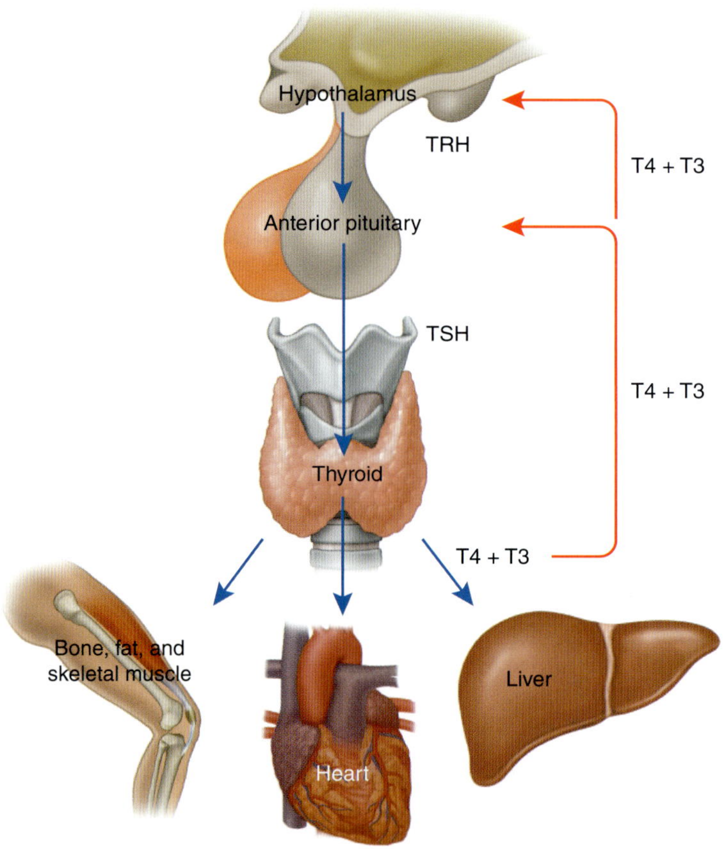

▲ **Figure 5–2.** Regulation of thyroid hormone by the hypothalamic-pituitary-thyroid axis. TRH, thyrotropin-releasing hormone; TSH, thyroid-stimulating hormone; T4, thyroxine; T3, triiodothyronine.

Table 5–1. Conditions associated with suppressed thyrotropin levels. Arrows indicate abnormality. Dashes represent values within the reference range.

Condition	Expected TSH (mU/L)	Free T4	Free T3	Clinical Thyroid Status
Hyperthyroidism	<0.1	↑	↑	↑
Excess exogenous T4	<0.1-0.5	↑	↑	-/↑
Thyroiditis	<0.1-0.5	-	↑	-/↑
High-dose glucocorticoids	0.1-0.5	-	↓	-/↑
Autonomous nodule or toxic multinodular goiter	0.2-0.5	-	↑	-/↑
Euthyroid Graves' disease	0.2-0.5	-	-/↑	-
First-trimester pregnancy	0.2-0.5	-	↑	-/↑
Elderly	0.2-0.5	-	-	-
Excess biotin supplementation	↓	-	-	-
Congenital TSH deficiency	0-↓	↓	↓	↓

When a patient's TSH level is below the normal range, this may indicate primary hyperthyroidism or thyrotoxicosis. Patients with serum levels between 0.1 mU/L and 0.4 mU/L may be asymptomatic (subclinical hyperthyroidism). Patients with clinical hyperthyroidism typically have a TSH level of less than 0.1 mU/L and demonstrate symptoms (Table 5–1). The possible etiologies of TSH suppression include excessive exogenous replacement or increased endogenous production. The differential diagnosis includes Graves' disease, hormone-producing adenomas, toxic multinodular goiter, subacute or painless thyroiditis, excessive exogenous replacement, and rare hormone-secreting tumors. In asymptomatic patients with a serum TSH level below the reference range and high free T4 values, concomitant biotin (Vitamin B7) supplementation should be investigated. Biotin supplementation should be stopped 2 to 3 days prior to repeat TSH testing.

Primary hypothyroidism is suggested by elevations in TSH above the reference range (Table 5–2). The degree of elevation typically correlates with the severity of hypothyroidism. Worldwide, iodine deficiency is the most common cause of elevated TSH. In the United States, primary hypothyroidism and Hashimoto thyroiditis are the most common causes. A diagnosis of subclinical hypothyroidism is made in symptomatic patients with normal serum concentrations of free T4 and an elevated serum concentration of TSH. Elevated levels of serum TSH may also be seen in adrenal insufficiency. TSH levels tend to normalize with adequate glucocorticoid replacement. Alternatively, thyrotrophin-secreting tumors in the pituitary gland may also demonstrate elevated levels of TSH, but in the setting of clinical hyperthyroidism.

Direct Assessment

A. T3 & T4 Concentrations

Serum levels of T3 and T4 are often measured after an abnormality is detected in TSH to help confirm the diagnosis. Thyroid status tends to correlate more with free T4 than with total hormone concentrations (bound hormone and

Table 5–2. Conditions associated with elevated thyrotropin levels. Arrows indicate abnormality. Dashes represent values within the reference range.

Condition	Expected TSH (mU/L)	Free T4	Free T3	Clinical Thyroid Status
Primary hypothyroidism	6-500	↓	↓	-/↓
Iodine deficiency	6-150	↓	-	↓/-
Recovery from severe illness	5-30	-/↓	-/↓	-
Adrenal insufficiency	5-30	-	-/↓	-
Thyroid hormone resistance	1-20	↑	↑	↑/-/↓
Hypothalamic-pituitary disease	1-20	↓	↓	↓
Thyrotroph-secreting tumor	0.5-50	↑	↑	↑

free hormone). The degree to which free T4 is abnormal is associated with the severity of disease. A euthyroid adult will typically have a serum T4 concentration of 64 to 142 nmol/L (5-11 μg/dL) and T3 levels between 1.1 and 2.9 nmol/L (70-190 ng/dL). Robotic assays directly measure serum concentrations of T3 and T4.

Certain conditions can create artifacts in the results of these assays, including patients with antibodies to T4 and patients with abnormal binding proteins or severe illness. Pregnancy is another condition where falsely low results may be observed due to alterations in thyroid hormone-binding proteins. Multiplying the normal serum T4 concentration by 1.5 can be used as an alternative to an automated free T4 assay for pregnant patients.

B. Free T4 Index

To calculate the free T4 index, the amount of bound and free thyroid hormone must first be determined. Assays use labeled T4, which is exposed to T4 antibody and allowed to bind in serum. The bound labeled T4 is then directly measured. The thyroid hormone binding ratio is multiplied by total T4 to determine the free T4 index. A normal thyroid hormone binding ratio is in the range of 0.8 to 1.1.

Many factors can affect thyroid hormone binding. Increased binding of thyroid hormone is observed in pregnant patients and neonates; with the use of tamoxifen, estrogen, and oral contraceptives; in patients with hepatitis, biliary cirrhosis, HIV, porphyria, and related genetic factors. Reduced thyroid hormone binding is seen in patients with excess androgens and glucocorticoids; nephrotic syndrome, acromegaly, major systemic illnesses, and related to genetic factors.

C. Radioiodine Uptake

RAIU uses radioactive iodine (I-123) to directly measure iodine uptake by the thyroid gland. Due to the improvement in TSH and thyroid hormone assays, RAIU is less commonly used, though it is still an essential part of the workup for determining the etiology of hyperthyroidism. Iodine-123 delivers gamma radiation with a very short half-life of 0.55 days compared to iodine-131 which has half-life of 8.1 days. Measurements are usually taken 24 hours after radioiodine administration when levels have plateaued. Normal uptake is 5% to 25% in a euthyroid patient. RAIU is contraindicated in pregnant and breastfeeding patients.

Abnormalities in RAIU are associated with specific clinical conditions but may also be aberrant related to iodine excess or deficiency. Diffuse uptake is observed in patients with Graves' disease, while focal uptake is observed in patients with toxic thyroid nodules. Increased uptake is observed in patients with acute or chronic iodine deficiency after withdrawal of antithyroid medications, thyroiditis, or conditions associated with increased loss of thyroid hormone, such as nephrotic syndrome. Decreased RAIU is observed in patients taking excessive amounts of exogenous thyroid hormone, subacute thyroiditis, and in patients with excess amounts of iodine as seen with recent administration of iodinated contrast media and/or amiodarone.

Evaluating the Effects of Thyroid Hormone on Peripheral Tissues

A. Basal Metabolic Rate

Thyroid hormone acts on peripheral tissues to increase energy expenditure and heat production. These effects can be quantified through the basal metabolic rate (BMR), which measures oxygen consumption under specific conditions. Twenty-five percent of oxygen consumption is attributed to visceral organs under normal resting conditions with 10% consumed by brain, 10% by respiratory effort, and the remainder by skeletal muscle. Patients with severe hypothyroidism may exhibit a BMR as low as −40% of normal, while patients with thyrotoxicosis may demonstrate a BMR of 25% to 50% in excess of the reference range.

Thyroid Markers

A. Thyroglobulin

Thyroglobulin is a protein synthesized in follicular cells of the thyroid that is essential to thyroid hormone synthesis and storage. It is also normally present in serum in concentrations of 20 to 50 ng/mL. Assays for the detection of thyroglobulin have been developed with a sensitivity of 1 ng/mL or less. Neonates with thyroid agenesis will have undetectable levels of thyroglobulin. Elevated levels of thyroglobulin may be present in patients with goiter, hypothyroidism, and thyroiditis. Patients with benign or malignant follicular cell tumors may also exhibit elevated serum concentrations of thyroglobulin. Since it is specific to the thyroid gland, thyroglobulin is used as a marker for thyroid cancer surveillance after total thyroidectomy. If thyroglobulin levels are detectable in the early postoperative period, it may suggest persistent disease. Subsequent increases in thyroglobulin levels from an undetectable concentration suggest recurrence of thyroid cancer.

B. Calcitonin

Calcitonin is a peptide synthesized in parafollicular, or "C" cells of the thyroid gland. It is cleaved from the pro-hormone, procalcitonin, to its active form. Calcitonin helps regulate serum calcium levels by inhibiting bone resorption at the level of osteoclasts. Calcitonin is a reliable tumor marker for surveillance in patients with medullary thyroid carcinoma (MTC) with serum levels correlating directly to C-cell mass. As such, a basal serum calcitonin level is routinely measured in patients with a nodule that is biopsy-proven MTC and again after surgical resection. It is also used in cytopathology of fine-needle aspiration of thyroid nodules to aid in the diagnosis of MTC. Levels of calcitonin may also be elevated in patients with C-cell hyperplasia, hyperparathyroidism, other neuroendocrine tumors, and malignancies such as breast, pancreas, and small-cell carcinoma of the lung. Calcitonin has a biphasic half-life that is concentration-dependent with a rapid and slower component (15 minutes and 40 minutes at normal concentrations, 3 hours and 30 hours at elevated concentrations).

C. Anti-thyroid Autoantibodies

Autoimmune thyroid disorders are characterized by the presence of circulating autoantibodies to one or more thyroid antigens, which result in overstimulation or destruction of the thyroid gland. These autoantibodies may play a role in activating thyroid-specific T cells. Many assays directly measure the interaction between the antibody in the antigen. Some euthyroid patients will exhibit low levels of thyroid antibodies before a disorder becomes clinically apparent. Higher levels of circulating antibodies improve the specificity of the test. Different commercial assays may vary considerably in their affinity and recognition of antigens. Therefore, it is important to use the same antibody assay when serially checking titers.

Almost all patients with Hashimoto thyroiditis will exhibit autoantibodies to thyroglobulin and TPO. Thyroid autoantibodies are five times more common in women and have been associated with an increased risk of early pregnancy losses. They may also be present in patients with other autoimmune disorders, goiter, thyroid nodules, and thyroid cancer. Autoantibodies to thyroglobulin and TPO are seen in 50% to 90% of patients with Graves' disease. TSH receptor antibodies are also vital to the evaluation of patients with hyperthyroidism with concern for Graves' disease.

THYROID HORMONE REPLACEMENT

Effective and reliable treatment for primary and surgical hypothyroidism is available. The goal of thyroid hormone replacement is to achieve a euthyroid state, which is defined as normalization of thyroid hormone levels (TSH, T4, and T3) with absence of the signs and symptoms associated with hypothyroidism. Most reliably, this is accomplished with normalization of serum TSH (0.4-4 mIU/L). Different forms of thyroid hormone replacement will be discussed.

Levothyroxine (LT4)

Levothyroxine is synthetic T4 and is considered the standard of care for thyroid hormone replacement. Advantages of LT4 replacement over other forms include a long half-life (approximately 7 days) and administration of prohormone, which allows for normal physiologic control by conversion of T4 to T3 in peripheral tissues. In addition, it is available in oral and intravenous formulations. LT4 takes approximately 6 weeks for LT4 levels to reach equilibrium. The long half-life provides ease of administration with once-daily preparations and also adds a level of safety for patients who may miss any doses.

Table 5–3. Recommendations for levothyroxine dosing based on patient sex, BMI, and weight in kilograms.

BMI Category (kg/m^2)	Male (μg/kg)	Female (μg/kg)
<21	2.1	1.8
22-26	1.9	1.7
27-32	1.7	1.6
33-40	1.5	1.4
>40	1.3	1.2

Source: Reproduced with permission from Elfenbein DM, Schaefer S, Shumway C, Chen H, Sippel RS, Schneider DF. Prospective intervention of a novel levothyroxine dosing protocol based on body mass index after thyroidectomy. *J Am Coll Surg*. 2016;222(1):83-88.

LT4 is absorbed in the jejunum and ileum with 70% to 80% absorption in most adults. Consistent time of administration is recommended, ideally 1 hour before breakfast or at bedtime (at least 3 hours after eating).[3] Although the FDA regulates LT4 manufacturing and quality, the variability between formulations may vary in effectiveness and make it difficult to titrate the dose and achieve a euthyroid state.

Initial dosing should be calculated based on lean body weight. A dose of 1.6 to 1.8 μg/kg is recommended. Patients who have undergone thyroidectomy often require higher doses of LT4 to achieve a euthyroid state. Elderly and obese patients tend to require lower doses of LT4 to achieve a normal TSH (Table 5–3).[4] Medications may interfere with achieving TSH goal such as calcium carbonate, proton pump inhibitors, cholestyramine, phosphate binders, ferrous sulfate, antacids containing aluminum and sucralfate, androgens, and estrogens.

Liothyronine (LT3)

Patients on T4 monotherapy may demonstrate T3 levels that are below the reference range or are low-normal; however, the clinical significance of this is unknown. T3 binds nuclear thyroid hormone receptors within the nucleus to affect gene transcription. Liothyronine monotherapy requires dosing 3 times a day due to its shorter half-life. In addition, T3 monotherapy often requires significantly higher levels to achieve the goal of a normal TSH.

Combination Therapy

Various formulations of combination T4/T3 therapy have been studied and compared to T4 therapy alone.

Combination therapy may lead to excess levels of circulating thyroid hormone when using serum TSH levels to compare effectiveness. In comparison with patients receiving LT4 replacement, the ratio of T3:T4 is approximately 20% lower than in an individual who is euthyroid and does not require thyroid hormone replacement.

No clear advantages have been observed regarding combination therapy over T4 monotherapy alone. Interestingly, one study looking at patients with hypothyroidism with and without D2 polymorphisms demonstrated greater improvements in measures of well-being on T4/T3 combination therapy in patients with D2 polymorphisms. However, additional studies are needed to confirm these results. The American Thyroid Association (ATA) recommends against routine use of combination therapy.

Desiccated Thyroid

Historically, extracts from desiccated animal thyroid glands were used for thyroid hormone replacement. Desiccated thyroid preparations often have a 2 to 3-fold higher ratio of T3:T4 found in normal human thyroglobulin.

Special Considerations

A. Pregnancy

Adequate levels of thyroid hormone are necessary for normal fetal development. Pregnant patients typically require an increased dose of levothyroxine during the first trimester. This also depends on to what extent the patient has residual thyroid function and whether the patient is athyreotic. The dose of levothyroxine may need to be increased by more than 30% from the patient's pre-pregnancy dose.[3] Thyrotropin should be assessed every 4 weeks during the first half of pregnancy to ensure TSH levels are maintained within the normal range. After delivery of the fetus, levothyroxine requirements typically return to the dose needed prior to pregnancy within a few weeks.

B. Myxedema Coma

Patients with severe longstanding hypothyroidism may develop myxedema coma. Patients may exhibit hypothermia, severe myxedema, bradycardia, and hypotension. Areflexia or delayed deep tendon reflexes may be present. Patients may also suffer from seizures. Timely diagnosis and initiation of treatment is essential as delays in treatment are associated with increased rates of mortality.

Intravenous thyroid hormone replacement is recommended in myxedema coma as absorption of therapeutic agents through other routes may be unpredictable related to poor circulation and severe hypometabolism. A single IV dose of levothyroxine (between 200 to 400 μg) is initially given to help replete the peripheral hormone pool and stimulate prompt improvement in the patient's condition. Subsequent doses of IV levothyroxine are reduced to approximately 100 μg daily or 75% of weight-based dosing (1.6 μg/kg).[3] Due to concerns for relative adrenal cortical insufficiency as the patient's metabolic rate increases, hydrocortisone infusion is often also administered in doses of 5 to 10 mg/h.

C. Differentiated Thyroid Cancer

Thyrotropin suppression is recommended in patients with differentiated thyroid cancer who are deemed high risk for recurrence; however, the length and extent of TSH suppression vary based on professional practice guidelines. The ATA guidelines for the management of differentiated thyroid cancer recommend that the TSH be maintained at normal levels (0.5-2 mU/L) for patients undergoing thyroid lobectomy or for those with low-risk disease and have undergone thyroidectomy with undetectable levels of thyroglobulin (Table 5–4).[5] For patients with low- or intermediate-risk disease who have undergone remnant ablation with detectable, but low levels of serum thyroglobulin, it is recommended that TSH be slightly suppressed (0.1-0.5 mU/L). TSH suppression below 0.1 mU/L is recommended for patients with high-risk thyroid cancers.[5] Thyrotropin suppression was proposed for differentiated thyroid cancer based on the hypothesis that suppressed levels of TSH would slow growth and spread of thyroid cancer cells. Support for this hypothesis includes that suppression of TSH results in minimal uptake of radioiodine. In addition, TSH is known to stimulate growth and differentiated differentiation of thyroid follicular cells. Multiple studies have demonstrated that TSH suppression is associated

Table 5–4. Recommendations for TSH suppression in patients with differentiated thyroid cancer per the 2015 American Thyroid Association guidelines.

Patient Risk Category	Target Serum TSH (mU/L)	Level of Evidence
Lobectomy	0.5-2	Low
Low risk, underwent RAI, undetectable Tg	0.5-2	Low
Low risk, underwent RAI, low Tg	0.1-0.5	Low
Low risk, no RAI	0.1-0.5	Low
Intermediate risk	0.1-0.5	Low
High risk	<0.1	Moderate

RAI, radioiodine ablation; Tg, thyroglobulin.
Source: Data from Haugen BR, Alexander EK, Bible KC, et al. 2015 American Thyroid Association Management Guidelines for Adult Patients with Thyroid Nodules and Differentiated Thyroid Cancer: The American Thyroid Association Guidelines Task Force on Thyroid Nodules and Differentiated Thyroid Cancer. *Thyroid*. 2016;26(1):1-133.

with reduced thyroid cancer recurrence and cancer-related death in patients who are at increased risk for recurrence.[6]

Long-term TSH suppression is not without its own risks. It can lead to signs and symptoms of hyperthyroidism as well as cardiovascular effects, bone effects, and poor quality of life. TSH suppression is associated with increased heart rate, left-ventricular mass, myocardial strain, and impaired diastolic dysfunction. Patients of advanced age are more likely to experience adverse events associated with TSH suppression. Thyrotropin suppression accelerates bone turnover placing patients at increased risk of osteoporosis and reduced bone density.[7] Patients may also experience emotional changes, mood disorders, and cognitive dysfunction that poorly affect their quality of life.

REFERENCES

1. De Felice M, Di Lauro R. Thyroid development and its disorders: genetics and molecular mechanisms. *Endocr Rev.* 2004;25(5): 722-746.
2. Alexander EK, Pearce EN, Brent GA, et al. 2017 Guidelines of the American Thyroid Association for the Diagnosis and Management of Thyroid Disease during Pregnancy and the Postpartum. *Thyroid.* 2017;27(3):315-389.
3. Jonklaas J, Bianco AC, Bauer AJ, et al. Guidelines for the treatment of hypothyroidism: prepared by the American Thyroid Association Task Force on Thyroid Hormone Replacement. *Thyroid.* 2014;24(12):1670-1751.
4. Elfenbein DM, Schaefer S, Shumway C, Chen H, Sippel RS, Schneider DF. Prospective intervention of a novel levothyroxine dosing protocol based on body mass index after thyroidectomy. *J Am Coll Surg.* 2016;222(1):83-88.
5. Haugen BR, Alexander EK, Bible KC, et al. 2015 American Thyroid Association Management Guidelines for Adult Patients with Thyroid Nodules and Differentiated Thyroid Cancer: The American Thyroid Association Guidelines Task Force on Thyroid Nodules and Differentiated Thyroid Cancer. *Thyroid.* 2016;26(1):1-133.
6. McGriff NJ, Csako G, Gourgiotis L, Guthrie LC, Pucino F, Sarlis NJ. Effects of thyroid hormone suppression therapy on adverse clinical outcomes in thyroid cancer. *Ann Med.* 2002;34(7-8): 554-564.
7. Grani G, Ramundo V, Verrienti A, Sponziello M, Durante C. Thyroid hormone therapy in differentiated thyroid cancer. *Endocrine.* 2019;66(1):43-50.

6

Thyroid Anatomy

Paladino Nunzia Cinzia, MD, PhD
Taïeb David, MD, PhD
Sebag Frédéric, MD

The thyroid is an endocrine gland located in the anterior part of the neck under the hyoid bone,[1] inferior to the laryngeal thyroid cartilage, approximately at the level of the C5-T1 vertebrae,[2,3] in front of and lateral to the larynx and the first tracheal ring.[3]

The thyroid is the first endocrine gland in the body to develop and, when fully developed, typically consists of two lobes joined by the isthmus (Figure 6–1). However, the thyroid gland is known to have many morphological variations. Usually, the gland is asymmetrical with a more voluminous right lobe.[1] A residual parenchymal extension of the thyroglossal duct, known as the *pyramidal lobe* or *pyramid of Morgagni-Lalouette* (Figure 6–1), is found at the upper margin of the isthmus,[3] but it can arise from either lobe,[3] though more commonly from the left.[2] The pyramidal lobe can be separated entirely from the thyroid gland and can even be bilateral.[2,3] Sometimes the pyramidal lobe may arise from the hyoid bone.[1] The pyramidal lobe is present in approximately 30% to 55%[2,4] of individuals, though a recent publication[5] suggests that it may be present in up to 65.7% of individuals.

Another common extension of the thyroid is found at the posterior aspect of each thyroid lobe and is known as the *tubercle of Zuckerkandl* (Figure 6–1).

The thyroid is found within the visceral compartment of the neck and is bound by pretracheal fascia.[2]

Three fascias are distinguished in the neck:

- **Superficial cervical fascia:** This surrounds the sternocleidomastoid muscles, salivary, maxillary, and parotid glands.
- **Middle cervical fascia:** This lies between the infrahyoid muscles.
- **Deep cervical or vertebral fascia:** This separates the prevertebral muscles from the retropharyngeal space.

The thyroid gland has its own capsule and a pseudocapsule which is a thickening of the middle cervical fascia. It is covered by the *pre-thyroid muscles* (sternothyroid, sternohyoid, and omohyoid muscles). Laterally, the two lobes are covered by the sternocleidomastoid muscles and posteriorly the thyroid is attached to the larynx, the first tracheal rings, and the laryngeal portion of the pharynx via the perithyroid sheath.[4]

The thyroid gland is held in place by the sternothyroid muscle and "ligaments" attaching the thyroid to the trachea. The ligaments are thickenings of the perithyroid sheath and include the following:

- The *median ligament*, called the **Grüber ligament**, is stretched between the posterior surface of the isthmus and the medial part of the cricoid cartilage. It is devoid of vessels.
- *Internal lateral ligaments* are the most tenacious means of fixation of the thyroid gland. They attach the upper third of the thyroid lobes to the cricoid cartilage and the first two tracheal rings. They are divided into an anteromedial portion called the **ligament of Grüber and Sappy** and a posteromedial portion called the **Berry ligament**. The latter is richly vascularized and it is an important landmark for the identification of the laryngeal recurrent nerve (RLN).
- The external lateral **ligaments of Sébileau** are related to the periadventitial component of the vascular pedicles of the superior and inferior thyroid arteries.[6]

PARATHYROID GLANDS

The parathyroid glands are responsible for parathyroid hormone secretion and are typically found in close proximity to the thyroid gland. There are usually four glands, two on each side of the central neck, although there may be supernumerary parathyroid glands. Parathyroid glands are commonly in contact with the posterior surface of the lobes, and can occasionally be under the capsule of the thyroid (or rarely intrathyroidal), though typically are loosely attached to the thyroid in their own fat pad.

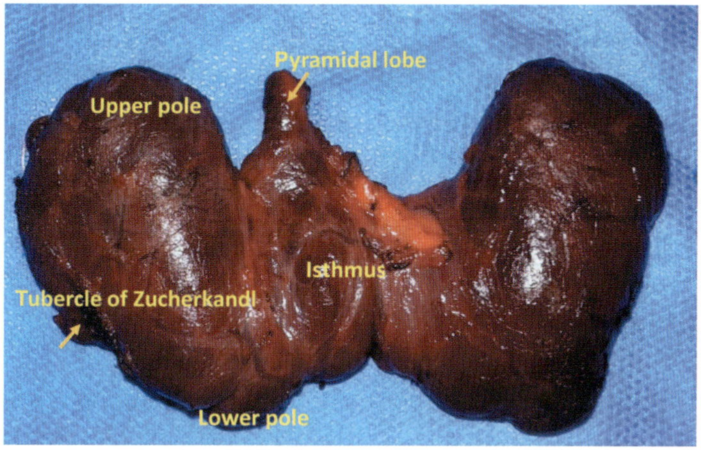

▲ **Figure 6–1.** Thyroid gland after surgical removal.

About 85% of people have four parathyroid glands located along the posterolateral surface of the thyroid gland. Normal parathyroid glands are approximately 0.3 × 0.4 × 0.3 cm in size, 30 to 40 mg in weight, and are chamois in color. The upper parathyroid glands have a more posterior location and have a more constant position. The lower glands are more anterior with the recurrent laryngeal nerve being the anatomic structure defining anterior and posterior (Figure 6–2). Both the superior and inferior glands are vascularized by the inferior thyroid artery or an anastomotic branch between the inferior and superior thyroid arteries.[3]

Vascularization

The thyroid gland is highly vascularized and it is estimated to receive six times the blood flow of the kidney and three to four times the blood flow of the brain on a weight basis.[2]

The blood supply is derived from the superior and inferior thyroid arteries.

- *Superior thyroid artery* (STA) (Figure 6–3) is the first branch of the external carotid artery that arises near the level of the superior horn of the thyroid cartilage. It then ascends anteriorly, then descends inferiorly and toward the midline behind the sternothyroid muscle to

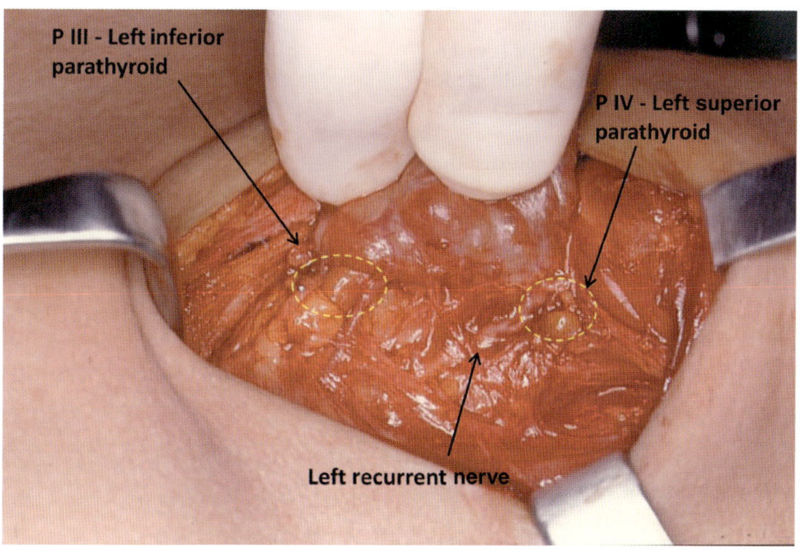

▲ **Figure 6–2.** Intraoperative photo of a left thyroid lobe with view of the recurrent nerve and the two parathyroid glands.

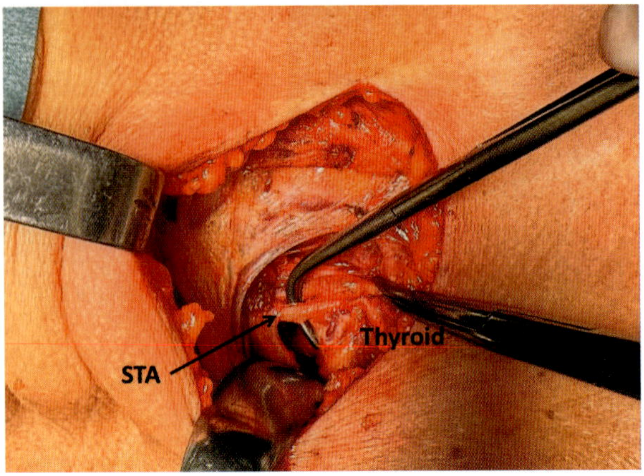

▲ **Figure 6–3.** Superior thyroid artery (STA), intraoperative view.

the superior pole of the thyroid gland. At this level, it branches out.

- The *inferior thyroid artery* is a branch of the thyrocervical trunk. The thyrocervical trunk arises from the anterosuperior surface of the subclavian artery and gives rise to three branches, one being the inferior thyroid artery. It branches at the inner border of the anterior scalene muscle and advances medially to the thyroid gland until reaches the posterior surface of the lateral lobe of the thyroid gland. The largest branch of the inferior thyroid artery is the ascending cervical branch.[2]

It has been reported that in 10% of the population, there is a *thyroid ima artery*, an inconstant branch that arises from the right common carotid, brachiocephalic trunk, aortic arch, transverse scapular, or internal thoracic artery. It vascularizes the isthmus and anterior surface of the thyroid gland. Some have doubted the existence of the thyroid ima artery and its clinical significance is questionable.

Venous drainage is provided by a diffuse plexus that consists of upper, middle, and lower veins that drain to the internal jugular vein (IJV). The *middle thyroid vein*, a relatively constant venous branch between the thyroid gland and the IJV, must be identified and controlled early in thyroid surgery.[5]

Lymphatic drainage involves deep cervical, prelaryngeal, and paratracheal lymph nodes.[2]

Lymphatic Drainage & Cervical Compartments

The neck lymphatic system consists of two compartments, one superficial and one deep, called the central and lateral lymphatic systems which are divided into certain compartments.

Knowledge of these areas is important for selective dissection during surgery for thyroid cancer; cervical metastasis of thyroid cancers occurs mainly in the deep lymphatic chain.

The lateral lymphatic system is divided into five compartments as Levels I, II, III, IV, and V, and some compartments are further divided into A and B groups (Figure 6–4).[7]

The compartments are defined as follows:

- Level I nodes comprise the submental and submandibular nodes.
  - Level IA is referred to as the submental group and contains the nodes located between the anterior bellies of the digastric muscles and the hyoid bone.
  - Level IB is referred to as the submandibular group and contains the nodes located between the inner side of the mandible, the anterior and posterior bellies of the digastric muscle, and the stylohyoid muscle.
- Level II nodes contain the upper jugular nodes located at the upper one-third of the IJV above the level of the hyoid bone to the base of the skull and between the sternohyoid muscle and stylohyoid muscle medially and the posterior border of the SCM laterally/posteriorly. Level II nodes are also divided into A and B groups:
  - Level IIA nodes are those anterior to the spinal accessory nerve.
  - Level IIB nodes are those found posterior to the spinal accessory nerve.
- Level III contains the middle jugular nodes located around the middle third of IJV. It extends from the caudal edge of the body of the hyoid bone to the caudal edge of the cricoid cartilage. The anterior limit is the

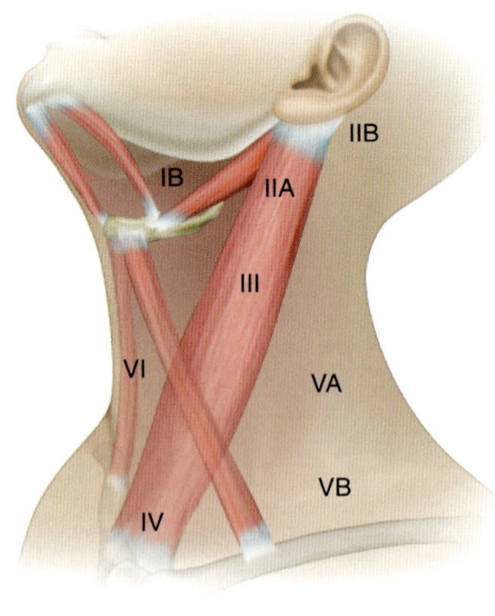

▲ **Figure 6–4.** Cervical compartments.

posterior border of the sternohyoid muscle, and the posterior limit is the posterior edge of the sternocleidomastoid muscle.

- Level IV contains the lower jugular lymph nodes located around the inferior third of the IJV from the caudal edge of the cricoid cartilage to the clavicle. The anterior and posterior borders are identical to Level III. Some further divide Level IV into A and B groups, though most commonly Level IV is considered as a single group of nodes.
- Level V nodes are considered the posterior triangle nodes and are located posterior to the sternocleidomastoid muscle from its attachment to the skull to the clavicle and are divided into A and B groups.[8,9]
  - Level VA nodes are those superior to the inferior border of the cricoid cartilage and include the spinal accessory nodes.
  - Level VB nodes are those inferior to the inferior border of the cricoid cartilage and include the transverse cervical artery nodes.

The central neck compartment (Figure 6–4) incorporates Level VI and VII lymph nodes and is bordered by the hyoid bone superiorly, the carotid arteries laterally, the prevertebral fascia posteriorly, the superficial layer of the deep neck fascia anteriorly, the innominate artery, and trachea on the right inferiorly.[7] Central compartment lymph nodes are further divided into prelaryngeal (Delphian), pretracheal, and right and left paratracheal lymph nodes. The inferior border of Level VI is the sternal notch, though the paratracheal lymphatic chains descend to the innominate artery at the inferior aspect of Level VI.[7] Level VII contains the upper anterior mediastinal lymph nodes which are found below the sternal notch and above the innominate artery.[8] The periglandular lymphatic network and tracheal lymphatic plexus provide drainage of the thyroid gland to the prelaryngeal, pre- and paratracheal lymph nodes. Superiorly, lymphatic vessels along the superior thyroid vessels drain to the deep cervical nodes; in addition, drainage is provided by the brachiocephalic nodes in the superior mediastinum toward the tracheobronchial nodes and finally to the thoracic duct.[8]

Innervation

The innervation of the thyroid gland is supplied by the **inferior laryngeal, or recurrent laryngeal nerve** (RLN) (Figure 6–2) and **superior laryngeal nerve** (SLN) (Figure 6–5).

- The **RLN** is a branch of the vagus nerve deputed to the motor innervation of the intrinsic muscles of the larynx. The vagus nerve provides the main parasympathetic fibers, while sympathetic fibers originate from the inferior, middle, and superior ganglia of the sympathetic trunk.[2,10] The RLN innerves all intrinsic laryngeal muscles, except for the cricothyroid muscles.[11]

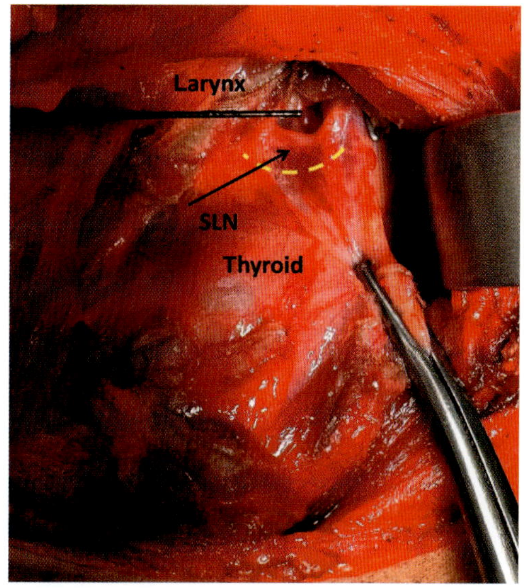

Figure 6–5. Superior laryngeal nerve.

The RLN is called "recurrent" because it descends into the chest passing from anterior to posterior around the aortic arch on the left, and around the subclavian artery on the right, and then ascends upward into the tracheaesophageal groove where it crosses the inferior thyroid artery. The RLN may pass anteriorly, posteriorly, or between the dividing branches of the artery. It continues its upward path until it enters the larynx passing behind the cricothyroid muscle. Before entering the larynx, it typically divides into two branches, an anterior and a posterior branch.[4] The anterior branch is considered the more critical branch providing the main motor innervation to the vocal cords. The distal portion of RLN is usually found posterior to the tubercle of Zuckerkandl, which can often be utilized as a point of identification, and the ligament of Berry.[2]

- The **SLN** often runs next to the STA. During surgery, selective ligation of the branches of the STA on the capsule of the thyroid is recommended to avoid accidental injury to the SLN. Careless use of electrocautery during surgery may also result in thermal damage to the SLN (as well as to the RLN). Care must also be taken not to damage the cricothyroid muscle itself during dissection of the anterior suspensory ligament.[2]

EMBRYOLOGY

The thyroid parenchyma is derived from the endoderm, between the first and second pharyngeal pouches. It originates from the foramen caecum, a pit at the posterior one-third of the tongue.

Around 20 to 24 days of development, endodermal cells of the primitive pharynx proliferate and create the thyroid diverticulum. At the fifth week of gestation, the thyroid diverticulum migrates caudally along the midline.[3] Also during the fifth week, the ultimobranchial bodies arise from the fourth/fifth pharyngeal pouches. These later differentiate into parafollicular C cells. Recent studies suggest C cells may originate from endoderm, challenging the traditional thinking of origin from neural crest cells.

The ultimobranchial bodies fuse with the superior dorsolateral aspect of the developing thyroid, forming the Zuckerkandl tubercle.[3,12] Parafollicular C-cells remain limited to the superolateral aspects of the thyroid gland.[3] Early in gestation, the thyroid gland begins to descend anteriorly to the pharynx. It descends anteriorly to the hyoid bone and laryngeal cartilages.[2] Division of the thyroid into right and left lobes occurs in the fifth week of gestation.[3] By the seventh week, the thyroid gland reaches its destination midline and anterior to the upper trachea. The thyroglossal duct maintains the connection of the thyroid gland to the base of the tongue until involution and disappearance of the duct.[2,3] Incomplete obliteration of the duct can lead to abnormalities such as thyroglossal duct cysts or lingual thyroid, and more commonly result in the finding of a pyramidal lobe. Cellular differentiation and maturation then continue until the thyroid is functionally mature by the 12-h gestational week.[3] Descent abnormalities during embryogenesis lead to anatomical variants including a rare subisthmic accessory gland, the absence of an isthmus and ectopic thyroid tissue. These occur secondary to failure of normal embryologic descent and the most common location is at the base of the tongue resulting in a lingual thyroid; however, ectopic thyroid tissue can be present anywhere along the thyroglossal duct tract. Conversely, excessive migration can lead to superior mediastinal or pericardiac thyroid tissue. Less commonly, ectopic thyroid tissue can be found in the adrenal or pituitary glands, in the gastrointestinal tract, within the female reproductive system, and in the iris of the eye.[3]

The **parathyroid glands** arise from the third and fourth branchial pouches.

The dorsal end of the fourth pouch gives rise to the superior glands, while the ventral end of the fourth pouch, the ultimobranchial body, gives rise to the cells that are arranged at the laterosuperior ends of the primitive thyroid, forming the parafollicular cells or C cells. These cells secrete calcitonin. This origin explains the possibility, although rare, of finding intrathyroidal ectopias in the upper parathyroid, termed P4.

The inferior parathyroid glands arise from the dorsal part of the third branchial pouch. From the ventral part of the same pouch derives the thymus. During embryological development, the two dorsal and ventral parts of the third pocket descend together for a long distance in a plane ventral to the fourth pocket. This is the reason why the lower parathyroid glands are located in a more anterior plane than the upper parathyroid glands. During the descent, the two different parts of the third pocket divide: The lower parathyroid glands stop their descent at the lower pole of the thyroid gland while the thymus continues its descent.

The migration of the lower parathyroid gland varies greatly; in fact, it can stop or continue in a much larger area. In case of no migration downward, the lower parathyroid may be positioned cranially at the upper pole of the thyroid gland. In such a case it can be confused with the upper parathyroid gland.

Usually, the P3 parathyroid would be anteriorly located, compared to the P4 gland. Alternatively, when the inferior parathyroid does not detach from the thymus, it can descend into the superior mediastinum with the thymus. Therefore, because of their embryological pathway, the glands that are ectopically located are most frequently the lower parathyroids.[4]

ANATOMICAL VARIANTS

In about 1% (or less) of cases, it is possible to find a **nonrecurrent laryngeal nerve** on the right as a branch that comes directly from the vagus without descent into the chest (Figure 6–6); the incidence on the left side is 0.004%.[2,13] A nonrecurrent laryngeal nerve was first described by Steadman in 1923.[13] This anatomic variant is commonly related to subclavian artery anatomical variation. Normally, the right subclavian artery originates from the fourth arch and the RLN originates from the sixth arch. When the heart descends during embryogenesis, it drags the sixth arch structure along; so, in case of abnormal descent of the right subclavian artery,

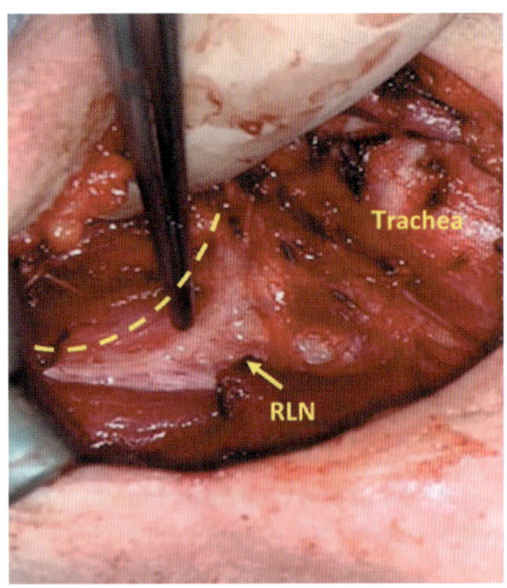

▲ **Figure 6–6.** Nonrecurrent laryngeal nerve after total thyroidectomy.

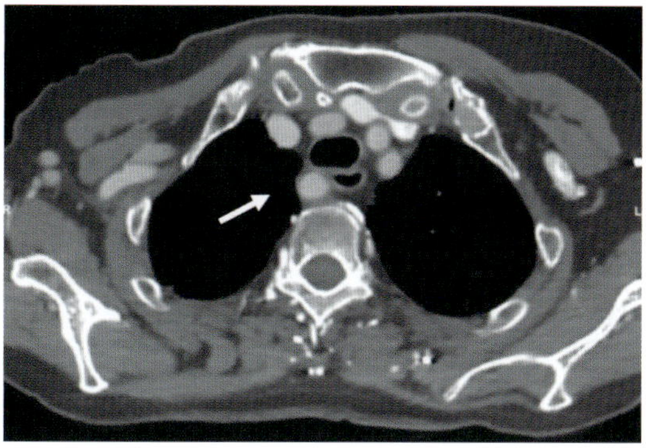

Figure 6–7. Lusoria artery.

an associated failure in the descent of RLN can be expected. In 80% of cases, the right subclavian artery is behind the esophagus, 15% between the esophagus and trachea, and in 5% of the cases it courses in front of the trachea. This is called **arteria lusoria** and occurs in 0.5% to 2% of the population[11,12] (Figures 6–7 and 6–8).

Anatomical variances of the origin and the branching pattern of **superior thyroid artery** (STA) have been reported frequently in the literature. Correct identification and ligation of this artery is important because of its close proximity to the superior laryngeal nerve. The typical origin of STA is the external carotid artery (30%-70%) but it may also arise from the common carotid artery and the common carotid bifurcation.[9,14] According to Toni et al., the STA arises most frequently from the external carotid artery in Caucasian individuals as opposed to East Asians, in which the most frequent origin is from the common carotid artery.[15] Double and unilateral STA are also described.

The STA gives off five arterial branches: terminal arterial branches for the thyroid and parathyroid glands, the superior laryngeal, infrahyoid, sternocleidomastoid, and cricothyroid artery.[16]

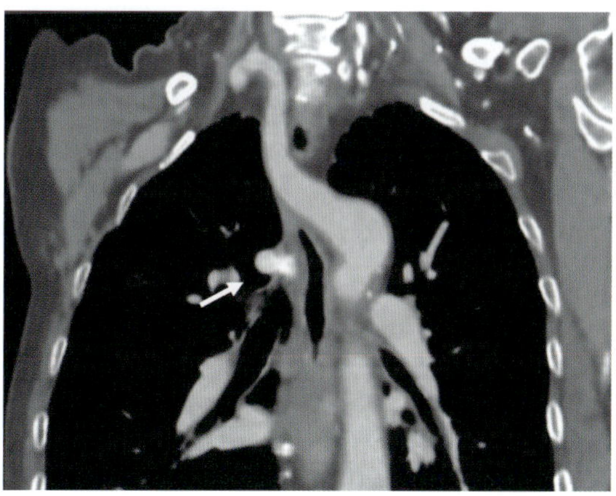

Figure 6–8. Lusoria artery.

REFERENCES

1. Di Frank H. Netter. *Commento ragionato all'atlante di anatomia umana*, Novartis Edizioni 2000.
2. Allen E, Fingeret A. *Anatomy, Head and Neck, Thyroid*. Book, StatPearls Publishing, Treasure Island; 2022.
3. Rosen RD, Sapra A. *Embryology, Thyroid*. StatPearls. Treasure Island (FL): StatPearls Publishing; 2022.
4. Miccoli P, Iacconi P. Chirurgia del Collo, Tiroide e Paratiroide. Grande Atlante di Tecnica Chirurgica. Utet.
5. Gurleyik E, Gurleyik G, Dogan S, Cobek U, Cetin F, Onsal U. Pyramidal lobe of the thyroid gland: surgical anatomy in patients undergoing total thyroidectomy. *Anat Res Int*. 2015; 2015:384148.
6. Avenia N, Rosato L, Fonsi GB. Cenni di anatomia chirurgica del collo, La patologia chirurgica della Tiroide e delle Paratiroidi, CLUB delle UEC, 2000:19-33.
7. Aygun N, Kostek M, Isgor A, Uludag M. Role and extent of neck dissection for neck lymph node metastases in differentiated thyroid cancers. *Sisli Etfal Hastan Tip Bul*. 2021;55(4):438-449.
8. Giuliano G, Proh M, Gibelli B, et al. Central neck dissection in differentiated thyroid cancer: technical notes. *Acta Otorhinolaryngol Ital*. 2014;34(1):9-14.
9. Grégoire V, Ang K, Budach W, et al. Delineation of the neck node levels for head and neck tumors: a 2013 update. DAHANCA, EORTC, HKNPCSG, NCIC CTG, NCRI, RTOG, TROG consensus guidelines. *Radiother Oncol*. 2014:110(1):172-181.
10. Roman BR, Randolph GW, Kamani D. Conventional thyroidectomy in the treatment of primary thyroid cancer. *Endocrinol Metab Clin North Am*. 2019;48(1):125-141.
11. Le QV, Ngo DQ, Ngo QX. Non-recurrent laryngeal nerve in thyroid surgery: a report of case series in Vietnam and literature review. *Int J Surg Case Rep*. 2018;50:56-59.
12. Nilsson M, Williams D. On the origin of cells and derivation of thyroid cancer: C cell story revisited. *Eur Thyroid J*. 2016;5(2):79-93.
13. Wang Y, Wang Z, Zhang H, Zhang P, Liang H, Dong W. Preoperative CT diagnosis of right nonrecurrent inferior laryngeal nerve. *Head Neck*. 2011;33(2):232-238.
14. Zarokosta M, Foutsitzi A, Mpartziotas I, Manthas A, Tsiaoussis J, Mariolis-Sapsakos T. Anomalous anatomic trajectory of the superior thyroid artery encountered during thyroidectomy. A rare case report. *J Surg Case Rep*. 2021;2021(4):rjab030.
15. Toni R, Della Casa C, Castorina S, et al. A meta-analysis of superior thyroid artery variations in different human groups and their clinical implications. *Ann Anat*. 2004;186:255-262.
16. Skandalakis J. *Skandalakis' Surgical Anatomy. The Embryologic and Anatomic Basis of Modern Surgery*. Athens: PMP; 2004: 7-108.

7 Thyroglossal Duct Cyst

Rhea Udyavar, MD
Aarti Mathur, MD, PhD

GENERAL CONSIDERATIONS

Thyroglossal duct cysts (TDCs) are the most common congenital neck mass, accounting for more than 75% of all midline neck masses in children and also present in about 7% of the adult population.[1] The thyroglossal tract results from the embryologic path of the developing thyroid gland as it descends from the primordial pharynx into its final position in the anterior neck, leaving behind a trail of epithelium that normally atrophies by 10 weeks' gestation.[2] When this epithelial tract fails to involute, its remnants can form a TDC. Therefore, a TDC can occur anywhere from the base of the tongue to the thyroid gland. Most are found near the hyoid bone, with 20% to 25% located in the suprahyoid region, 15% to 20% at the hyoid, and 25% to 65% below the hyoid.[3,4]

TDC commonly presents as a painless, mobile, midline neck mass that moves with swallowing and tongue protrusion. These lesions are usually benign, although papillary thyroid carcinoma is found in approximately 1% to 1.5% of TDCs.[5-8] Rarely, an ectopic lingual thyroid can be misdiagnosed as a TDC. Ectopic lingual thyroid occurs when the embryologic precursor of the thyroid gland fails to make its descent into its native position in the neck and remains in its embryologic position below the foramen cecum. Occasionally, this lingual thyroid can represent the patient's only functioning thyroid tissue.

Management of a symptomatic TDC is surgical resection via the Sistrunk procedure, which involves complete removal of the cyst and its contents, the central portion of hyoid bone, and a circumferential core of tissue between the hyoid bone and foramen cecum.[9] The most common complication of this procedure is recurrence of the TDC due to incomplete excision. Therefore, clinicians must be cognizant of the anatomy, embryology, physiology, and epidemiology of this disease process to ensure its adequate diagnosis and treatment.

PATHOGENESIS

Embryology

The embryology of the primordial tongue, thyroid gland, and hyoid bone is salient to the development and surgical management of a TDC. During the third week of gestation, the tongue begins to develop from the three cranial branchial arches. The first of these arches forms the anterior two-thirds of the tongue. The ventral portions of the second and third cranial branchial arches merge into paired anterior and posterior segments which then form the base of the tongue, as well as what will ultimately become the foramen cecum. The invagination of endodermal cells between these regions develops into the median anlage of the thyroid gland which begins to descend into the neck.[10-12]

As the thyroid gland descends along the midline into the anterior neck, the diverticulum formed by this invagination elongates into what is then known as the thyroglossal duct (Figure 7–1). Failure to descend may lead to ectopic lingual thyroid. The median thyroid anlage continues to migrate caudally, generally anterior to the region of the hyoid bone, until it establishes its anatomic position in the anterior neck. The lateral thyroid anlage fuses with the posterior aspect of the median thyroid anlage.

By the end of the eighth week of gestation, the thyroglossal duct atrophies, leaving a remnant proximally at the base of the tongue called the foramen cecum. The distal portion of the atrophied duct becomes the pyramidal lobe of the thyroid gland. Microscopic nests of thyroid follicular cells can be distributed anywhere along the tract of the atrophied thyroglossal duct.

The thyroglossal duct's migration path is variable and intimately associated with the hyoid bone, which develops from the mesodermal components of the second and third branchial arches. The primordial hyoid bone rotates as it matures and the two lateral components of the hyoid bone

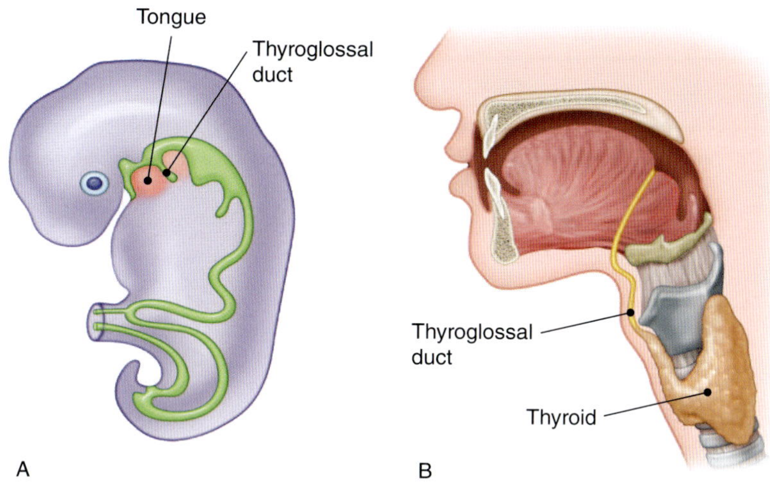

▲ **Figure 7–1.** Embryologic development and relevant anatomy of the thyroglossal duct. **(A)** Development of the thyroglossal duct in an embryo. **(B)** Extension of the patent thyroglossal duct extending from the foramen cecum to the thyroid.

fuse, in parallel with the descent of the thyroglossal duct in the midline of the neck.[11] If the migration path of the thyroglossal duct courses posterior or through the eventual fusion site of the hyoid bone, a thyroglossal duct remnant can become entrapped within the bone—thus the need to remove a portion of the hyoid bone when resecting a TDC.

CLINICAL FINDINGS

Symptoms & Signs

Classically, a TDC presents as a painless midline neck mass, close to the hyoid bone, that elevates with swallowing and protrusion of the tongue, although immobility does not rule out the diagnosis.[13] The location can be further categorized as intralingual, suprahyoid and/or submental, thyrohyoid, or suprasternal.[14]

In approximately one-third of cases, tenderness and associated lymphadenopathy can be present due to a secondary infection of the cyst, a sinus tract, or fistula accompanied by fluid drainage through a cutaneous opening.[15] The lining of the TDC is not always intact as it is frequently disrupted by an associated inflammatory process. TDCs are most frequently unilocular, but can also be multilocular.[16] Instead of a cyst, the remnant of the thyroglossal duct tract can form a fistula, generally the result of an inciting infectious, inflammatory, or traumatic process. A preceding infection was implicated in up to 35% of cases of thyroglossal duct fistulae.[17] Oral bacteria are believed to be transmitted through the foramen cecum and into the thyroglossal duct remnant, causing inflammatory fluid secretion and drainage through the new cutaneous orifice.

Although TDCs are typically diagnosed in childhood, and at least 60% are diagnosed by the age of 20, 7% are diagnosed in adults.[18,19] When TDCs present in adulthood, the size of the cysts tend to be larger and more likely to be off the midline than those that present in childhood.[20] Numerous studies report that diagnosis in adulthood is more common in males.[2,15,20-23] Table 7–1 summarizes the key clinical and imaging features of the common manifestations of TDCs.

Laboratory Findings

Laboratory testing, specifically thyroid function tests, are not routinely obtained as part of the diagnostic evaluation of a TDC. However, obtaining at least a TSH level prior to surgery may rarely diagnose hypothyroidism due to an ectopic lingual thyroid, rather than a TDC, which can be treated with a trial of levothyroxine.[24] This is of particular significance in children, as hypothyroidism in children under the age of 3 can result in permanent cognitive disability.

Imaging Studies

In children, ultrasound is the ideal imaging modality to diagnose a TDC because of its low cost, ease of administering without the need for sedation, sensitivity in detecting mural nodules and calcifications, and ability to detect normal functional thyroid tissue.[25] However, preoperative imaging is not universally performed in children, as clinical examination may be sufficient.[26] On ultrasound, a TDC generally appears anechoic and well circumscribed, often splaying the strap muscles apart. It can have a pseudosolid appearance due to the gelatinous material that may be contained in the cyst.[27] When prior or current infection is associated with the cyst or tract, sonographic appearance may be characterized

Table 7–1. Clinical manifestations of thyroglossal duct cysts.

	Relevant History	Diagnostic Ultrasound Features
Simple cyst	Midline, painless, fluid-filled neck mass	Anechoic, thin-walled, well-circumscribed unilocular cyst
Fistula	Often associated with prior infectious symptoms such as tenderness and lymphadenopathy	Fistula tract with increased heterogeneity and soft tissue edema on ultrasound
Ectopic lingual thyroid	May have clinical manifestations of hypothyroidism	Absent cervical thyroid*
Thyroglossal duct cyst carcinoma	Rapid enlargement of the mass, history of prior neck irradiation	Mural mass with calcification on ultrasound

*In these cases, radioisotope thyroid scan can be used to identify uptake of thyroid tissue near the foramen cecum.

by increased heterogeneity, complex cystic structures with internal echoes, or soft tissue edema.[27,28]

A TDC can be mistaken for an ectopic lingual thyroid at the base of the tongue, which may actually represent the patient's only functional thyroid tissue in an ectopic position, or it may be a focus of additional ectopic thyroid tissue in addition to the normal thyroid gland. The actual incidence of ectopic thyroid tissue masquerading as a TDC is estimated to be around 1% to 2%.[29] Radioisotope thyroid scanning can detect the presence of normal thyroid tissue caudal to the midline neck mass. However, this is not typically performed as it requires injection of a radiopharmaceutical compound.[30,31]

Cross-sectional imaging with a CT scan can assist in diagnosis and surgical planning for adult patients with cystic midline neck masses. Intravenous contrast-enhanced CT will typically show a smooth, well-circumscribed, thin-walled cyst within 2 cm of the midline and closely abutting the hyoid bone (Figure 7–2).

Preoperative MRI has also been described as being of limited utility in identifying the extent of the thyroglossal tract, which may have accessory tracts and pouches off the main tract in approximately 8% of cases.[32,33] However, it is not clear that these accessory tracts are associated with incomplete resection or cyst recurrence. The role of MRI may be limited to defining the residual tracts that are implicated in cases of cyst recurrence to ensure adequate removal of the tract on reoperation.[34]

Special Tests

Fine-needle aspiration cytology (FNAC) has limited utility in the preoperative evaluation of TDCs because cytology is typically nonspecific and rarely shows thyroid cells.[35] Controversy still exists regarding the necessity of FNAC for establishing a diagnosis of TDC as some argue that FNAC can help to preoperatively diagnose a malignancy in the cyst.[36,37] The sensitivity of FNAC for preoperative diagnosis of a malignancy in a TDC varies widely from 53% to 100%.[35,38,39]

Differential Diagnosis

The differential diagnosis for a midline or cystic, anterior neck mass includes both benign and malignant etiologies (Table 7–2).

Benign etiologies include congenital lesions such as branchial cleft cysts, dermoid cysts, lymphatic malformations, and laryngoceles, which mimic TDC.[40,41] Branchial cleft cysts also present as an anterior cystic mass; however, they tend to be more lateral and not associated with the hyoid bone. Additional differential diagnoses include masses originating from the thyroid gland, such as colloid

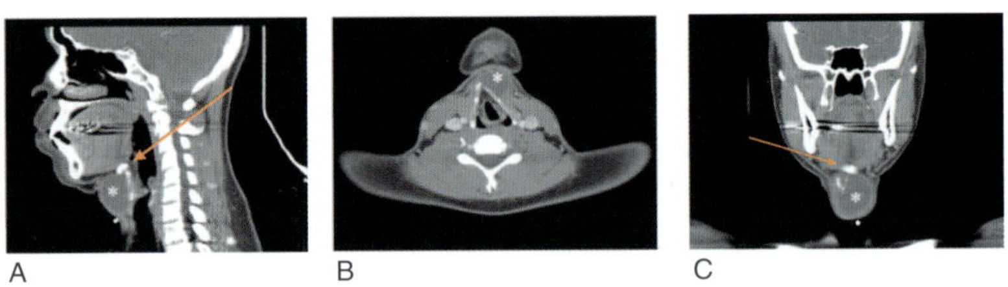

Figure 7–2. CT findings for a thyroglossal duct cyst (TDC) in an adult patient. **(A)** Sagittal view illustrating the relationship of the TDC, the anterior cystic structure (asterisk), to the hyoid bone (arrow). **(B)** Axial view illustrating the inferior extent of the TDC laterally displacing the thyroid cartilage by the TDC in the anterior neck (asterisk). **(C)** Coronal view demonstrating the position of the cyst (asterisk) within 2 cm of the midline of the neck, near the hyoid bone (arrow).

Table 7–2. Differential diagnosis for a cystic neck mass mimicking a thyroglossal duct cyst.

Diagnosis	Distinguishing Features
Benign	
Ectopic lingual thyroid	May present with dyspnea and stridor; ultrasound shows no thyroid tissue in the normal location
Midline branchial cleft cyst	Usually identified at birth as an ulcerated skin lesion in the midline, with a sinus tract pointing inferiorly from the cutaneous portion
Dermoid cyst	Superficial cyst usually in close proximity to the hyoid bone; no mesodermal attachments and therefore no movement with tongue protrusion or swallowing
Lymphatic malformation	Imaging findings of traversing vessels, presence of fluid levels from hemorrhage within the lesion
Laryngocele	Dilated saccule communicating with the laryngeal ventricle; may be fluid-filled or contain air-fluid levels
Cystic hygroma	Soft, fluctuant, fluid-filled cyst that transilluminates; secondary infection can occur
Hashimoto's thyroiditis	Thin-walled cystic lesions associated with antithyroid peroxidase or antithyroglobulin antibodies
Cystic thyroid adenoma	Fluid-filled, may rapidly enlarge and cause compressive symptoms, usually round and well circumscribed; often "cold" (non-functioning) nodules
Primary cystic parathyroid tumor	Often associated with hyperparathyroidism
Abscess	Often heterogeneous, may contain gas and demonstrate peripheral enhancement on imaging
Malignant	
Papillary thyroid cancer	Punctate calcifications, irregular central cystic changes on ultrasound
Metastatic Delphian lymph node from papillary thyroid cancer	Presence of central cystic necrosis, irregular borders, and punctate calcifications with disruption of normal fatty hilar architecture on ultrasound

nodules, cystic Hashimoto thyroiditis involving the isthmus or pyramidal lobe, or primary cystic parathyroid tumors.[42] An important diagnosis to recognize is an ectopic lingual thyroid, which can resemble a TDC, but is often also associated with elevated thyroid stimulating hormone.[43] A soft tissue abscess may also present as a cystic or fluctuant midline anterior neck mass, and may be difficult to distinguish from an infected TDC.

Malignant processes include a cystic variant of a papillary thyroid carcinoma or a metastatic cystic Delphian lymph node.

Associated Malignancy

Malignancy is present in 1% to 1.5% of TDCs, typically within an adenoma in the cyst wall. TDC carcinoma is believed to be either a sequela of ectopic thyroid tissue contained within the cyst or metastasis from a primary thyroid malignancy within the gland itself.[44,45] Therefore, establishing a diagnosis of a primary TDC carcinoma is contingent upon histological identification of an epithelial lining with normal thyroid follicles within the wall of the cyst or the duct, as well as normal thyroid tissue adjacent to the tumor.[46] The presence of an associated thyroid gland malignancy does not negate the diagnosis of a primary thyroglossal duct carcinoma, but does suggest a distinctive tumor biology.

Histologically, these tumors are most often of papillary thyroid, mixed papillary and follicular thyroid, or squamous cell origin.[47] The presentation of a thyroglossal duct carcinoma is difficult to distinguish preoperatively from that of a benign TDC. A rapidly growing mass in an adult may be more suggestive of malignancy, as is the presence of a mural mass with calcification on ultrasound, lymphadenopathy on physical examination, or a history of head and neck irradiation in childhood.[48-50]

TDC carcinoma is a rare process, with accordingly limited data from which to derive reliable epidemiologic features. It appears to affect predominantly adult female patients, with very few cases reported in the pediatric population.[5,51] Importantly, carcinoma diagnosed within a lingual thyroid is a distinct clinical entity from a TDC carcinoma.[46]

The majority of patients with incidentally diagnosed TDC carcinoma undergo Sistrunk procedure alone. These patients have an equivalent risk of having an incidental synchronous thyroid carcinoma as the general population.[52,53] In the rare instances in which a synchronous lesion is detected on ultrasound preoperatively in the thyroid gland, simultaneous total or partial thyroidectomy is warranted at the time of the Sistrunk procedure.[54] If there is no known thyroid gland malignancy detected at the time of diagnosis of a TDC carcinoma, most authors would suggest performing Sistrunk procedure alone. However, it remains clear that the minimum extent of resection for TDC carcinoma is performing wide excision via the Sistrunk procedure, and

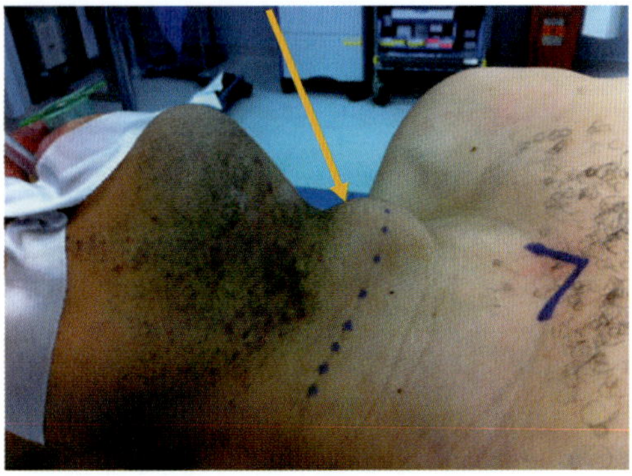

▲ **Figure 7–3.** Patient with thyroglossal duct cyst (TDC) positioned with neck extended for Sistrunk procedure for TDC (arrow).

the indications for total thyroidectomy with lymph node dissection, and postoperative adjuvant radioactive iodine remain under debate.[55]

Operative Treatment

The Sistrunk procedure was first described by Walter E. Sistrunk in 1920 and has since been minimally refined.

The patient is positioned supine with the neck hyperextended, or in the modified semi-Fowler's position (Figure 7–3). An incision is made transversely across the anterior neck, approximately at the level of the hyoid bone. Subplatysmal flaps are raised and the median raphe between the sternohyoid muscles are divided to expose the TDC. The cyst is dissected free of the surrounding soft tissue to the level of the hyoid bone. The sternohyoid muscles are separated from the central portion of the hyoid bone, and an approximately a 1/4-inch segment of central hyoid bone is excised. Superior to the hyoid bone, the thyroglossal tract is excised en bloc with an approximately 1/8-inch core of surrounding soft tissue to the level of the foramen cecum (Figure 7–4). To ensure an adequate resection margin, the base of tongue can be palpated through the mouth. The Sistrunk procedure is well tolerated and has few associated complications.

Complications & Prognosis

The Sistrunk procedure, when performed by experienced surgeons, is associated with low rates of major postoperative complications. The most commonly reported complications are infections, poor scarring (including keloid or hypertrophic scar formation), and cyst recurrence.[56-60]

Rarely, more significant complications such as hematoma or injury to the larynx, trachea, vocal cords, and hypoglossal nerve can occur.[38] The thyroid cartilage can be misidentified as the hyoid bone, leading to inadvertent resection of the anterior thyroid cartilage and transection of the anterior vocal folds. In those cases, immediate surgical

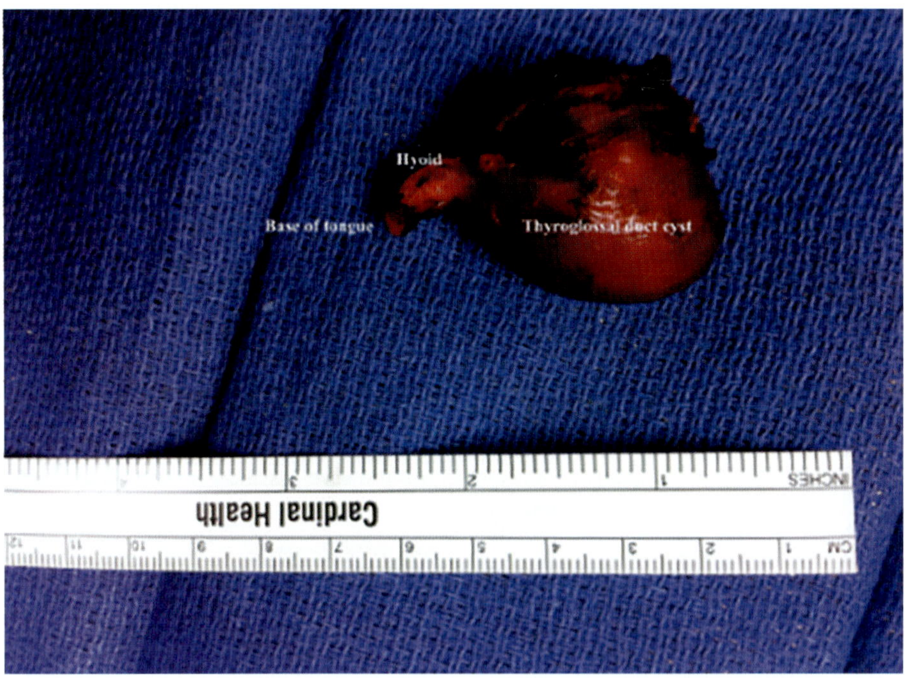

▲ **Figure 7–4.** Sistrunk procedure specimen containing the cyst and the central portion of the hyoid bone.

repair and tracheostomy placement is recommended. If a minor tracheal puncture occurs, drain placement and facilitation of healing by secondary intention is sufficient.[57] Neurovascular injury due to dividing the hyoid bone too laterally has also been reported. The hypoglossal nerve, lingual artery, and lingual vein are located in the submandibular region in close proximity to the lateral portions of the hyoid bone; failure to recognize these anatomic positions can result in hypoglossal nerve injury and/or postoperative hematoma.[38]

Cyst recurrence can occur in up to 27%. Clinical evidence of preoperative infection associated with the TDC is a known predictor of TDC recurrence, likely due to the predominance of inflammatory mediators that can attenuate tissue plains and preclude complete excision of the thyroglossal duct remnant.[3,61]

However, the best predictor for postoperative recurrence of a TDC is the extent of resection performed; specifically, whether a true Sistrunk procedure with removal of the central portion of the hyoid bone was completed. While it is clear that simple cyst excision is associated with a 40% to 50% recurrence rate, variation in the extent of suprahyoid dissection accounts for the Sistrunk procedure's recurrence rate of approximately 15.8%.[58,61] Some advocate for a suprahyoid dissection in all patients, even when the tract is not clearly identified, to completely excise the small, arborized ducts and multiple tracts that are often present between the hyoid bone and the base of the tongue, while others do not.[59,62] Slight variations in surgical technique and aggressiveness of the suprahyoid dissection may explain this ongoing controversy regarding the appropriate application of the Sistrunk procedure.

Conclusion

TDCs represent a common congenital cause of a painless, mobile, midline anterior neck mass that can be diagnosed in adults. Knowledge of the embryologic origins of the thyroid gland, as well as an understanding of the anatomic relations of the hyoid bone and the thyroglossal duct remnant, is central to the accurate diagnosis and surgical treatment of a TDC. Described over 100 years ago, the Sistrunk procedure remains the only definitive treatment for a TDC. When performed by experienced surgeons, outcomes are generally excellent.

REFERENCES

1. Brousseau VJ, Solares CA, Xu M, Krakovitz P, Koltai PJ. Thyroglossal duct cysts: presentation and management in children versus adults. *Int J Pediatr Otorhinolaryngol.* 2003;67(12):1285-1290.
2. Pollock WF, Stevenson EO. Cysts and sinuses of the thyroglossal duct. *Am J Surg.* 1966;112(2):225-232.
3. Ross J, Manteghi A, Rethy K, Ding J, Chennupati SK. Thyroglossal duct cyst surgery: a ten-year single institution experience. *Int J Pediatr Otorhinolaryngol.* 2017;101:132-136.
4. Thompson LDR, Herrera HB, Lau SK. A clinicopathologic series of 685 thyroglossal duct remnant cysts. *Head Neck Pathol.* 2016;10(4):465-474.
5. Rayess HM, Monk I, Svider PF, Gupta A, Raza SN, Lin HS. Thyroglossal duct cyst carcinoma: a systematic review of clinical features and outcomes. *Otolaryngol - Head Neck Surg (United States).* 2017;156(5):794-802.
6. Heshmati HM, Fatourechi V, Van Heerden JA, Hay ID, Goellner JR. Thyroglossal duct carcinoma: report of 12 cases. *Mayo Clin Proc.* 1997;72(4):315-319.
7. Patel SG, Escrig M, Shaha AR, Singh B, Shah JP. Management of well-differentiated thyroid carcinoma presenting within a thyroglossal duct cyst. *J Surg Oncol.* 2002;79(3):134-139.
8. Luna-Ortiz K, Hurtado-Lopez LM, Valderrama-Landaeta JL, Ruiz-Vega A. Thyroglossal duct cyst with papillary carcinoma: what must be done? *Thyroid.* 2004;14(5):363-366.
9. Sistrunk WE. The surgical treatment of cysts of the thyroglossal tract. *Ann Surg.* 1920;71(2):121.
10. Sugiyama S. *The Embryology of the Human Thyroid Gland Including Ultimobranchial Body and Others Related.* Springer Science & Business Media; 2012.
11. Mondin V, Ferlito A, Muzzi E, et al. Thyroglossal duct cyst: personal experience and literature review. *Auris Nasus Larynx.* 2008;35(1):11-25.
12. Gray SW, Skandalakis JE, Akin JT Jr. Embryological considerations of thyroid surgery: developmental anatomy of the thyroid, parathyroids and the recurrent laryngeal nerve. *Am Surg.* 1976;42(9):621-628.
13. Brunicardi F, Andersen D, Billiar T, et al. *Schwartz's Principles of Surgery.* 10th ed. New York, NY: McGraw-Hill; 2014.
14. Shah R, Gow K, Sobol SE. Outcome of thyroglossal duct cyst excision is independent of presenting age or symptomatology. *Int J Pediatr Otorhinolaryngol.* 2007;71(11):1731-1735.
15. Ostlie DJ, Burjonrappa SC, Snyder CL, et al. Thyroglossal duct infections and surgical outcomes. *J Pediatr Surg.* 2004;39(3):396-399.
16. Agnoni AA. Thyroglossal duct cyst. *Pediatr Surg Diagnosis Treat.* Published online 2014:237-240.
17. Deane SA, Telander RL. Surgery for thyroglossal duct and branchial cleft anomalies. *Am J Surg.* 1978;136(3):348-353.
18. Dedivitis RA, Camargo DL, Peixoto GL, Weissman L, Guimarães AV. Thyroglossal duct: a review of 55 cases. *J Am Coll Surg.* 2002;194(3):274-277.
19. Gorlin RJ, Goldman HM, Hurt W. Thoma's oral pathology. *J Periodontol.* 1972;43(9):575-577.
20. Lin ST, Tseng FY, Hsu CJ, Yeh TH, Chen YS. Thyroglossal duct cyst: a comparison between children and adults. *Am J Otolaryngol - Head Neck Med Surg.* 2008;29(2):83-87.
21. Hsieh Y-Y, Hsueh S, Hsueh C, et al. Pathological analysis of congenital cervical cysts in children: 20 years of experience at Chang Gung Memorial Hospital. *Chang Gung Med J.* 2003;26(2):107-113.
22. Ren W, Zhi K, Zhao L, Gao L. Presentations and management of thyroglossal duct cyst in children versus adults: a review of 106 cases. *Oral Surgery, Oral Med Oral Pathol Oral Radiol Endodontology.* 2011;111(2):e1-e6.
23. Zaman SU, Ikram M, Awan MS, Hassan NH. A decade of experience of management of thyroglossal duct cyst in a Tertiary Care Hospital: differentiation between children and adults. *Indian J Otolaryngol Head Neck Surg.* 2017;69(1):97-101.
24. Lilley JS, Lomenick JP. Delayed diagnosis of hypothyroidism following excision of a thyroglossal duct cyst. *J Pediatr.* 2013;162(2):427-428.

25. Ahuja AT, Wong KT, King AD, Yuen EHY. Imaging for thyroglossal duct cyst: the bare essentials. *Clin Radiol.* 2005;60(2):141-148.
26. Bhama AR, Smith RJ, Robinson RA, et al. Preoperative evaluation of thyroglossal duct cysts: children versus adults—is there a difference? *Am J Surg.* 2014;207(6):902-906.
27. Ahuja AT, King AD, Metreweli C. Sonographic evaluation of thyroglossal duct cysts in children. *Clin Radiol.* 2000; 55(10):770-774.
28. Kepertis C, Anastasiadis K, Lambropoulos V, Mouravas V, Spyridakis I. Diagnostic and surgical approach of thyroglossal duct cyst in children: ten years data review. *J Clin diagnostic Res JCDR.* 2015;9(12):PC13.
29. Radkowski D, Arnold J, Healy GB, et al. Thyroglossal duct remnants: preoperative evaluation and management. *Arch Otolaryngol Neck Surg.* 1991;117(12):1378-1381.
30. Leung AKC, Wong AL, Robson LM. Ectopic thyroid gland simulating a thyroglossal duct cyst: a case report. *Can J Surg.* 1995;38(1):87.
31. Tunkel DE, Domenech EE. Radioisotope scanning of the thyroid gland prior to thyroglossal duct cyst excision. *Arch Otolaryngol Neck Surg.* 1998;124(5):597-599.
32. King AD, Ahuja AT, Mok CO, Metreweli C. MR imaging of thyroglossal duct cysts in adults. *Clin Radiol.* 1999;54(5):304-308.
33. Al-Dousary S. Current management of thyroglossal-duct remnant. *J Otolaryngol.* 1997;26(4):259-265.
34. Patel NN, Hartley BEJ, Howard DJ. Management of thyroglossal tract disease after failed Sistrunk's procedure. *J Laryngol Otol.* 2003;117(9):710-712.
35. Shahin A, Burroughs FH, Kirby JP, Ali SZ. Thyroglossal duct cyst: a cytopathologic study of 26 cases. *Diagn Cytopathol.* 2005;33(6):365-369.
36. Chandan VS, Faquin WC, Wilbur DC, Khurana KK. The utility of GLUT-1 immunolocalization in cell blocks: an adjunct to the fine needle aspiration diagnosis of cystic squamous lesions of the head and neck. *Cancer Cytopathol Interdiscip Int J Am Cancer Soc.* 2006;108(2):124-128.
37. Weiner MF, Miranda RN, Bardales RH, et al. Diagnostic value of GLUT-1 immunoreactivity to distinguish benign from malignant cystic squamous lesions of the head and neck in fine-needle aspiration biopsy material. *Diagn Cytopathol.* 2004;31(5):294-299.
38. Oomen KPQ, Modi VK, Maddalozzo J. Thyroglossal duct cyst and ectopic thyroid: surgical management. *Otolaryngol Clin North Am.* 2015;48(1):15-27.
39. Lancini D, Lombardi D, Piazza C. Evidence and controversies in management of thyroglossal duct cyst carcinoma. *Curr Opin Otolaryngol Head Neck Surg.* 2021;29(2):113-119.
40. Patel S, Bhatt AA. Thyroglossal duct pathology and mimics. *Insights Imaging.* 2019;10(1):1-12.
41. Booth R, Tilak AM, Mukherjee S, Daniero J. Thyroglossal duct cyst masquerading as a laryngocele. *BMJ Case Reports CP.* 2019;12(3):e228319.
42. Massoll N, Nizam MS, Mazzaferri EL. Cystic thyroid nodules: diagnostic and therapeutic dilemmas. *Endocrinologist.* 2002;12(3). https://journals.lww.com/theendocrinologist/Fulltext/2002/05000/Cystic_Thyroid_Nodules__Diagnostic_and_Therapeutic.6.aspx
43. Foley DS, Fallat ME. Thyroglossal duct and other congenital midline cervical anomalies. *Semin Pediatr Surg.* 2006;15(2):70-75.
44. Pellegriti G, Lumera G, Malandrino P, et al. Thyroid cancer in thyroglossal duct cysts requires a specific approach due to its unpredictable extension. *J Clin Endocrinol Metab.* 2013;98(2):458-465.
45. Naik C, Basu S. Synchronous malignancies of thyroglossal duct cyst and thyroid gland. *Natl Med J India.* 2017;30(2):76-77.
46. Widström A, Magnusson P, Hellqvist H, Hallberg O, Ruber H. Adenocarcinoma originating in the thyroglossal duct. *Ann Otol Rhinol Laryngol.* 1976;85(2):286-290.
47. Motamed M, McGlashan JA. Thyroglossal duct carcinoma. *Curr Opin Otolaryngol Head Neck Surg.* 2004;12(2):106-109.
48. Tarnaris A, Giridharan W, Aird DW. Lymphoma mimicking a thyroglossal duct cyst in an adolescent. *J Laryngol Otol.* 2005; 119(3):216-218.
49. Doshi SV, Cruz RM, Hilsinger RL Jr. Thyroglossal duct carcinoma: a large case series. *Ann Otol Rhinol Laryngol.* 2001;110(8):734-738.
50. Alatsakis M, Drogouti M, Tsompanidou C, Katsourakis A, Chatzis I. Invasive thyroglossal duct cyst papillary carcinoma: a case report and review of the literature. *Am J Case Rep.* 2018;19:757-762.
51. Thompson LDR, Herrera HB, Lau SK. Thyroglossal duct cyst carcinomas in pediatric patients: report of two cases with a comprehensive literature review. *Head Neck Pathol.* 2017;11(4):442-449.
52. Martinez-Tello FJ, Martinez-Cabruja R, Fernandez-Martin J, Lasso-Oria C, Ballestin-Carcavilla C. Occult carcinoma of the thyroid. A systematic autopsy study from Spain of two series performed with two different methods. *Cancer.* 1993;71(12):4022-4029.
53. Bakkar S, Macerola E, Aljarrah Q, et al. BRAF(V600E) mutation: a potential predictor of more than a Sistrunk's procedure in patients with thyroglossal duct cyst carcinoma and a normal thyroid gland. *Updates Surg.* 2019;71(4):701-704.
54. Zizic M, Faquin W, Stephen AE, et al. Upper neck papillary thyroid cancer (UPTC): a new proposed term for the composite of thyroglossal duct cyst-associated papillary thyroid cancer, pyramidal lobe papillary thyroid cancer, and Delphian node papillary thyroid cancer metastasis. *Laryngoscope.* 2016;126(7):1709-1714.
55. Ramírez Plaza CP, López MED, Carrasco CEG, Meseguer LM, Perucho ADLF. Management of well-differentiated thyroglossal remnant thyroid carcinoma: time to close the debate? Report of five new cases and proposal of a definitive algorithm for treatment. *Ann Surg Oncol.* 2006;13(5):745-752.
56. Gioacchini FM, Alicandri-Ciufelli M, Kaleci S, Magliulo G, Presutti L, Re M. Clinical presentation and treatment outcomes of thyroglossal duct cysts: a systematic review. *Int J Oral Maxillofac Surg.* 2015;44(1):119-126.
57. Maddalozzo J, Venkatesan TK, Gupta P. Complications associated with the Sistrunk procedure. *Laryngoscope.* 2001;111(1):119-123.
58. Bratu I, Laberge J-M. Day surgery for thyroglossal duct cyst excision: a safe alternative. *Pediatr Surg Int.* 2004;20(9): 675-678.
59. Geller KA, Cohen D, Koempel JA. Thyroglossal duct cyst and sinuses: a 20-year Los Angeles experience and lessons learned. *Int J Pediatr Otorhinolaryngol.* 2014;78(2):264-267.
60. Lekkerkerker I, van Heurn ELW, van der Steeg AFW, Derikx JPM. Pediatric thyroglossal duct cysts: post-operative complications. *Int J Pediatr Otorhinolaryngol.* 2019;124:14-17.
61. Rohof D, Honings J, Theunisse HJ, et al. Recurrences after thyroglossal duct cyst surgery: results in 207 consecutive cases and review of the literature. *Head Neck.* 2015;37(12):1699-1704.
62. Kim MK, Pawel BR, Isaacson G. Central neck dissection for the treatment of recurrent thyroglossal duct cysts in childhood. *Otolaryngol Neck Surg.* 1999;121(5):543-547.

Thyroid Nodules & Multinodular Goiter

8

Rachel Liou, MD
James A. Lee, MD

GENERAL CONSIDERATIONS

Thyroid nodules are extremely common, occurring in up to 68% of a randomly selected population, with increasing prevalence in women and with increasing age.[1,2] Thyroid nodules can be found in patients who are euthyroid, hyperthyroid, or hypothyroid. Despite how common thyroid nodules are, only around 5% to 10% of thyroid nodules are malignant.[3] The term "goiter" denotes an enlarged thyroid which is present in approximately 5% of the population living in an iodine-sufficient area. There are many factors contributing to the formation of a goiter, including genetic as well as environmental causes, such as iodine deficiency and goitrogenic medications.

Clinical Findings

A. Symptoms and Signs

Detection of a thyroid nodule(s) occurs in a variety of different ways. Nodules are often asymptomatic and detected incidentally on imaging done for another reason or detected on physical exam. However, symptoms that may be associated with thyroid nodules are nonspecific and include voice changes, dysphagia, dyspnea, and a choking sensation among other compressive symptoms. Globus sensation is more prominent in patients with nodules greater than 3 cm and location anterior to the trachea or causing tracheal and/or esophageal impingement.[4] On evaluation, one must determine when and how the nodule(s) was identified and the speed of growth, as rapid growth may be concerning for malignancy. It is also important to obtain a thorough history, including signs and symptoms of thyroid hormone dysfunction. Hyperthyroid symptoms include anxiety, palpitations, insomnia, weight changes, visual changes, and heat intolerance. Hypothyroid symptoms include cold intolerance, fatigue, weight gain, and constipation. While these symptoms are nonspecific, they often present as the first clue that prompts a workup of thyroid disease. Significant radiation exposure should also be ascertained, as it is a risk factor for thyroid nodules, thyroid cancer, and hypothyroidism. Younger age at exposure and history of radiation dose above 40 mGy have been shown to increase the risk of developing radiation-induced thyroid nodules.[5,6] A family history of thyroid cancer, as well as thyroid cancer-associated syndromes (MEN 2A/B, Cowden complex, Gardner syndrome, familial adenomatous polyposis, and other syndromes), may increase the risk of thyroid disease. While over 90% of thyroid cancers are sporadic, 3% to 9% of thyroid cancers are familial nonmedullary type.[7] Twenty-five percent of medullary thyroid cancers are hereditary.[8] While rare, nonthyroid malignancies can metastasize to the thyroid gland and are most frequently seen with renal cell carcinoma, lung, colon, breast, melanoma, and ovarian cancers.[2]

Due to its higher sensitivity and diagnostic power, ultrasound has largely replaced physical exam in the evaluation of thyroid nodules. However, thyroid nodules are often palpable on physical exam. Solitary, firm, fixed nodules are more concerning for malignancy. Substernal goiters may be accompanied by the Pemberton sign which indicates vascular obstruction when the patients raise their arms over their head. Hyperthyroid patients may demonstrate signs suggesting hyperthyroidism, such as tachycardia, exophthalmos, and tremor while hypothyroid patients may present with delayed tendon reflexes, bradycardia, and hair loss.

B. Laboratory Findings

All patients with suspected thyroid nodules should undergo laboratory evaluation consisting of a serum TSH level. Suppressed TSH levels should prompt further testing with a free T4 to confirm hyperthyroidism and occasionally a total T3 to determine the severity of hyperthyroidism. In addition, a thyroid antibody panel may help elucidate the cause of the hyperthyroidism. The diagnosis of hyperthyroidism should prompt thyroid scintigraphy, as explained later. An elevated

Table 8–1. Data from ATA nodule sonographic patterns, risk of malignancy, size criteria for FNA.

Sonographic Pattern	Ultrasound Features	Estimated Risk of Malignancy %	FNA Size Cutoff (Largest Dimension)
High suspicion	Solid hypoechoic nodule/solid hypoechoic component of partially cystic nodule **with** one or more of the following: irregular margins, microcalcifications, taller than wide shape, rim calcifications with small extrusive soft tissue component, or evidence of extrathyroidal extension	>70-90	Recommend FNA at ≥1 cm
Intermediate suspicion	Hypoechoic solid nodule with smooth margins **without** microcalcifications, extrathyroidal extension, or taller than wide shape	10-20	Recommend FNA at ≥1 cm
Low suspicion	Isoechoic or hyperechoic solid nodule, or partially cystic nodule with eccentric solid areas **without** microcalcification, irregular margin or extrathyroidal extension, or taller than wide shape	5-10	Recommend FNA at ≥1.5 cm
Very low suspicion	Spongiform or partially cystic nodule **without** any of the sonographic features described in low, intermediate, or high suspicion patterns	<3	Consider FNA at >2 cm or observation
Benign	Purely cystic nodules	<1	No FNA

TSH level suggests hypothyroidism. Most patients with thyroid nodules are euthyroid and have normal thyroid function tests. Serum thyroglobulin levels are nonspecific and are not recommended during the initial evaluation of a thyroid nodule. However, serial thyroglobulin and thyroglobulin antibody levels are useful in postthyroidectomy surveillance in a patient with thyroid cancer. Calcitonin and CEA levels should be measured in patients with a personal or family history of medullary thyroid cancer, MEN 2, or in patients from areas with a higher baseline prevalence of medullary thyroid cancer.

C. Imaging Studies

Ultrasonography is the most important test in the evaluation of thyroid nodules. The ultrasound provides information regarding the size of the thyroid, the number of nodules, the size of the nodules, sonographic features of the nodules, and suspicious cervical lymph nodes. The American Thyroid Association (ATA) has classified the risk of malignancy of thyroid nodules into high, intermediate, low, and very low suspicion categories based on their ultrasound characteristics.[9] This, in turn, guides practitioners in determining which nodules to biopsy. For example, highly suspicious features (estimated risk of malignancy >70%-90%) include hypoechogenicity, irregular margins, microcalcifications, rim calcifications, taller than wide shape, and evidence of extrathyroidal extension, which would prompt biopsy at a size greater than or equal to 1 cm. Subcentimeter nodules are not usually biopsied unless there is a suspicion of metastasis (nodal or distant), local invasion, or if the nodule is posteriorly located which may raise the concern for invasion into posterior structures such as the recurrent nerve, trachea, and/or esophagus. See Table 8–1 for the ATA recommendations. The American College of Radiology (ACR) stratifies the need for biopsy of a thyroid nodule using the ACR Ti-RADS system (Table 8–2A, B).[10]

Fine-needle aspiration (FNA) is the most effective approach to determining the risk of cancer in thyroid nodules.[11] In this test, a small gauge needle (eg, 25 gauge) is placed into the nodule, most often under ultrasound guidance, and cellular material is aspirated. Typically, at least two passes are obtained to sample multiple regions of the nodule to ensure adequacy of the specimen and representative sampling of the nodule. A cytotechnologist may also be at the bedside to help determine the adequacy of the sample to avoid nondiagnostic samples. The most common complications of FNAs include bruising, soreness, and extremely rarely, hematoma formation, which could potentially affect the airway. It is ideal to hold anticoagulation and antiplatelet agents prior to the procedure to reduce the likelihood of a hematoma as well as to avoid diluting the cytologic sample with blood.

The Bethesda System for Reporting Thyroid Cytopathology is the most widely used standardized system for interpreting FNA and stratifies results into six risk categories: nondiagnostic (Bethesda I), benign (II), follicular lesion of undetermined significance/atypia of undetermined significance (III), follicular neoplasm/suspicious for follicular neoplasm (IV), suspicious for malignancy (V), and malignant (VI) (Table 8–3).[12] These classifications help with the clinical management of the thyroid nodule, given their associated risk of malignancy. A Bethesda I category generally indicates

Table 8–2. Data from the American College of Radiology: ACR TI-RADS. (A) scoring system (B) FNA recommendations.

A.

Category	Points			
	0	1	2	3
Composition	Cystic/almost completely cystic or spongiform	Mixed cystic and solid	Solid or almost completely solid	
Echogenicity	Anechoic	Hyperechoic or isoechoic	Hypoechoic	Very hypoechoic
Shape	Wider-than-tall			Taller-than-wide
Margin	Smooth or ill-defined		Lobulated	Extra-thyroidal extension
Echogenic Foci	None or large comet-tail artifacts	Macrocalcifications	Rim calcifications	Punctate echogenic foci

B.

Total Points	Classification	FNA Recommendation
0	TR1: Benign	No FNA
2	TR2: Not suspicious	No FNA
3	TR3: Mildly suspicious	FNA if ≥2.5cm Follow if ≥1.5 cm
4-6	TR4: Moderately suspicious	FNA if ≥1.5 cm Follow if ≥1 cm
≥ 7	TR5: Highly suspicious	FNA if ≥1 cm Follow if ≥0.5 cm

Table 8–3. Data from the 2017 Bethesda System for Reporting Thyroid Cytopathology.

Diagnostic Category	Risk of Malignancy (%)	Usual Management
I: Nondiagnostic	5-10	Repeat FNA
II: Benign	0-3	Ultrasound surveillance
III: Atypia of undetermined significance/ follicular lesion of undetermined significance	6-18	Repeat FNA, molecular testing, or lobectomy
IV: Follicular neoplasm or suspicious for a follicular neoplasm	10-40	Molecular testing, lobectomy
V: Suspicious for malignancy	45-60	Lobectomy or total thyroidectomy
VI: Malignant	94-96	Lobectomy or total thyroidectomy

an inadequate specimen and warrants a repeat FNA. The majority of FNAs are benign and patients typically only require ultrasound surveillance. The Bethesda III and IV categories carry a risk of malignancy ranging from 10% to 30%. These nodules may undergo a repeat biopsy, although nodules with suspicious ultrasound features should be considered for a diagnostic lobectomy or thyroidectomy. More recently, molecular testing that examines gene expression to determine cancer risk is being used to help guide treatment in Bethesda III, IV, and V lesions. Despite the potential benefit of molecular testing in the management of indeterminate cytology, it is important to note that it currently plays a limited role in the management of Hürthle cell lesions because studies have demonstrated a concerning false positive rate for medullary thyroid cancer.[13] Currently, histologic evaluation on surgically resected specimens looking for vascular or capsular invasion remains the most effective method of distinguishing Hürthle cell carcinomas from adenomas.

Computed tomography (CT), preferably with intravenous contrast, is used preoperatively as an adjunct to determine the mediastinal extent of a substernal goiter and extrathyroidal invasion. CT also helps to visualize extent of LN disease in advanced thyroid cancer. It is important to note that the iodine bolus associated with intravenous contrast may delay the administration of therapeutic radioactive iodine, and the multidisciplinary care team should discuss whether or not it is necessary on an individual basis.

Thyroid scintigraphy is indicated in hyperthyroid patients to determine if the thyrotoxicosis is due to destructive processes like lymphocytic thyroiditis or functional excess from toxic adenomas, toxic multinodular goiters, or Graves' disease. In this exam, radioactive iodine (I-123 or I-131) is taken by mouth or technetium TC-99m pertechnetate is injected intravenously, and radiotracer uptake is measured to determine if there are specific changes in uptake compared to normal thyroid.

D. Special Tests

Patients should undergo a preoperative vocal cord assessment prior to thyroidectomy when there is concern for potential impairment of the recurrent laryngeal nerves. Patients who are most at risk for recurrent laryngeal nerve dysfunction are those who have had previous thyroid/parathyroid surgery or other neck surgery. Flexible laryngoscopy, direct laryngoscopy, and laryngeal ultrasonography may aid in the diagnosis of vocal cord paralysis.

Differential Diagnosis

The differential diagnosis of a thyroid nodule and goiter is broad and includes the following: cystic lesions, adenomas, colloid nodules, well-differentiated and poorly differentiated thyroid cancers, thyroid lymphoma, thyroiditis, and metastases to the thyroid. In addition, a number of lesions may initially be thought to be a thyroid nodule such as lymphadenopathy, parathyroid adenoma, and paraganglioma.

Treatment

A. Surveillance

Asymptomatic benign thyroid nodules and indeterminate nodules deemed low risk via molecular profiling may be monitored with surveillance ultrasonography at 6 to 12 months and repeat FNA if the nodule(s) increases in size by greater than 50% and/or demonstrates worrisome features. Stable nodules may allow for longer intervals between follow-up. Papillary microcarcinomas (ie, < 1.5 cm in size) may be considered for a program of active surveillance with an experienced team of specialists.

B. Surgery

Thyroid surgery is indicated for Bethesda V and VI nodules and as a diagnostic/therapeutic modality for select Bethesda III and IV lesions, as previously discussed. Large goiters may benefit from a thyroidectomy if they cause compressive symptoms, if the burden of nodularity that precludes adequate evaluation is high, or if there is evidence of substernal growth or tracheal/esophageal compromise. Several factors go into determining the extent of thyroidectomy and should be discussed in a shared decision-making model with the patient and the rest of the medical team. A few factors favor total thyroidectomy including nodule size greater than 4 cm, history of radiation exposure, strong family history of thyroid cancer, certain genetic mutations, worrisome ultrasound characteristics, contralateral nodularity, concomitant hyperthyroidism, lymph node disease, and/or patient preference.

Complications of thyroid surgery are overall uncommon but may cause life-threatening or life-altering circumstances. The incidence of postsurgical hematoma formation is typically less than 2%, with the vast majority occurring within 24 hours of the operation.[14] Prompt evaluation of the hematoma and a very low threshold to evacuate the hematoma in controlled circumstances are critical to prevent airway compromise, which may have lethal consequences. Recurrent laryngeal nerve injury is also a well-known complication from thyroid surgery, most often manifesting as hoarseness and potentially aspiration after thyroidectomy. The incidence of temporary nerve injury ranges from 3% to 15% and the risk of permanent nerve injury ranges from ≤1% to 5%. A concern for nerve injury should lead to a laryngeal evaluation and, if present, should prompt referral to a voice specialist. Hypoparathyroidism is a concern after total thyroidectomy or completion thyroidectomy, in which there is a potential for all four parathyroid glands to be affected during surgery. The rate of temporary hypoparathyroidism ranges from 5% to 38% and the risk of permanent hypoparathyroidism ranges from 0% to 3%. Hypoparathyroidism leads to hypocalcemia and may result in a spectrum of symptoms ranging from mild perioral numbness and tingling to as severe as seizures and arrhythmias. Routine postoperative oral calcium administration has been shown in some series to reduce the rate of symptomatic hypocalcemia.[15,16]

C. Radiofrequency Ablation

Select institutions in the United States have begun to offer radiofrequency ablation (RFA) as a percutaneous option for treating benign thyroid nodules. In this technique, the probe is inserted into the thyroid nodule under ultrasound guidance, and the thyroid nodule is ablated using alternating current to generate ablative heat zones. International and emerging US data demonstrate shrinkage of nodules up to 80% in a 5-year follow-up. Despite being minimally invasive, there are documented risks associated with RFA. Major complications include recurrent nerve damage, which occurs in approximately 1% to 2% of cases and nodule rupture, with patients experiencing a sudden onset of pain and neck bulging. Minor risks include pain, hematoma, skin burn, and postprocedure vasovagal reaction.[17-21]

D. Ethanol Ablation

Ethanol ablation can serve as an alternative for symptomatic, recurrent, and/or large thyroid cysts. In this procedure, a needle is introduced into the cyst under ultrasound guidance, the cyst fluid is aspirated, and then 99% ethanol is instilled into the cyst cavity, causing fibrosis to the cavity lining, reducing the cyst volume over 50% to 80% as well as reducing the risk of recurrence of the cyst.[18]

When to Refer/When to Admit

Patients with a thyroid nodule or goiter should be referred to a specialist such as an endocrinologist or endocrine surgeon to determine the best diagnostic and treatment pathway. Patients who require resection should be referred to a high-volume thyroid surgeon since there is a clear volume-outcome relationship demonstrating that surgeons who consistently perform 25 to 50 thyroidectomies a year have significantly lower complication rates and better patient outcomes.[2]

REFERENCES

1. Guth S, Theune U, Aberle J, Galach A, Bamberger CM. Very high prevalence of thyroid nodules detected by high frequency (13 MHz) ultrasound examination. *Eur J Clin Invest.* 2009; 39(8).
2. Patel KN, Yip L, Lubitz CC, et al. The American association of endocrine surgeons guidelines for the definitive surgical management of thyroid disease in adults. *Ann Surg.* 2020; 271(3).
3. Bomeli SR, LeBeau SO, Ferris RL. Evaluation of a thyroid nodule. *Otolaryngol Clin North Am.* 2010;43(2):229-238.
4. Nam IC, Choi H, Kim ES, Mo EY, Park YH, Sun D Il. Characteristics of thyroid nodules causing globus symptoms. *European Archives of Oto-Rhino-Laryngology.* 2015;272(5).
5. Veiga LHS, Holmberg E, Anderson H, et al. Thyroid cancer after childhood exposure to external radiation: an updated pooled analysis of 12 studies. *Radiat Res.* 2016;185(5).
6. Veiga LHS, Lubin JH, Anderson H, et al. A pooled analysis of thyroid cancer incidence following radiotherapy for childhood cancer. *Radiat Res.* 2012;178(4):365-376.
7. Yang SP, Ngeow J. Familial non-medullary thyroid cancer: unraveling the genetic maze. *Endocr Relat Cancer.* 2016;23(12).
8. Wells SA, Asa SL, Dralle H, et al. Revised American Thyroid Association guidelines for the management of medullary thyroid carcinoma. *Thyroid.* 2015;25(6):567-610.
9. Haugen BR, Alexander EK, Bible KC, et al. 2015 American Thyroid Association Management Guidelines for Adult Patients with Thyroid Nodules and Differentiated Thyroid Cancer: The American Thyroid Association Guidelines Task Force on Thyroid Nodules and Differentiated Thyroid Cancer. *Thyroid.* 2016;26(1).
10. Tessler FN, Middleton WD, Grant EG, et al. ACR thyroid imaging, reporting and data system (TI-RADS): white paper of the ACR TI-RADS Committee. *Journal of the American College of Radiology.* 2017;14(5).
11. Sosa JA, Hanna JW, Robinson KA, Lanman RB. Increases in thyroid nodule fine-needle aspirations, operations, and diagnoses of thyroid cancer in the United States. *Surgery (United States).* 2013;154(6).
12. Cibas ES, Ali SZ. The 2017 Bethesda system for reporting thyroid cytopathology. *Thyroid.* 2017;27(11).
13. Brauner E, Holmes BJ, Krane JF, et al. Performance of the afirma gene expression classifier in Hürthle cell thyroid nodules differs from other indeterminate thyroid nodules. *Thyroid.* 2015;25(7).
14. Dehal A, Abbas A, Hussain F, Johna S. Risk factors for neck hematoma after thyroid or parathyroid surgery: ten-year analysis of the nationwide inpatient sample database. *Perm J.* 2015;19(1):22-28.
15. Edafe O, Antakia R, Laskar N, Uttley L, Balasubramanian SP. Systematic review and meta-analysis of predictors of post-thyroidectomy hypocalcaemia. *British Journal of Surgery.* 2014; 101(4).
16. Arer IM, Kus M, Akkapulu N, et al. Prophylactic oral calcium supplementation therapy to prevent early post thyroidectomy hypocalcemia and evaluation of postoperative parathyroid hormone levels to detect hypocalcemia: a prospective randomized study. *International Journal of Surgery.* 2017;38.
17. Muhammad H, Santhanam P, Russell JO, Kuo JH. RFA and benign thyroid nodules: review of the current literature. *Laryngoscope Investig Otolaryngol.* 2021;6(1).
18. Baek JH, Ha EJ, Choi YJ, Sung JY, Kim JK, Shong YK. Radiofrequency versus ethanol ablation for treating predominantly cystic thyroid nodules: a randomized clinical trial. *Korean J Radiol.* 2015;16(6).
19. Spiezia S, Garberoglio R, Milone F, et al. Thyroid nodules and related symptoms are stably controlled two years after radiofrequency thermal ablation. *Thyroid.* 2009;19(3).
20. Cesareo R, Pasqualini V, Simeoni C, et al. Prospective study of effectiveness of ultrasound-guided radiofrequency ablation versus control group in patients affected by benign thyroid nodules. *Journal of Clinical Endocrinology and Metabolism.* 2015;100(2).
21. Faggiano A, Ramundo V, Assanti AP, et al. Thyroid nodules treated with percutaneous radiofrequency thermal ablation: a comparative study. *Journal of Clinical Endocrinology and Metabolism.* 2012;97(12).

9 Hyperthyroidism: Graves' Disease

Anna Z. Fashandi, MD
Paul G. Gauger, MD

GENERAL CONSIDERATIONS

Graves' disease is the most common cause of hyperthyroidism in the United States, with an incidence of approximately 20 to 50 cases per 100,000 persons. Patients of all ages can be affected, though the incidence peaks in the fourth to sixth decades of life with females being five times more likely to carry the diagnosis than men.[1]

PATHOGENESIS

Graves' disease is an autoimmune disease in which TSH receptor antibodies (TRAbs) stimulate the TSH receptor, which leads to hyperthyroidism from increased thyroid hormone production and release from thyroid cells. In the eye, the circulating TSH and TRAbs stimulate orbital cells to release hydrophilic mucopolysaccharides in addition to inflammatory cytokines.[2-5] This can ultimately lead to edema, congestion, and exophthalmos, which is referred to as Graves' orbitopathy (GO).

CLINICAL FINDINGS

Symptoms & Signs

The symptoms and signs of Graves' disease are similar to those of hyperthyroidism in general, with the addition of ocular symptoms caused by GO in those patients who experience that specific manifestation of Graves' disease (Table 9–1). There is moderate correlation between the degree of thyroid hormone (T4 and T3) elevation and the clinical symptoms a patient experiences.[6]

Laboratory Findings

The laboratory evaluation of Graves' patients shows suppressed TSH with elevated free T3/T4, consistent with hyperthyroidism. The free T3 levels are usually elevated earlier and to a greater degree than the free T4 levels.[7] Testing for autoantibodies typically reveals elevated TRAbs and thyroid-stimulating immunoglobulins (TSI).

Imaging Studies

Radioactive iodine (RAI) uptake scan ($^{123/131}I$) or ^{99m}Tc pertechnetate scan can be used to quantitate the overall metabolism of the thyroid by measuring how much orally ingested iodide is concentrated in the thyroid gland. In Graves' disease, there will be increased uptake above the normal level of 3% to 16% at 6 hours or 8% to 25% at 24 hours.[8] This uptake is diffuse and homogenous throughout the entire thyroid gland. This differs from uptake scans seen in other causes of hyperthyroidism including toxic multinodular goiter, which has increased but heterogeneous uptake, as well as toxic adenoma, which has increased uptake in a single nodule.

DIFFERENTIAL DIAGNOSIS

Aside from Graves' disease, the differential diagnosis for hyperthyroidism includes toxic adenoma, toxic multinodular goiter, amiodarone toxicity, iodine-induced toxicity (Jod-Basedow effect), pregnancy, TSH-secreting pituitary tumor, thyrotoxicosis factitia, and human chorionic gonadotropin-secreting tumor.

COMPLICATIONS

The main complications from untreated Graves' disease are cardiac or ophthalmologic in nature. Uncontrolled hyperthyroidism can lead to dysrhythmias including sinus tachycardia and supraventricular tachycardia, most commonly atrial fibrillation. GO can have symptoms ranging from mild discomfort to severe visual disturbances including blindness.

Table 9–1. Symptoms and signs of Graves' disease.

System	Symptoms	Signs
Neurologic	Anxiety Nervousness Irritability Insomnia Weakness Fatigue	Tremor Hyperreflexia
Ophthalmologic	Diplopia Blurred vision Photophobia Grittiness	Conjunctival injection Lid lag Lid retraction Stare Proptosis/Exophthalmos Strabismus
Cardiovascular	Palpitations	Tachycardia Arrhythmia Murmur
Respiratory	Dyspnea	
Gastrointestinal	Increased frequency of bowel movements Diarrhea	
Endocrine	Weight loss Increased appetite Heat intolerance Menstrual changes Erectile dysfunction Decreased libido	Thyromegaly with bruit Diaphoresis Hair loss Gynecomastia Pretibial myxedema

TREATMENT

Antithyroid drugs (ATDs), RAI, and thyroidectomy are all options in the management of Graves' disease. Strategically, ATDs are often an appropriate initial step to achieve clinical euthyroidism but have not been considered the ideal long-term strategy. Each modality has its own advantages and disadvantages and patients should be counseled about the risks and benefits, side effects, and costs of the various treatment modalities.[6,7] Historically in the United States, RAI has been the preferred option by endocrinologists in the treatment for Graves' disease, though in more recent years the continued use of ATDs (ie, methimazole in particular) has been increasing to reduce the use of RAI.[9] Importantly for the patient, long-term quality of life has not been shown to be affected by the choice of treatment strategy.[10,11]

Antithyroid Drugs

ATDs work to decrease thyroid hormone synthesis by interfering with the binding of iodine and coupling of iodotyrosines within the thyroid gland, without destroying the gland itself. The goal of using ATDs is to make the patient euthyroid; the Graves' disease is not cured, but rather symptomatically controlled by these medications. The T4 level typically normalizes before the T3 level, so T3 is usually followed to determine when a euthyroid state has been reached. Given the known side effects of these drugs which are reviewed below, baseline complete blood count (CBC) with differential and liver function tests (LFTs) should be obtained prior to initiation of ATD treatment.[7] In the United States, methimazole (MMI) and propylthiouracil (PTU) are available for the treatment of hyperthyroidism. Outside the United States, an additional ATD called carbimazole is also used. This drug is a precursor of MMI which is rapidly converted in the serum to MMI. Table 9–2 shows a rough guide for recommended dosing of ATDs in the treatment of Graves' disease.[7]

Table 9–2. American Thyroid Association recommending dosing of ATDs in the treatment of Graves' disease.

Medication	Baseline Laboratory Levels	Recommended Initial Dosing
Methimazole (MMI)	Free T4 1-1.5 times upper limit of normal	5-10 mg daily
	Free T4 1.5-2 times upper limit of normal	10-20 mg daily
	Free T4 2-3 times upper limit of normal	30-40 mg daily
Propylthiouracil (PTU)		50-100 mg TID

mg, milligrams; T4, thyroxine; TID, three times daily.
Typical ATD dosing for Graves' disease taken from the ATA guidelines for management of hyperthyroidism.[7]

Methimazole

MMI is usually initiated at a dose of 10 to 30 mg daily in single or divided doses, with titration down to a maintenance dose usually around 5 to 10 mg daily, once a euthyroid state has been achieved. The most common side effects from MMI use are pruritis and rash. Patients can also experience agranulocytosis, vasculitis, and hepatocellular injury which is usually cholestatic. There is less risk of major side effects with MMI than with PTU overall. The American Thyroid Association (ATA) therefore recommends MMI for virtually every patient who chooses ATD therapy for Graves' disease. Those who should not receive MMI include patients who are in the first trimester of pregnancy due to the severe teratogenic effects associated with MMI. In addition, patients who present with thyroid storm or who have had a prior reaction to MMI but do not wish to proceed with RAI or surgery for treatment of their Graves' disease should be treated with PTU rather than MMI.[7]

Propylthiouracil

In addition to preventing thyroid hormone synthesis, PTU has the additional effect of inhibiting peripheral conversion of T4 to T3, the more potent form of thyroid hormone. PTU has a shorter duration of action than MMI and is therefore dosed two to three times daily starting at 50 to 150 mg TID. It is titrated down to a dose typically around 50 mg BID/TID for maintenance of euthyroidism.[7] The most common side effect of PTU is, similar to MMI, rash. Patients can, however, also experience fevers, hepatic injury, agranulocytosis, and vasculitis, as with MMI. The risk of hepatotoxicity has resulted in a "black box warning" for the drug. The liver damage is most often hepatocellular in nature, though fulminant hepatic necrosis and death have also occurred. PTU is the most effective ATD in lowering hormone levels during thyroid storm and is also the drug of choice during the first trimester of pregnancy, to avoid the teratogenic effects of MMI. However, PTU should be stopped after the first trimester to avoid the potential for severe hepatotoxic effects.

The most common adverse events that occur with ATDs are minor cutaneous and allergic reactions like rash, pruritis, and urticaria. These events typically occur early and can occur with arthralgias as well as gastrointestinal side effects including dyspepsia and nausea.[12] Agranulocytosis presents with abrupt onset of fever and severe pharyngitis. Although it is uncommon, it can be life-threatening and appears to be dose related with MMI but not with PTU.[12,13] No consensus exists regarding the utility of monitoring CBCs for detecting early onset of agranulocytosis as this serious side effect often occurs suddenly.[7] Many endocrinologists do follow CBCs, however, with the maximum benefit of this practice occurring in the first 90 days of initiation of an ATD, when the majority of these adverse events occur.[7,14] Similarly, routine monitoring of LFTs has not been shown to prevent severe hepatotoxicity; if monitoring is performed, the benefit occurs in the first 120 days of initiation of an ATD. In patients taking PTU, this drug should be discontinued if the transaminases reach more than three times the upper limit of normal or if baseline elevated LFTs, a phenomenon that can accompany hyperthyroidism in general, worsen after initiation of PTU. If these levels do not improve after cessation, prompt referral to a gastroenterologist or hepatologist is recommended.[7] It should be noted that there is cross-reactivity between MMI and PTU. Patients who experience serious side effects with one ATD should not simply be switched to the other unless they are experiencing life-threatening thyrotoxicosis; they should be considered for more definitive therapy.[7,15]

During treatment with ATDs, the ATA recommends following the TRAb levels, as lower levels typically indicate a greater chance of remission. The ATA recommends using ATDs for 12 to 18 months, with cessation if TSH and TRAb normalize. Patients should be monitored for relapse with thyroid function tests (TFTs) and TRAb every 3 months for 6 months, followed by every 6 months for 6 months and finally every 6 to 12 months. If patients remain or become hyperthyroid after cessation of ATDs, they can be safely continued, though most endocrinologists tend to refer the patient for definitive treatment with RAI or surgery at that time.

ATDs are best for use in those with small goiters who are reliable with medication compliance. They should be considered in those patients with mild Graves' disease with low or negative TRAb titer. They are recommended as first line for pregnant patients as RAI is contraindicated and thyroidectomy can be associated with risks to both the mother and fetus. ATDs are also useful in elderly patients with limited life expectancies, significant comorbidities precluding surgery, and those who live in care facilities who cannot comply with the radiation safety guidelines required for RAI. ATDs are recommended over thyroidectomy when Graves' patients have had prior thyroid or neck surgery or irradiation, or when a high-volume thyroid surgeon is not available to perform the surgery. They are safe for use in those with limited or even moderate-to-severe GO as well.[6,7]

Radioactive Iodine

RAI (I-131) is taken up by follicular thyroid cells and then causes focal tissue necrosis over the following 6 to 18 weeks. Patients are on a low iodine diet for at least 7 days prior to treatment to maximize uptake of the RAI. The goal of treatment of Graves' disease with RAI is to create a hypothyroid state to control the signs and symptoms of hyperthyroidism.[7] A perfectly euthyroid state can be difficult to attain and even more difficult to maintain with this treatment as further decline in thyroid function tends to occur over time in most patients. The hyperthyroidism typically resolves in 4 to 8 weeks and thyroid hormone replacement is initiated once the patient becomes hypothyroid.[6,7] RAI is administered as a single oral dose with the mean dose being 10 to 15 mCi (millicuries). The dose can be fixed or calculated based on the size of the thyroid gland and its ability to trap RAI, with both options having equal success in achieving hypothyroidism.[7,16] Because RAI crosses the placenta and has been demonstrated in breast milk of lactating mothers, it is contraindicated in pregnant and lactating patients.

RAI is generally well tolerated, though there are several important side effects of the treatment. Patients can suffer from sialadenitis and dry mouth secondary to effects on the salivary glands. They can also experience radiation thyroiditis with transient worsening hyperthyroidism secondary to release of thyroid hormones during tissue necrosis. Rarely, this release can lead to thyroid storm. For these reasons, care should be used in patients with cardiovascular disease and elderly patients who are prone to arrhythmia.[6] Physicians should consider initiation of beta blockade prior to RAI treatment in those who are at risk, and even in those who are asymptomatic.[7] Beta blockade can then be tapered off, once the free thyroid hormone levels normalize. Consideration should also be given to pretreatment with MMI in patients at high risk for complications from worsening hyperthyroidism including elderly patients and those with severe hyperthyroidism. Patients with high-risk comorbidities including atrial fibrillation, congestive heart failure, pulmonary hypertension, renal failure, infection, trauma, poorly controlled diabetes, and cerebrovascular and pulmonary disease may also benefit from pretreatment with MMI.[7] If this strategy is employed, MMI is typically discontinued 2 to 3 days prior to RAI dosing and then resumed 3 to 7 days after treatment to help prevent the typical worsening hyperthyroidism the week following treatment; it can be tapered later as free T3/T4 begins to improve. Although ATDs are useful in preventing the risks of poorly controlled hyperthyroidism in this population, they have been shown to decrease the efficacy of RAI treatment in some studies, and therefore the risks and benefits of pretreatment should be weighed and discussed with patients.[17] RAI can also be associated with keratoconjunctivitis and worsening or *de novo* orbitopathy in 15% to 20% of patients.[7,12,18,19] RAI should therefore not be used in those with evidence of moderate-to-severe GO.[6]

During treatment with RAI, patients should be monitored with regular T3/T4 and TSH levels every 4 to 6 weeks for 6 months or until the patient becomes hypothyroid and stable on thyroid hormone replacement. Hormone replacement should be initiated once free T4 is below normal limits; TSH should not be used as evidence of hypothyroidism as these levels take longer to respond to therapy than the free thyroid hormone levels do.[7] The size of the thyroid gland should also be monitored, along with clinical signs/symptoms to detect worsening clinical hyperthyroidism. Consideration can be given to re-treatment with RAI if hyperthyroidism persists 6 months after initial RAI dosing.[7] Excretion of I-131 occurs in the saliva, urine, perspiration, stool, and tears of patients being treated with RAI, so these patients must follow radiation precautions to reduce radiation exposure to others. It is particularly critical to avoid pregnant patients and young children given the higher risks of radiation exposure in these populations. Patients are also advised to avoid public transportation and working in offices or other densely populated areas. They should sleep away from family members and should not prepare food for or share eating utensils with any other persons.

RAI is best used in those with recurrent or uncontrolled hyperthyroidism or those with contraindications to ATDs. Those who are poor surgical candidates including patients with prior neck surgery or irradiation, or patients without access to a high-volume thyroid surgeon, are also good candidates for RAI. RAI is contraindicated in pregnant and lactating women but can be used for those patients wishing to have a child in the future; conception is permitted 6 months after RAI treatment in both male and female patients.[7,19] Those who wish to conceive should not undergo RAI treatment. RAI is also contraindicated in patients with known or suspected thyroid cancer by imaging features as these patients should be treated surgically for oncologic control of the cancer.[7] Therefore, Graves' disease accompanied by significant thyroid nodules should give some pause as to both the diagnosis and the inherent malignancy risk of the individual nodules.

Thyroidectomy

If a patient is referred for surgical treatment of Graves' disease, total or near-total thyroidectomy should be performed by a high-volume thyroid surgeon to maximize the chance for definitive cure while minimizing the risks of surgical complications.[6,7] Hyperthyroidism resolves within 2 to 6 weeks of thyroidectomy, depending on severity of disease and the associated preoperative thyroid hormone levels. Surgery is preferred over RAI in patients who are pregnant or desire pregnancy within 6 months, though surgery should be delayed until the second trimester to minimize risk of miscarriage or fetal demise.[6,7] Thyroidectomy is also recommended for those with poorly controlled hyperthyroidism in need of rapid normalization, compressive symptoms, or airway compromise. Patients with suspected thyroid cancer or with other cervical disease potentially requiring surgery, such as hyperparathyroidism, goiter more than 80 g estimated mass, thyroglossal duct cyst, and thyroid nodules should be referred for surgical treatment of their Graves' disease. Patients who have previously been treated unsuccessfully with RAI or with low iodine uptake on scanning are often referred for surgical management. Surgery may also be the best treatment for those with certain social situations preventing RAI treatment and adherence to radiation precautions after RAI therapy.[6,7] Relative contraindications to thyroidectomy include pregnancy (particularly in first or third trimester), end-stage cancer, lack of a high-volume thyroid surgeon to perform the surgery, and those patients with high-risk comorbidities precluding safe administration of general anesthesia.[7]

A. Preoperative Preparation

Once a Graves' patient has opted to undergo thyroidectomy, they should be treated with ATDs to render the patient clinically and biochemically euthyroid when possible. This is recommended to prevent thyroid storm which can be precipitated by the stress of anesthesia and surgery itself, in addition to thyroid manipulation during the procedure.[6,7] If the patient cannot be rendered euthyroid, the most important factor to address is tachycardia; beta blockade is used to control the heart rate to less than 90 beats per minute (bpm) to mitigate the cardiac effects of hyperthyroidism.[6] Propranolol is used most commonly given its dual effects of heart rate control and prevention of peripheral conversion of T4 to T3, though other beta blockers can be used as well. The typical propranolol dose is 10 to 40 mg three to four times daily.[7] The ATA recommends the use of preoperative potassium iodide (SSKI) or Lugol's solution for 1 week before surgery to decrease thyroid blood flow, vascularity, and intraoperative blood loss, although there are conflicting results in studies about these intended benefits.[7,20-22] These drugs transiently inhibit thyroid iodide organification and block conversion of T4 to T3, though administration for longer than 7 to 10 days can worsen hyperthyroidism as organification resumes at that time. The recommended dosing is 5 to 7 drops (0.25-0.35 mL) of Lugol's solution (8 mg iodide/drop) or 1 to 2 drops (0.05-0.1 mL) of SSKI (50 mg iodide/drop) TID for 7 to 10 days prior to surgery.[7] As Vitamin D deficiency and Graves' disease itself have been identified as risk factors for postoperative hypocalcemia,[23] the ATA recommends assessing calcium and 25-hydroxy Vitamin D levels preoperatively with repletion if the patient is found to have deficient levels.[7] Graves' patients treated with preoperative, prophylactic calcium had significantly less biochemical and symptomatic hypocalcemia than untreated Graves' patients.[24]

If surgery is emergent or the patient can't be rendered euthyroid prior to surgery, they should receive preoperative beta blockers, SSKI, steroids, and cholestyramine to decrease the risk of thyroid storm. Rarely, plasmapheresis is performed.[6,7] Although the ATA preoperative guidelines have been in place and followed by many high-volume thyroid surgeons, the utility of compliance with these guidelines has been called into question by studies showing no difference in intraoperative hypertension, OR time, or postoperative complications in those patients who were not euthyroid or receiving SSKI and beta blockade preoperatively.[25]

B. Postoperative Considerations

After thyroidectomy, all preoperative ATDs can be discontinued and beta blockade should be weaned over several days to prevent rebound tachycardia and headache.[6] The ATA recommends checking postoperative serum calcium, with discharge of the patient if the corrected level is more than 8 mg/dL and the patient is asymptomatic. Patients should receive 500 to 1000 g of elemental calcium QID to prevent postoperative hypocalcemia; this can be tapered over time.[7] Weight-based levothyroxine hormone replacement of 1.6 μg/kg should be started the following day unless the patient is hyperthyroid at the time of surgery. In this case, holding thyroid hormone replacement for 1 week will help prevent worsening symptoms of hyperthyroidism. TSH should be measured at 6 to 8 weeks after surgery, with adjustment to the levothyroxine dosing at that time, if the patient is not euthyroid.[6,7]

Complications

Although thyroidectomy is considered safe in the treatment of Graves' disease, there are several known complications which should be discussed with patients preoperatively. Graves' patients have a relatively higher risk of intraoperative blood loss and postoperative hematoma secondary to the glands being larger and more vascular and inflamed than normal thyroid tissue.[6,26] They have also been shown to have high rates of temporary hypocalcemia which is thought to be aggravated by thyrotoxic osteodystrophy or bone-hunger from long-standing hyperthyroidism.[6,27,28] The recurrent laryngeal nerve (RLN) can be more prone to stretch injury secondary to difficult medial rotation of the gland as well as increased intraoperative bleeding which decreases visualization during dissection. There are conflicting studies regarding whether RLN injury is more common in thyroidectomy performed for Graves' disease versus other pathologies, however.[6] Thyroid storm can also be precipitated by the stress of anesthesia and surgery for Graves' disease. It presents with tachycardia or arrhythmia, hyper- or hypotension, heart failure, fever, diaphoresis, nausea and vomiting, hepatic failure, and mental status change ranging from delirium to stupor or coma.[6]

Special Patient Populations

A. Pregnant Patients

Graves' disease affects 0.1% to 0.2% of all pregnancies with risks to both the mother and child.[12,29,30] Women are often diagnosed with Graves' disease when displaying typical clinical findings like GO and elevated TRAb in the setting of new hyperthyroidism. Graves' patients previously in remission are also at risk of relapse both during and immediately after pregnancy, and they therefore should be closely monitored throughout pregnancy with thyroid function tests.[30,31] As RAI is contraindicated in pregnant patients, ATDs are the therapy of choice. During the first trimester, PTU is preferred as MMI has been associated with a 2% to 4% risk of birth defects when used early in pregnancy. Once a patient has reached the second trimester, they are typically switched to MMI to prevent the higher risk of hepatotoxicity associated with PTU. After the first trimester, there is less risk of development of MMI-associated severe fetal defects including aplasia cutis, esophageal and gastrointestinal atresias, and various defects of the eye, heart, abdominal wall, and urinary tract.[7] ATDs and TRAbs can cross the placenta and affect the fetal thyroid, potentially leading to fetal hypothyroidism in addition to teratogenic effects.[7,12] Graves' patients should therefore receive the lowest dose of ATD possible to reduce the risk of goiter and hypothyroidism in the fetus. Once diagnosed in pregnancy, TRAb should be measured again at 18 to 22 weeks and 30 to 34 weeks gestation, with reduction or cessation of ATDs if the levels become negative. Rising TRAb levels are associated with a higher risk of fetal hyperthyroidism.[7] Although beta blockade can be used for tachycardia, atenolol should be avoided secondary to possible fetal growth restriction.[6,7] If patients with preexisting Graves' disease require high-dose ATDs to maintain a euthyroid state, they should be counseled regarding definitive management with RAI or thyroidectomy to reduce the risk of fetal hypothyroidism. Patients on lower maintenance doses of MMI can be switched to PTU before or soon after conception. The MMI can also be withdrawn followed by weekly TFTs for the first trimester and then monthly after, to monitor for worsening hyperthyroidism.[7,30] If medical management is unsuccessful in controlling hyperthyroidism or if ATDs are contraindicated in a pregnant patient, a second-trimester thyroidectomy can be considered. A high-risk obstetric consultation should be made prior to surgery and fetal thyroid ultrasound allows for evaluation of the risk of goiter or airway obstruction upon delivery.[6,32]

B. Pediatric Patients

Although children can be treated with all three mainstays of therapy for Graves' disease, definitive therapy with RAI or thyroidectomy is usually reserved for older children (age >5). The majority of pediatric patients will not achieve remission with MMI use, however, and will eventually require RAI or surgery. These patients are often treated medically until they are old enough to receive definitive treatment.[7] Typical MMI dosing is 0.2 to 0.5 mg/kg daily, though it can range from 0.1 to 1.0 mg/kg in some patients. Once TFTs normalize, doses can be reduced by 50% with monitoring for worsening symptoms and hyperthyroidism. Side effects include excessive weight gain as well as the more serious complications seen in adults. As side effects from ATDs are usually dose related, it is important to maintain children on the lowest doses possible since they have been shown to be more susceptible than adults to the complications of hepatotoxicity and vasculitis, particularly if receiving PTU.[7,33] Most recommend against using PTU altogether in children, except in situations when the course will be short or MMI is contraindicated, as the risk of hepatotoxicity has been shown to be unacceptably high.[7,19] RAI can be administered once a patient is over the age of 5; this age cutoff was chosen to reduce the theoretical risk of subsequent thyroid cancer, though there is little data describing a definitive cancer risk in children receiving RAI.[7,34] The ATA recommends administering doses less than 10 mCi in a single dose to obtain a hypothyroid state. Dose reduction based only on age is not recommended; the dose should be calculated based on the size of gland and uptake to avoid the need for additional RAI doses and irradiation.[7] The ATA also recommends pretreating pediatric Graves' patients with MMI and beta blockade to decrease the risk of thyroid storm with treatment. This can be withdrawn 2 to 3 days prior to RAI dosing and usually is not restarted after RAI is administered.[7] If children ultimately require thyroidectomy, this should be performed by a high-volume endocrine surgeon as children have been shown to have longer operative time, intraoperative blood loss, and temporary postoperative hypocalcemia requiring calcium infusion.[7,35,36] Preoperative preparation with MMI and SSKI is recommended and is similar to adult recommendations.

C. Patients With Graves' Orbitopathy

GO can present with many symptoms including pain behind the globe or with eye movement, redness in the conjunctiva and eyelids, chemosis, swollen caruncle, proptosis, decreased eye motion or visual acuity, lid retraction, stare, or diplopia.[7] It can develop before biochemical evidence of Graves' disease, though usually occurs simultaneously. Referral for ophthalmologic evaluation should be made for all patients as the symptoms can be quite subtle and easily missed.[6] GO occurs more frequently in women but is more severe in men and patients with advanced age. The highest prevalence is in Caucasian patients and it is uncommon in Asians. Smoking is a significant risk factor for GO and decreases the efficacy of treatment; smoking cessation is, therefore, critical for all smokers with Graves'.[7,37] Secondhand smoke also increases the risk of development of ocular symptoms and patients should be advised to avoid exposure to smoke. The eyes should be protected from light and dust irritants with dark glasses, eye shields, and methylcellulose or guanethidine eye drops. Edema can be improved with elevation of the head of bed and diuretics. GO is worsened in activity and severity in both a hypothyroid state with elevated TSH as well as a hyperthyroid state with elevated TRAb.[38,39] Resolution of symptoms is rare before hyperthyroidism is treated, and the goal of therapy is therefore prompt establishment of a euthyroid state while avoiding hypothyroidism. RAI is a risk factor for the development and worsening of GO, so its use should be weighed against these risks. The ATA recommends steroid use with RAI to prevent the risk of worsening GO in those with active, mild disease and those with risk factors for GO progression including tobacco use, disease progression over the previous 3 months, and high TRAb levels (>8.8 IU/L).[7] The use of steroids is also considered in those without risk factors for progression, when there is low risk of developing glucocorticoid side effects including poorly controlled diabetes, hypertension, osteoporosis, psychiatric disease, and infection. Those patients with active and moderate-to-severe disease should not be treated with RAI with or without steroids to prevent the risk of disease progression. These patients should be treated with thyroidectomy or ATDs.[6,7] Surgery has been associated with improvement in GO symptoms in some patients which may be more rapid and significant than treatment with ATDs alone.[7,40] The European Group on Graves' Orbitopathy and the European Thyroid Association recommend Selenium for mild GO and high-dose IV glucocorticoid (IVGC) pulses for active, moderate-to-severe disease.[18,41] If there is worsening GO, patients can be treated with lateral tarsorrhaphy, retrobulbar irradiation for diminished eye motility, or surgical decompression of the orbit for severe and persistent disease.

The insulin-like growth factor 1 receptor (IGF-1R) inhibitor teprotumumab (Tepezza) has recently been introduced to treat GO. IGF-1R has been implicated as a factor in GO pathogenesis and IGF-1R antibodies have been observed in those with Graves' and GO.[42,43] In vitro, teprotumumab inhibits activation of IGF-1R and its downstream signaling in addition to causing degradation of the receptor itself.[44] It also reduces TSH-stimulated release of proinflammatory cytokines and expression of TSH receptor and IGF-1R in fibrocytes.[45,46] Two randomized, multicenter, placebo-controlled trials showed rapid improvement of all signs and symptoms of disease with improvement in disease-specific quality of life after the first cycle of eight infusions over 24 weeks.[47,48] It has been approved by the FDA for adults with severe and active GO but it is expensive, only available in the United States and more trials are needed to compare it to IVGC.[12] Its ideal role as an alternative or adjunct to thyroidectomy has yet to be defined and an experienced ophthalmologist will provide significant expertise to these complicated therapy decisions.

PROGNOSIS

Graves' disease has an excellent prognosis with varying cure rates with the three mainstay treatment options. ATDs are used most commonly but induction of lasting remission is only moderately common and varies in worldwide studies from 20% to 68%.[7,49-51] Lower remission rates are seen in young patients, men, smokers, and those patients with large (>80 g) goiters or persistently elevated TRAb levels after 1 year of MMI treatment.[7,52-55] Although RAI can fail to completely treat Graves' disease in some patients, success rates are higher if higher doses of RAI are administered.[6,7] One study compared 10 mCi dosing to 15 mCi dosing and showed a 74% success rate with the lower dose compared to 81% in the higher dose group, though this did not reach statistical significance. Those with larger thyroid glands had a lower chance of going into remission at lower doses, however.[56] In one retrospective study, ATDs had a 48% failure rate, RAI had an 8% failure rate, and thyroidectomy had no failures to cure.[57] The extent of surgery performed does impact the success rate; there is a near 0% risk of recurrence after total thyroidectomy versus 8% risk of persistent or recurrent hyperthyroidism with subtotal thyroidectomy.[58] For this reason, total thyroidectomy is the preferred surgical strategy in developed nations with ready access to hormone replacement. Thyroidectomy has been shown to have better outcomes when performed by high-volume thyroid surgeons with lower average complication rates, length of stay, and costs when compared to lower-volume thyroid surgeons.[7,59]

WHEN TO REFER

Endocrinologists and primary care physicians are the usual frontline providers when Graves' disease is diagnosed. These physicians should present all options for treatment to the patient while remaining impartial about treatment strategy. They should refer newly diagnosed Graves' patients to nuclear medicine and high-volume thyroid surgeons so that the patients may discuss the risks and benefits of RAI and thyroidectomy, respectively, with these experts. In addition, referral for ophthalmologic evaluation should be made in all Graves' patients for baseline examination since the signs and symptoms of GO can be subtle and easily missed.

WHEN TO ADMIT

Patients with Graves' disease rarely require hospitalization for their treatment, aside from the surgical episode of care. However, those with frank signs of uncontrolled thyrotoxicosis with dysrhythmia should be hospitalized to allow for safe treatment with fluids, high-dose ATDs, beta blockers, steroids, and possible SSKI/Lugol's solution.

REFERENCES

1. Smith TJ, Hegedüs L. Graves' disease. *N Engl J Med*. 2016;375(16):1552-1565.
2. Davies TF, Andersen S, Latif R, et al. Graves' disease. *Nat Rev Dis Primers*. 2020;6(1):52.
3. Taylor PN, Zhang L, Lee RWJ, et al. New insights into the pathogenesis and nonsurgical management of Graves orbitopathy. *Nat Rev Endocrinol*. 2020;16(2):104-116.
4. Diana T, Ponto KA, Kahaly GJ. Thyrotropin receptor antibodies and Graves' orbitopathy. *J Endocrinol Invest*. 2021;44(4):703-712.
5. Kahaly GJ, Diana T, Olivo PD. TSH receptor antibodies: relevance & utility. *Endocr Pract*. 2020;26(1):97-106.
6. Patel KN, Yip L, Lubitz CC, et al. The American Association of Endocrine Surgeons guidelines for the definitive surgical management of thyroid disease in adults. *Ann Surg*. 2020;271(3):e21-e93.
7. Ross DS, Burch HB, Cooper DS, et al. 2016 American Thyroid Association guidelines for diagnosis and management of hyperthyroidism and other causes of thyrotoxicosis. *Thyroid*. 2016;26(10):1343-1421.
8. Iqbal A, Rehman A. Thyroid uptake and scan. In: *StatPearls*. StatPearls Publishing; 2021. http://www.ncbi.nlm.nih.gov/books/NBK555978/. Accessed August 29, 2021.
9. Burch HB, Burman KD, Cooper DS. A 2011 survey of clinical practice patterns in the management of Graves' disease. *J Clin Endocrinol Metab*. 2012;97(12):4549-4558.
10. Abraham-Nordling M, Törring O, Hamberger B, et al. Graves' disease: a long-term quality-of-life follow up of patients randomized to treatment with antithyroid drugs, radioiodine, or surgery. *Thyroid*. 2005;15(11):1279-1286.
11. Conaglen HM, Tamatea JAU, Conaglen JV, Elston MS. Treatment choice, satisfaction and quality of life in patients with Graves' disease. *Clin Endocrinol*. 2018;88(6):977-984.
12. Kahaly GJ. Management of Graves thyroidal and extrathyroidal disease: an update. *J Clin Endocrinol Metab*. 2020;105(12):dgaa646.
13. Takata K, Kubota S, Fukata S, et al. Methimazole-induced agranulocytosis in patients with Graves' disease is more frequent with an initial dose of 30 mg daily than with 15 mg daily. *Thyroid*. 2009;19(6):559-563.

14. Tajiri J, Noguchi S, Murakami T, Murakami N. Antithyroid drug-induced agranulocytosis. The usefulness of routine white blood cell count monitoring. *Arch Intern Med.* 1990;150(3): 621-624.
15. Ahmed K, Rao S, Simha V. Antineutrophil cytoplasmic antibody-positive vasculitis in a patient with Graves disease: cross-reaction between propylthiouracil and methimazole. *Endocr Pract.* 2010;16(3):449-451.
16. de Rooij A, Vandenbroucke JP, Smit JWA, Stokkel MPM, Dekkers OM. Clinical outcomes after estimated versus calculated activity of radioiodine for the treatment of hyperthyroidism: systematic review and meta-analysis. *Eur J Endocrinol.* 2009;161(5):771-777.
17. Walter MA, Briel M, Christ-Crain M, et al. Effects of antithyroid drugs on radioiodine treatment: systematic review and meta-analysis of randomised controlled trials. *BMJ.* 2007; 334(7592):514.
18. Bartalena L, Baldeschi L, Boboridis K, et al. The 2016 European thyroid Association/European group on Graves' orbitopathy guidelines for the management of Graves' orbitopathy. *Eur Thyroid J.* 2016;5(1):9-26.
19. Kahaly GJ, Bartalena L, Hegedüs L, Leenhardt L, Poppe K, Pearce SH. 2018 European Thyroid Association guideline for the management of Graves' hyperthyroidism. *Eur Thyroid J.* 2018;7(4):167-186.
20. Ansaldo GL, Pretolesi F, Varaldo E, et al. Doppler evaluation of intrathyroid arterial resistances during preoperative treatment with Lugol's iodide solution in patients with diffuse toxic goiter. *J Am Coll Surg.* 2000;191(6):607-612.
21. Erbil Y, Ozluk Y, Giriş M, et al. Effect of lugol solution on thyroid gland blood flow and microvessel density in the patients with Graves' disease. *J Clin Endocrinol Metab.* 2007; 92(6):2182-2189.
22. Shinall MC, Broome JT, Baker A, Solorzano CC. Is potassium iodide solution necessary before total thyroidectomy for Graves disease? *Ann Surg Oncol.* 2013;20(9):2964-2967.
23. Edafe O, Antakia R, Laskar N, Uttley L, Balasubramanian SP. Systematic review and meta-analysis of predictors of post-thyroidectomy hypocalcaemia. *Br J Surg.* 2014;101(4): 307-320.
24. Oltmann SC, Brekke AV, Schneider DF, Schaefer SC, Chen H, Sippel RS. Preventing postoperative hypocalcemia in patients with Graves disease: a prospective study. *Ann Surg Oncol.* 2015; 22(3):952-958.
25. Akram S, Elfenbein DM, Chen H, Schneider DF, Sippel RS. Assessing American Thyroid Association guidelines for total thyroidectomy in Graves' disease. *J Surg Res.* 2020;245:64-71.
26. Campbell MJ, McCoy KL, Shen WT, et al. A multi-institutional international study of risk factors for hematoma after thyroidectomy. *Surgery.* 2013;154(6):1283-1289; discussion 1289-1291.
27. Phitayakorn R, Morales-Garcia D, Wanderer J, et al. Surgery for Graves' disease: a 25-year perspective. *Am J Surg.* 2013;206(5): 669-673.
28. Wilkin TJ, Isles TE, Paterson CR, Crooks J, Beck J. Post-thyroidectomy hypocalcaemia: a feature of the operation or the thyroid disorder? *Lancet.* 1977;1(8012):621-623.
29. Cooper DS, Laurberg P. Hyperthyroidism in pregnancy. *Lancet Diabetes Endocrinol.* 2013;1(3):238-249.
30. Alexander EK, Pearce EN, Brent GA, et al. 2017 Guidelines of the American Thyroid Association for the diagnosis and management of thyroid disease during pregnancy and the postpartum. *Thyroid.* 2017;27(3):315-389.
31. Amino N, Tada H, Hidaka Y. Postpartum autoimmune thyroid syndrome: a model of aggravation of autoimmune disease. *Thyroid.* 1999;9(7):705-713.
32. Ferianec V, Papcun P, Grochal F, Schenková K, Bártová M. Prenatal diagnosis and successful intrauterine treatment of severe congenital hypothyroidism associated with fetal goiter. *J Obstet Gynaecol Res.* 2017;43(1):232-237.
33. Rivkees SA, Szarfman A. Dissimilar hepatotoxicity profiles of propylthiouracil and methimazole in children. *J Clin Endocrinol Metab.* 2010;95(7):3260-3267.
34. Freitas JE, Swanson DP, Gross MD, Sisson JC. Iodine-131: optimal therapy for hyperthyroidism in children and adolescents? *J Nucl Med.* 1979;20(8):847-850.
35. Breuer CK, Solomon D, Donovan P, Rivkees SA, Udelsman R. Effect of patient Age on surgical outcomes for Graves' disease: a case-control study of 100 consecutive patients at a high volume thyroid surgical center. *Int J Pediatr Endocrinol.* 2013;2013(1):1.
36. Sosa JA, Tuggle CT, Wang TS, et al. Clinical and economic outcomes of thyroid and parathyroid surgery in children. *J Clin Endocrinol Metab.* 2008;93(8):3058-3065.
37. Pfeilschifter J, Ziegler R. Smoking and endocrine ophthalmopathy: impact of smoking severity and current vs lifetime cigarette consumption. *Clin Endocrinol.* 1996;45(4):477-481.
38. Bartalena L. Diagnosis and management of Graves disease: a global overview. *Nat Rev Endocrinol.* 2013;9(12):724-734.
39. Kahaly GJ, Bartalena L, Hegedüs L. The American Thyroid Association/American Association of Clinical Endocrinologists guidelines for hyperthyroidism and other causes of thyrotoxicosis: a European perspective. *Thyroid.* 2011;21(6):585-591.
40. De Bellis A, Conzo G, Cennamo G, et al. Time course of Graves' ophthalmopathy after total thyroidectomy alone or followed by radioiodine therapy: a 2-year longitudinal study. *Endocrine.* 2012;41(2):320-326.
41. Marcocci C, Kahaly GJ, Krassas GE, et al. Selenium and the course of mild Graves' orbitopathy. *N Engl J Med.* 2011;364(20): 1920-1931.
42. Wang Y, Smith TJ. Current concepts in the molecular pathogenesis of thyroid-associated ophthalmopathy. *Invest Ophthalmol Vis Sci.* 2014;55(3):1735-1748.
43. Marinò M, Rotondo Dottore G, Ionni I, et al. Serum antibodies against the insulin-like growth factor-1 receptor (IGF-1R) in Graves' disease and Graves' orbitopathy. *J Endocrinol Invest.* 2019;42(4):471-480.
44. Smith TJ, Janssen JAMJL. Insulin-like growth factor-I receptor and thyroid-associated ophthalmopathy. *Endocr Rev.* 2019;40(1):236-267.
45. Chen H, Shan SJC, Mester T, Wei Y-H, Douglas RS. TSH-mediated TNFα production in human fibrocytes is inhibited by teprotumumab, an IGF-1R antagonist. *PLoS One.* 2015;10(6): e0130322.
46. Chen H, Mester T, Raychaudhuri N, et al. Teprotumumab, an IGF-1R blocking monoclonal antibody inhibits TSH and IGF-1 action in fibrocytes. *J Clin Endocrinol Metab.* 2014;99(9): E1635-1640.
47. Smith TJ, Kahaly GJ, Ezra DG, et al. Teprotumumab for thyroid-associated ophthalmopathy. *N Engl J Med.* 2017;376(18): 1748-1761.
48. Douglas RS, Kahaly GJ, Patel A, et al. Teprotumumab for the treatment of active thyroid eye disease. *N Engl J Med.* 2020; 382(4):341-352.
49. Klein I, Becker DV, Levey GS. Treatment of hyperthyroid disease. *Ann Intern Med.* 1994;121(4):281-288.

50. Mazza E, Carlini M, Flecchia D, et al. Long-term follow-up of patients with hyperthyroidism due to Graves' disease treated with methimazole. Comparison of usual treatment schedule with drug discontinuation vs continuous treatment with low methimazole doses: a retrospective study. *J Endocrinol Invest.* 2008;31(10):866-872.
51. Konishi T, Okamoto Y, Ueda M, et al. Drug discontinuation after treatment with minimum maintenance dose of an anti-thyroid drug in Graves' disease: a retrospective study on effects of treatment duration with minimum maintenance dose on lasting remission. *Endocr J.* 2011;58(2):95-100.
52. Bolaños F, González-Ortiz M, Durón H, Sánchez C. Remission of Graves' hyperthyroidism treated with methimazole. *Rev Invest Clin.* 2002;54(4):307-310.
53. Nedrebo BG, Holm PI, Uhlving S, et al. Predictors of outcome and comparison of different drug regimens for the prevention of relapse in patients with Graves' disease. *Eur J Endocrinol.* 2002;147(5):583-589.
54. Kimball LE, Kulinskaya E, Brown B, Johnston C, Farid NR. Does smoking increase relapse rates in Graves' disease? *J Endocrinol Invest.* 2002;25(2):152-157.
55. Allahabadia A, Daykin J, Holder RL, Sheppard MC, Gough SC, Franklyn JA. Age and gender predict the outcome of treatment for Graves' hyperthyroidism. *J Clin Endocrinol Metab.* 2000; 85(3):1038-1042.
56. Santos RB, Romaldini JH, Ward LS. A randomized controlled trial to evaluate the effectiveness of 2 regimens of fixed iodine (^{131}I) doses for Graves disease treatment. *Clin Nucl Med.* 2012; 37(3):241-244.
57. Sundaresh V, Brito JP, Thapa P, Bahn RS, Stan MN. Comparative effectiveness of treatment choices for Graves' hyperthyroidism: a historical cohort study. *Thyroid.* 2017;27(4): 497-505.
58. Palit TK, Miller CC, Miltenburg DM. The efficacy of thyroidectomy for Graves' disease: a meta-analysis. *J Surg Res.* 2000; 90(2):161-165.
59. Sosa JA, Bowman HM, Tielsch JM, Powe NR, Gordon TA, Udelsman R. The importance of surgeon experience for clinical and economic outcomes from thyroidectomy. *Ann Surg.* 1998; 228(3):320-330.

10 Hyperthyroidism: Toxic Multinodular Goiter (Plummer's Disease)

Allison Keane, MD
David Goldenberg, MD

GENERAL CONSIDERATIONS

Epidemiology

Hyperthyroidism affects 1% to 2% of the population. The most common cause of hyperthyroidism is Graves' disease (GD), followed by toxic multinodular goiter (TMNG), and thirdly autonomous functioning thyroid nodules (AFTN).[1] A rare etiology of hyperthyroidism is Marine-Lenhart syndrome or the co-occurrence of GD and TMNG.

The incidence of GD and TMNG varies by geographical location and patient population. GD is most common in iodine-sufficient regions, accounting for about 65% of hyperthyroidism. In iodine-deficient regions, GD accounts for about 15% of hyperthyroidism, and the prevalence of TMNG increases. Correction of iodine deficiency results in a decrease in the prevalence of TMNG, which implies iodine deficiency plays a role in the etiology of TMNG. However, TMNG occurs in iodine-sufficient locations as well, and not all iodine-deficient populations develop TMNG.[2]

In patients under 50 to 60 years old, hyperthyroidism is more commonly related to GD, while TMGs are predominant in older patients with hyperthyroidism. In TMNG, thyroid nodules form and subsequently become autonomous in function. The disease progresses gradually over many years, thus making TMNG less common in younger patients. Nodules may be present earlier in life, but hyperthyroidism secondary to TMNG peaks at 50 to 60 years of age.

Risk factors for TMNG are similar to those for other thyroid nodular diseases. Smoking contributes to a higher prevalence of thyroid goiters and nodules. Environmental, occupational, or accidental exposure to radiation increases the risk of developing thyroid disease, both malignant and benign. TMNG has a female predominance, although it does occur in both males and females. There is an increased incidence of TMNG in patients with a family history, but not all TMNG is inherited.[3]

Pathogenesis

A. Thyroid Hormone Homeostasis

Thyroid hormone production at a cellular level begins with iodide influx across the basal membrane of the thyrocyte via the sodium-iodide symporter. Next, a protein, pendrin, transports iodide across the apical membrane into a thyroid follicle. Iodide is then oxygenated and transferred to thyroglobulin. The enzyme responsible for this is thyroperoxidase. Finally, triiodothyronine (T3) and thyroxine (T4) are formed and transported back to the circulation.[4]

Thyrotropin-releasing hormone (TRH) is secreted from the hypothalamus, which stimulates the secretion of thyroid-stimulating hormone (TSH) from the pituitary gland. TSH increases the expression of sodium-iodide symporter, which increases thyrocyte uptake of iodide. In addition, TSH stimulates the production of thyroglobulin, hydrogen peroxide, and thyroperoxidase to increase the production of both T3 and T4. Thus, T3 and T4 contribute to a negative feedback loop suppressing TRH and TSH release from the hypothalamus and the pituitary gland (Figure 10–1).

The Etiology of TMNG

Thyroid nodules are follicular hyperplasia. In TMGs, multiple nodules of follicular hyperplasia develop that produce excessive amounts of T3 and T4. Increased T3 and T4 levels decrease TSH levels through a negative feedback loop. Over time, the nodules become autonomous by mechanisms not clearly understood, continually producing thyroid hormones despite decreased TSH levels and negative feedback. Nontoxic multinodular goiters are distinguished from TMGs by laboratory studies. Nontoxic thyroid nodules are also follicular hyperplasia. However, TSH, T3, and T4 levels remain within normal ranges. Thus, the nodules are not hyperfunctioning or autonomous. Nontoxic multinodular goiters may become TMNG if multiple nodules develop autonomous function.

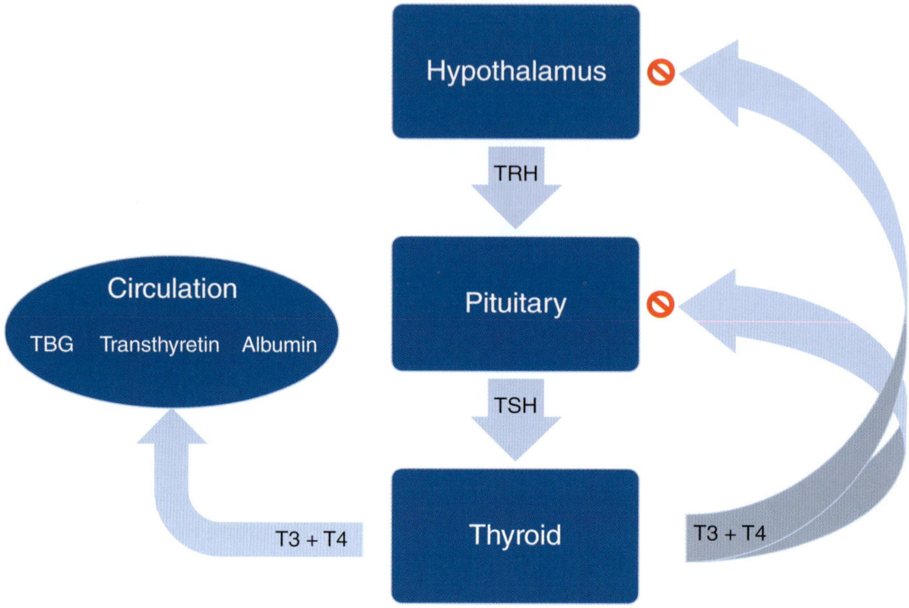

▲ **Figure 10–1.** Graphical depiction of the hypothalamic-pituitary-thyroid axis, thyroid hormone homeostasis, and the negative feedback loop.

The biochemical driving force behind autonomous thyroid nodules is a mutation in the TSH receptor resulting in a continually active TSH receptor. This leads to continuous cAMP downstream signaling and nodule autonomy. Nodules will grow in size, but the speed of growth and which nodules grow is variable. There is no association of nodule growth rate with thyroid malignancy reported; however, there have been reports of the correlation between nodule size and the development of hyperthyroidism. TSH receptor mutations occur spontaneously due to environmental factors or may have a genetic component as there can be a familial predisposition to thyroid disease.[4]

Clinical Findings

A. Signs and Symptoms

The signs and symptoms of TMGs (Table 10–1) are related to the systemic effects of increased thyroid hormones and the mass effect of an enlarged thyroid gland. Thyroid hormones increase basal metabolic rate, resulting in elevated body temperature and increased caloric expenditure. In addition, the skeletal system responds to thyroid hormones by increased bone resorption, raising the risk of osteoporosis and fracture. The effects of thyroid hormone on the cardiovascular system have been well studied. Hypertension, tachycardia, and arrhythmias are common cardiovascular manifestations of hyperthyroidism. Patients with TMNG have a higher risk of developing atrial fibrillation. Gastrointestinal effects include increased motility and diarrhea. Symptoms are reversible once hyperthyroidism is treated and a euthyroid state is restored.[5]

Visual inspection of the neck may reveal an enlarged thyroid in patients with TMG. The presence of multiple discrete nodules may be palpable on physical exam, and enlargement of the gland results in increased pressure on surrounding structures such as the esophagus or trachea. The mass effect can result in a globus sensation or dysphagia. Rarely, nodules can sufficiently enlarge and compress the recurrent laryngeal nerve or trachea, causing hoarseness or airway compromise.

Table 10–1. Symptoms of toxic multinodular goiters.*

Symptoms of Excess Thyroid Hormone	Symptoms of Goiter Mass Effect
Palpitations	Dysphagia
Tremors	Globus sensation
Fatigue	Orthopnea
Anxiety	Dyspnea
Weight loss	Dysphonia
Insomnia	Pain and pressure
Heat intolerance	Otalgia (referred pain)
Polydipsia	

*Including those related to the excessive thyroid hormone systemic circulation and those related to the enlarged, nodular thyroid gland.

Table 10–2. Differential diagnoses corresponding to the thyroid function test results.*

Differential Diagnosis	TSH	T3	T4
Euthyroid sick syndrome, central hypothyroidism	Low	Low	Low
Subclinical hyperthyroidism	Low	Normal	Normal
Overt hyperthyroidism	Low	High	High
Exogenous thyroid (T3) hormone	Low	High	Low/Normal
Exogenous thyroid (T4) hormone, thyroiditis	Low	Low/Normal	High
TSH producing mass	High	High	High
Primary hypothyroidism	High	Low	Low
Subclinical hypothyroidism	High	Normal	Normal

*Obtained as part of the initial diagnostic evaluation for hyperthyroidism symptoms.

B. Laboratory Findings

The first step in diagnostic evaluation for presumed hyperthyroidism is thyroid function tests. The diagnoses correlating with thyroid function tests are summarized in Table 10–2. An elevated TSH level indicates hypothyroidism. A decreased TSH level indicates hyperthyroidism. Overt hyperthyroidism is defined as low TSH levels with elevated T3 and T4 levels. Subclinical hyperthyroidism is defined as low TSH levels with normal T3 and T4 levels.[5]

Patients presenting with symptoms of hyperthyroidism require initial diagnostic evaluation with thyroid function tests. TSH, T3, and T4 levels are included in thyroid function tests. T3 and T4 are present in circulation bound to proteins (Figure 10–1). Seventy-five percent of T3 and T4 are bound to thyroxine-binding globulin, with one hormone-binding site and a higher affinity for T4. Transthyretin and albumin additionally bind about 20% of T3 and T4 in circulation. Transthyretin has two hormone-binding sites. Albumin has a low affinity for T3 and T4, but there is a comparative abundance of albumin in the circulation. Only 0.2% of T4 and 0.3% of T3 are unbound in circulation. The quantity of thyroxine-binding globulin, transthyretin, and albumin in circulation affects T3 and T4 levels. The T3:T4 ratio provides additional information regarding the etiology of hyperthyroidism. Overt hyperthyroidism from GD, TMNG, or AFTN has a higher T3:T4 ratio, while thyroiditis etiologies have lower T3:T4 ratios.

Adjunctive laboratory tests that provide further diagnostic information regarding thyroid disease are thyroglobulin, anti-TPO, and TRAb levels. Thyroglobulin level measures the thyroglobulin released from thyrocytes into the systemic circulation with T3 and T4. Low thyroglobulin level in combination with elevated thyroid hormones indicates exogenous thyroid hormone ingestion. Anti-TPO level measures thyroperoxidase antibodies and is elevated in autoimmune causes of thyroid disease, including GD and Hashimoto's thyroiditis. TRAb level measures thyrotropin receptor antibiotics, and a positive TRAb level in the setting of hyperthyroidism is indicative of GD.

C. Imaging Studies

The most appropriate imaging studies for TMNG include thyroid scintigraphy or ultrasound (US). In some cases, a computed tomography (CT) neck may be performed.

Thyroid scintigraphy is performed to evaluate thyroid function. It is indicated in patients with thyroid function tests revealing hyperthyroidism or patients identified with thyroid nodules of unknown function. The patient receives a radioactive tracer (^{123}I, ^{131}I-iodide, or ^{99m}Tc-pertechnetate) which is ingested or administered intravenously. At different time intervals, the thyroid gland's radioactivity is measured and reported as a percentage of the tracer ingested. Typical time intervals are at 6 hours and 24 hours. Normal radiotracer levels at 6 hours are 3% to 16% and at 24 hours are 8% to 25%. Radioactivity above the expected levels indicates hyperthyroidism; radioactivity below the expected levels indicates hypothyroidism. The radioactivity throughout the thyroid gland varies with the presence of nodules. The radioactivity of thyroid nodules indicates whether a nodule is considered "hot" (hyperfunctioning) or "cold" (hypofunctioning).

Thyroid scintigraphy assists in differentiating the etiologies of hyperthyroidism. A GD scan reveals diffuse thyroid gland radioactivity. Thyroid scintigraphy in toxic adenomas reveals a single localized area of increased radioactivity amongst normal or hypofunctioning thyroid tissue. In TMNG, thyroid scintigraphy shows areas of increased radioactivity interspersed in hypofunctioning tissue or tissue without radioactive uptake. However, radioactive uptake in TMNG can become high enough that it is indistinguishable from GD.

The radiotracer is excreted over 24 to 48 hours after the scan. Lactating patients are advised not to breastfeed after a thyroid scintigraphy scan. Patients are also advised against pregnancy for 6 months following the use of radioactive iodine as a treatment for hyperthyroidism. Thyroid scintigraphy is contraindicated during pregnancy due to the toxicity to the fetus.[6]

For patients for whom a thyroid scintigraphy scan is unable to be performed, an US is an alternative imaging modality to consider for patients with hyperthyroidism. US provides information on nodule presence, location, consistency, borders, and size. Specific findings on US may also raise suspicion for malignancy, including irregular borders, solid consistency, microcalcifications, central vascularization, and hypoechogenicity.[7,8]

US assists in differentiating the etiology in a hyperthyroid patient. GD on US imaging reveals increased blood flow diffusely typically in an otherwise homogeneous gland. Toxic nodular disease shows varying amounts of blood flow throughout the thyroid gland. Increased blood flow may signify a hyperfunctioning nodule, and decreased blood flow correlates with a hypofunctioning nodule. US utility may be limited by nodule location. Goiters that extend into the mediastinum are unable to be adequately assessed using US.[7]

CT scans are not necessary for the diagnostic evaluation of hyperthyroidism and TMNG. However, if surgical management is expected, CT imaging can be beneficial in cases of large nodules and hypertrophic glands. In addition, extension to the mediastinum, anatomy of surrounding structures and vessels, and tracheal or esophageal compression can be evaluated via CT imaging and provide pertinent information for preoperative planning.

Differential Diagnosis

The most common cause of hyperthyroidism in the United States is GD, followed by TMNG and AFTN. Rarely, hormone-producing tumors such as TSH-producing pituitary tumors and struma ovarii tumors affect the TRH-TSH-Thyroid hormone axis. Pituitary tumors can secrete TSH outside the pituitary-thyroid axis resulting in TSH-stimulated excessive production of T3 and T4.[9] Struma ovarii tumors are ovarian masses composed partly of thyroid tissue which can be hormone producing, resulting in hyperthyroidism. Exogenous thyroid hormone intake can result in sustained T3 or T4 elevation, contributing to symptoms of hyperthyroidism.

Thyroiditis can be iatrogenic, infectious, or medically induced, and all may result in inflammation of the thyroid gland. Depending on the etiology and phase of thyroiditis, patients may present with hyperthyroidism. Thyroiditis results in temporary hyperthyroidism with the release of excess thyroid hormone but no sustained hormone overproduction. History and physical exam may provide enough information to differentiate between thyroiditis and TMNG. Alternatively, the US can assist with differentiation as the thyroid will be diffusely inflamed in thyroiditis. The hyperthyroid phase of thyroiditis is typically temporary, whereas hypothyroidism from TMNG is usually sustained.

Complications

A. Risk of Malignancy

Hyperfunctioning thyroid nodules on thyroid scintigraphy were historically thought to have a low risk for malignancy. As such, a fine-needle aspiration (FNA) of hyperfunctioning nodules is not typically recommended.[10] If performed, pathologic analysis reveals hyperplasia and increased cellularity, possibly with atypia. Findings can be misinterpreted as a follicular neoplasm. That being said, more recent studies have demonstrated a higher malignancy rate than previously reported in hyperfunctioning nodules. In a meta-analysis of the malignancy risk in hyperfunctioning nodules, Lau et al. found the incidence of malignancy to be 10% to 34%.[7] The odds of malignancy in toxic nodules are 50% lower than in nontoxic nodules. In a systematic review of the incidence of thyroid carcinoma in patients who underwent thyroidectomy for hyperthyroidism, the overall rate of malignancy was 8%, but 12% in patients with TMNG. Of patients undergoing thyroidectomy for hyperthyroidism, TMNG patients had the highest incidence of thyroid carcinoma on pathology.[8]

B. TMNG in Pregnancy

Hyperthyroidism in pregnancy increases the risk of maternal and fetal complications.[6] Subclinical hyperthyroidism in pregnancy does not typically require management, but overt hyperthyroidism has been shown to increase the risk of complications and requires management. There is also a physiological increase in thyroid hormone secondary to pregnancy which must be distinguished from a pathological cause such as GD or TMNG. Human chorionic gonadotropin is synthesized in the placenta, and due to structural similarities, stimulates TSH receptors, increasing T3 and T4 production. This occurs in the first trimester. Additional changes in thyroid hormone homeostasis during pregnancy include increased activity of type 3 deiodinase and an increase in thyroxine-binding globulin. Type 3 deiodinase inactivates T3 and T4, resulting in increased TSH. In addition, increased estrogen in pregnancy increases thyroxine-binding globulin which results in increased T3 and T4 levels.[11]

The most common pathological cause of overt hyperthyroidism in pregnancy is GD. TMNG in pregnancy is rare due to the later age of onset of TMNG. Diagnosis of a pathological cause of hyperthyroidism during pregnancy is complicated due to the normal physiological changes in thyroid hormone synthesis during pregnancy. "Normal" reference ranges in pregnancy for TSH, T3, and T4 may differ from reference ranges in nonpregnant patients. In addition, a thyroid scintigraphy scan is contraindicated in pregnant patients due to the potential fetal toxicity of radioactive iodine.

Therefore, an US is the best imaging option available for further evaluation of hyperthyroidism in pregnancy.[11]

For patients with laboratory-confirmed hyperthyroidism and US consistent with TMNG, treatment options during pregnancy include antithyroid medications or surgery. While medical therapy is typically avoided during pregnancy due to possible increased incidence of birth defects, if there is no alternative, propylthiouracil (PTU) is recommended as medical therapy in the first trimester. Methimazole (MMI) is not used due to reported birth defects. However, after the first trimester, MMI is preferred due to the liver damage risk with PTU. Surgical intervention is a secondary option. If necessary, surgery is recommended in the second trimester to avoid fetal toxicity from anesthetics in the first trimester and the risk of preterm delivery in the third trimester. I-131 is contraindicated due to fetal toxicity.[11]

Treatment

Multiple treatments for TMNG are available with similar success rates but different patient criteria and risks. Treatment options include radioactive iodine, surgery, and thionamide medications.[12] The advantages and disadvantages of each treatment are presented in Table 10–3.

A. Radioactive Iodine

Radioactive iodine (RAI), most commonly I-131, is a widely used treatment for hyperthyroidism of multiple etiologies. RAI is absorbed into the bloodstream and then concentrated in the thyroid cells. Radiation causes cell death. Treatment with RAI is indicated as first-line therapy for poor surgical candidates, advanced age, or multiple medical comorbidities. RAI is also indicated in patients with persistent hyperthyroidism despite surgery.[11]

An increased hyperthyroid state may result initially after treatment, followed by a euthyroid or hypothyroid state. TSH, T3, and T4 serum levels are monitored every 4 to 6 weeks after treatment. A 50% response rate is reported at about 3 months after RAI treatment, and an 80% response rate is reported at about 6 months. Hyperthyroidism can take up to 24 months to resolve after RAI treatment. RAI has reported a cure rate for TMNG of about 80%, with 20% requiring re-treatment. The 2016 American Thyroid Association (ATA) guidelines recommend re-treatment with RAI if hyperthyroidism persists beyond 6 months following initial treatment. Higher T3 levels before RAI treatment are correlated with recurrence of hyperthyroidism after treatment.[11]

I-131 dosage is determined based on gland weight. TMNG is associated with higher-weight thyroid glands due to the mechanism of the disease. Therefore, TMNG treated with I-131 tends to require higher dosages than other hyperthyroidism etiologies. Higher I-131 dosage correlates with higher cure rates for TMNG and higher risks of treatment side effects.[11]

Thyrotoxicosis following RAI is common. Those at highest risk for complications related to exacerbated hyperthyroidism, such as cardiovascular complications, may benefit from beta-blocker administration pretreatment or MMI or PTU medical therapy before RAI, although antithyroid medications are associated with decreased efficacy of RAI. Permanent hypothyroidism is a risk of RAI, and risk correlates with treatment dosage, with reports of 14% for those receiving a high dose for TMNG. In addition, the development of secondary cancer due to exposure to radiation from treatment has been reported, although overall cancer mortality is not increased in patients treated with RAI.[12]

If patients with TMNG treated with RAI develop recurrence of hyperthyroidism, the most likely cause is the development of autonomously functioning nodules. However, there is an increased risk of developing GD in patients with TMNG treated with RAI. A thyroid scintigraphy scan and evaluation of the pattern of uptake can be diagnostic.

B. Surgical

Surgery is considered as an initial treatment for TMNG or secondary treatment for TMNG refractory to RAI. If surgical

Table 10–3. The advantages and disadvantages of the three main treatment modalities for TMNG.

Radioactive Iodine		Total Thyroidectomy		Thionamide Medications	
Advantages	Disadvantages	Advantages	Disadvantages	Advantages	Disadvantages
High success	Radiation exposure	High success	Risks of surgery	Comparable success rates	Medication dependent
Avoid surgery	Risk of thyrotoxicosis	Minimal morbidity	Risks of hypocalcemia or recurrent laryngeal nerve injury	Avoid surgery	Recurrence with stopping medications
Tolerable for medically complex or elderly	Risk of secondary Graves' disease		Dependent on thyroid hormone supplementation	Option for poor surgical candidates	Medication side effects

treatment is pursued, the ATA recommends a near-total or total thyroidectomy.[11] A total thyroidectomy prevents the possibility for recurrence or persistent hyperthyroidism due to TMNG. However, this approach requires the patient to take supplemental thyroid hormone indefinitely which may burden the patient. A near-total thyroidectomy involves the removal of both thyroid lobes except for a small amount of thyroid tissue on either side. This approach has a risk of recurrent TMNG as thyroid tissue remains but avoids the need for thyroid hormone supplementation.

If surgical treatment is pursued, the ATA recommends preoperative medical treatment optimization of overt hyperthyroidism.[11] Patients should receive MMI and have laboratory confirmation of a euthyroid state prior to surgical intervention. In addition, β-adrenergic blockage (beta-blocker) therapy should be considered preoperatively in patients with tachycardia and hypertension secondary to overt hyperthyroidism.

The most common complications associated with total or near-total thyroidectomy are hypocalcemia (transient or permanent) and recurrent laryngeal nerve injury (transient or permanent). Unintentional removal or devascularization of parathyroid glands can result in hypocalcemia. Most instances are transient, and all can be treated with appropriate medications when identified. Recurrent laryngeal nerve palsy can similarly be transient or permanent depending on the mechanism of injury to the nerve. Neuropraxia can cause hoarseness, dyspnea, and dysphagia. Complications related to thyroid surgery are minimized in the hands of high-volume surgery centers. However, due to the chronic inflammation and fibrosis of the thyroid gland associated with TMNG, postoperative complications are speculated to be higher in this population.[11]

C. Medical

Methimazole (MMI) and propylthiouracil (PTU) are thionamide medications that inhibit thyroid hormone synthesis. MMI and PTU inhibit iodide oxygenation and thyroperoxidase, which are necessary for the production of thyroid hormone synthesis. T3 is a more potent and active hormone. Deiodinases convert T4 to T3 in peripheral tissues. Type 1 deiodinase is active in the liver, kidney, and thyroid. Type II deiodinase is active in the central nervous system, pituitary, and cutaneous tissue. The conversion of T4 to T3 by type I deiodinase in liver, kidney, and thyroid tissue is also inhibited by PTU.

PTU and MMI are selectively used in TMNG as primary therapy or bridging therapy before more definitive treatment with RAI or surgery. Antithyroid medications as primary therapy are considered for patients whose risks of RAI or surgery are too high: elderly, cardiovascular comorbidities, or significant surgical risk. For TMNG, treatment options such as radiofrequency or alcohol ablation are less effective. Therefore, antithyroid drugs are a third-line treatment option in TMNG. When utilized as primary therapy for TMNG, PTU and MMI are lifelong medications. Discontinuation of antithyroid medications results in the return of hyperthyroidism in TMNG.[11]

A prospective study by Aziz et al. compared outcomes among TMNG patients under 60 years old who underwent either RAI or MMI treatment.[12] Treatment success, defined as a euthyroid or hypothyroid state, was similar between the RAI and MMI groups, reaching about 96%. The MMI group reached a euthyroid state sooner than the RAI group. Side effects for the MMI group were minimal and occurred within the first few months of treatment, consistent with other reports regarding the safety of MMI. The MMI dose was decreased over the years, and relapse of hyperthyroidism occurred in only 3.8% of patients. The RAI group had a more significant decrease in gland size than the MMI group.

Antithyroid medications also have a role as a bridging therapy before definitive treatment with RAI or surgery.[12] Antithyroid medication use prior to RAI therapy depletes thyroid hormone stores and potentially prevents the RAI-induced hyperthyroid exacerbation. However, PTU and MMI use before RAI therapy have also been associated with a higher failure rate of RAI therapy, so their use is controversial. Sufficient evidence for either approach is lacking. Prior to RAI, consideration for PTU or MMI is based on the severity of hyperthyroidism, cardiovascular comorbidities, and risk of decreasing RAI effectiveness.

Antithyroid medications are not without risks and side effects. Pruritis, rash, and arthralgias are the most common side effects, occurring in about 5% of patients. Severe side effects include agranulocytosis, vasculitis, and hepatitis. Agranulocytosis occurs in less than 0.5% of patients taking PTU or MMI and typically occurs within the first 90 days of taking the medication. PTU has a higher risk of hepatitis, commonly occurring in the first 90 days of taking the medication. Cholestasis and cholestatic hepatitis are side effects of MMI.

D. Radiofrequency Ablation

Thrombosis, ischemia, and ultimately fibrosis result from radiofrequency ablation of thyroid tissue. Multiple sessions are conducted in which thyroid tissue is elevated to over 100°C by ultrasound-based energy. Evidence supports the use of radiofrequency ablation in patients with ATN, with reports of improvement in 75% of patients.[13] Side effects include pain at the site of ablation. There are no reports of worsened hyperthyroidism following radiofrequency ablation.[14] Success in TMNG has not been supported with data. Radiofrequency ablation is a consideration for TMNG treatment when other more efficacious treatment modalities have failed or been refused.

E. Percutaneous Laser Ablation

Percutaneous laser ablation (PLA) delivers laser energy through a large gauge needle into a thyroid nodule. The mechanism of tissue fibrosis is similar to radiofrequency ablation.

Multiple sessions are required. For TMNG, PLA requires repeated ablations in multiple locations within the thyroid gland due to the multinodular nature of TMNG. PLA of toxic thyroid nodules has resulted in normalization of thyroid function in 100% of ATN patients and 50% of TMNG patients in some studies. In a study comparing PLA followed by I-131 treatment with patients receiving only I-131 treatment for toxic nodules, Chianelli et al. found that 20% of the patients in the combined group no longer required I-131 treatment after PLA.[15] The combined treatment group had a 70% reduction in nodule size compared to the I-131 group, with a 47% nodule size reduction. The dose of I-131 required for the combined group was also lower than the dose required for the I-131 only group. PLA shows promise as an alternative treatment modality alone or in combination with other therapies for TMNG, but further investigation into the efficacy alone and practicality for multiple nodules is necessary.

F. Alcohol Ablation

Percutaneous ethanol injections are used for the ablation of cystic thyroid nodules and are not recommended for TMNG. Studies have shown persistent hyperthyroidism in patients undergoing alcohol ablation.[16] In addition, side effects of the injections included infiltration of surrounding tissues, fibrosis of surrounding tissues, and subcutaneous hematomas. Alternative treatment modalities provide better outcomes with a lower risk profile.

Prognosis

The prognosis for TMNG is excellent, with multiple options for medical and surgical management. Treatment is focused on the resolution or management of hyperthyroidism. RAI therapy is reported to have rates of 80% to 96% resolution of hyperthyroidism and reduction of nodule sizes. Total thyroidectomy offers a complete resolution of TMNG with the removal of the nodules and thyroid gland. Near-total thyroidectomy harbors a small risk of recurrence depending on the amount of remaining thyroid tissue. Pharmacological management with MMI or PTU reports similar success rates as RAI therapy, although hyperthyroidism can recur if medications are stopped. Thus, TMNG is a disease with multiple treatment avenues and good outcomes for disease control.

REFERENCES

1. Doubleday AR, Sippel RS. Hyperthyroidism. *Gland Surg.* 2020;9(I):124-135.
2. Leo S De, Lee SY, Braverman LE, Unit E, Sciences C. Hyperthyroidism. *Lancet.* 388(10047):906-918.
3. Krohn K, Fu D, Bayer Y, et al. Molecular pathogenesis of euthyroid and toxic multinodular goiter. *Endocr Rev.* 2005;26(4):504-524.
4. Dietrich JW, Landgrafe G, Fotiadou EH. TSH and thyrotropic agonists: key actors in thyroid homeostasis. *J Thyroid Res.* 2012;2012:351864.
5. Bel Lassen P, Kyrilli A, Lytrivi M, Corvilain B. Graves' disease, multinodular goiter and subclinical hyperthyroidism. *Ann Endocrinol.* 2019;80(4):240-249.
6. Anderson SL, Laurberg P. Managing hyperthyroidism in pregnancy: current perspectives. *Int J Womens Health.* 2016;8:497-504.
7. Lau LW, Ghaznavi S, Frolkis AD, et al. Malignancy risk of hyperfunctioning thyroid nodules compared with non-toxic nodules: systematic review and a meta-analysis. *Thyroid Res.* 2021;14(1):1-16.
8. Varadharajan K, Choudhury N. A systematic review of the incidence of thyroid carcinoma in patients undergoing thyroidectomy for thyrotoxicosis. *Clin Otolaryngol.* 2020;45(4):538-544.
9. Fu H, Cheng L, Jin Y, Chen L. Thyrotoxicosis with concomitant thyroid cancer. *Endocr Relat Cancer.* 2019;26:R395-R413.
10. Alvarez AL, Mulder M, Handelsman RS, Lew JI, Farra JC. High rates of underlying thyroid cancer in patients undergoing thyroidectomy for hyperthyroidism. *J Surg Res.* 2019;245(305):523-528.
11. Ross DS, Burch HB, Cooper DS, et al. 2016 American Thyroid Association guidelines for diagnosis and management of hyperthyroidism and other causes of thyrotoxicosis. *Thyroid.* 2016;26(10):1343-1421.
12. Azizi F, Takyar M, Madreseh E, Amouzegar A. Treatment of toxic multinodular goiter: comparison of radioiodine and long-term methimazole treatment. *Thyroid.* 2019;29(5):625-630.
13. Cesareo R, Palermo A, Pasqualini V, Manfrini S. Radiofrequency ablation on autonomously functioning thyroid nodules: a critical appraisal and review of the literature. *Front Endocrinol.* 2020;11:317.
14. Sung JY, Baek JH, Jung SL, et al. Radiofrequency ablation for autonomously functioning thyroid nodules: a multicenter study. *Thyroid.* 2015;25(1):112-117.
15. Chianelli M, Bizzarri G, Todino V, et al. Laser ablation and 131-Iodine: a 24-Month pilot study of combined treatment for large toxic nodular goiter. *J Clin Endocrinol Metab.* 2014;99:1283-1286.
16. Papini E, Gugliemi R, Maurizio C. Laser, radiofrequency, and ethanol ablation for the management of thyroid nodules. *Curr Opin Endocrinol Diabetes Obes.* 2016;23(5):400-406.

11 Thyroiditis

Terry C. Lairmore, MD, FACS
Rajini K. Yatavelli, MD
Kamal Bhusal, MD, FACE

GENERAL CONSIDERATIONS

The term thyroiditis encompasses several clinicopathologically distinct disorders caused by autoimmune, infectious, and inflammatory processes affecting the thyroid gland. Except for Hashimoto thyroiditis (HT), these are uncommon disorders, and they are frequently not recognized or misdiagnosed by clinicians owing to nonspecific or insidious symptoms.[1] The recognition and accurate diagnosis of these disorders is of interest to primary care physicians, as well as to the specialists in endocrinology and endocrine surgery who are often involved in determining the most appropriate and current management. Many of these conditions are primarily treated medically. However, endocrine surgeons should have a clear understanding of the essential elements of differential diagnosis, current evidence-based treatments, and the unique subset of these conditions, or their complications that require surgical intervention.

This clinical review will focus on the important features of the epidemiology, predisposing conditions, risk factors, and essentials of diagnosis for the various forms of thyroiditis. The defining clinical features of each type of thyroiditis will be emphasized, as well as the physical examination and laboratory findings that differentiate between the separate diagnoses. Accurate diagnosis is a prerequisite for selecting the most appropriate management and determining the prognosis and expected clinical course. Although the scope of this chapter is not to exhaustively review the pathophysiology of the different forms of thyroiditis, recent findings that shed light on the important etiologic factors will be included (Table 11–1). Importantly, the role of diet, heredity, and medications in the development or predisposition to unique forms of thyroiditis are now more clearly understood. These associations are important for the diagnostic evaluation and recognition of the specific types of thyroiditis.

Finally, the current clinical management of the various forms of thyroiditis will be emphasized in this review. Guidelines for the management of patients who have a diagnosis of one of the forms of thyroiditis will be covered, as well as up-to-date evidence from the most current clinical studies. A practical and updated clinical approach to the evaluation, diagnosis, and treatment of the various types of thyroiditis will be provided, emphasizing the essential elements in the differential diagnosis and management that are of value to the primary care or specialist physician managing these uncommon disorders. A flow diagram summarizing the diagnostic evaluation of a thyroid mass in the context of thyroiditis is depicted in Figure 11–1.

HASHIMOTO THYROIDITIS

General Considerations

HT, also called autoimmune thyroiditis or chronic lymphocytic thyroiditis, is the leading cause of hypothyroidism in iodine-sufficient areas of the world. The incidence of HT is reported to be about 0.3 to 1.5 cases per 1000 people and has female preponderance with female to male ratio of 4-10:1.[2] HT is characterized by chronic lymphocytic infiltration of the thyroid parenchyma with resultant follicular destruction, fibrosis, and atrophy of the thyroid gland. Thyroid antibodies, particularly thyroid peroxidase antibodies (TPO antibodies) are present in 80% to 90% of patients, and thyroglobulin (TgAb) antibodies may be seen in 60% to 80% of patients.

The condition bears the name of the Japanese physician, Haraku Hashimoto, who in the beginning of the 20th century first reported patients with atrophy of thyroid follicular cells, lymphocyte infiltration with increased volume of the gland, naming this disease as "struma lymphomatosa."[3]

HT is the leading cause of hypothyroidism but can present with transient hyperthyroidism. While "silent" or "painless thyroiditis" is the most commonly seen clinical variant, "painful forms of HT" have also been described.[4,5]

Table 11–1. Classification and features of thyroiditis.[*]

Subtype	Clinical History	Etiology	TPO Antibodies	Treatment
Hashimoto thyroiditis[†]	Family history of thyroid disorder, absence of neck pain Triphasic course with initial thyrotoxicosis followed by euthyroid or permanent hypothyroidism	Autoimmune	+++	Symptoms are usually self-limited and improve in 1-3 months Beta-blockers for bothersome symptoms
Postpartum	History of pregnancy or miscarriage in the past year, painless, family history of thyroid disease	Autoimmune	+++	Symptoms are usually self-limited and improve in 1-3 months Beta-blockers for bothersome symptoms
Subacute[‡]	Subacute onset with neck pain and tenderness	Post viral inflammation	+/–	NSAIDs +/corticosteroids
Suppurative	Fever, neck pain, immunocompromised state	Acute bacterial thyroiditis	+/–	Surgery + antibiotics
Riedel thyriodities	Neck tightness, dysphonia, dysphagia, diffuse hard goiter	Extensive fibrosis, IgG4-related disease	++	Corticosteroids, tamoxifen, and surgery in selected cases
Drug Induced	History of offending drug	Induced autoimmunity or direct cytotoxicity to thyroid	+/–	Symptomatic management; weigh the risks and benefits of discontinuing the offending drug.

[*]Radioactive iodine uptake is low in thyroiditis.
[†]Silent thyroiditis or chronic autoimmune thyroiditis or painless thyroiditis.
[‡]de Quervain or granulomatous thyroiditis.

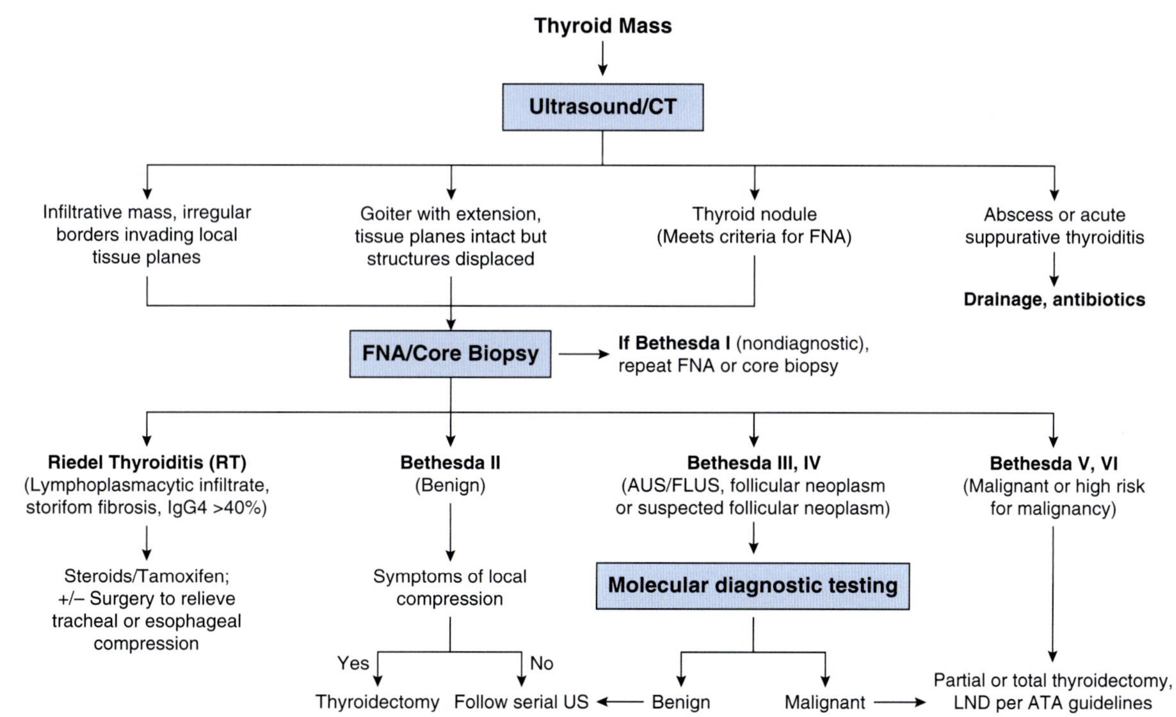

Figure 11–1. Evaluation and management of thyroid mass.

The characteristic diagnostic features of the disease include thyroid function abnormalities, ultrasonographic features of a heterogenous, hypoechoic gland, and presence of thyroid antibodies.

Pathogenesis & Risk Factors

HT is an autoimmune disease and pathogenesis is not completely defined; however, loss of immune tolerance to autoantigens in the thyroid gland is presumed to be the principal feature. HT is widely considered to be a thyroid helper cell 1 (Th1)-mediated autoimmune disease. The regulatory T cells (Treg) play an important role in maintaining the immune balance and studies have shown a decrease in the percentage of Treg cells in HT.[6] Another pathway—PD1/PDL1—is important for peripheral immune tolerance, and aberrant expression of PD1 is thought to play an important role in autoimmune damage to the thyroid cells.[7] Although the pathogenesis is not completely understood, it is suggested that genetic and environmental factors along with epigenetic effects result in the loss of self-tolerance and activation of $CD4^+$ T lymphocytes.

Lymphocytic infiltration of the thyroid gland leads to fibrosis and parenchymal atrophy of the thyroid gland. Histopathological features are not unique, and several variants of fibrosis have been identified. In the goitrous form, thyroid tissue is completely replaced by fibrous tissue resulting in a goiter, but the fibrous tissue does not extend beyond the thyroid capsule. In the atrophic variant, thyroid gland volume is reduced and replaced by fibrous tissue resulting in atrophy of the gland.[2,3]

An increased incidence of autoimmune thyroid disease in siblings, high concordance rate in monozygotic twins, and presence of circulating thyroid antibodies in 50% of siblings of affected parents supports the role of genetic susceptibility.[2] Environmental factors such as excess iodine exposure, insufficient selenium intake, vitamin D deficiency, and viral infections as triggers for autoimmunity have been areas of interest for many researchers, and while the results are preliminary they call for more extensive validated studies.[2,3]

Clinical Findings

HT (silent or painless thyroiditis) generally follows a triphasic course with an initial thyrotoxic phase followed by a hypothyroid phase and eventually returns to either euthyroidism or a permanent hypothyroid state.

A. Transient Thyrotoxicosis From HT

Systemic symptoms from thyrotoxicosis are usually mild and self-limiting. Symptoms of palpitations, heat intolerance, weight loss, and menstrual irregularities can be seen that typically resolve in 1 to 3 months. Hypothyroidism symptoms of fatigue, weight gain, and cold intolerance ensue in the hypothyroid state and the severity of symptoms depends on the degree of hypothyroidism. Local symptoms of dysphagia and dysphonia can be seen in patients with large goiters. A firm and enlarged gland can be felt in the goitrous form and the thyroid gland is barely palpable in atrophic form. Neck pain and tenderness are generally absent. HT is usually painless, but a much rarer entity of painful HT has been described.[5] A recent literature review by Munir et al. reported 70 published cases of painful HT over the past 70 years, which accounts for a minor prevalence compared to classic silent thyroiditis. The patients reported had an either insidious onset of progressive pain or acute intolerable pain in one lobe or the whole thyroid. The clinical course of the disease was reported to be fluctuating in terms of pain and size of the thyroid gland, and response to NSAIDs or corticosteroids was not as favorable as in subacute thyroiditis. A small percentage who underwent total thyroidectomy had 100% relief of pain.[4] Although the reports are retrospective in nature over a long duration of time with inherent selection and reporting bias, one should be aware of the rare and peculiar presentation of painful HT.[4,5]

B. Hypothyroidism From HT

After the initial thyrotoxic phase the patients may have a brief period of hypothyroidism with either recovery to euthyroid state or may develop permanent hypothyroidism. Patients may be asymptomatic or present with various symptoms of hypothyroidism such as fatigue, weight gain, mood disturbances, cold intolerance, etc., depending on the severity of hypothyroidism. On clinical examination, patients are often found to have dry skin, hoarse voice, bradycardia, diastolic hypertension, and delayed relaxation of tendon reflexes. The thyroid gland may be nodular with a large goiter or found to be atrophic and barely palpable.

Laboratory & Imaging Findings

Thyroid function tests may reveal a suppressed TSH with normal or elevated free thyroid hormone levels in the thyrotoxic phase. Overt or subclinical hypothyroidism with elevated TSH and normal or decreased free thyroid hormone levels are seen in the hypothyroid state. TPOs are present in 95% of patients with HT and higher titers are associated with elevated risk of progression to overt hypothyroidism. Thyroglobulin antibodies are seen in 60% to 80% of patients. Thyrotropin receptor antibodies (TRAB) or thyroid-stimulating immunoglobulin (TSI) can be checked based on clinical suspicion, and if positive are strongly suggestive of concomitant Graves' disease.

Other inflammatory markers, like ESR, are usually not elevated. ^{123}I radioactive iodine-uptake (RAIU) scan can readily differentiate thyroiditis from Graves' disease and should be obtained when the diagnosis is uncertain. RAIU scan shows less than 1% uptake in thyroiditis.

An ultrasound of the thyroid gland is not routinely recommended but can be obtained if there is any suspicion of a nodular goiter. Ultrasonograms show a diffuse hypoechoic heterogenous gland with decreased echogenicity and decreased vascularity.

Cytological evaluation is rarely needed and is only obtained if there are nodules that are suspicious for thyroid cancer. Cytology shows lymphocyte predominance in contact with thyroid cells.[8]

Differential Diagnosis

The differential diagnosis for thyroiditis is broad and includes subacute thyroiditis, suppurative thyroiditis, Riedel thyroiditis, drug-induced thyroiditis, and Graves' disease. Absence of neck pain or ophthalmopathy, positive TPO antibodies, normal ESR, and decreased or absent radioactive iodine uptake, as well as a family history of Hashimoto disease are suggestive of HT.

Treatment

A. Medical Management

Hyperthyroidism in painless thyroiditis is due to destruction of the thyroid gland and the release of preformed hormones, hence thionamides, which predominantly decrease new hormone synthesis, do not have a role in the management. Thyrotoxicosis is mild and self-limited, and treatment is mainly supportive with beta-blockers.[9] Since the hypothyroid phase is transient, levothyroxine replacement is indicated in hypothyroid patients who are symptomatic. If started on levothyroxine, consider stopping after several months as it is likely the hypothyroid phase has resolved. Some may develop permanent hypothyroidism and require life-long replacement with levothyroxine.

NSAIDs and/or corticosteroids have been used in painful HT, but the response has not shown to be as favorable as in subacute thyroiditis.

B. Surgical Treatment

Thyroidectomy is rarely indicated in HT and is usually limited to patients with compressive symptoms from the goiter, progressive increase in size of nodules, or malignant transformation of nodules.[10] In patients with painful HT with pain refractory to medical treatment, reports of total thyroidectomy with complete resolution of pain have been recorded.[4] Despite being euthyroid on adequate levothyroxine replacement a subset of HT patients can have persistent symptoms of chronic fatigue, weakness, nervousness, anxiety, and poor quality of life and many studies indicate that patients with high circulating TPO antibodies are more prone to these symptoms.[2,11] Total thyroidectomy to alleviate the symptoms has been explored and a recent randomized trial from Norway on a subset of 150 similar patients showed improved parameters in quality of life and significant decrease in TPO titers in those who underwent surgery.[12] Although the study was limited only to a subgroup of patients and follow-up was limited to 18 months, it raises the question as to whether TPO titers independently have any role in Hashimoto symptomatology and further studies to validate surgical exploration are needed.

Primary thyroid lymphoma is a rare malignancy that accounts for less than 5% of all thyroid malignancies with women being more commonly affected than men, and occurs with increased frequency in those with HT. The typical presentation is that of a woman, in her seventh or eighth decade of life, presenting with a rapidly enlarging thyroid mass (over a period of days to weeks). Men often present at a relatively younger age. Surgery and radiation therapy (RT) were traditionally considered to be the standard of treatment but with the advent of immunotherapy with favorable responses, the frequency of surgical approaches has declined.[13,14]

Thyroidectomy has the risk of recurrent laryngeal nerve injury and permanent hypoparathyroidism. When needed it is generally agreed that it should be performed by a high-volume thyroid surgeon with the risks versus benefits weighed and discussed with the patient.

RIEDEL THYROIDITIS

General Considerations

Riedel thyroiditis (RT) is a very uncommon condition with a unique clinical presentation and physical findings.[15] The disorder is a result of a rare chronic inflammatory disease involving progressive dense fibrosis that replaces the normal thyroid parenchyma. This fibrotic process extends through the normal anatomic border of the thyroid capsule and directly invades surrounding structures. The essential features of its clinical presentation include a rapidly enlarging and usually painless mass in the neck. Symptoms of local compression including progressive dysphagia, stridor, pressure sensation, dyspnea, and change in voice are frequently noted. The physical findings include a very firm, diffusely infiltrating mass in the anterior neck, often described as "woody" or fibrotic. The mass is characteristically fixed on physical exam and may not move with swallowing, as is often demonstrable in benign goiters or solitary thyroid nodules. The condition bears the name of Bernhard Moritz Carl Ludwig Riedel, who first described its clinical features in 1893.

RT has been recognized to occur as a component of a broader systemic disease termed IgG4 syndrome,[16] including idiopathic fibrosis of the retroperitoneum and mediastinum, sclerosing cholangitis, and lymphocytic infiltration of the salivary gland, lacrimal glands, and the extraocular orbital muscles (orbital pseudotumor). Patients may also develop interstitial pneumonia and autoimmune pancreatitis.

Table 11–2. Essential features of IgG4-related disease.

- Elevation of serum IgG4 (>110 mg/dL)
- Infiltration of tissue target with IgG4-positive lymphoplasmacytic cells
- Infiltrating IgG4-bearing plasma cells account for more than 40% of all IgG-producing B cells
- Pathologic findings of storiform fibrosis, obliterative phlebitis in end organ
- Associated spectrum of complex fibroinflammatory disorders involving multiple organs (autoimmune pancreatitis, retroperitoneal fibrosis, sialadenitis, Riedel thyroiditis)

Pathogenesis & Risk Factors

RT is currently understood to be a member of a broader spectrum of pathologic changes termed IgG4-related disease (Table 11–2). The defining histopathologic features in the thyroid parenchyma and other involved organs are lymphoplasmacytic infiltration, storiform fibrosis, and obliterative phlebitis (Figure 11–2). The end-organ damage and destructive or disabling fibrosis is mediated largely by CD4+ T and B cells.[17] Although the precise initiating factors and pathogenesis are not known, CD4+ CTLs are likely the major source of inflammatory, cytotoxic, and profibrotic cytokines that result in end-organ damage. Tobacco use has been identified as a potential risk factor for this rare disorder.[18] The cessation of smoking has not been associated with an impact on severity or clinical course of RT. Females predominate in most series, accounting for between 75% and 85% of patients.

Clinical & Radiographic Findings

Fatourechi and colleagues reviewed the experience at Mayo Clinic for 21 patients over a 32-year period (1976 through 2008) who met the inclusion criteria for a pathologic diagnosis of invasive fibrous thyroiditis.[18] In their series, 81% of patients were female, with a mean age of 42 years. The most frequent presenting symptoms were stridor due to tracheal narrowing (48%), dysphagia (33%), and vocal cord paralysis (29%). Less than one-quarter of patients (24%) presented with pain. Interestingly, three (14%) patients had associated hypoparathyroidism. These investigators noted a high frequency of tobacco use in affected patients. Signs of systemic disease and extracervical fibrosis were frequent (38% of patients overall), including mediastinal fibrosis in four patients, retroperitoneal fibrosis in three patients, and one patient each with orbital and pancreatic fibrosis. Importantly, surgical intervention was associated with frequent complications (injury to the recurrent laryngeal nerve and parathyroid glands). In this series, there was no cause-specific mortality noted, and the fibrotic process stabilized or partially resolved in all patients.

The correct diagnosis of RT is hampered by the rarity of the condition, and clinical findings that overlap with other more common conditions. The essential features of the clinical presentation are a firm, fixed goiter with local compressive symptoms. The mass may be painless or cause pain, and dysphagia, dyspnea, or new hoarseness may reflect direct local invasion of tissues. Enlarging benign goiters can cause symptoms of local compression, although the development is usually more insidious. An aggressive thyroid malignancy,

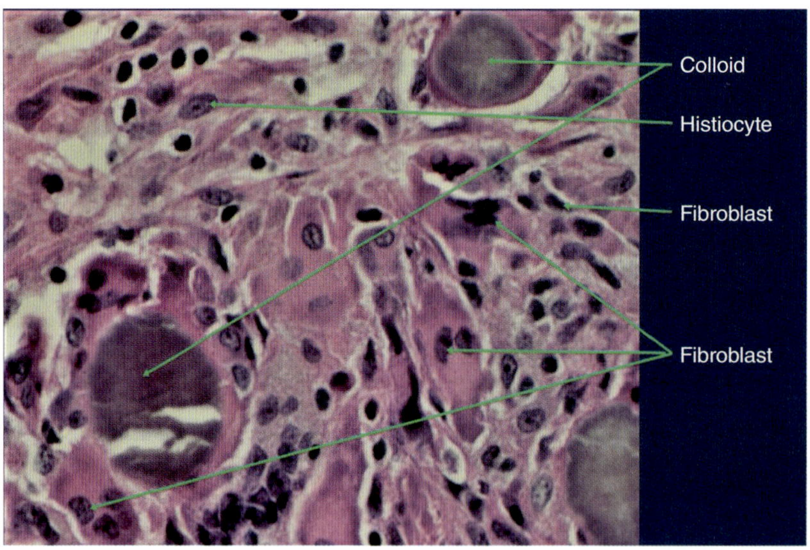

Figure 11–2. Photomicrograph of Riedel thyroiditis. (Image courtesy of Joshua D. Maier, MD, FACP, FACE, Endocrinology, Diabetes and Metabolism, Overton Brooks VA Medical Center, Shreveport, LA.)

notably anaplastic thyroid cancer (ATC), can also present with a rapidly enlarging thyroid mass that is locally invasive and results in marked symptoms of local compression. Patients with ATC can present with a very rapidly growing mass (visibly enlarging over days or a week), which may arise in a preexisting goiter or papillary thyroid cancer. Impending airway compromise and a fixed goiter that appears to invade surrounding tissues are frequently evident.

Imaging can provide initial information on which to base subsequent diagnostic evaluations. Benign goiters may extend into the mediastinum and push surrounding structures away without invading tissue planes directly. The typical findings of RT that have been described on CT include local advancement into surrounding structures and failure to respect anatomic planes. The presence of local invasion or indistinct borders suggests malignancy, and much less frequently a fibroinflammatory process such as RT. Therefore, local invasion on CT does not provide distinction between RT and malignancy. The features of RT on ultrasound include a homogeneously hypoechoic thyroid parenchyma with poor demarcation of borders and extension beyond the thyroid capsule. The sonographic findings may suggest an infiltrative pattern resulting from the expansion of fibrosis directly into the perithyroidal soft tissues.

If malignancy is strongly suspected, FDG-PET scanning is often considered. However, there are reports of intense hypermetabolic uptake on PET in both RT and ATC.[19] After characterization of a rapidly expanding neck mass with cross-sectional imaging such as CT, as well as ultrasonography to evaluate the thyroid parenchyma and surrounding lymph nodes, fine-needle aspiration (FNA) biopsy is the gold standard diagnostic test for most thyroid masses. Due to its rarity, there is little available literature on FNA diagnosis of RT. However, a recent report and review of the literature[20] emphasized image-guided biopsy from multiple foci using thin needles yielded moderate cellularity with follicular cells, lymphoplasmacytic infiltrate, scant colloid, and fibrous tissue fragments. These findings, in conjunction with clinical and radiographic presentation, were suggestive of RT. The absence of Hürthle cells pointed to an etiology for chronic thyroiditis other than Hashimoto's. A core biopsy or open procedure for thyroid biopsy may provide the best pathologic material for a definitive diagnosis.

Thyroid function tests may reveal a euthyroid state or hypothyroidism with an elevated TSH. Antithyroid antibodies, thyroid peroxidase (TPO), and thyroglobulin may also be elevated but do not establish a specific diagnosis. The most specific features, after recognizing the clinical presentation, physical findings of a firm infiltrating mass, and radiographic characteristics above, include laboratory and pathology findings that are diagnostic. These include elevation of serum IgG4, ratio of thyroid infiltrating IgG4/S-IgG4 in plasma more than 40%, and the presence of lymphoplasmacytic IgG4-positive plasma cells and storiform fibrosis in thyroid parenchyma. Although the unique clinical presentation and physical manifestations, serologic and pathologic features are all components of the classification of IgG4-related disease, none of these alone fulfills the classification criteria to establish the diagnosis of RT.[21] The definitive diagnosis of RT is made by a biopsy and pathologic evaluation.

Differential Diagnosis

There are diverse causes for firm thyroid enlargement that should be differentiated from RT as a possible etiology. The fibrosing variant of HT can present with similar clinical findings. Others have emphasized the need to identify features that separate the fibrosing variant of Hashimoto's from RT. The distinguishing features of this condition include increased vascular flow on Doppler ultrasound and presence of Hürthle cell metaplasia on pathology. The presence of these sonographic and pathologic features suggests fibrosing Hashimoto's as the cause. The presence of giant cells on FNA or pathology in surgical specimens suggests de Quervain thyroiditis (discussed later). A goiter with very rapid growth, direct invasion, and impending airway compromise suggests anaplastic thyroid cancer. This diagnosis can usually be readily established on FNA or core biopsy. FDG-PET may demonstrate hypermetabolic findings in both thyroid malignancy and RT. Other rare causes of a rapidly expanding firm thyroid goiter include thyroid lymphoma or primary thyroid sarcoma. It is important to recognize these conditions because many are not treated surgically. Anaplastic thyroid carcinoma is typically treated with chemoradiation as a first-line therapy, and surgical intervention is palliative and largely limited to tracheostomy to prevent impending airway obstruction. Although some have advocated surgical resection for Stage IVA and some IVB tumors, anaplastic thyroid cancer is often found to be markedly invasive of surrounding structures despite suggestion of limitation to thyroid on imaging. ATC very infrequently presents in an organ-confined fashion. Occasionally, a large papillary cancer that is surgically resected will have the finding of a focus of ATC arising from the background well-differentiated cancer. In many cases these patients will have a clinical course determined by the ATC. The prognosis for ATC is poor despite treatment. Thyroid lymphoma is also treated with chemotherapy and not surgical resection.

Recent advances in the management of ATC include tumor genomic profiling to identify specific molecular targets. BRAF mutation analysis and broader assessment of tumor mutational status with next-generation sequencing may be performed, with tailoring of therapy according to the genetic findings. Systemic therapy with multitarget tyrosine kinase inhibitors—TKIs (Lenvatinib, Sorafenib, Sunitinib, and Vandetanib), or single-target TKIs (Dabrafenib plus Trametinib and Vemurafenib against BRAF), Everolimus targeting mTOR, and immunotherapy such as Pembrolizumab for anti-PD-1/PD-L1 targeting have been utilized.[22]

Treatment

A. Medical Therapy

The mainstay of treatment for patients with RT is medical therapy with steroids for the manifestation related to fibrosclerosis and levothyroxine for hypothyroidism if present. Glucocorticoid therapy to decrease inflammation and the fibrotic effects of local mediators is often continued long term, and the disease process is controlled with stabilization or partial resolution in the majority of patients. Patients have also been treated with tamoxifen alone or in combination with steroids. Tamoxifen may act to inhibit fibroblast proliferation, and patients who do not tolerate or respond to steroids may be initiated on tamoxifen. Additional medical therapies that have been described include mycophenolate mofetil and rituximab. Levothyroxine is used to correct hypothyroidism associated with RT but it rarely has any ameliorating effect on the goiter or fibrosclerosis.

B. Surgical Treatment

Patients with recognized RT should be initiated on medical therapy with steroids as the first-line treatment. Other medical therapies may be added or initiated if there is no response to steroids. In the available series, most patients have either stabilization or partial resolution of their disease with long-term medical therapy. The disease-specific mortality is very low in available reports, but there are few comprehensive series, and most evidence is derived from case reports. Surgery should be limited to treatment of airway compromise, or specific goals of relieving local compression that does not respond to medical treatment. An additional potential role for surgical intervention is to obtain tissue to establish a diagnosis with a core or open biopsy if required. The thyroid fibrosis is nonprogressive in most patients. Attempts at surgical resection in patients with stable compensated disease may be associated with increased complications, specifically postoperative hypoparathyroidism and injury to the recurrent laryngeal nerves. The surgical procedures that may be required in well-selected patients include tracheostomy or partial thyroid resection.

ACUTE SUPPURATIVE THYROIDITIS

General Considerations

Acute suppurative thyroiditis (AST) is an infection of the thyroid gland that progresses to an abscess. Suppurative thyroiditis is a rare condition that can be associated with significant morbidity and mortality if not correctly diagnosed and treated appropriately.[23] The disorder is a result of a local infection of the thyroid parenchyma that arises either in association with predisposing congenital anatomic defects, by direct extension of a soft tissue infection, or iatrogenic introduction of pathogens. Congenital defects involving direct connections between the aerodigestive tract and the thyroid gland account for the higher incidence of AST in children compared to adults. The essential features of its clinical presentation include fever, localized pain over the thyroid gland in the anterior neck, sore throat, pain with swallowing, and dysphagia. Fluctuance over the thyroid is uncommonly detected on exam, but key elements of the history including the presence of associated risk factors should alert the physician to the possibility of the diagnosis. Diagnostic imaging with ultrasound of the thyroid or computed tomography (CT) of the neck will detect the presence of an abscess, and culture of the abscess following aspiration or drainage establishes the diagnosis.

Pathogenesis & Risk Factors

Infections of the thyroid gland are very uncommon owing to a number of anatomic and physiologic factors. The thyroid gland is encapsulated and protected by dense cervical fascial planes that act as a physical barrier to local extension of soft tissue infections. The increased vascularity of the thyroid parenchyma, high iodine content, and extensive lymphatic drainage also make the gland relatively resistant to invasion and growth of pathogenic organisms. It is estimated that only 8% of cases of AST occur in adults, and suppurative thyroiditis due to bacterial pathogens accounts for less than 1% of thyroid diseases.[23]

In children, the presence of a piriform sinus fistula (PSF) associated with a third or fourth branchial arch anomaly predisposes to the occurrence of AST, especially on the left side of the neck. A fistulous tract resulting in direct communication from the piriform fossa in the pharynx to the thyroid gland provides a pathway for direct extension of bacterial pathogens. Piriform sinus tract anomalies are rare and can be difficult to diagnose due to a nonspecific presentation. Children with PSFs present with recurrent neck abscesses or suppurative thyroiditis, especially following an upper respiratory tract infection. While soft tissue infections or abscesses of the neck are common in children, PSFs are rarely the cause. Many children undergo incision and drainage of recurrent neck abscesses prior to establishing the eventual diagnosis of a PSF. Neonates may present with respiratory distress, stridor, dysphagia, or feeding difficulties due to tracheal compression from a neck abscess. The occurrence of recurrent left-sided anterior neck abscesses or identification of thyroid gland involvement on imaging suggests an underlying PSF. The diagnosis is confirmed by direct laryngoscopy or barium swallow.

Underlying thyroid conditions including HT, large goiter, or thyroid cancer[24] may predispose to the development of

AST in rare cases. Patients with an immunocompromised state due to systemic lupus erythematosus (SLE), HIV infection,[25] Hodgkin lymphoma, chemotherapy, or immunosuppressive medications following transplantation may be more vulnerable to AST. Although the most common pathogens cultured from patients with AST are *Staphylococcus aureus* and *Streptococci* species, other organisms may be causative in immunocompromised patients including *Mycobacterium tuberculosis* (especially HIV patients), *Candida*, *Escherichia coli*,[26] *Klebsiella*, *Acinetobacter*, and *Salmonella*.[27] Very infrequently, suppurative thyroid infection can be iatrogenic after FNA,[23,28] or AST may occur by direct lymphatic or hematogenous spread from a local or systemic process.[23]

Clinical & Radiographic Findings

AST can be diagnosed by the clinical history and physical exam findings, in conjunction with appropriate radiographic imaging tests. Patients who present with neck pain, fever, dysphagia, or anterior neck mass are often evaluated initially with ultrasound or cross-sectional imaging tests such as CT. The characteristic ultrasound findings in AST include ill-defined hypoechoic areas of low vascularization in the thyroid, particularly the left upper lobe which can be related to the piriform sinus. These findings can progress to a loculated abscess, or in more advanced cases may extend to more superficial anterior tissue planes of the neck or extend to a deep cervical space infection. Reactive enlarged regional lymph nodes are often seen. Contrast studies with esophagography, followed immediately with concomitant CT, have been shown to improve the success rate for the diagnosis of a PSF.[29,30] Confirmation of the diagnosis is usually made by direct endoscopic identification of the fistulous tract.

Patients with AST typically have fever and pain with swallowing, tachycardia, and mild systemic illness or malaise. The erythrocyte sedimentation rate (ESR) and C-reactive protein (CRP) are frequently elevated. A serum thyroglobulin level may be elevated but is not diagnostic. Patients with AST are commonly euthyroid. However, some patients are reported to have thyrotoxicosis due to bacterial invasion and destruction of thyroid parenchyma, while other patients demonstrate biochemical hypothyroidism. Aspiration of the thyroid or anterior neck abscess with culture of the pathogenic organism establishes the diagnosis and allows directed antimicrobial therapy.

Differential Diagnosis

The differential diagnosis for acute neck swelling and pain associated with the thyroid gland is broad and includes subacute thyroiditis, rapid growth from an aggressive thyroid cancer or lymphoma, infarction of a thyroid nodule, hemorrhagic thyroid cyst, amiodarone-induced thyrotoxicosis, or neck trauma. The presence of fever and neck pain on swallowing suggests the diagnosis of AST, particularly with recurrent left-sided anterior neck abscess in children which suggests the occurrence of a predisposing congenital anomaly of the third or fourth branchial pouch.

Treatment

A. Medical Therapy

The mainstay of initial treatment for patients with AST is source control with incision and drainage of the thyroid and surrounding soft tissue infection, culture of the abscess fluid and/or blood, and treatment with appropriate antibiotic therapy directed against the specific etiologic organisms. Adequate surgical drainage and effective antimicrobial treatment usually results in prompt clinical improvement. Extensive thyroid parenchyma destruction as a sequela of AST can result in permanent hypothyroidism. Delay in diagnosis and institution of effective treatment can result in severe illness and high mortality.

B. Surgical Treatment

Treatment of suppurative thyroiditis associated with a PSF and a neck abscess extending to the thyroid gland parenchyma involves initial source control with incision and drainage and appropriate antibiotic therapy.[31] The gold standard for control of the local soft tissue infection is prompt and adequate open surgical drainage. CT-guided drainage may be utilized for smaller localized abscesses as an initial step, but if the patient does not respond promptly, surgical drainage should be immediately undertaken. Inadequately drained thyroid abscesses can dissect into the retropharyngeal space or chest, and rupture into the esophagus or trachea in rare cases. Finally, progression to uncontrolled systemic sepsis can result in patient death. Surgical excision or endoscopic closure techniques are utilized for definitive management of fistulous tracts or PSFs.[32] Complete surgical removal of the sinus tract and a portion of the thyroid gland is typically curative and has been the conventional standard approach historically. Endoscopic treatment approaches including suture ligation, electrocautery, or chemo-cauterization followed by application of fibrin sealants[33] have also been described. Incomplete surgical excision can result in recurrence, and potential complications of treatment include injury to the recurrent laryngeal nerve or branches of the facial nerve, salivary fistulas, hemorrhage, and wound infection.

SUBACUTE THYROIDITIS

General Considerations

Subacute thyroiditis (de Quervain's or granulomatous) is a self-limiting, painful inflammatory disease of the thyroid gland resulting in transient thyrotoxicosis often followed by a transient phase of hypothyroidism. Historically the disease was first recognized in the early 19th century and was named after a Swiss surgeon de Quervain.[34] It is believed that viral infections are the triggering factors in genetically susceptible individuals with subsequent cytotoxic T-cell activation infiltrating the thyroid and causing a form of destructive thyroiditis with release of preformed thyroid hormones. The characteristic clinical features include anterior neck pain, fever, fatigue, and associated thyrotoxic symptoms such as palpitations and nervousness, which are usually self-limited, and recovery is expected within 1 to 3 months.

Clinically there is a very tender, firm thyroid gland on examination, and laboratory findings are typical of hyperthyroidism with suppressed TSH and normal or elevated free thyroid hormone levels. Inflammatory markers like ESR or CRP are usually elevated. RAIU scan shows diffusely low uptake, and ultrasonogram may show a dyshomogenous gland with decreased vascularity. NSAIDs or corticosteroids are commonly used to alleviate the pain, and beta blockers help reduce adrenergic symptoms and tachycardia.[35]

Pathogenesis & Risk Factors

Subacute thyroiditis is thought to be a viral or postviral inflammatory process with activation of cytotoxic T cells in genetically susceptible individuals. Many viruses like Coxsackie virus, Echoviruses, adenoviruses, influenza viruses, measles, mumps, rubella, parvovirus B19, orthomyxovirus, HIV, Hep B, and Hep E have been implicated in triggering the insult. Most recently numerous reports of SARS-CoV-2-associated subacute thyroiditis have been reported.[36] Genetic predisposition in individuals with HLA-B35 haplotypes has been confirmed in many studies and in a more recent study HLA-B 18*:01;HLA-DRB1*01;HLA-C*04:01 have been associated with subacute thyroiditis.[37]

The typical cytological characteristics are multinucleated giant cells, epithelioid cell granulomas, inflammatory cells, degenerated follicular epithelial cells, and the nomenclature "*giant cell thyroiditis*" or "*granulomatous thyroiditis*" are interchangeably used with de Quervain's or subacute thyroiditis.[34]

Subacute thyroiditis quite often presents in middle-aged persons, around 40 years, and like other autoimmune thyroid disorders has a higher female preponderance.

Clinical Features & Diagnosis

Subacute thyroiditis typically has a clinical course of an initial thyrotoxic phase followed by subsequent hypothyroidism and eventually returning to a euthyroid state and less commonly permanent hypothyroidism. The classic symptoms of neck pain radiating to the jaw, ears, and upper mediastinum are reported by majority of patients; however, painless forms of subacute thyroiditis have been described. Other nonspecific symptoms such as fever, malaise, dysphagia, and myalgias can be observed. Palpitations, weight loss, heat intolerance, nervousness, and other hyperthyroid symptoms are seen depending on the degree of thyrotoxicosis. Exophthalmos is generally absent and if present should raise the suspicion that the patient has Graves' disease rather than subacute thyroiditis.

Inflammatory markers ESR or CRP are generally elevated and thyroid function tests during the initial thyroiditis phase show a suppressed TSH and normal or elevated free thyroid hormone levels. More recently there has been a growing interest to look at other surrogate markers like neutrophil-lymphocyte ratio (NLR); platelet-lymphocyte ratio (PLR); monocyte-eosinophil ratio (Mo/Eo) combined with free T3 to free T4 ratio (fT3/fT4) to differentiate subacute thyroiditis from Graves' disease. It is postulated that these tests might be helpful when resources are limited or other diagnostic tests are not available.[36,38,39] Thyroid antibodies were thought to be typically absent in subacute thyroiditis, but more recent studies have shown that thyroid peroxidase antibodies (anti-TPO) and thyroglobulin antibodies (Tg antibodies) can be seen in one-third of patients and coexistence of TRAB has been demonstrated in a minor fraction. It is postulated that some patients may have underlying autoimmune thyroid disease or the release of thyroglobulin likely triggers an antigenic response.[36,40]

I-123 radioactive iodine uptake and scan shows a diffusely low uptake and is a valuable tool to differentiate subacute thyroiditis from Graves' disease or a toxic nodular goiter. Ultrasonography findings of a heterogenous gland with hypoechogenicity and decreased vascularity are typical. Fine-needle aspiration biopsy (FNAB) is usually not indicated but sometimes the clinical presentation of subacute thyroiditis may be similar to that of primary thyroid malignancies (anaplastic thyroid cancer), nonthyroid malignancies with metastases to the thyroid, or amyloidosis infiltrating the thyroid. However, these presentations are very rare and FNAB can be considered in selected cases when the diagnosis is inconclusive or there is suspicion for other etiologies.[41,42]

Differential Diagnosis

The differential diagnosis of anterior neck pain and fever is broad. In addition to subacute thyroiditis, the clinician needs to consider suppurative thyroiditis, infarction or hemorrhage into a thyroid nodule or cyst, and aggressive malignancies. Suppurative thyroiditis presents with fever, neck pain, tenderness, elevated inflammatory markers, and ultrasonographic findings of a localized pus collection which can help differentiate this from subacute thyroiditis. Graves' disease, toxic nodular goiter can present with thyrotoxicosis and rarely compressive symptoms from a goiter. A high radioactive iodine uptake, distribution of iodine on a scan, increased vascularity on ultrasonography, and positive TSI/TRAB antibodies are useful in differentiating these problems from subacute thyroiditis. Anaplastic thyroid cancer or metastases from other cancers can mimic the clinical picture of subacute thyroiditis and an ultrasonogram of the thyroid is useful in distinguishing these from the more benign subacute thyroiditis. FNAB can be obtained in doubtful cases.[41] Ultrasonogram of the thyroid is a noninvasive, safe, and effective modality which is very helpful to rule out other serious conditions.

Treatment

Subacute thyroiditis is a self-limited disease with mild thyrotoxic phase lasting for approximately 2 to 8 weeks followed by hypothyroid phase which may last up to 6 months. Most of the patients regain normal thyroid function by the end of 1 year but about 5% to 15% may develop permanent hypothyroidism. Recurrence rates of 1% to 4% have been reported.[43] NSAIDs are typically used for pain control and resolution of pain is expected within 5 weeks. With more severe presentations or in patient's refractory to NSAIDs, corticosteroids are found to be very effective and usually provide relief within 2 weeks. If corticosteroids are required, the general recommendations are to use prednisone 40 mg/day for 1 to 2 weeks followed by a gradual taper over 2 to 4 weeks depending on clinical response. Levothyroxine may be used during the hypothyroid phase but a trial off medication should be tried in 3 to 6 months to assess if there has been spontaneous recovery of the thyroid function.

DRUG-INDUCED THYROIDITIS

General Considerations

Several drugs are known to cause thyroid dysfunction and the association of thyroid dysfunction with medications like lithium, amiodarone, interferon alfa, interleukin 2, and iodinated contrast agents is well established. Emerging cancer drugs, especially tyrosine kinase inhibitors and immune checkpoint inhibitors, have been consistently shown to be associated with thyroid dysfunction. Amiodarone can cause hypothyroidism and two distinctive types of thyrotoxicosis—amiodarone-induced thyrotoxicosis (AIT) Type 1 which is autoimmune mediated and Type 2 which is a form of destructive thyroiditis.

Treatment is usually supportive and the risks of discontinuing the offending agent should be weighed against the benefits of continuing the drug for the preexistent condition.[44,45]

A brief list of drugs causing thyroiditis is presented in Table 11–3.

Table 11–3. Drugs causing thyroiditis and thyroid dysfunction.

Drugs	Mechanism/Type of Thyroid Dysfunction
Amiodarone	Iodine-induced hyperthyroidism or destructive thyroiditis
Immune checkpoint inhibitors PD-1 inhibitors • Nivolumab (Opdivo) • Pembrolizumab (Keytruda) • Cemiplimab (Libtayo) PD-L1 inhibitors • Atezolizumab (Tecentriq) • Avelumab (Bavencio) • Durvalumab (Imfinzi) CTLA-4 inhibitors • Ipilimumab	Destructive thyroiditis or immune induced
Interferon-alpha	Immune effects and direct cytotoxic effects
Interleukin	Induces lymphoid thyroiditis
Lithium	Hypothyroidism is more common but hyperthyroidism can occur
Tyrosine kinase inhibitors Sunitinib (Sutent) Sorafenib (Nexavar)	Destructive thyroiditis Likely a class effect

Pathogenesis & Risk Factors

A. Amiodarone

Amiodarone is a Class III antiarrhythmic agent which is widely prescribed in the management of atrial and ventricular arrhythmias. It is rich in iodine; each 200 mg tablet contains 75 mg of iodine providing approximately 20 times the daily iodine content found in the average American diet. Amiodarone is lipophilic and has long half-life of approximately 60 to 142 days which explains the long-lasting effects even after discontinuation of the drug. It reduces the conversion of T4 to T3 by inhibiting the deiodinase enzymes, inhibits the binding of T3 to nuclear receptors, and is known to be directly cytotoxic to thyroid follicular cells. All these combined effects contribute to the various forms of thyroid dysfunction seen with amiodarone (Table 11–4).[46]

Amiodarone-induced thyroid dysfunction can be broadly classified as follows:

(a) Amiodarone-induced hypothyroidism
(b) Amiodarone-induced thyrotoxicosis (AIT)
    i. Amiodarone-induced thyrotoxicosis Type 1 (due to excess thyroid hormone synthesis)
    ii. Amiodarone-induced thyrotoxicosis Type 2 (destructive thyroiditis)

It is important to understand the pathophysiology and attain a diagnosis of the type of AIT to provide appropriate treatment.

1. Amiodarone-induced hypothyroidism (AIH)—AIH has a female preponderance (female to male: 1.5:1), and a higher

Table 11–4 Characteristics of amiodarone-induced thyrotoxicosis (AIT).

	Type 1 AIT	Type 2 AIT
Pathogenesis	Iodine-induced thyrotoxicosis	Destructive thyroiditis
Time of onset	3.5 months	30 months
Goiter	Diffuse or nodular	Sometimes small firm goiter
Thyroid antibodies	TSI or TRAB may be present	Generally absent
Radioactive iodine uptake	Low or normal	Low or absent
CFDS	High vascularity	Decreased vascularity
^{99m}Tc-sestamibi	High uptake	Low uptake
Treatment	Methimazole	Corticosteroids
Subsequent hypothyroidism	Unlikely	Likely

CFDS = color flow doppler study; ^{99m}Tc-sestamibi = technetium 99m sestamibi scintigraphy; TRAB = Thyrotropin receptor antibody; TSI = Thyroid-stimulating immunoglobulin.

prevalence in patients with an underlying autoimmune thyroid disease and those who live in iodine-deficient areas. The median time of onset of hypothyroidism is generally within 3 months (10%-20% of cases); however, a late presentation of up to 1 year has been reported in 5% to 10% of cases.[46] Iodine overload inhibits the physiologic thyroid iodine organification, thereby diminishing hormone synthesis, a phenomenon referred to as the Wolff-Chaikoff effect. A normal thyroid gland would usually have an escape phenomenon and resumes normal thyroid hormone synthesis in few days to weeks, but in patients with thyroid autoimmunity, there is failure to escape from the Wolff-Chaikoff effect which results in hypothyroidism.[45,46] Lab findings show elevated TSH and normal or low free thyroid hormone levels.

2. Type 1 Amiodarone-induced thyrotoxicosis (Type 1 AIT)—Type 1 AIT is due to increased thyroid hormone synthesis. Subjects with underlying predisposition to autonomous thyroid function like Graves' disease or toxic multinodular goiter are more susceptible and there is a higher prevalence in areas with iodine deficiency. The excess iodine load from amiodarone serves as a substrate which results in overproduction of thyroid hormones, a phenomenon referred to as the Jod-Basedow effect. Although the median time of onset of amiodarone-induced thyrotoxicosis is unpredictable, one retrospective study showed a median time of 3.5 months for Type 1 AIT compared to 30 months for Type 2 AIT, from the time of initiation of amiodarone.[47]

3. Type 2 Amiodarone-induced thyrotoxicosis (Type 2 AIT)—Type 2 AIT is a destructive form of thyroiditis which is believed to be due to direct cytotoxic effect of amiodarone resulting in the release of preformed thyroid hormones. It can occur months to years after amiodarone initiation or even after discontinuation of the drug and the natural course of disease either results in permanent hypothyroidism or restoration of euthyroid state. Type 2 AIT is more common than Type 1. A mixed Type 1 and Type 2 form can be seen in a subset of patients which leads to diagnostic and therapeutic challenges.

Clinical Findings & Diagnosis

Patients with amiodarone-induced hypothyroidism may remain asymptomatic or present with hypothyroid symptoms depending on the degree of hypothyroidism. Amiodarone has antiadrenergic activity and prevents the conversion of T4 to T3, so the classic symptoms of thyrotoxicosis may not be evident and patients may exhibit apathetic thyrotoxicosis. Unexplained weight loss, heat intolerance, new onset, or exacerbation of preexisting arrhythmias, angina, or heart failure should raise the clinical suspicion for AIT. Goiter or neck pain may or may not be present. Orbitopathy is usually absent and if noted, the patient likely has underlying Graves' disease.

Laboratory results may show overt or subclinical hyperthyroidism with suppressed TSH and elevated or normal free thyroid hormone levels. It is especially important to differentiate Type 1 AIT from Type 2 AIT as the management and clinical course of each condition is different, but it can be challenging as sometimes both forms may coexist, or the distinction may not be obvious. Thyroid-stimulating antibodies (TSI) or TRAB should be checked and if positive are more suggestive of a Type 1 AIT. Inflammatory markers like CRP and IL-6 have been studied but found to have limited clinical utility. Radioactive iodine uptake scan *with I-123* or *Tc99 Pertechnetate scan* does not readily differentiate Type 1 or Type 2 AIT as the uptake is low in both conditions. *99m Tc-sestamibi* scan has reportedly shown some promising results but the number of patients studied was small and large studies are needed for further validation.[48] Color flow Doppler sonography (CFDS) is a safe, noninvasive modality and provides real-time assessment of thyroid vascularity. CFDS is the preferred investigation to differentiate Type 1 AIT from Type 2 AIT, with the former showing increased vascularity and the latter decreased or no vascularity.[49]

Treatment

A. Amiodarone-Induced Hypothyroidism

Treatment is usually straightforward with levothyroxine replacement. Amiodarone need not be stopped as it has long half-life and effects of the drug persist even after discontinuation. If it is stopped, the thyroid function tests may need to be monitored closely as it can be reversible in some patients.

B. Type 1 Amiodarone-Induced Thyrotoxicosis (Type 1 AIT)

Type 1 AIT is due to increased production of thyroid hormone and thionamides are the drug of choice. Thionamides (methimazole, propylthiouracil, carbimazole) work by inhibiting thyroid peroxidase enzyme and decrease thyroid hormone synthesis. High doses of methimazole up to 40 to 60 mg a day are usually needed. Propylthiouracil can also be used but is more hepatotoxic and methimazole is the preferred drug. Amiodarone has a long half-life and even if the drug were to be stopped, the effects can last up to a year. Beta-blockers are indicated to counteract the hyperadrenergic state of thyrotoxicosis.

In refractory cases, sodium or potassium perchlorate, which blocks the sodium/iodine symporter and further transport of iodine into thyroid gland, may be used. But perchlorate is highly toxic and can cause agranulocytosis, aplastic anemia, and nephrotic syndrome. Potassium perchlorate is currently unavailable in the United States.[45] Lithium blocks release of T4 and T3 and inhibits coupling of iodotyrosine residues to form T4 and T3. Lithium has been used in small number of patients but has a narrow therapeutic index and use is limited due to the associated toxicities.

C. Type 2 Amiodarone-Induced Thyrotoxicosis (Type 2 AIT)

Type 2 AIT is due to destruction of thyroid gland and the release of preformed thyroid hormones, so thionamides have limited utility in treatment. Glucocorticoids in high doses inhibit deiodinases, have anti-inflammatory and membrane-stabilizing effects. Prednisone in doses of 40 to 60 mg/day is recommended and may need to be continued for 1 to 3 months. A small subset of patients may have overlapping features of Type 1 AIT and Type 2 AIT, or it may be difficult to differentiate between the two types. Combined therapy with thionamides and glucocorticoids is usually preferred in such scenarios.

Plasmapheresis can be used in cases refractory to medical management.

Surgical Treatment

Total thyroidectomy can be considered in patients who fail to respond to aggressive medical therapy, have severe underlying cardiac disease, very low ejection fraction, or if there is a progressive deterioration of cardiac function.[50,51]

A recent retrospective study by a group in Italy compared the mortality rates of surgical versus medical therapy in patients with AIT and reduced ejection fraction (EF). The subgroup with moderate to severely reduced EF who underwent surgery had a lower mortality rate as compared to those who were medically managed but the same was not observed in patients with normal or mildly reduced EF suggesting total thyroidectomy could be considered as a therapeutic choice in patients with severe systolic dysfunction.[52]

The decision to operate on patients with serious underlying cardiac disease who are also thyrotoxic is quite complex. In challenging cases of amiodarone-induced thyrotoxicosis, a multidisciplinary approach involving cardiologist, endocrinologist, and a thyroid surgeon should be considered for achieving best possible outcomes.

Tyrosine Kinase Inhibitors & Immune Checkpoint Inhibitors

Immune checkpoint inhibitors (ICPi) are being increasingly used to treat many cancers with promising results, and thyroid dysfunction is one of the most commonly reported ICPi-related endocrinopathy. Thyroid dysfunction is relatively more common with anti-PD-1 agents such as nivolumab and pembrolizumab or in combination with ipilimumab (anti-CTLA4).[53,54] Tyrosine kinase inhibitors have also been shown to be increasingly associated with thyroid dysfunction. Destructive thyroiditis with transient thyrotoxicosis has been reported to be the most common pathology.[55]

Treatment

The thyroid dysfunction associated with drugs is usually transient with mild thyrotoxicosis and symptomatic management with beta-blockers is helpful. Levothyroxine replacement is recommended if patient develops permanent hypothyroidism. As the symptoms are usually mild and transitory, discontinuation of the lifesaving drug is not recommended and close collaboration between endocrinologists and oncologists is needed to make critical decisions.

POSTPARTUM THYROIDITIS

General Considerations

Postpartum thyroiditis (PPT) is defined as the occurrence of autoimmune thyroid dysfunction, excluding Graves' disease, in the first year after pregnancy or miscarriage in a previously euthyroid women.[56,57] The reported prevalence varies markedly from 1.1% to 16.7%; a higher risk is seen in women with other autoimmune diseases; for example, the prevalence is 3 to 4 times higher in women with type 1 diabetes mellitus.[56-58] PPT is an autoimmune disease and almost all the affected women have thyroid autoantibodies—either thyroid peroxidase antibodies (Anti-TPO) and or thyroglobulin antibodies. The clinical presentation of PPT is often subtle depending on the severity of thyroid dysfunction and some of the symptoms could easily be attributed to the stress of being a mother with a newborn child. In its classic form, an initial transient thyrotoxic phase develops 1 to 3 months postpartum, lasting for 2 to 3 months followed by a transient hypothyroid phase and return to euthyroid state by the end of 1 year. However, 20% to 30% of women who experience the hypothyroid phase may not return to the euthyroid state.[58,59]

Pathogenesis & Factors

PPT is an autoimmune disease with majority of patients being positive for thyroid antibodies (TPO antibodies and/or thyroglobulin antibodies). As compared to general population, women with positive TPO antibodies have 33% to 50% chance of developing PPT and a higher TPO titer is associated with much greater risk.[58] Women with other autoimmune disease such as lupus, type1 diabetes, chronic viral hepatitis, and multiple sclerosis were also observed to be at an increased risk.[59] Pregnancy is a relatively immunosuppressed state and the rebound of selective immunogenicity in the postpartum period contributes to the exacerbation of autoimmune thyroid disease. Histologically a lymphocyte predominance like HT has been described. An initial destructive phase by infiltrating lymphocytes leads to the release of preformed thyroid hormones followed by either a transient or permanent fall in thyroid hormone synthesis.[58,60]

Clinical Findings

A. Symptoms & Signs

The classic presentation of PPT is transient thyrotoxicosis (2-6 months postpartum) followed by a transient hypothyroid phase (3-12 months postpartum) with either complete recovery back to a euthyroid state or permanent hypothyroidism. The initial hyperthyroid phase may be subtle and go unrecognized or realized retrospectively when patients present with hypothyroidism. Symptoms are often mild and most frequently reported symptoms include fatigue, heat intolerance, palpitations, nervousness, and irritability. Neck pain or tenderness is usually absent. Clinical examination may reveal tachycardia, elevated blood pressure, brisk tendon reflexes, and other signs of hyperthyroidism. PPT is not associated with orbitopathy, and any findings of eye disease should raise the suspicion for Graves' disease.

In the hypothyroid phase, fatigue, generalized aches, dry skin, impaired concentration or memory, depression, cold intolerance, or mood changes are frequently reported. Breastfeeding can be affected in the hyper- or hypothyroid phase.[58,59,61] Bradycardia, delayed relaxation of tendon reflexes, and other signs of hypothyroidism may be elucidated clinically.

Laboratory Findings & Imaging Studies

Thyroid function tests obtained in the hyperthyroid phase would show suppressed TSH and normal or elevated free T4/free T3 levels depending on the degree of thyrotoxicosis. TPO antibodies are positive in the majority of patients and thyroglobulin antibodies may also be positive. TSI or TRAB should be obtained to rule out Graves' disease. Imaging studies are rarely indicated and should be obtained only if the diagnosis is uncertain from clinical history and physical exam. RAIU is not advisable in breastfeeding women but if obtained, nursing should be avoided for 2 to 3 days.[56] RAIU scan would show a very low iodine uptake. ^{123}I has lower radiation exposure and is preferred over ^{131}I for radioactive uptake scan. Systemic markers of inflammation like ESR are usually normal and not indicated. In the hypothyroid phase, elevated TSH and normal or low free thyroid hormone levels are seen.

Differential Diagnosis

Graves' disease may recur in the postpartum period, but the degree of hyperthyroidism is usually more severe. Orbitopathy if noted on clinical examination is pathognomonic of Graves' disease and it is essential to rule it out as the management is different. Hyperthyroidism due to any other pathology such as toxic nodule, drug-induced thyroiditis, and painful thyroiditis should be ruled out based on clinical history and exam. Studies looking at the association between postpartum thyroid dysfunction and depression have yielded mixed results, but it is reasonable to obtain thyroid function tests in postpartum women with depressive symptoms.[56,58]

Treatment

A. Medical Therapy

The thyrotoxic phase is transient, symptoms are usually mild, and treatment is often not required. In patients with bothersome symptoms, beta-blockers (propranolol 10-20 mg q 6 h) can be used to alleviate the adrenergic symptoms and titrated based on the severity of symptoms. The thyrotoxicosis is due to the release of preformed hormones and thionamides are not indicated. As it is a transient phase, radioactive iodine treatment or surgery should be avoided. Levothyroxine if initiated for severe and symptomatic hypothyroidism should be reassessed with repeat labs in 3 to 6 months to see if there is any recovery.

OTHER RARE FORMS OF THYROIDITIS

Palpation Thyroiditis

Palpation thyroiditis refers to the transient hyperthyroidism following surgical manipulation or direct trauma to the normal thyroid gland. Mostly documented in patients following parathyroidectomy, it can also occur following blunt trauma to the anterior cervical region, strangulation, and vigorous palpation of the thyroid gland. Thyrotoxicosis is usually transient and beta blockers can be used for symptomatic management.[62,63]

Radiation Thyroiditis

Radioactive iodine treatment used for thyroid ablation in Graves' disease or thyroid cancer can cause radiation thyroiditis. High doses of ^{131}I used for remnant ablation of thyroid cancer can cause radiation thyroiditis but case reports following treatment of Graves' disease have been documented. Radiation thyroiditis is usually self-limited; neck pain being the commonly reported symptom usually responds to NSAIDs. A short course of corticosteroids can be used in refractory cases.[64]

REFERENCES

1. Zala A, Berhane T, Juhlin CC, Calissendorff J, Falhammar H. Riedel thyroiditis. *J Clin Endocrinol Metab*. 2020;105(9): dgaa468.
2. Ragusa F, Fallahi P, Elia G, et al. Hashimotos' thyroiditis: epidemiology, pathogenesis, clinic and therapy. *Best Pract Res Clin Endocrinol Metab*. 2019;33(6):101367.
3. Ralli M, Angeletti D, Fiore M, et al. Hashimoto's thyroiditis: an update on pathogenic mechanisms, diagnostic protocols, therapeutic strategies, and potential malignant transformation. *Autoimmun Rev*. 2020;19(10):102649.
4. Peng CC, Huai-En Chang R, Pennant M, Huang HK, Munir KM. A literature review of painful Hashimoto thyroiditis: 70 published cases in the past 70 years. *J Endocr Soc*. 2020;4(2):bvz008.
5. Rotondi M, Capelli V, Locantore P, Pontecorvi A, Chiovato L. Painful Hashimoto's thyroiditis: myth or reality? *J Endocrinol Invest*. 2017;40(8):815-818.
6. Hu Y, Zhang L, Chen H, et al. Analysis of regulatory T cell subsets and their expression of helios and PD-1 in patients with Hashimoto thyroiditis. *Int J Endocrinol*. 2019;2019:5368473.
7. Alvarez-Sierra D, Marin-Sanchez A, Ruiz-Blazquez P, et al. Analysis of the PD-1/PD-L1 axis in human autoimmune thyroid disease: insights into pathogenesis and clues to immunotherapy associated thyroid autoimmunity. *J Autoimmun*. 2019;103:102285.
8. Harvey AM, Truong LD, Mody DR. Diagnostic pitfalls of Hashimoto's/lymphocytic thyroiditis on fine-needle aspirations and strategies to avoid overdiagnosis. *Acta Cytol*. 2012;56(4):352-360.
9. Sharma A, Stan MN. Thyrotoxicosis: diagnosis and management. *Mayo Clin Proc*. 2019;94(6):1048-1064.
10. Gan T, Randle RW. The role of surgery in autoimmune conditions of the thyroid. *Surg Clin North Am*. 2019;99(4):633-648.
11. Djurovic M, Pereira AM, Smit JWA, et al. Cognitive functioning and quality of life in patients with Hashimoto thyroiditis on long-term levothyroxine replacement. *Endocrine*. 2018;62(1):136-143.
12. Guldvog I, Reitsma LC, Johnsen L, et al. Thyroidectomy versus medical management for euthyroid patients with Hashimoto disease and persisting symptoms: a randomized trial. *Ann Intern Med*. 2019;170(7):453-464.
13. Ollila TA, Olszewski AJ. Extranodal diffuse large B cell lymphoma: molecular features, prognosis, and risk of central nervous system recurrence. *Curr Treat Options Oncol*. 2018;19(8):38.
14. Stein SA, Wartofsky L. Primary thyroid lymphoma: a clinical review. *J Clin Endocrinol Metab*. 2013;98(8):3131-3138.
15. Falhammar H, Juhlin CC, Barner C, Catrina SB, Karefylakis C, Calissendorff J. Riedel's thyroiditis: clinical presentation, treatment and outcomes. *Endocrine*. 2018;60(1):185-192.
16. Stan MN, Sonawane V, Sebo TJ, Thapa P, Bahn RS. Riedel's thyroiditis association with IgG4-related disease. *Clin Endocrinol*. 2017;86(3):425-430.
17. Maehara T, Moriyama M, Nakamura S. Pathogenesis of IgG4-related disease: a critical review. *Odontology*. 2019;107(2):127-132.
18. Fatourechi MM, Hay ID, McIver B, Sebo TJ, Fatourechi V. Invasive fibrous thyroiditis (Riedel thyroiditis): the Mayo Clinic experience, 1976-2008. *Thyroid*. 2011;21(7):765-772.
19. Mansberg R, Bency R, Shen L, Bui C, Park K. Riedel's thyroiditis with intense FDG uptake demonstrated on FDG PET/CT. *Mol Imaging Radionucl Ther*. 2015;24(1):29-31.
20. Kumar N, Gupta R, Sayed S, Moloo Z, Vinayak S, Ahmed M. Difficulties in diagnosis of Riedel's thyroiditis on aspiration cytology: a case report and brief review of the literature. *Diagn Cytopathol*. 2019;47(5):512-516.
21. Hsieh SC, Shen CY, Liao HT, et al. The cellular and molecular bases of allergy, inflammation and tissue fibrosis in patients with IgG4-related disease. *Int J Mol Sci*. 2020;21(14):5082.
22. De Leo S, Trevisan M, Fugazzola L. Recent advances in the management of anaplastic thyroid cancer. *Thyroid Res*. 2020; 13(1):17.
23. Falhammar H, Wallin G, Calissendorff J. Acute suppurative thyroiditis with thyroid abscess in adults: clinical presentation, treatment and outcomes. *BMC Endocr Disord*. 2019; 19(1):130.
24. Otani H, Notsu M, Koike S, et al. Acute suppurative thyroiditis caused by thyroid papillary carcinoma in the right thyroid lobe of a healthy woman. *Thyroid Res*. 2018;11:4.
25. Yedla N, Pirela D, Manzano A, Tuda C, Lo Presti S. Thyroid abscess: challenges in diagnosis and management. *J Investig Med High Impact Case Rep*. 2018;6:2324709618778709.
26. Siddiqui N, Deletic N, Raal F, Mohamed F. Acute suppurative thyroiditis secondary to *Escherichia coli* infection. *Eur J Case Rep Intern Med*. 2021;8(11):003009.
27. Khoo KS, Koh PS, Ng KL. Salmonella thyroid abscess-two case reports. *Gland Surg*. 2020;9(6):2198-2203.
28. Htet ZW, Tai ES, Yang SP. Acute bacterial suppurative thyroiditis following fine needle aspiration: a case report and review of the literature. *Case Rep Endocrinol*. 2020;2020:7104806.
29. Chen T, Ge G, Chen J, et al. Pyriform sinus fistula in children: preferred imaging modality and risk factors for diagnostic delay. *Front Pediatr*. 2020;8:575812.
30. Pan J, Zou Y, Li L, Yang TY, Yang JL, Hu C. Clinical and imaging differences between neonates and children with pyriform sinus fistula: which is preferred for diagnosis, computed tomography, or barium esophagography? *J Pediatr Surg*. 2017;52(11):1878-1881.
31. Josephson GD, Black K. A review over the past 15 years of the management of the internal piriform apex sinus tract of a branchial pouch anomaly and case description. *Ann Otol Rhinol Laryngol*. 2015;124(12):947-952.
32. Zhao L, Chen L, Li W, Ni K, Chen W, Li X. Retrospective review of 70 cases of pyriform sinus fistula. *Int J Pediatr Otorhinolaryngol*. 2021;150:110904.
33. Chen W, Chen J, Chen F, et al. Endoscopic coblation treatment for congenital pyriform sinus fistula in children. *Medicine*. 2021;100(19):e25942.
34. Lamichaney R, Sherpa M, Das D, Bhutia CT, Laishram S. Fine-needle aspiration of de Quervain's thyroiditis

(subacute granulomatous thyroiditis): a cytological review of 20 cases. *J Clin Diagn Res.* 2017;11(8):EC09-EC11.
35. Sharma A, Stan MN. Thyrotoxicosis: diagnosis and management. *Mayo Clin Proc.* 2019;94(6):1048-1064.
36. Brancatella A, Ricci D, Viola N, Sgro D, Santini F, Latrofa F. Subacute thyroiditis after Sars-COV-2 infection. *J Clin Endocrinol Metab.* 2020;105(7):dgaa276.
37. Stasiak M, Tymoniuk B, Michalak R, Stasiak B, Kowalski ML, Lewinski A. Subacute thyroiditis is associated with HLA-B*18:01, -DRB1*01 and -C*04:01—the significance of the new molecular background. *J Clin Med.* 2020;9(2):534-541.
38. Calapkulu M, Sencar ME, Sakiz D, et al. The prognostic and diagnostic use of hematological parameters in subacute thyroiditis patients. *Endocrine.* 2020;68(1):138-143.
39. Cengiz H, Varim C, Demirci T, Cetin S. Hemogram parameters in the patients with subacute thyroiditis. *Pak J Med Sci.* 2020;36(2):240-245.
40. Stasiak M, Michalak R, Stasiak B, Lewinski A. Clinical characteristics of subacute thyroiditis is different than it used to be: current state based on 15 years own material. *Neuro Endocrinol Lett.* 2019;39(7):489-495.
41. Jonklaas J. Infiltration of the thyroid gland by non-thyroid malignancy: a literature review reveals this to be an unusual cause of hyperthyroidism. *J Clin Transl Endocrinol.* 2020;20:100221.
42. Stasiak M, Michalak R, Lewinski A. Thyroid primary and metastatic malignant tumours of poor prognosis may mimic subacute thyroiditis—time to change the diagnostic criteria: case reports and a review of the literature. *BMC Endocr Disord.* 2019;19(1):86.
43. Alexander EK, Pearce EN, Brent GA, et al. 2017 Guidelines of the American Thyroid Association for the diagnosis and management of thyroid disease during pregnancy and the postpartum. *Thyroid.* 2017;27(3):315-389.
44. Sharma A, Stan MN. Thyrotoxicosis: diagnosis and management. *Mayo Clin Proc.* 2019;94(6):1048-1064.
45. Trohman RG, Sharma PS, McAninch EA, Bianco AC. Amiodarone and thyroid physiology, pathophysiology, diagnosis and management. *Trends Cardiovasc Med.* 2019;29(5):285-295.
46. Ylli D, Wartofsky L, Burman KD. Evaluation and treatment of amiodarone-induced thyroid disorders. *J Clin Endocrinol Metab.* 2021;106(1):226-236.
47. Tomisti L, Rossi G, Bartalena L, Martino E, Bogazzi F. The onset time of amiodarone-induced thyrotoxicosis (AIT) depends on AIT type. *Eur J Endocrinol.* 2014;171(3):363-368.
48. Wang J, Zhang R. Evaluation of (99m)Tc-MIBI in thyroid gland imaging for the diagnosis of amiodarone-induced thyrotoxicosis. *Br J Radiol.* 2017;90(1071):20160836.
49. Theodoraki A, Vanderpump MPJ. Thyrotoxicosis associated with the use of amiodarone: the utility of ultrasound in patient management. *Clin Endocrinol.* 2016;84(2):172-176.
50. Bartalena L, Bogazzi F, Chiovato L, Hubalewska-Dydejczyk A, Links TP, Vanderpump M. 2018 European Thyroid Association (ETA) guidelines for the management of amiodarone-associated thyroid dysfunction. *Eur Thyroid J.* 2018;7(2):55-66.
51. Ross DS, Burch HB, Cooper DS, et al. 2016 American Thyroid Association guidelines for diagnosis and management of hyperthyroidism and other causes of thyrotoxicosis. *Thyroid.* 2016;26(10):1343-1421.
52. Cappellani D, Papini P, Pingitore A, et al. Comparison between total thyroidectomy and medical therapy for amiodarone-induced thyrotoxicosis. *J Clin Endocrinol Metab.* 2020;105(1):dgz041.
53. Chang LS, Barroso-Sousa R, Tolaney SM, Hodi FS, Kaiser UB, Min L. Endocrine toxicity of cancer immunotherapy targeting immune checkpoints. *Endocr Rev.* 2019;40(1):17-65.
54. Elia G, Ferrari SM, Galdiero MR, et al. New insight in endocrine-related adverse events associated to immune checkpoint blockade. *Best Pract Res Clin Endocrinol Metab.* 2020;34(1):101370.
55. Makita N, Iiri T. Tyrosine kinase inhibitor-induced thyroid disorders: a review and hypothesis. *Thyroid.* 2013;23(2): 151-159.
56. Nguyen CT, Mestman JH. Postpartum thyroiditis. *Clin Obstet Gynecol.* 2019;62(2):359-364.
57. Alexander EK, Pearce EN, Brent GA, et al. 2017 Guidelines of the American thyroid association for the diagnosis and management of thyroid disease during pregnancy and the postpartum. *Thyroid.* 2017;27(3):315-389.
58. Stagnaro-Green A. Approach to the patient with postpartum thyroiditis. *J Clin Endocrinol Metab.* 2012;97(2):334-342.
59. Epp R, Malcolm J, Jolin-Dahel K, Clermont M, Keely E. Postpartum thyroiditis. *BMJ.* 2021;372:n495.
60. Moleti M, Mauro MD, Alibrandi A, Vita R, Benvenga S, Vermiglio F. Postpartum thyroiditis in women with euthyroid and hypothyroid Hashimoto's thyroiditis antedating pregnancy. *J Clin Endocrinol Metab.* 2020;105(7):dgaa197.
61. Di Bari F, Granese R, Le Donne M, Vita R, Benvenga S. Autoimmune abnormalities of postpartum thyroid diseases. *Front Endocrinol.* 2017;8:166.
62. Ross DS, Burch HB, Cooper DS, et al. 2016 American Thyroid Association guidelines for diagnosis and management of hyperthyroidism and other causes of thyrotoxicosis. *Thyroid.* 2016;26(10):1343-1421.
63. Yatavelli RK, Levine SN. Transient hyperthyroidism induced by thyroid ultrasound. *Ann Otol Rhinol Laryngol.* 2018;127(8):558-562.
64. Mizokami T, Hamada K, Maruta T, Higashi K, Tajiri J. Painful radiation thyroiditis after (131)I therapy for Graves' hyperthyroidism: clinical features and ultrasonographic findings in five cases. *Eur Thyroid J.* 2016;5(3):201-206.

Follicular Thyroid Adenoma & Hürthle Cell Adenoma

12

Amanda R. Doubleday, DO, MBA
Alexander S. Chiu, MD
Rebecca S. Sippel, MD

INTRODUCTION

Thyroid nodules are very common in the adult population and most are asymptomatic. According to some autopsy reports, nodules have been found in almost 50% of examinations in otherwise asymptomatic patients. The American Thyroid Association defines a thyroid nodule as a lesion that is discretely separate from the surrounding parenchyma by either palpable or sonographic evidence. Incidental thyroid nodules have been found more frequently over the last few decades due to an overall increase in imaging studies, while the mortality from these nodules has not significantly changed. Over 80% of thyroid nodules are benign and the majority of thyroid nodules arise from the follicular cell of the thyroid gland. Risk factors for developing a thyroid nodule include older age, radiation exposure (particularly to the head and neck), and iodine deficiency.[1,2] This chapter will discuss two types of benign thyroid nodules, follicular adenomas and Hürthle cell adenomas, both of which have malignant counterparts. The following sections will highlight recognition of these nodules, appropriate workup, and the recommended treatment and surveillance approaches.

CLINICAL PATHOPHYSIOLOGY

Anatomy & Physiology

The thyroid gland is a midline structure in the neck that primarily makes thyroid hormone, a vital hormone for almost every organ system's function in the body. Thyroid hormone is made and stored in follicular cells, which form a single-cell layer in a circular pattern to create a follicle. These follicles encircle colloid where thyroglobulin (TG) is stored, an important protein needed in the synthesis of thyroid hormone. The remainder of the thyroid glandular tissue between follicles contains parafollicular cells (C cells) which secrete calcitonin, connective tissue, nerves, and blood vessels (Figure 12–1).[3]

The hypothalamus makes and secretes thyroid-releasing hormone which will stimulate the anterior pituitary to make and secrete thyroid-stimulating hormone (TSH). TSH will stimulate the thyroid follicular cells to produce and release thyroid hormones by binding to a TSH receptor. Approximately 80% of the hormone released from the follicular cells of the thyroid gland is in the form of thyroxine (T4) and approximately 20% triiodothyronine (T3). Thyroid hormone production requires TSH stimulation, the building block of TG, and iodine molecules. Thyroxine contains four iodine molecules while triiodothyronine contains three iodine molecules (Figure 12–2). Once T4 and T3 are in circulation and in particular cells, deiodination occurs converting T4 to T3, the more biologically active form of thyroid hormone. Each hormone can exert negative feedback on its stimulant, thus creating the hypothalamic-pituitary-thyroid axis. Different thyroid pathology includes developmental anomalies, functional abnormalities such as a hyper- or hypothyroid state, thyroiditis from many different etiologies, or the development of either functional or nonfunctional, benign or malignant nodules.[2]

Etiology

The follicular cells of the thyroid are most commonly the source of thyroid nodules, which are four times more common in women. Over half of these thyroid nodules are asymptomatic and are only characterized on ultrasound (US), while approximately 5% are discovered on palpation. Most (80%-85%) of the follicular nodules are benign, while the remaining 15% to 20% are malignant.[2,4] Follicular neoplasms or cellular nodules include papillary thyroid cancer, follicular adenomas (FAs), and follicular carcinoma. FAs are benign thyroid neoplasms that can form sporadically, from iodine deficiency, genetic alterations, or radioactive iodine exposure.[1,5]

Another form of thyroid neoplasms called Hürthle cell neoplasms are growths of predominantly oncocytic or

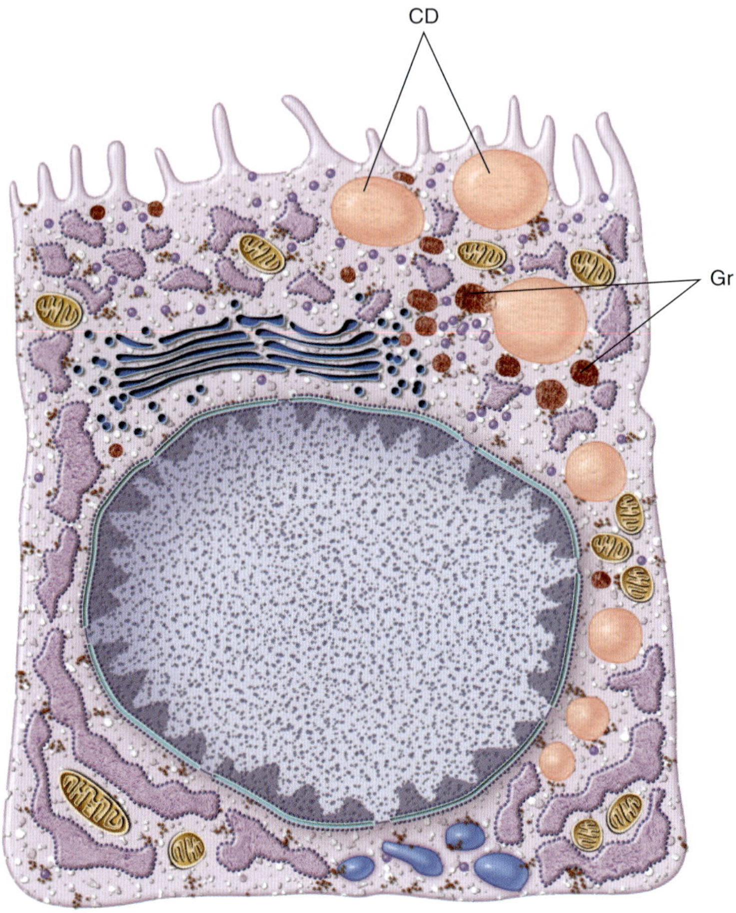

▲ **Figure 12–1.** Illustration of high-power view of a thyroid follicular cell. The cell contains dense granules (Gr) and colloid droplets (CD), where thyroglobulin is stored. (Reproduced with permission from Norman AW, Litwack G. Thyroid Hormones. In: Norman AW, Litwack G, eds. *Hormones*. 2nd ed. San Diego: Academic Press; 1997.)

"Hürthle" cells. They can be associated with malignancy but are also often associated with autoimmune thyroiditis. Similar oncocytic tumors have been reported in other organs including the pituitary gland, salivary glands, parathyroid glands, lacrimal glands, pancreas, liver, and kidney. The history of the name Hürthle cell is misleading as in 1894, Karl Hürthle first described intrafollicular thyroid cells from canine thyroid tissue that later were defined as C cells. Thyroid oncocytic cells were first accurately described by Max Askanazy in 1898 in Graves' disease, yet oncocytic thyroid tumors were later described as Hürthle cell tumors. Sometimes these tumors are referred to as Askanazy cell tumors crediting the correct German scientist but are more commonly referred to as Hürthle cell tumors. Thus, not only is the terminology a misnomer, but the origin of these cells has also been controversial. The most likely theory is that these cells arise from follicular cells because they can secrete TG and the TSH receptor-adenylate cyclase system is present, yet another theory is that they arise from parafollicular cells. The most recent World Health Organization classification of Hürthle cell neoplasms considers them separate from follicular neoplasms. Hürthle cell neoplasms may present as a benign Hürthle cell adenoma (HCA) or a Hürthle cell carcinoma. A higher percentage of Hürthle cell neoplasms are malignant (up to 65% in some studies), and they tend to be more aggressive than follicular carcinomas, especially when they grow large (>4 cm) or are present in older males.[6,7]

Toxic adenomas are one of the most common causes of hyperthyroidism. Nodules or multinodular goiters may initially develop sporadically but can become autonomous over time presenting as clinical hyperthyroidism. The chance of

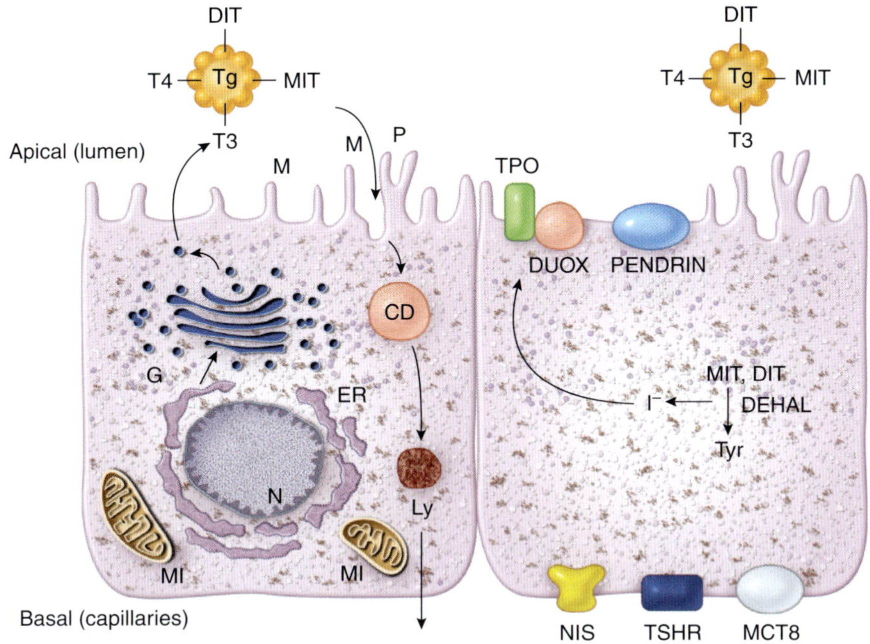

Figure 12–2. Process of thyroid hormone biosynthesis and secretion by a thyroid follicular cell. The organelles and major proteins involved in thyroid hormone synthesis are depicted on the left and right, respectively. The arrows on the left depict the direction of hormone synthesis, re-uptake into the follicle, and then eventual secretion into capillaries. CD, colloid droplets; DHEAL, iodotyrosine dehalogenase; DIT, Diiodotyrosine; DUOX, supplier of peroxide for reaction; ER, endoplasmic reticulum; G, Golgi apparatus; Ly, lysosome; M, microvilli; MI, mitochondria; MCT8; monocarboxylate transporter 8; MIT, monoiodotyrosine; N, nucleus; NIS, sodium/iodine transporter; P, pseudopods; Tg, thyroglobulin; TPO, thyroid peroxidase; TSHR; receptor for thyroid stimulating hormone. (Reproduced with permission from Norman AW, Henry HL. Thyroid Hormones. In: Norman AW, Henry HL, eds. *Hormones*. 3rd ed. San Diego: Academic Press; 2015.)

developing a toxic, hyperfunctioning nodule or goiter can increase with age and iodine deficiency.[2,8]

Cytologic Features

Follicular lesions that do not contain a capsule but are well circumscribed are often identified as hyperplastic nodules. In contrast, neoplastic follicular lesions grow within a capsule and on histology are usually classified as normofollicular, microfollicular, macrofollicular, solid, and/or trabecular patterned. They will have a follicular architecture but it may appear abnormal in varying degrees. The follicular pattern may contain smaller or larger than normal amounts of colloid, some may have large amounts of connective tissue making follicles appear more spread out, or increased cellularity which is often called architectural crowding. FAs tend to have normofollicular or macrofollicular patterns with a background of watery colloid (Figure 12–3). Follicular carcinomas tend to have a solid, microfollicular trabecular pattern, with more cellularity and architectural crowding.

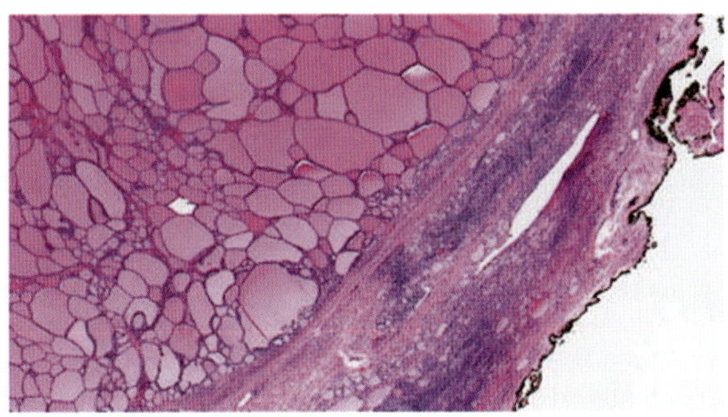

Figure 12–3. Histology of a follicular adenoma. There is evidence of increased amount of colloid, but no evidence of invasion or other irregularities. (Adapted from LiVolsi VA, Baloch ZW. Follicular-patterned tumors of the thyroid: the battle of benign vs. malignant vs. so-called uncertain. *Endocr Pathol*. 2011;22(4):184-189.)

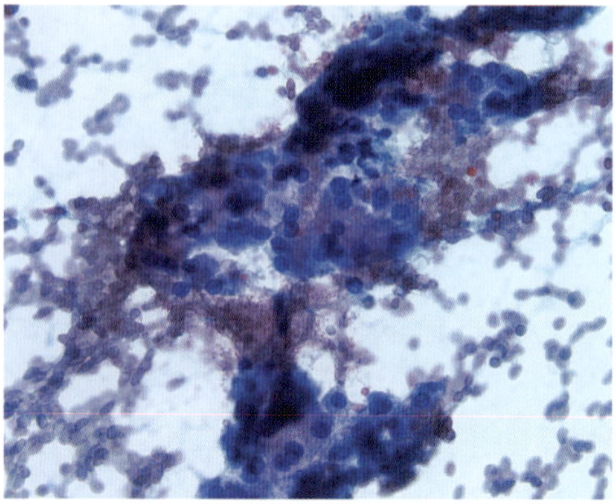

▲ **Figure 12–4.** Fine-needle aspiration cytology demonstrating polygonal-shaped Hürthle cells with pleomorphic hyperchromatic nuclei and granular cytoplasm.

The defining characteristic between a benign FA and its malignant counterpart is capsular and/or vascular invasion.[5,9]

Hürthle cells contain a large amount of eosinophilic and acidophilic, granular cytoplasm due to high amounts of mitochondria with a hyperchromatic nucleus and a large nucleolus. Individual Hürthle cells that are not clustered and/or encapsulated are not necessarily neoplastic. Encapsulated Hürthle cell nodules similarly exist as HCA if not invasive and Hürthle cell carcinoma if capsular and/or vascular invasion exists. In the case of an HCA, follicular-appearing oncocytic cells may be enlarged with large amounts of acidophilic cytoplasm, colloid or lymphocytes (Figure 12–4). Conversely, Hürthle cell carcinomas more often contain cells with very prominent nucleoli, a high nucleo-cytoplasm ratio, small- or large-cell dysplasia, cellular crowding, intracellular inclusions, or cellular dyshesion.[7,9]

Molecular Pathogenesis

FAs may contain mutations that can be associated with both benign and malignant nodules, most notably RAS mutations. PAX8-PPAR genetic rearrangements may cause a loss of growth inhibition and perpetuate the growth of follicular neoplasms. Multiple adenomas may be present in familial adenomatous polyposis, Carney complex syndrome, and PTEN hamartoma tumor syndrome due to mutations causing an inactivation of PTEN tumor suppressor gene. Up to 20% of FAs with such mutations will eventually evolve into follicular carcinoma.[5]

Radioactive iodine exposure is a risk factor for developing thyroid nodules. The 1986 Chernobyl nuclear power plant accident in Ukraine exposed many people to radioactive contamination. Although this event has been studied in the context of papillary thyroid cancer, it did prove that environmental radioactive iodine exposure causes dose-dependent DNA double-strand breaks including less common mutations in *BRAF* (like the K601 mutation) and *RET* genes that can be present in FAs.[5,10]

The abnormal genetic profile of Hürthle cell neoplasms is distinctly different from that of thyroid follicular neoplasms.[6] Hürthle cells contain high amounts of mitochondria, and thus mutations in mitochondrial DNA are commonly found in these tumors. Various types of genetic alterations specific to Hürthle cell neoplasms include mitochondrial DNA deletion mutations, somatic missense mutations in GRIM19, altered membrane transporter TRMM44, and polymorphisms of the G protein beta-3 subunit.[7]

Toxic hyperfunctioning adenomas or toxic multinodular goiters produce thyroid hormone in excess. This may be due to monoclonal activation of the TSH receptor, genetic mutations affecting thyroid hormone synthesis regulation and adenylate cyclase-stimulating G protein resulting in thyroid hormone access without TSH stimulation.[3,8]

CLINICAL PRESENTATION

Most follicular lesions present as a single nodule, but they may also be part of a multinodular goiter or be present in patients with autoimmune thyroiditis. Follicular neoplasms may present at any age or sex but are most common in younger adults, while Hürthle cell neoplasms are most commonly seen in the fifth to sixth decade of life and are more common in women.[4-6,11,12]

When an FA or HCA is symptomatic due to size, it is usually a slow-growing nodule and a progressive process that becomes palpable, visible, or causes compressive symptoms. Common compressive symptoms from tracheoesophageal compression include dysphagia or odynophagia, pressure or globus sensation, choking, dyspnea or shortness of breath when lying flat, and voice changes. These symptoms may or may not be associated with thyroiditis or tracheal deviation. Family history of thyroid nodules, thyroid cancer, autoimmune thyroiditis, or other familial syndromes should be investigated. Rarely, a patient may present with spontaneous acute pain and swelling, and this can be from a spontaneous bleed into the nodule. On physical exam, a nodule may not be palpable but all nodules can be identified with US.[2,5]

Most smaller nodules are asymptomatic and are nonfunctional, thus most patients are euthyroid. However, if a nodule is functional, the patient may present with clinical hyperthyroidism with low or undetectable TSH and high T3 and T4. Symptoms include constitutional (weight loss, fatigue, heat intolerance), integument changes (moist skin, thin hair), musculoskeletal manifestations (weakness, osteoporosis), gastrointestinal symptoms (diarrhea, increased hunger), and cardiovascular manifestations (hypertension, tachycardia).[5,8]

Prevention

Known risk factors for developing nodules that could be avoided, if possible include head and neck radiation and iodine deficiency. The ATA does not recommend for or against screening individuals with a family history of differentiated thyroid cancer with US.[1,5]

IMAGING STUDIES, LABORATORY TESTS, & DIAGNOSIS

Imaging Studies

Ultrasound is the most common imaging modality to assess thyroid nodules and is the first-line imaging modality recommended by the ATA.[1] Ultrasonography can be operator-dependent, but should evaluate the characteristics of the thyroid parenchyma, overall gland size, nodule size and characteristics, the location of the nodule, and any abnormal cervical lymph nodes in both the transverse and longitudinal views. When evaluating imaging of a nodule, it is important to identify any previous imaging that may allow for comparison and show potential interval change.[1,11]

Several universal characteristics of thyroid nodules are used in radiologic reporting systems. The American College of Radiology (ACR) and the ATA both have developed systems to standardize how thyroid nodules are interpreted and followed or treated. Some general concerning US characteristics of thyroid nodules include hypoechogenicity, irregular borders, solid appearance, taller than wide shape, and calcifications. Unfortunately, these characteristics are not specific for follicular or Hürthle cell lesions, and are often associated with papillary thyroid cancer. FAs and HCAs can look similar to their malignant counterparts on US, and tend to be solid, hypervascular, and well circumscribed (Figure 12–5).[1,4,11-13]

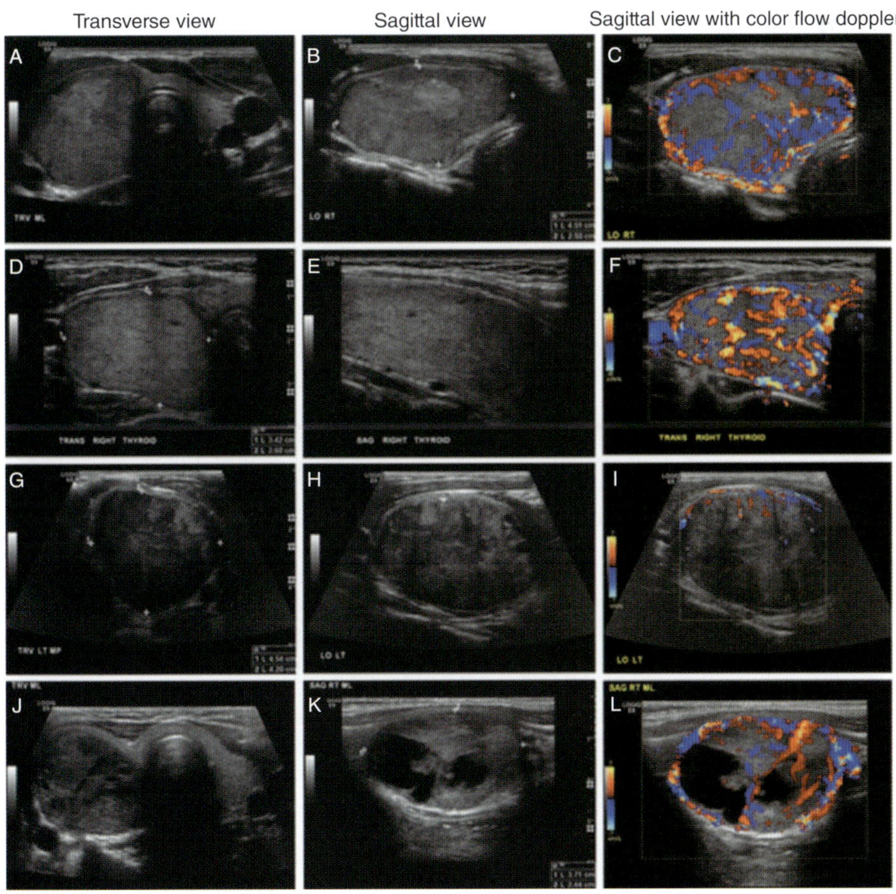

▲ **Figure 12–5.** Ultrasound of follicular adenoma **(A-C)**, Hürthle cell adenoma **(D-F)**, follicular thyroid carcinoma **(G-I)**, and Hürthle cell carcinoma **(J-L)**. (Adapted from Nilubol N, Keutgen X, Kebebew E. Follicular and Hürthle Cell Carcinoma. In: Roman SA, Sosa JA, Solórzano CC, eds. *Management of Thyroid Nodules and Differentiated Thyroid Cancer: A Practical Guide.* Cham: Springer International Publishing; 2017:379-393.)

Some studies have compared benign FA characteristics to follicular carcinoma on US to try to predict malignancy. A common finding in these studies is a characteristic halo that often appears as a hypoechoic ring around a follicular nodule likely representative of the capsule. Capsular invasion in the case of a carcinoma can result in an interrupted, thick halo ring while an FA appears to have a thin, well-circumscribed halo if present. Other US characteristics of follicular nodules that are suspicious for malignancy include larger size, hypoechogenicity, heterogeneous features (possibly due to necrosis, hemorrhage, or fibrosis), internal or rim calcifications, cluster of grapes sign (multiple solid nodules separated by hypoechoic bands), and hypervascularity. Rim or eggshell calcification can be seen in benign thyroid lesions but may appear in follicular carcinomas due to thickening of the capsule. Benign characteristics of a follicular nodule include an ovoid or round shaped, a smooth well-demarcated border with a thin halo, homogeneous with or without cystic change, isoechogenicity, no calcification, and minimal vascularity.[1,4,11]

Other studies have compared thyroid Hürthle cell neoplasms and found no preoperative characteristics to confidently discriminate HCA from Hürthle cell carcinoma. Some features consistent in Hürthle cell malignancy that should raise suspicion are similar to those of follicular carcinomas and papillary thyroid carcinomas including: larger size more than 4 cm, solid, hypoechogenicity, calcifications, irregular borders, and taller when compared to wide (Figure 12–5). Such findings, however, are never definitive to establish a diagnosis. Furthermore, US examination and interpretation are subjective, so one must consider this investigative tool as just one component of the diagnosis algorithm.[12]

Incidental thyroid nodules are found on many imaging studies including US, computed tomography (CT), magnetic resonance imaging (MRI), fluorodeoxyglucose positron emission tomography (FDG-PET) scans, nuclear medicine studies, and chest radiography. Up to 25% of contrast CT and MRI scans will identify an incidental thyroid nodule. With the exception of US, these other studies have limited roles in evaluating malignant versus benign thyroid nodules, yet a thyroid nodule with increased activity on an FDG-PET scan or the presence of significant lymphadenopathy may raise suspicion for a malignant process. The next step after an incidental thyroid nodule is found, per ATA guidelines, should be US for better characterization. One situation where CT is useful in benign disease is in the case of a very large nodule or goiter. Characterizing the borders of a large thyroid gland may not be possible with US due to its limited ability to penetrate sound waves through bone or air. Therefore, a CT scan may be very helpful to identify any tracheal deviation or to identify a retrotracheal, retroclavicular, substernal, or intrathoracic component of a very large FA, HCA, or goiter (Figure 12–6).[1,13]

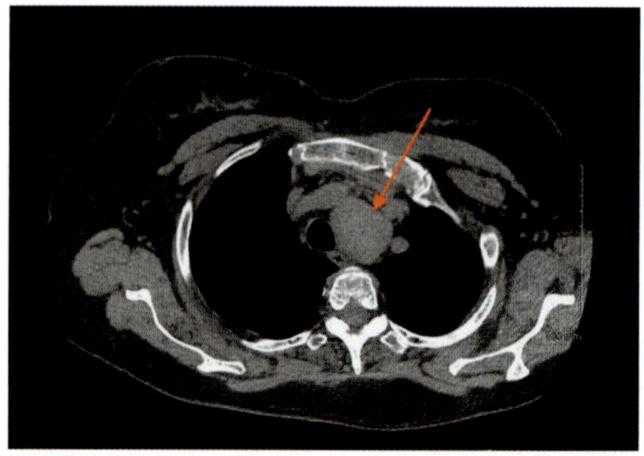

Figure 12–6. Computed tomography scan of substernal thyroid gland. This shows a left-sided nodule (red arrow) at the level of the sternum deviating the trachea to the right.

Laboratory Tests

Laboratory evaluation for a newly discovered thyroid nodule should include a TSH level. If the TSH is low, further workup includes a T4 and T3 level to characterize the severity of the dysfunction. In addition, low TSH warrants a radionuclide Iodine-123 uptake scan to determine if the nodule is hyperfunctioning. A toxic adenoma will show a localized area of uptake while a multinodular toxic goiter will show irregular uptake patterns.[1,5,8]

Diagnosis

Newly discovered thyroid nodules can either be followed with imaging surveillance or further evaluated with a biopsy. Imaging surveillance is appropriate for small nodules less than 1 cm with benign features, extremely poor surgical candidates, and individuals with significant comorbidities that will limit life expectancy. Any nodule with concerning features should be further evaluated with US-guided fine-needle aspiration (FNA). This is the most common diagnostic test in the workup of thyroid nodules as it is cost effective, sensitive and specific, usually well-tolerated, and performed on an outpatient basis. FNA is usually performed with a 25- or 27-gauge needle and obtains groups of cells that are analyzed for cytopathology (Figure 12–7). In some select cases, core needle biopsy is considered for follicular lesions, aggressive variants of thyroid cancer, or lymphoma because it provides histology and can be sent for flow cytometry. However, these needles are larger at 14, 16, or 18-gauge which increases the risk of bleeding, pain, and disruption of a final histopathologic diagnosis. Therefore, it is not considered the first-line diagnostic technique.[1,2,9]

The ACR developed the thyroid imaging reporting and data system (TI-RADS) in 2017 which uses a point system based on nodule sonographic characteristics to help

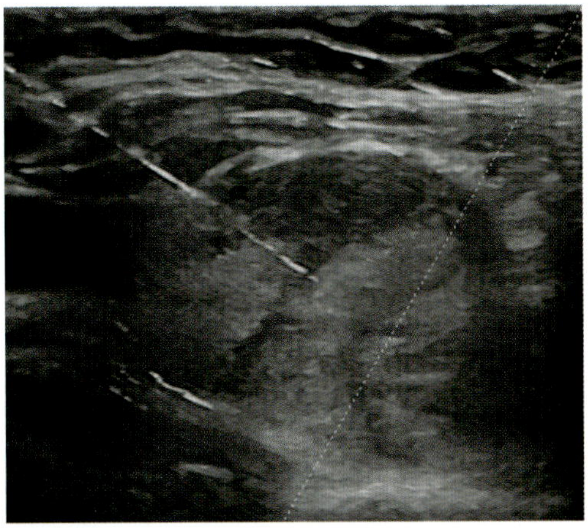

▲ **Figure 12–7.** Ultrasound image showing a fine-needle aspiration of a follicular nodule depicting the needle within the nodule.

determine next steps. Conversely, the ATA uses a nodule sonographic pattern-based system which may be more user friendly to the experienced clinician, but perhaps harder to apply by the nonspecialist because this pattern recognition does not allow for individual nodule characteristics to be scored independent of each other. Both systems, however, are designed to evaluate the same set of nodule characteristics including size, composition of the nodule (cystic vs solid), echogenicity, margins, echogenic foci that may represent calcifications, and width versus height. These systems help to guide the clinician when it is appropriate to discontinue workup, follow closely with repeat imaging, or perform FNA. While both systems yield a fair number of benign FNA results, TI-RADS does generate a higher rate of malignancy (14%) compared to the ATA system (10%).[1,12]

Once a thyroid nodule is identified and determined to meet criteria for FNA biopsy, this can be performed by experienced clinicians in interventional radiology, endocrinology, or endocrine surgery. Over 600,000 FNA biopsies are performed in the United States every year with the ultimate goal to distinguish benign from malignant nodules.[14,15] FNA will yield a cytopathologic diagnosis based on individual cells obtained in the aspirate and is reported based on The Bethesda System for Reporting Thyroid Cytopathology (Table 12–1). Nondiagnostic cytology is reported when the sample did not include the required 10 follicular cells per group with at least six groups of cells per slide. US-guided FNA should then be repeated, preferably with immediate cytology evaluation, at least 3 months after the first biopsy. If cytology is reported as benign, no further workup is needed immediately, keeping in mind the false-negative rate is approximately 3%. If cytology is reported as malignant or suspicious for malignancy, surgical intervention is recommended in surgically appropriate patients.[1,2]

Table 12–1. Bethesda criteria.

Category	Description	Risk of Malignancy (%)
I	Nondiagnostic or unsatisfactory	5-10
II	Benign	0-3
III	Atypia of undetermined significance or follicular lesion of undetermined significance	6-18
IV	Follicular neoplasm or suspicious for a follicular neoplasm	10-40
V	Suspicious of malignancy	45-60
VI	Malignant	94-96

Source: Data from Cibas ES, Ali SZ. The 2017 Bethesda system for reporting thyroid cytopathology. *Thyroid*. 2017;27(11):1341-1346.

Approximately 20% to 25% of nodules that undergo FNA will report indeterminate cytology. Indeterminate cytology reported in Bethesda III or IV means there is cytological architecture that is atypical but no nuclear features consistent with carcinoma. These diagnoses render a 6% to 40% risk of malignancy depending on the institution. If the cytopathology is reported as a follicular neoplasm, about 80% to 90% of these will be FAs and about 10% to 20% will be carcinoma.[1,2,16]

Cytology among FA, HCA, their malignant counterparts, and other follicular-patterned thyroid nodules have many overlapping features. The differential diagnosis of an FA or HCA includes follicular carcinoma, Hürthle cell carcinoma, nodular hyperplasia, noninvasive follicular thyroid neoplasm with papillary-like nuclear features (NIFTP), and follicular variant of papillary thyroid cancer.[5,9] The distinction between benign FA/HCA and malignancy is invasiveness. The hallmark findings of follicular or Hürthle cell carcinomas are varying degrees of capsular invasion and/or vascular invasion within the thyroid gland, invasion extending outside the gland to adjacent tissues, or metastases. These features cannot be determined on cytopathology from FNA or frozen section; thus, definitive diagnosis requires a surgically resected specimen. Therefore, in the case of indeterminate cytology, the ATA guidelines recommend either repeat FNA, diagnostic surgery, or molecular testing. Repeating the FNA can occasionally give more information, but approximately 10% to 30% of the time will render a repeat indeterminate result.[1,4,9,11,12]

Molecular Testing

Historic management of indeterminate cytology reports was repeat FNA or diagnostic surgery (either with a total thyroidectomy or thyroid lobectomy), but now molecular testing has become the adjunct diagnostic tool of choice for many clinicians. Indeterminate cytology reported in Bethesda III and IV is now being sent for molecular testing up to 33% of the time. Molecular testing in the United States is done with one of several current platforms. These techniques analyze either messenger RNA or DNA to detect genetic mutations associated with malignancy and there are five classes of molecular alterations: point mutations, insertions or deletions, gene fusions, copy number alterations, and gene-expression alterations. Final results of these techniques report nodules as benign, suspicious for malignancy, or detect a specific mutation with a corresponding risk of malignancy.[14,17]

Identifying such mutations or changes in gene expression, or lack thereof, has helped to clarify which nodules are likely benign versus malignant, and thus has helped surgeons determine that it is safe to avoid diagnostic surgery for up to 90% of patients with negative molecular reports. The most current form of the DNA-RNA test is ThyroSeq v3 multigenomic classifier (CBLPath) which analyzes 112 genes. The most current RNA-based test is Afirma genomic sequencing classifier (Veracyte). The most current combination test is the ThyGeNEXT/ThyraMIR (Table 12–2). Certain mutations such as BRAF V600E, RET fusions, and TERT promoter are strong predictors of thyroid cancer, while other common mutations such as RAS are weaker predictors of malignancy and are commonly found in both benign and malignant follicular nodules. Finally, many other mutations and fusions included in these panels are rare and therefore difficult to study due to lack of long-term data.[14,15,18]

Table 12–2. Commercially available molecular testing for indeterminate thyroid nodules and their attributes.

Test	Method Used	Utility and Accuracy
ThyroSeq Genomic Classifier version 3	Detection of thyroid cancer-associated alterations in DNA and RNA. Analysis of 112 genes regarding >12,000 mutations and >150 fusion types	Sensitivity: 94%-97% Specificity: 82%-85%
Afirma	RNA only whole transcriptome sequencing	Sensitivity: 91%-100% Specificity: 68%-80%
ThyGeNext/ ThyraMIR	Evaluation for common RNA and DNA mutations with microRNA markers	Sensitivity: 95% Specificity: 90%

Source: Data from information from ThyroSeq for Physicians. Accessed October 1, 2021; https://www.thyroseq.com/physicians/, Why Afirma? Accessed October 1, 2021; https://www.afirma.com/physicians/why-afirma/, and Performance. Accessed October 1, 2021; and https://thygenext-thyramir.com/performance/.

A recent prospective, blinded, multicenter study found that the Thyroseq v3 multigenomic classifier test was very sensitive (94%) and relatively specific (82%) for distinguishing between benign and malignant (including premalignant NIFTP) nodules. There was a 3% false negative rate, comparable to the 3.7% cancer risk in nodules with benign cytology. All cancers in this false negative category were considered low risk per ATA criteria. Of the false positives with benign surgical pathology, 94% did show one or more type of molecular alteration, thus representing benign neoplastic nodules. Furthermore, Thyroseq showed promising use in Hürthle cell nodules. Historically, molecular testing for Hürthle cell carcinoma has shown low specificity; yet this study found correct identification in all 10 Hürthle cell carcinomas, and 53% of all types of Hürthle cell nodules were reported as negative meaning no or low probability of cancer. Thus, Thyroseq could allow for avoidance of surgery in approximately half of Hürthle cell nodules biopsied. The authors concluded that using Thyroseq multigenomic classifier can prevent diagnostic surgery in up to 61% of all Bethesda III and IV indeterminate nodules. This is beneficial to reduce patient anxiety, improve quality of life, and decrease healthcare costs.[15]

Another recent prospective randomized study compared the most current RNA test (Afirma genomic sequencing classifier [Veracyte]) to the most current DNA-RNA test (ThyroSeq v3 multigene classifier [CBLPath]). The authors found both tests to have high sensitivities (RNA 100.0%, DNA-RNA 96.9%) with relatively high specificities (RNA 79.6%, DNA-RNA 84.8%) with no statistically significant difference. A subanalysis was done for nodules with Hürthle cell cytology and found comparable high sensitivities (RNA 100.0%, DNA-RNA 100.0%) and specificities (RNA 83.3%, DNA-RNA 57.9%). The overall benign call rate was comparable and resulted in 48.6% of patients able to avoid diagnostic surgery. Both of these tests are best used to rule out malignancy, with a satisfactory ability to rule in malignancy. The authors concluded that both the most current RNA and DNA-RNA tests are valid to analyze molecular behavior of nodules and guide surgical decision-making. The choice of molecular test may come down to provider or institution-specific factors.[14]

Finally, a recent blinded, retrospective multicenter study also evaluated the ThyGeNEXT/ThyraMIR test which is a combination test. The first platform evaluates a mutation panel and if found to be negative, a secondary platform tests for micro-RNA markers which are short, single-stranded RNA segments that do not code for anything; yet their abnormal expression has been found to be associated with thyroid cancer. This two-step process is designed to enhance both sensitivity and specificity, and reports results as either negative, moderate, or positive. This study was unique in that it retrospectively evaluated indeterminate thyroid nodules that did not undergo molecular testing by sending cytology slides still viable for ThyGeNEXT/ThyraMIR and comparing these results to final surgical pathology. The authors found that the false positives identified in the first platform were mostly (95%) due to RAS mutations found in benign adenomas. Thus, rendering specimens through the second microRNA platform was much better at ruling in malignancy with RAS mutations, other weaker predictor mutations, and those with Hürthle cells. Overall, this last combination test was found to be very sensitive (93%) and specific (90%). Due to the retrospective nature of this study, it included more benign nodules than the previously discussed prospective studies so results were prevalence adjusted. After this adjustment, the authors concluded that this combination two-step platform performed comparable or slightly superior to other commercial platforms available. Finally, the authors caution that decisions for close surveillance versus surgery cannot be made solely on the presence of an RAS mutation or other weak predictors of malignancy that would be reported at moderate risk.[18]

There are several benefits and limitations to molecular testing. Molecular markers offer assistance in management with indeterminate cytology and have decreased the number of diagnostic surgical interventions for benign disease. However, it is very difficult to study direct comparisons between cohorts and types of tests, and while each new version of a test offers more comprehensive data, no test will ever be perfect. Future advances in molecular profiling will be required to further clarify the behavior of certain mutations. Providers should always consider other clinical and imaging findings, as well as the patient on an individualized basis, to make a shared clinical or surgical decision.[14,15,17,18]

TREATMENT

Surgery for Diagnosis & Treatment

Diagnostic surgical excision may be indicated for a suspected follicular or Hürthle cell neoplasm to obtain a definitive diagnosis. The defining characteristic to delineate an FA and HCA from carcinoma is capsular or vascular invasion.[12,19] As discussed earlier, molecular testing may suggest benign versus malignant disease in the case of an indeterminate cytology, but diagnostic surgical excision allows for interpretation of the cellular behavior at the capsular or vascular interface and thus it is the only definitive way to get a final histopathologic diagnosis (Figure 12–8). This distinction remains challenging for pathologists for many reasons.[4,11] Follicular carcinomas tend to have a thicker, even calcified capsule compared to FAs. An adenoma may have irregular fibrinous deposition and thus any irregularity in the capsule may be indistinguishable from minimal invasion into the capsule. There may be irregularities in the capsule from cells pushing on or embedded in the inner portion of the capsule, or an adjacent cellular reaction from incomplete capsular

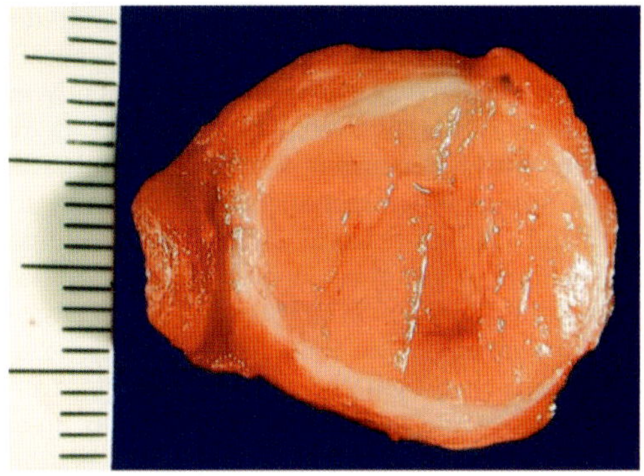

Figure 12–8. Gross specimen of a follicular adenoma. (Adapted from Sakr MF. Solitary Thyroid Nodule. In: *Thyroid Disease: Challenges and Debates.* Cham: Springer International Publishing; 2020:193-303.)

penetration by tumor cells. There is no consensus on whether partial or complete penetration of the capsule is sufficient for a malignant diagnosis. Vascular invasion is identified as blood vessels within or outside the capsule that demonstrate tumor cells extending into the vessel lumen which may or may not have an attached fibrin thrombus. Tumors with any vascular invasion are considered more aggressive, especially if invasion is seen in four or more blood vessels, and therefore is sufficient evidence for a malignant diagnosis. Complicating this diagnostic dilemma is the recent development of a novel nomenclature for a follicular lesion that is lined with cells with nuclear features associated with papillary thyroid cancer, but no capsular invasion present. This lesion, which historically was termed an encapsulated follicular variant of papillary thyroid cancer, has now been renamed a noninvasive follicular thyroid neoplasm with papillary-like nuclear features (NIFTP). The elimination of the word cancer aimed to help minimize overtreatment of this low-grade lesion that usually behaves in a benign fashion.[16,19]

Another indication for surgical excision is the size of a nodule. If a patient has developed significant compressive symptoms, regardless of cytology, thyroid lobectomy or total thyroidectomy is typically recommended. Compressive symptoms from increased tracheoesophageal compression can vary in severity. Mild dysphagia may not interrupt daily life compared to severe esophageal compression interrupting daily nutritional intake resulting in weight loss. Some patients report dyspnea causing abrupt awakening from sleeping on the opposite side of a large nodule due to tracheal compression. Furthermore, if tracheal compression is associated with tracheal deviation, this could result in a highly morbid situation in the event of acute respiratory failure due to infection, trauma, or cardiac arrest. Emergent intubation is difficult with a deviated airway, so in the event that the endotracheal tube cannot be passed, a surgical airway may be indicated which could also be difficult with a large thyroid nodule or goiter. Voice changes could indicate that the nodule is compressing the recurrent laryngeal nerve and over time, the nerve may become permanently injured if compression is not relieved.[1,2] Autoimmune thyroiditis may present with a concurrent FA, HCA, or other benign nodules. Chronic inflammation can result in a fibrotic thyroid gland causing tracheal compression among other systemic symptoms and thus, in select cases thyroidectomy may be indicated and beneficial.[20] Finally, once a large single FA, HCA, or other nodule thought to be benign on FNA becomes greater than 4 cm, the sensitivity of FNA decreases. The false negative rate can increase exponentially up to 50% due to sampling error, so diagnostic lobectomy is indicated. In such nodules, preoperative FNA would still be indicated because if it is proven to be a cancer greater than 4 cm, a total thyroidectomy would be indicated upfront.[1]

Other indications for surgery for an FA or HCA include a toxic, hyperfunctioning nodule causing hyperthyroidism. If this is a solitary nodule, thyroid lobectomy would be appropriate. A multinodular goiter in the setting of a family history of thyroid cancer or history of radiation may raise suspicion or anxiety for cancer, so in select cases total thyroidectomy may be appropriate.[2,8]

Complications of Surgery

Commonly reported surgical complications such as mortality, surgical site infections, deep vein thrombosis, stroke, or pneumonia are not common in routine thyroidectomy, so it is more appropriate to discuss surgical complications in terms of procedure-specific outcomes. The American College of Surgeons' National Surgical Quality Improvement Program has modified their program to track this surgery-specific data. Over 70,000 thyroidectomies are performed every year in the United States, and surgeon experience and hospital volume vary greatly.[21] It is well accepted that high-volume surgeons in specific procedures will have lower complication rates compared to lower-volume surgeons. The most common complications in thyroid surgery include hypocalcemia from parathyroid disruption, recurrent laryngeal nerve injury, and postoperative neck hematoma.[21-23]

Hypocalcemia from hypoparathyroidism is the most common complication after thyroidectomy. This is because the parathyroid glands are anatomically in very close proximity to the thyroid gland, they are very small, and often times receive some or all of their blood supply from the thyroid gland (Figure 12–9). In the case of a thyroid lobectomy, only two of the four parathyroid glands will be at risk and so hypocalcemia will not occur from an initial operation. In a total thyroidectomy, however, hypocalcemia is more likely, especially in the setting of a large nodule or goiter when the typical anatomy is altered. Transient hypoparathyroidism will recover in weeks to months postoperatively and is reported anywhere from 3% to 53%, while approximately 2% of patients will experience permanent hypoparathyroidism lasting longer than 6 months. This variability in rates is due to the fact that there is no standard definition of hypoparathyroidism. Some institutions define hypoparathyroidism by postoperative biochemical values of calcium and/or parathyroid hormone, some monitor for symptoms of hypocalcemia, while others use a combination of labs and symptoms. In addition, there is no universal treatment protocol for such cases which further contributes to the ambiguity of this reported complication rate. Studies have shown that in certain institutions that treat postoperative hypoparathyroidism aggressively with oral calcium supplementation and additional vitamin D (if needed in severe cases), the patients do very well, and the condition will usually resolve within weeks as the parathyroid glands recover.[24,25]

Recurrent laryngeal nerve injury can occur in approximately 3% to 11% of thyroidectomies.[21] Most variation exists due to surgeon volume or distorted anatomy from large nodules which can cause the course of the nerve to be displaced from its normal anatomic position in the tracheoesophageal groove. Like hypoparathyroidism, this complication is usually transient from a traction injury to the nerve causing temporary vocal cord paresis. However, in approximately 0.3% to 3% of cases the injury will be permanent from nerve severance and this results in permanent vocal cord paralysis. Transient nerve injuries usually recover at a rate of about 1 mm per day from the point of the injury. Patients with permanent unilateral injuries can still achieve normal oral intake and voice with time as the contralateral vocal cord compensates, with voice therapy, and interventions such as vocal cord injection. Continuous and intermittent nerve monitoring does aid the surgeon in recognizing a recurrent laryngeal nerve injury on one side. This can prevent dissection and risk of injury to the contralateral side that could result in a devastating bilateral nerve injury requiring tracheostomy.[21,26]

Postoperative neck hematoma occurs in approximately 1% to 2% of cases. This condition does not appear to vary much among surgeon experience or hospital volume like hypoparathyroidism or recurrent laryngeal nerve injury does. This complication can be a true emergency due to compression of the airway from a hematoma and does require return to the operating room for control of the bleed. High-risk patients include those on anticoagulation, large thyroid nodules or goiters, and chronic cough which increases intrathoracic and neck pressure postoperatively.[21]

Medical Therapy

The ATA does not recommend TSH suppression for benign thyroid nodules. This practice is characterized by initiating thyroid hormone supplementation to suppress natural TSH secretion to a subnormal level using the hypothalamic-pituitary-thyroid axis. The goal is to suppress the trophic effects of TSH and halt growth of thyroid follicular or cancer cells. This is a widely used treatment algorithm in postoperative

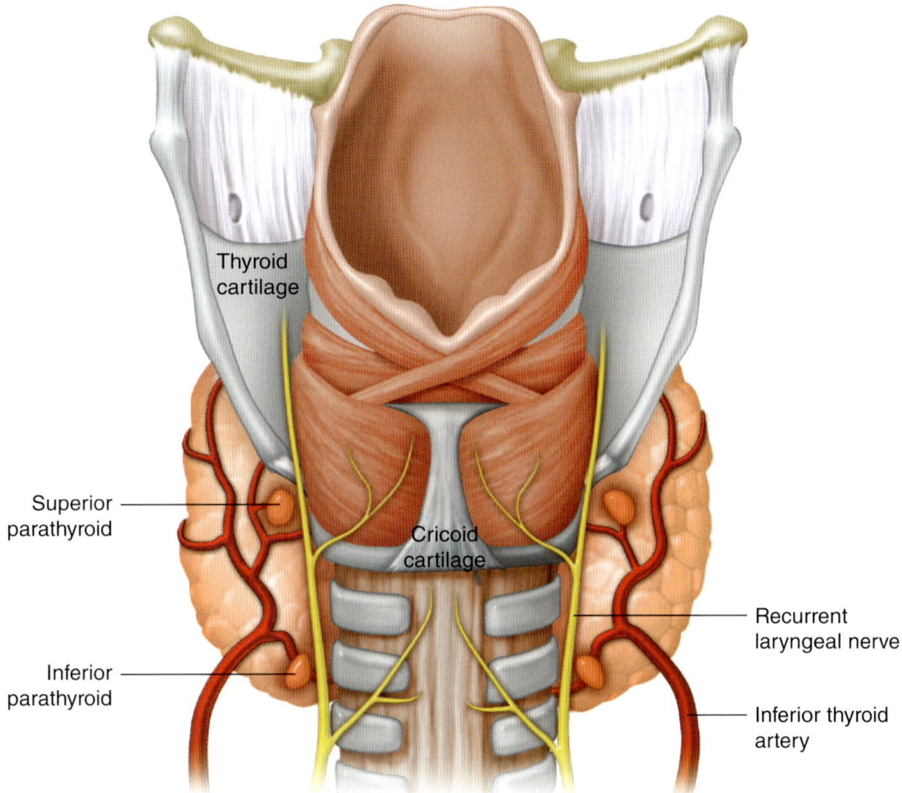

Figure 12–9. A posterior view of thyroid anatomy demonstrating the relationship of the parathyroid glands and recurrent laryngeal nerves to the thyroid gland. (Adapted from Norman AW, Henry HL. Chapter 5, Thyroid Hormones. In: Norman AW, Henry HL, eds. *Hormones*, 3rd ed. San Diego: Academic Press; 2015:89-107.)

thyroid cancer patients, but no data exist to recommend this strategy in benign nodules and in fact, it has been proven not to be effective.[1]

One of the risk factors for developing thyroid nodules is iodine deficiency. If a benign nodule is found in the setting of iodine deficiency, iodine supplementation can be offered at approximately 150 μg daily.[1,5]

SURVEILLANCE & FOLLOW-UP

If an FNA cytology report returns benign, or a molecular testing report returns negative, the nodule will require monitoring based on the US characteristics. At this time, we do not have long-term follow-up data for nodules reported as negative on molecular tests, especially for Hürthle cell nodules, but we do have data showing the risk of malignancy increases with size. Likely, these follicular and Hürthle cell nodules represent a spectrum of disease, and an initial negative report on molecular testing does not eliminate the possibility that the nodule could grow, develop further mutations or changes in the future and become malignant. Certain FAs may possess a mutation that can later evolve into follicular carcinoma, specifically NRAS and KRAS, so any nodules with suspicious US features should have continued surveillance.[1,5,18]

The ATA recommends that nodules with highly suspicious US characteristics should have a repeat US and FNA within 1 year. Nodules with a low or intermediate suspicion should undergo a repeat US within 1 to 2 years. Repeat FNA can be considered in the case of growth, specifically a 20% increase in two dimensions (a minimum of 2 mm) or greater than 50% volume increase, or the development of new highly suspicious US characteristics. Nodules with very low suspicion on US can undergo repeat US in 2 years. If a US-guided FNA yields benign cytology twice, no further surveillance is necessary.[1,2]

REFERENCES

1. Haugen BR, Alexander EK, Bible KC, et al. 2015 American Thyroid Association Management guidelines for adult patients with thyroid nodules and differentiated thyroid cancer: the American Thyroid Association guidelines task force on thyroid nodules and differentiated thyroid cancer. *Thyroid.* 2016; 26(1):1-133.
2. Detweiler K, Elfenbein DM, Mayers D. Evaluation of Thyroid Nodules. Sippel RS, Schneider DF, eds. *Surgical Management of Endocrine Disease: Surgical Clinics*. 1st ed. Elsevier; 2019: 571-586.
3. Pirahanchi Y, Tariq MA, Jialal I. Physiology, Thyroid. [Updated 2021 Feb 25]. In: StatPearls [Internet]. Treasure Island (FL): StatPearls Publishing; 2021 Jan. Available from: https://www.ncbi.nlm.nih.gov/books/NBK519566/.
4. Li W, Song Q, Lan Y, et al. The value of sonography in distinguishing follicular thyroid carcinoma from adenoma. *Cancer Manag Res.* 2021;13:3991-4002.
5. Norris JJ, Farci F. Follicular Adenoma. [Updated 2021 Jul 30]. In: StatPearls [Internet]. Treasure Island (FL): StatPearls Publishing; 2021 Jan. Available from: https://www.ncbi.nlm.nih.gov/books/NBK559320/.
6. Coca-Pelaz A, Rodrigo JP, Shah JP, et al. Hürthle cell carcinoma of the thyroid gland: systematic review and meta-analysis. *Adv Ther.* 2021;38(10):5144-5164.
7. Kure S, Ohashi R. Thyroid Hürthle cell carcinoma: clinical, pathological, and molecular features. *Cancers.* 2020;13(1):26.
8. Doubleday AR, Sippel RS. Hyperthyroidism. *Gland Surg.* 2020;9(1):124-135.
9. Na HY, Moon JH, Choi JY, et al. Preoperative diagnostic categories of fine needle aspiration cytology for histologically proven thyroid follicular adenoma and carcinoma, and Hürthle cell adenoma and carcinoma: analysis of cause of under- or misdiagnoses. *PLoS One.* 2020;15(11):e0241597.
10. Morton LM, Karyadi DM, Stewart C, et al. Radiation-related genomic profile of papillary thyroid carcinoma after the Chernobyl accident. *Science.* 2021;372(6543):eabg2538.
11. Lai X, Jiang Y, Zhang B, et al. Preoperative sonographic features of follicular thyroid carcinoma predict biological behavior: a retrospective study. *Medicine.* 2018;97(41):e12814.
12. Santana NO, Freitas RMC, Marcos VN, et al. Diagnostic performance of thyroid ultrasound in Hürthle cell carcinomas. *Arch Endocrinol Metab.* 2019;63(3):300-305.
13. Nguyen XV, Job J, Fiorillo LE, Sipos J. Thyroid incidentalomas: practice considerations for radiologists in the age of incidental findings. *Radiol Clin North Am.* 2020;58(6):1019-1031.
14. Livhits MJ, Zhu CY, Kuo EJ, et al. Effectiveness of molecular testing techniques for diagnosis of indeterminate thyroid nodules: a randomized clinical trial. *JAMA Oncol.* 2021;7(1):70-77.
15. Steward DL, Carty SE, Sippel RS, et al. Performance of a multigene genomic classifier in thyroid nodules with indeterminate cytology: a prospective blinded multicenter study. *JAMA Oncol.* 2019;5(2):204-212.
16. Sauter JL, Lehrke H, Zhang X, et al. Assessment of the Bethesda system for reporting thyroid cytopathology. *Am J Clin Pathol.* 2019;152(4):502-511.
17. Nasar C. Thyroid health—molecular testing in thyroid nodules: it is all about risk of malignancy. American Thyroid Association. https://www.thyroid.org/molecular-testing. Updated September 21, 2020. Accessed July 7, 2021.
18. Lupo MA, Walts AE, Sistrunk JW, et al. Multiplatform molecular test performance in indeterminate thyroid nodules. *Diagn Cytopathol.* 2020;48(12):1254-1264.
19. Suster S. Controversies regarding the interpretation of follicular thyroid nodules. *Arch Pathol Lab Med.* 2019;143(12): 1472-1476.
20. Guldvog I, Reitsma LC, Johnsen L, et al. Thyroidectomy versus medical management for euthyroid patients with hashimoto disease and persisting symptoms: a randomized trial. *Ann Intern Med.* 2019;170(7):453-464.
21. Liu JB, Sosa JA, Grogan RH, et al. Variation of thyroidectomy-specific outcomes among hospitals and their association with risk adjustment and hospital performance. *JAMA Surg.* 2018;153(1):e174593.
22. Sosa JA, Bowman HM, Tielsch JM, Powe NR, Gordon TA, Udelsman R. The importance of surgeon experience for clinical and economic outcomes from thyroidectomy. *Ann Surg.* 1998; 228(3):320-330.
23. Kandil E, Noureldine SI, Abbas A, Tufano RP. The impact of surgical volume on patient outcomes following thyroid surgery. *Surgery.* 2013;154(6):1346-1353.
24. Doubleday AR, Robbins SE, Macdonald CL, Elfenbein DM, Connor NP, Sippel RS. What is the experience of our patients with transient hypoparathyroidism after total thyroidectomy? *Surgery.* 2021;169(1):70-76.
25. Mazotas IG, Wang TS. The role and timing of parathyroid hormone determination after total thyroidectomy. *Gland Surg.* 2017;6(Suppl 1):S38-S48.
26. Paniello RC, Park AM, Bhatt NK, Al-Lozi M. Recurrent laryngeal nerve recovery patterns assessed by serial electromyography. *Laryngoscope.* 2016;126(3):651-656.

SUGGESTED READINGS

Cibas ES, Ali SZ. The 2017 Bethesda system for reporting thyroid cytopathology. *Thyroid.* 2017;27(11):1341-1346.

National Comprehensive Cancer Network (NCCN) Clinical Practice Guidelines in Oncology. Thyroid Carcinoma. Version 2.2021-September 1, 2021. https://www.nccn.org/professionals/physician_gls/pdf/thyroid_blocks.pdf.

Nikiforov YE, Seethala RR, Tallini G, et al. Nomenclature revision for encapsulated follicular variant of papillary thyroid carcinoma: a paradigm shift to reduce overtreatment of indolent tumors. *JAMA Oncol.* 2016;2(8):1023-1029.

Tessler FN, Middleton WD, Grant EG, et al. ACR Thyroid imaging, reporting and data system (TI-RADS): white paper of the ACR TI-RADS committee. *J Am Coll Radiol.* 2017;14(5):587-595.

Papillary Thyroid Microcarcinoma

13

Iwao Sugitani, MD, PhD

INTRODUCTION

In recent years, the incidence of thyroid carcinoma has been increasing rapidly worldwide. This is interpreted as an increase in the incidental detection of small papillary thyroid carcinomas (PTCs) by the widespread use of high-resolution imaging techniques, such as ultrasound. However, the mortality rates of thyroid carcinoma have not changed, suggesting that small PTCs may be overdiagnosed and overtreated.[1-4] Currently, thyroid carcinoma screening using ultrasound is not recommended for asymptomatic adults.[5] In addition, recent management guidelines set a lower limit on the diameter of tumors to be examined with fine-needle aspiration cytology (FNAC) in cases where PTC is suspected based on ultrasound findings.[6]

Prospective clinical trials of active surveillance for papillary thyroid microcarcinomas (PTMCs) without apparent clinical metastasis and invasion have been conducted at two Japanese institutions since the 1990s.[7,8] Based on the favorable outcomes of these trials, active surveillance has been gradually adopted worldwide as an alternative to immediate surgery.

General Considerations

PTC is a malignant epithelial tumor with follicular cell origin characterized by distinctive nuclear features like nuclear grooves and pseudoinclusions. FNAC has a high accuracy (>90%) in the diagnosis of PTC. The term PTMC is used for a PTC that measures 1 cm or less in maximal diameter, regardless of lymph node metastasis (LNM), distant metastasis, and extrathyroidal extension (ETE).

Hitherto, most PTMCs were detected incidentally on postoperative pathological examinations of other thyroid diseases such as Graves' disease or benign tumor. These incidental PTMCs are usually harmless and remain innocuous throughout the life of the patient and do not need further treatment. On the other hand, some PTMCs are found occasionally as primary lesions as the root cause of symptoms due to metastasis or invasion. The prognosis of such patients is not always favorable even after aggressive treatment with total thyroidectomy and radioactive iodine. Based on a meta-analysis regarding the treatment outcomes of incidental and nonincidental PTMC,[9] the recurrence rate for incidental carcinoma (854 cases; mean tumor size, 4.6 mm) diagnosed on postoperative pathological examination was 0.5%, significantly better than the 7.9% for nonincidental carcinoma (2669 cases; mean tumor size, 6.9 mm) diagnosed preoperatively (odds ratio 14.7, 95% confidence interval 5.6-54.8).

Clinically apparent LNM, distant metastasis, and ETE are significant risk factors for poor prognosis in patients with PTMC. PTMCs with these features are classified into "high-risk" ones; while those without high-risk features (clinical T1aN0M0 PTC) are considered "low-risk" PTMCs.[8] It should be noted that small LNM or minimal ETE can often be found during surgery or by histopathological examination even in PTMC patients diagnosed as having no clinical LNM or ETE. PTMC has a 12.4% to 33% risk of pathological LNM when lymph node dissection is performed for patients without clinical LNM. The frequency of minimal ETE was reported to range from 6.3% to 48%. However, LNM and ETE diagnosed only histopathologically have not been shown to be significant risk factors for cancer mortality.[10] Moreover, from the results of active surveillance, progression of these potential LNM into clinical problems appears rare, and if surgery is performed when these metastases become detectable on ultrasound, treatment outcomes are generally favorable.[7,8]

Epidemiology

The clinical incidence of PTC is only about 0.05% to 0.1% in the general population, but many autopsy series from various countries have shown a very high prevalence of latent PTC, ranging from 5.6% to 35.6% among patients dying from diseases other than thyroid cancer. The prevalence increases steeply from birth to adulthood and remains relatively constant thereafter. Likewise, incidental PTCs can be found in up to 24% of surgical specimens of thyroidectomies conducted for disorders unrelated to thyroid cancer.

The incidence of thyroid carcinomas has increased worldwide since the 1980s. The histopathological type was mostly PTC, especially small PTC with tumor diameter less than 20 mm. Mortality from thyroid carcinomas during the period has remained almost unchanged.[1] The increased incidence of small PTC is interpreted as an increased frequency of thyroid examinations—mainly by ultrasound—that has a high sensitivity in detecting small, suspicious thyroid nodules. Indeed, active screening for thyroid carcinoma using ultrasound and FNAC could reportedly find PTC in 3.5% of adult women subjects.[10] In the United States, the number of ultrasound examinations has increased 5-fold and the number of FNAC procedures increased 7-fold, resulting in a 2-fold increase in the incidence of thyroid carcinoma in 2012 compared to 2000.[4] In Korea, the policy of general cancer screening with no charge has led to the active use of thyroid ultrasound, resulting in a 15-fold increase in the incidence of PTC between 1993 and 2011, and most of those cases involved a tumor less than 10 mm in maximal diameter.[2] Again, penetration of thyroid cancer screening with ultrasound coincided with the incidence of PTC.

Recently, computed tomography (CT), magnetic resonance imaging, and fluorodeoxyglucose-positron emission tomography/CT carried out for screening or evaluation of other diseases have also led to the increased detection of incidental thyroid carcinoma.

According to a meta-analysis of 35 studies covering 12,834 autopsies of patients with no known history of thyroid pathology in 38 regions of 25 countries from 1949 to 2007, the prevalence of differentiated thyroid cancer among whole gland examination was 11.2% (95% confidence interval, 6.7-16.1%). This prevalence stabilized from 1970 onward, and no time effect was observed.[11] Thus, current increasing incidence of thyroid cancer is unlikely to reflect a true increase in tumorigenesis.

Imaging Studies & Diagnosis of PTMC

Ultrasound findings are useful to differentiate PTC from benign nodules. Common malignant features include hypoechoic solid nodules with irregular borders, taller-than-wide shape, microcalcifications, and internal blood flow. However, to prevent overdiagnosis and overtreatment, active search for PTMC in health screenings is not recommended. In 2017, the United States Preventive Service Task Force published a statement that thyroid carcinoma screening using cervical palpation or ultrasound was not recommended for asymptomatic adults without a history of radiation exposure to the neck or a family history of thyroid carcinoma.[5]

Recent management guidelines set a lower limit on the diameter of tumors to be examined with FNAC in cases where PTC is suspected based on ultrasound finding.[6,12,13] The criteria for FNAC according to the tumor size in various guidelines are summarized in Table 13–1. In all guidelines, FNAC is recommended for thyroid nodules >10 to 15 mm in size that have ultrasound findings suspicious of malignancy, and FNAC is not recommended for thyroid nodules with diameter ≤10 mm in principle. However, FNAC should be considered when there is clinically suspicious LNM, ETE, or distant metastasis.

Clinically evident LNM and ETE are evaluated mainly by ultrasound. Contrast-enhanced CT can be added if needed. When LNM is suspected, FNAC with measurement of thyroglobulin on the washout of the needle is recommended. Lymph node swelling is frequently observed in cases with chronic thyroiditis, requiring careful consideration of the individual case.[14]

For tumors on the dorsal side near the thyroid capsule, not only ultrasound, but also CT may be useful to evaluate the relationship between tumor and the trachea and recurrent laryngeal nerve (RLN). Laryngoscopy is also used to evaluate vocal cord paralysis. As for evaluation of tracheal invasion, the angle formed by the tumor and the surface of the trachea is important. An obtuse angle between the tumor and trachea carries a high risk of invasion (Figure 13–1). To assess involvement of the RLN, particular attention should be given to the presence of a normal rim of thyroid tissue between the tumor and the course of the RLN. If no normal rim of the thyroid was apparent, the RLN was at risk of invasion (Figure 13–2).[15] ETE only to the strap muscles is not considered to be an independent risk factor for cancer mortality.

Although distant metastasis is an important poor prognostic factor for PTMC, the frequency of distant metastases to the lung, bone, and brain in PTMC was reported to be 0.14% to 0.50%. Distant metastasis is extremely rare in PTMC without LNM or ETE. There is a report reviewing 1000 consecutive patients with low-risk PTMC who underwent chest CT as a routine preoperative study. They reported that none of these patients showed metastatic lesions on chest CT.[16] Evaluation of distant metastases in incidentally found PTMC is not regarded as mandatory.

Surgical Treatment & Outcomes

Surgery has been a cornerstone for the treatment of PTC. Postoperative outcomes for PTC with tumor size ≤10 mm and no clinical invasion or metastasis are excellent. Ten-year disease-specific survival rate was reported as 99.5% to 100%. Recurrence in lymph nodes can be seen in 3% to 6%; however, distant recurrence is extremely rare. The recurrence rate for PTC with tumor size ≤5 mm was slightly lower than that for PTC with tumor size 5 to 10 mm.

A report from Kuma Hospital compared the frequency of unfavorable events for patients with PTMC between active surveillance (n = 1179, including 94 patients who underwent conversion surgery) and immediate surgery

Table 13–1. Indication of fine-needle aspiration cytology on thyroid nodule according to the size in various guidelines.

Guidelines	5-10 mm	10-15 mm	15-20 mm	>20 mm
ATA (2016)	Can be observed except for nodules with evidence of extrathyroidal extension or sonographically suspicious lymph nodes	High-suspicion pattern (Solid hypoechoic nodule or solid component of a partially cystic nodule with one or more suspicious US features) Intermediate-suspicion pattern (Hypoechoic solid nodule)	Low-suspicion pattern (Iso- or hyperechoic solid nodule, or partially cystic nodule with eccentric solid areas)	Very low-suspicion pattern (Spongiform pattern or partially cystic nodule without suspicious US features)
NCCN (2019)	Not recommended	Solid nodule with suspicious US features Mixed cystic-solid nodule with suspicious US features if solid component >1 cm	Solid nodule without suspicious US features Mixed cystic-solid nodule without suspicious US features of solid component >1.5 cm	Spongiform nodule
ACR (2017)	Not recommended	Highly suspicious (≥7/14 points*)	(15-25 mm) Moderately suspicious (4–6/14 points*)	(≥25 mm) Mildly suspicious (3/14 points*)
ETA (2017)	Nodules with highly suspicious US features and no abnormal lymph nodes can have the choice of FNAC or observation. In case of proven growth or detection of a suspicious lymph node, FNAC should be performed.	Nodule with high-risk US features	Nodule with intermediate-risk US features	Nodule with low-risk US features
JABTS (2016)	Highly suspicious (Meets most suspicious US findings including shape, boundary, internal echo, high echo level, and halo sign)	Suspicious (Meets any suspicious US features) (Except for spongiform)	Recommend FNAC	Recommend FNAC

*Sum of points from each category including composition, echogenicity, shape, margin, and echogenic foci determines the Thyroid Imaging, Reporting and Data System (TI-RADS) level.

ACR: American College of Radiology; ATA: American Thyroid Association; ETA: European Thyroid Association; FNAC: fine-needle aspiration cytology; JABTS: Japan Association of Breast and Thyroid Sonology; NCCN: National Comprehensive Cancer Network; US: ultrasound.

($n = 974$, 575 underwent lobectomy, 399 had a total thyroidectomy, all had central lymph node dissection). Patients who chose active surveillance had less incidence of transient vocal cord paralysis (0.6% vs 4.1%, $p < 0.0001$), transient hypoparathyroidism (2.8% vs 16.7%, $p < 0.0001$), and permanent hypoparathyroidism (0.08% vs 1.6%, $p < 0.0001$) than those who underwent immediate surgery. Permanent vocal cord paralysis was observed in 0.2% of patients who underwent immediate surgery.[17] Surgery performed for low-risk PTMC does little to affect the incidence of recurrence or spread; however, surgical complications still occur, albeit rarely, even when surgery is performed by well-trained thyroid surgeons. They recently reported that there were no differences in the incidence of unfavorable events between patients with immediate surgery and those who had conversion surgery after progression during active surveillance.[18]

Active Surveillance

Clinical trials of active surveillance for low-risk PTMC have been conducted at two Japanese institutions (Kuma Hospital, Kobe and Cancer Institute Hospital, Tokyo) since the 1990s.[7,8,19,20] Those studies showed favorable outcomes: (1) the incidence of tumor enlargement and new LNM was low; (2) no patients who underwent conversion surgery after the appearance of these progression signs showed life-threatening recurrence or died of thyroid carcinoma; and (3) no patients developed distant metastases or died of thyroid carcinoma during active surveillance. Based on these findings, the 2015 American Thyroid Association guidelines for adult patients with thyroid nodules and differentiated thyroid cancer have acknowledged a policy of active surveillance for low-risk PTMC.[6] Subsequently, reports on active

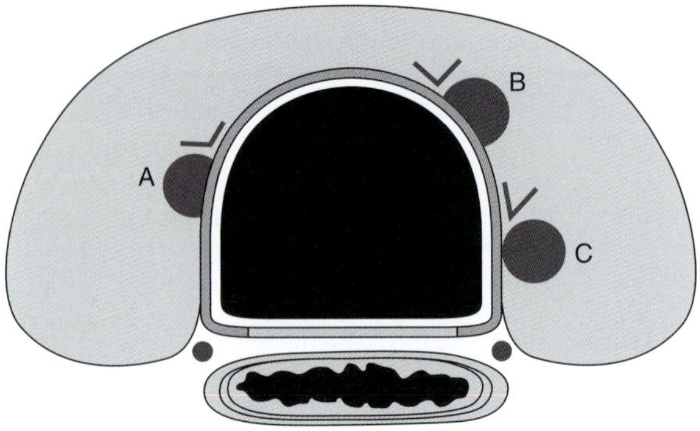

▲ **Figure 13–1.** Risk evaluation of tracheal invasion according to the location of papillary thyroid microcarcinoma. **(A)** Tumor attaching to the trachea wall forming obtuse angle (high-risk of tracheal invasion). **(B)** Tumor attaching to the trachea wall with right angle (intermediate-risk of tracheal invasion). **(C)** Tumor attaching to the trachea wall with acute angle (low-risk of tracheal invasion).

surveillance from several countries have been published.[21-24] The outcomes of these trials are also favorable as shown in Table 13–2. In this way, this new management policy to prevent overtreatment of low-risk PTMC has gradually spread worldwide as an alternative to immediate surgery.

To implement a proper program of active surveillance, the Memorial Sloan Kettering Cancer Center group collaborated with the Kuma Hospital group and proposed a clinical framework for active surveillance (Table 13–3).[25] It evaluated the risk of active surveillance using three domains namely: tumor characteristics as assessed largely by ultrasound, patient characteristics, and medical team characteristics. Then, it classified candidates into three categories (ie, ideal, appropriate, and inappropriate). Active surveillance should be performed through a multidisciplinary team including highly experienced ultrasound examiners who can accurately evaluate primary tumors and lymph nodes. Moreover, an adequate shared decision should be made with individual patients. In 2021, the Japan Association of Endocrine Surgery task force on management for PTMC published consensus statements on indications and strategy for active surveillance of adult low-risk PTMC to facilitate the implementation of this management alternative appropriately.[14]

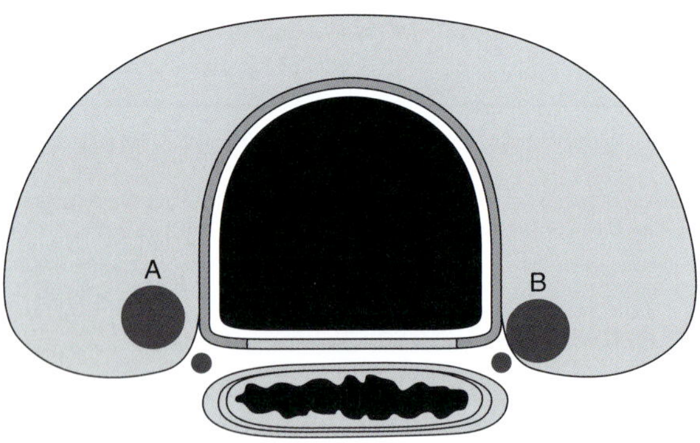

▲ **Figure 13–2.** Risk evaluation of recurrent laryngeal nerve (RLN) invasion according to the location of papillary thyroid microcarcinoma. **(A)** Normal rim is present between the tumor and course of the RLN (low-risk of invasion). **(B)** Normal rim is absent between the tumor and course of the RLN (high-risk of invasion). Attention should be paid to difference in the path of the RLN between sides. Left RLN usually runs through the tracheoesophageal groove; however, the path of right RLN is more oblique and tumor located in the dorsal region, away from the tracheoesophageal groove still has a risk of invasion of the RLN.

A. Indications for Active Surveillance

Candidates for active surveillance are adult patients with low-risk PTMC; namely, clinical T1aN0M0 PTC. PTMCs with high-risk features including clinically apparent LNM, distant metastasis, and invasion to adjacent organs (particularly the trachea and RLN) should undergo immediate surgery and postoperative radioactive iodine therapy if indicated. In addition, FNAC features suggestive of aggressive subtypes of PTC, such as tall cell variant, are recommended for immediate surgery. Immediate surgery is also recommended for tumors adhering to the trachea or located along the course of the RLN. Evidence for the safety of active surveillance in patients under 20 years old is lacking at present. Table 13–4 shows indications for immediate surgery without active surveillance recommended by the Japan Association of Endocrine Surgery.[14]

B. Factors Affecting Decision-Making in Management of Adult Patients With PTMC

At present, age is the most significant factor to predict progression of low-risk PTMC under active surveillance. The risk of tumor progression decreases with age. A report from Kuma Hospital enrolling 1235 cases of low-risk PTMCs under observation showed that the 10-year rate of progression to clinical disease (enlargement of tumor diameter to ≥12 mm or appearance of LNM) was 2.5% in patients ≥60 years old, 4.9% in those 40 to 59 years old, and 22.5% in those less than 40 years old. Multivariate analysis revealed young age (≤40 years) as an independent risk factor for PTMC becoming clinical disease.[19] Furthermore, they estimated that the lifetime probability of disease progression was 48.6% for patients in their 20s at presentation, 25.3% in the 30s, 20.9% in the 40s, 10.3% in the 50s, 8.2% in the 60s, and 3.5% in the 70s.[26] Recent systematic review and meta-analysis including five studies reported that risk ratio for a ≥3-mm increase in tumor diameter for patients ≥40 and <40 was 0.55

Table 13–2. Outcomes of active surveillance for patients with low-risk papillary thyroid microcarcinoma.

Site, Country (Year)	Number of Patients	Duration of Follow-up (months)	Tumor Enlargement (maximum diameter ≥3 mm)	Tumor Enlargement (tumor volume ≥50%)	Appearance of Lymph Node Metastasis	Development of Extrathyroidal Extension	Appearance of Distant Metastasis
Kuma Hospital, Japan (2014)	1235	Mean, 60 (range 18-227)	4.6% 4.9%/5 years 8.0%/10 years	ND	1.5% 1.7%/5 years 3.8%/10 years	0.16%	0%
Cancer Institute Hospital, Japan (2016)	409	Mean, 81.6 (range 1-23)	6.0% 6.3%/5 years 7.3%/10 years	ND	1.0%	0%	0%
Memorial Sloan Kettering Cancer Center, United States (2017)	291*	Mean, 25 (range 6-166)	3.8% 2.5%/2 years 12.1%/5 years	12.4% 11.5%/2 years 24.8%/5 years	0%	0%	0%
Asan Medical Center, Samsung Medical Center, Seoul St. Mary's Hospital, Korea (2018)	370	Median 32.5 (IQR 21.5-47.6)	3.5%	23.2%	1.4%	ND	0%
University Hospital of Pisa, Italy (2020)	93	Median, 19 (range 6-54)	2.1%	16%	1.1%	ND	0%
Neck Cancer Center in Medellin, Colombia (2020)	102*	Median, 13.9 (range 0.2-112)	10.8%	25.5%	ND	ND	ND

*Included patients with papillary thyroid carcinoma >10 mm in diameter.
ND: no data; IQR: interquartile range.

(95% confidence interval, 0.36-0.82).[27] Older patients with low-risk PTMC are ideal candidates for active surveillance. Although tumors in young patients are more likely to progress, these patients can be candidates for active surveillance since the outcomes of conversion surgery are excellent and the lifetime probability of progression is estimated as less than 50% even among patients in their 20s at presentation. Active surveillance could be considered as a way to identify patients who need surgery, since no difference in prognosis exists between conversion surgery after active surveillance and immediate surgery.

A report from Cancer Institute Hospital described that degree of calcification was associated with the enlargement of PTMCs. They divided tumors into four categories of calcification: none; micro; macro; and rim. The degree of calcification correlated significantly with patient age, and tumors with coarse (macro or rim) calcification were less likely to enlarge. Also, during active surveillance, 25.1% and 51.8% of lesions showed an increase in degree of calcification at 5- and 10-year follow-up, respectively. On multivariate analysis, cases with coarse calcification in the most recent examination showed a significantly lower enlargement rate compared to cases with weak (none or micro) calcification (odds ratio, 0.34; 95% confidence interval, 0.11-0.87; $p = 0.022$).[20] In contrast, a report from South Korea studied 273 low-risk PTMCs observed for ≥1 year and demonstrated that cases with macrocalcification at initiation were more likely to show an enlargement of tumor volume by ≥50% compared to those with microcalcification.[28] Although low-risk PTMCs with fine or no calcification may be more likely to progress than those with coarse calcification, calcification is reported to become strong with time. PTMCs with fine or no calcification remain candidates for active surveillance.

A study from Cancer Institute Hospital also demonstrated the relationship between change in vascularity over time in each tumor and progression during active surveillance.[20] According to the data, 14.6% of 70 lesions with rich vascularity at initiation of active surveillance enlarged by ≥3 mm, significantly higher than the rate of enlargement in 410 lesions with poor vascularity (4.6%). Also, vascularity became poor during active surveillance in 61.4% of PTMCs with rich vascularity at the beginning. On multivariate analysis, cases

Table 13–3. Risk-stratified management of papillary thyroid microcarcinoma proposed by the Memorial Sloan Kettering Cancer Center group.

Candidates for Active Surveillance	Tumor, Neck US Characteristics	Patient Characteristics	Medical Team Characteristics
Ideal	Solitary nodule Well-defined margins Surrounded by normal thyroid parenchyma No evidence of ETE No clinical LNM No distant metastasis	Older patients (>60 years) Willingness and compliance for active surveillance Understands that a surgical intervention may be necessary in the future Life-threatening comorbidities	Experienced multidisciplinary management team High-quality neck US Prospective data collection Tracking/reminder program to ensure proper follow-up
Appropriate	Multifocal PTMCs Subcapsular locations not adjacent to RLN Ill-defined margins Background US findings that will make follow-up difficult FDG-avid PTMCs	Middle-aged patients (18-59 years) Strong family history of thyroid cancer Child-bearing potential	Experienced endocrinologist or thyroid surgeon Neck US routinely available
Inappropriate	Evidence of aggressive cytology on FNAC Subcapsular locations adjacent to RLN Evidence of ETE Clinical evidence of invasion of RLN or trachea Clinically apparent LNM Distant metastasis	Young patients (<18 years) No willingness for active surveillance Not compliant with active surveillance	Reliable neck US not available Little experience with thyroid cancer management

ETE: extrathyroidal extension; FDG: fluorodeoxyglucose; FNAC: fine-needle aspiration cytology; LNM: lymph node metastasis; PTMC: papillary thyroid microcarcinoma; RLN: recurrent laryngeal nerve; US: ultrasound.
Source: Modified from Brito JP, Ito Y, Miyauchi A, et al. A clinical framework to facilitate risk stratification when considering an active surveillance alternative to immediate biopsy and surgery in papillary microcarcinoma. *Thyroid.* 2016;26:144-149.

with poor vascularization as of the most recent examination showed significantly lower tumor enlargement rates than cases with rich vascularity (odds ratio, 0.17; 95% confidence interval, 0.07-0.43; $p = 0.0004$). Tumors with rich vascularity seem to have a higher possibility of enlarging than those with poor vascularity; however, vascularity in low-risk PTMCs is suggested to decrease over time very often.

Multiplicity is sometimes regarded as a risk factor for recurrence in patients with PTC; however, no evidence has suggested multiple PTMCs are related to tumor progression during active surveillance.[29] Patients with multiple lesions can still be candidates for active surveillance. This recommendation can help to avoid total thyroidectomy and the resulting increased risk of surgical complications for those patients.

Patients with a family history of PTC are more likely to have multifocal disease and have LNMs, and possibly have a higher incidence of postoperative recurrence. However, the relationship between outcomes of active surveillance and family history of PTC has not been adequately studied. The presence of a family history does not override the indications for active surveillance. However, familial PTC may be more aggressive. If conversion surgery becomes necessary in patients with familial PTC, total thyroidectomy should be considered.

Controversial results were reported about the risk of progression under active surveillance for patients during pregnancy. However, since careful and constant surveillance enables safe management of low-risk PTMC during pregnancy, patients planning pregnancy and actively pregnant patients can be candidates for active surveillance.

C. Methods of Active Surveillance

Small numbers of PTMCs under active surveillance show progression—specifically tumor enlargement or novel LNM appearance. Periodic checkup examinations are mandatory to avoid missing the appropriate time for conversion surgery. The conditions to move onto conversion surgery recommended by the Japan Association of Endocrine Surgery are shown in Table 13–4.[14]

1. Interval between examinations—Although no comparative studies have been published regarding the optimal interval, ultrasound evaluation for changes in tumor size, the appearance of novel thyroid lesions, and LNM are recommended to be performed every 6 months for 1 to 2 years after initiation of active surveillance, and once a year thereafter, if no disease progression is detected. No evidence is available regarding when the interval between examinations can be further extended, such as to every 2 to 3 years.

Table 13–4. Papillary thyroid microcarcinoma indicated for immediate surgery without active surveillance and indicated for conversion surgery after active surveillance recommended by the consensus statements from the Japan Association of Endocrine Surgery.

Indication of immediate surgery without active surveillance for papillary thyroid microcarcinoma
1. Presence of clinical lymph node metastasis or distant metastasis (rare)
2. Clinically apparent invasion to the recurrent laryngeal nerve or trachea
3. Diagnosis of aggressive subtype of papillary thyroid carcinoma on cytology (rare)
4. Tumors adhering to trachea, possibly invading
5. Tumors located along course of the recurrent laryngeal nerve
6. Associated other thyroid or parathyroid disease indicated for surgery
7. Age <20 years (no current evidence)
Indication of conversion surgery after active surveillance for papillary thyroid microcarcinoma
1. Tumor diameter reaches 13 mm
2. Appearance of novel lymph node metastasis
3. Alteration of patient preference
4. Appearance of other thyroid disease or parathyroid disease indicated for surgery

Source: Modified from Sugitani I, Ito Y, Takeuchi D, et al. Indications and strategy for active surveillance of adult low-risk papillary thyroid microcarcinoma: consensus statements from the Japan Association of Endocrine Surgery Task Force on management for papillary thyroid microcarcinoma. *Thyroid.* 2021;31:183-192.

2. Definition of tumor enlargement and timing for conversion surgery—During active surveillance, enlargement of the tumor has been defined as an "increase in maximal diameter by ≥3 mm" in most studies. According to this definition, no study has reported cases in which RLN paralysis or distant metastasis occurred, or conversion surgery was too late. Evaluation based on maximal diameter is considered as a simple and sufficient method in the daily practice.

On the other hand, some researchers defined enlargement as a "50% increase in tumor volume" by measuring three dimensions.[21,28,30,31] The advantages are that tumor volume and its doubling time can accurately reflect changes in tumor size and can be used as a potential prognostic marker of future growth. However, this approach is sometimes overly sensitive and is subject to a high degree of observer variability.

A decision for surgery when maximal diameter exceeds 10 mm is not always necessary. A kinetic analysis of low-risk PTMC under active surveillance showed that growth activity after enlargement decreased significantly compared with before enlargement, and many cases fell into a stabilized stage or showed tumor shrinkage.[32,33] Active surveillance could be allowed to continue until tumor diameter reaches 13 mm, since a 3-mm increase in the largest PTMC (ie, 10 mm in maximum diameter) makes a 13-mm tumor; however, tumor location (possibility of invasion to the RLN and trachea), velocity of growth, and patient preference should also be considered for such cases.

3. Thyroid-stimulating hormone (TSH) suppression during active surveillance—No randomized prospective studies have been published about TSH-suppression therapy during active surveillance for low-risk PTMC, but some reports have been published regarding the relationship between TSH levels and tumor enlargement. A study from Cancer Institute Hospital reported that TSH levels at diagnosis and average TSH levels during active surveillance did not differ between the enlargement group (≥3 mm) and the nonenlargement group. On multivariate analysis, TSH at diagnosis was not regarded as a significant predictor of tumor enlargement, and average TSH level during active surveillance did not correlate significantly with change in tumor volume.[34] In contrast, another study from South Korea described that the high-TSH group had a higher incidence of tumor volume increasing by ≥50% than the other groups among patients who underwent active surveillance. They claimed that high TSH level as an independent risk factor for PTMC enlargement, and progression-free survival rates were significantly worse for low-risk PTMC with TSH more than 2.50 mIU/L than for other groups.[35] The possibility of high TSH level affecting low-risk PTMC progression cannot be ruled out, but at present, it is impossible to conclude that TSH suppression therapy is beneficial for patients. Active TSH suppression might have adverse effects on the heart or bone, particularly for old patients. Setting the TSH level at a low normal to avoid excess stimulation could be acceptable for young patients in whom PTMCs are more likely to enlarge.

4. Termination of active surveillance—The incidence of low-risk PTMC progression could become lower with age. However, in clinical PTC, old age is one of the most important factors predicting poor prognosis. Thus, if PTMCs in old patients turn into clinical disease and it is not detected in the early phase by constant surveillance, that could result in a life-threatening situation. At present, there is no evidence regarding after how many years active surveillance can be terminated. Active surveillance throughout life is recommended as far as circumstances permit.[14]

Ongoing & Future Tasks for the Management of Patients With PTMC

A. Molecular Markers to Differentiate Progressive PTMC From Others

Genetic abnormalities found in PTC include mutations in *BRAF*, *RET/PTC*, and *APC* in relation to tumor occurrence and *p53*, *TERT*, and *CTNNB1* relating to tumor progression.

Some investigators have reported that *BRAF* gene mutations in PTMC are related to characteristics such as ETE, LNM, and recurrence. However, there has been no reliable molecular marker to predict progression of low-risk PTMC at initiation of active surveillance.

B. Cost Analysis Comparing Active Surveillance With Immediate Surgery

Several studies were carried out to analyze the cost-effectiveness of active surveillance for PTMC compared with immediate surgery. A study from Hong Kong reported that active surveillance could reduce medical costs for the first 16 years compared to immediate surgery.[36] A report from Australia indicated that active surveillance had lower medical costs than immediate surgery during the first 16.2 years, but immediate surgery offered economic advantages for young people who need long-term follow-up.[37] Another study from the United States had shown that lobectomy was more cost-effective than active surveillance for patients in whom nonoperative management would be associated with at least a modest decrement in quality of life (QOL).[38] From Kuma Hospital, the 10-year total cost of immediate surgery was reported to be 4.1 times more expensive than active surveillance.[39] Of course, it is important to remember the influence of the differing costs of care in the insurance systems of each country when interpreting these results. In addition, the interval and duration of postoperative follow-up varies in actual clinical practice depending on the patient and facilities. It is also important to note that young people require long-term follow-up and often undergo conversion from active surveillance to surgery.

C. Patient-reported Outcome (PRO) Study Comparing Active Surveillance With Immediate Surgery

When deciding the management strategy for patients with PTMC, it is important to take into account PROs, such as other health problems and anxiety, that would be experienced by patients who undergo medical care. In many reports of active surveillance, a substantial percentage of patients undergo conversion surgery as a result of patient preference related to anxiety and not due to tumor progression. According to a qualitative study on the perspective of patients who underwent active surveillance at Kuma Hospital, 37% of patients worried about cancer progression; however, 60% reported that their anxiety had decreased over time.[40]

There are some cross-sectional and longitudinal PRO studies comparing patients who underwent immediate surgery and those who decided to undergo active surveillance (Table 13–5).[41-46] While active surveillance generally appeared superior to immediate surgery in terms of physical QOL, psychological QOL was reported to sometimes be worse than surgery. However, patient anxiety generally gradually diminishes with the lapse of time. Previous studies of PRO on PTMC management have been hampered by limitations such as a biased period from diagnosis to investigation, small number of cases, and a short observation period. The evidence regarding PRO in PTMC remains insufficient, and long-term comparative studies regarding PROs are required.

D. Active Surveillance for T1bN0M0 PTC

A study using the National Cancer Database and the Surveillance, Epidemiology and End Results program showed that adjusted overall and disease-specific survival were not different significantly between T1a (-10 mm) and T1b (11-20 mm) differentiated thyroid carcinoma. A report from Cancer Institute Hospital showed that disease progression rates of 61 patients with T1bN0M0 PTC were not significantly different from those of 360 patients with T1aN0M0 for an average of 7.9 years of active surveillance. No postoperative recurrence was seen in patients who underwent immediate or conversion surgery with tumors less than 15 mm in diameter. Select patients with T1bN0M0 PTC might be candidates for active surveillance.[47]

E. Thermal Ablation Techniques for Low-Risk PTMC

Recent studies evaluated the efficacy and safety of thermal ablation techniques including radiofrequency ablation, laser ablation, and microwave ablation for patients with low-risk PTMC. A Korean group conducted ultrasound-guided radiofrequency ablation on 84 nodules from 74 patients. All patients tolerated the ablation, and the mean follow-up duration was 72 months. After the therapy, complete disappearance rates of 98.8% and 100% were achieved at 24- and 60-month follow-up, respectively. The major complication rate was 1.4% (1/74), and there was no delayed complication or procedure-related death.[48] A report from China showed that ultrasound-guided microwave ablation reduced tumor volume from 1.87 ± 1.03 mL immediately after ablation to 0.01 ± 0.04 mL at the final evaluation, with a mean volume reduction ratio of 99.4 ± 2.2% and 107 cases (93.9%) had complete remission (119 unifocal low-risk PTMC; mean follow-up duration after ablation, 37.2 ± 20.9 months). No delayed complications associated with the technique were encountered.[49] Thermal ablation can be done safely and with excellent local control rates at specialized centers. It can be useful, particularly for patients with significant comorbidities that increase the risk of surgical intervention and for patients who are unwilling to choose either the surgical or active surveillance option. However, additional studies are needed to address which specific thermal ablation modality is optimal for individual patients and to analyze long-term efficacy, QOL, and cost compared with active surveillance or surgery.

Table 13–5. Patient-reported outcome studies comparing immediate surgery and active surveillance in patients with low-risk papillary thyroid microcarcinoma.

Site, Country (Year)	Number of Patients	Period From Diagnosis to Investigation	Instrument of Measurement	Main Outcomes
Cross-sectional studies				
Asan Medical Center, Korea (2019)	Surgery: 148 AS: 43	Median: 38.0 months Median: 29.6 months	SF-12v2 THYCA-QOL FoP	Psychological problems were less frequent in AS group. AS group had fewer problems involving the nerves, muscles, pharynx, oral symptoms, and wounds. No differences about fear of cancer progression between groups.
Tokyo Women's Medical University, Japan (2020)	Surgery: 30 AS: 20	Median 4.25 years Median 4.05 years	STAI VAS (originally developed to measure symptoms and concerns)	AS group showed deeper anxiety, but the degree of anxiety correlated with the trait anxiety of each patient, not with the choice of the management. Anxiety correlated inversely with the observation time. Symptoms of "discomfort in the neck," "weak voice," and "nervousness about neck appearance" were favorable in AS group.
Kuma Hospital, Japan (2020)	Surgery: 49 AS: 298	Median: 84 months Median: 56.5 months	THYCA-QOL HADS	AS group had less complaints about "voice," "psychological," "problems with scar," and "gained weight." AS group had significantly better anxiety and depression.
Cancer Institute Hospital & Nippon Medical School, Japan (2023)	Surgery: 32 AS: 249	Median: 4.0 years Median: 7.9 years	STAI SF-36v2 VAS (originally developed to measure symptoms and concerns)	After matching, AS group showed better trait anxiety and mental health than surgery group. Surgery group displayed worse neck symptoms than AS group. Among AS group, better trait anxiety and longer time from the onset were significant predictors of better state anxiety.
Longitudinal studies				
Seoul National University Hospital, Seoul National University Bundang Hospital, National Cancer Center, Korea (2019)	Surgery: 203 AS: 192	Mean: 7.1 ± 4.2 months Mean: 9.3 ± 4.8 months	Thyroid-specific QOL questionnaire	AS group was superior in psychological health at baseline, and in physical and psychological health at after a mean follow-up of 8.2 months.
Seoul National University Hospital, Seoul National University Bundang Hospital, National Cancer Center, Korea (2021)	Surgery: 381 AS: 674	Median: 24.6 months Median: 24.0 months	Thyroid-specific QOL questionnaire	2-year QoL was good in order of AS, lobectomy, and total thyroidectomy group after adjustment for age, sex, baseline tumor size, and baseline QOL scores. Among patients who changed their treatment from AS to surgery during the follow-up period, patients who changed treatment due to disease progression had better QOL than who had no disease progression.

AS: active surveillance; FoP: fear of progression questionnaire; HADS: hospital anxiety and depression scale; QOL: quality of life; SF-12v2: 12-item short-form health survey version 2.0; SF-36v2: 36-item short-form health survey version 2.0; STAI: state-trait anxiety inventory; THYCA-QOL: thyroid cancer-specific health-related quality of life questionnaire; VAS: visual analog scale.

F. Insights Into the Natural History of PTMC

Accumulated evidence on active surveillance has shed light on the natural history of low-risk PTMC. Age is the most important predictive factor of tumor progression for low-risk PTMC under active surveillance. The proportion of patients having higher growth activity significantly decreased with age. In most cases, tumor calcification becomes stronger and the vascularity gets poorer over time and the tumor loses its potential to progress. Most low-risk PTMCs are thought to grow rapidly to some extent at first, but decelerate in their growth rate and become stable or even decrease in size afterward. The management strategy for individual patients with PTMC should be optimized considering the natural history of the disease.

REFERENCES

1. Davies L, Welch HG. Increasing incidence of thyroid cancer in the United States, 1973-2002. *JAMA*. 2006;295:2164-2167.
2. Ahn HS, Kim HJ, Welch HG. Korea's thyroid-cancer "epidemic"—screening and overdiagnosis. *N Engl J Med*. 2014;371: 1765-1767.
3. Vaccarella S, Maso LD, Laversanne M, et al. The impact of diagnostic changes on the rise in thyroid cancer incidence: a population-based study in selected high-resource countries. *Thyroid*. 2015;25:1127-1136.
4. Zevallos JP, Hartman CM, Kramer JR, et al. Increased thyroid cancer incidence corresponds to increased use of thyroid ultrasound and fine-needle aspiration: a study of the Veterans Affairs health care system. *Cancer*. 2015;121:741-746.
5. Bibbins-Domingo K, Grossman DC, Curry SJ, et al. Screening for thyroid cancer: US Preventive Services Task Force recommendation statement. *JAMA*. 2017;317:1882-1887.
6. Haugen BR, Alexander EK, Bible KC, et al. 2015 American Thyroid Association management guidelines for adult patients with thyroid nodules and differentiated thyroid cancer: the American Thyroid Association Guidelines Task Force on thyroid nodules and differentiated thyroid cancer. *Thyroid*. 2016; 26:1-133.
7. Ito Y, Uruno T, Nakano K, et al. An observation trial without surgical treatment in patients with papillary microcarcinoma of the thyroid. *Thyroid*. 2003;13:381-387.
8. Sugitani I, Toda K, Yamada K, et al. Three distinctly different kinds of papillary thyroid microcarcinoma should be recognized: our treatment strategies and outcomes. *World J Surg*. 2010;34: 1222-1231.
9. Mehanna H, Al-Maqbili T, Carter B, et al. Differences in the recurrence and mortality outcomes rates of incidental and nonincidental papillary thyroid microcarcinoma: a systematic review and meta-analysis of 21,329 person-years of follow-up. *J Clin Endocrinol Metab*. 2014;99:2834-2843.
10. Horiguchi K, Yoshida Y, Iwaku K, et al. Position paper from the Japan Thyroid Association task force on the management of low-risk papillary thyroid microcarcinoma (T1aN0M0) in adults. *Endocr J*. 2021;68:763-780.
11. Furuya-Kanamori L, Bell KJL, Clark J, et al. Prevalence of differentiated thyroid cancer in autopsy studies over six decades: a meta-analysis. *J Clin Oncol*. 2016;34:3672-3679.
12. Tessler FN, Middleton WD, Grant EG, et al. ACR thyroid imaging, reporting and data system (TI-RADS): white paper of the ACR TI-RADS committee. *J Am Coll Radiol*. 2017;14:587-595.
13. Russ G, Bonnema SJ, Erdogan MF, et al. European Thyroid Association guidelines for ultrasound malignancy risk stratification of thyroid nodules in adults: the EU-TIRADS. *Eur Thyroid J*. 2017;6: 225-237.
14. Sugitani I, Ito Y, Takeuchi D, et al. Indications and strategy for active surveillance of adult low-risk papillary thyroid microcarcinoma: consensus statements from the Japan Association of Endocrine Surgery task force on management for papillary thyroid microcarcinoma. *Thyroid*. 2021;31:183-192.
15. Ito Y, Miyauchi A, Oda H, et al. Revisiting low-risk thyroid papillary microcarcinomas resected without observation: was immediate surgery necessary? *World J Surg*. 2016;40:523-528.
16. Kawano S, Miyauchi A, Ito Y. Routine chest CT at presentation does not identify distant metastasis in cT1aN0 papillary thyroid carcinoma. *Thyroid*. 2020;30:1620-1624.
17. Oda H, Miyauchi A, Ito Y, et al. Incidences of unfavorable events in the management of low-risk papillary microcarcinoma of the thyroid by active surveillance versus immediate surgery. *Thyroid*. 2016;26:150-155.
18. Sasaki T, Miyauchi A, Fujishima M, et al. Comparison of postoperative unfavorable events in patients with low-risk papillary thyroid carcinoma: immediate surgery versus conversion surgery following active surveillance. *Thyroid*. 2023;45:2769-2776.
19. Ito Y, Miyauchi A, Kihara M, et al. Patient age is significantly related to the progression of papillary microcarcinoma of the thyroid under observation. *Thyroid*. 2014;24:27-34.
20. Fukuoka O, Sugitani I, Ebina A, et al. Natural history of asymptomatic papillary thyroid microcarcinoma: time-dependent changes in calcification and vascularity during active surveillance. *World J Surg*. 2016;40:529-537.
21. Tuttle RM, Fagin JA, Minkowitz G, et al. Natural history and tumor volume kinetics of papillary thyroid cancers during active surveillance. *JAMA Otolaryngol Head Neck Surg*. 2017;143:1015-1020.
22. Oh HS, Ha J, Kim HI, et al. Active surveillance of low-risk papillary thyroid microcarcinoma: a multi-center cohort study in Korea. *Thyroid*. 2018;28:1587-1594.
23. Molinaro E, Campopiano MC, Pieruzzi L, et al. Active surveillance in papillary thyroid microcarcinomas is feasible and safe: experience at a single Italian center. *J Clin Endocrinol Metab*. 2020;105:e172-e180.
24. Sanabria A. Experience with active surveillance of thyroid low-risk carcinoma in a developing country. *Thyroid*. 2020;30:985-991.
25. Brito JP, Ito Y, Miyauchi A, et al. A clinical framework to facilitate risk stratification when considering an active surveillance alternative to immediate biopsy and surgery in papillary microcarcinoma. *Thyroid*. 2016;26:144-149.
26. Miyauchi A, Kudo T, Ito Y, et al. Estimation of the lifetime probability of disease progression of papillary microcarcinoma of the thyroid during active surveillance. *Surgery*. 2018;163:48-52.
27. Koshkina A, Fazelzad R, Sugitani I, et al. Association of patient age with progression of low-risk papillary thyroid carcinoma under active surveillance: a systematic review and meta-analysis. *JAMA Otolaryngol Head Neck Surg*. 2020;146:552-560.
28. Oh HS, Kwon H, Song E, et al. Tumor volume doubling time in active surveillance of papillary thyroid carcinoma. *Thyroid*. 2019;29:642-649.
29. Nagaoka R, Ebina A, Toda K, et al. Multifocality and progression of papillary thyroid microcarcinoma during active surveillance. *World J Surg*. 2021;45:2769-2776.
30. Kwon H, Oh HS, Kim M, et al. Active surveillance for patients with papillary thyroid microcarcinoma: a single center's experience in Korea. *J Clin Endocrinol Metab*. 2017;102:1917-1925.

31. Jin M, Kim HI, Ha J, et al. Tumor volume doubling time in active surveillance of papillary thyroid microcarcinoma: a multicenter cohort study. *Thyroid*. 2021;31(10):1494-1501.
32. Miyauchi A, Kudo T, Ito Y, et al. Natural history of papillary thyroid microcarcinoma: kinetic analyses on tumor volume during active surveillance and before presentation. *Surgery*. 2019;165:25-30.
33. Ito Y, Miyauchi A, Kudo T, et al. Kinetic analysis of growth activity in enlarging papillary thyroid microcarcinomas. *Thyroid*. 2019;29:1765-1773.
34. Sugitani I, Fujimoto Y, Yamada K. Association between serum thyrotropin concentration and growth of asymptomatic papillary thyroid microcarcinoma. *World J Surg*. 2014;38: 673-678.
35. Kim HI, Jang HW, Ahn HS, et al. High serum TSH level is associated with progression of papillary thyroid microcarcinoma during active surveillance. *J Clin Endocrinol Metab*. 2018;103:446-451.
36. Lang BH, Wong CK. A cost-effectiveness comparison between early surgery and non-surgical approach for incidental papillary thyroid microcarcinoma. *Eur J Endocrinol*. 2015;173:367-375.
37. Lin JF, Jonker PKC, Cunich M, et al. Surgery alone for papillary thyroid microcarcinoma is less costly and more effective than long-term active surveillance. *Surgery*. 2020;167:110-116.
38. Venkatesh S, Pasternak JD, Beninato T, et al. Cost-effectiveness of active surveillance versus hemithyroidectomy for micropapillary thyroid cancer. *Surgery*. 2017;161:116-126.
39. Oda H, Miyauchi A, Ito Y, et al. Comparison of the costs of active surveillance and immediate surgery in the management of low-risk papillary microcarcinoma of the thyroid. *Endocr J*. 2017;64:59-64.
40. Davies L, Roman BR, Fukushima M, et al. Patient experience of thyroid cancer active surveillance in Japan. *JAMA Otolaryngol Head Neck Surg*. 2019;145:363-370.
41. Jeon MJ, Lee YM, Sung TY, et al. Quality of life in patients with papillary thyroid microcarcinoma managed by active surveillance or lobectomy: a cross-sectional study. *Thyroid*. 2019;29:956-962.
42. Yoshida Y, Horiuchi K, Okamoto T. Patients' view on the management of papillary thyroid microcarcinoma: active surveillance or surgery. *Thyroid*. 2020;30:681-687.
43. Nakamura T, Miyauchi A, Ito Y, et al. Quality of life in patients with low-risk papillary thyroid microcarcinoma: active surveillance versus immediate surgery. *Endocr Pract*. 2020;26:1451-1457.
44. Kazusaka H, Sugitani I, Toda K, et al. Patient-reported outcomes in patients with low-risk papillary thyroid carcinoma: cross-sectional study to compare active surveillance and immediate surgery. *World J Surg*. 2023;47:1190-1198.
45. Kong SH, Ryu J, Kim MJ, et al. Longitudinal assessment of quality of life according to treatment options in low-risk papillary thyroid microcarcinoma patients: active surveillance or immediate surgery (interim analysis of MAeSTro). *Thyroid*. 2019;29:1089-1096.
46. Moon JH, Ryu CH, Cho SW, et al. Effect of initial treatment choice on 2-year quality of life in patients with low-risk papillary thyroid microcarcinoma. *J Clin Endocrinol Metab*. 2021;106:724-735.
47. Sakai T, Sugitani I, Ebina A, et al. Active surveillance for T1bN0M0 papillary thyroid carcinoma. *Thyroid*. 2019;29:59-63.
48. Cho SJ, Baek SM, Lim HK, et al. Long-term follow-up results of ultrasound-guided radiofrequency ablation for low-risk papillary thyroid microcarcinoma: more than 5-year follow-up for 84 tumors. *Thyroid*. 2020;30:1745-1751.
49. Yue WW, Qi L, Wang DD, et al. US-guided microwave ablation of low-risk papillary thyroid microcarcinoma: longer-term results of a prospective study. *J Clin Endocrinol Metab*. 2020 Jun 1;105(6):dgaa128.

14 Papillary Thyroid Carcinoma

Alison P. Woods, MD, MHS
Frederick Thurston Drake, MD, MPH
Ashok R. Shaha, MD

GENERAL CONSIDERATIONS

Thyroid cancer is among the most common cancers in the United States. Recent Surveillance, Epidemiology, and End Results Program (SEER) data show that over 43,000 new cases are estimated to be diagnosed in 2023, and Americans face a lifetime risk of developing thyroid cancer of about 1.2%.[1] Both incidence and mortality rates for thyroid cancer increased significantly from the 1970s through at least the first decade of the 2000s with an approximate increase in incidence of 3% per year (Figure 14–1).[2] Though recent SEER-based studies have reported a stabilization or small decrease in thyroid cancer diagnoses over the past 10 years, thyroid cancer mortality has continued to increase.[3]

Papillary thyroid carcinoma (PTC) is by far the most common subtype of thyroid cancer and represents 80% to 90% of all diagnoses.[2,3] Radiation exposure early in life is the most significant risk factor for PTC, though a family history of PTC is also a risk factor. Approximately 75% of thyroid cancer diagnoses occur in women, though a recent analysis by LeClair et al. found that this gender disparity is driven largely by small (≤2 cm) PTC with excellent prognosis; moreover, mortality was similar between genders. The same study's meta-analysis of autopsy data showed a similar prevalence of subclinical PTC across genders, suggesting that the predominance of PTC among women may in fact be rooted in differences in detection rather than biological incidence.[4] PTC diagnoses are widely distributed in age, with a median around age 50.

PATHOGENESIS

PTC arises from differentiated follicular epithelial cells, as does follicular thyroid carcinoma (FTC). Mutations, rearrangements, and fusions of genes causing constitutive activation in the mitogen-activated protein kinase signaling pathway, particularly in the *BRAF*, *RAS*, and *RET* genes, are found in a majority of PTC. Alterations in the telomerase reverse transcriptase (TERT) promoter region may also be present. PTC tumors often harbor a relatively small number of mutations, suggesting that tumorigenesis is driven by a limited number of key genetic alterations.[5,6]

PREVENTION

The majority of patients diagnosed with PTC do not have any major risk factors. Limiting childhood radiation exposure and ensuring judicious use of radiation in pediatric medical care are likely beneficial in preventing PTC at the societal level. Family history of thyroid cancer or inherited conditions such as familial adenomatous polyposis (FAP), excess iodine intake (notably different from the association between FTC and dietary iodine deficiency), and obesity have also been identified as risk factors for PTC.[7,8]

CLINICAL FINDINGS

Symptoms & Signs

PTC may be discovered incidentally on imaging or based on clinical symptoms. Symptomatic patients often present with a palpable neck mass, representing either primary tumor or metastatic lymph nodes. Those with larger tumors may report a globus sensation, dysphagia, or dysphonia. Dyspnea is also possible, though it is associated more often with large goiter than malignancy.

Initial Clinical Evaluation

Initial evaluation begins with a history and physical exam. In particular, patients should be asked about any history of ionizing radiation exposure. In the present-day United States, this is often related to a history of radiation treatment, as was common in Hodgkin lymphoma. Prior environmental exposures (eg, from nuclear incidents) are also relevant. A thorough family history, particularly of malignancies in general and of thyroid cancer in particular, should be gathered.

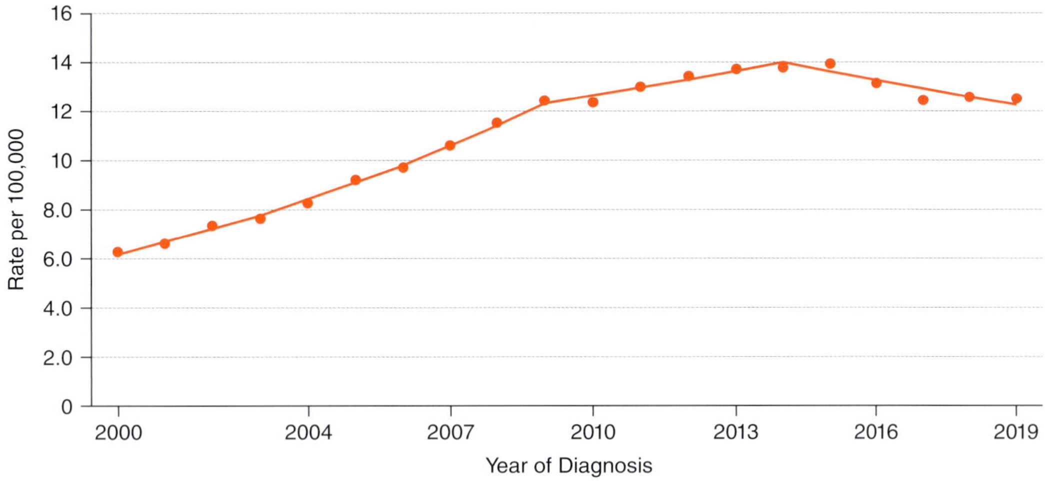

Figure 14–1. Papillary thyroid carcinoma age-adjusted incidence rates, 2000-2019. (Data from SEER*Explorer: An interactive website for SEER cancer statistics [Internet]. Surveillance Research Program, National Cancer Institute. [Cited 2022 August 24]. Available at: https://seer.cancer.gov/statistics-network/explorer/.)

Though authoritative definitions vary slightly, familial nonmedullary thyroid cancer is typically defined as nonmedullary thyroid cancer in at least two or three first-degree relatives. However, patients with a family history that does not meet these criteria are likely still at higher risk than the general population; a large study of the Utah Population Database found an increased PTC risk among PTC patients' first-degree (5.4-fold), second-degree (2.2-fold), and third-degree (1.8-fold) relatives.[9] Finally, several familial syndromes that are nonspecific to thyroid cancer have also been associated with increased risks of nonmedullary thyroid cancers such as PTC, including familial adenomatous polyposis, Cowden syndrome, Carney complex, and Werner syndrome.[10] PTC related to familial syndromes may be associated with more extensive disease.

Laboratory Evaluation

Before a diagnosis of thyroid cancer is made, patients frequently present with a thyroid nodule. As part of any thyroid nodule workup, initial laboratory studies should include thyroid-stimulating hormone (TSH). If TSH is suppressed, free thyroxine (T4) and triiodothyronine (T3) should be evaluated. A so-called "cold" nodule—that is, a nodule on a thyroid radioactive iodine (RAI) uptake scan that has lower RAI uptake compared to the surrounding thyroid parenchyma—should be considered more suspicious for malignancy than a hormonally active "hot" nodule. Generally speaking, however, unless a patient is hyperthyroid, this scan is not part of the evaluation of suspected thyroid cancer. Physicians may also consider obtaining a serum calcium level to rule out comorbid parathyroid disease prior to potential operative intervention in the neck for PTC, though the cost-effectiveness of this strategy is debated.[11,12] In addition, in our own practices, we routinely check and optimize 25-hydroxy vitamin D levels, especially prior to total thyroidectomy.

Imaging Studies & Image-Guided Biopsy

Initial imaging of suspected PTC is by neck ultrasonography. Fine-needle aspiration (FNA) is then performed to evaluate suspicious nodule(s), with cytology reported using the Bethesda classification system (see Table 8–2, Chapter 8). In the contemporary evaluation, it is most common for FNA to be performed under ultrasound guidance, but some centers perform palpation-guided biopsy, and retrospective, single-center data has previously supported the equivalence of both methods.[13] Most lesions that are ultimately found to be PTC were classified as Bethesda 5 (suspicious for malignancy) or 6 (malignant) on the preoperative evaluation.

Special Tests & Exams

For patients with a nodule that may be PTC who receive a Bethesda 1 cytologic result (nondiagnostic), repeat FNA is generally indicated unless there are other indications for thyroidectomy. Those with a lesion classified as Bethesda 3 (atypia of undetermined significance/follicular lesion of undetermined significance) or Bethesda 4 (suspicious for follicular neoplasm) have several different management options according to American Thyroid Association (ATA) guidelines: diagnostic lobectomy, molecular testing of the original FNA sample or repeat FNA with molecular testing of indeterminate result, or close observation with short-interval ultrasound. Several types of molecular-testing technologies are commercially available and covered by most medical insurance plans, including testing for certain mutations or testing for gene expression within tumors. Indications, benefits, and limitations of molecular testing are discussed in detail in Chapter 25. Given the multiple options available to patients with Bethesda 3 or 4 nodules, individualized decision-making remains critical.

DIFFERENTIAL DIAGNOSIS

When presenting as a neck mass, PTC must first be differentiated from other thyroid masses as well as nonthyroid neck masses. In the case of nonthyroid masses, acute-onset and associated constitutional symptoms are more suggestive of infectious lymphadenopathy. A combination of patient risk factors, exam findings, and imaging is often helpful to rule out nonthyroid malignancies, such as lymphoma, aerodigestive tract squamous cell carcinoma, or metastatic cancer. Though rare, parathyroid carcinoma should also be considered, especially in the presence of profound hypercalcemia. Physical exam alone can also suggest a likely diagnosis in some benign masses. For instance, thyroglossal duct cysts are midline and fluid-filled on palpation, and lipomas of the neck are characteristically soft and mobile in the subcutaneous tissues. In general, unless a neck mass is acute and can be attributed to an infectious process, imaging is indicated to aid in diagnosis. We start with ultrasound if the mass is suspected to originate in the thyroid gland.

Once a neck mass is confirmed to be originating from the thyroid on imaging, PTC must be differentiated from benign thyroid nodules, goiter (generalized glandular enlargement with or without distinct nodules), and other types of thyroid cancer. FNA results are often critical to defining the presence and subtype of malignancy, and final surgical pathology (if obtained) provides definitive diagnosis. In particular, PTC should be distinguished from other differentiated thyroid cancers (ie, follicular carcinoma), medullary thyroid carcinoma, poorly differentiated carcinoma, anaplastic carcinoma, and thyroid lymphoma. Classic PTC is defined by its nuclear features, including enlarged, elongated, oval-shaped, and/or overlapping nuclei (Figure 14–2). Papillary architecture and psammoma bodies are also typically present, but not strictly required for diagnosis. Over 10 variants of PTC have been defined based on histologic variations from "classic" or "conventional" PTC. Several variants, including tall cell, columnar, diffuse sclerosing, and hobnail variant PTC, are thought to represent more aggressive disease.[14] Notably, in 2015, noninvasive encapsulated follicular variant PTC was re-termed "noninvasive follicular thyroid neoplasm with papillary-like nuclear features" (NIFTP) to better reflect its low-risk nature. Another lower-risk diagnosis, the "well-differentiated tumor of uncertain malignant potential" (WDT-UMP), applies to well-circumscribed lesions that have some nuclear features consistent with PTC, but—unlike the noninvasive NIFTP—do have questionable capsular or vascular invasion after a thorough pathologic investigation.[15] Finally, even if nuclear features consistent with PTC are present, nodules less than 1 cm in size are considered micropapillary cancers and have multiple acceptable treatment options, including observation, as discussed in Chapter 13.

TREATMENT

Preoperative Workup

In addition to the aspects of a general thyroid nodule history and physical detailed earlier, a preoperative visit should include documentation of the patient's and surgeon's assessment of voice quality. For patients with preoperative voice abnormalities, prior neck or upper chest surgery, or extensive

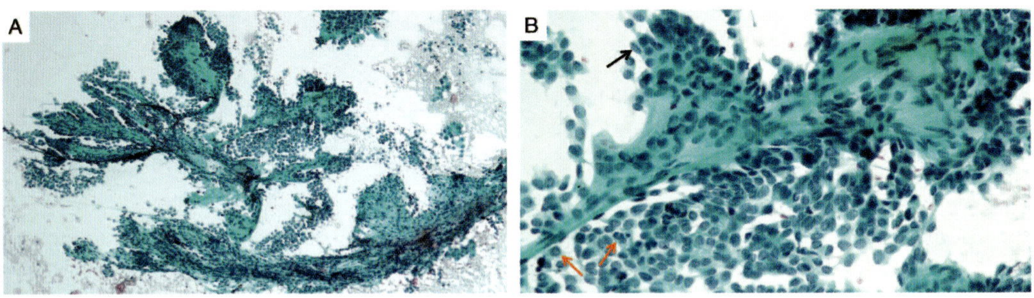

Figure 14–2. Pathological image of Bethesda 6 papillary thyroid cancer. **(A)** PTC with classical fibrovascular cores lined by neoplastic cells (Papanicolaou stain, ×100). **(B)** The neoplastic cells are arranged around a fibrovascular core and show nuclear features of PTC including nuclear enlargement with pale powdery chromatin, nuclear grooves (black arrow), and scattered nuclear inclusions (red arrows) (Papanicolaou stain, ×400). (Reproduced with permission from Dr. Sandra Cerda, Boston University School of Medicine and Boston Medical Center Department of Pathology & Laboratory Medicine.)

local disease including posterior extrathyroidal extension or bulky central neck nodal metastases, we recommend performing fiberoptic laryngoscopy to assess vocal fold movement.

If not already performed as part of the initial thyroid nodule evaluation, cervical ultrasound with visualization of the entirety of the thyroid gland as well as central and lateral cervical lymph node compartments is an essential preoperative step. Radiographically suspicious central and lateral lymph nodes with diameter ≥8 to 10 mm should be biopsied by FNA if results would change clinical management. Measurement of thyroglobulin (Tg) in washout fluid can also be considered among patients with insufficient cells for cytology or if there is discordance between the cytologic findings and worrisome sonographic features.[16] Alternatively, some surgeons elect to forgo FNA for any sonographically suspicious central neck nodes and simply resect these at the time of index operation. If a patient appears to have locally advanced disease, contrast-enhanced computed tomography (CT) or magnetic resonance imaging (MRI) can be a useful adjunct to evaluate the extent of primary tumor invasion or nodal metastases, especially beyond superficial cervical locations. Although IV contrast introduces significant iodine, the benefits of improved imaging accuracy typically outweigh the potential for a short delay in postoperative RAI therapy waiting for iodine clearance.[17] Regardless of apparent disease stage, there is generally no role for preoperative positron emission tomography (PET) scan or measurement of serum Tg.

Surgical Resection

Once malignancy has been established and preoperative workup and staging is completed, upfront surgery is recommended in the vast majority of cases of PTC. Well-differentiated thyroid cancers such as PTC are somewhat unusual in that the presence of metastatic disease does not preclude surgical resection. Potential exceptions to initial surgical resection include papillary microcarcinoma (<1 cm) without aggressive features or invasion, for which active surveillance may be considered, or PTC in patients with such extensive comorbidities or limited expected life span that the risks of surgical treatment outweigh the potential benefits.[16] Whether active surveillance protocols might be safely expanded beyond microcarcinomas to small PTC is an area of active investigation. However, tumor growth data suggest that it may eventually be possible to identify a population appropriate for active surveillance. For instance, a US-based prospective cohort of patients with small PTC (<1.5 cm) by Tuttle et al. demonstrated that among 59 patients with a tumor diameter of 1.1 to 1.5 cm and follow-up of at least 6 months, no meaningful increase in tumor size occurred in over 80% of patients.[18] Nevertheless, no long-term clinical outcomes are currently available for active surveillance in PTC, and upfront surgery remains the standard of care. Broadly speaking, the goals of initial surgery are to remove all disease within the thyroid and all clinically significant nodal metastases. Complete surgical resection reduces the risk of disease recurrence, allows for final pathologic staging, and—in cases of total thyroidectomy—enables the use of therapeutic RAI ablation and disease surveillance using serum Tg levels.

For patients undergoing surgery, the American Association of Endocrine Surgeons (AAES) guidelines recommend against routine antimicrobial prophylaxis, given the low rates of surgical site infection in clean head and neck surgeries. In addition, pharmacologic venous thromboembolism (VTE) prophylaxis should be given only in select patients with high risk for VTE.[19] Thyroid lobectomy and total thyroidectomy may be performed as inpatient procedures or, increasingly, as outpatient procedures among appropriately selected patients. A patient's extent or complexity of disease, overall comorbidity status, bleeding proclivity, home environment and support network, proximity to medical care, and personal preferences should all be taken into account when considering the setting of his or her operation. Reassuringly, a recent meta-analysis of 10 observational studies by Lee et al.[20] and large review of American College of Surgeons National Surgical Quality Improvement Program (ACS-NSQIP) data by McLaughlin et al.[21] found similar rates of reoperation and readmission after inpatient or outpatient operations. Finally, referral to a high-volume surgeon should be especially considered in the case of extensive, complex, or recurrent PTC. One large retrospective study of patients undergoing total thyroidectomy using the National Inpatient Sample found that the likelihood of complications diminished as surgeon volume increased up to a threshold of 26 cases per year, and accordingly proposed a threshold of more than 25 total thyroidectomies per year to define a high-volume thyroid surgeon.[22] Decision-making surrounding the extent of thyroidectomy and nodal dissection is detailed in the following discussion, while technical aspects of surgery are discussed in Chapter 21.

A. Extent of Thyroid Resection

Whether patients are candidates for thyroid lobectomy or should be recommended for total thyroidectomy depends on several factors, and surgical aggressiveness in the extent of resection has varied over the past several decades.[23] Patients with PTC more than 4 cm, gross extrathyroidal extension (clinical T4 disease), clinically positive nodes (clinical N1a or N1b disease), or concurrent distant metastases (M1 disease) should be recommended for total or near-total thyroidectomy. (For this chapter, use of the term "total thyroidectomy" includes "near-total" thyroidectomy, which refers to preservation of a very small thyroid remnant at the Ligament of Berry left only when necessary to preserve the recurrent laryngeal nerve [RLN].)

For patients with PTC that is 1 to 4 cm in size with no extrathyroidal extension, no clinical or radiographic evidence of nodal disease, and no evidence for distant metastases, either thyroid lobectomy or total thyroidectomy can be considered. This represents a major shift in practice, and only recently was included as part of the official ATA guidelines in 2015.[16] For its part, the 2020 AAES guidelines list the management of low-risk 1 to 4 cm PTC as an area of "no consensus."[19]

The choice of thyroid lobectomy versus total thyroidectomy requires consideration of oncologic outcomes as well as the need for reoperation/completion thyroidectomy and a consideration of the potential for complications. In terms of major oncologic outcomes, the literature largely supports similarly excellent survival and recurrence for lobectomy and thyroidectomy. Among studies that found equivalent survival and recurrence, as well as among those that showed small advantages for total thyroidectomy, 10-year survival was typically 90% or higher, and 10-year recurrence less than 10% in both groups.[24-26] Several large database studies were used to develop the recommendation that both thyroid lobectomy and total thyroidectomy are acceptable treatments for patients with low-risk 1 to 4 cm differentiated thyroid cancers. These large studies are at risk of bias by indication, and have been criticized for that reason. However, in four studies, Adam et al. used the National Cancer Database (NCDB),[27] while Barney et al.,[25] Haigh et al.,[28] and Mendelsohn et al.[29] used SEER data, to demonstrate no difference in overall survival among patients undergoing lobectomy versus total thyroidectomy after employing multivariable adjustment techniques to address problems of confounding in these observational data. Because survival is so high, many thyroid cancer clinicians focus their decision-making on reducing the risk of locoregional recurrence. Though data on locoregional recurrence rates are less definitive, recurrence in low-risk PTC occurs in relatively few patients and remains highly treatable. Reassuringly, a recent meta-analysis by Bojoga et al. incorporating 175,000 patients with differentiated thyroid cancer found no difference in overall survival, disease-free survival, and disease-specific survival between patients who underwent lobectomy and those who underwent total thyroidectomy.[30]

Based on the updated 2015 ATA recommendations, some patients who undergo thyroid lobectomy have findings on final pathology for which a total thyroidectomy would have been recommended, had these findings been known at the time of surgery. For example, high-risk pathologic features such as angioinvasion may be present. In these cases, completion thyroidectomy is recommended except in cases of clear surgical contraindications. The proportion of patients who will ultimately need a completion thyroidectomy remains controversial. Though ATA guidelines state that completion thyroidectomy rates with a lobectomy approach in properly selected patients can be less than 10%, AAES guidelines suggest that high-risk pathologic features may be present in over 40% of patients. An early retrospective study by Kluijfhout et al. looked at total thyroidectomy patients who hypothetically would have been eligible for lobectomy; they found that nearly 20% of potential lobectomy patients would have needed to undergo completion total thyroidectomy to receive RAI.[31] Data from the post-2015 era are still limited. In a single-institutional study by Kuo et al. examining early implementation of the new ATA guidelines, 25% of patients who underwent thyroid lobectomy in 2016 to 2018 for low-risk, 1 to 4 cm differentiated thyroid cancer ultimately underwent completion thyroidectomy.[32] However, a study of ACS-NSQIP data from 2009 to 2017 by Ullman et al. showed that the proportion of patients undergoing thyroid lobectomy after 2015 increased without a corresponding increase in completion thyroidectomy, which remained at approximately 8%.[33] To our knowledge, no prospective studies have yet examined completion thyroidectomy rates or long-term oncologic outcomes between patients undergoing lobectomy versus total thyroidectomy in a post-2015 US-based population.

Regardless of the exact number of patients who require completion thyroid surgery, it seems clear that clinical practice is changing. When thyroid lobectomy is selected, intraoperative assessment of tumor invasiveness and surrounding lymph nodes is of utmost importance to enable conversion to total thyroidectomy when appropriate and thus avoid a second operation. One retrospective analysis by Craig et al. found that 21% of total thyroidectomy patients who would have been potentially eligible for lobectomy under the 2015 guidelines had synoptic operative notes that described high-risk features intraoperatively, which would have led the surgeon to adjust plans from lobectomy to total thyroidectomy.[34] Such ability to recognize high-risk features intraoperatively, perhaps combined with preoperative risk-assessments that guide higher-risk patients toward initial total thyroidectomy, may account for some of the discrepancy between hypothetical completion thyroidectomy rates and actual completion thyroidectomy rates observed in our clinical practices and the ACS-NSQIP data cited earlier.

Finally, in addition to considering oncologic and reoperation outcomes, surgeons and patients should also consider the complication rates of total thyroidectomy as compared to thyroid lobectomy. Though complication rates vary by underlying thyroid disease etiology and may be globally reduced among high-volume surgeons, total thyroidectomy confers increased risk of both transient and permanent complications. Given the relatively excellent survival and recurrence outcomes after treatment of low-risk PTC, avoidance of permanent complications and optimization of quality of life are of especially high importance during surgical decision-making in this population. A recent prospective study of differentiated thyroid cancer patients in China by Chen et al. noted lower postoperative health-related quality of life at 1 and 3 months, but not 6 and 12 months, after total thyroidectomy compared to thyroid lobectomy, suggesting that long-term quality of life is likely to be similar regardless of operation choice.[35] A summary of the pros and

Table 14–1. Considerations when selecting thyroid lobectomy versus total thyroidectomy in low-risk PTC.

	Thyroid Lobectomy	Total Thyroidectomy
Pros	• Guideline-concordant • Improved early (<6 months) health-related quality of life • Lower risk of transient and permanent surgical complications (hypoparathyroidism, voice changes) • Avoidance of lifelong thyroid replacement therapy in many patients	• Guideline-concordant • Some studies support lower recurrence and/or slight survival advantage • Single operation • Enables radioactive iodine treatment, if needed • Allows use of thyroglobulin for disease surveillance
Cons	• Potential need for completion thyroidectomy • Some studies support higher recurrence rates and/or slight survival disadvantage	• Higher risk of transient and permanent surgical complications (hypoparathyroidism, voice changes) • Lower early (<6 months) health-related quality of life • Mandates lifelong thyroid replacement therapy • Potentially altered quality of life related to management of thyroid replacement therapy

cons related to extent of surgery for total thyroidectomy and thyroid lobectomy is provided in Table 14–1. Overall, both surgeons and patients should understand that neither procedure is currently recommended above the other for low-risk 1 to 4 cm PTC. As the medical community continues to accumulate more data on this change in practice, shared decision-making remains essential.

B. Extent of Nodal Dissection

The management of clinically positive nodes in PTC is relatively straightforward. Patients with clinically suspected central compartment (level VI) metastatic disease, whether based on imaging or intraoperative inspection, should undergo therapeutic compartmental neck dissection at the time of thyroidectomy. For suspected disease in the lateral cervical lymph nodes (levels II-V), compartmental dissection is also recommended after confirming metastatic disease on preoperative lymph node biopsy. Traditionally, lateral nodal metastases were addressed with modified radical neck dissection, which includes compartments II, III, IV, and V and preserves the internal jugular vein, sternocleidomastoid muscle, and spinal accessory nerve (Figure 14–3). Today, a therapeutic selective neck dissection is performed

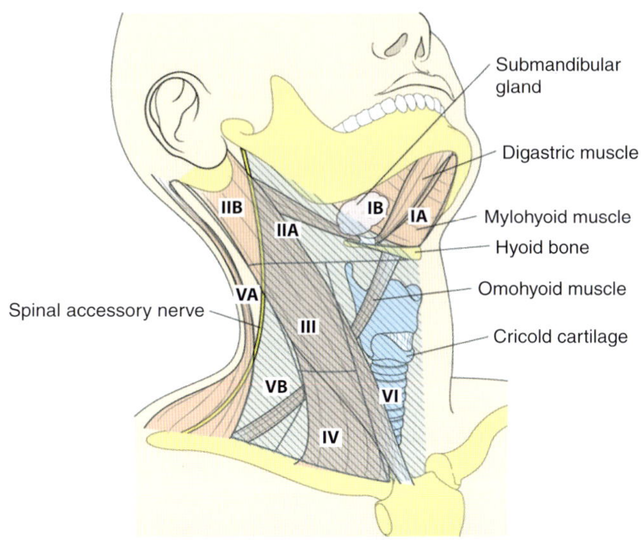

Figure 14–3. Cervical lymph node compartments and the lateral neck. (Reproduced with permission from Sang-Wook Kang et al. Initial experience with robot-assisted modified radical neck dissection for the management of thyroid carcinoma with lateral neck node metastasis. *Surgery*. 2010;148(6):1214-1221.)

more commonly; this omits at least some of the lateral nodal compartments to reduce morbidity. Compartments IIb and Va are most frequently left undissected in this procedure due to their lower propensity to harbor metastases and proximity to the spinal accessory nerve.[19] Patients noted to have lateral neck nodal metastases typically have central neck metastases, though a minority of upper pole tumors can exhibit "skip" metastases directly to the lateral compartments.[36] Regardless, the central compartment (level VI) should routinely be included in the dissection for any patient undergoing a lateral neck dissection. Though only a small proportion of patients with PTC present with extensive and/or large cervical lymph node metastases, this subset of patients with aggressive disease frequently require substantial, careful surgical dissection to ensure all disease is resected (Figure 14–4).

For the majority of patients with PTC who do not present with preoperatively identified nodal metastases, decision-making regarding whether to perform prophylactic central neck dissection (CND) is more complex and represents an ongoing and vigorous controversy in thyroid surgery. Central nodal micrometastases are now known to be present in most patients with PTC, but their clinical significance is likely low. The presence of these micrometastases has created controversy over whether central neck dissections should be done prophylactically (ie, for all patients with PTC) or selectively,

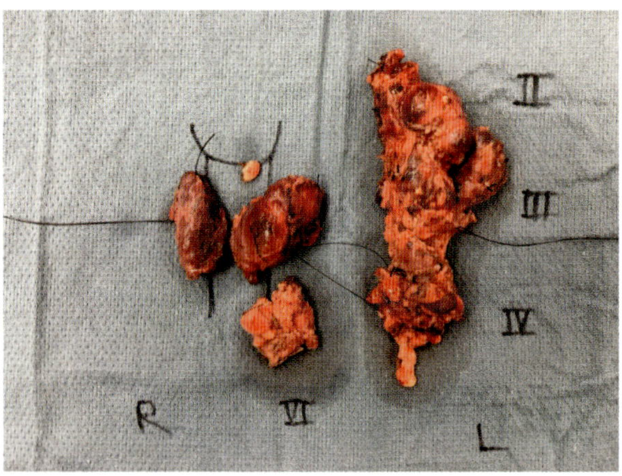

Figure 14–4. N1b papillary thyroid carcinoma with extensive lateral neck nodal metastases. Photograph of a surgical specimen including the resected thyroid placed atop a surgical marker drawing showing its position relative to the trachea and cricoid cartilage superiorly. The left-sided central (VI) and lateral (II-IV) compartments exhibited gross nodal metastases, which have also been resected. (Reproduced with permission from Dr. F. Thurston Drake, Boston University School of Medicine and Boston Medical Center Department of Surgery.)

either in the case of clinically apparent disease or when selected high-risk factors are present. In general, CND can be omitted for T1 and T2 PTC without any clinically apparent metastatic lymph nodes. However, it may be reasonably considered for patients with T3 or T4 disease. Evidence is mixed regarding whether prophylactic CND reduces recurrence rates, though recent studies have suggested that recurrence rates may remain unchanged. A large single-institution series of 11,000 patients in South Korea by Kim et al. showed no decrease in locoregional recurrence among patients who underwent prophylactic CND.[37] Similarly, a study of 1800 total thyroidectomy patients at Memorial Sloan Kettering Cancer Center by Nixon et al. who did not undergo prophylactic CND, but did undergo therapeutic excision of any clinically suspicious lymph nodes, found more than 99% 5-year central neck recurrence-free survival. With a median follow-up of just under 4 years, these patients had 100% disease-specific survival.[38] Prospective data concerning prophylactic CND in total thyroidectomy are limited. Viola et al.'s randomized trial of 181 patients found comparable rates of biochemical and structural disease after a median of 5 years of follow-up, but noted that more total thyroidectomy-only patients required more than one RAI treatment. However, patients in the CND group had significantly higher rates of permanent hypoparathyroidism.[39] Another randomized trial by Sippel et al., which included 60 patients and was powered to primarily examine hypoparathyroidism, showed comparable 1-year oncologic outcomes and similar postoperative complication rates between groups undergoing and not undergoing CND.[40] Finally, relatively little data exist to guide whether prophylactic CND should be performed in patients undergoing thyroid lobectomy, a scenario that is likely to become more common given recent recommendation changes. The potential use of intraoperative frozen section to guide CND is an area of active investigation.[41] In general, we omit CND in patients undergoing lobectomy. However, it may occasionally be preferable to perform a unilateral prophylactic CND ipsilateral to the lobectomy so that, should a completion thyroidectomy become necessary, the entire side of the neck will not require reoperation; patients with previous ipsilateral neck operations, challenging anatomy, or concern for temporary RLN injury are the clearest candidates for considering this approach.

Complications

Complications of PTC can be related either to the disease process itself or to its treatment. Tumor invasion of or surgical injury to surrounding structures can have serious clinical consequences due to the proximity of so many critical structures within the neck. Because of the symmetrical nature of most cervical structures, complications related to surgery are more likely, and may be more severe, among patients undergoing total thyroidectomy as opposed to thyroid lobectomy.

A. Vocal Cord Paralysis

Vocal cord paralysis represents one of the most feared complications of PTC and its treatment, and is most commonly rooted in injury to the RLN. This type of injury can result in hoarseness, cough, or—in bilateral cases—potential for airway compromise and aphonia. In contrast, injury to the external branch of the superior laryngeal nerve (EBSLN) often presents as more subtle voice alterations, including in pitch or volume. These may be noticeable primarily in those who spend time singing or doing public speaking. The superior laryngeal nerve has an internal and external branch and originates from the vagus nerve; its external branch travels in a caudal direction to the cricothyroid muscle. This nerve is substantially more variable in its anatomic course than the RLN.[42] The possibility of a nonrecurrent laryngeal nerve, which branches directly from the vagus nerve and travels to the larynx without first coursing through the upper chest, should always be considered when the RLN is not readily identified in its usual anatomic position (Figure 14–5). Estimated to be present in up to 1% of the population, nonrecurrent laryngeal nerves are overwhelmingly right sided. In the modern era, the use of intraoperative nerve monitoring for assistance in identifying and preserving the RLN is common. Though we personally make use of nerve monitoring, high-quality data supporting this practice remains lacking. A retrospective study by Liu et al. employing ACS-NSQIP data noted an overall RLN injury rate of 5.7% and found that use of intraoperative nerve monitoring was more prevalent at best-performing hospitals, as opposed to the worst-performing hospitals with regard to RLN injury; however, no causal link could be drawn in this observational dataset.[43] A recent Cochrane review determined there was no conclusive evidence about the value of intraoperative nerve monitoring over visual nerve identification.[44] There are data to support the assertion that use of the nerve monitor does prevent bilateral nerve injuries, because total thyroid operations are aborted after lobectomy when a nerve injury is identified.[45] Since most RLN palsies recover spontaneously, this scenario can generally be managed with a completion thyroidectomy a few months after the index operation. Our clinical experience, supported by published data from other high-volume centers,[46,47] suggests that RLN injuries remain permanent in approximately 1% of operations.

B. Neck Hematoma

In the early postoperative period, all patients should be monitored or counseled to monitor for a neck hematoma. Neck hematoma requiring intervention—typically advanced airway management, bedside evacuation, and/or reoperation—may occur in up to 1% of patients. Previously identified risk factors include older age, male sex, Graves' disease, use of antiplatelet or anticoagulation therapies, and a variety of markers likely signaling technical challenge in the operation, such as prior neck operation, use of hemostatic adjuncts, and larger extent of resection. Drain usage has not been associated with a reduction in neck hematomas requiring intervention, and we do not use drains routinely during thyroidectomy without lateral neck dissection. In management of neck

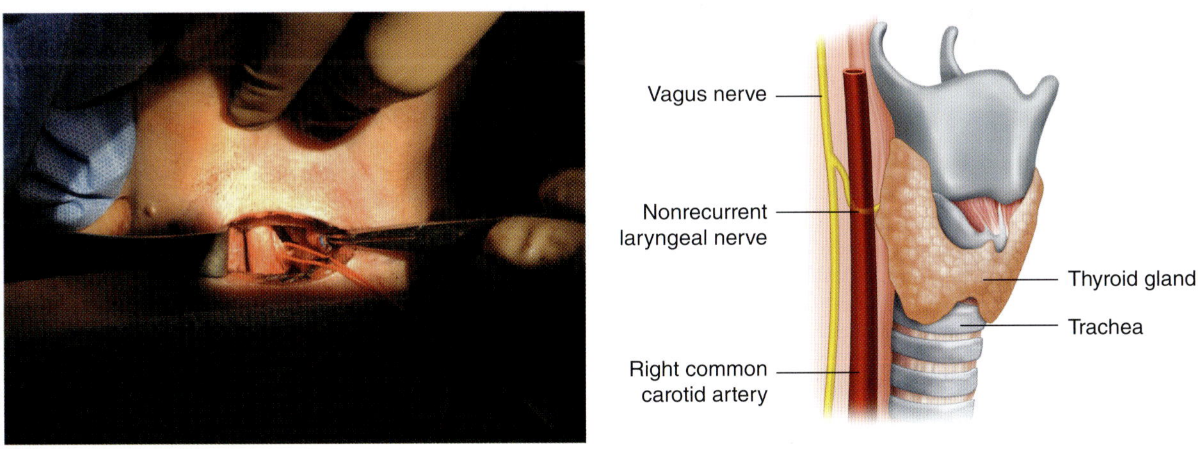

▲ Figure 14–5. Right-sided nonrecurrent laryngeal nerve. Intraoperative photograph from a "lateral approach" superior parathyroid operation. The red vessel loop surrounds the vagus nerve. The branching white structure is the nonrecurrent laryngeal nerve, coursing directly from the vagus to the larynx. The surgical peanut is reflecting the right thyroid lobe medially, the army/navy retractor is exposing the jugular vein and the carotid artery (medial to the jugular vein). (Personal photograph obtained with patient permission from Dr. F. Thurston Drake, Boston University School of Medicine and Boston Medical Center Department of Surgery. Line art adapted from Henry BM, Sanna S, Graves MJ, et al. The non-recurrent laryngeal nerve: a meta-analysis and clinical considerations. *Peer J.* 2017;5:e3012.)

hematomas, airway status takes primacy and may worsen with supine positioning due to pressure from the overlying hematoma. In addition, edema of the larynx and pharyngeal wall is often present in the postoperative setting. Intubation of these patients is often challenging and should be performed by an experienced clinician. Bedside intubation or evacuation of the hematoma can be warranted to maintain airway patency, but when possible, we strive to return emergently to the operating room and address the hematoma under optimally controlled conditions. In the case of an unstable airway, many surgeons prefer to drape and prep the patient's neck and be gowned and gloved with appropriate equipment in hand prior to the induction of general anesthesia in case of an airway emergency during attempted intubation.

C. Hypoparathyroidism

Hypoparathyroidism, which typically presents as hypocalcemia, is another important potential complication of thyroidectomy; it is almost always transient but can also be permanent. Patients undergoing total thyroidectomy with neck dissection are at the highest risk for hypoparathyroidism. Conversely, patients with no prior neck surgery undergoing a thyroid lobectomy are at virtually zero risk of hypoparathyroidism. A recent investigation by Kazaure et al. using ACS-NSQIP found that severe hypocalcemia requiring intravenous calcium, emergent evaluation, or readmission occurred in 5.8% of patients undergoing total thyroidectomy, subtotal thyroidectomy, or completion thyroidectomy.[48] Similarly, a large claims database analysis by Powers et al. included patients undergoing complete or partial thyroidectomy, parathyroidectomy, or neck dissection, and found a 7.6% rate of hypoparathyroidism, with 25% of those cases considered permanent.[49] For high-volume surgeons, we estimate that about 5% of routine total thyroidectomy operations are complicated by temporary hypoparathyroidism, and about 1% result in permanent hypoparathyroidism.

Every effort should be made to identify and preserve the parathyroid glands during thyroidectomy. If a suspected parathyroid is devascularized over the course of the operation, we confirm its identity as a parathyroid gland (and not a lymph node that could represent metastatic PTC) on frozen section and then proceed with autotransplantation into the sternocleidomastoid muscles. The parathyroid tissue should be minced into fragments smaller than 1×1 mm as the tissues are initially oxygenated via imbibition until they undergo development of a neovascular supply. The muscle pocket must be hemostatic, as parathyroid fragments implanted into a hematoma will not survive to become functional. Regardless of intraoperative course, all post-thyroidectomy patients should be observed for and counseled on the symptoms of hypocalcemia, including perioral numbness, muscle tetany, carpopedal spasm, and paresthesias. Though individual surgeon practices vary, patients often have serum calcium and/or PTH checked in the early postoperative period to guide calcium and vitamin D supplementation postoperatively. Alternative approaches include empiric calcium and vitamin D supplementation in all patients for 1 to 3 weeks. The ATA recommends that patients with a PTH value of <15 pg/mL measured 20 minutes or more postoperatively may require further serum monitoring or supplementation, while a PTH value of ≥15 pg/mL signals a low risk of hypocalcemia such that intensive calcium monitoring or supplementation may be unnecessary.[50] Optimal cutoff values and timelines of early postoperative PTH measurement remain under active investigation,[51,52] and progress in this area may facilitate wider adoption of outpatient total thyroidectomy.

D. Complications of Lateral Neck Dissection

When lateral neck dissection is performed, additional complications are possible. Injury to the spinal accessory nerve, which is exposed as it courses from the sternocleidomastoid to the trapezius, is perhaps the most feared complication (Figure 14–3). Clinically, this results in trapezius muscle dysfunction and difficulty with shoulder abduction. Though 10% or more of lateral neck dissection patients have transient shoulder dysfunction postoperatively, only a fraction of these patients have permanent deficits. Less commonly reported peripheral nervous system complications include Horner syndrome, injury to the brachial plexus, and injury to the hypoglossal nerve. On the left side in particular, patients are also at risk for chyle leak after neck dissection near the thoracic duct, which is located where the left internal jugular vein joins the subclavian vein. If identified intraoperatively, the duct may be ligated with nonabsorbable sutures or hemoclips. If a chyle leak is identified postoperatively based on copious chylous drainage, conservative management with fat-free or medium-chain fatty acid diet and consideration of pressure dressing and octreotide therapy is successful in most patients without high-output leaks. Neck re-exploration, thoracoscopic ligation, or interventional radiologic embolization can all be considered in the extremely rare cases of patients for whom conservative management is unsuccessful.

Postoperative Treatment

In most cases, patients are able to leave the hospital on the day of or the day following their operation. As discussed earlier, education and monitoring surrounding the potential for early complications are critical. For patients who have undergone total thyroidectomy, levothyroxine can be initiated immediately at a starting dose of approximately 1.6 μg/kg.[19] TSH should be checked at postoperative weeks 6 to 8 and dosing is then adjusted by the patient's endocrinologist as needed. In the setting of thyroid cancer, slightly supraphysiologic doses of levothyroxine are sometimes employed to decrease recurrence risk. ATA guidelines propose that in the absence of contraindications (such as atrial fibrillation or excessive bone loss), high-risk patients should be maintained at a TSH level of less than 0.1 mU/L, intermediate-risk patients at 0.1 to 0.5 mU/L, and low-risk patients in the low reference range of TSH at approximately 0.5 to 2 mU/L (Table 14–2).[16]

Postoperative RAI treatment is not routinely performed in low-risk PTC patients, may be considered in intermediate-risk patients, and is frequently recommended for patients with high-risk PTC. Serum Tg may be measured to help assess appropriateness for RAI at approximately 3 to 4 weeks post-thyroidectomy. Decision-making surrounding RAI is complex and discussed in more detail in Chapter 16. Finally, there is no routine role for postoperative external beam radiation therapy or adjuvant cytotoxic chemotherapy in PTC. However, tyrosine kinase inhibitors are increasingly playing a role in the management of advanced PTC with BRAF-V600E mutations, and referral to a medical oncologist with expertise in this treatment modality is warranted for patients with such cancers.[53-55]

Postoperative Staging & Risk Stratification

Postoperative risks among patients with PTC include mortality and recurrence, and several classification systems aid in patient stratification with regard to these risks. Staging designation systems are based on pathologic review of the surgical specimen and have been designed with mortality risk primarily in mind. The most widely used staging system is the American Joint Commission on Cancer (AJCC) TNM system. The eighth edition AJCC system, published in 2016 and adopted clinically in 2018, incorporates patient age (<55 vs ≥55 years), tumor size and degree of gross extrathyroidal extension (T1: ≤2 cm, T2: >2 cm and ≤4 cm, T3: >4 cm or extension into the strap muscles, T4: extension into major neck structures), presence and location of nodal metastases (N1: any regional nodal metastasis), and presence of distant metastasis.[56] Notably, thyroid cancer staging is the only solid-tumor staging system to incorporate patient age. Compared to the seventh edition guidelines, changes included an increase in the staging age cut point from 45 to 55 years, a revised classification of extrathyroidal extension, the explicit grouping of pNX and pN0 status together, and reclassification of metastatic level VII nodes from N1b to N1a. Compared to prior staging systems, these changes improved the ability of staging categories to accurately predict survival, which is the goal of a staging system. In a study of SEER and NCDB cohorts by Pontius et al., about 20% to 25% of patients were downstaged under the current eighth edition compared to the seventh edition, primarily from stage III to stage II or I, and from stage II to stage I.[57]

Table 14–2. ATA risk stratification definitions and treatment.

Risk Category	Characteristics	Likelihood of NED After TT and RAI Ablation, %	Minimal Extent of Thyroidectomy	RAI?	Goal TSH, mUL/L
Low	Intrathyroidal, completely resected PTC or encapsulated FV-PTC No local or distant metastasis No aggressive histology (tall cell, hobnail, or columnar cell) Intrathyroidal FTC with capsular and/or <4 foci vascular invasion Clinical N0 or ≤5 pathologic N1 micrometastasis (<2 mm)	78–91	Lobectomy	Usually no	0.5–2
Intermediate	PTC with microscopic extrathyroidal extension, vascular invasion Incomplete response to treatment Clinical N1 or >5 pathologic N1 <3 cm	52–54	Total	Strongly considered esp with aggressive histologies, older age, and/or lateral LNM	0.1–0.5
High	Gross extrathyroidal extension Incomplete tumor resection Distant metastases Nodal metastasis ≥3 cm FTC with extensive vascular invasion	31–32	Total	Yes	<0.1

NED indicates no evidence of disease; for example, Tg undetectable and no radiographic evidence of disease.

Source: Reproduced with permission from Patel KN, Yip L, Lubitz CC et al. The American Association of Endocrine Surgeons Guidelines for the Definitive Surgical Management of Thyroid Disease in Adults. *Ann Surg*. 2020;271(3):e21-e93.

In addition to considering mortality risk as reflected by TNM staging, prediction of recurrence risk is also critical for patients and clinicians. ATA guidelines for recurrence risk stratification in differentiated thyroid cancer separate patients into low, intermediate, and high risk as shown in Table 14–2.

Finally, as patients who have undergone total thyroidectomy and RAI move further into the postoperative period, their response to therapy can also be stratified into four categories to guide ongoing recurrence surveillance, as originally proposed by Tuttle and Leboeuf.[58] Under this system, "excellent response" is reserved for patients with no evidence of disease by any metric, "biochemical incomplete response" refers to the presence of abnormal serum Tg but no evidence of disease on imaging, "structural incomplete response" describes persistent or new disease, generally noted on sonographic surveillance, and "indeterminate response" includes patients with biochemical or imaging findings that do not clearly suggest the absence of disease or generate clear evidence of persistent or recurrent disease.

Metastatic or Locally Advanced Disease

Decision-making surrounding recurrent or persistent disease is individualized. For patients discovered to have metastatic or locally advanced disease in the cervical region, whether on initial workup or as a recurrence, locoregional surgery remains the oncologically optimal initial treatment when feasible. When not possible, RAI ablation, alternative ablation techniques (such as radiofrequency or ethanol ablation), radiation therapy, supraphysiologic levothyroxine therapy, and, for BRAF-mutated tumors, systemic treatment with tyrosine kinase inhibitors remain potential options. These therapies may also be considered as adjunctive therapies after resection of particularly invasive or aggressive cancers. Neoadjuvant tyrosine kinase inhibitor treatment may allow less extensive surgical resection among patients with locally invasive thyroid cancer, though this remains an experimental strategy.[59] For iodine-avid pulmonary and bone metastases, and among patients with rising Tg but without localizable metastases, RAI is the generally recommended initial strategy.[16] In all cases of metastatic and locally advanced PTC, both multidisciplinary discussion and incorporation of patient preferences are warranted.

One relatively common scenario is the patient with prior total thyroidectomy for PTC who presents with nodal metastases but no evidence of distant disease. In these cases, the AAES suggests the following criteria for reoperation: central lymph node metastasis of more than 8 mm, lateral lymph node metastasis of more than 10 mm, growth of more than 3 to 5 mm/year, or increasing Tg levels, in addition to consideration of patient and endocrinologist preference and comorbidity status.[19] When possible, a compartmental dissection should be performed in the presence of metastatic lymph nodes; however, a "berry-picking" approach may be utilized if a full compartmental dissection cannot be safely completed or was previously done.

For all patients in whom reoperation is planned, all available information from the patient's prior operation should be reviewed along with current and prior imaging. Current laboratory values for TSH, Tg (if the prior operation was a total thyroidectomy), and serum calcium should also be obtained. A formal fiberoptic laryngeal exam should be performed to evaluate for vocal fold dysfunction. Patients should also be counseled about increased risks for hypoparathyroidism and vocal fold dysfunction following reoperation, each of which may range as high as 1% to 10%.[19]

Long-Term Surveillance

Patients who are disease free after initial treatment of their PTC should continue to be followed. Following total thyroidectomy, ATA guidelines recommend assessment of serum Tg to detect potential recurrence among patients who have undergone RAI.[16] Thyroglobulin antibodies, which are present in a substantial minority of thyroid cancer patients, should also be measured to rule out spuriously low Tg. Though patients who have not undergone RAI may have normal residual thyroid tissue (and appropriate Tg levels are not well defined in this situation), rising Tg values may still provide useful information. Initially, serum Tg can be measured every 6 to 12 months, with eventual spacing to every 1 to 2 years. Patients on long-term levothyroxine replacement therapy should have at least annual serum TSH to aid in appropriate dosing and reduce endogenous thyroid tissue stimulation.

Surveillance imaging typically consists of cervical ultrasound of the central and lateral neck performed at 6 to 12 months post-thyroidectomy and should be repeated regularly for all but the lowest-risk patients at an interval that reflects the patient's likelihood of recurrence.[16] Suspicious lymph nodes ≥8 mm should be biopsied with FNA. CT and MRI are used less commonly but play a role in the evaluation of bulky or distant recurrence and can also provide improved visualization of the central neck and potential involvement of the cancer with the aerodigestive tract. Whole-body RAI scans and PET/CT as surveillance imaging are generally used only among patients who are at highest risk for recurrent or persistent disease or who have Tg antibodies and may have falsely negative Tg laboratory surveillance results.

PROGNOSIS

In general, both disease-specific and overall survival are highly favorable in PTC. Among patients less than 55 years of age with classic, tall cell, or diffuse sclerosing PTC, Feng et al. found that 10-year disease-specific survival exceeds 95%.[60] Current SEER Explorer application data for papillary thyroid cancer demonstrate more than 99% 5-year survival for patients with local or regional disease at diagnosis, and 74% 5-year survival for patients with distant disease at diagnosis.[61] Additional recent data from the NCDB show that aggressive variants of PTC are more commonly associated with invasive features (eg, extrathyroidal extension or metastasis, multifocality, lymphovascular invasion), but that histology alone does not confer worse overall survival in the absence of these features.[62] Factors associated with decreased survival include advanced age, larger tumor size, positive margins, extrathyroidal extension, lymphovascular invasion, and distant metastases. Data on the association between lateral neck metastases and survival are mixed, and the association between certain molecular mutations, such as BRAF or TERT mutations, and survival also remains unclear. Overall, in the context of over 60,000 incident cases of PTC annually in the United States, approximately 1000 deaths are expected to occur. Survival may still be prolonged: among patients with PTC who ultimately die of thyroid cancer, over 1 in 4 can expect to survive more than 10 years after initial diagnosis.[2]

REFERENCES

1. Cancer of the Thyroid–Cancer Stat Facts. SEER. Accessed May 25, 2022. https://seer.cancer.gov/statfacts/html/thyro.html
2. Lim H, Devesa SS, Sosa JA, Check D, Kitahara CM. Trends in thyroid cancer incidence and mortality in the United States, 1974-2013. *JAMA*. 2017;317(13):1338-1348.
3. Megwalu UC, Moon PK. Thyroid cancer incidence and mortality trends in the United States: 2000-2018. *Thyroid*. 2022;32(5):560-570.
4. LeClair K, Bell KJL, Furuya-Kanamori L, Doi SA, Francis DO, Davies L. Evaluation of gender inequity in thyroid cancer diagnosis: differences by sex in us thyroid cancer incidence compared with a meta-analysis of subclinical thyroid cancer rates at autopsy. *JAMA Intern Med*. 2021;181(10):1351-1358.
5. Agrawal N, Akbani R, Aksoy BA, et al. Integrated genomic characterization of papillary thyroid carcinoma. *Cell*. 2014;159(3):676-690.
6. Prete A, Borges de Souza P, Censi S, Muzza M, Nucci N, Sponziello M. Update on fundamental mechanisms of thyroid cancer. *Front Endocrinol*. 2020;11.
7. Kim K, Cho SW, Park YJ, Lee KE, Lee DW, Park SK. Association between iodine intake, thyroid function, and papillary thyroid cancer: a case-control study. *Endocrinol Metab*. 2021;36(4):790-799.
8. Kitahara CM, Pfeiffer RM, Sosa JA, Shiels MS. Impact of overweight and obesity on us papillary thyroid cancer incidence trends (1995-2015). *JNCI J Natl Cancer Inst*. 2020;112(8):810-817.
9. Oakley GM, Curtin K, Pimentel R, Buchmann L, Hunt J. Establishing a familial basis for papillary thyroid carcinoma using the Utah Population Database. *JAMA Otolaryngol Neck Surg* 2013;139(11):1171-1174.
10. Hińcza K, Kowalik A, Kowalska A. Current knowledge of germline genetic risk factors for the development of non-medullary thyroid cancer. *Genes*. 2019;10(7):E482.
11. Rosário PW, Mourão GF, Calsolari MR. Screening for hyperparathyroidism by measurement of calcium in patients undergoing thyroid surgery: a prospective study. *Horm Metab Res*. 2016;48(10):673-676.
12. Denizot A, Dadoun F, Meyer-Dutour A, Alliot P, Argème M. Screening for primary hyperparathyroidism before thyroid surgery: a prospective study. *Surgery*. 2002;131(3):264-269.
13. Choong KC, Khiyami A, Tamarkin SW, McHenry CR. Fine-needle aspiration biopsy of thyroid nodules: is routine ultrasound-guidance necessary? *Surgery*. 2018;164(4):789-794.
14. Asa SL. The current histologic classification of thyroid cancer. *Endocrinol Metab Clin North Am*. 2019;48(1):1-22.
15. Baloch ZW, Asa SL, Barletta JA, et al. Overview of the 2022 WHO classification of thyroid neoplasms. *Endocr Pathol*. 2022; 33(1):27-63.
16. Haugen BR, Alexander EK, Bible KC, et al. 2015 American Thyroid Association management guidelines for adult patients with thyroid nodules and differentiated thyroid cancer: the American Thyroid Association guidelines task force on thyroid nodules and differentiated thyroid cancer. *Thyroid*. 2016;26(1): 1-133.
17. Yeh MW, Bauer AJ, Bernet VA, et al. American Thyroid Association statement on preoperative imaging for thyroid cancer surgery. *Thyroid Off J Am Thyroid Assoc*. 2015;25(1):3-14.
18. Tuttle RM, Fagin JA, Minkowitz G, et al. Natural history and tumor volume kinetics of papillary thyroid cancers during active surveillance. *JAMA Otolaryngol Neck Surg*. 2017;143(10): 1015-1020.
19. Patel KN, Yip L, Lubitz CC, et al. The American Association of Endocrine Surgeons guidelines for the definitive surgical management of thyroid disease in adults. *Ann Surg*. 2020; 271(3):e21.
20. Lee DJ, Chin CJ, Hong CJ, Perera S, Witterick IJ. Outpatient versus inpatient thyroidectomy: a systematic review and meta-analysis. *Head Neck*. 2018;40(1):192-202.
21. McLaughlin EJ, Brant JA, Bur AM, et al. Safety of outpatient thyroidectomy: review of the American College of Surgeons National Surgical Quality Improvement Program. *The Laryngoscope*. 2018;128(5):1249-1254.
22. Adam MA, Thomas S, Youngwirth L, et al. Is there a minimum number of thyroidectomies a surgeon should perform to optimize patient outcomes? *Ann Surg*. 2017;265(2):402-407.
23. Yeh MW. The rise and fall of surgical aggressiveness for known or suspected differentiated thyroid cancer. *Cancer Cytopathol*. 2020;128(7):435-439.
24. Bilimoria KY, Bentrem DJ, Ko CY, et al. Extent of surgery affects survival for papillary thyroid cancer. *Ann Surg*. 2007;246(3): 375-384.
25. Barney BM, Hitchcock YJ, Sharma P, Shrieve DC, Tward JD. Overall and cause-specific survival for patients undergoing lobectomy, near-total, or total thyroidectomy for differentiated thyroid cancer. *Head Neck*. 2011;33(5):645-649.
26. Chan S, Karamali K, Kolodziejczyk A, et al. Systematic review of recurrence rate after hemithyroidectomy for low-risk well-differentiated thyroid cancer. *Eur Thyroid J*. 2020;9(2):73-84.
27. Adam MA, Pura J, Gu L, et al. Extent of surgery for papillary thyroid cancer is not associated with survival: an analysis of 61,775 patients. *Ann Surg*. 2014;260(4):601-605; discussion 605-607.
28. Haigh PI, Urbach DR, Rotstein LE. Extent of thyroidectomy is not a major determinant of survival in low- or high-risk papillary thyroid cancer. *Ann Surg Oncol*. 2005;12(1):81-89.
29. Mendelsohn AH, Elashoff DA, Abemayor E, St John MA. Surgery for papillary thyroid carcinoma: is lobectomy enough? *Arch Otolaryngol Head Neck Surg*. 2010;136(11):1055-1061.
30. Bojoga A, Koot A, Bonenkamp J, et al. The impact of the extent of surgery on the long-term outcomes of patients with low-risk differentiated non-medullary thyroid cancer: a systematic meta-analysis. *J Clin Med*. 2020;9(7):E2316.
31. Kluijfhout WP, Pasternak JD, Drake FT, et al. Application of the new American Thyroid Association guidelines leads to a

substantial rate of completion total thyroidectomy to enable adjuvant radioactive iodine. *Surgery*. 2017;161(1):127-133.
32. Kuo LE, Angell TE, Pandian TK, et al. Completion thyroidectomy is less common following updated 2015 American Thyroid Association guidelines. *Ann Surg Oncol*. 2021;28(1):484-491.
33. Ullmann TM, Gray KD, Stefanova D, et al. The 2015 American Thyroid Association guidelines are associated with an increasing rate of hemithyroidectomy for thyroid cancer. *Surgery*. 2019;166(3):349-355.
34. Craig SJ, Bysice AM, Nakoneshny SC, Pasieka JL, Chandarana SP. The identification of intraoperative risk factors can reduce, but not exclude, the need for completion thyroidectomy in low-risk papillary thyroid cancer patients. *Thyroid Off J Am Thyroid Assoc*. 2020;30(2):222-228.
35. Chen W, Li J, Peng S, et al. Association of total thyroidectomy or thyroid lobectomy with the quality of life in patients with differentiated thyroid cancer with low to intermediate risk of recurrence. *JAMA Surg*. 2022;157(3):200-209.
36. Fraser S, Zaidi N, Norlén O, et al. Incidence and risk factors for occult level 3 lymph node metastases in papillary thyroid cancer. *Ann Surg Oncol*. 2016;23(11):3587-3592.
37. Kim SK, Woo JW, Lee JH, et al. Prophylactic central neck dissection might not be necessary in papillary thyroid carcinoma: analysis of 11,569 cases from a single institution. *J Am Coll Surg*. 2016;222(5):853-864.
38. Nixon IJ, Wang LY, Ganly I, et al. Outcomes for patients with papillary thyroid cancer who do not undergo prophylactic central neck dissection. *Br J Surg*. 2016;103(3):218-225.
39. Viola D, Materazzi G, Valerio L, et al. Prophylactic central compartment lymph node dissection in papillary thyroid carcinoma: clinical implications derived from the first prospective randomized controlled single institution study. *J Clin Endocrinol Metab*. 2015;100(4):1316-1324.
40. Sippel RS, Robbins SE, Poehls JL, et al. A randomized controlled clinical trial: no clear benefit to prophylactic central neck dissection in patients with clinically node negative papillary thyroid cancer. *Ann Surg*. 2020;272(3):496-503.
41. Raffaelli M, De Crea C, Sessa L, et al. Modulating the extension of thyroidectomy in patients with papillary thyroid carcinoma pre-operatively eligible for lobectomy: reliability of ipsilateral central neck dissection. *Endocrine*. 2021;72(2):437-444.
42. Morton RP, Whitfield P, Al-Ali S. Anatomical and surgical considerations of the external branch of the superior laryngeal nerve: a systematic review. *Clin Otolaryngol*. 2006;31(5):368-374.
43. Liu JB, Sosa JA, Grogan RH, et al. Variation of thyroidectomy-specific outcomes among hospitals and their association with risk adjustment and hospital performance. *JAMA Surg*. 2018; 153(1):e174593.
44. Cirocchi R, Arezzo A, D'Andrea V, et al. Intraoperative neuromonitoring versus visual nerve identification for prevention of recurrent laryngeal nerve injury in adults undergoing thyroid surgery. *Cochrane Database Syst Rev*. 2019;1:CD012483.
45. Fontenot TE, Randolph GW, Setton TE, Alsaleh N, Kandil E. Does intraoperative nerve monitoring reliably aid in staging of total thyroidectomies? *The Laryngoscope*. 2015;125(9):2232-2235.
46. Joliat GR, Guarnero V, Demartines N, Schweizer V, Matter M. Recurrent laryngeal nerve injury after thyroid and parathyroid surgery. *Medicine (Baltimore)*. 2017;96(17):e6674.
47. Lo CY, Kwok KF, Yuen PW. A prospective evaluation of recurrent laryngeal nerve paralysis during thyroidectomy. *Arch Surg*. 2000;135(2):204-207.
48. Kazaure HS, Zambeli-Ljepovic A, Oyekunle T, et al. Severe hypocalcemia after thyroidectomy: an analysis of 7366 patients. *Ann Surg*. 2021;274(6):e1014.
49. Powers J, Joy K, Ruscio A, Lagast H. Prevalence and incidence of hypoparathyroidism in the United States using a large claims database. *J Bone Miner Res Off J Am Soc Bone Miner Res*. 2013;28(12):2570-2576.
50. Orloff LA, Wiseman SM, Bernet VJ, et al. American Thyroid Association statement on postoperative hypoparathyroidism: diagnosis, prevention, and management in adults. *Thyroid Off J Am Thyroid Assoc*. 2018;28(7):830-841.
51. Mattoo S, Agarwal A, Mayilvaganan S, et al. Role of postoperative intact serum PTH as an early predictor of severe post-thyroidectomy hypocalcemia: a prospective study. *J Endocrinol Invest*. 2021;44(9):1961-1970.
52. Košec A, Hergešić F, Matovinović F, Rašić I, Vagić D, Bedeković V. Identifying early postoperative serum parathyroid hormone levels as predictors of hypocalcaemia after total thyroidectomy: a prospective non-randomized study. *Am J Otolaryngol*. 2020;41(3):102416.
53. Huang J, Harris EJ, Lorch JH. Treatment of aggressive thyroid cancer. *Surg Pathol Clin*. 2019;12(4):943-950.
54. Raue F, Frank-Raue K. Thyroid cancer: risk-stratified management and individualized therapy. *Clin Cancer Res Off J Am Assoc Cancer Res*. 2016;22(20):5012-5021.
55. White PS, Pudusseri A, Lee SL, Eton O. Intermittent dosing of dabrafenib and trametinib in metastatic BRAFV600e mutated papillary thyroid cancer: two case reports. *Thyroid*. 2017;27(9):1201-1205.
56. Tuttle M, Morris LF, Haugen B, et al. Thyroid—differentiated and anaplastic carcinoma. In: Amin MB, Edge S, Greene F, et al., eds. *AJCC Cancer Staging Manual*. 8th ed. 2017, Corr. 3rd printing 2018 edition. Springer; 2016.
57. Pontius LN, Oyekunle TO, Thomas SM, et al. Projecting survival in papillary thyroid cancer: a comparison of the seventh and eighth editions of the American Joint Commission on Cancer/Union for International Cancer Control staging systems in two contemporary national patient cohorts. *Thyroid Off J Am Thyroid Assoc*. 2017;27(11):1408-1416.
58. Tuttle RM, Leboeuf R. Follow up approaches in thyroid cancer: a risk adapted paradigm. *Endocrinol Metab Clin North Am*. 2008;37(2):419-435.
59. Hartl DM, Guerlain J, Bresuskin I, et al. Surgery in the context of kinase inhibitor therapy for locally invasive thyroid cancer. *Eur J Surg Oncol*. 2020;46(4):650-655.
60. Feng J, Shen F, Cai W, Gan X, Deng X, Xu B. Survival of aggressive variants of papillary thyroid carcinoma in patients under 55 years old: a SEER population-based retrospective analysis. *Endocrine*. 2018;61(3):499-505.
61. Surveillance, Epidemiology, and End Results Program. Thyroid SEER 5-Year Relative Survival Rates, 2012-2018. SEER*Explorer Application. Accessed August 28, 2022. https://seer.cancer.gov/statistics-network/explorer/application.html?site=80&data_type=4&graph_type=5&compareBy=subtype&chk_subtype_80=80&chk_subtype_651=651&chk_subtype_650=650&series=9&sex=1&race=1&age_range=1&stage=101&advopt_precision=1&advopt_show_ci=on&hdn_view=1
62. Limberg J, Ullmann TM, Stefanova D, et al. Does aggressive variant histology without invasive features predict overall survival in papillary thyroid cancer? A National Cancer Database analysis. *Ann Surg*. 2021;274(3):e276-e281.

Follicular Thyroid Carcinoma

15

Alessandra L. Moore, MD
Gerard M. Doherty, MD

INTRODUCTION

Of the subtypes of thyroid neoplasms, follicular thyroid carcinomas represent the most challenging to distinguish pathologically from their benign counterparts, with serious implications to the patient in regard to treatment algorithms, clinical outcomes, and 5-year survival. Despite years of research and major advancements in molecular diagnostics, follicular thyroid cancers still cannot be distinguished without a definitive surgical pathology specimen. As a result, many people will undergo unnecessary diagnostic surgery to secure a benign diagnosis for a relatively rare, and certainly poorly understood malignant thyroid condition.

Generally, follicular thyroid carcinomas (FTC) are thought to imbue an excellent prognosis owing to its well-differentiated pathology. Derived from the thyroid follicular epithelium, FTCs, like papillary thyroid carcinoma (PTC), can concentrate iodine and, therefore, have favorable treatment options even with advanced local and metastatic disease. However, with the reclassification and acknowledgment of the follicular variant of papillary thyroid carcinoma (FV-PTC), previous assumptions about prognosis of follicular thyroid cancers and their response to therapy have been called into question; as prior large-scale publications erroneously included this subtype of papillary thyroid carcinoma in the analysis of follicular thyroid carcinomas. What is certain, however, is that compared to PTC, follicular thyroid carcinomas are much less prevalent, representing 10% or less of thyroid malignancies in the United States, making a deep understanding of their disease progression and tumor biology more challenging. In this chapter, we discuss the various clinical presentations, diagnostic workup modalities, and treatment options for patients with FTC based on the most recent evidence.

Clinical Pathophysiology

A multistep tumorigenic pathway leading to FTC was recently uncovered with the aid of high-throughput next-generation sequencing methods. With it, aberrant activation of mitogen-activated protein kinase (MAPK) and phosphoinositide 3-kinase–PTEN–AKT signaling pathways were identified as the culprit molecular alterations leading to carcinogenesis. In addition, molecular alterations appear to be stepwise, with a distinct correlation between genotype and phenotype. This stepwise acquisition of genetic alterations permits tumor genetic testing as a method of prognostication in patients with both papillary and follicular cancers.[1] With the data from next-generation sequencing, we also gained clarity as to the reason that follicular adenomas and FTC cannot be distinguished by molecular targets, or cytology; namely, because these thyroid neoplasms exist in a biologic continuum.[2] For instance, follicular adenomas with PAX8-PPARG rearrangements will show atypia and hypercellularity like their PAX8-PPARG carcinoma counterparts, and those with *RAS* point mutations will grow similarly quickly as benign and malignant neoplasms. Histologically, the two are only distinguished by the presence or absence of tumor capsular and true vascular invasion, otherwise being morphologically identical. Thus, to this date, despite the presence of modern tumor-molecular diagnostic tools, follicular thyroid neoplasms obligate whole surgical pathologic specimen evaluation to arrive at a diagnosis.[2]

Of the molecular alterations known to follicular thyroid carcinoma, *RAS* mutations are particularly significant. *RAS* mutations with oncogenic potential function by altering the downstream GTP binding domain, or GTPase domain, rendering GTP in an activated form within tumor cells. These mutations are known to occur in any of the *RAS* proteins (*NRAS, KRAS, HRAS*), but *NRAS* is the most common. Accumulation of additional mutations, such as *TERT*, *PTEN*, and *AKT*, are thought to underpin the progression of tumorigenesis from well-differentiated to poorly differentiated thyroid tumors, as shown in Figure 15–1.[3]

Chromosomal alternations such as hypodiploidy and rearrangements are also common in FTCs and may be

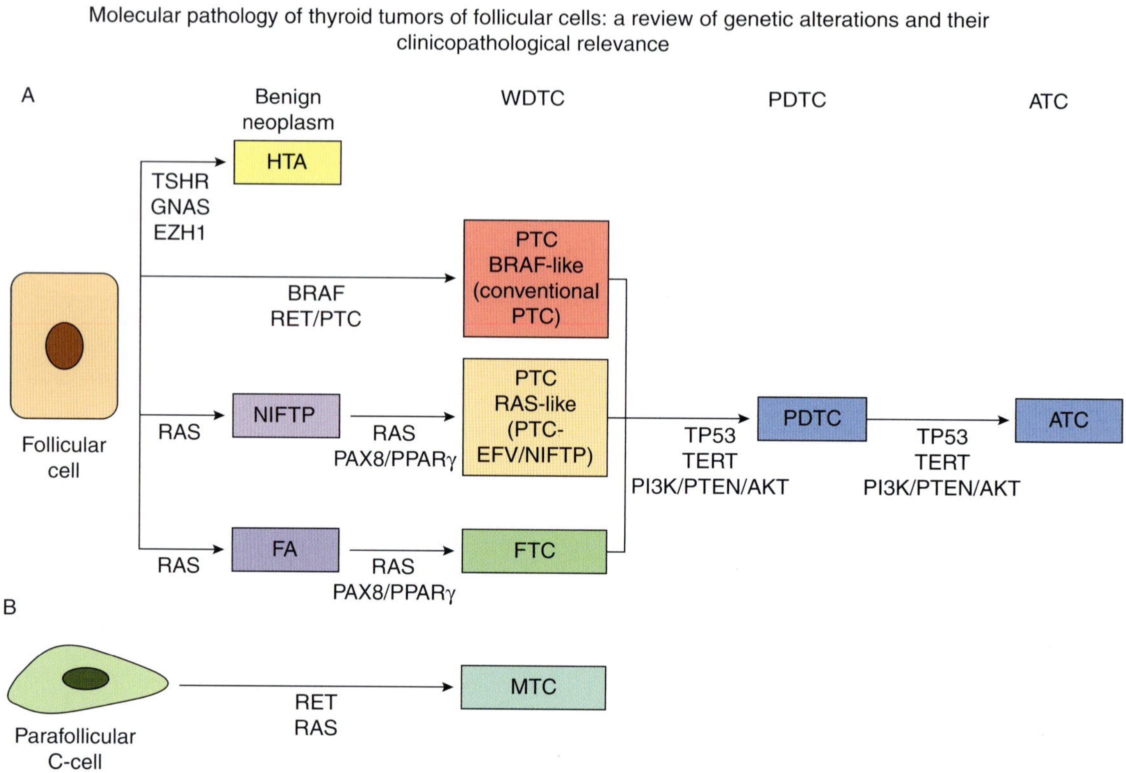

Figure 15–1. **Schematic of multistep tumorigenic pathway in thyroid cancer.** (Reproduced with permission from Acquaviva G, Visani M, Repaci A, et al. Molecular pathology of thyroid tumours of follicular cells: a review of genetic alterations and their clinicopathological relevance. *Histopathology*. 2017;72(1):6-31.)

associated with environmental insults such as radiation exposure. Based on these cytogenetic aberrations, FTCs can be divided into two molecular and pathologic groups. For FTCs with aneuploidy and chromosomal gains, tumor specimens often show a solid and/or trabecular phenotype. FTCs with chromosome losses and diploid or near diploid-chromosome content, architecture is characteristically normofollicular, albeit with an invasive component.

Some genetic alterations leading to FTC are likely inherited as well. Germline *PTEN* mutations, as in patients with Cowden syndrome, are also correlated with an increased risk for FTC, and should be suspected in patients with rapidly recurrent disease after total or near total thyroidectomy, or FTC co-occurring with multiple follicular adenomas, microadenomas, and adenolipomas. Other nonmedullary familial thyroid cancers and cancer syndromes have been described but are mostly associated with papillary thyroid cancers. Familial adenomatous polyposis (*FAP*), Cowden syndrome (*PTEN*), LiFraumani (*p53*), DICER 1 (*DICER 1*), Lynch syndrome (DNA mismatch repair genes *MLH1*, *MSH2*, *MSH6*, *PMS2*, or *EPCAM*), Werner syndrome (*WRN*), and Carney complex (*PRKAR1A*) represent the most commonly inherited mutations leading to thyroid cancer; however, that is specifically measured as a papillary thyroid cancer risk, and the risk of follicular thyroid cancer is mostly theoretical.

In addition to radiation exposure, iodine deficiency is associated with the development of follicular thyroid cancers. In areas of the world with endemic iodine deficiency, the incidence of goiter and other follicular thyroid neoplasms is increased; however, the exact causative mechanism is not understood. Female gender and age are two predominant risk factors for the development of FTC, with oncogenic abnormalities found in the background non-neoplastic thyroid tissue of older individuals.[2,4]

Etiology

Like papillary malignancies, follicular thyroid cancers confer a low disease-specific mortality (DSM) of about 8%. This is higher than PTC (approximately 2% for classical type), but due to sensitivity of FTC to radioactive iodine (RAI) therapy, the DSM of FTC remains favorable. FTCs with development of distant metastasis (DM) have a closer association of DSM compared to PTC, and DM are more common in recurrent FTC (3%) than PTC (1%). For those patients with DM, radioiodine treatment can slow disease progression even in patients with widespread metastasis, with the exception being those patients with bulky disease. DM in FTC tends to occur in the bone and lungs, with liver and brain being secondary, and other sites less common, though reported. When DM is identified in FTC, 5- and 10-year survival is 40% and 30%, respectively.

Lymph node metastasis (LNM) is rare and only observed in follicular thyroid cancers with unique, papillary-like features. For this reason, ultrasound of the lymph node basins of the neck is not typically useful as a screening tool for recurrence, except in those patients with incomplete resections or significant extrathyroidal extension (ETE). The value of LNM in predicting DSM in FTC is also unclear.

Separating FTCs into those with capsular invasion (CI), capsular invasion and less than four vessel vascular invasion (VI), and those with CI and more than four vessels VI or those with extensive ETE can accurately stratify risk for recurrence and DSM. However, the current ATA guidelines on staging (TNM) system takes none of these pathologic findings into account for FTC. Practitioners should recognize that the current TNM system is only validated for PTCs. Increasing age (>60 years old), male gender, and increasing tumor size (>4 cm) are all associated with decreased DSM in follicular thyroid cancer, and to some degree in PTCs; however, it should be noted that these may be surrogates for CI and VI. Ultimately, the ATA staging system does not take these factors into account (other than age) in predicting disease-specific survival (DSS) and therefore may over- and under-predict DSS based on significant tumor and patient-associated characteristics.[2,3,7,9]

Epidemiology

The incidence of FTC is increasingly challenging to estimate. In general, FTC is thought to represent 10% to 30% of thyroid malignancies, depending on geographic location, with a greater incidence endorsed by iodine-deficient locations. However, now that the follicular variant of papillary thyroid carcinoma (FVPTC) has largely supplanted FTC, the validity of previous studies must be called into question. In addition, geographic disparities in FTC raise questions about access to experienced thyroid pathologists who can accurately distinguish between FVPTC and FTC. Several studies report that the annual incidence of FTC is increasing with time; however, this is challenging to discern definitively with the prevalence and sensitivity of modern imaging modalities. Regardless, the recent body of literature would suggest a net increase in the incidence and disease-specific mortality for FTC, like other forms of differentiated thyroid cancer. The incidence of FTC in the United States is now estimated at 0.88 cases per 100,000 person-years.

The increased incidence and disease-specific mortality associated with thyroid carcinoma (inclusive of papillary thyroid carcinoma) may be related to the obesity epidemic and smoking, which are thought to account for nearly 40% of new cases. Interestingly, however, active smoking has repeatedly shown to have a protective effect against the development of thyroid carcinoma. Lastly, endocrine-disrupting chemicals, such as pesticides and bisphenol A, are also implicated in the net increase in incidence and disease-specific mortality of thyroid carcinomas. Challenges with studying net exposures limit evidence to support these claims.[5,6]

Clinical Presentation

FTC, like other thyroid neoplasms, can present as either asymptomatic or symptomatic thyroid nodules. In the first scenario, a nodule may be palpated by a patient, or during an annual physical exam, or may be brought to the attention of a patient by an observer. FTC may also be identified on imaging obtained for other pathologies. The most concerning clinical presentations include those with symptomatic nodules, who may report voice changes, neck pressure, dysphagia, shortness of breath, or a bulky neck mass, as these are more likely to represent locally advanced disease. Rarely, FTC presents with symptomatic metastasis, for instance to the bone. While overall the prognosis for FTC is excellent (>80% 5-year survival) and comparable to PTC, it should be noted that compared to PTC, FTC is more likely to spread hematogenously, as well as present with clinically relevant distant metastases. Regardless of these facts, FTC remains under the umbrella of well-differentiated thyroid carcinoma and those that are radioactive-iodine sensitive; therefore, prognosis is excellent.[2]

Diagnosis, Laboratory, & Imaging Studies

A. Diagnosis

There is a significant emphasis on avoiding overtreatment of malignant thyroid neoplasms due to their often-indolent progression. However, the mere process of arriving at a diagnosis of FTC is likely to result in overtreatment. Unlike PTC, for which the hallmark nuclear features permit identification by cytology, follicular thyroid neoplasms cannot be properly classified without a surgical specimen. FTC does not display cellular or nuclear atypia with the same degree as PTC, thus making its identification by fine-needle aspiration (FNA) challenging and unreliable. Follicular adenoma and FTC both display thick tumor capsule but lack many of the features associated with PTC (hypoechoic, taller than wide, microcalcifications, irregular borders) making their distinction by ultrasonography also a challenge. Clinicians are then left with thyroid lobectomy as the diagnostic and treatment mechanism for follicular thyroid neoplasms otherwise categorized as Bethesda III and IV lesions. To conclusively arrive at a diagnosis of FTC at the time of surgery, gross extension beyond the tumor or thyroid gland capsule must be appreciated. Pathologically, gross extension beyond the tumor capsule, often "mushrooming" beyond the tumor capsule, is required for diagnosis.[6] Tumor cells within the tumor capsule are considered artifactual that may be related to a prior FNA. True vascular invasion is defined as veins containing tumor cells adherent to the vascular endothelium or encapsulated within fibrin or thrombus within the vessel wall. To avoid misdiagnosis as minimally invasive FTC, clinical pathologists recommend examining the entirety of the tumor capsule and specimen. Indeed, failure to do so may result in misclassification, inappropriate follow-up, and is associated with a greater incidence of DM (Fig. 15–2)[3,6,8].

When FTC is associated with concurrent lymph node metastases, misdiagnosis of follicular variant of PTC must be entertained. Previous studies have highlighted the rare association of FTC with lymph node metastases, or with multifocality. True multifocal FTC should alert clinicians to the possibility of Cowden syndrome, as most "multifocal" FTC are in actuality specimens with coexisting papillary microcarcinoma.

The World Health Organization (WHO) and Armed Forces Pathology Unit agree that the degree of tumor capsular invasion as well as angioinvasion are important for risk stratification as well as clinical management. While there are several guidelines suggesting between three to four categories of FTC, most clinicians in the United States abide by the standards set previously by the American Thyroid Association (ATA), which permits three subdivisions of FTC. In the 2015 ATA guidelines, FTCs were subdivided into three categories as defined by their tumor capsular invasion (CI) and vascular invasion (VI). Specifically, those categories include, in order of disease severity: FTC with CI alone, with CI and with minimal VI (less than four blood vessels), and with CI and extensive VI (more than four blood vessels). Since 2015, inclusion of the degree of ETE has also made its way into pathology reports, though its effectiveness in categorizing patient risk is yet to be fully understood.[2,3,6,8]

B. Laboratory

There are no specific laboratory tests that can definitively diagnose FTC. Clinicians are advised to check a serum thyrotropin (TSH) after the discovery of a thyroid nodule. A suppressed TSH would be anticipated in those with an autonomous adenoma (a typically benign process); however, there are reports of rarely occurring metabolically active follicular thyroid cancer. Normal or elevated TSH is more suspicious for malignant pathology, though 90% of identified thyroid nodules with a normal or elevated serum TSH are benign. Nodules exceeding 1 cm in size generally meet criteria for FNA biopsy.

It can be helpful to understand the molecular profiles of FTC to determine if a follicular adenoma should be treated as a "pre-malignant" lesion. The genetic landscape of FTC is altogether different than PTC. In general, FTC harbors *RAS* mutations (*KRAS, NRAS, HRAS*) in 40% to 50% of tumors, with *PAX8/PPRγ* in 20% to 30% of FTC. Follicular adenoma (FA) can harbor the same mutations, though to a much lesser frequency (20%-40%, 2%-13% respectively), and when encountered, consideration of the malignant potential of the lesion should influence treatment recommendations.

Thyroglobulin (Tg), the majority glycoprotein produced by thyroid follicular cells, is also produced by differentiated thyroid cancers including FTC. In patients with prior total thyroidectomy or prior thyroid lobectomy and contralateral lobe radioactive iodine-ablation, serum Tg levels trended over time can be useful in predicting local and distant recurrences.

C. Imaging

The gold standard of imaging thyroid neoplasms is dedicated thyroid gland ultrasound and evaluation of the central and lateral lymph node compartments. In the hands of experienced technicians, most clinically significant pathology can be identified. It should be noted, however, that TIRADS

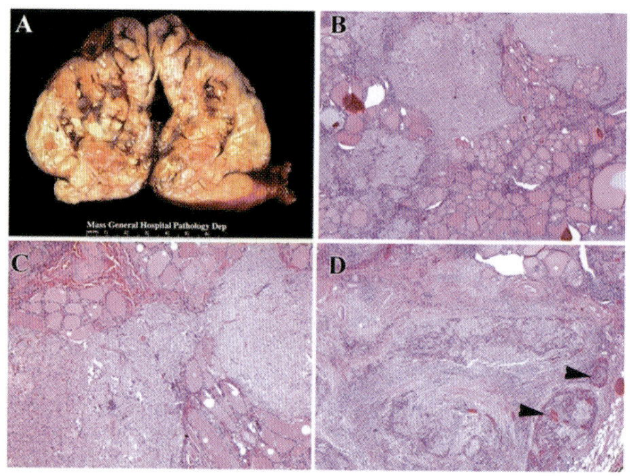

Figure 15–2. Widely invasive follicular thyroid carcinoma. The gross tumor (**A**), bisected, shows multinodular replacement of the thyroid lobe grossly with yellow foci of necrosis (most clearly center). Low-power H7E (x40) image of the tumor (**B**) demonstrates nodular and branching infiltration of normal thyroid by tumor, with the grossly normal patches of macrofollicular thyroid tissue between intervening tumor clusters, seen also at higher power (×200, **C**). There is extensive vascular invasion of the tumor, including at the tumor periphery (arrowheads) at low power (×40 H&E, **D**). (Reproduced with permission from Glomski K, Nose V, Faquin WC, Sadow PM. Metastatic follicular thyroid carcinoma and the primary thyroid gross examination: institutional review of cases from 1990 to 2015. *Endocr Pathol*. 2017;28(2):177-185.)

scoring was developed to identify PTC. FTC tends to be larger at diagnosis, rounded, and less often has hallmarks of papillary malignancies, such as hypoechogenicity, internal microcalcifications, taller than wide appearance, and irregular borders. FTC may display border irregularity and possibly extracapsular extension during diagnostic imaging; however, this is less often the case and may imply a locally advanced disease process.

For patients with suspicious imaging findings, [^{18}F] fluorodeoxyglucose positron emission tomography (^{18}FDG-PET) with focal uptake in a thyroid nodule is associated with an increased risk of thyroid carcinoma (one in three will have a malignancy). For those patients with nodules greater than 1 cm in size and ^{18}FDG-PET positive, FNA is recommended. ^{18}FDG-PET is not recommended as a first-line imaging study for thyroid nodules; however, more are being performed each year for other malignancies, with an increasing percentage identifying incidental uptake in the thyroid gland.

Cross-sectional imaging may play a role in the diagnosis of FTC by identifying asymptomatic lesions in patients imaged for other pathology. It may also be helpful in planning operative interventions or deciding care algorithms in patients with locally advanced and/or metastatic disease. Should lymph node metastases be identified during a workup for follicular thyroid cancer, this should immediately alert the clinician to potential misdiagnosis of follicular variant of PTC, or alternatively, simultaneous pathology (FTC and PTC).

Thyroid scintigraphy can identify metabolically active thyroid nodules, though FTC generally presents as a "cold" nodule (ie, less metabolically active than the surrounding normal thyroid tissue). For patients with suspected metastatic disease, whole body radioiodine scanning may also be useful. This imaging modality can identify distant metastases by their unique uptake of radioactive iodine (I^{123} or I^{131}). However, this can be challenging to obtain for some patients, as it requires no recent (in the last 60 days) intravenous contrast loads, and thyrotropin stimulation by either exogenous recombinant human TSH (rhTSH/Thyrogen) injections or withdrawal of exogenous thyroxine (T4). If there is a lack of clinical experience with this imaging technique as a surgeon, whole body radioiodine scanning should be obtained in concert with an experienced thyroid endocrinologist.[2,7,9]

Medical Management & Treatment

Medical management of FTC largely depends on the size and grade of the tumor.[6,7] The current ATA guidelines regarding the management of thyroid carcinomas are largely based on studies in PTC. In addition, many of those studies wrongly categorized FVPTC as a subtype of FTC, thus biasing data. For instance, FTC cannot be identified as a "microFTC" based on challenges associated with FNA cytology (unlike microPTC).[2] Thus, serial imaging and follow-up of less than 1 cm FTC, to treat only clinically significant disease, does not present itself as a clinical option. Also, due to the paucity of medical treatment options, surgical resection remains the standard of care. Postresection, TSH suppression with supplemental exogeneous thyroxine (T4) is often performed for moderate- to high-risk patients, such as those with higher risk for recurrence by molecular profiling, male gender, and young age (<40 y/o). In addition, radioactive-iodine treatment should be considered in patients with high-risk disease, as defined by extensive capsular invasion and angioinvasion (more than four vessels) on pathologic examination.[2]

For those patients with radioiodine refractory disease and/or distant metastases, there are several ongoing clinical trials examining the efficacy of oral kinase inhibitor therapy. Lenvatinib is one such therapeutic agent with a response rate of approximately 60%.[10] Pembrolizumab, an anti-PD-1 antibody, has also emerged as a treatment option for iodine refractory differentiated thyroid carcinoma patients with PD-L1 positive tumors.[11] Lastly, an exhaustive list of recommendations for a variety of clinical scenarios may be found in the 2015 American Thyroid Association Management Guidelines for Adult Patients with Thyroid Nodules and Differentiated Thyroid Cancer.[9] These may be viewed at www.thyroid.org.

Surgical Treatment

For patients with FTC less than 4 cm in size, thyroid lobectomy is considered an acceptable diagnostic approach and treatment option in those with low-risk disease as defined by final pathologic examination. This is based on consensus opinion from the 2015 ATA guidelines, which lumped recommendations for PTCs and FTCs as "differentiated thyroid carcinomas." Benefits of thyroid lobectomy over total thyroidectomy include a reduced risk of recurrent laryngeal nerve injury, reduced need for thyroid hormone supplementation, and avoidance of hypoparathyroidism (transient or permanent). However, lobectomy commits patients to lifelong surveillance imaging (thyroid ultrasound) which may not be practical for everyone. In addition, those patients with high-risk pathologic features (CI + VI) should be offered completion thyroidectomy, thus obligating a second surgical operation.

Central and lateral lymph node dissections, either therapeutic or prophylactic, are not recommended for FTC as metastases to lymph nodes are rare. As mentioned previously, FTC coexisting with pathologic lateral or central neck adenopathy should be concerning for a second or misclassified malignancy (namely PTC).

For patients with locally advanced tumors, R0 resection is optimal to prevent recurrence. In experienced hands, aerodigestive tract and tracheal involvement can be resected without profound morbidity to the patient. If R0 resection is not possible, either due to extensive disease burden, or perhaps recurrent nerve involvement in a patient unwilling experience nerve sacrifice, external beam radiation therapy can augment local control, particularly in radioiodine refractory tumors.

Lastly, for patients with extensive local disease as well as distant metastases, surgical resection continues to be a viable treatment option. In this scenario, palliating neck disease can prevent an untimely passing by asphyxiation and permit ongoing alimentation *per ora*.[9]

Prognosis

Prognosis for FTC is generally excellent, with an 80% or better 5-year survival.[2] Preventing local and distant disease recurrence is paramount, as there is a less than 10% 5-year survival after the detection of distant disease. After determining the extent of capsular invasion (CV) as well as vascular invasion (VI) in tumor specimens, they are typically subdivided into following categories: those with CI alone, CI with less than four foci VI, and CI with more than four foci VI (Table 15–1).

For the first category, the estimated recurrence risk (ERR, inclusive of local and distant disease) is low at around 2% to 5%. For the second category, ERR is estimated around 15% to 20%, and for the third more than 20%. For individuals with widely invasive disease or more than four foci VI, ERR ranges from 33% to 55%. Lastly, those FTC patients with presumed DM at diagnosis (by serum Tg level), confirmed metastasis, or an incomplete resection, recurrences are virtually guaranteed. Taken together, patients with favorable histology and complete surgical resection can anticipate a relatively low risk of recurrence and an exceptionally low disease-specific mortality, similar to PTC. However, additional studies are necessary to improve our understanding of the etiology of FTC and prove our assumptions. With the reclassification of FVPTC, and subsequent realization that our prior body of literature on FTCs was contaminated with papillary cancers, a critical eye on our patients will be required until stronger evidence-based recommendations emerge.[2,9]

Table 15–1. Risk stratification system for the prediction of persistent or recurrent disease in DTC patient.

Level of Risk (ERR)	Histology	Definition	Estimated Risk of Recurrence (ERR)
Low (<5%)	NIFTP	Noninvasive follicular thyroid neoplasm with papillary-like nuclear features, formerly referred to as "non-invasive encapsulated follicular-variant PTC"	<1%
	PTC	With all the following: • No macroscopic tumor-tissue remnants after resection • No locoregional invasion or local metastases • Clinical N0 or pathological N1 disease (<5 micrometastases, each measuring <0.2 cm) • No distant metastases • No RAI-avid metastatic foci outside the thyroid bed on first post-treatment whole-body RAI scan (if ^{131}I is given) • No vascular invasion • Nonaggressive histology BRAF V600E-mutated PTCs can be assigned to the low-risk category only if the tumor is <1 cm	1%-6%
	FTC	Intrathyroidal, well-differentiated FTC with capsular invasion and minimal (<4 foci) or no vascular invasion	2%-3%
Intermediate (6%-20%)	PTC	Microscopic invasion of perithyroidal soft tissues	3-8%
		Tumor-related symptoms	9%
		Intrathyroidal tumor measuring <4 cm, BRAF V600E-mutated (if known)	10%
		Aggressive histology	~15%
		Vascular invasion	15%-30%
		Multifocal papillary microcarcinoma with ETE and known BRAF V600E mutation	20%
		Clinical N1 or pathological N1 disease (>5 involved lymph nodes, each measuring <3 cm)	20%
		RAI-avid metastatic foci in the neck on the first post-treatment whole-body RAI scan	—
	FTC	Clinical N1 or pathological N1 disease (>5 involved lymph nodes, each measuring <3 cm)	20%
		RAI-avid metastatic foci in the neck on the first post-treatment whole-body RAI scan	—

(Continued)

Table 15–1. Risk stratification system for the prediction of persistent or recurrent disease in DTC patient. (Continued)

Level of Risk (ERR)	Histology	Definition	Estimated Risk of Recurrence (ERR)
High (>20%)	PTC	Gross ETE (macroscopic invasion of perithyroidal soft tissues)	30%-40%
		Pathological N1 disease: one or more nodal metastases measuring >3 cm	30%
		Extranodal extension	40%
		Concomitant BRAF V600E and TERT mutations	>40%
		Postoperative serum Tg suggestive of distant metastases	Virtually 100%
		Incomplete tumor resection	100%
		Distant metastases	100%
	FTC	Widely invasive or extensive vascular invasion (>4 foci)	30%-55%
		Postoperative serum Tg suggestive of distant metastases	Virtually 100%
		Incomplete tumor resection	100%
		Distant metastases	100%

Source: Reproduced with permission from Filetti S, Durante C, Hartl D, et al. Thyroid cancer: ESMO Clinical Practice Guidelines for diagnosis, treatment and follow-updagger. *Ann Oncol*. 2019;30(12):1856-1883.

REFERENCES

1. Acquaviva G, Visani M, Repaci A, et al. Molecular pathology of thyroid tumours of follicular cells: a review of genetic alterations and their clinicopathological relevance. *Histopathol.* 2018;72(1):6-31.
2. Daniels GH. Follicular thyroid carcinoma: a perspective. *Thyroid*. 2018;28(10):1229-1242.
3. Xu B, Ghossein R. Evolution of the histologic classification of thyroid neoplasms and its impact on clinical management. *Eur J Surg Oncol*. 2018;44(3):338-347.
4. Lim H, Devesa SS, Sosa JA, Check D, Kitahara CM. Trends in thyroid cancer incidence and mortality in the United States, 1974-2013. *JAMA*. Apr 4 2017;317(13):1338-1348.
5. Sajisevi M, Caulley L, Eskander A, et al. Evaluating the rising incidence of thyroid cancer and thyroid nodule detection modes: a multinational, multi-institutional analysis. *JAMA Otolaryngol Head Neck Surg*. Sep 1 2022;148(9):811-818.
6. Lang BH, Shek TW, Wu AL, Wan KY. The total number of tissue blocks per centimetre of tumor significantly correlated with the risk of distant metastasis in patients with minimally invasive follicular thyroid carcinoma. *Endocrine*. 2017;55(2):496-502.
7. Baloch ZW, Asa SL, Barletta JA, et al. Overview of the 2022 WHO classification of thyroid neoplasms. *Endocr Pathol*. 2022;33(1):27-63.
8. Glomski K, Nose V, Faquin WC, Sadow PM. Metastatic follicular thyroid carcinoma and the primary thyroid gross examination: institutional review of cases from 1990 to 2015. *Endocr Pathol*. 2017;28(2):177-185.
9. Haugen BR, Alexander EK, Bible KC, et al. 2015 American Thyroid Association Management Guidelines for Adult Patients with Thyroid Nodules and Differentiated Thyroid Cancer: The American Thyroid Association Guidelines Task Force on Thyroid Nodules and Differentiated Thyroid Cancer. *Thyroid*. 2016;26(1):1-133.
10. Schlumberger M, Tahara M, Wirth LJ, et al. Lenvatinib versus placebo in radioiodine-refractory thyroid cancer. *N Engl J Med*. 2015;372(7):621-630.
11. Mehnert JM, Varga A, Brose MS, et al. Safety and antitumor activity of the anti-PD-1 antibody pembrolizumab in patients with advanced, PD-L1-positive papillary or follicular thyroid cancer. *BMC Cancer*. 2019;19(1):196.

16 Hürthle Cell Carcinoma

Polina V. Zmijewski, MD, MA
Herbert Chen, MD
Kimberly M. Ramonell, MD

GENERAL CONSIDERATIONS

Hürthle cell neoplasms arise from follicular cells of the thyroid. They are characterized by the presence of Hürthle cells, which are eosinophilic, oxyphilic cells with round to oval nuclei. They contain prominent nucleoli as well as small, densely packed mitochondria that have a granular appearance in the otherwise empty cytoplasm. Hürthle cells are often referred to as oncocytes, derived from the Greek word "onkos," meaning "swelling."[1] The characteristic histologic appearance of Hürthle cell carcinoma (HCC) is demonstrated in Figure 16–1.

The first published scientific description of what is now known as a Hürthle cell was written in 1898 by Dr. Max Askanzy, who identified these unusually enlarged follicular cells in patients with Graves' disease. Askanzy's oncocytic cells were largely unrecognized by the scientific community until James Ewing published a description in his 1919 textbook *Neoplastic Diseases* and called them "Hürthle cells" after the German histologist, Karl Hürthle. This, however, was a misnomer as the cells Karl Hürthle discovered in 1894 were in fact parafollicular C cells.[2,3]

HCC accounts for approximately 3% of all differentiated thyroid cancers[4] and historically was classified as an oncocytic variant of follicular thyroid carcinoma.[5] However, genomic analysis data performed by Ganly et al. in 2013 demonstrated that HCC is its own distinct genomic entity with three distinct subtypes: adenoma, minimally invasive carcinoma, and widely invasive carcinoma.[6] In light of these findings, the World Health Organization revised their classification of follicular thyroid cancers in 2017 and recognized HCC as a distinct type of differentiated thyroid cancer.[7]

Histologically, a benign Hürthle cell adenoma is differentiated from an HCC by the absence of vascular or capsular invasion. This histologic differentiation is demonstrated in Figure 16–2. Minimally invasive HCCs are encapsulated with only microscopic foci of capsular or vascular invasion, while widely invasive tumors have more extensive vascular invasion and extrathyroidal extension.[2,8] These subtypes and their associated prognostic implications will be discussed with greater granularity later in this chapter. The diagnostic evaluation of HCC is similar to papillary and follicular thyroid carcinomas per the 2015 American Thyroid Association (ATA) guidelines and will be reviewed in this chapter.[8]

The treatment of HCC involves a multidisciplinary approach combining surgery with adjuvant medical and radiotherapy. Adjuvant therapies can include thyroid suppression, radioactive iodine ablation, external beam radiation, and systemic therapy, similar to the management of other differentiated thyroid cancers. HCC, like follicular carcinoma, spreads primarily via the hematogenous route.[9] Incidence of locoregional metastasis to lateral cervical lymph nodes at the time of presentation ranges from 17.7% to 33.5% and warrants a therapeutic ipsilateral lateral neck dissection.[10-12] Routine ultrasound evaluation of the lateral cervical nodes is essential in preoperative evaluations and for ongoing structural surveillance.

PREVENTION

As HCC is a rare malignancy, few studies identify modifiable and nonmodifiable risk factors contributing specifically to HCC development. A number of small, single-center studies exist that identify potential drivers of carcinoma.

A 2003 case-control study of 244 men with differentiated thyroid cancer (180 papillary and 24 follicular and Hürthle cell) identified tobacco use, history of thyroid goiter/nodules, history of non-thyroid malignancies, diabetes mellitus, and external beam radiotherapy of the head and neck as potential risk factors for differentiated thyroid cancer development.[13] A study by Arduc et al. of 244 women who underwent thyroidectomy for Bethesda Category IV thyroid nodules in 2015 demonstrated a significant link between waist circumference and high body mass index and final pathologic diagnosis of thyroid carcinoma.[14] A 2008 study of 55 patients with Hürthle cell neoplasms by Zhang et al. demonstrated

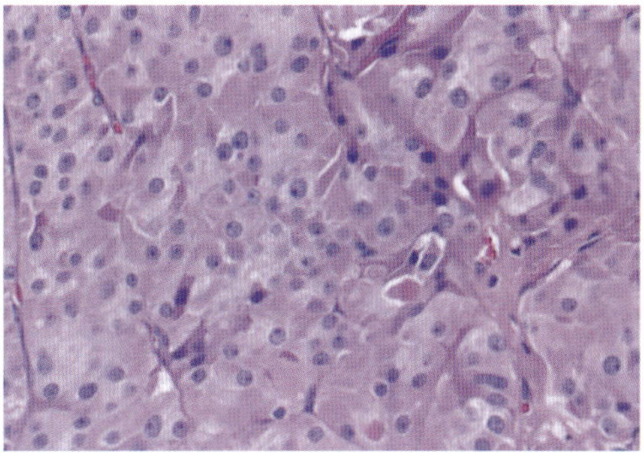

Figure 16–1. Hürthle cell carcinoma (hematoxylin and eosin, ×40). (Figure provided by M. Zheng, MD, PhD and A. Shifrin, MD.)

that older age (66 vs 52 years of age) and large tumor size (>2 cm) were factors predictive of HCC rather than adenoma diagnosis.[15] Others have also demonstrated that the risk of malignancy increases with increasing size of a Hürthle cell neoplasm.[16] Age has consistently been associated with diagnosis of HCC and other differentiated thyroid cancers in a number of other small studies.[17]

While HCC is overwhelmingly a sporadic disease, familial risk factors have been considered. A small study by Hemminki et al. demonstrated that development of Hürthle cell cancers was associated with a familial presence of Hodgkin's and non-Hodgkin's lymphoma.[18]

CLINICAL FINDINGS

Symptoms & Signs

HCC most commonly presents as a painless nodule, which is either palpable or incidentally discovered on imaging. Additional symptoms related to mass effect of the tumor in the neck have been reported, including hoarseness and dysphagia. Alterations in thyroid function are uncommon; most patients are euthyroid on presentation. Thyrotoxicosis as an initial presenting symptom is rare, but has also been reported in the literature.[19]

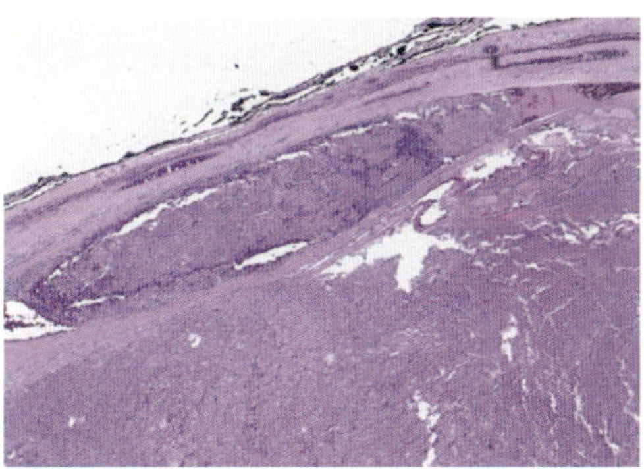

Figure 16–2. Vascular invasion in a Hürthle cell carcinoma (hematoxylin and eosin). (Figure provided by M. Zheng, MD, PhD and A. Shifrin, MD.)

Laboratory Findings

Patients with HCC most commonly present with normal TSH and T3/T4 levels. While there is no diagnostic role for serum thyroglobulin (Tg) levels prior to surgical treatment of HCC, post-thyroidectomy Tg and anti-Tg antibody levels are monitored as part of routine surveillance similar to other differentiated thyroid cancer subtypes.

Imaging Studies

Ultrasonography of a thyroid nodule is an essential first step to establishing a diagnosis. The most commonly used classification system of thyroid nodules for malignancy concern include the ATA classification system[8] and the Thyroid Imaging Reporting & Data System (TIRADS) system, more commonly employed by radiologists.[20]

On ultrasound, HCC lesions appear solid, hypoechoic, and frequently larger in size, but none of these features are unique to Hürthle cell compared to papillary or follicular carcinomas. A small center study by Lee et al. demonstrated that hypoechogenicity of nodules and size more than 2.5 cm were the factors most predictive of a malignant HCC lesion.[21] Unlike papillary carcinoma, HCC is less likely to contain microcalcifications.[21,22]

For locally advanced disease presenting with symptomatic dysphagia or hoarseness, direct laryngoscopy prior to operation may be indicated, as well as preoperative CT scan or MRI to assess for aerodigestive or vascular invasion. Preoperative neck CT may be useful in the evaluation of bulky, invasive disease as well as recurrent or persistent locoregional disease. A study by Debnam et al. demonstrated the usefulness of neck CT to differentiate thyroid carcinoma recurrence from residual nonmalignant thyroid tissue.[23] In addition, a meta-analysis of nine studies with an overall patient sample size of 1691 patients found that adjunct CT in addition to standard ultrasonography had higher sensitivity than ultrasound alone at detecting cervical metastases, suggesting its usefulness as a complementary diagnostic method.[24]

Though ultrasonography is currently the gold standard for preoperative evaluation of cervical lymph node metastasis, FDG-PET scan has been investigated as a potential adjunct to preoperative workup. A meta-analysis of nine studies demonstrated a low sensitivity but a high specificity of FDG-PET for detection of metastatic lymph nodes. Current evidence does not support the routine use of FDG-PET.[25]

Special Tests

HCC can only be definitively diagnosed on surgical pathology because it requires evaluation of the thyroid capsule and vasculature for presence of invasion, which cannot be seen on a fine-needle aspiration (FNA). FNA results can therefore only suggest the presence of an HCC. The FNA results of an HCC lesion most commonly fall into Bethesda Categories III or IV. Bethesda Category III lesions will be described in the pathology report as follicular lesions of undetermined significance and atypia of undetermined significance with Hürthle cell features. This FNA result is associated with a 5% to 15% risk of malignancy. Follicular or Hürthle Cell Neoplasm of Undetermined Significance is associated with a higher rate of malignancy (15%-30%) and can also be the result obtained from an aspirate of an HCC.[26]

HCC, as previously stated, cannot be definitively diagnosed without surgical pathology. FNA biopsies suggestive of Hürthle cell neoplasm can be managed in a number of ways. Patients can proceed to surgery based on patient preference and provider assessment of malignancy risk based on patient factors and ultrasonographic appearance. Alternatively, FNA can be repeated or coupled with molecular testing.[8]

Examples of commonly utilized molecular tests for thyroid genomic profiling includes the Afirma® Gene Expression Classifier (Veracyte, Inc) and the ThyroSeq® Thyroid Genomic Classifier (Sonic Healthcare USA). The clinical usefulness of molecular testing in differentiating benign from malignant Hürthle cell neoplasms, however, has been questioned. Hürthle cell predominance may lead to a higher rate of suspicious Afirma Gene Expression results, causing overtreatment of a lesion that has low risk of malignancy.[27] Thyroseq has been similarly shown to have limited clinical usefulness due to relatively low pretest probability of accurately identifying malignant Hürthle cell neoplasms.[28]

As previously stated, patients may elect to undergo surgery for definitive pathologic diagnosis, as this remains the gold standard for differentiating benign from malignant Hürthle cell neoplasms.[8] Patient preference and provider assessment of malignancy risk may dictate a treatment plan of close follow-up with active surveillance for benign appearing, low-risk lesions.

TREATMENT

Operative Management

Surgery is the gold standard of treatment for HCC. Decision to proceed with a diagnostic lobectomy (with plan for return to the operating room for completion thyroidectomy if patient demonstrates carcinoma on final pathology) versus an initial total thyroidectomy is a complex decision based on clinical appearance of the nodule, ultrasonographic features, molecular diagnostic testing (if available), and patient preference. Total thyroidectomy and thyroid lobectomy can be performed safely as an outpatient procedure, with same day patients demonstrating similar rates of neck hematoma and transient hypocalcemia as inpatients in a large single-center study.[29] Patients without restrictive underlying comorbidities are scheduled for same day discharge after thyroidectomy at our institution. For total thyroidectomy, a parathyroid hormone (PTH) testing protocol has been shown in multiple studies to predict hypoparathyroidism and allow for effective outpatient management.[30-33]

Some consideration should be given to thyroid lobectomy as definitive management of HCC if it is a low-risk lesion per ATA and NCCN criteria. In a study by Chindris et al. of 39 minimally invasive, low-risk HCCs, thyroid lobectomy alone was sufficient, with no evidence of recurrence of disease-specific mortality after 69.8 months of follow-up.[11]

Though HCC uncommonly metastasizes to the lymph nodes, cervical lymph nodes must be evaluated preoperatively. Suspicious lymph nodes should undergo FNA biopsy, with plan for thyroidectomy and compartment-oriented neck dissection if biopsy confirms locoregional metastasis. Frozen section should not be utilized for the evaluation of follicular or Hürthle cell neoplasms.[34,35] In a single-center study performed by Mallick et al. in 2019, only 2.1% of patients who had intraoperative frozen sections had a significant change in operative management, suggesting that frozen section analysis adds cost without value to thyroid operations.[36]

Adjuvant Therapies

Radioactive iodine ablation therapy (RAI) has been studied as an adjuvant therapy complementing treatment for HCC after thyroidectomy in a number of retrospective observational studies. These studies were overall equivocal. A study of 239 HCC patients by Oluic et al. found that there was no difference in cancer-specific survival. However, a study of HCC patients by Jillard et al., which included patients with high-risk features, demonstrated improvements in survival. These studies indicate that RAI may be helpful in patients with high-risk features of HCC, perhaps including those of the maximally invasive subtype, though further research in this area is necessary.[12,37,38]

RAI is the most commonly used adjuvant therapy for high-risk localized disease or presence of locoregional or distant metastatic HCC. In select cases of RAI refractory disease when not amenable to surgical resection or of prohibitive risk, external beam radiation therapy (EBRT) may be indicated, as part of a multimodal treatment regimen as discussed later. A study of 18 patients by Foote et al. demonstrated that HCC is a radiosensitive tumor, and suggested that EBRT can prevent recurrence in aggressive, widely metastatic disease and successfully provide palliative pain relief for patients with intractable disease burden.[39]

Patients with RAI refractory disease may benefit from systemic immunologic and receptor-targeted therapy as well. The SELECT trial in 2015 investigated the use of levantanib, a tyrosine kinase and growth factor inhibitor, in the treatment of metastatic, poorly differentiated Hürthle and follicular cell cancers. This study demonstrated increased progression-free survival in the levantanib group relative to the placebo group. This clinical trial was unique in that it included a large subset of HCC patients (18%) suggesting that their results may be applicable to this population.[40]

PROGNOSIS

The prognosis of HCC is much poorer than that of papillary and follicular thyroid carcinoma, likely due to its lower rate of responsiveness to RAI and its overall more aggressive disease profile.[10] Prognosis of patients with HCC is dependent on stage as well as categorization in widely or minimally invasive subtypes. The TNM Classification system for staging differentiated thyroid carcinoma can be seen in Table 16–1.[41] A study by Bhattacharyya et al. included 602 nonmetastatic HCC patients reported 5- and 10-year survivals as 85.1% and 71.1%, respectively.[42]

Per the ATA, low-risk HCC patients include those who have less than four foci of capsular or vascular invasion, less than five metastatic lymph nodes, tumors that are intrathyroidal and encapsulated, and those who have foci of metastases less than 0.2 cm (micrometastases). Intermediate-risk lesions include those that do have vascular invasion, exhibit some degree of extrathyroidal extension and have more than five metastatic lymph nodes. The highest risk group of patients with HCC have macroscopic extrathyroidal disease, those who undergo surgery but have inadequate margin of resection, those with distant metastatic disease, and lymph nodes with evidence of metastatic disease that are more than 3 cm in size.[8]

Patients with widely invasive HCC (>4 foci of invasion) have a worse prognosis than patients with a minimally invasive (<4 foci) subtype. In a study by Xu et al., 276 thyroid cancers, including 16 HCC were examined. They found that more than four foci of vascular invasion predicted recurrence in patients with differentiated thyroid carcinoma. The risk of recurrence in this patient population was found to be 42%, versus 1% in the no vascular or focal invasion group.[43] A study of 50 HCC patients by Ghossein et al. similarly demonstrated that more than four foci of vascular invasion was the most predictive pathologic factor for recurrence. Patients with less than four foci had 100% recurrence-free survival at 5 years versus 20% of patients with more than four foci of vascular invasion.[44]

Other factors associated with reduced overall survival include large size of tumor, extrathyroidal extension, older age, and inability to undergo surgery.[45,46] Male sex and cancers staged III and IV (per American Joint Committee on Cancer TNM system) were risk factors associated with death and recurrence.[11]

Table 16–1. TNM staging classification system for differentiated thyroid cancers.[41]

Stage	Age <55 Y	Age ≥55 Y
I	TanyNanyM0	T1-2 N0 M0
II	TanyNanyM1	T1 N1 M0 T2 N1 M0 T3 a-b N_{any} M0
III		T4a N_{any} M0
IVA		T4b N_{any} M0
IVB		T_{any} N_{any} M1

WHEN TO REFER/ADMIT

Management of HCC requires a multidisciplinary approach including surgery, endocrinology, and radiation oncology teams familiar with the disease and capable of appropriate treatment and surveillance. All patients with HCC should be referred to a high-volume thyroid surgeon.

While outpatient thyroidectomy and neck dissections can be safely performed in the appropriate patient and setting, postoperative admission after thyroidectomy should be considered based on complexity of surgery, patient preoperative risk stratification, and postoperative readiness for discharge.

REFERENCES

1. Mete O, Asa SL. Oncocytes, oxyphils, Hürthle, and Askanazy cells: morphological and molecular features of oncocytic thyroid nodules. *Endocr Pathol.* 2010;21(1):16-24.
2. Ahmadi S, Stang M, Jiang XS, Sosa JA. Hürthle cell carcinoma: current perspectives. *Onco Targets Ther.* 2016;9:6873-6884.
3. Caturegli P, Ruggere C. Karl Hürthle! Now, who was he? *Thyroid.* 2005;15(2):121-123.
4. Hundahl SA, Fleming ID, Fremgen AM, Menck HR. A National Cancer Data Base report on 53,856 cases of thyroid carcinoma treated in the U.S., 1985-1995. *Cancer.* 1998;83(12):2638-2648.
5. DeLellis RA, Lloyd RV, Heitz PU. *World Health Organization Classification of Tumors. Pathology and Genetics: Tumors of Endocrine Organs.* Lyon, France: IARC Press; 2004:69-72.
6. Ganly I, Ricarte Filho J, Eng S, et al. Genomic dissection of Hürthle cell carcinoma reveals a unique class of thyroid malignancy. *J Clin Endocrinol Metab.* 2013;98(5):E962-E972.
7. Lloyd RV, Osamura RY, Klöppel G, Rosai J. *WHO Classification of Tumours of Endocrine Organs.* 4th ed. Lyon, France: IARC, 2017.
8. Haugen BR, Alexander EK, Bible KC, et al. 2015 American Thyroid Association Management Guidelines for adult patients with thyroid nodules and differentiated thyroid cancer: the American Thyroid Association Guidelines task force on thyroid nodules and differentiated thyroid cancer. *Thyroid.* 2016;26(1):1-133.
9. Kushchayeva Y, Duh QY, Kebebew E, D'Avanzo A, Clark OH. Comparison of clinical characteristics at diagnosis and during follow-up in 118 patients with Hürthle cell or follicular thyroid cancer. *Am J Surg.* 2008;195(4):457-462.
10. Mills SC, Haq M, Smellie WJ, Harmer C. Hürthle cell carcinoma of the thyroid: retrospective review of 62 patients treated at the Royal Marsden Hospital between 1946 and 2003. *Eur J Surg Oncol.* 2009;35(3):230-234.

11. Chindris AM, Casler JD, Bernet VJ, et al. Clinical and molecular features of Hürthle cell carcinoma of the thyroid. *J Clin Endocrinol Metab*. 2015;100(1):55-62.
12. Grani G, Lamartina L, Durante C, Filetti S, Cooper DS. Follicular thyroid cancer and Hürthle cell carcinoma: challenges in diagnosis, treatment, and clinical management. *Lancet Diabetes Endocrinol*. 2018;6(6):500-514.
13. Zivaljevic V, Slijepcevic N, Sipetic S, et al. Risk factors for well-differentiated thyroid cancer in men. *Tumori*. 2013; 99(4):458-462.
14. Arduc A, Dogan BA, Tuna MM, et al. Higher body mass index and larger waist circumference may be predictors of thyroid carcinoma in patients with Hürthle-cell lesion/neoplasm fine-needle aspiration diagnosis. *Clin Endocrinol*. 2015;83(3):405-411.
15. Zhang YW, Greenblatt DY, Repplinger D, et al. Older age and larger tumor size predict malignancy in Hürthle cell neoplasms of the thyroid. *Ann Surg Oncol*. 2008;15(10):2842-2846.
16. Chen H, Nicol TL, Zeiger MA, et al. Hürthle cell neoplasms of the thyroid: are there factors predictive of malignancy? *Ann Surg*. 1998;227(4):542-546.
17. Strazisar B, Petric R, Sesek M, Zgajnar J, Hocevar M, Besic N. Predictive factors of carcinoma in 279 patients with Hürthle cell neoplasm of the thyroid gland. *J Surg Oncol*. 2010; 101(7):582-586.
18. Hemminki K, Eng C, Chen B. Familial risks for nonmedullary thyroid cancer. *J Clin Endocrinol Metab*. 2005;90(10):5747-5753.
19. Russo D, Wong MG, Costante G, et al. A Val 677 activating mutation of the thyrotropin receptor in a Hürthle cell thyroid carcinoma associated with thyrotoxicosis. *Thyroid*. 1999;9(1):13-17.
20. Tessler FN, Middleton WD, Grant EG, et al. ACR thyroid imaging, reporting and data system (TI-RADS): white paper of the ACR TI-RADS committee. *J Am Coll Radiol*. 2017;14(5): 587-595.
21. Lee SK, Rho BH, Woo SK. Hürthle cell neoplasm: correlation of gray-scale and power Doppler sonographic findings with gross pathology. *J Clin Ultrasound*. 2010;38(4):169-176.
22. Sippel RS, Elaraj DM, Khanafshar E, et al. Tumor size predicts malignant potential in Hürthle cell neoplasms of the thyroid. *World J Surg*. 2008;32(5):702-707.
23. Debnam JM, Guha-Thakurta N, Sun J, et al. Distinguishing recurrent thyroid cancer from residual nonmalignant thyroid tissue using multiphasic multidetector CT. *AJNR Am J Neuroradiol*. 2020;41(5):844-851.
24. Suh CH, Baek JH, Choi YJ, Lee JH. Performance of CT in the preoperative diagnosis of cervical lymph node metastasis in patients with papillary thyroid cancer: a systematic review and meta-analysis. *AJNR Am J Neuroradiol*. 2017;38(1):154-161.
25. Kim DH, Kim SJ. Diagnostic role of F-18 FDG PET/CT for preoperative lymph node staging in thyroid cancer patients: a systematic review and metaanalysis. *Clin Imaging*. 2020;65:100-107.
26. Cibas ES, Ali SZ. The 2017 Bethesda system for reporting thyroid cytopathology. *Thyroid*. 2017;27(11):1341-1346.
27. Brauner E, Holmes BJ, Krane JF, et al. Performance of the Afirma gene expression classifier in Hürthle cell thyroid nodules differs from other indeterminate thyroid nodules. *Thyroid*. 2015;25(7):789-796.
28. Schatz-Siemers N, Brandler TC, Oweity T, Sun W, Hernandez A, Levine P. Hürthle cell lesions on thyroid fine needle aspiration cytology: molecular and histologic correlation. *Diagn Cytopathol*. 2019;47(10):977-985.
29. Mazeh H, Khan Q, Schneider DF, Schaefer S, Sippel RS, Chen H. Same day thyroidectomy program: eligibility and safety evaluation. *Surgery*. 2012;6:1133-1141.
30. Dream S, Wang R, Lovell K, Iyer P, Chen H, Lindeman B. Outpatient thyroidectomy in the pediatric population. *Am J Surg*. 2020;219(6):890-893.
31. Obiarinze R, Fazendin J, Iyer P, Lindeman B, Chen H. Intraoperative parathyroid hormone measurement facilitates outpatient thyroidectomy in children. *Am J Surg*. 2021;221(4): 683-686.
32. Youngwirth L, Benavidez J, Sippel R, Chen H. Postoperative parathyroid hormone testing decreases symptomatic hypocalcemia and associated emergency room visits after total thyroidectomy. *Surgery*. 2010;148(4):841-844; discussion 844-6.
33. Carter Y, Chen H, Sippel RS. An intact parathyroid hormone (iPTH) based protocol for the prevention and treatment of symptomatic hypocalcemia after thyroidectomy. *J Surg Res*. 2014;186:23-28.
34. Chen H, Nicol TL, Udelsman R. Follicular lesions of the thyroid. Does frozen section evaluation alter operative management? *Ann Surg*. 1995;222(1):101-106.
35. Callcut RA, Selvaggi SM, Mack E, Ozgul O, Warner T, Chen H. The utility of frozen section evaluation for follicular thyroid lesions. *Ann Surg Oncol*. 2004;11(1):94-98.
36. Mallick R, Stevens TM, Winokur TS, et al. Is frozen-section analysis during thyroid operation useful in the era of molecular testing? *J Am Coll Surg*. 2019;228(4):474-479.
37. Jillard CL, Youngwirth L, Scheri RP, Roman S, Sosa JA. Radioactive iodine treatment is associated with improved survival for patients with Hürthle cell carcinoma. *Thyroid*. 2016;26(7):959-964.
38. Oluic B, Paunovic I, Loncar Z, et al. Survival and prognostic factors for survival, cancer specific survival and disease free interval in 239 patients with Hürthle cell carcinoma: a single center experience. *BMC Cancer*. 2017;17(1):371.
39. Foote RL, Brown PD, Garces YI, McIver B, Kasperbauer JL. Is there a role for radiation therapy in the management of Hürthle cell carcinoma? *Int J Radiat Oncol Biol Phys*. 2003;56(4): 1067-1072.
40. Schlumberger M, Tahara M, Wirth LJ, et al. Lenvatinib versus placebo in radioiodine-refractory thyroid cancer. *N Engl J Med*. 2015;372(7):621-630.
41. Townsend CM, Beauchamp RD, Evers BM, Mattox KL. *Sabiston Textbook of Surgery: The Biological Basis of Modern Surgical Practice*. 20th ed. Ch. 36: Thyroid. Philadelphia, PA: Elsevier Saunders; 2017.
42. Bhattacharyya N. Survival and prognosis in Hürthle cell carcinoma of the thyroid gland. *Arch Otolaryngol Head Neck Surg*. 2003;129(2):207-210.
43. Xu B, Wang L, Tuttle RM, Ganly I, Ghossein R. Prognostic impact of extent of vascular invasion in low-grade encapsulated follicular cell-derived thyroid carcinomas: a clinicopathologic study of 276 cases. *Hum Pathol*. 2015;46(12):1789-1798.
44. Ghossein RA, Hiltzik DH, Carlson DL, et al. Prognostic factors of recurrence in encapsulated Hürthle cell carcinoma of the thyroid gland: a clinicopathologic study of 50 cases. *Cancer*. 2006;106(8):1669-1676.
45. Goffredo P, Roman SA, Sosa JA. Hürthle cell carcinoma: a population-level analysis of 3311 patients. *Cancer*. 2013; 119(3):504-511.
46. Guerrero MA, Suh I, Vriens MR, et al. Age and tumor size predicts lymph node involvement in Hürthle cell carcinoma. *J Cancer*. 2010;1:23-26.

SUGGESTED READINGS

Cibas ES, Ali SZ. The 2017 Bethesda system for reporting thyroid cytopathology. *Thyroid*. 2017;27(11):1341-1346.

Ganly I, Ricarte Filho J, Eng S, et al. Genomic dissection of Hürthle cell carcinoma reveals a unique class of thyroid malignancy. *J Clin Endocrinol Metab*. 2013;98(5):E962-E972.

Haugen BR, Alexander EK, Bible KC, et al. 2015 American Thyroid Association Management Guidelines for adult patients with thyroid nodules and differentiated thyroid cancer: the American thyroid association guidelines task force on thyroid nodules and differentiated thyroid cancer. *Thyroid*. 2016;26(1):1-133.

Lloyd RV, Osamura RY, Klöppel G, Rosai J. *WHO Classification of Tumours of Endocrine Organs*. 4th ed. Lyon, France: IARC, 2017.

Tessler FN, Middleton WD, Grant EG, et al. ACR thyroid imaging, reporting and data system (TI-RADS): white paper of the ACR TI-RADS committee. *J Am Coll Radiol*. 2017;14(5):587-595.

17 Medullary Thyroid Carcinoma

Uriel Clemente, MD
Danica M. Vodopivec, MD
Catherine M. Skefos, MA, MS
Nancy D. Perrier, MD

GENERAL CONSIDERATIONS

Medullary thyroid carcinoma (MTC) is a neuroendocrine tumor arising from the parafollicular C cells of the thyroid gland. This histology accounts for approximately 2% of thyroid cancers in the United States and has a variety of clinical behaviors and prognosis ranging from indolent to aggressive tumors, with reported 10-year survival rates ranging from 69% to 89%.

Approximately 75% of MTC cases are sporadic, while 25% present as part of familial syndromes, specifically Multiple Endocrine Neoplasia type 2A and 2B (MEN2A and MEN2B)

PATHOGENESIS

The parafollicular C cells are present in the thyroid gland and form part of the neuroendocrine system. Parafollicular C cells originate from ectoderm neural crest cells which migrate to the ultimobranchial bodies. By the end of thyroid embryonic development, they locate mainly in the junction of the top and middle third of each thyroid lobe. Parafollicular cells secrete calcitonin, which is a hormone involved in calcium homeostasis, as well as carcinoembryonic antigen (CEA) and chromogranin.

The Rearranged during Transfection (*RET*) protooncogene is located on chromosome 10q11.2 and encodes a single-pass transmembrane receptor of the tyrosine kinase family. The *RET* gene is expressed in cells arising from the neural crest, branchial arches, and urogenital system. It also plays a role in the regulation of the hematopoietic cells and spermatogenesis. Thus, *RET* functions in a wide range of tissue types and has been associated with the development of not only sporadic and hereditary MTC, but other conditions including Hirschsprung disease (HD), follicular cell-derived thyroid carcinoma, lung adenocarcinoma, and chronic myelomonocytic leukemia. The presence of a *RET* germline mutation causes progression from C-cell hyperplasia to MTC. It is known that all patients with MEN2 have *RET* germline mutations and that nearly 45% of sporadic MTC patients have somatic *RET* mutations.[1]

CLINICAL FINDINGS

Sporadic MTC is most often diagnosed between ages 30 and 50. The most common clinical presentation is that of a solitary thyroid nodule. In this context, a detailed physical exam is fundamental. This examination should always be complimented with a neck ultrasound (US) and fine-needle aspiration (FNA) biopsy. Once diagnosed, serum calcitonin and CEA levels should be obtained.

Inherited MTC presents as part of MEN2A or MEN2B, each one with specific clinical manifestations. When MTC is diagnosed in the setting of a hereditary syndrome, this may present as a palpable thyroid nodule with or without calcitonin excess symptoms in index cases. On the other hand, when the diagnosis is made by screening a member of a known hereditary MTC syndrome family, this might present as an asymptomatic or nonpalpable thyroid nodule.[2]

MEN2A accounts for 95% of MEN2 cases, and there are four variants of this syndrome:

- Classical MEN2A: This is considered the most common variant. All patients will present with MTC and some will develop pheochromocytoma (50%) or PHPT (20%-30%). In this variant, the majority of mutations occur in codons 609, 611, 618, or 620 of exon 10 or codon 634 of exon 11, with the latter accounting for about 85% of cases. Additional mutations in exons 8, 10, 11, 13, 14, 15, and 16 have also been observed. The penetrance of pheochromocytoma and PHPT development differs based on the specific mutation detected.
- MEN2A CLA: The association of cutaneous lichen amyloidosis (CLA) and MEN2A develops in patients with mutations in the *RET* codon 634, although some case reports of codon 804 mutations have been described. CLA presents as a consequence of notalgia paresthetica involving the dorsal spinal nerves. This sensory neuropathy leads to intense pruritus in the subscapular region, with secondary hyperpigmented lesions, caused by

scratching (Figure 17–1A). It is important to mention that in this MEN2A subtype, pheochromocytoma and PHPT are present in the same frequency as in classical MEN2A.

- MEN2A with HD: In most cases, HD will be noticed soon after birth. Nevertheless, older patients with MEN2A caused by exon 10 *RET* mutations (including codons 609, 611, 618, and 620) should be evaluated if they have gastrointestinal symptoms concerning for HD (Figure 17–1B). Hirschsprung disease is diagnosed with histologic findings of hypertrophic nerve trunks and absence of ganglion cells in the colonic submucosa. In some patients, pathology may not show decreased or absent ganglion cells; however, the presence of ganglioneuromas may lead to loss of normal bowel tone, distention, segmental dilation and megacolon.
- Familial MTC: In past years, familial MTC was considered a separate syndrome from MEN2A. Most recent consensus guidelines suggested including familial MTC as a variant along the spectrum of MEN2A. This variant is characterized by the presence of a *RET* germline mutation in families with MTC who do not develop pheochromocytoma or hyperparathyroidism. The absence of pheochromocytoma and hyperparathyroidism must be documented and adequate family history with long-term follow-up should be addressed to consider this diagnosis.

MEN2B accounts for 5% of MEN2 cases, and this is mainly associated with *RET* germline mutations in exon 16 codon 918 and less frequently in exon 15 codon 883. It has the most aggressive clinical presentation with early onset of MTC, approximately 50% risk of development of pheochromocytoma, and unique physical features like marfanoid body habitus and ganglioneuromas affecting the aerodigestive tract, lacrimal duct, and eyelids (Figure 17–2).

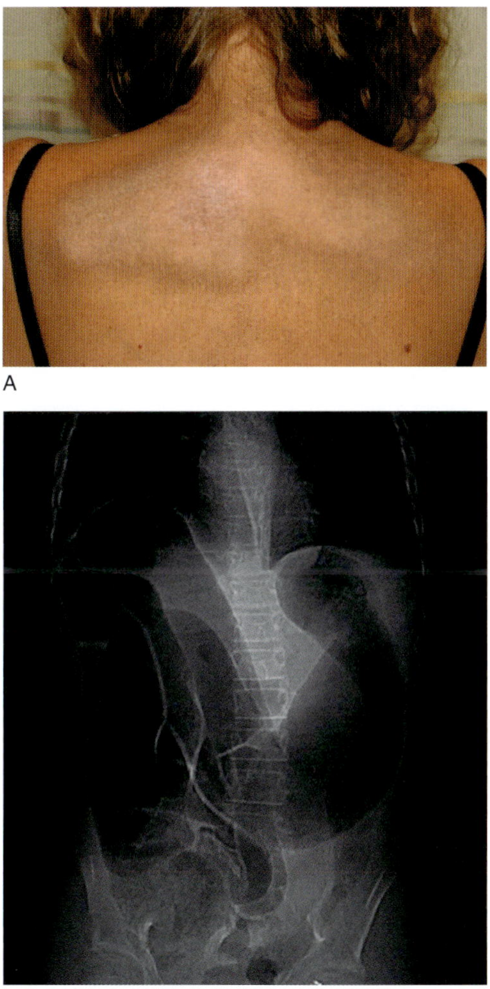

A

B

▲ **Figure 17–1.** Clinical characteristics of MEN2A. **(A)** CLA in a patient with MEN2A usually seen in the interscapular region, characterized by popular and pigmented lesions. **(B)** Abdomen X-ray showing colon dilation in MEN2A.

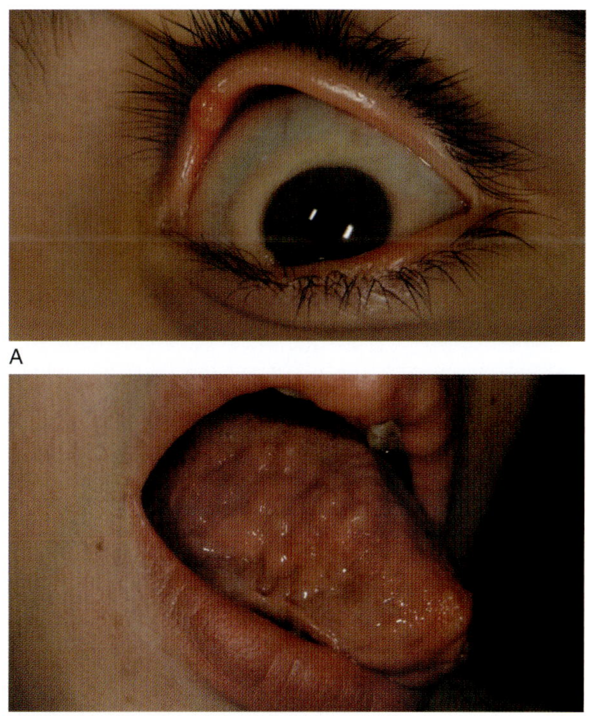

A

B

▲ **Figure 17–2.** Clinical characteristics of MEN2B. **(A)** Ganglioneuroma of the eyelid. **(B)** Ganglioneuromas of the tongue.

DIAGNOSIS, LABORATORY, & IMAGING STUDIES

The first step for MTC diagnosis is to obtain a detailed history and physical exam. Sporadic and index cases in hereditary MTC usually present as a solitary thyroid nodule with or without palpable cervical lymphadenopathy. Asking about compressive symptoms, which represent local signs of invasion (ie, hoarseness of voice, dysphagia, dry cough, shortness of breath), is crucial. Signs and symptoms concerning excess of calcitonin secretion or metastatic disease should be evaluated, specifically flushing, diarrhea, and bone pain. All cases require a clinical and biochemical evaluation for PHPT and pheochromocytoma. Obtaining family history is a key element for hereditary MTC diagnosis.

Laboratory evaluation is useful when MTC is suspected. Secretory products of parafollicular C cells are used as tumor markers, especially calcitonin and CEA. Calcitonin is a 32 amino acid hormone deeply involved in calcium homeostasis. This hormone is produced as a result of procalcitonin cleavage. In normal physiology, calcitonin secretion is stimulated by serum calcium elevation with subsequent inhibition of bone resorption and renal tubular reabsorption of calcium to oppose hypercalcemia. Some pathologic conditions may lead to high calcitonin levels, such as chronic kidney disease, hypercalcemia, papillary and follicular thyroid carcinomas, goiter, chronic autoimmune thyroiditis, and diverse hormonally active neuroendocrine tumors (ie, gastrinoma).[3] In addition, certain medications (ie, prolonged use of proton pump inhibitors, beta blockers, glucocorticoids) and heterophilic antibodies to calcitonin can falsely elevate serum calcitonin levels.[4,5] The routine use of calcitonin as a screening tool in all patients with a thyroid nodule is not warranted due to the low prevalence of MTC and should be reserved for patients with concerning family history of hereditary MTC or suggestive cytology in the FNA.[6] Basal serum calcitonin concentrations in MTC often correlate with tumor load, though normal calcitonin levels with high CEA levels could reflect tumor dedifferentiation. Though there is no established calcitonin cutoff value for MTC diagnosis, some studies have found that levels more than 46 pg/mL in males and more than 35 pg/mL in females have a positive predictive value of 97% and 98%, respectively. Other studies describe a positive predictive value of 100% in patients with calcitonin levels of 100 pg/mL or above. Pentagastrin stimulation test is mainly mentioned for historic purposes and was used to promote calcitonin secretion when tumor burden was still low. This test is rarely performed in some countries (ie, United States and Canada) where pentagastrin is largely unavailable; however, European consensus suggests using pentagastrin stimulation tests when basal calcitonin levels are found ≥10 pg/mL. If the stimulation test prompts a calcitonin level ≥100 pg/mL, a total thyroidectomy is indicated, while if stimulated calcitonin levels are 30 to 100 pg/mL, reevaluation after 4 to 6 months is suggested. Calcium stimulation is another option to evaluate borderline calcitonin levels; however, few studies have used calcium stimulation tests and cut points to determine the presence or absence of C-cell hyperplasia or MTC are not standardized for calcium stimulation.[7]

Calcitonin and CEA are also useful for evaluating disease progression and during follow-up after thyroidectomy. The biomarker CEA is not specific for MTC and can also be elevated in smokers or gastrointestinal carcinomas.

One of the most important diagnostic tools in MTC is the cervical (neck) US. This will help to evaluate the extension of the disease within the thyroid gland, lymph nodes, and adjacent structures (Figure 17–3). When baseline serum calcitonin is above 500 pg/mL, metastatic disease should be suspected; thus, additional radiologic studies are indicated. Chest computed tomography (CT) is used to evaluate lung and mediastinal lymph node metastases, abdominal imaging with CT or magnetic resonance

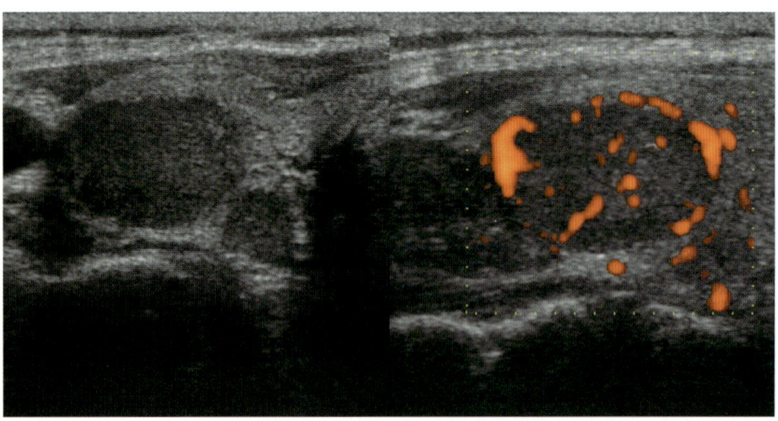

Figure 17–3. Ultrasonographic findings in MTC showing a 1.9 cm hypoechoic nodule with increased vascular flow.

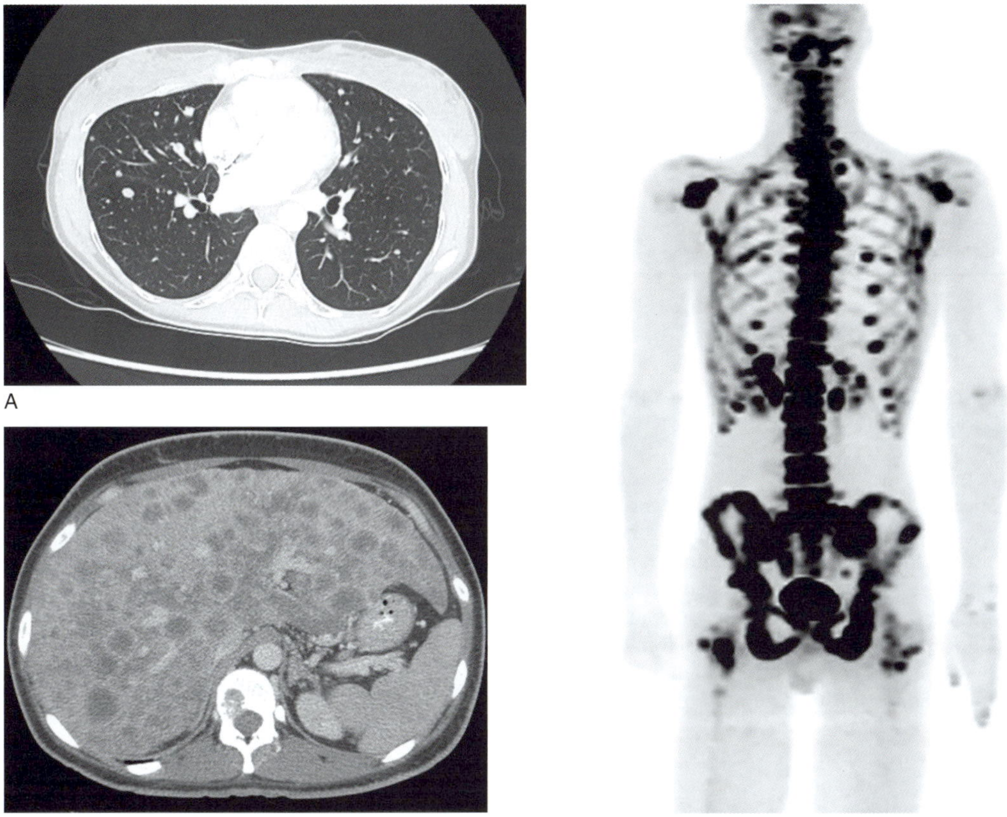

A B C

▲ **Figure 17–4.** Staging imaging studies for MTC. **(A)** Chest CT scan showing multiple lung metastases from MTC. **(B)** Abdomen CT scan demonstrating multiple liver metastases from MTC. **(C)** ^{111}In-octreotide somatostatin receptor scintigraphy showing bone metastases from MTC.

imaging (MRI) is indicated to evaluate liver metastasis, and bone metastasis can be evaluated with axial bone MRI or bone scintigraphy (Figure 17–4).

Genetic Testing

Over 100 mutations involving *RET* have been identified in patients with hereditary MTC. Different guidelines have described the disease phenotypes associated with specific *RET* mutations. The most recent guidelines from the American Thyroid Association (ATA) suggest classifying these mutations by aggressiveness of the MTC, based on age at diagnosis and association with metastatic disease. The M918T mutation is considered highest risk, while C634 and A883F are considered high risk, and all other mutations are considered moderate risk (Table 17–1).

Since 25% of MTC cases are hereditary, it is recommended that genetic screening be performed in all newly identified cases of MTC.[8] Because up to 7% of patients with apparently sporadic MTC are found to have a germline *RET* mutation, genetic counseling and testing should be offered to all patients with MTC. Historically, patients with suspected hereditary MTC underwent genetic testing via a tiered approach, beginning with the most commonly mutated "hotspots" and then proceeding to analysis of other exons if needed. More recently, due to the increasing availability of genetic testing and decreasing cost of next-generation sequencing, commercial genetic testing labs instead offer sequencing of the entire coding region (and some noncoding regions) of the gene with or without deletion and duplication analysis.

When a *RET* mutation is identified, genetic counseling should be pursued not only for the benefit of the patient in understanding and adapting to their genetic diagnosis, but also to aid in identifying, notifying, and coordinating testing for at-risk family members. When a familial mutation

Table 17–1. Genotype-phenotype correlations in hereditary medullary thyroid carcinoma syndromes and American Thyroid Association recommended age for early thyroidectomy.

MTC Risk Level	RET Mutation	MEN2 Subtype	ATA Recommended Age for Early Surgery
Moderate	533, 609, 611, 618, 620, 630, 631, 666, 768, 790, 804, 891, 912	MEN2A	Based on the detection of an elevated calcitonin level. Surveillance starting at 5 years.
High	634, 883	MEN2A	Before or around 5 years
Highest	918	MEN2B	Before 1 year

MEN, multiple endocrine neoplasia; MTC, medullary thyroid carcinoma; RET, rearranged during transfection.

is known, targeted testing can be offered to a patient to identify the presence or absence of the known mutation. Screening and early surgery can then be offered to asymptomatic family members who test positive, depending on age and the specific *RET* mutation that is identified. In families with a codon 918 (highest risk) mutation, predictive genetic testing should be offered in infancy so that thyroidectomy can be pursued in the first months of life, whereas testing for high and moderate risk mutations can take place around age 3.[2] Genetic counselors can also discuss family planning considerations, including the availability of prenatal testing and preimplantation genetic diagnosis.

Some reports have described rare variants, referred to as variants of unknown significance (VUS), whose biological significance is still unknown; to the extent possible, their pathogenic potential should be defined before testing family members of the index case. When a variant of unknown significance is identified, patients should be managed based on available clinical and family history data since the associated risk of the variant is unknown.[9]

STAGING & PROGNOSIS

The 8th edition of the American Joint Committee on Cancer TNM (AJCC-TNM) Staging for MTC is the most widely used tool for staging and establishing prognosis for patients with MTC diagnosis (Tables 17–2 and 17–3).[10] The 10-year survival rates for patients with stages I, II, III, and IV are 100%, 93%, 71%, and 21%, respectively.

The AJCC-TNM staging system provides prognosis but is not used to guide clinical therapy because it lacks important prognostic factors like age, gender, rapidly increasing CEA level, postoperative residual hypercalcitoninemia, and even codon analysis. Other staging systems like the European Organization for Research and Treatment of Cancer, National Thyroid Cancer Treatment Cooperative Study and Surveillance, Epidemiology and End Results program include other prognostic factors and can also be used.

Table 17–2. American Joint Committee on Cancer Tumor, Node, Metastasis Staging for Medullary Thyroid Carcinoma (8th ed., 2017).

T	Primary tumor
TX	Primary tumor cannot be assessed
T0	No evidence of primary tumor
T1	Tumor ≤2 cm or less in greatest dimension limited to the thyroid
T1a	Tumor ≤1 cm in greatest dimension limited to the thyroid
T1b	Tumor >1 cm but ≤2 in greatest dimension limited to the thyroid
T2	Tumor >2 cm but ≤4 cm in greatest dimension limited to the thyroid
T3	Tumor ≥4 cm or with extrathyroidal extension
T3a	Tumor ≥4 cm in greatest dimension limited to the thyroid
T3b	Tumor of any size with gross extrathyroidal extension invading only strap muscles
T4	Advanced disease
T4a	Moderately advance disease (gross extrathyroidal extension into the nearby tissues of the neck including subcutaneous soft tissue, larynx, trachea, esophagus, or RLN)
T4b	Very advanced disease (tumor of any size with extension toward the spine or into nearby large blood vessels, gross extrathyroidal extension invading the prevertebral fascia, or encasing the carotid artery or mediastinal vessels)
N	Regional lymph nodes
NX	Regional lymph nodes cannot be assessed
N0	No evidence of locoregional lymph node metastasis
N0a	One or more cytologically or histologically confirmed benign lymph nodes
N0b	No radiologic or clinical evidence of locoregional lymph node metastasis
N1	Metastasis to regional nodes
N1a	Metastasis to central lymph nodes
N1b	Metastasis to unilateral, bilateral, or contralateral neck lymph nodes
M	Distant metastasis
M0	No distant metastasis
M1	Distant metastasis

Table 17–3. AJCC prognostic stage groups.

	T	N	M
Stage I	T1	N0	M0
Stage II	T2-T3	N0	M0
Stage III	T1-T3	N1a	M0
Stage IVA	T4a T1-T3	Any N N1b	M0 M0
Stage IVB	T4	N0	M0
Stage IVC	Any T	Any N	M1

AJCC, American Joint Committee on Cancer.

TREATMENT

Surgical Treatment

The standard treatment for patients with sporadic or hereditary MTC is total thyroidectomy and dissection of cervical lymph node compartments.[11] This lymphadenectomy should be directed depending on preoperative serum calcitonin levels and neck US findings (Figure 17–5).[12,13]

Lymph node metastases in MTC depend on the size and location of the primary lesion in the thyroid. Tumors located in the upper part of the thyroid lobes usually lead to metastases in the upper lateral cervical compartment, while tumors in the middle or lower portion of the thyroid

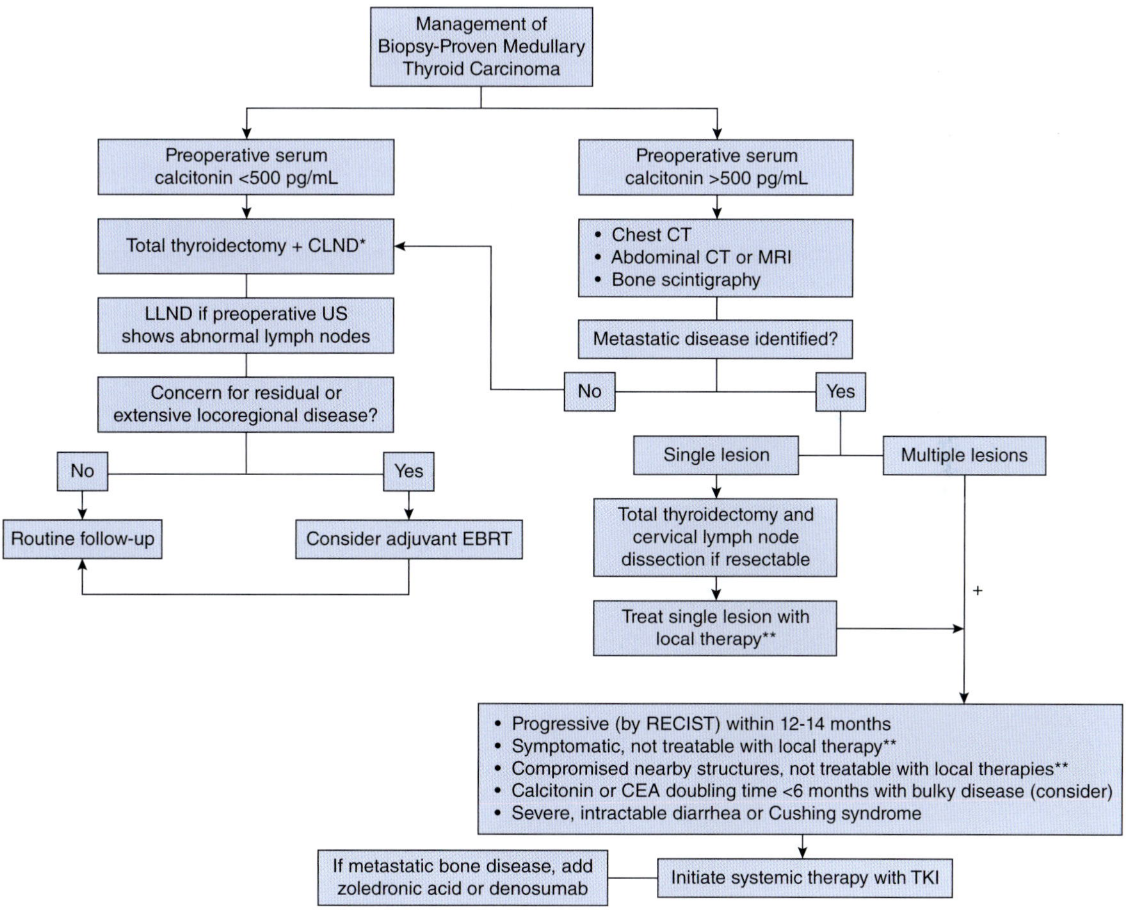

▲ **Figure 17–5.** Suggested algorithm for management of biopsy-proven patients with MTC.

*Extent (unilateral vs bilateral) requires judgment of age, mutation, biochemical profile, intraoperative findings, and coexisting factors.

**Includes metastasectomy, radiotherapy, cryotherapy, embolization, etc.

CLND: central lymph node dissection; EBRT: external beam radiation therapy; LLND: lateral lymph node dissection; MTC: medullary thyroid carcinoma; TKI: tyrosine kinase inhibitors.

tend to spread to the central compartment of the neck. Lymph nodes in the central compartment are the most often affected, in more than 70% of cases, followed by lateral compartment on the ipsilateral side of the tumor. Contralateral lymph node involvement has been observed frequently when preoperative calcitonin levels are more than 200 pg/mL. Regardless of the low cure rates in patients with regional lymph node metastases, resecting all involved lymph nodes decreases the risk of local recurrence. For these reasons, for patients with biopsy-proven disease with no evidence of neck lymph node involvement and absence of distant metastases, total thyroidectomy and consideration of prophylactic level VI compartment dissection is usually recommended. The extent of the central neck dissection, unilateral versus bilateral, and degree of aggressiveness of the parathyroid pedicle require judgment based on age, mutation, biochemical profile, intraoperative findings, and coexisting factors. Dissection of the lateral compartments (levels II, III, IV, and V) is indicated when abnormal lymph nodes are identified with the preoperative neck US. In case of unilateral, bulky lateral neck lymphadenopathy documentation, contralateral prophylactic lymph node dissection can be considered based on preoperative calcitonin levels (above 200 pg/mL) (Figure 17–6).

To be more granular, intraoperative prognostic factors have been evaluated in different studies to determine if prophylactic cervical lymph node dissection could be omitted in a subgroup of patients. These studies have concluded that lymph node surgery may be individualized based on intraoperative analysis of desmoplastic stromal reaction; if this is not present, prophylactic lymph node neck dissection does not add any benefit.[14] Recently, specific *RET* mutations have been associated with a higher risk of cervical lymph node metastases, and it has been suggested that patients with mutations in exons 11 and 13 may benefit from prophylactic ipsilateral lymphadenectomy in addition to central neck dissection, even without ultrasonographic evidence of lateral cervical lymph node metastases.[15]

When an advanced disease is identified, the goals of surgery are palliative rather than curative, and it is worth noting that less aggressive surgery is indicated to minimize complications. In the presence of MTC invading adjacent structures such as trachea, thyroid cartilage, esophagus, carotid artery, jugular vein, or recurrent laryngeal nerve, the extent of surgery is dictated by the overall prognosis and maintaining speech and swallowing must be balanced with the patient's life expectancy. In this scenario, systemic medical therapy should be considered to achieve local tumor control. Neoadjuvant treatment is much more mainstream for advanced disease (see section below on medical management). External beam radiation is reserved for those in whom surgical extirpation has been excluded and the patient is deemed a nonoperative candidate.

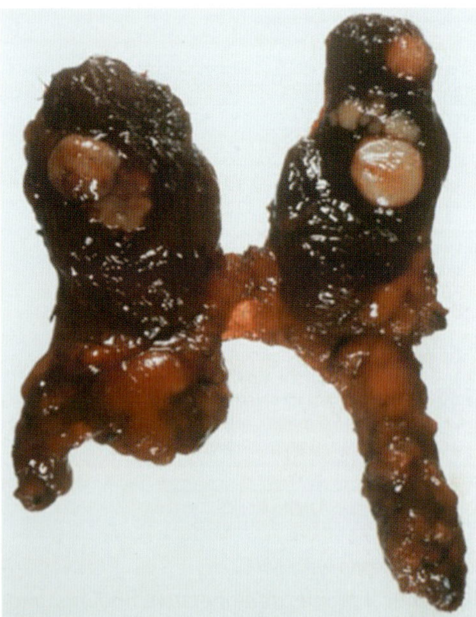

Figure 17–6. Therapeutic thyroidectomy surgical specimen demonstrating tumors in the upper third of both thyroid lobes.

A. Special Considerations in Surgical Treatment of Hereditary MTC

Pheochromocytoma increases cardiovascular and intraoperative risk. This neuroendocrine tumor has an incidence of up to 50% in patients with MEN2A and MEN2B, depending on the specific *RET* mutation. Pheochromocytoma may develop as early as 8 years of age in children with highest-risk *RET* mutations,[16] 12 years of age when associated with high-risk *RET* mutations, and around 19 years of age in patients with moderate-risk *RET* mutations. For this reason, screening for pheochromocytoma is recommended by age 11 years for children in the ATA high-risk and ATA highest-risk categories and by age 16 years in children in the ATA moderate-risk category. When MTC is diagnosed in a patient with MEN2A or MEN2B, pheochromocytoma must be excluded prior to surgical treatment of MTC and if detected, this should be medically blocked and preferably surgically removed prior to the neck operation. Surgical resection of pheochromocytoma in hereditary syndromes is performed by laparoscopic or retroperitoneoscopic approach and cortical sparing adrenal surgery can be considered to preserve adrenal cortical function, especially when there is risk of developing bilateral pheochromocytomas.[17,18] The details about surgical treatment of hereditary pheochromocytoma are beyond the scope of this chapter and will not be discussed further.

B. Role of Timing of Early Surgery

The presence of a *RET* germline mutation causes progression from C-cell hyperplasia to MTC. From this point, the natural progression of disease continues into locoregional expansion with cervical lymph node involvement and ultimately, distant metastases (lungs, liver, and bone). The aggressiveness and velocity of this progression depends on the mutated *RET* allele. As mentioned before, the ATA has proposed a classification based on the aggressive risk potential of MTC in MEN2 syndromes. Mutation in codon M918T is considered highest risk, while codons C634 and A883F are considered high risk and all other mutations are considered moderate risk. This classification is useful to establish an adequate timing for early thyroidectomy in hereditary MTC (Figure 17–7).[2]

Patients in the ATA highest-risk category are treated with early thyroidectomy during the first year of life. Neck dissection is indicated if any lymphadenopathy is identified during preoperative imaging studies or intraoperatively.

Children classified as ATA high-risk category will benefit from having a early thyroidectomy based on age, mutation status, calcitonin trend, and family preference. The discussion usually begins in the kindergarten time frame, around age 5 or 6. Performing it electively when it is least stressful for life parameters such as school and family dynamics is important for the psychological welfare of the child. If calcitonin is found to be elevated or the trend is rising before this age, thyroidectomy will be performed earlier. In the setting of early thyroidectomy, central neck dissection is not performed unless enlarged or worrisome lymph nodes are identified intraoperatively. If incidentally noted, unilateral central neck dissection is performed. Protection of the parathyroid glands is critical and requires discernment of thymic tissue, brown fat, and any reactive lymphadenopathy.

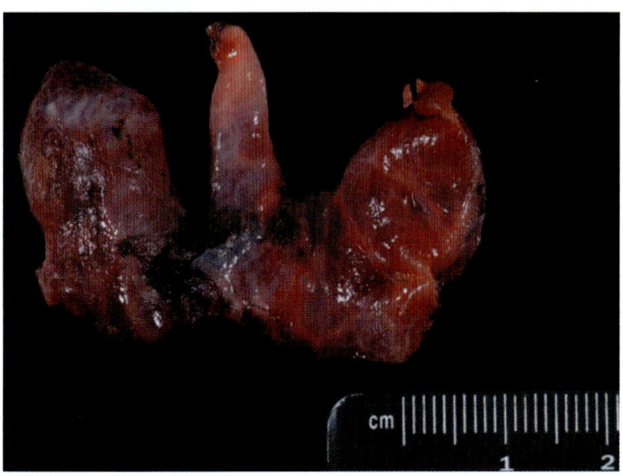

Figure 17–7. Prophylactic thyroidectomy surgical specimen.

Finally, those children with ATA moderate-risk category should be screened on a 6-month to annual cycle beginning around 5 years of age. The screening consists of physical exam, neck US, and calcitonin levels. Thyroidectomy is indicated based on the detection of an elevated or rising trend of serum calcitonin level or abnormalities noted on US examination. In this group of patients, parents who are concerned about long-term screening can decide on early thyroidectomy based on timing that is deemed appropriate for the family, pediatric endocrinologist, and endocrine surgeon. Often these are planned and electively performed during summer or school breaks.

C. Post-operative Follow-Up

After the initial surgical treatment, where thyroidectomy is performed, and given the fact that MTC is not a follicular-derived thyroid neoplasm, levothyroxine replacement therapy should aim to maintain serum TSH levels in the euthyroid range rather than suppressed.

Biochemical postoperative evaluation is fundamental for follow-up.[19] Serum levels of calcitonin and CEA should be measured 3 months after surgical resection of MTC. If these levels are undetectable or within the normal range, new serum levels should be measured every 6 months for 1 year, and then yearly thereafter.

In patients with calcitonin levels above normal range but below 150 pg/mL, physical examination and US of the neck should be obtained. If there is no evidence of structural disease in the neck US, follow-up can be done with imaging studies and biochemical evaluation every 6 months. If calcitonin levels are found above 150 pg/mL, extensive workup should be done to exclude metastatic disease, including neck US, chest CT, liver imaging (contrast-enhanced MRI or three-phase CT), bone scintigraphy/MRI of the pelvis and axial skeleton. Positron emission tomography/computed tomography (PET/CT) using fluorine-18-fludeoxyglucose (^{18}F-FDG), fluorine-18-L-dihydroxyphenylalanine (^{18}F-DOPA), or 68-gallium DOTATATE (^{68}Ga-DOTATATE) has demonstrated utility when evaluating metastatic/recurrent MTC with previous negative anatomic imaging (conventional CT or US).[20,21] The sensitivity of these nuclear medicine imaging modalities ranges from 14% to 100% and it is directly proportional to the differentiation of the tumor and calcitonin levels.

In case of persistent or recurrent locoregional MTC localized to the neck, surgical resection should include compartmental dissection of sites that are image or biopsy proven to be positive. Selective lymph node dissection or "berry picking" is not recommended unless previous extensive surgery has been performed in the involved neck compartment.

Microscopic or macroscopic residual MTC, extrathyroidal extension, and extensive lymph node metastases have proven to be high risk for local recurrence. In the past, this group of patients would have been more likely to consider postoperative adjuvant external beam radiotherapy to the neck and mediastinum, with a typical postoperative dose of 60 to 66 Gy, delivered to the thyroid bed over 6 weeks. A multidisciplinary team approach is even more necessary than before because of the multitude of pharmacologic therapies that are now available, several of which are FDA approved for this indication.

Medical Management

Surgery is the only curative treatment for MTC. However, the cure rate is low when there are cervical lymph node metastases involved at the time of initial surgery, with 90% of patients demonstrating either structural or biochemical residual disease. Patients with persistent or recurrent locoregional disease with progression over time can undergo a repeat surgery. Certain single-focus metastases may be treated with local or symptom-specific therapies like external beam radiation, surgical resection, embolization, or ablation. This is also the case with bone metastases (painful or to prevent skeletal-related events, ie, spinal cord compression, fracture) or metastatic disease to the liver. Bone metastases also should be considered for intravenous zoledronic acid or denosumab injection. Localized treatments may be beneficial to decrease tumor burden, alleviate pain, or to treat refractory diarrhea. Many patients with distant metastases have indolent disease, with stable or slowly rising calcitonin and/or CEA levels, that require active surveillance without the need for systemic therapy for years. Initiating treatment with chemotherapeutic agents should not be taken lightly as they confer toxicities, are not curative, and require chronic use for disease control. As a result, they are reserved for metastatic disease with at least one of the following characteristics: (1) progressive (by RECIST) within 12 to 14 months; (2) symptomatic and not treatable with local or symptom-specific therapies; (3) threatening or compromising nearby structures and not treatable with localized therapies; (4) calcitonin or CEA doubling time less than 6 months with structural evidence of clinically significant disease; and (5) severe, intractable MTC-related diarrhea or Cushing syndrome with lack of an alternative efficacious treatment. Most recently, the use of tyrosine kinase inhibitors (TKIs) as neoadjuvant therapy for locally advanced MTC has been described, with greater than 50% response, allowing complete surgical resection and avoiding significant upfront surgical morbidity, although there is no recommendation about neoadjuvant use of these agents in current guidelines.

With the advent of precision oncology, TKIs replaced cytotoxic chemotherapy as first-line treatment in unresectable, advanced, and progressive MTC. Currently, vandetanib, cabozantinib, pralsetinib, and selpercatinib are preferred (Table 17–4).[22]

Vandetanib and cabozantinib are multikinase inhibitors (MKIs) with predominant vascular endothelial growth factor (VEFGR) inhibition ("antiangiogenics"). In addition, vandetanib blocks epidermal growth factor receptor (EGFR) and cabozantinib, mesenchymal epithelial transition factor (MET). ZETA (NCT00410761 for vandetanib) and EXAM (NCT00704730 for cabozantinib) were the phase 3 clinical trials that led to approval by the US Food and Drug Administration (FDA) and the European Medical Agency (EMA).[23-25] Vandetanib showed an increase of 11.2 months in progression-free survival (PFS) compared to placebo and an overall response rate (ORR) of 45% (all partial responses [PRs]). Cabozantinib showed an increase of 7.2 months in median PFS compared to placebo and an ORR of 28% (all PRs). Responses were seen regardless of *RET* mutation status; however, responses were statistically significant in the M918T subgroup when compared with placebo, and there is suggested benefit in *RAS* mutated patients when compared with placebo, but this was not statistically significant due to the small number of patients analyzed. The cabozantinib trial required a radiological progression before enrollment, whereas the vandetanib study did not. The overall survival (OS) for vandetanib was not reached at the study cut-off date; however, it is likely to be confounded due patients on placebo crossing over to vandetanib at disease progression. There was a 5.5-month improvement in median OS with cabozantinib over placebo (26.6 vs 21.1 months) that was not statistically significant. Patients receiving placebo were not allowed to cross over to cabozantinib at the time of disease progression. The most common adverse events (AEs) for vandetanib and cabozantinib are listed in Table 17–4. AEs prompting dose reductions or withdrawals occurred in 35% and 12% of patients receiving vandetanib, respectively. Vandetanib has a black box warning listing QTc prolongation, Torsades de pointes, and sudden cardiac death, which is why only certified individuals under a Risk Evaluation and Mitigation Strategy (REMS) program can prescribe vandetanib. Cabozantinib had dose reduction, interruption, and discontinuation rates of 79%, 65%, and 16% of patients, respectively. Cabozantinib has a black box warning listing gastrointestinal perforations, fistulas, and hemorrhage. Clinically relevant QTc prolongation more than 500 ms was not appreciated with cabozantinib, as it was with vandetanib.

The lack of specificity of MKIs results in a higher rate of drug-related toxicities leading to dose reduction, interruption, or discontinuation. In addition, MKIs are subject to drug resistance by Val804 residue gatekeeper mutations. To overcome these deficiencies, highly selective RET-inhibitors were developed (Table 17–4). LIBRETTO-001 (NTC03157128 for selpercatinib) and ARROW (NCT03037385 for pralsetinib) were the phase 1/2 clinical trials that led to approval by the US FDA and EMA.[26,27] Selpercatinib showed an ORR of 69% (complete response, CR 9% [n = 5], PR 60% [n = 33], SD 25% [n = 14]) and a 1-year PFS of 82% in *RET*-mutant MTCs previously treated with vandetanib and/or cabozantinib. In *RET*-mutant MTCs not previously treated with

Table 17–4. Efficacy and safety of tyrosine kinase inhibitors for the treatment of medullary thyroid carcinoma.

Agent (Target)	References	Trial Design (Name)	Subjects (n)/ Cancer Type	ORR n (%)	CR n (%)	PR n (%)	SD n (%)	PFR	OS	Most Common Adverse Effects
Nonselective multikinase-inhibitors										
Vandetanib (VEGFR, EGFR, RET)	Wells Jr. et al.	Phase 3 trial (ZETA)	331 MTC (2:1; 231:100)	73/231 patients were analyzed 33 (45%)	None	33 (45%)	NR	Vandetanib predicted 30.5 months vs Placebo 19.3 months[×]	NR	Diarrhea, rash, dermatitis acneiform/acne, nausea, hypertension, headache, fatigue, decreased appetite, abdominal pain, dry skin, vomiting, QT prolongation, photosensitivity, hypocalcemia *Black box warning for QTc prolongation.*
Cabozantinib (VEFGR, MET, RET)	Elisei et al.	Phase 3 trial (EXAM)	330 MTC (2:1; 219:111)	28%	None	28%	NR	Cabozantinib 11.2 months vs 4 months placebo[×]	Cabozantinib 26.6 months vs placebo 21.1 months■	Diarrhea, stomatitis, hand-foot skin reaction, weight loss, decreased appetite, nausea, fatigue, dysgeusia, hair color changes, hypertension, constipation, abdominal pain, vomiting dysphonia *Black box warning for perforation, fistula, and hemorrhage.*

(Continued)

Table 17–4. Efficacy and safety of tyrosine kinase inhibitors for the treatment of medullary thyroid carcinoma. (*Continued*)

Agent (Target)	References	Trial Design (Name)	Subjects (n)/ Cancer Type	ORR n (%)	CR n (%)	PR n (%)	SD n (%)	PFR	OS	Most Common Adverse Effects
Selective RET inhibitors										
Selpercatinib (RET)	Wirth et al.	Phase 1/2 trial (LIBRETO-001)	55 RET+ MTC previously treated[*] 88 RET+ MTC treatment naive 19 RET fusion+ thyroid cancer[^]	38 (69%)[×] 64 (72%)[×] 15 (79%)[×]	5 (9%) 10 (11%) 1 (5%)	33 (60%) 54 (61%) 14 (74%)	14 (25%) 20 (23%) 4 (21%)	82%-1 year 92%-1year 64%-1 year	NR NR NR	Dry mouth, hypertension, increased AST/ALT, fatigue, peripheral edema, diarrhea, constipation, nausea, increased creatinine, headache, QT prolongation
Pralsetinib (RET)	Subbiah/ Hu et al.	Phase 1/2 trial (ARROW)	55 RET+ MTC previously treated[*] 21 RET+ MTC treatment naïve 9 RET fusion+ thyroid cancer[°]	33 (60%)[×] 15 (71%)[×] 8 (89%)[×]	1 (2%) 1 (5%) 0	32 (58%) 14 (67%) 8 (89%)	18 (33%) 6 (29%) 0	75%-1 year 91%-1 year 81%-1 year	89%-1 year 91%-1 year 91%-1 year	Leukopenia, neutropenia, increased ALT, hypertension, anemia, constipation, asthenia, increased ALT, hyperphosphatemia, lymphopenia, increased creatinine, muscle/joint pain, dysgeusia, diarrhea, low platelets, edema, headache, dry mouth

CR, complete response; NR, not reported; m, months; ORR, objective response rate; OS, overall survival; PFR, progression free survival; PR, partial response; SD, stable disease.

■Not statistically significant; however, reached significance in the M918T subgroup; [×]primary outcome; [*]with vandetanib and/or cabozantinib; [^]13 papillary thyroid carcinoma, 3 poorly differentiated thyroid carcinoma, 2 anaplastic thyroid carcinoma, 1 Hürthle cell carcinoma; [°]10 papillary thyroid carcinoma, 1 poorly differentiated thyroid carcinoma (9/11 response-evaluable patients).

vandetanib or cabozantinib, selpercatinib showed an ORR of 73% (CR 11% [n = 10], PR 61% [n = 54], SD 23% [n = 20]] and a 1-year PFS of 92% (95% CI, 82-97). Pralsetinib showed an ORR of 60% (n = 33/55; 95% CI 46-73) with 2% CR (n = 1/55), an estimated 1-year PFS of 75% after a median follow-up of 14.9 months, and an estimated 1-year OS of 89% after median follow-up of 16.5 months in *RET*-mutant MTC patients previously treated with cabozantinib and/or vandetanib. In treatment naïve *RET*-mutant MTC patients, pralsetinib showed an ORR of 71% (n = 15/21; 95% CI 48-89) with 5% CR (n = 1/21), an estimated 1-year PFS of 81% after a median follow-up of 15.1 months, and an estimated 1-year OS of 91% after median follow-up of 18.5 months. Responses were observed regardless of the *RET* mutation type, including gatekeeper mutations V804L/M. The most common AEs for selpercatinib and pralsetinib are listed in Table 17–4. AEs prompting dose reductions or withdrawals occurred in 30% and 2% of patients receiving selpercatinib, respectively. Pralsetinib had dose reduction, interruption, and discontinuation rates of 46%, 54%, and 4% in patients, respectively.

In addition to *RET* V804M/L gatekeeper mutations, new mutations affecting other portions of the RET receptor kinase domain have evolved, such as *RET* solvent front mutations (SFMs) G810A/C/S/R/V.[28] Mutations contribute to diminished drug efficacy, underlying the need to develop the selective second-generation RET inhibitors. TPX-0046 has the benefit to overcome SFMs; however, it is not effective against the gatekeeper V804 mutations. BOS172738 and TAS0953/HM06 are other selective RET inhibitors in development.

As a general concept, systemic therapy with TKIs may be considered for patients with progressive, unresectable, locally advanced, or metastatic MTC. Selective RET inhibitors are the treatment of choice when a targetable *RET*-activating mutation is identified. On the other hand, advanced thyroid cancers with *RAS* or other nontargetable mutations can be treated with the approved nonselective MKIs. Furthermore, there has been intensive research in new therapies like immunotherapy, tumor vaccines, radioimmunotherapy, and radiolabeled octreotide with less efficacious results.

REFERENCES

1. Kouvaraki MA, Shapiro SE, Perrier ND, et al. RET proto-oncogene: a review and update of genotype-phenotype correlations in hereditary medullary thyroid cancer and associated endocrine tumors. *Thyroid*. 2005;15(6):531-544.
2. Wells SA Jr, Asa SL, Dralle H, et al. Revised American Thyroid Association guidelines for the management of medullary thyroid carcinoma. *Thyroid*. 2015;25(6):567-610.
3. Toledo SP, Lourenço DM Jr, Santos MA, Tavares MR, Toledo RA, Correia-Deur JE. Hypercalcitoninemia is not pathognomonic of medullary thyroid carcinoma. *Clinics (Sao Paulo)*. 2009;64(7):699-706.
4. Erdogan MF, Gursoy A, Kulaksizoglu M. Long-term effects of elevated gastrin levels on calcitonin secretion. *J Endocrinol Invest*. 2006;29(9):771-775.
5. Preissner CM, Dodge LA, O'Kane DJ, Singh RJ, Grebe SK. Prevalence of heterophilic antibody interference in eight automated tumor marker immunoassays. *Clin Chem*. 2005;51(1):208-210.
6. Karges W, Dralle H, Raue F, et al. Calcitonin measurement to detect medullary thyroid carcinoma in nodular goiter: German evidence-based consensus recommendation. *Exp Clin Endocrinol Diabetes*. 2004;112(1):52-58.
7. Colombo C, Verga U, Mian C, et al. Comparison of calcium and pentagastrin tests for the diagnosis and follow-up of medullary thyroid cancer. *J Clin Endocrinol Metab*. 2012;97(3):905-913.
8. Hyde SM, Cote GJ, Grubbs EG. Genetics of multiple endocrine neoplasia type 1/multiple endocrine neoplasia type 2 syndromes. *Endocrinol Metab Clin North Am*. 2017;46(2):491-502.
9. Innella G, Rossi C, Romagnoli M, et al. Results and clinical interpretation of germline RET analysis in a series of patients with medullary thyroid carcinoma: the challenge of the variants of uncertain significance. *Cancers (Basel)*. 2020;12(11):3628-3639.
10. National Comprehensive Cancer Network. Thyroid Carcinoma (Version 1.2021). 2021.
11. Viola D, Elisei R. Management of medullary thyroid cancer. *Endocrinol Metab Clin North Am*. 2019;48(1):285-301.
12. Jin LX, Moley JF. Surgery for lymph node metastases of medullary thyroid carcinoma: a review. *Cancer*. 2016;122(3):358-366.
13. Moses LE, Oliver JR, Rotsides JM, et al. Nodal disease burden and outcome of medullary thyroid carcinoma. *Head Neck*. 2021;43(2):577-584.
14. Niederle MB, Riss P, Selberherr A, et al. Omission of lateral lymph node dissection in medullary thyroid cancer without a desmoplastic stromal reaction. *Br J Surg*. 2021;108(2):174-181.
15. Wang S, Wang B, Xie C, Ye D. RET proto-oncogene gene mutation is related to cervical lymph node metastasis in medullary thyroid carcinoma. *Endocr Pathol*. 2019;30(4):297-304.
16. Rowland KJ, Chernock RD, Moley JF. Pheochromocytoma in an 8-year-old patient with multiple endocrine neoplasia type 2A: implications for screening. *J Surg Oncol*. 2013;108(4):203-206.
17. Hasse-Lazar K, Zeman M, Kotecka-Blicharz A, et al. Laparoscopic cortical-sparing adrenal surgery in pheochromocytomas associated with hereditary neoplasia syndromes. *Endokrynol Pol*. 2020;71(6):518-523.
18. Grubbs EG, Rich TA, Ng C, et al. Long-term outcomes of surgical treatment for hereditary pheochromocytoma. *J Am Coll Surg*. 2013;216(2):280-289.
19. Mathiesen JS, Kroustrup JP, Vestergaard P, et al. Survival and long-term biochemical cure in medullary thyroid carcinoma in Denmark 1997-2014: a nationwide study. *Thyroid*. 2019;29(3):368-377.
20. Ganeshan D, Paulson E, Duran C, Cabanillas ME, Busaidy NL, Charnsangavej C. Current update on medullary thyroid carcinoma. *AJR Am J Roentgenol*. 2013;201(6):W867-W876.
21. Yamaga LYI, Cunha ML, Campos Neto GC, et al. ^{68}Ga-DOTATATE PET/CT in recurrent medullary thyroid carcinoma: a lesion-by-lesion comparison with ^{111}In-octreotide SPECT/CT and conventional imaging. *Eur J Nucl Med Mol Imaging*. 2017;44(10):1695-1701.
22. Cabanillas ME, Hu MI, Jimenez C. Medullary thyroid cancer in the era of tyrosine kinase inhibitors: to treat or not to treat–and with which drug–those are the questions. *J Clin Endocrinol Metab*. 2014;99(12):4390-4396.

23. Wells SA Jr, Robinson BG, Gagel RF, et al. Vandetanib in patients with locally advanced or metastatic medullary thyroid cancer: a randomized, double-blind phase III trial. *J Clin Oncol.* 2012;30(2):134-141.
24. Elisei R, Schlumberger MJ, Müller SP, et al. Cabozantinib in progressive medullary thyroid cancer. *J Clin Oncol.* 2013;31(29):3639-3646.
25. Schlumberger M, Elisei R, Müller S, et al. Overall survival analysis of EXAM, a phase III trial of cabozantinib in patients with radiographically progressive medullary thyroid carcinoma. *Ann Oncol.* 2017;28(11):2813-2819.
26. Wirth LJ, Sherman E, Robinson B, et al. Efficacy of selpercatinib in *RET*-altered thyroid cancers. *N Engl J Med.* 2020;383(9):825-835.
27. Subbiah V, Hu MI, Wirth LJ, et al. Pralsetinib for patients with advanced or metastatic RET-altered thyroid cancer (ARROW): a multi-cohort, open-label, registrational, phase 1/2 study. *Lancet Diabetes Endocrinol.* 2021;9(8):491-501.
28. Subbiah V, Shen T, Terzyan SS, et al. Structural basis of acquired resistance to selpercatinib and pralsetinib mediated by non-gatekeeper RET mutations. *Ann Oncol.* 2021;32(2):261-268.

Anaplastic & Undifferentiated Thyroid Carcinoma

18

Jina Kim, MD
Sanziana A. Roman, MD
Julie A. Sosa, MD, MA

GENERAL CONSIDERATIONS

Globally, anaplastic thyroid carcinoma (ATC) accounts for less than 5% of all thyroid cancers. While it is the least common type of thyroid cancer, it is the most lethal, with a 1-year overall survival of 20%. Due to the high mortality associated with ATC, prompt diagnostic evaluation and multidisciplinary decision-making are essential to management.

ATC typically is diagnosed by biopsy, which can be performed by either fine-needle aspiration (FNA) or core-needle biopsy. As 50% of patients will present with distant metastases, cross-sectional imaging can help determine extent of disease. Adjunctive studies such as laryngoscopy and esophagoscopy also can delineate tumor invasion into nearby structures. Workup of patients presenting with a rapidly expanding neck mass should be accomplished in less than a week from the time of presentation (Figure 18–1).

Management of ATC should follow the key principles outlined in the 2021 American Thyroid Association (ATA) guidelines (Table 18–1).[1] In patients with nonmetastatic disease, surgical resectability of the primary tumor should be assessed. Surgery aims to resect all visible tumor, as studies suggest that R0/R1 resection is associated with improved survival. Surgery is then followed by adjuvant chemoradiation. More recently, targeted molecular therapies are being used to treat patients with ATC harboring certain genetic mutations. In patients with unresectable or metastatic disease, radiotherapy, chemotherapy, and targeted molecular therapy all can be considered, but the treatment plan should reflect the patient's overall performance status and goals of care.

Compared to the original 2012 ATA guidelines for ATC, the updated 2021 ATA guidelines highlight the growing role of molecular targeted therapy for patients with ATC. Recently approved drugs such as dabrafenib and trametinib have improved patient outcomes and made neoadjuvant therapy possible for patients with ATC. Especially in patients with unresectable ATC who desire aggressive care, assessment of actionable genetic mutations now should be part of the management algorithm (Figure 18–2).

PATHOGENESIS

ATC derives from follicular thyroid cells. It is hypothesized that anaplastic thyroid cancer develops from well-differentiated tumors. As the tumor develops more genetic mutations, dedifferentiation occurs. ATC commonly has multiple genetic abnormalities. Mutations in ATC have been reported in p53, RAS, BRAF, β-catenin, PIK3CA, and others. Since mutations in BRAF and RAS are seen in well-differentiated thyroid cancer (DTC) as well as ATC, these mutations are thought to be earlier events in the dedifferentiation process. Late events may include mutations in p53, β-catenin, and PIK3CA, as these typically are not seen with well-differentiated tumors.

CLINICAL FINDINGS

The mean patient age at diagnosis is 65 years, and like other thyroid cancers, women are disproportionately affected. Risk factors associated with ATC include goiter, lower education level, and type B blood group. Only 10% of patients with ATC will present with an intrathyroidal tumor, and 40% will have extrathyroidal invasion and/or locoregional metastases. Half of patients will have metastatic disease at time of presentation, with pulmonary metastases being the most common. Among patients with ATC, about 20% will have a history of DTC, and another 20% to 30% will have a synchronous DTC. Most synchronous thyroid cancers are papillary.

The most common presentation of ATC is a rapidly enlarging neck mass, which can cause neck pain. Rarely, thyroiditis or hemorrhage from the rapidly growing tumor can manifest as severe neck pain. Patients may also experience local compression symptoms such as dysphagia, cough, dyspnea, and hoarseness.

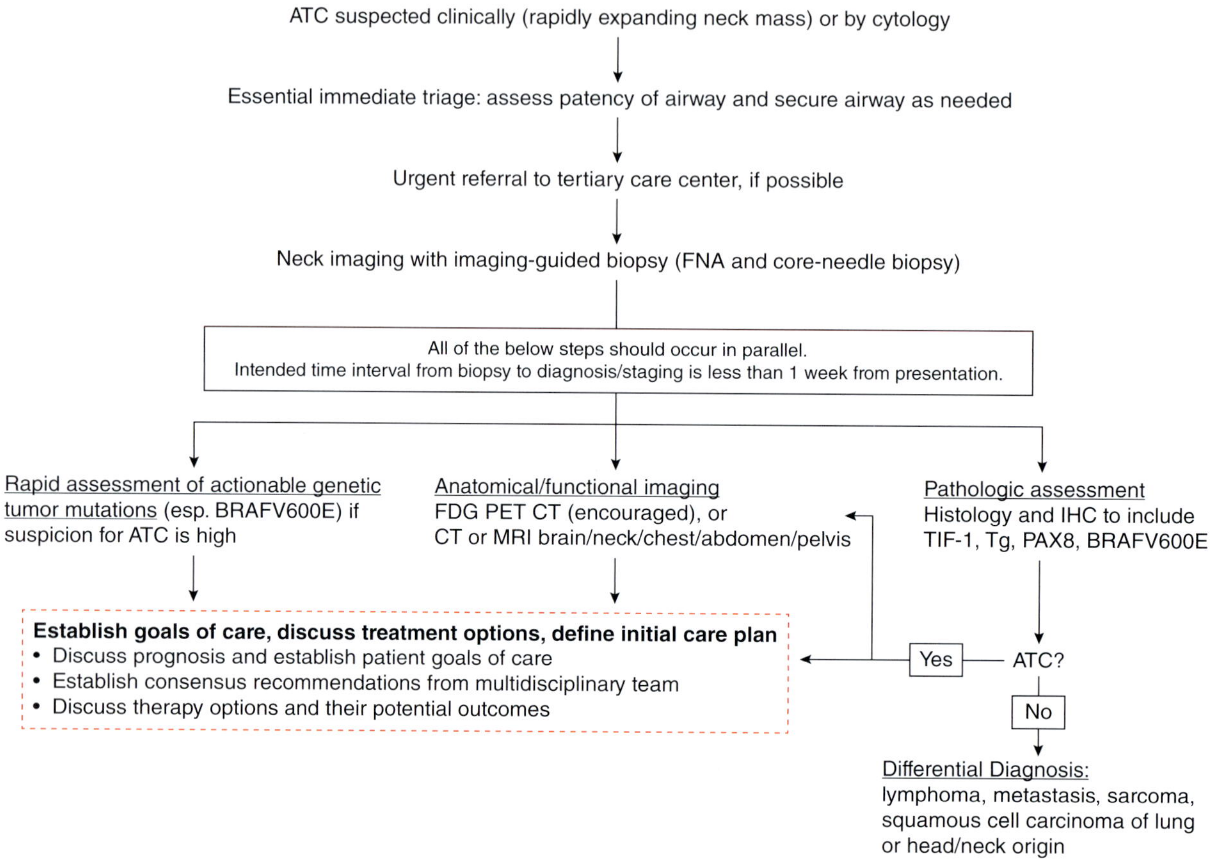

Figure 18–1. Initial evaluation for suspected anaplastic thyroid cancer. (Adapted from Bible KC. (2021, Sep 30-Oct 3). *Update in Management of Anaplastic Thyroid Cancer: 2021 ATA Guidelines* [Conference session]. American Thyroid Association, virtual.)

On physical exam of the neck, the thyroid is typically enlarged, hard, and fixed. A dominant nodule may be palpable. About 50% of patients will have palpable cervical lymphadenopathy. Other exam findings such as stridor or hoarseness suggest local tumor invasion. Focal neurologic findings may indicate brain metastases.

DIAGNOSIS

The diagnostic evaluation for ATC should occur expeditiously (within no more than a week from presentation) and accurately, as appropriate treatment of this aggressive tumor relies on accurate histopathology, labs, and imaging (Table 18–2). In the histopathologic evaluation, tumor morphology and immunohistochemistry can help diagnose ATC. Thyroid function tests and thyroglobulin level should be measured if ATC is diagnosed. For staging, which is discussed in more detail later, PET/CT whole body using ^{18}F-fluorodeoxyglucose (FDG) is preferred, but CT neck, chest, abdomen, and pelvis with IV contrast is acceptable if PET/CT is unavailable. It is important to note that the imaging studies should occur simultaneously with pathologic assessment and evaluation for actionable gene mutations to expedite care (Figure 18–3).

Histopathology

Histopathologic diagnosis of ATC can be challenging, but often a diagnosis can be made with percutaneous biopsy. Biopsies, either FNA or CNB, should be performed with ultrasound guidance to identify more solid areas of the tumor and avoid necrotic or inflamed areas that may yield nondiagnostic results. FNA may be adequate if the aspirate has sufficient cellularity, and immunohistochemistry (IHC) can be performed. While molecular testing can be performed on FNA samples, CNB often allows for a greater range of molecular tests. The 2021 ATA guidelines for ATC recommend that the diagnosis of ATC be established

Table 18–1. Key steps in the management of anaplastic thyroid cancer.

1. **Establish the diagnosis, quickly and definitively.**
   - Due to the rapid growth of ATC, early diagnosis and assessment of tumor mutations is critical.
   - Differential diagnosis also includes thyroid lymphoma, head/neck squamous cell carcinoma, and secondary metastasis to the thyroid.
2. **Engage a multidisciplinary team** that includes surgeons, radiation and medical oncologists, endocrinologists, and palliative care specialists.
3. **Determine extent of disease.**
   - Staging is best done with FDG PET/CT and/or alternatively, dedicated body CT or MRI.
   - Local invasion can be assessed with endoscopic studies, such as laryngoscopy.
4. **Understand patient's goals of care to individualize patient counseling.**
   - Patient counseling should be provided by members of the multidisciplinary team who are experienced in management of complex thyroid cancer.
   - Engage both the patient and their support individuals/family members in the care plan.
   - Risks and benefits of treatment should be discussed in the context of the patient's goals of care.
5. **Determine surgical options.**
   - In patients with stages IVA and IVB ATC, treatment goals may include complete resection with transition to adjuvant definitive-intention therapy. There is limited benefit to surgery in stage IVC ATC.
   - In assessing resectability of the primary tumor, consider extent of thyroidectomy, neck dissection, need for tracheotomy, and need to avoid laryngectomy, esophageal resection, or major vessel reconstruction.
   - Potential surgical morbidity should be discussed in the context of the patient's goals of care and expected prognosis. Surgery should not cause wounds or complications significantly delay systemic treatment or radiation.
6. **Determine nonsurgical options for management.**
   - Mutational status of the tumor should be determined expeditiously for possible targeted therapies.
   - Systemic therapy, radiation, or best supportive care plan should be planned while considering the patient's goals of care and performance status.
   - In cases of locally advanced cancer without extensive distant metastasis, consider systemic therapy with determination of disease response that could downstage the tumor and allow the patient to be reconsidered for surgical resection.
7. **Maintain palliative care/hospice/end-of-life discussions as part of the care plan.**

Source: Adapted from Bible KC, Kebebew E, Brierley J, et al. 2021 American Thyroid Association guidelines for management of patients with anaplastic thyroid cancer. *Thyroid*. 2021;31:337-384, Table 1.

before proceeding with surgical resection, as resection may be inappropriate in certain cases such as primary thyroid lymphoma.

While the histopathologic presentation of ATC can be variable, there are certain recognized morphological subtypes: sarcomatoid or spindle cell, giant cell, and squamoid or epithelial (Figure 18–4). Other histopathological characteristics include chronic inflammation, high cellular proliferation, and atypical mitoses. If DTC is identified alongside an undifferentiated component, the diagnosis of ATC is straightforward.

Generally, IHC is essential for diagnosis of ATC. Thyroid-specific proteins are absent due to the undifferentiated character of ATC. On the other hand, immunoreactivity for BRAF V600E can support a diagnosis of ATC in the appropriate clinical setting, as somatic BRAF mutations are common in both ATC and PTC. Abnormal p53 immunoreactivity also can support a diagnosis of ATC; somatic mutations of TP53 are characteristic of ATC.

Laboratory Findings & Imaging Studies

Once ATC is diagnosed, initial lab studies should include thyroid function tests, thyroglobulin (Tg)/Tg antibody, complete blood count with differential, comprehensive metabolic panel and coagulation studies. Thyroid function tests are important because large tumors can compromise thyroid function, and in rare cases, ATC has been associated with significant thyrotoxicosis. Also, the absence of Tg can help support a diagnosis of ATC. ATC can present with leukocytosis (due to secretion of lymphokines) or hypercalcemia of malignancy, and therefore blood counts and electrolytes should be measured.

Staging

According to the American Joint Committee on Cancer TNM staging system, all ATCs are stage IV. Stage IVA ATC remains localized within the thyroid gland and has not metastasized to the lymph nodes or distant locations. Stage IVB ATC has grown outside or through the thyroid and/or involve cervical lymph nodes, but has not spread to distant sites. Lastly, stage IVC ATC has spread to distant extra-cervical sites.

^{18}F FDG PET/CT whole body is preferred in the staging evaluation of ATC. However, if PET/CT is unavailable, IV contrast-enhanced CT of the neck, chest, abdomen, and pelvis can be obtained. CT neck can help determine extent

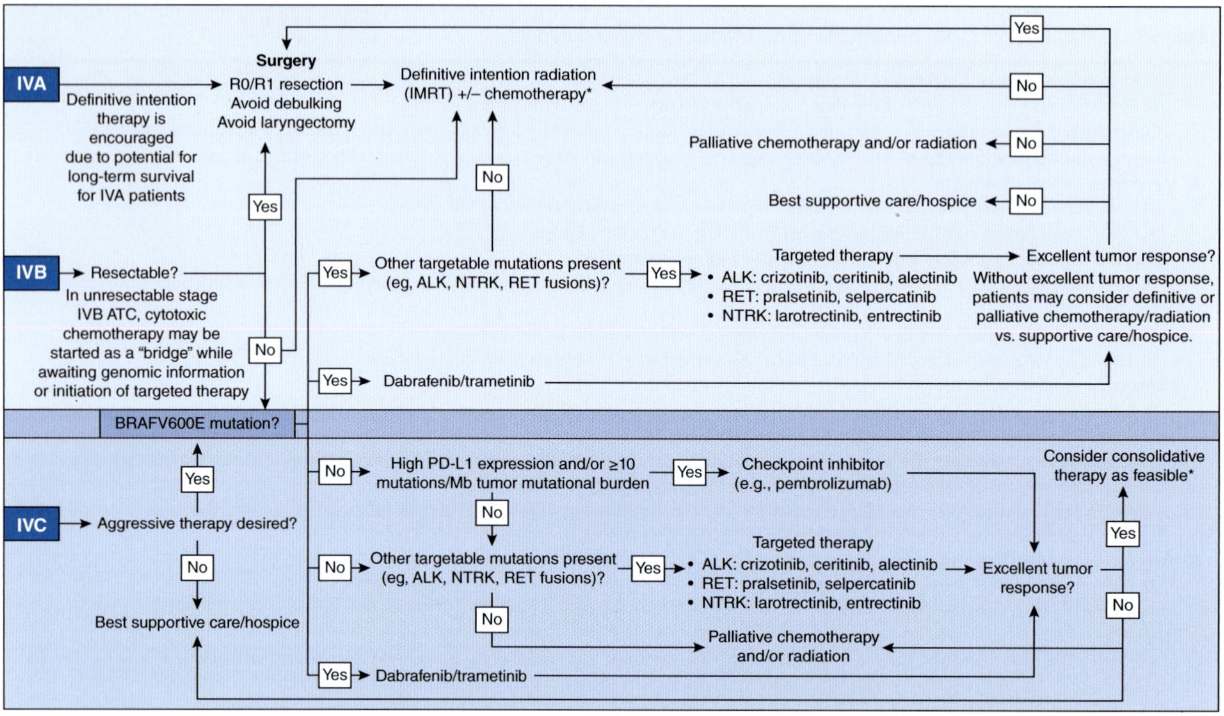

▲ Figure 18–2. Initial management of anaplastic thyroid cancer, by stage. Clinical trials are strongly recommended if available. Best supportive care/hospice option can be elected at any point.

*In stage IVC management, consolidative therapy refers to focal therapy intended to control residual macrometastatic disease among patients electing for aggressive therapy.

(Adapted from Bible KC, Kebebew E, Brierley J, et al. 2021 American Thyroid Association guidelines for management of patients with anaplastic thyroid cancer. *Thyroid*. 2021;31:337-384.)

Table 18–2. Initial evaluation for anaplastic thyroid cancer.

Laboratory tests
• Complete blood count with differential
• Comprehensive chemistry panel
• Thyroid function tests, thyroglobulin/thyroglobulin antibody
Imaging
• ^{18}F FDG PET/CT (preferred, whole body)
• CT neck, chest, abdomen, and pelvis with contrast or MRI (acceptable if PET unavailable)
• MRI brain with and without contrast (recommended and if clinically indicated)
Other
• Laryngoscopy +/– esophagoscopy as indicated
• BRAF assessment by immunohistochemistry and next-generation sequencing

CT, computed tomography; FDG, fluorodeoxyglucose; MRI, magnetic resonance imaging.
Source: From Bible KC, Kebebew E, Brierley J, et al. 2021 American Thyroid Association guidelines for management of patients with anaplastic thyroid cancer. *Thyroid*. 2021;31:337-384.

of disease to plan a surgical approach and/or radiation therapy. ^{18}F FDG PET/CT is useful in identifying metastases that are not appreciated on CT alone. If PET/CT is not available, a bone scan to identify bony metastases should be considered. Also, MRI or CT of the brain should be performed to assess for brain metastases, if clinically indicated. If imaging studies reveal distant metastases, biopsy is often unnecessary if adequate material for histopathologic diagnosis and molecular testing was obtained from the primary tumor.

Brain metastases are fairly uncommon at initial presentation, and they are associated with worse prognosis. In a retrospective study from a single cancer center, ATC patients with brain metastases were also likely to have locoregional invasion and locoregional lymph node metastases. Median time of disease-specific survival for ATC patients after diagnosis of brain metastases was 1.3 months. Therefore, the ATA guidelines recommend brain MRI as part of the initial staging for ATC and when symptoms concerning for brain metastases develop. If brain metastases are diagnosed, neurosurgery and

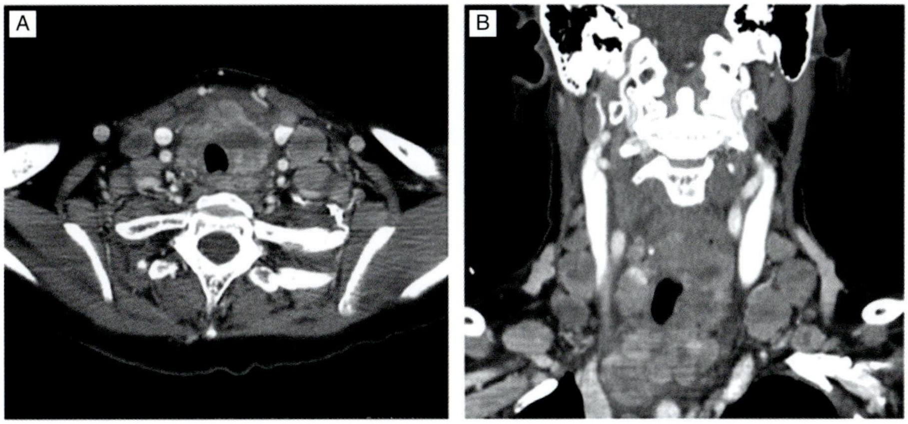

▲ **Figure 18–3.** In this patient diagnosed with anaplastic thyroid cancer, computed tomography—shown here in representative axial **(A)** and coronal **(B)** images—revealed a heterogeneous, partially necrotic thyroid mass with substernal extension and bilateral cervical lymphadenopathy. This patient also had distant metastases and proceeded with systemic treatment.

radiation oncology should be part of the patient's multidisciplinary care team.

Special Examinations

Because vocal cord paralysis is fairly common with ATC, patients should undergo laryngeal evaluation with fiberoptic or mirror laryngoscopy at initial presentation to assess vocal cord mobility. Fiberoptic laryngoscopy can also help evaluate whether the tumor involves the larynx and upper trachea. Subsequently, patients should undergo repeat laryngoscopy if their symptoms change.

Also, if a patient complains of dysphagia or has imaging suggestive of esophageal invasion, esophagoscopy should be performed. Endoscopic ultrasonography can help estimate the proximity of the cancer to the lumen of the esophagus.

SURGICAL MANAGEMENT

Once the diagnosis and appropriate evaluation for ATC are completed, resectability of the primary tumor should be established. Patients with stage IVA or IVB ATC may be surgical candidates. Surgery should aim to resect all visible tumor (R0 or R1 resection) in patients with ATC, rather than debulking (R2 resection). Most studies suggest that R0 or R1 resection is associated with longer disease-free survival and/or overall survival. Patients with ATC also should undergo a palliative care consultation, and discussion about goals of care should be started from the beginning.

Most commonly, the extent of surgery in ATC will involve total thyroidectomy with lymph node dissection; rarely, laryngectomy/pharyngectomy is performed as part

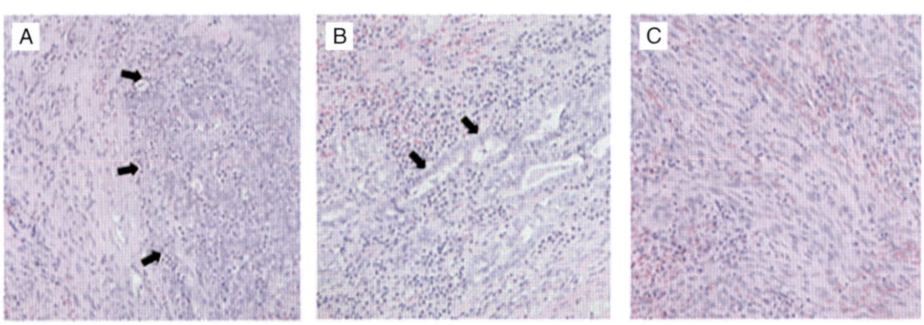

▲ **Figure 18–4.** Histopathologic features of anaplastic thyroid cancer (H&E, x200). Tumors can demonstrate areas of necrosis (indicated by arrows, **A**) as well as adjacent areas of more well-differentiated papillary thyroid carcinoma (indicated by arrows, **B**). Tumors also contain a mixture of spindled, epithelioid, and pleomorphic giant cells, and the most common histologic pattern is the spindle cell pattern **(C)**.

of the resection. Due to the poor prognosis of ATC, radical resection to include major vascular structures, mediastinum, esophagus, trachea, or larynx is generally not recommended and should be discussed in a multidisciplinary fashion with consideration of molecular testing results.

In 2% to 6% of cases, ATC will be diagnosed after thyroid surgery for a predominant, non-ATC tumor. If thyroid lobectomy was the initial surgery, completion thyroidectomy may be considered based more on the pathological characteristics of the non-ATC tumor. Intrathyroidal, completely resected ATC generally is associated with improved survival, but currently, there are no data to suggest a difference in survival based on extent of thyroidectomy for incidentally diagnosed ATC.

Neoadjuvant Therapy

If the primary tumor is considered unresectable, neoadjuvant therapy may be appropriate in select patients. Neoadjuvant radiation, chemotherapy, or chemoradiation have been shown to allow delayed primary resection in a minority of patients with ATC. In a 2016 multicenter prospective trial from Japan, 56 patients with ATC received weekly paclitaxel administration, and complete local tumor resection could be achieved in eight patients. These eight patients survived longer compared to those who did not undergo complete resection (7.6 months vs 5.4 months, $p = 0.018$).[2]

In patients with $BRAF^{V600E}$ mutated ATC, neoadjuvant dabrafenib and trametinib followed by complete resection and adjuvant chemoradiation has been described in a 2019 US case series of six patients. Overall survival at 1 year was 83%, and the locoregional control rate was 100%.[3]

Tracheostomy Placement

Need and timing of tracheostomy in patients with ATC remains equivocal. While tracheostomy helps prevent death by asphyxiation, it will also likely be permanent and significantly alter the patient's quality of life. Tracheostomy also may delay radiation and/or chemotherapy due to wound healing issues. Therefore, elective or prophylactic tracheostomy generally is not recommended for patients who do not have impending airway compromise.

If a patient presents with life-threatening airway distress, tracheostomy is best performed under anesthesia in an operating room. To perform tracheostomy, concomitant isthmusectomy or pretracheal tumor debulking may be necessary. This is not usually an easy operation, and therefore, an experienced surgeon and a controlled setting are imperative. Fiberoptic examination should be performed to confirm luminal position of the tracheotomy tube and a patent airway distally.

MEDICAL MANAGEMENT

Medical management of ATC includes locoregional approaches (radiotherapy with or without chemotherapy) and systemic treatments (cytotoxic chemotherapy and targeted therapies). The 2021 ATA guidelines for ATC recommend radiotherapy with systemic treatment in patients who have undergone resection and those who have unresectable but nonmetastatic disease. If medical management renders the primary tumor potentially resectable, surgery should be reconsidered.

Radiotherapy

Multiple studies have shown that both survival and local control are optimal with R0/R1 surgical resection followed by radiotherapy and chemotherapy. The ATA guidelines recommend standard fractionation intensity modulated radiation therapy (IMRT) after R0/R1 resection in patients who have good performance status and desire aggressive therapy. After R2 resection, IMRT or combined BRAF/MEK inhibitors (for $BRAF^{V600E}$ mutated ATC) can be considered. Generally, radiotherapy should aim to begin within 6 weeks after surgery.

In 2003, IMRT became available and allowed for more complete tumor coverage while reducing radiation to nearby critical structures such as the larynx, esophagus, and brachial plexus. In a 2010 US institutional retrospective study, 10 patients with stage IVA and IVB ATC were treated with multimodal therapy (surgery, IMRT, and docetaxel + doxorubicin). Median overall survival was 60 months. Five patients were cancer-free after more than 32 months of follow-up.[4] In an updated 2017 study from the same institution, median survival was 21 months if patients received multimodal therapy, compared to 4 months for patients undergoing palliative treatment only. Over half of patients undergoing multimodal therapy were hospitalized with complications, typically mucositis, dehydration, and failure to thrive. Other reasons for hospitalization included septic shock, respiratory failure, and venous thromboembolism.[5]

For patients with unresectable disease or R2 resection, radiation therapy can help local control. Retrospective studies have shown radiation dose to be related to outcome, but these data are subject to selection bias, as healthier patients with less extensive disease were more likely to receive high-dose radiation therapy. For example, in a 2006 retrospective study of 47 ATC patients who underwent radiotherapy, those who received a radiation dose more than 40 Gy experienced enhanced survival compared with those who received a radiation dose ≤40 Gy (median survival 11 months vs 3 months, respectively), but those receiving a dose more than 40 Gy were younger and had smaller primary tumors.

Chemotherapy

The 2021 ATA guidelines for ATC recommend cytotoxic chemotherapy involving a taxane, with or without anthracyclines or platin, in patients treated with definitive-intention radiation. Taxanes are radiosensitizing agents and may be more effective than chemotherapies traditionally used in ATC. Studies, albeit with small patient cohorts, have shown successful use of taxanes in combination with radiotherapy. In a 2010 institutional retrospective from Austria, six patients with ATC were treated with standard external beam radiation (60 Gy in 30 fractions) and docetaxel 100 mg every 3 weeks for six cycles. Of the six patients, four patients had complete remission, and two experienced a partial response to treatment.

Use of taxanes without concurrent radiation also has been studied in ATC patients. In a prospective phase 2 trial of paclitaxel in patients with ATC, there was a 53% total response rate (one complete response and nine partial responses among 19 evaluable patients). In a prospective feasibility trial of docetaxel in ATC patients, one of seven patients experienced complete response, and two patients experienced stabilized disease.

Doxorubicin, an anthracycline class medication, is the only cytotoxic chemotherapy agent approved by the FDA for use in ATC. Doxorubicin mostly has been studied in conjunction with surgery and radiation therapy, so the impact on survival is unclear in advanced disease. In a 1976-1982 trial by the Eastern Cooperative Oncology Group, 84 patients with advanced progressive thyroid cancer (not necessarily ATC) were randomized to doxorubicin alone or doxorubicin with cisplatin. Among 37 patients with ATC enrolled in the study, doxorubicin with cisplatin produced three complete responses and three partial responses, compared to doxorubicin alone, which produced no complete response and one partial response. Therefore, the 2021 ATA guidelines recommend cytotoxic chemotherapy (taxane with or without cis- or carbo-platin or taxane and/or anthracycline) in ATC patients who may desire aggressive therapy but lack other therapeutic options, including clinical trials.

Targeted Therapies

BRAF-targeted therapy can result in significant tumor regression among patients with $BRAF^{V600E}$ mutated ATC. In 2018, the US Food and Drug Administration approved use of dabrafenib and trametinib (BRAF/MEK inhibitor combination) to treat ATC with $BRAF^{V600E}$ mutation. If patients with unresectable stage IVB ATC have a contraindication or unwillingness to undergo chemoradiation, BRAF-directed therapy can be pursued. Also, neoadjuvant dabrafenib and trametinib have been studied as a means to convert an unresectable primary tumor to a resectable one. In an institutional retrospective cohort study, 20 patients who underwent neoadjuvant BRAF-directed therapy followed by surgery had a 94% 1-year survival rate.

For patients with a somatic neurotrophic tyrosine receptor kinase (NTRK) fusion, tyrosine receptor kinase (TRK) inhibitors (larotrectinib and entrectinib) are FDA-approved treatment options. In a phase 1/2 trial evaluating the efficacy and safety of larotrectinib in 55 patients with NTRK fusion solid tumors, five patients with thyroid cancer were included, although it is unclear whether any of these patients had ATC. All thyroid cancer patients did achieve response (four partial responses, one complete response).[6] Therefore, patients with ATC who are considering TRK inhibitors are recommended to participate in clinical trials if they are able to do so.

Selpercatinib is a selective RET inhibitor that received FDA approval in 2020 for patients with RET fusion thyroid cancers, including RET-mutated medullary thyroid carcinoma. In a phase 1/2 trial of 162 thyroid cancer patients, two patients with RET fusion anaplastic thyroid cancer were included, and one of these patients responded for 18 months to selpercatinib. Given these limited data, patients with stage IV RET fusion ATC also are recommended to consider RET inhibitor therapy in a clinical trial setting.

Anaplastic lymphoma kinase (ALK) is an oncogene initially associated with anaplastic large-cell lymphoma. ALK-rearranged anaplastic thyroid cancer has been treated with ALK inhibitors, albeit in a single published case. Therefore, ALK inhibitors also are recommended to be used in clinical trials.

Immunotherapy

Like molecular targeted therapy, immunotherapy for ATC is also under investigation. Spartalizumab is a humanized monoclonal antibody against the programmed death-1 (PD-1) receptor. By binding to PD-1, spartalizumab blocks interaction with its ligands, such as programmed death-ligand 1 (PD-L1), resulting in T-cell activation. In a phase 1/2 study of 42 patients with ATC, the overall response rate was 19% (three complete responses, five partial responses). Patients with PD-L1 expression ≥50% had the highest response rate of 35%, while those with PD-L1 expression less than 1% had no response.[7] The ATA recommends consideration of checkpoint inhibitors like spartalizumab in patients with high PD-L1 expression and no other targetable alterations, preferably in a clinical trial setting.

METASTATIC DISEASE

Data regarding the treatment of site-specific metastases in ATC are limited. Radiotherapy can be used to treat brain metastases or palliate pain from bony metastases. While surgery generally is not recommended, it may be considered in select patients with bony metastases that threaten spinal cord compression or musculoskeletal function.

Treatment decision-making for metastatic ATC should be considered in relation to the patient's goals of care and other comorbidities. Also, given the poor prognosis or metastatic and progressive ATC, goals of care and hospice should be discussed as part of the treatment plan.

PROGNOSIS

ATC patients have a median survival of about 5 months and a 1-year overall survival of 20%. Studies have found that certain patient and cancer characteristics such as younger age, smaller primary tumor size, and absence of metastases are associated with improved survival. Also, certain genetic mutational profiles can help predict outcome; for example, concomitant BRAF/RAS and TERT mutations in ATC are associated with worse prognosis than a mutation in only one of those genes.

In general, given the poor prognosis and rarity of ATC, every diagnosed patient should be managed by a multidisciplinary team of subspecialists, including those with palliative care expertise. The multidisciplinary team should aim to reach consensus rapidly on realistic treatment options, goals of care, and prognosis for the patient, and it is important for the patient to participate in these critical conversations.

REFERENCES

1. Bible KC, Kebebew E, Brierly J, et al. American Thyroid Association guidelines for management of patients with anaplastic thyroid cancer. *Thyroid*. 2021;31(3):337-386.
2. Onoda N, Sugino K, Higashiyama T, et al. The safety and efficacy of weekly paclitaxel administration for anaplastic thyroid cancer patients: a nationwide prospective study. *Thyroid*. 2016;26:1293-1299.
3. Wang JR, Zafareo ME, Dadu R, et al. Complete surgical resection following neoadjuvant dabrafenib plus trametinib in BRAF(V600E)-mutated anaplastic thyroid carcinoma. *Thyroid*. 2019;29:1036-1043.
4. Foote RL, Molina JR, Kasperbauer JL et al. Enhanced survival in locoregionally confined anaplastic thyroid carcinoma: a single-institution experience using aggressive multimodal therapy. *Thyroid*. 2011;21(1):25-30.
5. Prasongsook N, Kumar A, Chintakuntlawar AV, et al. Survival in response to multimodal therapy in anaplastic thyroid cancer. *J Clin Endocrinol Metab*. 2017;102(12):4506-4514.
6. Drilon A, Laetsch TW, Kummar S, et al. Efficacy of larotrectinib in TRK fusion-positive cancers in adults and children. *N Eng J Med*. 2018;178:731-739.
7. Capdevila J, Wirth LJ, Ernst T et al. PD-1 blockade in anaplastic thyroid carcinoma. *J Clin Oncol*. 2020;38(23):2620-2627.

Primary Thyroid Lymphoma

19

Caitlin T. Yeo, MD, FRCSC
Janice L. Pasieka, MD, FRCSC

GENERAL CONSIDERATIONS

Primary thyroid lymphoma (PTL) refers to lymphoma arising from the thyroid gland and is differentiated from secondary thyroid lymphoma which involves a nonthyroidal primary lymphoma that has metastasized to the thyroid gland. The treatment and prognosis of primary versus secondary thyroid lymphomas are different. PTL is rare and constitutes only 1% to 5% of all thyroid malignancies and 2% of extranodal lymphomas, with an incidence of 2 per 1 million. Approximately 98% of PTL are non-Hodgkin B-cell lymphomas, favoring women to men 2-3:1, and most often occurring in the sixth to seventh decade.[1,2] Men tend to present at a slightly younger age, and age less than 55 years has been associated with higher grade PTL.[3]

Due to its rarity, PTL is a challenging diagnosis and lacks randomized control trial-level evidence for treatment. The highest-level evidence to date is based on two large retrospective reviews of the Surveillance, Epidemiology, and End Results (SEER) database[2] and the National Cancer Database (NCDB),[1] and two meta-analyses combining small cohort studies.[3,4]

PTL usually presents as a painless rapidly growing neck mass in at least 88%. Local compressive symptoms, including dysphagia, hoarseness, and shortness of breath, are seen in 30% to 50% of patients.[5] PTL rarely presents with typical lymphoma B symptoms, such as night sweats, weight loss, or fevers, only occurring in 10% to 13%.[1,2,5] Patients with a history of Hashimoto lymphocytic thyroiditis are at a 70 to 80-fold increased risk of developing PTL, with 55% to 90% of PTL patients reported having clinical or pathologic findings of Hashimoto's.[1,2,4-6] Overall, only 0.5% of Hashimoto's patients will develop PTL.[7]

The acute presentation of PTL is similar to anaplastic thyroid cancer and must be distinguished, as prognosis and treatment are very different. Prognosis and treatment also depend on stage and histologic subtype, with diffuse large B-cell lymphoma (DLBCL) being the most aggressive and mucosa-associated lymphoid tissue (MALT) having a more indolent course.[2,3] Additional subtypes include mixed DLBCL/MALT (often grouped with DLBCL), follicular lymphoma, Hodgkin lymphoma, Burkitt lymphoma, mantle-cell lymphoma, and peripheral T-cell lymphoma.

Pathogenesis

The exact pathogenesis of PTL is unknown, but one theory involves the slow malignant transformation that occurs from chronic antigenic stimulation in Hashimoto thyroiditis.[8] It is thought that the chronic stimulation results in lymphocyte atypia and hyperplasia akin to other inflammatory-mediated malignancies. Moshynska et al.[8] demonstrated clonal similarity in the immunoglobulin gene sequence rearrangements in patients with PTL and Hashimoto thyroiditis. This pathogenic pathway is more commonly associated with the MALT subtype.[9,10] Some hypothesize that DLBCL arises from preexisting MALT with background lymphocytic thyroiditis that has undergone transformation to a higher grade.[6] However, a meta-analysis of studies from 2009 to 2018 found that Hashimoto's was identified more frequently in MALT than DLBCL (OR 2.18), and much more frequently in mixed DLBCL/MALT than pure DLBCL (OR 9.11).[4] A recent study identified a 92% frequency of Hashimoto's in MALT, but only 67% in DLBCL,[9] suggesting an alternate pathogenic pathway.

A second theory involves proto-oncogene aberrant somatic hypermutation, resulting in dysregulated B-cell lymphomagenesis. Hypermutations are found in almost all cases of follicular lymphoma subtype, 30% to 50% of DLBCL, and rarely in MALT.[11,12] These two theories are likely both involved with the development of PTL, with the first theory resulting in the development of most MALT and some DLBCL (likely mixed DLBCL/MALT subtype), and the second theory more consistently related to follicular lymphoma and pure DLBCL.

Prevention

There are no known preventative measures to date.

Clinical Findings

Symptoms & Signs

Patients most often present with a painless rapidly enlarging neck mass (88%) and symptoms of compression including dysphagia (45%), hoarseness (37%), and difficulty breathing (24%). Symptoms of rapid growth and compression are most often associated with DLBCL.[6] Only 10% to 13% of patients will have B symptoms such as weight loss, fevers, and night sweats.[1,2,5]

Investigations

Ultrasound is the first-line imaging modality for the thyroid and is considered an essential part of the thyroid physical exam. PTL imaging characteristics include a solid mass that is usually diffusely hypoechoic to adjacent thyroid and often very hypoechoic, described as less echogenic than adjacent muscle. The nodule has increased vascularity, variable border/margin characteristics (well to ill-defined), and rarely any calcifications. The average measured volume is 70 cubic cm.[5] One retrospective study of 32 PTL patients found that more than 96% of patients were classified as intermediate or high suspicion based on ultrasound findings.[13] Another prospective study of 165 patients suspected of PTL based on ultrasound found a positivity rate of 48%, with the positive predictive value being up to 65% in those with distinct nodules.[14]

Fine-needle aspirate (FNA) is often the first attempt at obtaining tissue diagnosis for thyroid nodules. However, FNA cytology for PTL can often be confused with benign lymphocytic thyroiditis, leading to a false negative diagnosis. In the setting of PTL, the sensitivity of FNA is only about 45% to 60% on cytology alone,[13,15] and increases to 71% to 75% with advancements in flow cytometry and immunohistochemistry.[5,9,15,16] If the clinical history involves a rapidly enlarging thyroid mass, an increased level of suspicion should prompt further investigation. Core-needle biopsy has a 93% sensitivity, especially with adjuncts such as flow cytometry, immunohistochemistry, and molecular testing. Core biopsy also provides architectural information and histologic subtype, and has predominantly replaced the need for open surgical biopsy.[5,13] Histologic subtype is important for treatment selection and prognosis. As PTL often requires a core biopsy to provide histologic subtype, it would be reasonable to forego FNA and start with core-needle biopsy in patients with a history highly suspicious for PTL, as this will prevent delays in diagnosis and treatment triage.[17] Biopsy tissue should not be preserved in alcohol or formalin as this affects flow cytometry results. Specimens should be handled in a similar fashion to the institution's histopathological lymphoma protocol.

Bloodwork should include standard chemistries (CBC, electrolytes, BUN, creatinine), thyroid indices (TSH, Free T3/T4, thyroid peroxidase antibodies), and tumor markers (lactate dehydrogenase [LDH], β-2 microglobulin). LDH and β-2 microglobulin levels have been identified as prognostic in PTL, with elevated levels conferring a worse prognosis.[18]

Anatomical/Functional Imaging & Staging

With the diagnosis of PTL, upfront staging with computed tomography (CT) head, neck, chest, abdomen, and pelvis is required as the extent of disease will affect treatment decisions and prognosis. CT imaging of PTL (Figure 19–1A) can better delineate the aerodigestive tract, regional lymph node status, and provide evidence of disease beyond the head and neck region. Staging is performed using the Ann Arbor staging system for non-Hodgkin lymphoma with the designation of "E" for extranodal location (Figure 19–2).[19] Stage IE represents disease confined to the thyroid, stage IIE involves regional lymph nodes above the diaphragm, stage IIIE includes lymph node spread on both sides of the diaphragm, and stage IVE is systemic dissemination. The majority of patients with PTL present with stage IE or IIE disease (55%-56% and 30%-32%, respectively), while few present with stage IIIE or IVE (2%-5% and 10%-11%, respectively) (Table 19–1).[1,2]

In a small series of 57 PTL patients that underwent FDG-PET, Sharma et al.[5] found that only 65% were PET avid. FDG-PET may be helpful in patients with DLBCL subtype for staging and assessing response to treatment, as this subtype is more PET avid and metabolic activity may decrease prior to radiographic tumor size. However, benign lymphocytic thyroiditis is an inflammatory state that may result in false positive FDG-PET, and because the MALT subtype often has low avidity that overlaps with lymphocytic thyroiditis, FDG-PET is less useful in this subtype.[20]

Differential Diagnosis

The differential diagnosis for an enlarging central neck mass is extensive and summarized in Table 19–2. The main differential diagnosis that must be distinguished from PTL is anaplastic thyroid cancer, which has a very different prognosis and treatment course. Other aggressive thyroid tumors in the differential would include medullary thyroid cancer and primary thyroid sarcoma. PTL can also be mislabeled as benign lymphocytic thyroiditis on FNA and requires further investigation if clinical history is suspicious. Immunohistochemical staining and flow cytometry are needed to establish monoclonality of the lymphocytes and to determine the subtype. Different subtypes confer different prognosis and potentially alters treatment course. The most common subtype is DLBCL (60%-70%), followed

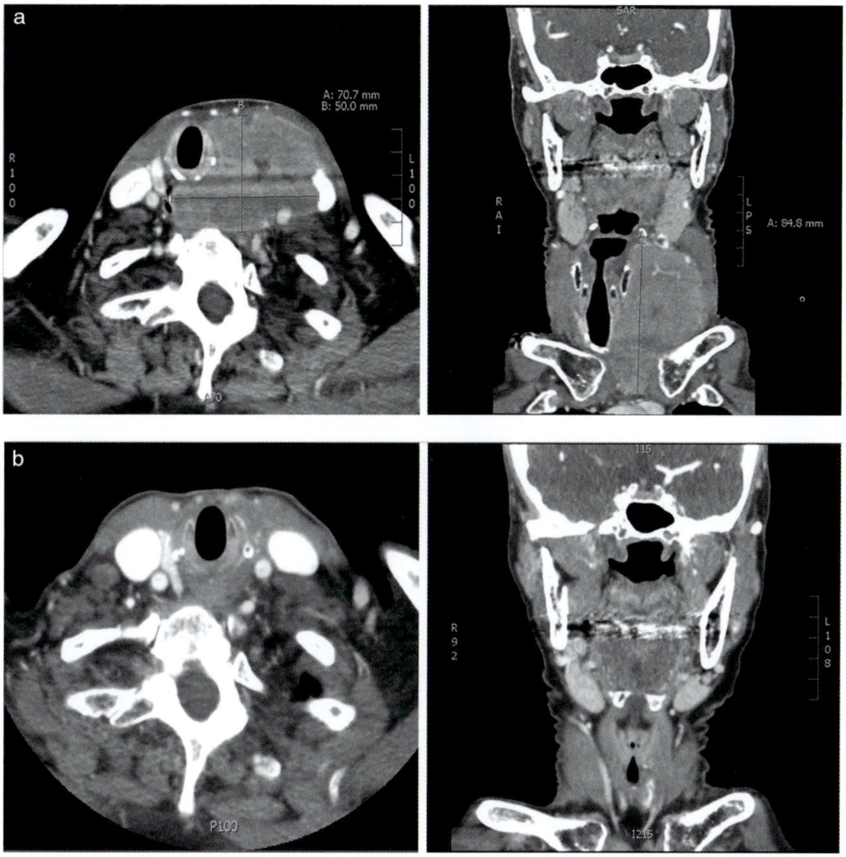

▲ **Figure 19–1** **A.** Axial and coronal CT neck images of PTL (DLBCL subtype) at time of diagnosis, presenting with symptoms of airway obstruction. Images demonstrate homogeneity, large size of thyroid mass, and tracheal deviation. Patient was stage IE. **B.** Axial and coronal CT neck images of the same patient 1 month after treatment shows significant resolution of thyroid mass and effect on airway after 3 cycles of R-CHOP and prior to initiation of radiation.

by MALT (10%-20%), and follicular (3%-10%). It is critical to distinguish between the high-grade DLBCL and the more indolent MALT subtypes. Immunochemical staining is usually positive for CD19, CD20, and CD45 in DLBCL and CD5, CD10, and CD23 are usually negative in MALT lymphomas.[21] Additional subtypes include mixed DLBCL/MALT (often grouped with DLBCL), Hodgkin lymphoma, Burkitt lymphoma, mantle-cell lymphoma, and peripheral T-cell lymphoma; each occurs with a frequency of 1% to 3% except the mixed subtype.[1,2,5]

Complications

The main life-threatening complication related to PTL is airway obstruction. If indicated, obtaining urgent airway control with intubation is appropriate. Tracheal stents can also be utilized for airway protection as a bridge to treatment. In a series of 30 patients with thyroid-related airway obstruction, 92% of patients had immediate relief of symptoms with stenting, although none had PTL.[22] Lee et al.[23] demonstrated successful stent removal without airway compromise after just one cycle of multiagent chemotherapy treatment for PTL. High-dose prednisone also aids in tumor regression and relief of symptoms in as quickly as 24 hours.[24] Less threatening complications include dysphagia, dysphonia, Horner syndrome, and superior vena cava syndrome.

Complications can also arise from the treatment of PTL. Surgical resection includes complications such as hypoparathyroidism and recurrent laryngeal nerve (RLN) palsy. Although data on rates of surgical complications are lacking, one small study showed 2 of 9 (20%) PTL patients sustained permanent RLN injury.[25] Given the size of the tumor in PTL, surgical risk is likely increased compared to other thyroid malignancies. Radiation therapy complications include acute toxicity leading to dermatitis, mucositis, and dysphagia. Late-phase toxicity includes pneumonitis, hypothyroidism,

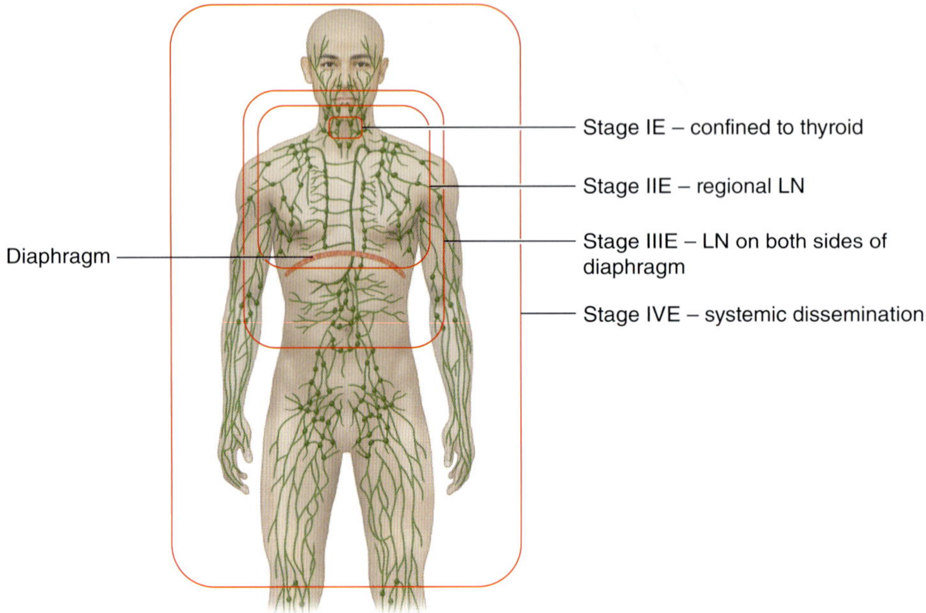

Figure 19–2. Stages of primary thyroid lymphoma.

and radiation-induced malignancy of the thyroid or adjacent organs.[26] Chemotherapy side effects are extensive but generally well tolerated, most are reversible with dose reduction or completion of therapy. Side effects include neutropenia, neuropathy, heart failure, esophagitis, mucositis, pneumonia, nausea, and vomiting.[27]

Treatment

Due to the rare occurrence of PTL no randomized trial data exists to direct treatment. Most recommendations are based on retrospective data or extrapolation from other extranodal lymphomas. Historically, surgery in the form of a total thyroidectomy was the main treatment modality, but with the advent of effective modern multiagent chemotherapy and immunotherapy that has changed significantly. Current recommendations are to tailor treatment to PTL subtype and stage of disease. All thyroid lymphomas should be treated by a multidisciplinary team of thyroid cancer experts whenever possible. Treatment options include surgery, radiation therapy, multiagent chemotherapy with or without immunotherapy, or a combination of the above.

Indolent & Localized PTL

Although surgery is no longer the predominant treatment recommendation for PTL, it may still have a role in treating PTL for some patients with indolent localized disease. There are studies demonstrating that patients with stage IE MALT lymphoma subtype can obtain prolonged remission and disease-free survival with surgery alone if completely resected.[6,28] However, studies have also shown that surgery plus radiation does not result in better outcomes than radiation alone, with remission rates approaching 100% with a

Table 19–1. Ann Arbor staging for primary thyroid lymphoma, stage at presentation, and survival data.

Stage	Stage at Presentation[1,2]	Mean OS (Years)[1]	5-year DSS[2]
IE–confined to thyroid	55%-56%	9.3	86%
IIE–regional lymph nodes	30%-32%	9	81%
IIIE–lymph nodes on both sides of diaphragm	2%-5%	8.1	64%
IVE–systemic dissemination	10%-11%	7.5	

DSS, disease specific survival; E, extranodal; OS, overall survival.

Table 19–2. Differential diagnosis of a central neck mass.

Condition	History/Risk Factors	Physical Findings
Benign		
Hematoma	Trauma	Bruising, tenderness
Hemorrhagic cyst	Sudden often painful enlargement	Firm, enlarged mass
Laryngocele	Repetitive nose blowing, coughing, or wind instrument use	Midline, superior to thyroid cartilage
Thyroglossal duct cyst	Waxing and waning history, often since childhood	Adjacent to hyoid bone, rises with deglutition
Thyroid goiter/benign nodules (MNG: multinodular goiter)	Hyperthyroid symptoms (Graves, toxic MNG), iodine deficiency (MNG)	Enlarged thyroid, findings of hyperthyroidism
Lipoma	Slow growth, usually asymptomatic	Soft, usually mobile mass
Malignant		
Well-differentiated thyroid cancer (papillary, follicular, etc.)	Family history, head/neck radiation, indolent history	Thyroid nodule, usually mobile
Anaplastic (undifferentiated) thyroid cancer	Rapid painless enlargement, may have compressive symptoms	Large thyroid mass, often firm and fixed
Primary thyroid lymphoma	Rapid painless enlargement, may have compressive symptoms, history of Hashimoto's	Large thyroid mass
Primary thyroid sarcoma	Painless large goiter, symptoms of compression	Can be unilateral or bilateral, often fixed
Parathyroid carcinoma	Hypercalcemic crisis	Palpable neck mass, decreased level of consciousness
Head and neck paraganglioma	Family history/genetic risk, multiple paragangliomas	Often more lateral neck mass, but can arise adjacent to thyroid
Metastatic cancer	Prior malignancy	Variable findings

median follow-up of 4.9 years.[29] In a review of older series, patients with disease localized to the neck (stage IE and early-stage IIE with neck-only lymphadenopathy), had similar outcomes from radiation alone compared to combined chemotherapy plus radiation, and both approaches were better than surgery alone. Patients with localized MALT subtype had improved remission rates of 70% with RT alone versus 55% for non-MALT subtypes.[30] Thus, in patients with stage IE MALT lymphoma, the risks of surgery versus radiation must be weighed against patient comorbidities and age, while in early-stage IIE (lymphadenopathy that has advanced beyond the thyroid but limited to the neck), radiation would be the preferred first-line treatment. If MALT lymphoma presents as stage IIE beyond the neck, stage IIIE, or stage IVE, then chemotherapy plus radiation is recommended.

Transformation of MALT into a high-grade, more aggressive lymphoma such as mixed DLBCL/MALT subtype has been documented and should be considered in patients with a diagnosis of MALT with more advanced stage or rapidly progressing disease.[17]

Aggressive & Disseminated PTL

Conversely DLBCL and other non-MALT subtypes are more aggressive and have higher risk for systemic recurrence. These patients are best treated with multiagent chemotherapy, immunotherapy, and radiation[30] and often have a significant response to treatment (Figures 19–1A and B). Standard multiagent chemotherapy consists of cyclophosphamide, doxorubicin, vincristine, and prednisone (CHOP), with the option of adding the immunotherapy agent rituximab, a B-cell specific anti-CD20 monoclonal antibody (R-CHOP). Rituximab is approved as first-line DLBCL treatment in combination with multiagent chemotherapy, with several phase 3 randomized control trials showing significant progression-free and overall survival for R-CHOP versus CHOP alone for nodal and extranodal DLBCL not restricted to PTL.[31,32] The efficacy of rituximab in PTL is unknown. One large retrospective database review suggested a lack of statistical benefit, but only 16% of patients in the study received immunotherapy.[1] A smaller international review demonstrated that for aggressive PTL, disease-free survival,

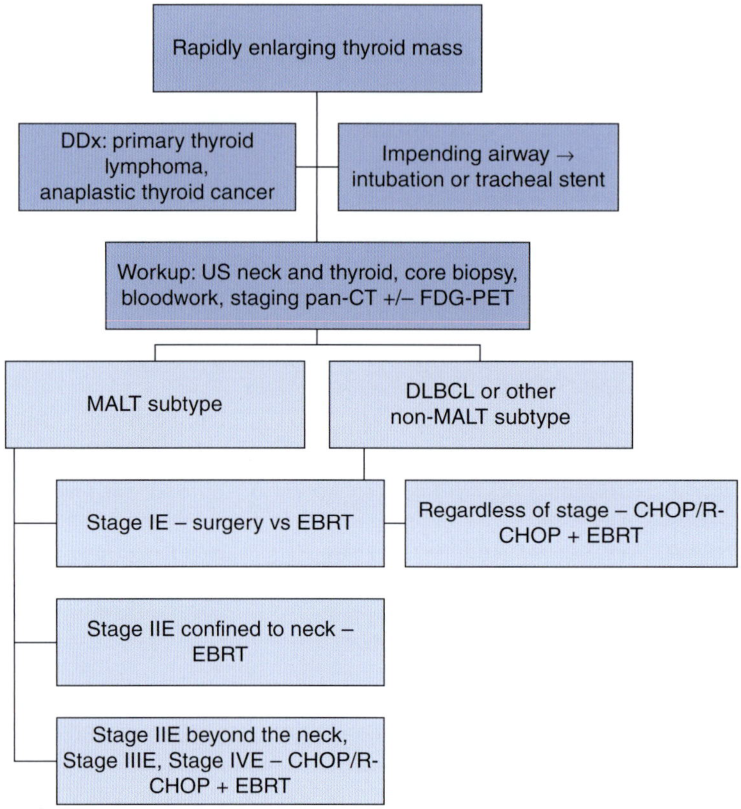

Figure 19–3. PTL workup and treatment algorithm.

overall survival, and local control is best with combined multiagent chemotherapy and external beam radiation, and the addition of rituximab further improved overall survival (92% versus 71%).[33]

In a recent retrospective review of 3466 patients from 2004 to 2015 using the NCDB,[1] 54% of patients underwent surgery (lobectomy or total thyroidectomy), 41% had external beam radiation, 62% had multiagent chemotherapy, 4% had single-agent chemotherapy, and 16% had immunotherapy. 22% of patients underwent combined surgery and radiation, and 34% had surgery followed by chemotherapy. Overall, multiagent chemotherapy had the greatest overall survival benefit (HR 0.40). Surgery and radiation also conferred a survival benefit (HR 0.58 and HR 0.67, respectively). When controlled for stage and histology, surgery maintained a significant benefit, but the retrospective database does not account for patient selection bias or incidental indolent MALT on final pathology and, therefore, this finding should be taken in context.

Palliative Surgery

Palliative surgery for debulking of PTL is no longer favored, as temporary tracheal stents can provide good airway protection, meanwhile response to steroids, chemotherapy, and radiation results in rapid tumor shrinkage and symptom relief.[22-24] In an evidenced-based review by Mack et al.,[34] no recommendations could be made as there is lack of evidence for or against palliative surgery. The current sentiment has moved away from palliative debulking for metastatic PTL.[17] There may still be a role for palliative debulking in the setting of persistent airway compression and minimal response to nonsurgical management. These decisions should be made in a multidisciplinary setting with a surgeon experienced in thyroidectomy.

Ongoing research is still required to determine the optimal treatment and treatment order according to PTL stage and histology. A general algorithm of current recommendations for workup and treatment of PTL according to stage and subtype can be found in Figure 19–3.

Prognosis

Based on the two large database reviews the median all-cause survival for PTL is between 9.3 to 11.6 years.[1,2] Prognosis of PTL is dependent on stage and subtype. Although advanced stages confer worse survival, the majority of patients present with early-stage disease (> 80% stage IE/IIE) (Table 19–1).

DLBCL subtype has the worst prognosis with a 5-year disease-specific survival of 75%, while follicular is 87%, and MALT has the best prognosis at 96%.[2] Additional poor prognostic factors include age greater than 60 years old, tumor size larger than 10 cm, rapid tumor growth, presence of obstructive symptoms, and elevated LDH and β-2 microglobulin levels.[2,18]

WHEN TO REFER/ADMIT

Any patient with a rapidly enlarging thyroid mass should be referred urgently to a thyroid specialist, this includes endocrinologists, medical oncologists, and surgeons who specialize in thyroid disorders. Do not delay referral while awaiting investigations or results. All patients should be discussed and treated in a multidisciplinary setting with experts in lymphoma and thyroid disease that include medical oncologists, radiation oncologists, thyroid surgeons, endocrinologists, pathologists, palliative care teams, primary care physician, and specialty care nurse. Patients with impending airway compromise will require hospital admission and airway protection while undergoing workup and treatment.

REFERENCES

1. Noble VV, Ermann DA, Griffin EK, Silberstein PT. Primary thyroid lymphoma: an analysis of the national cancer database. *Cureus*. 2019;11(2):e4088.
2. Graff-Baker A, Roman SA, Thomas DC, Udelsman R, Sosa JA. Prognosis of primary thyroid lymphoma: demographic, clinical, and pathologic predictors of survival in 1,408 cases. *Surgery*. 2009;146(6):1105-1115.
3. Travaglino A, Pace M, Varricchio S, et al. Clinical features associated with high pathological grade in primary thyroid lymphoma. *Pathology-Research and Practice*. 2020;216(3):152819.
4. Travaglino A, Pace M, Varricchio S, et al. Hashimoto thyroiditis in primary thyroid non-Hodgkin lymphoma: a systematic review and meta-analysis. *Am J Clin pathol*. 2020;153(2):156-164.
5. Sharma A, Jasim S, Reading CC, et al. Clinical presentation and diagnostic challenges of thyroid lymphoma: a cohort study. *Thyroid*. 2016;26(8):1061-1067.
6. Derringer GA, Thompson LD, Frommelt RA, Bijwaard KE, Heffess CS, Abbondanzo SL. Malignant lymphoma of the thyroid gland: a clinicopathologic study of 108 cases. *The American journal of surgical pathology*. 2000;24(5):623-639.
7. Watanabe N, Noh JY, Narimatsu H, et al. Clinicopathological features of 171 cases of primary thyroid lymphoma: a long-term study involving 24 553 patients with Hashimoto's disease. *Br J Haematol*. 2011;153(2):236-243.
8. Moshynska OV, Saxena A. Clonal relationship between Hashimoto thyroiditis and thyroid lymphoma. *J Clin Pathol*. 2008;61(4):438-444.
9. Suzuki A, Hirokawa M, Higashiyama T, et al. Flow cytometric, gene rearrangement, and karyotypic analyses of 110 cases of primary thyroid lymphoma: a single-institutional experience in Japan. *Endocr J*. 2019;66(12):1083-1091.
10. Hwang Y-C, Kim TY, Kim WB, et al. Clinical characteristics of primary thyroid lymphoma in Koreans. *Endocr J*. 2009:0902030237.
11. Troppan K, Wenzl K, Neumeister P, Deutsch A. Molecular pathogenesis of MALT lymphoma. *Gastroenterol Res Pract*. 2015;2015.
12. Takakuwa T, Miyauchi A, Aozasa K. Aberrant somatic hypermutations in thyroid lymphomas. *Leuk Res*. 2009;33(5):649-654.
13. Hirokawa M, Kudo T, Ota H, Suzuki A, Kobayashi K, Miyauchi A. Preoperative diagnostic algorithm of primary thyroid lymphoma using ultrasound, aspiration cytology, and flow cytometry. *Endocr J*. 2017:EJ17-0111.
14. Ota H, Ito Y, Matsuzuka F, et al. Usefulness of ultrasonography for diagnosis of malignant lymphoma of the thyroid. *Thyroid*. 2006;16(10):983-987.
15. Ha EJ, Baek JH, Lee JH, et al. Core needle biopsy could reduce diagnostic surgery in patients with anaplastic thyroid cancer or thyroid lymphoma. *Eur Radiol*. 2016;26(4):1031-1036.
16. Huang CG, Li MZ, Wang SH, Zhou TJ, Haybaeck J, Yang ZH. The diagnosis of primary thyroid lymphoma by fine-needle aspiration, cell block, and immunohistochemistry technique. *Diagn Cytopathol*. 2020;48(11):1041-1047.
17. Walsh S, Lowery AJ, Evoy D, McDermott EW, Prichard RS. Thyroid lymphoma: recent advances in diagnosis and optimal management strategies. *Oncologist*. 2013;18(9):994.
18. Peixoto R, Pinto JC, Soares V, Koch P, Gomes AT. Primary thyroid lymphoma: a case report and review of the literature. *Annal Med Surg*. 2017;13:29-33.
19. Armitage JO. Staging non-Hodgkin lymphoma. *Cancer J Clin*. 2005;55(6):368-376.
20. Nakadate M, Yoshida K, Ishii A, et al. Is 18F-FDG PET/CT useful for distinguishing between primary thyroid lymphoma and chronic thyroiditis? *Clin Nucl Med*. 2013;38(9):709-714.
21. Zhang S, Gong Y. From cytomorphology to molecular pathology: maximizing the value of cytology of lymphoproliferative disorders and soft tissue tumors. *American journal of clinical pathology*. 2013;140(4):454-467.
22. Noppen M, Poppe K, D'Haese J, Meysman M, Velkeniers B, Vincken W. Interventional bronchoscopy for treatment of tracheal obstruction secondary to benign or malignant thyroid disease. *Chest*. 2004;125(2):723-730.
23. Lee J, Won JH, Kim HC, Soh EY. Emergency dilation by self-expandable tracheal stent for upper airway obstruction in a patient with a giant primary thyroid lymphoma. *Thyroid*. 2009;19(2):193-195.
24. Czopnik P, Aporowicz M, Niepokój-Czopnik A, Wojtczak B, Domosławski P, Bolanowski M. Primary thyroid lymphoma: a rare but challenging diagnosis. *Pol Arch Intern Med*. 2017;127(5):361-364.
25. Kikuchi M, Shinohara S, Fujiwara K, et al. Clinical evaluation of 24 cases of primary thyroid malignant lymphoma. *Nihon Jibiinkoka Gakkai Kaiho*. 2011;114(11):855-863.
26. Ishibashi N, Maebayashi T, Aizawa T, et al. Hypothyroidism After Radiotherapy for Primary Thyroid Lymphoma. *Anticancer Res*. 2014;34(8):4427-4431.
27. Watanabe N, Narimatsu H, Noh JY, et al. Rituximab-including combined modality treatment for primary thyroid lymphoma: an effective regimen for elderly patients. *Thyroid*. 2014;24(6):994-999.
28. Wöhrer S, Kiesewetter B, Fischbach J, et al. Retrospective comparison of the effectiveness of various treatment modalities of extragastric MALT lymphoma: a single-center analysis. *Annal Hematol*. 2014;93(8):1287-1295.
29. Tsang RW, Gospodarowicz MK, Pintilie M, et al. Localized mucosa-associated lymphoid tissue lymphoma treated with

radiation therapy has excellent clinical outcome. *J Clin Oncol.* 2003;21(22):4157-4164.
30. Stein SA, Wartofsky L. Primary thyroid lymphoma: a clinical review. *J Clin Endocrinol Metab.* 2013;98(8):3131-3138.
31. Coiffier B, Thieblemont C, Van Den Neste E, et al. Long-term outcome of patients in the LNH-98.5 trial, the first randomized study comparing rituximab-CHOP to standard CHOP chemotherapy in DLBCL patients: a study by the Groupe d'Etudes des Lymphomes de l'Adulte. *Blood.* 2010;116(12): 2040-2045.
32. Pfreundschuh M, Schubert J, Ziepert M, et al. Six versus eight cycles of bi-weekly CHOP-14 with or without rituximab in elderly patients with aggressive CD20+ B-cell lymphomas: a randomised controlled trial (RICOVER-60). *Lancet Oncol.* 2008;9(2):105-116.
33. Onal C, Li Y, Miller R, et al. Treatment results and prognostic factors in primary thyroid lymphoma patients: a rare cancer network study. *Annal Oncol.* 2011;22(1):156-164.
34. Mack LA, Pasieka JL. An evidence-based approach to the treatment of thyroid lymphoma. *World J Surg.* 2007;31(5):978-986.

Pediatric Thyroid Carcinomas

20

Chad K. Sudoko, MD
Andrew J. Bauer, MD
Ken Kazahaya, MD, MBA

GENERAL CONSIDERATIONS

Thyroid carcinoma represents up to 3% of all pediatric malignancies and 7% of all pediatric head and neck tumors.[1,2] Over the last two decades, the incidence of pediatric thyroid carcinoma has steadily increased.[3,4] Although thyroid cancer in children is less common than in adults, there has been a similar annual increase in overall incidence per the Surveillance, Epidemiology, and End Results (SEER) database.[5] Most pediatric thyroid malignancies (approximately 85%-90%) are papillary thyroid carcinoma (PTC), with the remainder being divided between follicular thyroid carcinoma (FTC) and medullary thyroid carcinoma (MTC). In the pediatric population, most MTCs are associated with multiple endocrine neoplasia (MEN) type 2.[6] Following a diagnosis of thyroid cancer, surgical resection is the mainstay of treatment with consideration for radioactive iodine (RAI) pending the postoperative staging. Overall survival for pediatric differentiated thyroid cancer (DTC) is excellent with a greater than 91% rate at 30 years.[7]

PATHOGENESIS

Embryology & Anatomy

The primordial thyroid begins as an involution of the foregut on the midline of the embryonic mouth referred to as the *median anlage*. In humans, this anlage appears at embryonic day 20 to 22 with caudal migration through the thyroglossal duct to its mature location at the base of the neck starting at embryonic day 30 to 40. By the seventh week, the developing thyroid will reach the level of the larynx and form an attachment to the second and third tracheal rings, also known as the ligament of berry. During development and the descent of the thyroid, if the migration path does not involute, a residual tract may form as a thyroglossal duct or cyst which may also contain ectopic thyroid tissue.[8]

As a fully formed thyroid gland, there are two lobes located on either side of the trachea. In close proximity to the thyroid lobes are two branches of the vagus nerve, the superior laryngeal nerve (SLN) and the recurrent laryngeal nerve (RLN). The SLN splits into the internal and external branches approximately 1 to 2 cm above the superior thyroid pole. The internal branch enters through the thyrohyoid membrane and provides sensation to the supraglottis and larynx above the level of the vocal cords. The external branch is typically found just medial to the superior thyroid artery as it innervates the cricothyroid muscle. Injury to the external branch of the SLN during thyroid surgery can result in changes to vocal pitch and difficulty with vocal projection (Figure 20–1).

The RLNs branch off the vagus in the upper chest and have an indirect course back to the larynx (Figure 20–2). The right RLN branches from the vagus nerve around the level of T1-T2, travels around the right subclavian artery, and up through the neck, all the while taking a more oblique angle as it approaches the larynx. The left RLN branches at the level of the aorta and passes around the ductus arteriosus (ligamentum arteriosum), loops under the aorta, and courses almost vertically back into the neck in the tracheoesophageal groove. The nerves will then enter the larynx at the cricothyroid joint, where they will provide motor function to all the intrinsic muscles of the larynx, except for the cricothyroid muscle. Injury to a unilateral RLN will result in limited vocal cord abduction; however, a small amount of adduction may still be present as the interarytenoid muscles have bilateral innervation. Approximately 1% of the time, patients will have a nonrecurrent RLN. This is more common on the right side as it is associated with an aberrant retroesophageal subclavian artery (arteria lusoria).

The blood supply to the thyroid is made up of two arteries and three veins. The two arteries are the superior thyroid artery, a branch off of the external carotid artery, and the

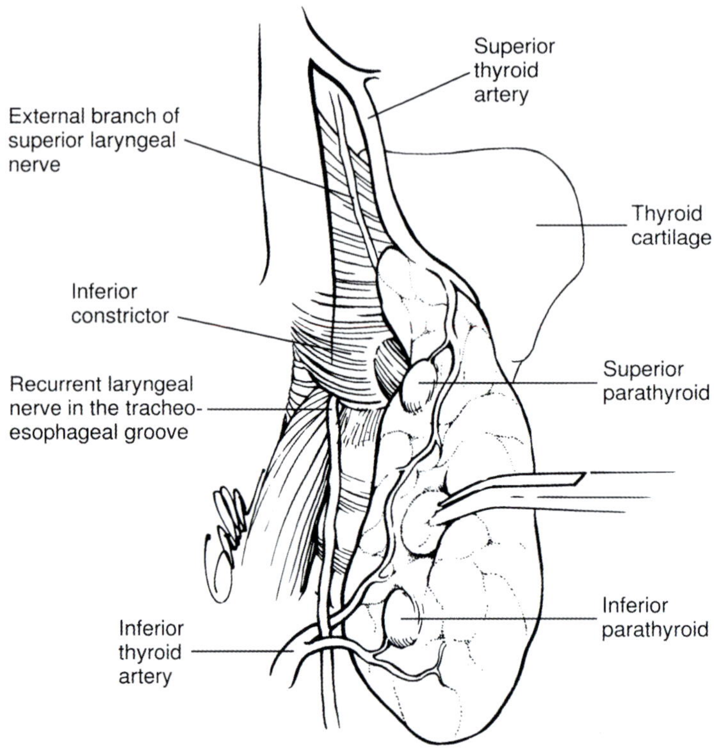

Figure 20–1. Laterally, the inferior thyroid artery and superiorly, the superior thyroid artery are followed to identify inferior and superior parathyroid glands. (Reproduced with permission from Chan Y, Goddard JC, eds. *K.J. Lee's Essential Otolaryngology: Head and Neck Surgery*. 12th ed. New York: McGraw Hill; 2019.)

inferior thyroid artery, a branch off of the thyrocervical trunk. Venous drainage is through the superior, middle, and inferior thyroid veins. In addition, the lymphatic drainage from the thyroid starts with the pretracheal, paratracheal, lower deep cervical nodes, and the Delphian node.

The superior parathyroid glands develop from the fourth pharyngeal pouch and are more consistent in their location at the posterolateral aspect of the superior pole. The inferior parathyroid glands develop from the third pharyngeal pouch and are more variable in their location due to further migration during development. The inferior glands are most commonly found about 1 to 2 cm from the entry of the inferior thyroid artery into the inferior thyroid pole but can also be found in the thymus, thyroid, and carotid sheath. When fully formed, the parathyroid glands are typically 30 to 35 g in size and appear yellow-brown.

Etiology

The majority of children and adolescents diagnosed with thyroid cancer are asymptomatic at the time of diagnosis and have no identifiable risk factor. In a small cohort of patients, there are identifiable risk factors, most notably ionizing radiation or genetic predisposition.

The most common identifiable risk factor associated with developing differentiated thyroid cancer is exposure to ionizing radiation.[9,10] An increased incidence of thyroid cancer has been seen from initial observations in Hiroshima and Nagasaki,[11,12] to medical exposure during a CT scan,[13] and childhood cancer survivors who received therapeutic radiation therapy (greatest risk when <10 years at the time of exposure). The standard incidence ratio for radiation-induced differentiated thyroid cancer ranges from 5 to 70-fold, with a younger age and higher dose of exposure correlating with the highest risk and the shortest latency for thyroid cancer to develop.[14] The increased risk of thyroid nodules and thyroid cancer in pediatric patients is likely due to the increased proliferative cellular activity in the thyroid that is observed during childhood as compared to an adult.[15]

The second most common identifiable risk factor for the development of thyroid cancer is genetic predisposition. Genetic predisposition can be organized into two broad categories: nonsyndromic and syndromic

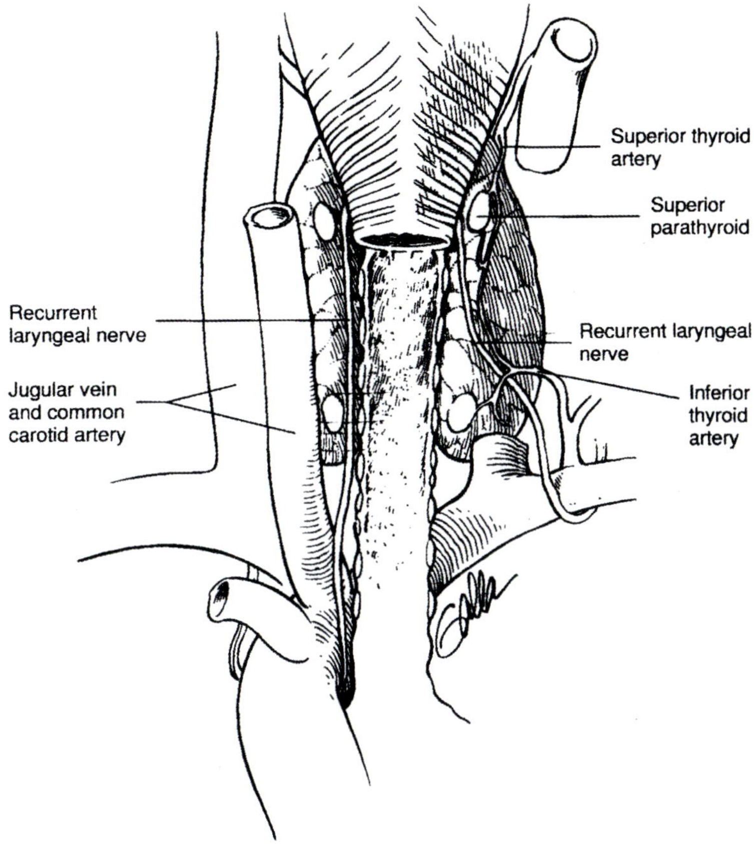

▲ **Figure 20–2.** Posterior view of thyroid showing superior and inferior thyroid arteries and their relationship to the RLNs. (Reproduced with permission from Chan Y, Goddard JC, eds. *K.J. Lee's Essential Otolaryngology: Head and Neck Surgery*. 12th ed. New York: McGraw Hill; 2019.)

(thyroid cancer associated with other tumors). Non-syndromic genetic predisposition is often referred to as familial nonmedullary thyroid cancer (FNMTC). This is defined by the presence of two or more first-degree relatives with either PTC or FTC with an inheritance pattern that most resembles an autosomal dominant mode of transmission. Compared to sporadic DTC, FNMTC generally presents at a younger age and exhibits clinical anticipation between generations, where subsequent generations of family members may present with earlier and more invasive disease.[16] Despite the inheritance pattern and clear genetic association, a single germline locus has not been identified.[17]

Syndromic forms of thyroid cancer are associated with mutations in several genes that result in an increased risk for thyroid and nonthyroid malignancies, in addition to phenotypic findings on physical exam. In DTC, these syndromes include PTEN hamartoma tumor syndrome (PHTS), DICER1 syndrome, familial adenomatous polyposis (FAP), and Carney complex.[18] In medullary thyroid cancer (MTC), the familial syndrome is MEN type 2.

A. Papillary Thyroid Cancer

Papillary thyroid cancer and its variants are the most common form of thyroid malignancy, with the most common subtypes being classic PTC (60%) and follicular variant PTC (20%). The remaining histological subtypes include diffuse sclerosing variant PTC (dsvPTC), widely invasive (diffuse) follicular variant PTC, solid-trabecular PTC (sPTC), and tall-cell variant PTC (tcvPTC). The histological appearance of PTC and its subtypes in children are similar to those in adults. Despite the similarities in appearance, pediatric PTC has a higher predilection to invade lymphatics compared to adults resulting in a higher rate of regional lymph node involvement (70%-90% of patients), multifocal disease (30%-80%), and distant metastasis, primarily to the lungs (8%-20%) at the time of diagnosis.[19,20]

For some variants, the presence of a capsule may correlate with the risk of metastasis. Encapsulated cPTC has a similar risk for lymph nodes metastasis when compared to unencapsulated cPTC. However, in encapsulated fvPTC there is a lower risk for multifocality and lymph node metastasis.[21,22] Variants such as dsvPTC, widely invasive follicular variant PTC, sPTC, and tcvPTC are all associated with an increased risk of regional and distant metastasis. dsvPTC is unusual in that it displays diffuse invasion of the thyroid rather than presenting as a distinct nodule.

Molecular testing for PTC is commonly performed for adults and the BRAF V600E mutation has been associated with poorer outcomes due to a higher recurrence and mortality rate.[23,24] Despite the strong association in adults, a correlation between the BRAF V600E mutation and a more invasive phenotype has not been shown in the pediatric population.[25] In contrast to the BRAF V600E mutation, the presence of a fusion oncogene in one of several tyrosine kinase receptors in PTC, that is, RET, NTRK, and others, has been associated with more extensive disease.[26]

B. Follicular Thyroid Cancer

FTC, like PTC, is a well-differentiated cancer; however, it represents less than 10% of thyroid cancer in children. FTCs produce thyroglobulin (Tg) and have the capacity to transport iodine across the cell membrane via the sodium-iodine symporter (NIS). In sporadic FTC, the most common somatic mutations are in DICER1, NRAS, PTEN, FGFR3, and STK11[18,27] and there is an increased incidence in iodine-deficient regions of the world.[28] In familial DTC, there is a higher incidence of FTC associated with PTEN hamartoma tumor syndrome. In pediatrics, the majority of FTC is minimally invasive; however, in contrast to PTC, FTC metastasizes hematogenously[29] with the risk of local and distant metastasis mostly determined by the extent of angioinvasion into both peri- and intracapsular blood vessels.[18] Minimally invasive FTC (miFTC) is defined as invasion of the tumor in less than four blood vessels and widely invasive FTC with invasion in more than four blood vessels. With widely invasive FTC, there is an increased risk of distant metastasis and associated higher rates of recurrence and worse outcomes.[30,31]

C. Medullary Thyroid Carcinoma

MTC originates from parafollicular C cells and account for approximately 5% of pediatric thyroid cancers. MTC can occur sporadically or in association with familial syndromes, with the bulk of adult cases being from sporadic causes. In pediatrics, MTC is generally associated with MEN type 2. MEN2 is caused by activating mutations in the *RET* proto-oncogene that are transmitted in an autosomal dominant pattern. In addition, the phenotype of the tumors that are associated with MEN2 correlate with the specific *RET* proto-oncogene mutation.[18]

CLINICAL PRESENTATION

Pediatric thyroid cancer can present in a number of different ways. Smaller thyroid masses can be incidentally found on imaging studies performed for a nonthyroid-related indication. Larger lesions can present as a neck mass noted on physical examination, usually by the patient's primary care provider. Palpable and symmetric level II lymph nodes are a common finding in healthy children; however, the presence of a thyroid nodule with cervical lymphadenopathy in level III or level IV is a concerning finding and a predictor for malignancy (Table 20–1).[32]

In pediatrics as well as the adult population, a low normal or suppressed TSH is associated with an autonomously functioning thyroid nodule that is correlated with a lower risk of malignancy. In these patients, thyroid ultrasound is warranted to evaluate for the presence of a nodule even if the patient has minimal signs or symptoms of hyperthyroidism. In patients with a family history of MEN2, if there are clinical features or a cytology suspicious for MTC, a serum calcitonin should be obtained.

A. Imaging

When suspicion for a thyroid nodule or malignancy arises, an ultrasound of the thyroid and neck is the best radiologic modality to assess the nodule's morphologic characteristics. In patients with moderate to high-risk thyroid lesions, assessment of the central and lateral neck lymph nodes for evidence of metastasis must be performed.[33,34] One of the grading scales with which to stratify thyroid nodules and determine whether a fine-needle aspiration (FNA) should be performed is the Thyroid Imaging Reporting and Data System (TI-RADS).[35] In many patients, ultrasound alone will provide sufficient imaging information. However, in patients with large thyroid lesions or metastatic lymphadenopathy seen on ultrasound, cross-sectional imaging with CT or MRI can provide useful information in the examination of the superior mediastinum, retropharynx, and subclavicular regions.[33,36] In patients with significant lymphadenopathy,

Table 20–1. Well-differentiated thyroid cancer.

	Pediatric	Adult
Thyroid nodules in the population[62,63]	5%	35%
Thyroid nodules and risk of malignancy[63,64]	25%	5%
Bilateral disease[65-68]	30%-40%	20%
Multifocal disease[69,70]	30%-80%	10%-42%
Nodal Disease[63,69]	70%-90%	20%-50%

chest imaging with CT should be considered to assess for pulmonary metastases.[33]

B. Fine-Needle Aspiration

Similar to adults, FNA in pediatrics has been shown to have the same accuracy and The Bethesda System for Reporting Thyroid Cytopathology (TBSRTC) is used to classify the results. However, in contrast to adults, there does appear to be an increased risk of malignancy for pediatric patients with indeterminate cytology, although the risk appears to be widely disparate between different institutes.[37] For pediatric patients with indeterminate cytology, the risk for malignancy in nodules with Bethesda Category III is similar compared to adults, approximately 15%; however, in nodules with Bethesda Category IV cytology, the risk for malignancy is higher in pediatrics, approximately 55% compared to 40% in adults.

C. Genetic Testing

Oncogenic testing has the clinical utility to predict an increased risk for malignancy in pediatric patients. As mentioned earlier, in pediatrics the presence of a BRAF mutation has not been shown to be associated with a more aggressive PTC phenotype; however, the presence of a BRAF mutation in an indeterminate FNA specimen is associated with a near 100% likelihood of PTC. Additional oncogene mutations and fusion genes with this predictive ability include RET/PTC and NTRK-fusion. Oncogenes that may be associated with either benign nodules or DTC with lower-risk for invasive behavior include PTEN, DICER1, RAS, and others[37] (Table 20–2).

In patients with a family history of a known tumor predisposition syndrome or a family pedigree that is consistent with such a syndrome, germline testing should be considered. If physical exam is concerning for MEN2 or cytology is suspicious for MTC, then serum calcitonin or calcitonin immunohistochemistry should be performed.

D. Vocal Cord Assessment

Evaluation of vocal cord function should be performed on all patients undergoing thyroid surgery and can be performed with a flexible fiberoptic laryngoscopy or a laryngeal ultrasound.[38] Confirming function of the vocal cords is essential to the preoperative workup as paresis of one or both of the vocal folds can occur due to RLN compromise from invasive disease. If paresis is seen during preoperative evaluation, then further discussion regarding the disease and surgical approach should be with consideration for systemic therapy if a targetable, somatic alteration is found in the tumor in an effort to determine if medical debulking can restore RLN function prior to surgery. Following surgery, reassessment of

Table 20–2. Oncogene mutations and thyroid cancer.

Somatic Driver Alteration	Histology	Invasive Potential*	Surgical Approach
RET fusions and mutations	PTC	High	Thyroidectomy with central neck lymph node dissection; lateral neck dissection based on US and FNA
	MTC	Based on RET codon	Based on calcitonin level, imaging, FNA
NTRK-fusion	PTC	High	Thyroidectomy with central neck lymph node dissection; lateral neck dissection based on US and FNA
ALK-fusion†	PTC	High	Thyroidectomy with central neck lymph node dissection; lateral neck dissection based on US and FNA
	MTC	Limited cases	Based on calcitonin level, imaging, FNA
BRAFV600E	PTC	Intermediate to high	Thyroidectomy with central neck lymph node dissection; lateral neck dissection based on US and FNA
RAS† PTEN DICER1† PAX8/PPARg†	PTC and FTC and benign	Low	Lobectomy if unilateral disease Consider thyroidectomy if thyroid cancer predisposition syndrome or autoimmune thyroiditis
TSHR GNAS	Benign	Not applicable	Lobectomy
TERT, EIF1X, CTNNB1, AKT1, others	PTC and FTC	Limited data in pediatrics	

*Invasive potential (1) Low—intrathyroidal, (2) Intermediate—intrathyroidal and N1a, (3) High—intrathyroidal, N1a/N1b, and M1.
†May be associated with poorly differentiated thyroid cancer; rare in pediatrics.
PTC: Papillary thyroid cancer, FTC: Follicular thyroid cancer, MTC: Medullary thyroid cancer

the vocal cords is useful to either confirm function or to help guide further options in the management of paresis.

SURGICAL MANAGEMENT

Papillary Thyroid Cancer

Surgical options for thyroid cancer include a thyroid lobectomy, a subtotal or near total thyroidectomy, and a total thyroidectomy. A thyroid lobectomy involves removal of the thyroid lobe along with the isthmus, a subtotal involves removal of the entire lobe and most of the remaining lobe to preserve the RLN and parathyroid glands, and a total thyroidectomy involves removal of the thyroid in its entirety. Due to the low incidence, most recommendations come from small cohorts, retrospective reviews, and extrapolations from adult studies. To standardize the evaluation and management of thyroid nodules and thyroid cancer, the American Thyroid Association (ATA) published guidelines for pediatric patients in 2015. In these guidelines, the recommendation for pediatric PTC is a total thyroidectomy (TT), regardless of tumor size.[39] This recommendation was based on data showing a high incidence of bilateral disease (30%-40%) and a reduced risk of recurrence (6% vs 30%) when a total thyroidectomy is performed rather than a lobectomy.[40] In addition, given the more advanced stage at presentation, a total thyroidectomy allows for the more accurate use of Tg levels in the postoperative period to monitor for persistent and recurrent disease.[39] More recently, there are pediatric studies showing that lobectomy may be considered in patients with DTC associated with low invasive potential, including encapsulated fvPTC as well as unifocal PTC less than 1 cm in size (N1a).[41,42]

A prophylactic central neck lymph node dissection should be considered for all pediatric patients undergoing surgery for PTC. Multiple studies have shown that the presence of nodal disease is an independent risk factor for recurrence and distant metastasis.[43,44] Because of this, the presence and extent of nodal disease is used to help stratify patients into a low, intermediate, or high risk according to the ATA.[39] Depending on the patient's risk level, RAI may be recommended. Lateral neck dissections should only be performed on FNA-proven metastasis to the lateral neck lymph nodes.

Thyroid surgery carries significant risks that could meaningfully impact a patient's quality of life, and unfortunately, the pediatric population carries a higher complication rate than their adult counterparts. Higher volume surgeons have been shown to have significantly lower complication rates with permanent nerve injury and hypocalcemia being reported as low as 0.4% and 0.6%.[45]

Intraoperative monitoring of the RLN should be performed during thyroid surgery. This can be performed with a nerve monitoring endotracheal tube (ETT), which will transmit a signal when the vocal cords are stimulated. The surgeon should be cognizant of the use of paralysis when neuromonitoring is being used. Unfortunately for infants and young children, an age-appropriate nerve-monitoring ETT may not be available. In such cases, direct laryngeal monitoring with hookwire electrodes or even stick-on electrodes can be used.[46]

All efforts should be taken to decrease the risk of permanent hypoparathyroidism by preserving the integrity of the parathyroid glands and their blood supply (inferior thyroid artery). Intraoperative parathyroid hormone can be measured to help identify patients at risk of hypoparathyroidism and to ensure early treatment, avoiding clinically symptomatic hypocalcemia.[47] In the postoperative setting, calcium levels should be monitored approximately every 4 to 8 hours after completion of a total thyroidectomy or completion of thyroid lobectomy. Early identification of hypoparathyroidism with initiation of calcium and calcitriol decreases the risk of symptomatic hypocalcemia and the duration of postoperative hospitalization.[48]

Follicular Thyroid Cancer

Unlike PTC, FTC is more often unifocal and metastasizes by a hematogenous route to the bone, liver, or lungs. Many patients ultimately diagnosed with FTC will have had indeterminate FNA cytology as FTC is distinguished from follicular adenoma by the presence of invasion through the capsule or angioinvasion on pathology rather than by nuclear features as in PTC. Once pathology is obtained, FTC can be defined as either minimally invasive or widely invasive. Given the challenge of diagnosis prior to surgery, many patients will undergo a thyroid lobectomy with plans for a staged completion thyroidectomy if pathology is consistent with FTC. Some exceptions to this staged approach include patients with an underlying thyroid disease, bilateral nodules, or a known diagnosis of a thyroid tumor predisposition syndrome. In patients with minimally invasive FTC that is less than 4 cm a lobectomy can be considered sufficient; however, for tumors with tumor metastasis into ≥4 capsular blood vessels or more than 4 cm in size a completion thyroidectomy should be performed with postoperative RAI therapy based on the findings from the diagnostic radioiodine whole body scan and TSH stimulated Tg level.[39]

Medullary Thyroid Cancer

The bulk of MTC cases in pediatric patients are hereditary and the ultimate goal is to remove the thyroid before onset of metastatic MTC. Historically, all patients with a germline *RET* proto-oncogene mutation were referred for surgical intervention; however, the more recent recommendations are that the timing for thyroidectomy should be based on the specific codon mutation.[49] In patients with the highest risk mutation, typically associated with MEN2B, a therapeutic thyroidectomy should be performed at diagnosis (ideally within the first year of life).[49,50] MEN2A is typically broken up into high and moderate-risk mutations. In those with a high-risk mutation, a thyroidectomy should be performed at or before 5 years of age. In a moderate-risk mutation, surgery is recommended when serum calcitonin levels show an upward trend or sooner if the parents do not want to undergo a potentially lengthy period of active surveillance. Following surgical removal, serum levels of calcitonin and carcinoembryonic antigen (CEA) should be monitored every 6 months for 1 year, then annually.

MEDICAL MANAGEMENT

Radioactive Iodine for Differentiated Thyroid Cancer

RAI is an effective medical therapy to treat persistent post-surgical disease. The benefits of RAI include destruction of thyroid cancer cells as well as any postoperative thyroid tissue, thus increasing the future sensitivity of surveillance thyroglobulin (Tg). For DTC, the ATA has stratified pediatric patients into three risk categories—low risk, intermediate risk, and high risk. These categories are based on the extent of the primary tumor, lymph node involvement, and distant metastasis to guide the use of RAI ablation in patients with more advanced disease.[51]

Postoperative assessment for evidence of postsurgical persistent disease is typically performed 6 to 12 weeks following surgery. In ATA pediatric low-risk patients, no further scans are needed and patients may be followed with TSH-suppressed Tg and neck ultrasound. In those patients with ATA pediatric intermediate and high-risk profiles, a TSH-stimulated Tg and a I^{123} diagnostic whole-body scan (DxWBS) should be performed to evaluate for persistent disease and to determine if I^{131} therapy would be beneficial.

Systemic Therapy

A small proportion of children and adolescents will develop progressive DTC that is refractory to ^{131}I therapy. Radioactive iodine refractory (RAIR) DTC is defined by (1) absence of initial RAI uptake in metastasis, (2) absence of RAI uptake in metastasis after treatment with RAI, (3) presence of RAI uptake in some metastasis, but absence in others (patchy uptake on WBS), and (4) progression despite RAI uptake in metastasis.[52] The main criteria for initiation of systemic therapy in adults include (1) large tumor burden with tumors greater than 1 to 2 cm in size, (2) Response Evaluation Criteria in Solid Tumors (RECIST) progressive disease over than 12 months, and (3) symptomatic disease and risk of local complications.[52,53] There are no pediatric age-specific definitions for RAIR, or criteria for when to initiate systemic therapy and there is a significant challenge when using the RECIST criteria, as the majority of pediatric patients with pulmonary metastasis have diffuse, micronodular disease.

Over the last decade, there are an increasing number of oral chemotherapies that have been incorporated into clinical practice for adults with RAIR. These agents target tyrosine-kinase receptors or constitutively activated protein kinases in the MAPK pathway.[54] The multitargeted tyrosine kinase inhibitors (TKIs) target the vascular endothelial growth factor receptors as well as other tyrosine kinase receptors, including the epithelial growth factor receptor, fibroblast growth factor receptor, platelet-derived growth factor receptor, and RET. There are currently two MKIs that have received FDA approval in the treatment of advanced DTC, sorafenib and lenvatinib.[55] These agents are not tumoricidal but they have been shown to slow progression and to decrease tumor burden. Unfortunately, in adults, the effect is often transient and many patients experience side effects, including hypertension, diarrhea, anorexia with weight loss, dermatitis, and fatigue.[55] Within pediatrics, there are several case reports where MKIs have been used; however, the data is quite limited and there is no consensus regarding the timing to initiate therapy or in the selection of which oral chemotherapeutic agent should be used.[56,57]

The newer oncogene-specific, targeted inhibitors have increased efficacy and less toxicity compared to the multityrosine inhibitors. Several of these agents have been in clinical use for several years, repurposed from the treatment of other nonthyroid malignancies but with the same molecular alterations. The most effective of these molecular targeted inhibitors have shown remarkable clinical efficacy with regression in tumors harboring *RET*, *NTRK*, and *ALK* fusion genes and the *BRAF*^{V600E} mutation. Larotrectinib (LOXO-101) is a selective *NTRK* inhibitor that has been approved for use in pediatric age patients. The Children's Oncology Group (COG) recently opened a phase II study with larotrectinib (ADVL1823, NCT03834961) for children with previously untreated TRK fusion solid tumors, including thyroid cancer. In addition, the National Cancer Institute and COG Pediatric MATCH (NCT03155620) is a phase II study that offers access to several agents based on knowledge of the oncogenic driver mutation, including BRAF alterations (vemurafenib), ALK fusions (ensartinib), and RET mutations/fusions (LOXO 292). One of the most exciting observations is that several of the oncogene-specific targeted therapies are associated with resensitization of tumors to RAI, both in adults and in pediatrics.[58]

A. Systemic Therapy for Medullary Thyroid Cancer

For patients with MTC who have progressive disease that is not amenable to surgery, systemic treatment with receptor tyrosine kinase inhibitors or oncogene-specific targeted therapies against *RET* may be indicated. The same criteria used for "initiation of systemic therapy" described in the preceding DTC section should be followed for patients with MTC within the context that the majority of patients with metastatic MTC will not achieve remission from disease. Vandetanib and cabozantinib have been FDA-approved for the treatment of adults with progressive, metastatic MTC.[54,59] Limited data suggest that vandetanib is effective and well tolerated in children with advanced MTC in the setting of MEN2B.[60] The selective *RET*-inhibitors (selpercatinib and pralsetinib) are currently in clinical trials with preliminary data demonstrating a very favorable response with low side effects.[61]

PROGNOSIS

When histology and tumor size are controlled for, children with DTC are more likely to have regional lymph node involvement, extrathyroidal extension, and pulmonary metastasis. However, despite more extensive disease at clinical presentation, children and adolescents are much less likely to die from the disease. In a review of nearly 1600 children with DTC of all stages, the 30-year survival was greater than 91%.[7] Even when pulmonary metastases are present, many patients will develop persistent but stable disease following RAI treatment. When compared to adults with persistent DTC, children also have a more favorable progression-free survival. Continued effort is needed to better understand pediatric thyroid cancer and their associated clinical, molecular, and pathological differences to optimize treatment plans and long-term outcomes.

Knowledge of the somatic oncogene driver mutation is increasingly important for the diagnosis of thyroid nodules with indeterminate cytology as well as for the prediction of clinical behavior, response to therapy, and for the selection of systemic therapy in both DTC and MTC. For patients that present with morbidly invasive disease, including evidence of RLN paralysis, encasement of great vessels, evidence of aerodigestive tract invasion, or with pulmonary metastasis associated with hypoxia, neoadjuvant systemic therapy for medical debulking should be considered. For patients with DTC, surgery and RAI should be pursued once the patient achieves improved clinical status associated with systemic therapy-induced tumor regression. For patients with MTC, surgery may be deferred if the systemic therapy is associated with significant regression as it is unlikely to achieve surgical remission once MTC metastasizes. For patients with progressive DTC or MTC that is not surgically resectable, or in patients with RAI-refractory DTC, adjuvant systemic therapy should be considered based on anatomic progression with early evidence showing a potential role for repeat RAI after oncogene-targeted therapy secondary to resensitization. Multicenter, collaborative studies are needed to better define the timing for initiation, selection of drug, monitoring, and adjustment of therapy so that we optimize outcome while minimizing the risk of side effects and adverse events.

REFERENCES

1. Thompson GB, Hay ID. Current strategies for surgical management and adjuvant treatment of childhood papillary thyroid carcinoma. *World J Surg.* 2004;28:1187-119804.
2. Palmer BA, Zarroug AE, Poley RN, et al. Papillary thyroid carcinoma in children: risk factors and complications of disease recurrence. *J Pediatr Surg.* 2005;40:1284-1288.
3. Holmes L Jr, Hossain J, Opara F. Pediatric thyroid carcinoma incidence and temporal trends in the USA (1973-2007): race or shifting diagnostic paradigm? *ISRN Oncol.* 2012;2012:906197.
4. Vergamini LB, Frazier AL, Abrantes FL, Ribeiro KB, Rodriguez-Galindo C. Increase in the incidence of differentiated thyroid carcinoma in children, adolescents, and young adults: a population-based study. *J Pediatr.* 2014;164(6):1481-1485.
5. Golpanian S, Perez EA, Tashiro J, et al. Pediatric papillary thyroid carcinoma: outcomes and survival predictors in 2504 surgical patients. *Pediatr Surg Int.* 2016;32(3):201-208.
6. Dermody S, Walls A, Harley EH Jr. Pediatric thyroid cancer: an update from the SEER database 2007-2012. *Int J Pediatr Otorhinolaryngol.* 2016;89:121-126.
7. Hogan AR, Zhuge Y, Perez EA, Koniaris LG, Lew JI, Sola JE. Pediatric thyroid carcinoma: incidence and outcomes in 1753 patients. *J Surg Res.* 2009;156(1):167-172.
8. Hanley P, Lord K, Bauer AJ. Thyroid disorders in children and adolescents: a review. *JAMA Pediatr.* 2016;170(10):1008-1019.
9. Meadows AT, Friedman DL, Neglia JP, et al. Second neoplasms in survivors of childhood cancer: findings from the Childhood Cancer Survivor Study cohort. *J Clin Oncol.* 2009;27(1)4:2356.
10. Ronckers CM, Sigurdson AJ, Stovall M, et al. Thyroid cancer in childhood cancer survivors: a detailed evaluation of radiation dose response and its modifiers. *Radiat Res.* 2006;166(4):618-628.
11. Hamilton TE, van Belle G, LoGerfo JP. Thyroid neoplasia in Marshall Islanders exposed to nuclear fallout. *JAMA.* 1987;258:629-635.
12. Yoshimoto Y, Ezaki H, Etoh R, et al. Prevalence rate of thyroid diseases among autopsy cases of the atomic bomb survivors in Hiroshima, 1951-1985. *Radiat Res.* 1995;141:278-286.
13. Schonfeld SJ, Lee C, Berrington de Gonzalez A. Medical exposure to radiation and thyroid cancer. *Clin Oncol.* 2011;23(4):244-250.
14. Clement SC, Kremer LCM, Verburg FA, et al. Balancing the benefits and harms of thyroid cancer surveillance in survivors of childhood, adolescent and young adult cancer. *Cancer Treat Rev.* 2018;63:28-39.
15. Saad AG, Kumar S, Ron E, et al. Proliferative activity of human thyroid cells in various age groups and its correlation with the risk of thyroid cancer after radiation exposure. *J Clin Endocrinol Metab.* 2006;91(7):2672-2677.
16. Bauer AJ. Clinical behavior and genetics of nonsyndromic, familial nonmedullary thyroid cancer. *Front Horm Res.* 2013;41:141-148.
17. Klubo-Gwiezdzinska J, Yang L, Merkel R, et al. Results of screening in familial non-medullary thyroid cancer. *Thyroid.* 2017;27(8):1017-1024.
18. Bauer AJ. Pediatric thyroid cancer: genetics, therapeutics and outcome. *Endocrinol Metab Clin.* 2020;49(4):589-611.
19. Balachandar S, La Quaglia M, Tuttle RM, Heller G, Ghossein RA, Sklar CA. Pediatric differentiated thyroid carcinoma of follicular cell origin: prognostic significance of histologic subtypes. *Thyroid.* 2016;26(2):219-226.
20. Golpanian S, Perez EA, Tashiro J, et al. Pediatric papillary thyroid carcinoma: outcomes and survival predictors in 2504 surgical patients. *Pediatr Surg Int.* 2016;32(3):201-208.

21. Rivera M, Tuttle RM, Patel S, et al. Encapsulated papillary thyroid carcinoma: a clinic-pathologic study of 106 cases with emphasis on its morphologic subtypes (histologic growth pattern). *Thyroid.* 2009;19(2):119-127.
22. Samuels SL, Surrey LF, Hawkes CP, et al. Characteristics of follicular variant papillary thyroid carcinoma in a pediatric cohort. *J Clin Endocrinol Metab.* 2018;103(4):1639-1648.
23. Xing M, Alzahrani AS, Carson KA, et al. Association between BRAF V600E mutation and mortality in patients with papillary thyroid cancer. *JAMA.* 2013;309(14):1493-1501.
24. Xing M, Alzahrani AS, Carson KA, et al. Association between BRAF V600E mutation and recurrence of papillary thyroid cancer. *J Clin Oncol.* 2015;33(1):42-50.
25. Mostoufi-Moab S, Labourier E, Sullivan L, et al. Molecular testing for oncogenic gene alterations in pediatric thyroid lesions. *Thyroid.* 2018;28(1):60-67.
26. Prasad ML, Vyas M, Horne MJ, et al. NTRK fusion oncogenes in pediatric papillary thyroid carcinoma in northeast United States. *Cancer.* 2016;122(7):1097-1107.
27. Bae J-S, Jung S-H, Hirokawa M, et al. High prevalence of DICER1 mutations and low frequency of gene fusions in pediatric follicular-patterned tumors of the thyroid. *Endocr Pathol.* 2021;32(3):336-346.
28. Nettore IC, Colao A, Macchia PE. Nutritional and environmental factors in thyroid carcinogenesis. *Int J Environ Res Public Health.* 2018;15(8):1735.
29. Lin X, Liu Y, Silverman JF. Follicular thyroid carcinoma invades venous rather than lymphatic vessels. *Diagn Pathol.* 2010;5:8.
30. Dionigi G, Kraimps JL, Schmid KW, et al. Minimally invasive follicular thyroid cancer (MIFTC): a consensus report of the European Society of Endocrine Surgeons. *Langenbecks Arch Surg.* 2015;399(2):165-184.
31. Haugen BR, Alexander EK, Bible KC, et al. 2015 American Thyroid Association management guidelines for adult patients with thyroid nodules and differentiated thyroid cancer. *Thyroid.* 2016;26(1):1-133.
32. Buryk MA, Simons JP, Picarsic J, et al. Can malignant thyroid nodules be distinguished from benign thyroid nodules in children and adolescents by clinical characteristics? A review of 89 pediatric patients with thyroid nodules. *Thyroid.* 2015;25(4):392-400.
33. Yeh MW, Bauer AJ, Bernet VA, et al. American Thyroid Association statement on preoperative imaging for thyroid cancer surgery. *Thyroid.* 2015;25(1):3-14.
34. Navallas M, Daneman A, Amirabadi A, Ngan B-Y, Wasserman J. Utility of sonography for identifying metastatic cervical adenopathy in children with differentiated thyroid carcinoma at presentation. *Pediatr Radiol.* 2021;51(2):273-281.
35. Martinez-Rios C, Daneman A, Bajno L, van der Kaay DCM, Moineddin R, Wasserman JD. Utility of adult-based ultrasound malignancy risk stratifications in pediatric thyroid nodules. *Pediatr Radiol.* 2018;48(1):74-84.
36. Francis GL, Waguespack SG, Bauer AJ, et al. Management guidelines for children with thyroid nodules and differentiated thyroid cancer. *Thyroid.* 2015;25(7):716-759.
37. Bauer AJ. Thyroid nodules in children and adolescents. *Curr Opin Endocrinol Diabetes Obes.* 2019;26(5):266-274.
38. Hamilton CE, Su E, Tawfik D, et al. Assessment of vocal cord motion using laryngeal ultrasound in children: a systematic review and meta-analysis. *Pediatr Crit Care Med.* 2021;22(10):e532-e539.
39. Francis GL, Waguespack SG, Bauer AJ, et al. Management guidelines for children with thyroid nodules and differentiated thyroid cancer: the American Thyroid Association guidelines task force on pediatric thyroid cancer. *Thyroid.* 2015;25(7): 716-759.
40. Hay ID, Gonzalez-Losada T, Reinalda MS, Honetschlager JA, Richards ML, Thompson GB. Long-term outcome in 215 children and adolescents with papillary thyroid cancer treated during 1940 through 2008. *World J Surg.* 2010;34(6):1192-1202.
41. Kluijfhout WP, Pasternak JD, van der Kaay D, Vriens MR, Propst EJ, Wasserman JD. Is it time to reconsider lobectomy in low-risk paediatric thyroid cancer? *Clin Endocrinol (Oxf).* 2017;86(4):591-596.
42. Sugino K, Nagahama M, Kitagawa W, et al. Risk stratification of pediatric patients with differentiated thyroid cancer: is total thyroidectomy necessary for patients at any risk? *Thyroid.* 2020;30(4):548-556.
43. Mercante G, Frasoldati A, Pedroni C, et al. Prognostic factors affecting neck lymph node recurrence and distant metastasis in papillary microcarcinoma of the thyroid: results of a study in 445 patients. *Thyroid.* 2009;19(7):707-716.
44. Chow S-M, Law SCK, Chan JKC, Au S-K, Yau S, Lau W-H. Papillary microcarcinoma of the thyroid—prognostic significance of lymph node metastasis and multifocality. *Cancer.* 2003;98(1):31-40.
45. Baumgarten HD, Bauer AJ, Isaza A, Mostoufi-Moab S, Kazahaya K, Adzick NS. Surgical management of pediatric thyroid disease: complication rates after thyroidectomy at the Children's Hospital of Philadelphia high-volume Pediatric Thyroid Center. *J Pediatr Surg.* 2019;54(10):1969-1975.
46. Stack BC Jr, Twining C, Rastatter J, et al. Consensus statement by the American Association of Clinical Endocrinology (AACE) and the American Head and Neck Society Endocrine Surgery Section (AHNS-ES) on Pediatric Benign and Malignant Thyroid Surgery. *Head Neck.* 2021;43(4):1027-1042.
47. Tsai SD, Mostoufi-Moab S, Bauer S, et al. Clinical utility of intraoperative parathyroid hormone measurement in children and adolescents undergoing total thyroidectomy. *Front Endocrinol (Lausanne).* 2019;10:760.
48. Patel NA, Bly RA, Adams S, et al. A clinical pathway for the postoperative management of hypocalcemia after pediatric thyroidectomy reduces blood draws. *Int J Pediatr Otorhinolaryngol.* 2018;105:132-137.
49. Wells SA Jr, Asa SL, Dralle H, et al. Revised American Thyroid Association guidelines for the management of medullary thyroid carcinoma: the American Thyroid Association Guidelines Task Force on medullary thyroid carcinoma. *Thyroid.* 2015;25(6):567-610.
50. Castinetti F, Waguespack SG, Machens A, et al. Natural history, treatment, and long-term follow up of patients with multiple endocrine neoplasia type 2B: an international, multicentre, retrospective study. *Lancet Diabetes Endocrinol.* 2019;7(3): 213-220.
51. Francis GL, Waguespack SG, Bauer AJ, et al. Management guidelines for children with thyroid nodules and differentiated thyroid cancer: the American Thyroid Association guidelines task force on pediatric thyroid cancer. *Thyroid.* 2015;25(7):716-759.
52. Berdelou A, Lamartina L, Klain M, Leboulleux S, Schlumberger M. Treatment of refractory thyroid cancer. *Endocr Relat Cancer.* 2018;25(4):R209-R223.

53. Eisenhauer EA, Therasse P, Bogaerts J, et al. New response evaluation criteria in solid tumours: revised RECIST guideline (version 1.1). *Eur J Cancer*. 2009;45(2):228-247.
54. Covell LL, Ganti AK. Treatment of advanced thyroid cancer: role of molecularly targeted therapies. *Target Oncol*. 2015; 10(3):311-324.
55. Rao SN, Cabanillas ME. Navigating systemic therapy in advanced thyroid carcinoma: from standard of care to personalized therapy and beyond. *J Endocr Soc*. 2018;2(10):1109-1130.
56. Mahajan P, Dawrant J, Kheradpour A, et al. Response to lenvatinib in children with papillary thyroid carcinoma. *Thyroid*. 2018;28(11):1450-1454.
57. Waguespack SG, Sherman SI, Williams MD, Clayman GL, Herzog CE. The successful use of sorafenib to treat pediatric papillary thyroid carcinoma. *Thyroid*. 2009;19(4):407-412.
58. Lee YA, Lee H, Im S-W, et al. NTRK- and RET-fusion-directed therapy in pediatric thyroid cancer yields a tumor response and radioiodine uptake. *J Clin Invest*. 2021;131(18):e144847.
59. Weitzman SP, Cabanillas ME. The treatment landscape in thyroid cancer: a focus on cabozantinib. *Cancer Manag Res*. 2015;7:265-278.
60. Fox E, Widemann BC, Chuk MK, et al. Vandetanib in children and adolescents with multiple endocrine neoplasia type 2B associated medullary thyroid carcinoma. *Clin Cancer Res*. 2013;19(15):4239-4248.
61. Thein KZ, Velcheti V, Mooers BHM, Wu J, Subbiah V. Precision therapy for RET-altered cancers with RET inhibitors. *Trends Cancer*. 2021;7(12):1074-1088.
62. Niedziela M. Thyroid nodules. *Best Pract Res Clin Endocrinol Metab*. 2014;28(2):245-277.
63. Haugen BR, Alexander EK, Bible KC, et al. 2015 American Thyroid Association management guidelines for adult patients with thyroid nodules and differentiated thyroid cancer: the American Thyroid Association guidelines task force on thyroid nodules and differentiated thyroid cancer. *Thyroid*. 2016; 26(1):1-133.
64. Mussa A, Andrea MD, Motta M, Mormile A, Palestini N, Corrias A. Predictors of malignancy in children with thyroid nodules. *J Pediatr*. 2015;167(4):886-892.e1.
65. Hay ID, Losada TG, Reinalda MS, Honetschlager JA, Richards ML, Thompson GB. Long-term outcome in 215 children and adolescents with papillary thyroid cancer treated during 1940 through 2008. *World J Surg*. 2010;34(6):1192-1202.
66. Macedo FI, Mittal VK. Total thyroidectomy versus lobectomy as initial operation for small unilateral papillary thyroid carcinoma: a meta-analysis. *Surg Oncol*. 2015;24(2):117-122.
67. Baumgarten H, Jenks CM, Isaza A, et al. Bilateral papillary thyroid cancer in children: risk factors and frequency of postoperative diagnosis. *J Pediatr Surg*. 2020;55(6):1117-1122.
68. Wang W, Su X, He K, et al. Comparison of the clinicopathologic features and prognosis of bilateral versus unilateral multifocal papillary thyroid cancer: an updated study with more than 2000 consecutive patients. *Cancer*. 2016;122(2):198-206.
69. Golpanian S, Perez EA, Tashiro J, Lew JI, Sola JE, Hogan AR. Pediatric papillary thyroid carcinoma: outcomes and survival predictors in 2504 surgical patients. *Pediatr Surg Int*. 2016;32(3):201-208.
70. Kim K-J, Kim S-M, Lee YS, et al. Prognostic significance of tumor multifocality in papillary thyroid carcinoma and its relationship with primary tumor size: a retrospective study of 2,309 consecutive patients. *Ann Surg Oncol*. 2015;22(1): 125-131.

SUGGESTED READINGS

Balachandar S, La Quaglia M, Tuttle RM, Heller G, Ghossein RA, Sklar CA. Pediatric differentiated thyroid carcinoma of follicular cell origin: prognostic significance of histologic subtypes. *Thyroid*. 2016;26(2):219-226.

Bauer AJ. Papillary and follicular thyroid cancer in children and adolescents: current approach and future directions. *Semin Pediatr Surg*. 2020;29(3):150920.

Christison-Lagay ER, Baertschiger RM, Dinauer C, et al. Pediatric differentiated thyroid carcinoma: an update from the APSA Cancer Committee. *J Pediatr Surg*. 2020;55(11):2273-2283.

Francis GL, Waguespack SG, Bauer AJ, et al. Management guidelines for children with thyroid nodules and differentiated thyroid cancer: the American Thyroid Association guidelines task force on pediatric thyroid cancer. *Thyroid*. 2015;25(7):716-759.

Graves CE, Gosnell JE. Medullary thyroid carcinoma in children. *Semin Pediatr Surg*. 2020;29(3):150921.

Martinez-Rios C, Daneman A, Bajno L, van der Kaay DCM, Moineddin R, Wasserman JD. Utility of adult-based ultrasound malignancy risk stratifications in pediatric thyroid nodules. *Pediatr Radiol*. 2018;48(1):74-84.

Niedziela M, Breborowicz D, Trejster E, Korman E. Hot nodules in children and adolescents in western Poland from 1996 to 2000: clinical analysis of 31 patients. *J Pediatr Endocrinol Metab*. 2002;15(6):823-830.

Wells SA Jr, Asa SL, Dralle H, et al. Revised American Thyroid Association guidelines for the management of medullary thyroid carcinoma: the American Thyroid Association Guidelines Task Force on medullary thyroid carcinoma. *Thyroid*. 2015;25(6):567-610.

Open Thyroidectomy: Principles for Performing Safe Thyroid Surgery

21

Jennifer T. Castle, MD
William B. Inabnet, III, MD, MHA

INTRODUCTION

Thyroidectomy is one of the most commonly performed surgical procedures. Thyroid surgery is often classified as a low-risk operation, yet adverse outcomes can greatly impair quality of life and the cost of health-care delivery. Though efforts are underway to decrease variability in the surgical management of thyroid disease, adherence to sound principles can minimize the chance of adverse outcomes. This chapter aims to discuss the essential foundational elements for performing safe thyroid surgery.

PREOPERATIVE EVALUATION

History & Exam

When evaluating a patient for thyroid surgery a detailed history and physical examination should be performed. An accurate account of prior neck surgeries and radiation is important for future surgical and medical treatment planning. Physical exam of the neck can assist a surgeon in better determining the relative size, texture, and shape of the gland which may influence surgical decision-making. Physical exam should also include evaluation of both sides of the neck for lymphadenopathy. A patient's voice is evaluated for character and strength as some patients may have preoperative dysfunction of their vocal cords from nerve involvement or injury from prior surgery. A flexible laryngoscopy is better suited to evaluate for any dysfunction by directly visualizing the movements of the vocal cords. Flexible laryngoscopy is discussed more thoroughly in Chapter 31.

Labs

No matter the disease process, all thyroidectomy patients should have their thyroid function evaluated prior to surgery to ensure that they are euthyroid. Lab studies for thyroid function include thyroid-stimulating hormone (TSH), free thyroxine (T4), and selective use of total triiodothyronine (T3) levels in the setting of suspected subclinical hyperthyroidism. Thyroid antibody testing can be useful not only in establishing or confirming an autoimmune diagnosis but also in obtaining informed consent when discussing the risks of surgery. For example, markedly elevated thyroid peroxidase (TPO) antibody levels correlate with the extent of Hashimoto thyroiditis; when these data are combined with physical examination and ultrasound findings, the surgeon may wish to discuss the higher incidence of temporary and permanent hypoparathyroidism in patients with severe Hashimoto thyroiditis.[1] If a diagnosis of Graves' disease has not been firmly established, TSH receptor antibodies should be measured. Routine thyroglobulin (Tg) testing prior to surgery is not advised; rather Tg levels are reserved for dynamic surveillance following total thyroidectomy for well-differentiated thyroid cancer.

Ultrasound

Ultrasound is an essential tool for evaluating the thyroid gland and plays an integral role in disease evaluation, operative planning, and surveillance. Surgeon-performed ultrasound evaluation of the thyroid and lateral neck is essential preoperatively. Surgeon-performed ultrasound has been associated with less incorrect index operations through more accurate evaluation of the lateral neck for lymph nodes as well as a more extensive evaluation of thyroid lesions.[2] Ultrasound helps the surgeon determine the size of the thyroid gland, evaluate for extrathyroidal extension of cancerous lesions, inspect the lateral neck for suspicious lymph nodes, perform fine-needle aspiration of suspicious nodules, or as a tool for monitoring nodules.

Having a firm understanding of the size, shape, and location of malignant or suspicious nodules assists with preoperative risk stratification and influences informed consent. For example, if a malignant nodule abuts the capsule of the posterior thyroid gland near the anatomical location of the recurrent laryngeal nerve (RLN), a more detailed discussion of operative strategies for managing recurrent nerve invasion may ensue. This scenario is particularly relevant if the nodule is located near the insertion site of the RLN. Ultrasound images can be viewed with the patient in real time, increasing their understanding of different operative scenarios. Moreover, developing such partnership with the patient whereby the patient participates in decision-making has been shown to decrease the incidence of litigation.[3]

PERIOPERATIVE CONSIDERATIONS

Antibiotics

Perioperative antibiotics are routinely used in general surgery procedures as well as head and neck procedures with antibiotic choice depending on the contamination status of the surgical procedure. Although they are useful in preventing surgical site infections and complications thereafter in surgeries at high risk for infection, their utility in thyroidectomies is less clear. According to the literature available, the incidence of surgical site infection following thyroidectomy via the typical anterior neck incision is 0.09% to 2%. Multiple studies have shown no statistical benefit from the administration of perioperative antibiotics in reducing postoperative infection rate in clean neck procedures. Although every patient should be evaluated individually for their risk of surgical site infection and need for perioperative antibiotics, in general, it is not recommended to use perioperative antibiotics in routine practice for clean thyroid cases.[4,5]

Venous Thromboembolism Prophylaxis

Appropriate use of chemical and mechanical venous thromboembolism prophylaxis is vital in every patient population. While some patients are at increased risk of thrombotic events, this risk must be weighed against their risk for bleeding before utilizing chemical prophylaxis. This is more pertinent in the thyroidectomy patient as even a small bleed in the operative field could be catastrophic postoperatively due to its compressive effects on the airway. Given the published rate of VTE following thyroidectomy is less than 0.2%, it is the strong recommendation from the American Association of Endocrine Surgeons to employ chemical VTE prophylaxis only in select patients at higher risk for VTE.[4] Every patient's thromboembolic versus bleed risk should be determined preoperatively and the decision for chemical prophylaxis made at that time. Whether or not chemical prophylaxis is given, mechanical prophylaxis with sequential compression devices on the legs and early ambulation should be used routinely as these prophylactic methods are not associated with increased operative bed bleeding.

Steroids

Postoperative nausea and vomiting (PONV) are well-known side effects of anesthetics with incidence as high as 84% in the thyroidectomy population.[6] Beyond just the general patient discomfort, PONV is associated with increased complications and health-care costs. A one-time dose of steroid, such as dexamethasone, preoperatively has been shown to decrease PONV after thyroidectomy. While some surgeons have concerns for steroid-induced complications postoperatively, these studies did not demonstrate any wound-healing issues nor steroid-induced diabetes.[7] Multimodal perioperative nausea prophylaxis is encouraged to reduce postoperative complications, the addition of single-dose steroid preoperatively is beneficial without increased risk of complication.

INTRAOPERATIVE CONSIDERATIONS

Patient Positioning

The patient position is crucial in assisting the surgeon in having the ideal exposure for dissection. The general goal of patient position is to fully expose the anterior neck without positioning the patient in a way that would cause postoperative pain or disability. Generally, the patient will be in a supine position with head extended and both arms tucked at the patient's sides. It is important to not overextend the neck as this can cause postoperative discomfort. If the neck is still not well exposed in this position, a roll can be tucked under the shoulders. While tucking the arms, make sure the thumbs are pointing up and the wrist is in a neutral position. It is also important to make sure anesthesia still has open access to any IVs placed in the arms after tucking them. The finer points to positioning include making sure the endotracheal tube and associated wires are not draping over the operative space and that all ECG leads are both placed outside of the operative area and without wires crossing this area. As detailed in the following discussion, all wires and probes used for nerve monitoring should be inserted and secured prior to prepping the patient and ensuring an appropriate signal is obtained. The patient should be prepped from their chin down to the nipple line and extend bilaterally to cover the entire exposed neck and shoulders. Draping technique is surgeon's preference and should facilitate a safe and sterile operation.

Intraoperative Nerve Monitoring

Intraoperative nerve monitoring (IONM) utilizes electrostimulation to test the functionality of the RLN throughout the operation by recording the vocal response to RLN stimulation. Although there are different probes on the market, they all essentially function the same way. The system requires an endotracheal tube with sensory electrodes to detect vocal cord movement attached to a monitor box to interpret the input data and provide the surgical team visual and/or auditory electromyographic (EMG) signal response. Also attached to the monitor box are grounding electrode inputs from needles placed in the skin of the patient (typically around the shoulders). These work in conjunction so that when the RLN is stimulated the vocal cords will move in response creating an EMG that is projected via the monitor box. It is important to note that the surgeon must coordinate with the anesthesiologist to not only use the appropriate endotracheal tube with electrodes positioned correctly between the vocal cords, but to also avoid use of long-acting paralytics throughout the case. Because this technology relies on EMG, neuromuscular blockade agents will impede response in the vocal cords to nerve stimulation.

IONM was originally used as an intermittent monitor in that the functionality of the nerve is only checked at various points through the procedure by the surgeon manually stimulating the nerve with the probe. There are other systems on the market that do continuous monitoring of the nerve throughout the procedure. These allow for more immediate surgical response to loss of signal; however, it requires a more extensive dissection of the nerves. Given the published data are conflicting in benefit versus risk of continuous monitoring it is not currently recommended to be used in routine practice.

There is not a consensus on the use of intermittent IONM in the published data on prevention of RLN injury. Various studies have suggested benefit in decreasing RLN injury; however, these have been hindered by statistical insignificance with larger systematic reviews and meta-analyses demonstrating no significant difference with use of IONM. IONM may be beneficial in reducing RLN injury and palsy, particularly in high-risk patients, but it should not replace direct visualization of the nerve and safe surgical dissection techniques.[8]

Incision

The Kocher or collar incision originally used for thyroidectomy is typically taught as an anterior mid-neck incision of approximately 8 to 10 cm in length. As surgical techniques have progressed, the length of the classically described incision is rarely required. Today, the standard incision is approximately 4 to 8 cm in length with minimally invasive open thyroidectomy incisions described at 2.5 to 3.5 cm in length. Many surgeons place the incision one fingerbreadth above the sternal notch while also attempting to place it within a natural skin crease for cosmetic effects.[1] As in other specialties of surgery, the drive for improved patient satisfaction has led to pushes for smaller and more discreet incisions. Accordingly, some surgeons, including the senior author of this chapter, prefer to place the incision higher in the neck. A more superior incision allows direct access to the superior pole vessels which are somewhat fixed in their location; after dividing the superior vascular pedicle, the inferior aspect of the gland, which is more mobile, can be elevated through the small incision permitting facile identification of the relevant nerve and parathyroid anatomy. Ultimately, the surgeon must decide what length and location incision is safest for each patient based on native neck anatomy, pathology of the disease, and size of the specimen to be removed.

Exposure

The incision is carried down through the subcutaneous tissue until the platysma is encountered. This is a superficial, thin, fan-shaped muscle that is divided along the entirety of the incision. Subplatysmal flaps are created on both sides of the incision. After this maneuver, you should have good visualization of the strap muscles which are then separated along the midline and retracted laterally or divided. It is not generally recommended to divide the strap muscles unless necessary to gain safe exposure to an enlarged thyroid or if strap resection is required due to gross involvement or adherence to the diseased thyroid. Once past the strap muscles, dissection and delivery of the thyroid from the neck can begin.

Dissection

Dissection of the thyroid gland sometimes depends on the etiology of the disease as well as the size of the gland. Necessities of disease-specific dissections will be discussed in their respective chapters.

A. Thyroid Gland and Recurrent Laryngeal Nerve

Whether doing a lobectomy or total thyroidectomy, dissection is begun by dissecting the anterior capsule of the thyroid from the overlying strap muscles starting at the isthmus and extending laterally. Once at the lateral border, the carotid sheath should be exposed, permitting stimulation of the vagus nerve. Dissection to the carotid sheath and identification of the vagus nerve prior to extensive dissection of the thyroid gland is paramount if utilizing IONM. This is particularly important on the right side where an aberrant innominate artery causes an atypical course of the RLN making it more prone to injury if not first identified. The middle thyroid vein will be encountered along the lateral edge of the thyroid lobe and should be ligated close to the thyroid capsule. The superior pole of the thyroid is also interrogated as the external branch of the superior laryngeal nerve usually runs with the superior pole vascular bundle. Once the superior pole is free, the thyroid lobe can be retracted anteriorly and medially. The RLN should be identified and traced until insertion in the larynx. While IONM assists the surgeon, it should not be a substitute for direct visualization. Throughout the dissection of the thyroid, all vessels should be ligated as close to the thyroid capsule as possible without violating the capsule while ensuring visualization of the RLN away from the tissue you intend to transect. This dissection is continued along the posterior border of the thyroid gland with division of the ligament of Berry. If performing a total thyroidectomy, the contralateral side is dissected in a similar fashion. If there is concern for injury or palsy to the ipsilateral RLN, continuation to the contralateral side is not advised. It is recommended that a completion thyroidectomy be performed as a staged procedure following investigation of vocal cord function with flexible laryngoscopy.

B. Parathyroid Glands

The parathyroid glands are typically located behind the thyroid, nearly adherent to the posterior capsule. Careful dissection along the posterior inferior and superior thyroid poles with identification of each gland assists in their preservation. The surgeon must also be aware of the parathyroid vascular pedicle and perform careful dissection to prevent devascularization of the parathyroid glands. If the parathyroid is intentionally or unintentionally removed or devascularized, it can be cut into multiple pieces and implanted in the sternocleidomastoid muscles.

Vessel Sealing Systems

There are many vessel sealing systems on the market that have been compared to conventional means for hemostasis. Conventional methods include suture tying, vascular clips, and electrocautery. Ultrasonic devices have been found to be associated with shorter operating room times without increase in complications compared to conventional methods and electrothermal bipolar devices. Although some smaller studies found the electrothermal bipolar device to be as expedient as ultrasonic devices, in all the published studies both forms of devices are faster than conventional methods and safe for the patient.[9,10]

Closure

A. Hemostasis

The key aspect of closing is to ensure hemostasis. As mentioned earlier and discussed in further detail later this chapter, postoperative bleeding can be deadly. Extensive irrigation to disrupt any unstable clots should be done. Hemostatic agents, both biologically active and physical agents, are readily available to help achieve hemostasis although costly. The published data regarding the utility of these hemostatic agents to prevent postoperative bleeding are conflicting. This was addressed in a meta-analysis in 2018 which studied multiple different biological and physical agents versus conventional hemostatic techniques and no difference in rate of hematomas, seromas, or infection was found. The authors did find operative time to be reduced with the use of physical agents and a decrease in drain output and hospital stay when biologically active agents were used.[11] Given the cost of these hemostatic agents without clear benefit, their use in routine practice during thyroidectomies is questionable and their use is certainly not a substitute for good surgical technique.

Prior to beginning the multilayer closure of the incision, the surgeon can ask the anesthesiologist to perform a Valsalva maneuver, increasing peak airway pressures (PAP) and thus increasing internal jugular vein pressure to help locate any bleeding. The value at which to raise the PAP to and duration of the maneuver to most effectively find any areas of bleeding while not causing harm to the patient has not yet been determined. While some studies report safe use of up to 50 cm H_2O for 30 seconds, most surgeons and anesthesiologists still have reservations going above 30 cm H_2O due to concern for barotrauma. While these studies do show increased bleed-point detection following Valsalva, postoperative hemorrhagic complications are unchanged thus throwing into question the actual benefit of this maneuver intraoperatively.[12]

B. Multilayer Closure

The incision is closed in layers. Whether the strap muscles were divided for access or simply separated at the midline, they should be reapproximated with absorbable suture. Traditionally, the platysma is also closed using absorbable suture, however, recent literature shows no comparable difference whether the platysma is closed or not with some suggestion that sutureless closure of the platysma has less immediate postoperative pain.

Like incisions elsewhere, the skin of the transverse neck incision can be closed in a multitude of ways including sutures, staples, adhesives, or skin glue. The high visibility of this incision makes cosmetic effect a major factor in closing technique. As staples are associated with poorer immediate postoperative cosmesis and painful removal, their use in neck incisions has fallen out of favor. Overall, the published data available has not demonstrated a clear method that is superior to the others regarding postoperative pain, cosmesis, and wound complications.[13]

C. Drain Placement

Prophylactic use of closed suction drainage in the postoperative thyroid patient has no impact on postoperative seroma or hematoma collection. Use of a drain is associated with increased pain, increased wound infection, prolonged hospital stays, and increased odds of hematoma formation. Use of drains in patients with large thyroids, preoperative use of anticoagulation, and intraoperative bleeding have also not been shown to be beneficial in prevention of postoperative fluid collections. Drain placement after open thyroidectomy is not routinely recommended.[14]

POSTOPERATIVE CONSIDERATIONS

Disposition

In 2013, the American Thyroid Association issued a statement outlining the safety of outpatient thyroidectomy in a select group of patients. This included patients with no major comorbidities, ASA less than 4, effective preoperative education, an adult at home able to help, and a home close to the care facility. Subsequent studies have shown outpatient thyroidectomy in clinically appropriate patients is as safe as inpatient thyroidectomy. Patients with more comorbidities such as dialysis dependence, coagulopathy (either native or medicine induced), and heart or lung disease, among others, should stay for at least a 23-hour observation period rather than same day surgery. Observation is typically recommended to watch for hematoma formation. As hematoma formation that requires operative intervention typically forms within the first 24 hours postoperatively, longer hospitalizations are rarely ever indicated. While cost should not influence a surgeon to go against what is safest for the patient, a study published in 2021 suggested a cost benefit to outpatient thyroidectomy but only on medically appropriate patients.[4,15]

Thyroid Hormone Replacement

The need for thyroid hormone replacement as well as the amount of replacement is dependent on the extent of surgery and the pathology of the disease. In general, thyroid hormone replacement following total thyroidectomy is patient weight dependent with starting dose of 1.6 μg/kg daily. Hormone replacement following hemithyroidectomy is rarely indicated and should be evaluated on a patient-by-patient basis.

Complications

A. Hematoma

One of the most feared complications for an endocrine surgeon is a postoperative hematoma in the neck. These patients present with severe respiratory distress rather than any symptoms of hemorrhagic shock. This is due to the compression imposed on the trachea by even a small amount of bleeding confined in the operative bed. Hematomas requiring operative intervention occur in less than 5% of neck surgeries with more recent publications reporting a rate closer to 1%. With the severity of consequences of this complication, it is important that patients are appropriately educated prior to surgery of the dangers and signs of hematoma formation and when to seek help. This is particularly important as outpatient surgery for thyroidectomies is growing in popularity. Signs of hematoma formation include swelling of the neck, tachypnea, stridor, and oxygen desaturation. Not all patients with impending airway collapse will exhibit all of these symptoms. The most important factor in management of these patients is achieving an airway. If the patient is unstable and you are unable to expeditiously get to the operating room, opening of the operative incision at bedside can be performed. To appropriately relieve the pressure from a forming hematoma all layers of the incision must be opened including the skin, the platysma, and the strap muscle closures. Although bedside decompression can be stressful for the patient, sedative medications should not be provided as this can cause loss of the airway. Similarly, if the patient can be transported to the operating room first, the incision should be opened, and hematoma evacuated prior to induction and intubation. Once the hematoma is evacuated, the wound should be explored, and hemostasis achieved.[16,17]

Historically, bleeding disorders including use of anticoagulants/antiplatelets, multiple comorbidities, male gender, bilateral dissection, neck dissection, and prior neck surgery are among the risk factors for hematoma formation. While some of the agents and devices mentioned earlier in this chapter may mitigate the bleeding risk in such patients, they do not replace careful dissection and adequate surgical technique ensuring hemostasis throughout the case and prior to closure.

B. Seroma

Seroma formation after thyroidectomy is usually benign and self-resolved. There is not much published on the management of seromas after thyroidectomy, but some studies utilized serial aspiration given its efficacy in resolution of seromas after breast surgery.[2] If the seroma is symptomatically manageable and without secondary signs of infection, it is reasonable to manage with observation alone. As stated earlier in this chapter, drain placement does not reduce the risk of fluid accumulation. Antibiotics should only be used if signs of infection are present.[18]

C. Chyle Leak

Chyle leak is typically associated more with lateral neck dissections; however, injury to the thoracic duct can occur in thyroidectomy with central lymph node dissection alone. The incidence of chyle leak is 0.5% to 1.4% after thyroidectomy, higher with neck dissections. Symptoms include bulging of the neck similar to what would be seen in hematoma or seroma; however, visualization of the fluid would reveal a milky fluid. Poorly controlled chyle leaks can lead to poor wound healing, respiratory compromise from chylothorax, electrolyte imbalances, and malnutrition. Prevention of injury to the thoracic duct involves careful dissection along the inferior thyroid particularly when the dissection extends toward the mediastinum. If injury to the duct is identified intraoperatively, it can be ligated during the index operation. Management of postoperatively identified chyle leaks depends on the output. Low-volume chyle leaks can be managed conservatively with a medium-chain fatty acid diet, nonfat diet, or nil per os (NPO) if a short course is suspected. For chyle leaks of high output, or those that fail conservative management, the thoracic duct can be embolized by interventional radiology or surgical reexploration can be employed to find and ligate the thoracic duct.[19]

D. Hypoparathyroidism and Hypocalcemia

Hypocalcemia secondary to hypoparathyroidism after thyroidectomy surgery is one of the most common complications after thyroidectomy. It is secondary to either removal or devascularization of the parathyroid glands during the thyroid dissection. Although meticulous dissection should be done with careful surveillance and preservation of the parathyroid glands, removal or devascularization may be unavoidable.

Symptoms of hypocalcemia range from mild (peripheral extremity and perioral paresthesia, muscle cramping, Chvostek sign, Trousseau sign) to severe (seizures, heart failure). Severely symptomatic hypocalcemia should be treated with intravenous calcium replacement. Mildly symptomatic forms can be treated with oral replacement, whereas asymptomatic hypocalcemia may not require any supplementation. As the majority of post-thyroidectomy parathyroid dysfunction is transient, the need for calcium supplementation should be reevaluated at each visit based on patient symptomatology and calcium levels. Magnesium levels should be checked and replaced if low in persistently hypocalcemic patients.

E. Nerve Injury

The nerves most at risk, and most clinically relevant, during a thyroidectomy are the RLN and the external branch of the superior laryngeal nerves (EBSLN). Injury of the EBSLN is clinically benign with symptoms of vocal fatigue, deeper voice, and difficulty with vocal intonation/projection. While none of these symptoms are life-threatening, they can be distressing to patients, particularly in those where voice and singing are a major part of their lives. Careful dissection and identification of the nerve at the superior pole of the thyroid helps prevent injury.

Injury of the RLNs can result in symptoms ranging from mild postoperative hoarseness to pulmonary obstruction requiring tracheostomy. The RLNs innervate the posterior cricoarytenoid muscles, the only muscle that abducts the vocal cords. Injury to the RLN causes medialization of the ipsilateral vocal cord. Injury to bilateral RLNs causes medialization and apposition of bilateral vocal cords which can lead to severe respiratory arrest and necessity for tracheostomy. IONM is gaining popularity in identifying the RLN; however, direct visualization of the nerve via careful dissection and conscientious traction by a skilled surgeon remains the most-effective method to prevent RLN injury.

F. Dysphagia

Postoperative dysphagia is a difficult symptom to evaluate after thyroidectomy as this is a frequent symptom of thyroid pathology preoperatively. The etiology of postoperative dysphagia is not well understood and likely multivariate. Dysphagia typically resolves within 6 months after surgery without intervention in patients where RLN injury was not the root cause of the dysfunction. It is important to support the patient if they are unable to maintain nutrition and hydration on their own.[20]

G. Tracheal Injury

Tracheal injuries that are identified intraoperatively should be repaired at that time with or without tracheostomy depending on extent of the injury. If not identified in the operating room, tracheal injuries can present as subcutaneous emphysema, pneumomediastinum, pneumothoraces, and wound infection. Delayed tracheal injury from tracheal necrosis, although rare, has been noted in the literature. Following identification of a delayed tracheal injury, reexploration with extensive wound irrigation and tracheostomy was reported. Given the rarity of tracheal injury, prevention and management of these injuries in the thyroidectomy population is not well documented.[21]

H. Esophageal Injury

Esophageal injury during thyroidectomy is extremely rare and not well reported in the literature. When noted intraoperatively, primary repair should be performed and drain placement may be appropriate. The cases of missed esophageal injury that present postoperatively are more complicated. Esophageal perforation is associated with high mortality and morbidity with early detection being imperative in limiting damage to surrounding tissue, as well as the systemic response. Esophageal injury can be managed in various ways with limited data indicating superiority in post-thyroidectomy patients. Reexploration, wound washout, esophageal repair, and wide drainage can be employed. Endoscopic interventions are advancing rapidly and may be helpful in small, easily manageable defects or subsequent esophageal stenosis. Contained injuries can also be managed with strict NPO with drainage of any fluid collections. Antibiotics and antifungals should be administered as soon as esophageal injury is detected postoperatively.[22]

REFERENCES

1. Thomusch O, Sekulla C, Billmann F, et al. Risk profile analysis and complications after surgery for autoimmune thyroid disease. *Br J Surg*. 2018;105(6):677-685.
2. Monteiro R, Han A, Etiwy M, et al. Importance of surgeon-performed ultrasound in the preoperative nodal assessment of patients with potential thyroid malignancy. *Surgery*. 2018;163(1):112-117.

3. Lagoo J, Berry WR, Miller K, et al. Multisource evaluation of surgeon behavior is associated with malpractice claims. *Ann Surg*. 2019;270(1):84-90.
4. Patel KN, Yip L, Lubitz CC, et al. The American Association of Endocrine Surgeons Guidelines for the Definitive Surgical Management of Thyroid Disease in Adults. *Ann Surg*. 2020;271(3):e21-e93.
5. Vamvakidis K, Rellos K, Tsourma M, et al. Antibiotic prophylaxis for clean neck surgery. *Ann R Coll Surg Engl*. 2017;99(5):410-412.
6. Cho YJ, Choi GJ, Ahn EJ, Kang H. Pharmacologic interventions for postoperative nausea and vomiting after thyroidectomy: a systematic review and network meta-analysis. *PLoS One*. 2021;16(1):e0243865.
7. Tarantino I, Warschkow R, Beutner U, et al. Efficacy of a single preoperative dexamethasone dose to prevent nausea and vomiting after thyroidectomy (the tPONV study): a randomized, double-blind, placebo-controlled clinical trial. *Ann Surg*. 2015;262(6):934-940.
8. Yang S, Zhou L, Lu Z, Ma B, Ji Q, Wang Y. Systematic review with meta-analysis of intraoperative neuromonitoring during thyroidectomy. *Int J Surg*. 2017;39:104-113.
9. Siu JM, McCarty JC, Gadkaree S, et al. Association of vessel-sealant devices vs conventional hemostasis with postoperative neck hematoma after thyroid operations. *JAMA Surg*. 2019;154(11):e193146.
10. Luo Y, Li X, Dong J, Sun W. A comparison of surgical outcomes and complications between hemostatic devices for thyroid surgery: a network meta-analysis. *Eur Arch Otorhinolaryngol*. 2017;274(3):1269-1278.
11. Khadra H, Bakeer M, Hauch A, Hu T, Kandil E. Hemostatic agent use in thyroid surgery: a meta-analysis. *Gland Surg*. 2018;7(Suppl 1):S34-S41.
12. Beyoglu CA, Teksoz S, Ozdilek A, et al. A comparison of the efficacy of three different peak airway pressures on intraoperative bleeding point detection in patients undergoing thyroidectomy: a randomized, controlled, clinical trial. *BMC Surg*. 2020;20(1):69.
13. Lee K, Ward N, Oremule B, Mani N. Optimal wound closure techniques for thyroid and parathyroid surgery: a systematic review of cosmetic outcomes. *Clin Otolaryngol*. Nov 2019; 44(6):905-913.
14. Soh TCF, Ong QJ, Yip HM. Complications of neck drains in thyroidectomies: a systematic review and meta-analysis. *Laryngoscope*. 2021;131(3):690-700.
15. Lee DJ, Chin CJ, Hong CJ, Perera S, Witterick IJ. Outpatient versus inpatient thyroidectomy: a systematic review and meta-analysis. *Head Neck*. 2018;40(1):192-202.
16. Mahoney RC, Vossler JD, Woodruff SL, Murayama KM. Predictors and consequences of hematoma after thyroidectomy: an American College of Surgeons National Surgical Quality Improvement Program Database Analysis. *J Surg Res*. 2021;260:481-487.
17. Fan C, Zhou X, Su G, et al. Risk factors for neck hematoma requiring surgical re-intervention after thyroidectomy: a systematic review and meta-analysis. *BMC Surg*. 2019;19(1):98.
18. Ramouz A, Rasihashemi SZ, Daghigh F, Faraji E, Rouhani S. Predisposing factors for seroma formation in patients undergoing thyroidectomy: cross-sectional study. *Ann Med Surg (Lond)*. 2017;23:8-12.
19. Delaney SW, Shi H, Shokrani A, Sinha UK. Management of chyle leak after head and neck surgery: review of current treatment strategies. *Int J Otolaryngol*. 2017;2017:8362874.
20. Marchese MR, Galli J, D'Alatri L, et al. Neck complaints before and after uncomplicated thyroidectomy: prevalence, postoperative outcome and relationships with thyroid weight and reflux like symptoms. *Endocrine*. 2021;73(1):98-106.
21. Shew M, Boyd C, Kraft S. Delayed multifocal tracheal injury following thyroidectomy: a case report and review of the literature. *Cureus*. 2020;12(5):e8164.
22. Chen S, Shapira-Galitz Y, Garber D, Amin MR. Management of Iatrogenic cervical esophageal perforations: a narrative review. *JAMA Otolaryngol Head Neck Surg*. 2020;146(5): 488-494.

22 Thyroidectomy Procedure: TOETVA & BABA

Gustavo Fernandez-Ranvier, MD, PhD
Benjamin Lieberman, DO
Elliot Scott, MD

TRANSORAL ENDOSCOPIC THYROIDECTOMY VESTIBULAR APPROACH

History & Development

The emergence of minimally invasive techniques and remote access technology has dramatically changed surgical approaches over the last 30 years, and thyroid surgery has been no exception to this trend. Avoiding an anterior cervical scar is the main advantage of minimally invasive techniques in thyroid surgery, but transoral thyroidectomy offers the chance to avoid all skin incisions.[1,2] For patients who have a tendency toward hypertrophic and keloid scarring, this offers a particular advantage. Beginning in 2008 with cadaveric and porcine studies, transoral endoscopic thyroidectomy (TOET) was introduced.[1] Access through intraoral mucosal incisions avoids any cutaneous scars; thus, TOET is a natural orifice transluminal endoscopic surgery (NOTES) procedure. In addition, by keeping all incisions to mucosal surfaces, there is no risk of hypertrophic or keloid scarring.[2]

The original description of TOET required a sublingual dissection through the floor of the mouth to access the thyroid gland. Early adoption of TOET was stymied by never-before-seen complications and the steep learning curve associated with violating the floor of the mouth. Patients had a high rate of mental nerve injury, causing temporary or permanent chin and lower lip numbness. The viewing port offered a relatively limited exposure and resulted in a high rate of conversion to open.[1]

In 2014, after further cadaveric studies, Dr Angkoon Anuwong modified the original sublingual dissection, dissecting over the chin via the lower vestibule of the lip to develop a subplatysmal plane with a top-down view of the thyroid. This would be called transoral endoscopic thyroidectomy vestibular approach (TOETVA).[3]

Indications & Contraindications

The most common reason for a patient to seek out TOETVA is to avoid having an anterior neck scar from a conventional open thyroidectomy (COT). The additional advantage of TOETVA is that it leaves no cutaneous scars.[3,4]

Most surgeons experienced in TOETVA have recognized certain patient characteristics that are associated with success of the TOETVA technique. In Dr Anuwong's original case series, inclusion criteria were thyroid gland diameter less than 10 cm, benign tumors (eg, cysts or multinodular goiters), follicular neoplasms, papillary microcarcinoma, and Graves' disease or other types of thyroiditis.[3,5,6]

Exclusion criteria were substernal goiters, previous neck surgery or radiation, and dental braces. In a later series, dental braces were no longer a contraindication. Surgeons point out other inclusion and exclusion factors to make TOETVA a success. For example, the patient must have sufficient cervical mobility to tolerate the extension required to insert the ports.[3]

Comparison to Conventional Thyroidectomy

A growing body of literature surrounding TOETVA establishes it as an efficacious alternative to the gold standard of COT.[7,8] In a recent meta-analysis comparing TOETVA and COT, differences in intraoperative and postoperative outcomes between the two groups were examined. For intraoperative outcomes, there were no significant differences found for blood loss. There was, however, a significant increase in operative time in the TOETVA cases compared with COT.[7] This is a common theme in studies comparing the two techniques, although the operative time does decrease with surgeon experience.[2] For postoperative outcomes, transient and permanent recurrent laryngeal nerve (RLN) injuries were rare in both TOETVA and COT groups and no significant difference was found between them. In addition, no significant difference in transient hypocalcemia was found between either group.[7,9,10]

TOETVA is establishing itself as a viable alternative to COT for both benign and malignant disease. In a retrospective study comparing TOETVA and COT in patients with benign pathology only, there was no significant difference found between blood loss, postoperative hypothyroidism, or RLN injury. Operative time, again, was found to be significantly longer in the TOETVA group.[11,12]

TOETVA also functions similarly to COT regarding length of stay (LOS). There are cultural differences globally that impact LOS in thyroid surgery patients.[2] In Asian countries, patients typically stay anywhere from 2 to 3 days while in North America patients may stay overnight, or even have thyroidectomy as an ambulatory procedure. While not standard practice globally, TOETVA has been shown to be safe as an ambulatory procedure as well. In a retrospective review of 70 TOETVA and 70 COT patients who underwent their surgery in an ambulatory setting, there was no difference in complication rates between the two groups.[13] The TOETVA patients were observed for multiple hours before discharge, but those who met strict criteria were safe when discharged home.

Interestingly, there was no significant difference between rates of infection in COT and TOETVA, despite there being a difference in wound class.[14] COT is classified as a clean procedure and as such its reported infection rate is exceedingly rare, between 0.09% and 2%. Prophylactic antibiotics are not routinely recommended for COT although they are often used.[8] TOETVA, as it violates the oral mucosa, is considered a clean-contaminated procedure.[2] Despite the difference in wound class, there does not appear to be a significant difference in rates of infection between TOETVA and COT. Routine use of prophylactic antibiotics is recommended and almost universally used for TOETVA cases.[3,5,6,9] However, antibiotic duration in a patient who underwent TOETVA is a question that is actively being explored. The only prospective randomized trial comparing prophylactic dosing (single preoperative dose) and extended dosing (7 days of PO amoxicillin-clavulanate) in TOETVA patients showed no significant difference in infection rate.[15]

Despite its similar complication profile and patient satisfaction, TOETVA does differ from COT with the introduction of novel—although generally mild—complications and an additional learning curve.[9,14,16] Temporary mental nerve injury, with the symptoms of lip and/or chin numbness, is seen in 0% to 27% of patients depending on the case series.[14,15,17] The mental nerve emerges from the mental foramen of the mandible at the site of the first premolar teeth. The mental nerve can be injured by the lateral vestibular ports if they are not kept medial to the canine teeth. In all cases, injury has not been permanent with mean time to recovery being 8 weeks.

Although safe and effective, TOETVA can be a challenging technique that requires confidence with laparoscopic surgery and familiarity with thyroid anatomy. TOETVA gives excellent exposure to the entire gland, but from a top-down perspective. As such, the learning curve for TOETVA is still being established. There are several published papers on the TOETVA learning curve, all of which focus on operative time as the primary outcome. The learning curve as described in these studies is between 11 and 53 cases.[14,16,17]

Technique[2,3,5,6]

The patient is nasotracheally intubated and positioned supine with the neck in extension. The patient is prepped from the nose superiorly to the sternal notch inferiorly, and the mouth is prepped with a chlorhexidine wash. Preoperative prophylactic antibiotics are administered, typically IV amoxicillin-clavulanic acid or ceftriaxone and metronidazole. The operating surgeon is positioned at the head of the patient, with the monitor at the patient's feed.

Three 5 mm incisions are then made at the vestibule of the lower lip. The central incision is transverse between the two inferior incisors. The lateral two incisions are medial to the inferior canines to avoid injury to the mental nerve. Electrocautery is used to create a working space through the mentalis muscle through each of the incisions. With great care not to puncture the skin, a Veress needle is inserted and a dilute 60 cc solution of NaCl and epinephrine (1 mg in 500 cc) is injected under the platysma for hydrodissection. This space is then dilated with a blunt dissector.

The original description is to use a 10 mm camera through the central viewing port, but given advances in laparoscopic technology, we find it adequate to use a 5 mm camera through the central port. This can be upsized later if needed for removal of the specimen. A 5 mm port is first placed through the central incision, over the mandible, advancing around 2 cm distal to the chin. The two lateral 5 mm ports are then placed. CO_2 insufflation is maintained at a 6 mm Hg. See Figure 22-1.

Using a 5 mm 30-degree scope through the central port, and a Maryland dissector and a bipolar or ultrasonic energy device through the lateral ports, a working space is dissected in the subplatysmal plane with the strap muscles forming the "floor" of your working space. This space is typically dissected down to the sternal notch. Once the strap muscles are visualized, they are separated at the midline and retracted laterally, allowing the thyroid gland to be visualized. See Figure 22-2. Starting from a "top-down" dissection, the blood vessels are identified and divided with the bipolar or ultrasonic device. Great care is taken to identify and maintain both the parathyroid glands and the RLN. We use intraoperative nerve monitoring in all of our cases. Once this is completed on one or both sides, depending on the surgery,

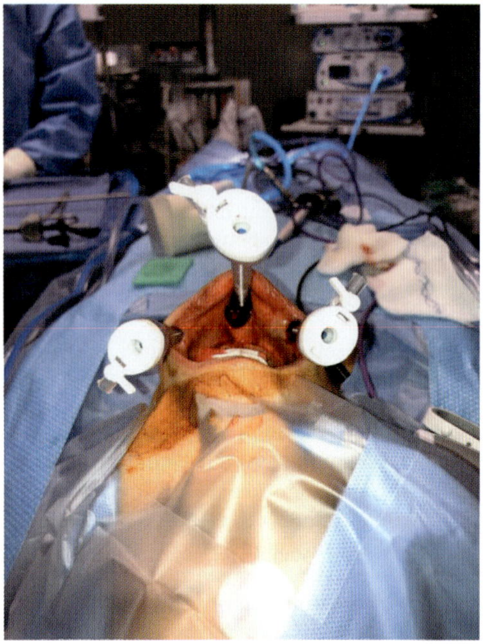

▲ **Figure 22–1.** Laparoscopic port placement in TOETVA. (From Dr. Gustavo Fernandez-Ranvier's collection.)

the thyroid gland is then freed circumferentially from all attachments and removed in a specimen bag through the central port. Hemostasis is confirmed; the strap muscles are reapproximated with absorbable self-locking suture. The original technique calls for drains to be placed but we no longer use them in our practice. After the ports are removed, the mucosal incisions are closed with 5-0 absorbable sutures.

BILATERAL AXILLO-BREAST APPROACH

History & Development

The bilateral axillo-breast approach for endoscopic thyroidectomy (BABA) was developed in Seoul National University Hospital in South Korea with the first published report in 2007.[18] Originally working with the axillobilateral breast approach (ABBA) for endoscopic thyroidectomy, the authors Choe et al. added an additional axillary port on the contralateral side. The addition of this contralateral port allowed for easy access to both sides of the thyroid gland, allowing for better visualization and central neck dissection. The first series of 110 patients had novel complications that will be expanded upon below, but the procedure was considered an overall success. Although feasible to do laparoscopically, the neck proved to be a difficult to access area endoscopically. The DaVinci Robotic Surgery system,

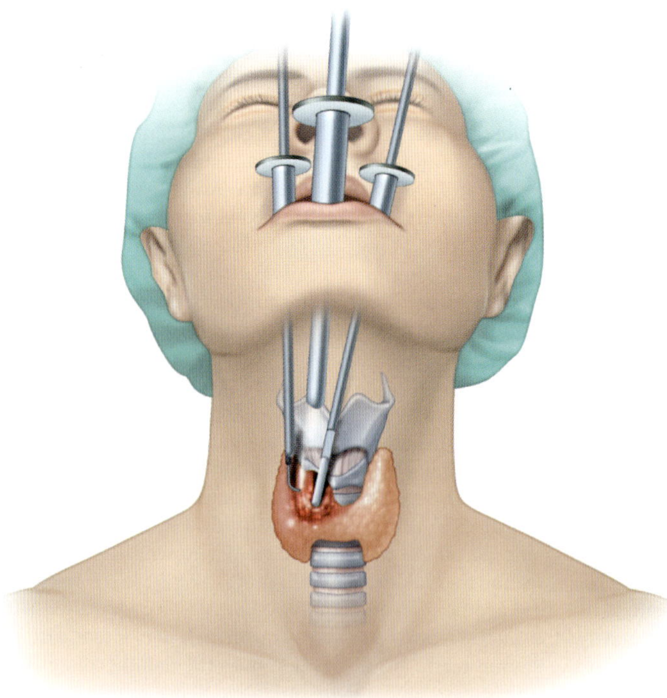

▲ **Figure 22–2.** Diagram of access to thyroid gland in TOETVA. (From Dr. Gustavo Fernandez-Ranvier's collection.)

with its three-dimensional image, increased dexterity of instruments, and tremor correcting technology was incorporated into the BABA procedure in 2009.[19,20] Now, BABA is one of the most widely used endoscopic thyroid surgery techniques, popular in Asia and especially in its birthplace, South Korea.[21]

Indications & Contraindications

As with TOETVA, patients desire endoscopic thyroid procedures like BABA to avoid an anterior cervical neck scar as seen in COT. BABA was perhaps the first endoscopic thyroid procedures, though, that could offer as near a "conventional" view of the thyroid gland as possible.[18,19]

In the original BABA series by Choe et al., the inclusion criteria were limited to benign thyroid masses, T1 thyroid carcinomas less than 1 cm, and follicular neoplasms less than 3 cm, all in patients with normal thyroid function tests.[18] Since the original series, and with the additional of robotic BABA, these inclusion criteria have been expanded: benign thyroid nodules up to 8 cm, low-risk differentiated thyroid carcinoma up to 4 cm, modified radical neck dissection, as well as Graves' disease can all be approached by BABA.[22-24]

Previous thyroid surgery and/or previous neck radiation are contraindications to BABA as well as TEOTVA. Neoplasms that invade nearby structures including the trachea, esophagus, and larynx are also contraindications. Although not a contraindication, obesity is considered by some surgeons to make the procedure more difficult. A retrospective series found no increased complications in patients with a BMI >25 kg/m^2 compared with <25 kg/m^2.[25]

Comparison to Conventional Thyroidectomy

The body of literature surrounding BABA is supportive and growing. In a 2018 meta-analysis, 11 publications comparing BABA with COT were analyzed.[26] All of these studies were performed in Korea or China. All but two of these studies were retrospective series. Of the 2733 patients accounted for, BABA was favored by female patients, younger patients, and patients with a lower BMI (although the mean BMI for all patients was relatively narrow, from 21 kg/m^2 to 24.7 kg/m^2). The meta-analysis showed that in terms of safety, there was no difference between BABA and COT in rates of postoperative hypocalcemia, RLN injury, infection, or bleeding. Both BABA and COT are clean procedures, unlike TOETVA above which is considered clean-contaminated. The reported rates of infection in BABA are very low, around 0.8% which shows no significant difference from COT. Tumor sizes of the two groups were equal, but the BABA patients retrieved on average 1.26 fewer lymph nodes than the COT group ($P < 0.00001$). The BABA group also had a significantly longer operative time, on average 110 minutes longer than the COT group ($P < 0.00001$). The authors attribute this to the time needed to create the necessary flaps as well as docking the robot system.

One oncologic-based study, which was included in the meta-analysis, looked at differentiated thyroid cancer patients who had tumors between 2 and 4 cm. This study of 86 patients did not see a significant difference in the number of retrieved central neck lymph nodes in these patients (P value 0.816). This study also included the amount of radioactive iodine needed to achieve ablation after the BABA and COT thyroidectomy. There was no significant difference between the BABA group and COT group in either the number of RAI treatments (1.9 vs 1.7, $P = 0.757$) or the total RAI dose (61.2 mCi vs 74.3 mCi $P = 0.290$). The authors concluded that in terms of oncologic completeness, BABA was a safe alternative to COT.[26]

Another retrospective study compared BABA with COT in benign or indeterminate disease only. Over a 7-year period, they compared 95 BABA patients with 262 COT patients. When controlling for the patient's age, sex, and benign tumor size, the researchers found no difference in infection, complications, or injury to a surrounding structure. They did find that BABA had an increased cost, as well as an increased operating time.[27]

Given that BABA is a remote access procedure for thyroidectomy, it required more extensive skin flaps than COT. The four access points, two in the axilla, two on the supra-areolar border and their subcutaneous flaps raise concerns about possible sensory changes to the anterior chest and breasts. In one study, 51 patient experiences were examined with monofilament testing after their BABA surgery. While 50% of patients had diminished light touch to bilateral nipples 1 month after surgery, by 3 months 81% of patients had normal nipple sensation. Risk factors for decreased nipple and anterior chest sensation were BMI and chest circumference. That being said, the sensation changes noted by the authors were minimal and did not change quality of life.[28]

Other, very rare, complications are possible given the nature of the distant trocar placement in BABA, including skin flap perforation and brachial plexus injury, but in the largest series the incidence of such complications was very low at 0.1%.[20]

Unlike TOETVA, BABA allows for a more conventional midline view of the thyroid gland. Despite this familiarity, like all procedures, there is a learning curve associated with BABA. In the original series, taking place in a high-volume center already working with other endoscopic thyroid techniques, the authors noticed that their operative times decreased after 15 cases, and so that was their estimated learning curve. In a 2015 series of 100 cases by a single surgeon, the operative time decreased significantly in 40 cases, with no significant difference in lymph nodes retrieved, complication rate, or tumor size in the cases before and after.[29]

Technique[18-20]

General anesthesia is induced and the patient is positioned supine, with the neck in gentle extension, and bilateral arms abducted slightly to allow access to the axilla. The patient is prepped and draped, allowing access to the neck, bilateral axilla, anterior chest, and breasts. The planned incisions are marked along the bilateral superior circumareolar border, and along existing skin folds of bilateral axillae (see Figure 22-3). Lines are then marked from the planned incision sites to the cricoid cartilage to facilitate the subcutaneous and subplatysmal injection of a dilute epinephrine solution, to aid in hydrodissection and hemostasis.

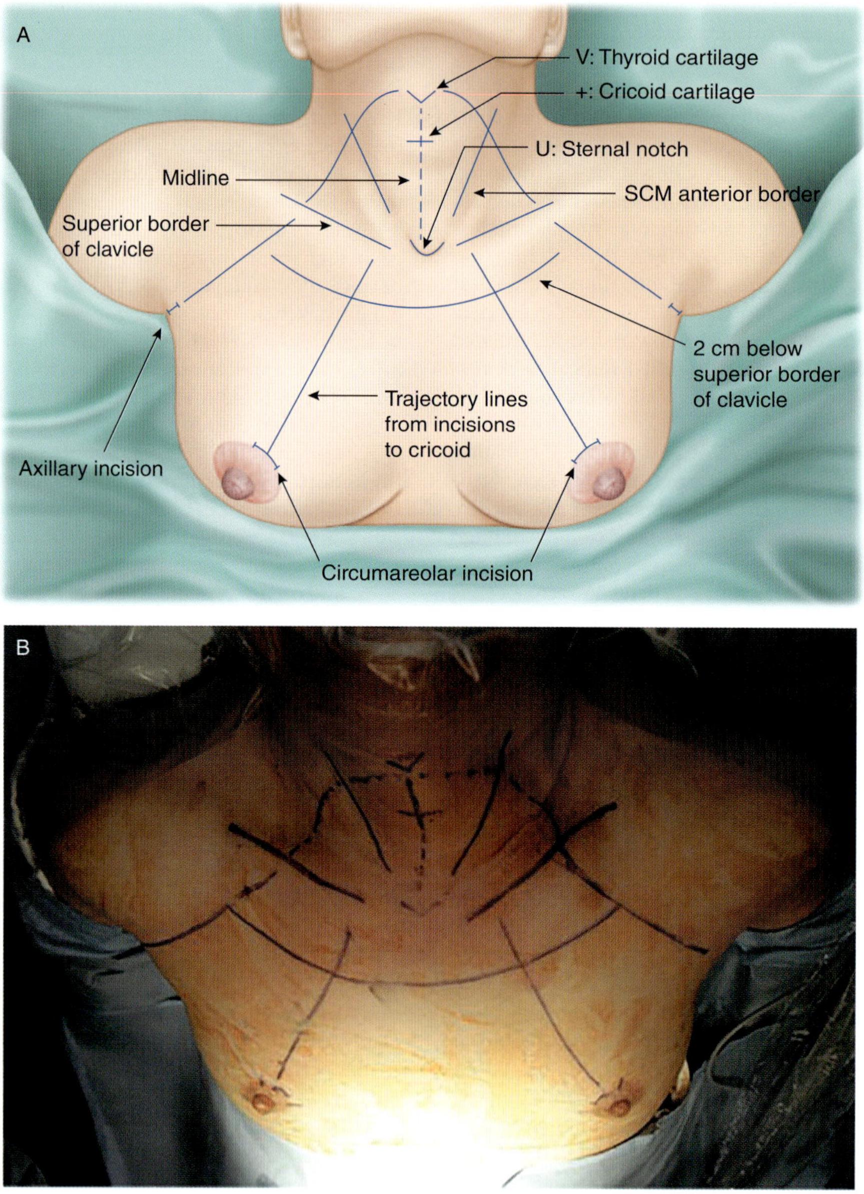

▲ **Figure 22–3.** Guidelines of BABA endoscopic thyroidectomy. **(A)** illustration, **(B)** photo. (Reproduced with permission from Youn YK, Lee KE, Choi J. Endoscopic Thyroidectomy: Bilateral Axillo-Breast Approach (BABA). In: *Color Atlas of Thyroid Surgery.* Springer, Berlin, Heidelberg; 2014.)

Once hydrodissection is complete, bilateral circumareolar incisions are made large enough to facilitate a 12 mm port on either side. Skin flaps from the circumareolar incisions to the working area of the thyroid are made using long clamps and a blunt tunneler. The 12 mm ports are then inserted to allow for the endoscope and an ultrasonic or electrocautery device. CO_2 insufflation is begun at 5 to 6 mm Hg. Incisions of 8 mm are made in the axilla bilaterally with similar skin flaps dissected to join at the cricoid cartilage. A subplatysmal working space is established from the thyroid cartilage superiorly, to the clavicle inferiorly, to the medial border of the sternocleidomastoid muscles bilaterally. At this point, a robot can be docked over either of the patient's shoulders, and the four arms attached. Otherwise, the surgery can continue laparoscopically.

Once the working space is established, the midline raphe is divided with electrocautery and the strap muscles are retracted laterally and dissected away from the thyroid capsule. This dissection is continued bilaterally to the lateral aspects of the thyroid. Once the thyroid is visualized, the isthmus is divided using a ultrasonic or electrocautery device. With gentle retraction on the thyroid gland, the inferior, middle, and superior thyroid arteries can be divided. Meticulous preservation of the parathyroid glands is sought. The recurrent laryngeal nerve should be identified and preserved. The use of neuromonitoring is recommended.

The specimen is removed in a specimen bag through one of the axillary incisions with an endoscopic retrieval bag. The operative field is irrigated and hemostasis is obtained. A closed suction drain is placed through one or both of the axillary incisions. The incisions are then closed and a postoperative brassier is placed to aid in compression of the skin flaps.

REFERENCES

1. Witzel K, von Rahden BH, Kaminski C, Stein HJ. Transoral access for endoscopic thyroid resection. *Surg Endosc.* 2008;22(8):1871-1875.
2. Fernandez-Ranvier G, Meknat A, Guevara DE, Inabnet WB. Transoral endoscopic thyroidectomy vestibular approach. *JSLS.* 2019;23(4).
3. Anuwong A. Transoral endoscopic thyroidectomy vestibular approach: a series of the first 60 human cases. *World J Surg.* 2016;40(3):491-497.
4. Zhang D, Park D, Sun H, et al. Indications, benefits and risks of transoral thyroidectomy. *Best Pract Res Clin Endocrinol Metab.* 2019;33(4):101280.
5. Anuwong A, Kim HY, Dionigi G. Transoral endoscopic thyroidectomy using vestibular approach: updates and evidences. *Gland Surg.* 2017;6(3):277-284.
6. Anuwong A, Sasanakietkul T, Jitpratoom P, et al. Transoral endoscopic thyroidectomy vestibular approach (TOETVA): indications, techniques and results. *Surg Endosc.* 2018;32(1):456-465.
7. Wang Y, Zhou S, Liu X, et al. Transoral endoscopic thyroidectomy vestibular approach vs conventional open thyroidectomy: meta-analysis. *Head Neck.* 2021;43(1):345-353.
8. Patel KN, Yip L, Lubitz CC, et al. The American Association of Endocrine Surgeons Guidelines for the Definitive Surgical Management of Thyroid Disease in Adults. *Ann Surg.* 2020;271(3):e21-e93.
9. Anuwong A, Ketwong K, Jitpratoom P, Sasanakietkul T, Duh QY. Safety and outcomes of the transoral endoscopic thyroidectomy vestibular approach. *JAMA Surg.* 2018;153(1):21-27.
10. Lira RB, Ramos AT, Nogueira RMR, et al. Transoral thyroidectomy (TOETVA): complications, surgical time and learning curve. *Oral Oncol.* Nov 2020;110:104871.
11. Chai YJ, Chung JK, Anuwong A, et al. Transoral endoscopic thyroidectomy for papillary thyroid microcarcinoma: initial experience of a single surgeon. *Ann Surg Treat Res.* 2017;93(2):70-75.
12. Fernández-Ranvier GG, Guevara D, et al. Transoral endoscopic thyroidectomy vestibular approach (TOETVA): treatment for benign thyroid diseases. *JSLS.* 2019 Oct-Dec;23(4):e2019.00036.
13. Fernández-Ranvier GG, Guevara D, Alawwa G, et al. Feasibility of the TOETVA as an ambulatory procedure. *J Surgical Endocrinol.* 2020:2(1):49-54.
14. Chai YJ, Chae S, Oh MY, Kwon H, Park WS. Transoral endoscopic thyroidectomy vestibular approach (TOETVA): surgical outcomes and learning curve. *J Clin Med.* 2021;10(4).
15. Yi JW, Kim SJ, Lee KE. Evaluation of the efficacy of postoperative antibiotic treatment in transoral endoscopic thyroidectomy: a prospective randomised controlled trial. *Br J Oral Maxillofac Surg.* 2020;58(3):334-340.
16. Luo JH, Xiang C, Wang P, Wang Y. The learning curve for transoral endoscopic thyroid surgery: a single surgeon's 204 case experience. *J Laparoendosc Adv Surg Tech A.* 2020;30(2):163-169.
17. Razavi CR, Vasiliou E, Tufano RP, Russell JO. Learning curve for transoral endoscopic thyroid lobectomy. *Otolaryngol Head Neck Surg.* 2018;159(4):625-629.
18. Choe JH, Kim SW, Chung KW, et al. Endoscopic thyroidectomy using a new bilateral axillo-breast approach. *World J Surg.* 2007;31(3):601-606.
19. Lee KE, Rao J, Youn YK. Endoscopic thyroidectomy with the da Vinci robot system using the bilateral axillary breast approach (BABA) technique: our initial experience. *Surg Laparosc Endosc Percutan Tech.* 2009;19(3):e71-e75.
20. Lee KE, Choi JY, Youn YK. Bilateral axillo-breast approach robotic thyroidectomy. *Surg Laparosc Endosc Percutan Tech.* 2011;21(4):230-236.
21. Park KN, Cho SH, Lee SW. Nationwide multicenter survey for current status of endoscopic thyroidectomy in Korea. *Clin Exp Otorhinolaryngol.* 2015;8(2):149-154.
22. Kwon H, Yi JW, Song RY, et al. Comparison of bilateral axillo-breast approach robotic thyroidectomy with open thyroidectomy for Graves' disease. *World J Surg.* 2016;40(3):498-504.
23. Liu SY, Kim JS. Bilateral axillo-breast approach robotic thyroidectomy: review of evidences. *Gland Surg.* Jun 2017;6(3): 250–257.
24. Chai YJ, Lee KE, Youn YK. Can robotic thyroidectomy be performed safely in thyroid carcinoma patients? *Endocrinol Metab (Seoul).* 2014;29(3):226-232.
25. Lee HS, Chai YJ, Kim SJ, Choi JY, Lee KE. Influence of body habitus on the surgical outcomes of bilateral axillo-breast approach robotic thyroidectomy in papillary thyroid carcinoma patients. *Ann Surg Treat Res.* 2016;91(1):1-7.
26. Shan L, Liu J. Meta-analysis comparison of bilateral axillo-breast approach robotic thyroidectomy and conventional thyroidectomy. *Surg Innov.* 2019;26(1):112-123.

27. Alramadhan M, Choe JH, Lee JH, Kim JH, Kim JS. Propensity score-matched analysis of the endoscopic bilateral axillo-breast approach (BABA) versus conventional open thyroidectomy in patients with benign or intermediate fine-needle aspiration cytology results, a retrospective study. *Int J Surg*. 2017;48:9-15.
28. Kim SJ, Lee KE, Myong JP, Kwon MR, Youn YK. Recovery of sensation in the anterior chest area after bilateral axillo-breast approach endoscopic/robotic thyroidectomy. *Surg Laparosc Endosc Percutan Tech*. 2011;21(5):366-371.
29. Kim WW, Jung JH, Park HY. The learning curve for robotic thyroidectomy using a bilateral axillo-breast approach from the 100 cases. *Surg Laparosc Endosc Percutan Tech*. 2015;25(5): 412-416.

23 Thyroid Replacement Therapy

Vivian Sobel, MD
Aaron Schulman, MD

GENERAL CONSIDERATIONS

The main function of the butterfly-shaped thyroid gland is the production of thyroid hormones, among the many factors regulating cellular metabolic rate. This role of the thyroid can be fully replaced by exogenous thyroid hormone, supported by the observation that in babies born without thyroid glands, a condition called congenital hypothyroidism, normal development ensues when these children are given thyroid hormone replacement from birth. Thyroidectomy is a common surgical procedure to treat both benign and malignant thyroid disease. The goal of thyroid hormone replacement postoperatively is, in most cases, to normalize thyroid function and therefore thyroidal metabolic regulation. The pituitary hormone thyrotropin, more commonly referred to as thyroid stimulating hormone (TSH), serves as an accurate physiologic indicator of thyroid hormone action in the peripheral tissues. When thyroid hormone levels are low, resulting in deficient thyroid hormone action, TSH levels measured in the peripheral blood will increase through negative feedback control. When there is excessive thyroid hormone signaling in the periphery, due to high thyroid hormone levels, serum TSH levels are, in turn, suppressed. In most circumstances, the goal of thyroid hormone replacement relates more to target levels of TSH and less to levels of thyroxine (T4) and triiodothyronine (T3), the biologically relevant thyroid hormones. In the case of benign disease, the goal of levothyroxine therapy after thyroid surgery is to restore TSH levels to the normal range. In the case of malignant thyroid disease with a significant risk of recurrence, the goal of thyroid hormone replacement after thyroidectomy is both to replace missing thyroid hormone, and in some cases, to suppress TSH to levels below the commonly accepted normative range, to eliminate the stimulus for residual or recurrent thyroid cancer growth. Thyroid hormone replacement is usually achieved using levothyroxine, due to its convenience, stability, and efficacy.

Physiology

Thyroid hormones play crucial roles in the differentiation, growth, function, and metabolism of nearly all tissues. The thyroid gland synthesizes two clinically relevant thyroid hormones: thyroxine (T4) and 3,5,3′-triiodothyronine (T3). T4 functions largely as a prohormone with little inherent biological activity, whereas T3 is more biologically active and has significantly higher binding affinity for nuclear receptors which mediate the physiological action of thyroid hormone.

Components required for the production of thyroid hormone include iodine, thyroglobulin (Tg)—a large glycoprotein synthesized in thyroid follicular cells, and thyroid peroxidase (TPO)—an enzyme that exerts its effects at the apical cell membrane of thyroid follicular cells. Iodide is actively transported into the thyroid by the Na^+/I^- symporter (NIS), an intrinsic protein which is located on the thyroid follicular cells' basolateral membrane. Upon diffusing to the apical membrane, iodide is transported into the follicular lumen by a chloride/iodide transporter called pendrin. At this point, iodide is oxidized and incorporated into tyrosine residues of Tg by TPO, producing monoiodotyrosine (MIT) and diiodotyrosine (DIT). TPO also catalyzes the coupling of MIT and/or DIT to produce T4 and T3, with the coupling of two DIT molecules leading to T4, and the coupling of one MIT and one DIT leading to T3.

Of note, only about 20% of daily T3 production results directly from thyroid synthesis and secretion. The remaining 80% derives from peripheral conversion of T4 via deiodination. Two enzymes are involved in the conversion of T4 to T3: Type 1 deiodinase (D1) and Type 2 deiodinase (D2). D1 is expressed in liver and kidney, and is responsible for the production of smaller amounts of T3. D2 is responsible for the predominance of T4-to-T3 conversion, and is expressed in multiple tissues, including the central nervous system, pituitary gland, thyroid, heart, brown adipose tissue, and skeletal muscle. A third deiodinase, known as Type 3 deiodinase (D3), is inactivating as it converts T4 to 3,3′,5′-triiodothyronine, known as reverse T3, which is biologically inactive.

The synthesis and secretion of thyroid hormone is under the control of a tightly regulated negative feedback system involving the hypothalamus, the pituitary, and the thyroid. Thyrotropin-releasing hormone (TRH), produced in the paraventricular nucleus of the hypothalamus, acts upon TRH receptors in pituitary thyrotropes leading to synthesis and release of TSH. TSH is the predominant regulator of thyroid hormone synthesis and secretion, and it causes thyroid growth and development, exerting its actions by binding to the TSH receptor. TRH and TSH secretion are both decreased by thyroid hormones via a negative feedback loop, with very small linear increases in serum T4 and T3 leading to inhibition of TSH secretion on a logarithmic scale. Conversely, very small decreases in serum T4 and T3 concentrations cause a dramatic increase in TSH secretion. Furthermore, each individual appears to have a genetically determined set-point for the hypothalamic-pituitary-thyroid axis.

Epidemiology

The incidence of thyroidectomy as a surgical procedure has increased in recent years along with rising rates of differentiated thyroid cancer, mainly papillary thyroid cancer (PTC). In a SEERS report, the incidence of PTC increased from 4.8 to 14.9/100,000 persons between 1975 and 2012, though it has since plateaued. The age- and gender-adjusted incidence increased faster for PTC than for any other malignancy. This rising incidence is largely due to increased detection of small, subclinical lesions by ultrasonography, as well as discovery of incidental thyroid cancers in surgical specimens, although increased rates of PTC are observed with all sizes of tumors, including those more than 4.0 cm.

Furthermore, the proportion of patients being treated with total thyroidectomy versus lobectomy for thyroid cancer increased between 2000 and 2014 according to a retrospective cohort study using the NCI SEERS database. Although the publication of the 2015 American Thyroid Association (ATA) guidelines on management of differentiated thyroid cancer may have reversed the trend in surgical practices back toward increasing use of hemithyroidectomy to treat low-risk thyroid cancers, the rising incidence of thyroid cancers requiring surgical intervention means that postsurgical thyroid hormone replacement is becoming an increasingly common form of therapy.

Thyroidectomy, both total and hemithyroidectomy, is also performed to treat benign thyroid diseases such as toxic thyroid nodules, multinodular goiter, benign thyroid nodules causing compressive symptoms, as well as Graves' disease. Thyroidectomy is used to treat Graves' disease in those who may have allergies, side effects, or contraindications to antithyroid drugs or radioiodine therapy. Some centers are reporting the increased use of thyroidectomy for benign diseases such as Graves' disease.

Clinical Presentation

Patients who have undergone either partial or total thyroidectomy may present with symptoms of hypothyroidism if they are receiving insufficient doses of levothyroxine, or they fail to start levothyroxine replacement after surgery. The symptoms of hypothyroidism are nonspecific, mostly relating to absence of the stimulatory effect of thyroid hormone on metabolism, and they can involve virtually every organ system. In addition, some hypothyroid symptoms are due to accumulation of glycosaminoglycans (GAG) in the interstitial spaces of the skin and oral mucosa. Symptoms of hypothyroidism relating to diminished metabolic rate include mental slowing, decreased memory, depression, fatigue, constipation, cold intolerance, fluid retention, dyspnea on exertion, and weight gain. Clinical signs include bradycardia, narrowed pulse pressure, delayed deep tendon reflexes, and slowing speech and movement. Signs and symptoms relating to GAG deposition include thinning and coarsening of hair, tongue enlargement, hoarseness, generalized edema including facial puffiness and periorbital edema, coarse skin, and peripheral loss of eyebrow. Severity of symptoms and signs often, but not always, relates to degree of hypothyroidism. Hypothyroid women may also complain of menorrhagia.

Those patients who have been given excessive amounts of thyroid hormone replacement after surgery may exhibit signs and symptoms of *hyperthyroxinemia*, or excessive peripheral thyroid hormone action, including palpitations, tachycardia, widened pulse pressure, weight loss, increased appetite, tremor, insomnia, anxiety/agitation, heat intolerance, and frequent bowel movements. However, these symptoms are rare in patients who merely have a suppressed TSH and normal levels of thyroxine. Usually, they are present in individuals receiving supratherapeutic doses of levothyroxine that raise thyroid hormone levels to above the normal range.

Diagnosis

As described in the preceding section, the clinical manifestations of hypothyroidism are remarkably nonspecific. Therefore, we must rely upon laboratory assessment to determine whether thyroid hormone replacement is indicated. As a result of the aforementioned negative feedback loop, in which very small changes in thyroxine induce large reciprocal changes in TSH, the most sensitive indicator of postoperative primary hypothyroidism is an elevated serum TSH. However, it is important to note that what would be considered to be an abnormally high TSH is influenced by the patient's age. An examination of National Health and Nutrition Examination Survey (NHANES) data revealed an age-related increase in the normal TSH reference range, such that slightly higher TSH values would be tolerated in elderly patients.

When TSH is found to be elevated, the patient's free T4 should be assessed next to distinguish between overt and subclinical hypothyroidism. By definition, *subclinical hypothyroidism* features a free T4 that is within normal limits, while the TSH is abnormally high. *Overt hypothyroidism* is significant for both an elevated TSH and a serum-free T4 that is below normal limits.

Since serum T3 largely derives from peripheral deiodination of T4 (and not as much from direct thyroid gland production), there is little utility to measuring serum T3 levels in the diagnosis of primary hypothyroidism.

Medical Management

Clearly, thyroid hormone replacement should be initiated immediately after total thyroidectomy. However, individuals who have undergone thyroid lobectomy, or hemithyroidectomy, may also require levothyroxine replacement depending on their baseline thyroid function, the volume of residual thyroid tissue, and the presence of underlying autoimmune thyroiditis. The incidence of hypothyroidism following a hemithyroidectomy depends on the precise definition of hypothyroidism, the duration of follow-up, and the extent of thyroid surgery. Hypothyroidism has been reported to occur in 5.6% to 48.9% of patients post-thyroid lobectomy, depending on the study. A recent retrospective study found hypothyroidism to occur in 55.8% of patients following hemithyroidectomy; however, most of these cases presented with subclinical hypothyroidism, with only 1% of patients developing overt hypothyroidism. In a recent meta-analysis, the pooled incidence of hypothyroidism following hemithyroidectomy was approximately 30%. Factors predicting future need for levothyroxine replacement following hemithyroidectomy or thyroid lobectomy included female sex, higher preoperative TSH level, lower preoperative free thyroxine (free T4) level, Hashimoto's thyroiditis (chronic lymphocytic thyroiditis), and lighter weight of the thyroid gland preoperatively. In another retrospective study of 276 patients following thyroid lobectomy, the overall percentage of patients taking levothyroxine was 23.6%; however, in those with preoperative TSH levels more than 2.5 and serologic markers of Hashimoto's, 77.8% required levothyroxine replacement. In the group with TSH less than 2.5 and negative thyroidal antibodies, the risk dropped to 7%. In patients who have undergone hemithyroidectomy, thyroid hormone levels should be checked approximately 1 month after surgery to assess need for thyroid hormone replacement, as this should allow time for stabilization of the hypothalamic-pituitary-thyroid axis.

Several pharmacological options exist to replace thyroid hormone in patients who are diagnosed with hypothyroidism. These include levothyroxine (T4), liothyronine (T3), and desiccated porcine thyroid extract. ATA guidelines recommend monotherapy with levothyroxine as the standard of care in the management of hypothyroidism. Factors that contribute to this recommendation include long-term experience in its use, a favorable side effect profile, long serum half-life, and ease of administration. The long half-life allows for once-daily dosing and stable serum levels of T4 and T3. Just as the majority of T3 in individuals without thyroid disease derives from peripheral conversion of T4 via deiodinase, adequate and stable serum T3 levels result from monotherapy with levothyroxine due to peripheral deiodinase.

When determining levothyroxine dose requirement, numerous factors should be considered including actual body weight, ideal body weight, degree of TSH elevation and TSH goal, etiology of hypothyroidism, pregnancy, age, and comorbidities. The full daily replacement dose of levothyroxine needed in individuals with minimal or absent endogenous thyroid function, such as in patients who are status post total thyroidectomy, is approximately 1.6 μg/kg ideal body weight. Because of potential adverse effects of excess thyroid hormone replacement, older individuals and those with a history of cardiac disease should initially be started at a lower levothyroxine dose, with the dose gradually increased until goal TSH is reached. Approximately 70% to 80% of an orally administered levothyroxine dose is absorbed while the patient is fasting. When levothyroxine is taken with food or coffee, absorption is significantly decreased. Therefore, it is advised that levothyroxine be administered at least 60 minutes before breakfast to ensure consistent and optimal absorption. When this is not possible, a reasonable alternative is administering the levothyroxine at bedtime, at least 3 hours after the evening meal. Levothyroxine absorption may also be affected by commonly used supplements including calcium carbonate and ferrous sulfate and therefore, it is recommended that levothyroxine be separated from these supplements by at least 4 hours. Based on its half-life, levothyroxine can take up to 6 weeks to reach steady-state levels. Therefore, it is recommended that serum TSH measurement be repeated 6 weeks after initiation of levothyroxine to allow for dose adjustment. It is important to note that TSH cannot be used as a parameter to adjust levothyroxine dose in the rare instances of patients with secondary (central) hypothyroidism from pituitary or hypothalamic disease, or peripheral thyroid hormone resistance.

Numerous studies have investigated the use of desiccated thyroid extract (DTE), or a combination of levothyroxine and liothyronine, in comparison to levothyroxine monotherapy in managing hypothyroidism. In one randomized, double-blind, crossover study, patients significantly preferred DTE over levothyroxine. However, this study was not powered for safety endpoints and the supraphysiologic and fluctuating T3 levels observed with DTE use remain concerning. Thirteen original randomized controlled trials and four systematic reviews/meta-analyses have investigated the use of a combination of levothyroxine and liothyronine as compared to levothyroxine alone. While there was great heterogeneity among these trials, overall they did not demonstrate superiority of combined levothyroxine/liothyronine over levothyroxine monotherapy with regard to quality of life, neurocognitive function, thyroid-specific symptom questionnaires, weight, or adverse effects. The data were not more compelling in patients with low serum T3 levels, or in those with a specific deiodinase gene polymorphism. Therefore, the ATA recommends against the routine use of combination levothyroxine and liothyronine treatment over monotherapy with levothyroxine.

In the course of adjusting levothyroxine dose, one's goal serum TSH will vary depending on the specific patient population being treated. Individuals with differentiated thyroid cancer, who are at higher risk for recurrence, or who have demonstrated an incomplete response to therapy, should be maintained at a lower TSH value. Higher TSH values should also be avoided in pregnant patients, particularly those who have positive thyroid peroxidase antibodies, in whom a goal TSH of less than 2.5 is generally used. Women with hypothyroidism who are planning for pregnancy are often maintained at TSH levels in the lower half of the normal range in anticipation of conception. Conversely, as mentioned before, goal serum TSH should often be higher in older individuals and those with cardiac disease.

Prognosis

The prognosis for patients on appropriate thyroid hormone replacement after undergoing surgical removal of thyroid tissue is not significantly different from the euthyroid population, independent of the risk of thyroid cancer itself. As long as serum TSH is restored to normal, and thyroid hormone levels maintained in the normal range, there should be no effect on patients' morbidity and mortality from exogenous thyroid hormone. Temporary lapses in compliance with thyroid hormone replacement, such as a day or two of skipped pills, do tend to be forgiving. Slightly under-dosing levothyroxine replacement therapy, in most cases, should not result in long-term harm.

Clinically overt hyperthyroidism is associated with increased overall mortality with increased cardiovascular events including venous thromboembolic events. Subclinical hyperthyroidism has also been associated with increased overall mortality as well as increased major adverse cardiovascular events. Patients with subclinical hyperthyroidism have been shown to have increased resting heart rate as compared with euthyroid controls, increased frequency of premature atrial and ventricular beats, increased carotid intimal media thickness, increased frequency of carotid plaques, and stroke. Rates of atrial fibrillation are higher in patients with subclinical hyperthyroidism as compared with individuals with normal TSH. In one population-based report, the risk of atrial fibrillation doubled across a 13-year follow-up in those with subclinical hyperthyroidism who were aged 65 and older, with similar risks whether serum TSH was less than 0.1 or 0.1 to 0.44.

Subclinical hyperthyroidism also has an effect on bone metabolism. Most studies find decreased bone mineral density in postmenopausal women with subclinical hyperthyroidism. One cohort study in 686 women aged 65 or older with subclinical hyperthyroidism found the rate of fractures to be four times higher for vertebral fractures, and three times higher for hip fractures, in women with baseline TSH less than 0.1 versus those with normal TSH.

Exogenous subclinical hyperthyroidism is common, occurring at one point in time in 20% to 40% of patients receiving levothyroxine therapy. In some cases, as in individuals with a personal history of thyroid cancer, the subclinical hyperthyroidism may be intentional and overall beneficial. In these cases, the risks of subclinical hyperthyroidism must be weighed against the risk of thyroid cancer recurrence.

Hypothyroidism has additionally been associated with an increased risk of major adverse cardiovascular events, and clinical hypothyroidism is associated with increased mortality. Most studies also find increased mortality in subclinical hypothyroidism with TSH more than 10; however, the data on mild, subclinical hypothyroidism are more conflicting with one retrospective study in a Danish cohort showing a reduction in all-cause mortality in subjects with subclinical hypothyroidism with TSH 5 to 10.

Some studies suggest that even minimal subclinical hypothyroidism is associated with worse pregnancy outcome, and therefore special attention should be paid to women of reproductive age, in whom pregnancy may lead to an increased levothyroxine requirement, even in those women who have undergone hemithyroidectomy.

Conclusion

Total thyroidectomy and thyroid lobectomy are common surgical procedures that are being performed with increasing frequency for both malignant and benign thyroid disease. As a result, the incidence of postsurgical hypothyroidism is rising with the accompanying need for thyroid hormone replacement. Patients who have undergone total thyroidectomy require immediate, weight-based treatment with thyroid hormone in the form of levothyroxine, with reassessment of TSH and thyroid hormone levels after at least 6 weeks, the amount of time for the hypothalamic-pituitary-thyroid axis to reach steady state. Alternate forms of thyroid hormone replacement in the form of desiccated thyroid products or liothyronine (T3) have not been shown to improve health outcome measures, and there are concerns about the safety and stability of these preparations. Patients who have undergone hemithyroidectomy should have an assessment of TSH and thyroid hormone levels approximately 1 month after surgery since a significant percentage of these patients will become subclinically or clinically hypothyroid. In the case of patients with thyroid cancer that has a significant risk of recurrence, the goal of thyroid hormone replacement is not only to restore TSH levels to the normal range, but to suppress TSH levels to reduce the risk of cancer recurrence and growth. There is significant morbidity from under- and overtreating patients with levothyroxine replacement therapy; however, thyroid hormone replacement that results in return of thyroid hormone levels to the normal range does not alter life expectancy and should not result in excess morbidity as compared to euthyroid individuals. Optimal thyroid hormone replacement should easily be achieved within a few months of thyroid surgery, leading to a euthyroid state and return to baseline state of health for the patient.

SUGGESTED READING

Ahn D, Sohn JH, Jeon JH. Hypothyroidism following hemithyroidectomy: incidence, risk factors, and clinical characteristics. *J Clin Endocrinol Metabol.* 2016;101(4):1429-1436.

Alexander EK, Pearce EN, Brent GA, et al. 2017 guidelines of the American Thyroid Association for the diagnosis and management of thyroid disease during pregnancy and the postpartum. *Thyroid.* 2017;27:315-389.

Andersen S, Pedersen KM, Bruun NH, Laurberg P. Narrow individual variation in serum T4 and T3 in normal subjects: a clue to the understanding of subclinical thyroid disease. *J Clin Endocrinol Metabol.* 2002;87:1068-1072.

Asban A, Anue A, Xie R, Chen H. Increasing use of thyroidectomy as definitive treatment for hyperthyroidism. *J Surg Res.* 2020;246:434-441.

Bauer DC, Ettinger B, Nevitt MC, Stone KL. Risk for fracture in women with low serum levels of thyroid-stimulating hormone. *Ann Intern Med.* 2001;134:561-568.

Campbell NRC, Hasinoff BB, Stilts H, et al. Ferrous sulfate reduces thyroxine efficacy in patients with hypothyroidism. *Ann Int Med.* 1992;117:1010-1013.

Canaris GJ, Manowitz NR, Mayor G, Ridgeway EC. The colorado thyroid disease prevalence study. *Arch Intern Med.* 2000;160:526-534.

Cooper DS, Biondi B. Subclinical thyroid disease. *Lancet.* 2012;379:1142-1154.

de los Santos ET, Starich GH, Mazzaferri EL. Sensitivity, specificity, and cost-effectiveness of the sensitive thyrotropin assay in the diagnosis of thyroid disease in ambulatory patients. *Arch Intern Med.* 1989;149:526-532.

Dekkers OM, Horvath-Puho E, Cannegieter SC, Vandenbroucke JP, Sorensen HT, Jorgensen JO. Acute cardiovascular events and all-cause mortality in patients with hyperthyroidism: a population-based cohort study. *Eur J Endocrinol.* 2017;176: 1-9.

Hansen PS, Brix TH, Sorensen TI, Kyvik KO, Hegedus L. Major genetic influence on the regulation of the pituitary-thyroid axis: a study of healthy Danish twins. *J Clin Endocrinol Metabol.* 2004;89:1181-1187.

Haugen BR, Alexander EK, Bible KC, et al. 2015 American Thyroid Association management guidelines for adult patients with thyroid nodules and differentiated thyroid cancer. *Thyroid.* 2016;26:1-133.

Hoang TD, Olsen CH, Mai VQ, et al. Desiccated thyroid extract compared with levothyroxine in the treatment of hypothyroidism: a randomized, double-blind, crossover study. *J Clin Endocrinol Metabol.* 2013;98:1982-1990.

Huang H-K, Wang J-H, Kao S-L. Association of hypothyroidism with all-cause mortality: a cohort study in an older adult population. *J Clin Endocrinol Metabol.* 2018;103:3310-3318.

James BC, Timsana L, Graham R, Angelos P, Haggerstrom DA. Changes in total thyroidectomy versus thyroid lobectomy for papillary thyroid cancer during the past 15 years. *Surgery.* 2019;166:41-47.

Jonklaas J, Bianco AC, Bauer AJ, et al. Guidelines for the treatment of hypothyroidism. *Thyroid.* 2014;24:1670-1751.

Krugman LG, Hershman JM, Chopra IJ, et al. Patterns of recovery of the HPT axis in patients taken off chronic thyroid therapy. *J Clin Endocrinol Metabol.* 1975;41(1): 70-80.

LaFranchi S. Treatment and prognosis of congenital hypothyroidism. In: Ross DL, Geffner, ME, Hoppin AG, ed. *www.uptodate.com.* 2021.

Lee DY, Seok J, Jeong WJ, Ahn SH. Prediction of thyroid hormone supplementation after thyroid lobectomy. *J Surg Res.* 2015;193:273-278.

Lee SY, Cabral HJ, Aschengrau A, Pearce EN, Associations between maternal thyroid function in pregnancy and obstetric and perinatal outcomes. *J Clin Endocrinol Metabol.* 2020;105: e2015-e2023.

Lee SY, Pearce EN. Testing, monitoring and treatment of thyroid dysfunction in pregnancy. *J Clin Endocrinol Metabol.* 2021;106:883-892.

Li Z, Qiu Y, Fei Y, et al. Prevalence of and risk factors for hypothyroidism after hemithyroidectomy: a systematic review and meta-analysis. *Endocrine.* 2020;70:243-255.

Mandel SJ, Brent GA, Larsen PR. Levothyroxine therapy in patients with thyroid disease. *Ann Intern Med.* 1993;119: 492-502.

Powers AE, Marcadis AR, Lee M, Morris LGT, Marti JL. Changes in trends in thyroid cancer incidence in the United States 1992 to 2016. *JAMA.* 2019;322(24):2440.

Rodondi N, den Elzen WPJ, Bauer DC, et al. Subclinical hypothyroidism and the risk of coronary heart disease and mortality. *JAMA.* 2010;304(12):1365-1374.

Ross DS. Subclinical hypothyroidism in nonpregnant adults. In: Cooper DS, ed. *www.uptodate.com.* 2021.

Ross DS. Thyroid hormone synthesis and physiology. In: Cooper DS, ed. *www.uptodate.com.* 2021.

Selmer C, Olesen JB, Hansen ML, et al. Subclinical and overt thyroid dysfunction and risk of all-cause mortality and cardiovascular events: a large population study. *J Clin Endocrinol Metabol.* 2014;99:2372-2382.

Singh N, Singh PN, Hershman JM. Effect of calcium carbonate on the absorption of levothyroxine. *JAMA.* 2000;283:2822-2825.

Spencer CA, Lo Presti JS, Patel A, et al. Applications of a new chemiluminometric thyrotropin assay to subnormal measurement. *J Clin Endocrinol Metabol.* 1990;70:453-460.

Spitzweg C, Heufelder AE, Morris JC. Thyroid iodine transport. *Thyroid.* 2000;10:321-330.

Surks MI, Hollowell JG. Age-specific distribution of serum thyrotropin and anti-thyroid antibodies in the U.S. population: implications for the prevalence of subclinical hypothyroidism. *J Clin Endocrinol Metabol.* 2007;92:4575-4582.

Surks MI. Clinical manifestations of hypothyroidism. In: Ross DS, ed. *www.uptodate.com.* 2021.

Ullman TM, Gray KD, Stefanova D, et al. The 2015 American Thyroid Association guidelines are associated with an increasing rate of hemithyroidectomy for thyroid cancer. *Surgery.* 2019;166(3):349-355.

Yen PM. Physiological and molecular basis of thyroid hormone action. *Physiological Reviews.* 2001;81:1097-1142.

Molecular Testing for Thyroid Nodules & Targeted Therapies for Thyroid Cancer

24

Martha E. Teke, MD
Tahsin M. Khan, MD
Martha A. Zeiger, MD

GENERAL CONSIDERATIONS

The incidence of thyroid cancer (TC) has increased exponentially from 4.9 to 14.3 per 100,000 people in the United States over the past three decades. The worldwide incidence has also increased sharply and currently ranges between 4.1 per 100,000 men and 18.6 per 100,000 women, making TC the ninth most common malignancy in the world. In addition, nearly 70% of adults have thyroid nodules detectable via ultrasound, and a further 5% have palpable lesions. These nodules may harbor aggressive malignancies or be benign lesions with minimal threat to a person's health, thus calling for markedly different treatment strategies. Therefore, accurate diagnosis, prognostication, and treatment of thyroid nodules and TC remain a key health-care need worldwide (Table 24–1).

Physical examination, radiographic characterization with ultrasonography, and fine-needle aspiration (FNA) with cytopathologic analysis remain the "gold standard" for the evaluation of thyroid nodules. Cytopathology is evaluated according to The Bethesda System for Reporting Thyroid Cytopathology (TBSRTC) which stratifies lesions into six main categories of various malignant potential. Accurate interpretation of FNA specimens must include at least six groups of follicular cells, each comprised of a minimum of 10 cells according to the Bethesda System. The cells are then evaluated for their arrangement, shape, background cytoplasmic features, nuclear features, as well as any special immunohistochemical stains as needed. Based on these, nodules can be classified into one of six categories (Table 24–2). The interpretations of Bethesda I (nondiagnostic cytology), II (benign), and VI (malignant) are straightforward. However, the management of lesions classified Bethesda III, IV, and V "indeterminate" or suspicious nodules (ITN) is more nuanced, since the frequency of malignancy detected on final pathology for these nodules ranges widely from 6% to up to 75%. This diagnostic ambiguity can lead to patients (1) undergoing surgical resection for ultimately benign pathology, contributing to overtreatment, unnecessary morbidity, and cost or (2) undergoing inadequate surgical resection for malignant lesions, resulting in the need for a second operation further leading to increased cost. The development of adjunctive diagnostic tests and their incorporation into the management schema for thyroid nodules has thus become a critical need in recent decades.

Concurrently, the advent of genome sequencing and advances in molecular biology in recent years have afforded insights into the biological underpinnings of this common malignancy. The broad classification of TC into differentiated (DTC, which includes papillary thyroid cancer [PTC] and follicular thyroid cancer [FTC]), poorly differentiated (PDTC), anaplastic (ATC), or medullary thyroid cancer (MTC) continues to become more discretely defined with the identification of driver mutations, characterization of pathway alterations, and consequent genetic classification of these tumors. Not surprisingly, the translation of these basic science advancements to the clinic has been the focus of many research and clinical endeavors. Nowhere are these efforts more apparent than in the fields of molecular testing (MT) of thyroid nodules, and molecular targeted therapies in TC.

As such, this chapter will discuss how TC diagnostics and treatment have been informed by our understanding of the molecular landscape of the disease. We will present a succinct summary of our current knowledge of the molecular aspects of TC and discuss both the rationale and limitations behind using MT to better characterize indeterminate or suspicious thyroid nodules. Lastly, we will highlight the existing therapeutic options and strategies for advanced TC based on molecular insights.

Table 24–1. List of abbreviations.

Term	Explanation
MT	Molecular testing
ITN	Indeterminate thyroid nodule
TC	Thyroid Cancer
DTC	Differentiated thyroid cancer
PTC	Papillary thyroid cancer
FTC	Follicular thyroid cancer
PDTC	Poorly differentiated thyroid cancer
ATC	Anaplastic thyroid cancer
MTC	Medullary thyroid cancer
HCN	Hürthle cell neoplasm
NIFTP	Noninvasive follicular thyroid neoplasm with papillary-like nuclear features
GEC	Afirma gene expression classified
GSC	Afirma genomic sequencing classified
v2	ThyroSeq version 2
v3	ThyroSeq version 3
NPV	Negative predictive value
PPV	Positive predictive value

GENETICS & MOLECULAR PATHOLOGY OF THYROID CANCER

TC comprises a heterogenous group of malignancies that is broadly categorized as DTC, PDTC/ATC, and MTC based on the tissue of origin and degree of differentiation. DTC, arising from endodermal follicular cells, comprises the largest group (90% of all TCs) and is further subdivided into PTC or FTC. TC aggressiveness increases with higher grades of de-differentiation, with ATC demonstrating rapid growth and metastasis leading to a dismal median survival of 5 to 12 months. MTC accounts for ~5% of all TCs, demonstrates aggressiveness falling between DTC and ATC, and is often associated with the familial MEN2A/B syndromes. Advances in sequencing and molecular biology over the past couple of decades have now revealed specific molecular and genomic signatures associated with each TC type (Figure 24–1). Furthermore, certain genetic alterations have now been linked with specific inherited syndromes as is the case with RET proto-oncogene in MEN2A/B syndromes. Much like other cancers, the genetic alterations in TC can be broadly classified into activating mutations in oncogenes/oncogenic pathways or inactivating mutations in tumor suppressors such as DNA repair and chromatin regulatory genes. In each TC subtype, these genetic alterations produce a complex interplay of downstream signaling pathways that promote carcinogenesis.

Differentiated Thyroid Cancer

DTCs harbor genetic alterations that lead to activation of a key oncogenic signal transduction cascade—the mitogen-activated protein kinase (MAPK) pathway. The mutational landscape of this pathway is heterogenous. The predominant MAPK pathway mutations occur in *BRAF*, where the activating valine to glutamic acid substitution at residue 600 ($BRAF^{V600E}$) has been reported in ~60% of PTC (range 36%-83%). This mutation results in phosphorylation and activation of BRAF kinase activity, leading to constitutive activation of the MAPK pathway. This in turn promotes uncontrolled cell proliferation and escape from apoptosis. An additional ~15% of PTCs demonstrate mutations in another canonical MAPK family member, *RAS*, with activating mutations having been observed in *HRAS*, *KRAS*, and *NRAS*. Intriguingly, despite belonging to the same MAPK signaling pathway, the presence of *BRAF* and *RAS* mutations appears to be mutually exclusive in PTC. Indeed, PTCs can be profiled according to the $BRAF^{V600E}$-RAS score (BRS), which categorizes tumors as either BRAF-like (BVL) or RAS-like (RL) based on expression levels of 71 associated genes. Each type has been associated with

Table 24–2. The Bethesda System for reporting thyroid cytopathology including associated malignancy risks (2017).

Diagnostic Categories	Risk of Malignancy	Recommended Management
I. Nondiagnostic/Unsatisfactory	5%-10%	Repeat ultrasound-guided FNA
II. Benign	0%-3%	Clinical and sonographic follow-up
III. Atypia of undetermined significance (AUS)/follicular lesion of undetermined significance (FLUS)	6%-18%	Repeat ultrasound-guided FNA, molecular testing, or lobectomy
IV. Follicular neoplasm/suspicious for a follicular neoplasm	10%-40%	Molecular testing, lobectomy
V. Suspicious for malignancy	45%-60%	Lobectomy or total thyroidectomy
VI. Malignant	94%-96%	Lobectomy or total thyroidectomy

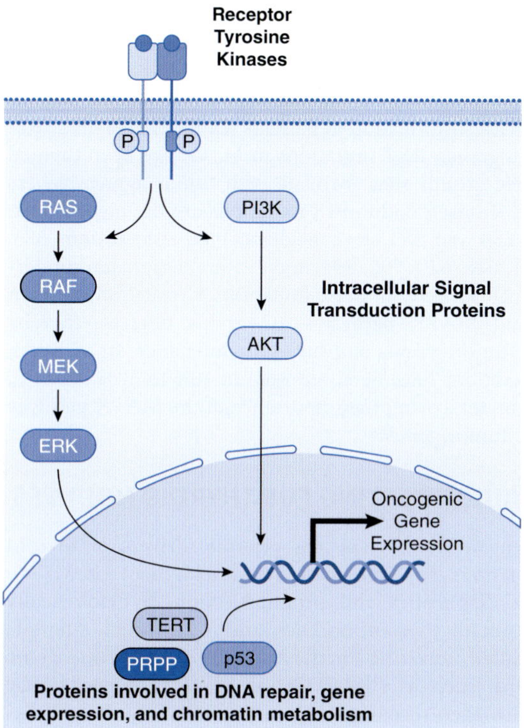

DTC	ATC	MTC
Receptor Tyrosine Kinases		
RET (5%-25%) *NTRK* (5%-25%)	*ALK* (11%)	*RET* (hereditary 95%, sporadic 40%-70%)
Intracellular Signal Transduction Proteins		
BRAF (40%-80%) *RAS* (15%-50%) *PTEN* (2%) *AKT1* (8%) *PIK3CA* (1%)	*BRAF* (10%-50%) *RAS* (10%-20%) *PTEN* (11%-15%) *AKT1* (19%) *PIK3CA* (18%)	*RAS* (10%-30%)
Proteins involved in DNA repair, gene expression, and chromatin metabolism		
TP53 (10%-35%) *TERT* (10%-30%) *PAX8-PPARγ* (30%-35%)	*TP53* (50%-80%) *TERT* (40%-70%) SWI-SNF complex (35%) Histone methyltransferase (24%) *MSH2, MSH6, MLH1(10%)*	
Miscellaneous		
	CTTNB1 (60%-65%)	

Figure 24–1. Key molecular pathways in thyroid cancer and common molecular alterations by thyroid cancer type.

specific biological patterns and different clinical outcomes, with BVL PTCs demonstrating poorer differentiation, increased aggressiveness, and worse outcomes. Finally, PTCs commonly demonstrate fusion mutations involving receptor tyrosine kinases (RTK) such as *RET-PTC* or *NTRK* (5%-25% of PTC). These fusions lead to constitutive, ligand-independent kinase activity of the receptors, which subsequently leads to activation of the downstream MAPK and PI3K signaling pathways. The presence of *RET-PTC* fusions is often associated with sporadic childhood and radiation-related DTCs.

Other genetic alterations in PTC include inactivating mutations in the tumor suppressor *TP53, PAX8-PPARγ* rearrangements, and promoter mutations in the *TERT* enzyme that also leads to its constitutive activation. The consequences of inactivating mutations in *TP53* and their role in oncogenesis via genomic instability are well described. The *PAX8-PPARγ* rearrangement is observed in up to 35% of FTC as well as in some follicular variant PTC, and entails a translocation event between chromosomes 2 and 3 (t(2;3)(q12;p25)). PAX8 and PPARγ are both transcription factors involved in normal thyroid development. The novel fusion product called PPFP resulting from this translocation functions as an oncoprotein by "rewiring" the transcriptional networks associated with these wild-type proteins. Activating mutations of the *TERT* promoter leads to constitutive expression of the catalytic component of telomerase (telomerase reverse transcriptase) which results in lengthening of telomeres at chromosomal ends, continued DNA replication, and thus persistent cell divisions beyond the Hayflick limit. In general, *TERT* alterations in PTC are associated with more aggressive phenotype and poorer outcomes.

Poorly Differentiated & Anaplastic Thyroid Cancer

The genomic landscape of PDTC and ATC overall mimic that of PTC, likely because of their shared origin from endodermal follicular cells. However, the frequencies of highly oncogenic mutations are much higher in these tumor types. For instance, in addition to the aforementioned MAPK pathway alterations in BRAF and RAS, ATCs demonstrate frequent alterations in *PIK3CA* (20%), *PTEN* (15%), and *AKT1* (20%). The latter mutations culminate in activation of the PI3K/AKT signaling pathway that promotes transformation, progression, and invasion. ATCs also frequently harbor activating mutations or gene fusions involving the *ALK* RTK, which has been shown to function as a strong oncogene in other tumor types (lymphoma, lung cancer) and imparts an aggressive phenotype by driving activation of PI3K-AKT and MAPK signaling cascades. Additional RTK mutations in ATC include *EGFR*, *FGFR2*, *FLT3*, *KIT*, *MET*, *PDGFRα/β*, and *VEGFR1/2*, all of which are known oncogenes. Another pathway more commonly altered in PDTC/ATC includes the WNT pathway, a major cell differentiation pathway, where gain of function mutations in *CTNNB1* or loss of function mutations in *Axin1* are observed in 25% and 60% of PDTC and ATC, respectively. Finally, PDTC/ATC appears to demonstrate more frequent alterations in genes involved in DNA integrity, replication, and organization compared to PTC. Inactivating *TP53* mutations, for instance, are seen in 50% to 80% of ATC, and *TERT* promoter mutations in 40% to 70% of ATC (compared to 10% of PTC). In addition, mutations in *MSH2*, *MSH6*, and *MLH1* DNA repair pathway proteins (2%-12%), histone methyltransferases (*HMTs*, 7%-24%), and SWI-SNF chromatin remodeling complexes (6%-36%) are also seen in PDTC/ATC. Taken together, these findings suggest that in addition to accumulating driver mutations as in DTC, the progression to PDTC/ATC also requires secondary mutations that interfere with maintenance and homeostasis of DNA elements and the genome.

Medullary Thyroid Cancer

Owing to their origin from neural crest-derived neuroendocrine cells, MTCs demonstrate a distinct genomic landscape compared to DTC/PDTC/ATC. The classic genetic alteration associated with MTC involves the *RET* RTK, where activating point mutations are observed in 40% to 70% of sporadic MTC and 95% of hereditary MTC (associated with MEN2A/B). While many MTC-associated mutations across seven key exons in *RET* (8, 10, 11, 13, 14, 15, and 16) have been reported, 90% of alterations in MEN2A-associated lesions occur at cystine at position 634, while 95% of MEN2B-associated and 75% to 95% of sporadic MTC involve mutations of the methionine at position 918.

Interestingly, the clinical presentation of MTC appears to vary according to the specific mutation, leading to strong genotype-phenotype correlations. Indeed, recommended timing for prophylactic thyroidectomy is based on codon-specific risk stratification in patients with heritable disease as well. Altogether, RET mutations in MTC have been divided into three groups that correlate with tumor aggressiveness and age of onset: codon 918 mutations are the highest risk; codons 634 and 883 are considered high risk; codons 533, 609, 611, 618, 620, 790, 804, and 891 are designated moderate risk. Ultimately, all these mutations activate downstream PI3K and MAPK pathways in various degrees, thereby driving tumorigenesis and tumor maintenance. In addition, *RAS* alterations have been reported in 10% to 30% of MTC, further underscoring the importance of the MAPK pathway in MTC tumorigenesis.

MOLECULAR TESTING FOR THYROID NODULES

The identification of specific genomic drivers of thyroid carcinogenesis has informed the development of MT to improve diagnostics and prognostication of cytologically indeterminate thyroid nodules and TC. Initial attempts were limited to testing for the presence of single oncogenic mutations, such as *BRAFV*^{600E} or *TERT* promoter mutations. However, recent years have seen the advent and dissemination of commercial molecular tests that incorporate assessment of multiple genetic alterations and gene expression panels to gauge malignancy risk. As such, the dual purpose of MT is improving oncologic risk stratification, as well as potentially reducing patient morbidity secondary to unnecessary diagnostic surgical interventions. Current commercially used tests include Afirma Genomic Sequencing Classifier (GSC), a microarray-based test evaluating gene expression, ThyroSeq v3 based on next-generation RNA and DNA sequencing (NGS) technology, and ThyraMIR and Rosetta GX Reveal which are based on microRNA expression (Table 24–3). These tests have evolved over time to keep up with technological advancements, identification of novel

Table 24–3. Description of currently available molecular testing platforms in thyroid cancer.

Platform	Afirma GSC/XA	ThyroSeq v3	ThyGeNEXT/ThyraMIR
Method	Microarray mRNA expression analysis	Next-generation RNA and DNA sequencing	Next-generation RNA and DNA sequencing/miRNA analysis
Evaluated molecular variant	• GSC—10,196 mRNA panel • XA—594 genes including 905 variants and 235 fusions	• 112 gene panel including >12,000 variants and 150 gene fusions	• 10 genes • 37 fusions • 10 miRNA
TERT testing?	No	Yes	Yes
Sensitivity-specificity	91%-68%	94%-82%	95%-90%
NPV-PPV	96%-47%	97%-66%	97%-79%

oncogenic mutations, and pathologic nomenclature revisions for TC. However, attempts at clinical implementation of the preceding generations of these tests—Afirma Gene Expression Classifier (GEC) and ThyroSeq v2—revealed limitations and challenges to the practical utility of MT which will be discussed herein.

Current Commercial Molecular Testing Platforms

A. Afirma Gene Sequencing Classifier

Afirma GSC, a product of Veracyte Inc (San Francisco, USA), is a microarray-based test designed to identify benign histology and "rule out" the presence of malignancy. Its initial version, the Afirma GEC, categorized ITNs as either benign or suspicious based on their mRNA expression of 167 genes. In a seminal study reported in 2012 by Alexander and colleagues, the GEC revealed a robust sensitivity of 92% and negative predictive value (NPV) of 95% and 94% for Bethesda III and Bethesda IV nodules respectively, deeming it a good "rule out" test for malignancy in ITN. To reduce the risk of missed malignancy, the newer GSC additionally incorporates testing for the presence of $BRAF^{V600E}$ mutation, *RET/PTC* mutations, MTC, Hürthle cell, and parathyroid tissue. This yielded an improved specificity and PPV, while sensitivity and NPV remained at 91% and 96%, respectively. An additional testing option offered by Afirma since 2018, the Afirma Xpression Atlas (XA), further evaluates expression of 905 variants, 235 fusions, and 593 genes, thereby expanding its utilization to guide selection of targeted therapies in the setting of metastatic TC.

B. ThyroSeq v3

In contrast to the "rule out" methodology of Afirma, ThyroSeq (Sonic Healthcare, NY, USA) adopted sequencing of a multigene panel to identify deleterious gene alteration and "rule in" ITN suspicious for malignancy. ThyroSeq has undergone multiple iterations starting from its original version. ThyroSeq v0 was a seven-gene panel detecting mutations/rearrangements in $BRAF^{V600E/K601E}$, *NRAS* codon 61, *HRAS* codon 61, and *KRAS* codons 12/13 and gene rearrangements in *PAX8/PPAR*, *RET/PTC1*, and *RET/PTC3*. Subsequent panels based on TCGA discoveries and advances in NGS technique yielded subsequent expansive iterations including ThyroSeq v1 (12-gene panel), ThyroSeq v2 (56-gene panel) and its current version, ThyroSeq v3 (112-gene panel). ThyroSeq v3 detects five categories of genetic data including (1) mutations; (2) gene fusions; (3) insertions and deletions; (4) copy number alterations; and (5) gene expression alterations. Initial studies have reported sensitivity and specificity of 91% and 85% for Bethesda III nodules, and 97% and 75% for Bethesda IV nodules, respectively. It had similarly favorable, NPV and PPV at 97% and 64% for Bethesda III and 98% and 68% in Bethesda IV lesions, respectively.

C. ThyraMIR/ThyGeNEXT and RosettaGX

The ThyraMIR/ThyGeNEXT multiplatform approach combines a 10-miRNA classifier test (ThyraMIR) with a mutational panel (ThyGeNEXT) detecting common oncogenic point mutations and fusion genes via a two-step approach. Samples initially undergo ThyGeNEXT oncogenic analysis where they are placed into three main categorizes: strong mutational profile (*BRAF*-like), weak profile (*RAS*-like), or no detectable mutations. Surgical resection is recommended for patients with lesions deemed as *BRAF*-like, while the latter categories are further stratified with the ThyraMIR miRNA classifier. The validation study for this platform revealed a 95% and 90% sensitivity and specificity, respectively, as well as a 97% NPV and 75% PPV. Lastly, RosettaGX, another miRNA classifier, utilizes a 24-miRNA panel to risk-stratify ITNs. Although preliminary studies are promising, prospective validation studies are necessary to support its integration into routine clinical practice.

Caveats & Considerations When Incorporating MT in Thyroid Nodule Classification

The initial reports of Afirma GSC and ThyroSeq v3 documented improved test performance (sensitivity, specificity, NPV, PPV) compared to the preceding versions, thereby promising improved clinical benefit on their implementation in clinical practice (Figure 24–2). Furthermore, retrospective, single-institution studies have reported a reduction in number of diagnostic thyroid lobectomies during recent years when GSC/v3 were implemented compared to period of GEC/v2 use (although these results may be confounded by concurrent shift in practice patterns by papillary-like nuclear features [NIFTP] designation change occurring around the same time). Regardless, there are some nuances to implementing and interpreting MT results in ITN diagnosis and management that should be considered. These caveats are highlighted by challenges encountered in the deployment and real-world use of the previous GEC/v2 tests and should be kept in mind as the utilization of GSC and v3 becomes more widespread, and are outlined as follows.

A. Variable Test Performance Depending on Population Prevalence of Thyroid Cancer

Like any diagnostic test, the NPV/PPV of thyroid nodule MTs has been found to depend on the population prevalence of TC in the tested population. For instance, when initially described in 2012, the GEC was touted as able to "rule out" malignancy (and thus spare diagnostic surgery) in over 90% of indeterminate nodules. Subsequent studies have observed, however, that the NPV of GEC varies greatly depending on the institution and thus the malignancy prevalence within the evaluated populations. Most of the initial publications reporting on test performance were from

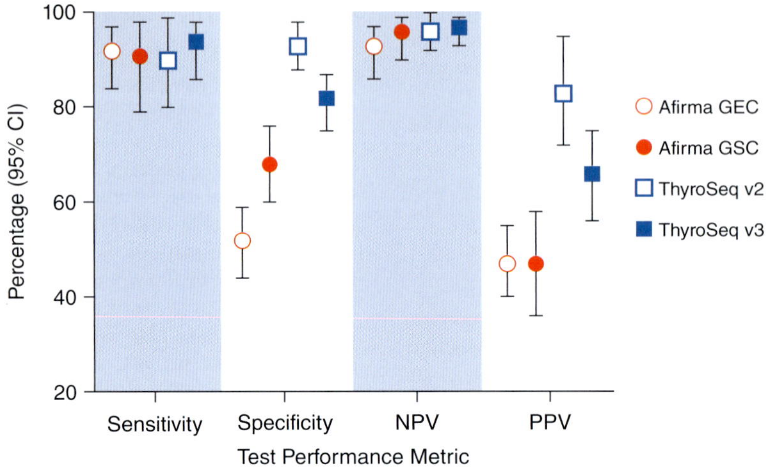

▲ **Figure 24–2.** Diagnostic performance of widely used molecular tests. (Reference values for this figure obtained from: Alexander et al. *NEJM*. 2012 [Afirma GEC]; Patel et al. *JAMA*. Surgery 2018 [Afirma GSC]; Nikiforov et al. *Cancer* 2014 [ThyroSeq v2]; Steward et al. *JAMA*. Oncology 2019 [ThyroSeq v3].)

tertiary academic institutions and had relatively small sample sizes, leading to high rates of selection bias.

Interinstitutional variability was also observed with the ThyroSeq v2, where paltry positive predictive values of 22% to 43% (compared to initially reported PPV of 83%) have been reported. These numbers significantly undermine this "rule in" test's ability to accurately identify malignant nodules that require surgical intervention. Thus, while the more current GSC and v3 present improvements in the NPV/PPV compared to the older GEC and v2, these new data are again derived from academic institutions with unique referral patterns. The true NPV/PPV for the newer tests still needs to be validated in larger studies incorporating more community/nonacademic institutions, where most of MT will ultimately be performed.

B. Impact of Varying Genetic Landscape of Thyroid Cancer and Nodules on Test Performance

Further confounding the diagnostic utility of MTs is their differential emphasis on what constitutes a "driver mutation" in TC. For instance, while its role in thyroid carcinogenesis has been well defined, the positive predictive value of isolated *RAS* mutations has been reported to be only 7% to 25% primarily because *RAS* mutations also frequently occur in benign thyroid nodules. Thus, MTs that consider *RAS* mutations as a strong indicator of malignancy may overestimate the risk from an otherwise benign ITN.

Another example of this was observed with initial studies of GEC in samples containing a predominance of Hürthle cell nodules (HCNs). Since HCNs have slightly different genetic landscape relative to other PTC subtypes (eg, less frequent *RAS* [15% vs 30%] and more frequent *TERT* [30% vs 20%] alterations), it was noted that the GEC did not accurately capture the true malignancy potential of ITNs when utilized in populations with higher frequency of HCNs. The newer GSC has been improved to incorporate our updated understanding of HCN genetic landscape, and thus performs more accurately for samples with a Hürthle cell background. Nevertheless, the fact that MT performance metrics are dependent on the underlying histopathology should be kept in mind when interpreting their results.

C. Updates to Thyroid Cancer Nomenclature That Confounds Test Performance

The introduction of a new thyroid pathological entity, noninvasive follicular thyroid neoplasm with NIFTP, in 2016 was noted to significantly alter the performance and accuracy of GEC/v2 MTs that were already in use at that time. This NIFTP category, originally considered as encapsulated follicular variant of PTC and estimated to have an estimated average prevalence of 61% amongst indeterminate thyroid nodules, is now considered either benign or at most an indolent tumor. Given that the computational algorithms for GEC/v2 MTs were developed and validated prior to this redesignation (and thus originally designed to classify this potential benign pathology as malignant), their performance measures deteriorated considerably on the description of NIFTP. For instance, the NPV of GEC declined from 96% to 81% and the PPV of v2 decreased from 42% to 33% when the NIFTP designation was retrospectively applied to previously studied cohorts. Again, while GSC/v3 have been improved to incorporate this updated thyroid pathological entity, any interpretation of MT results should be tempered by the fact that improvements in our understanding of TC cytopathology and natural history may confound and supplant MT results estimating malignancy potential.

D. MT Results Have Limited Impact on Practical Surgical Decision-Making

Despite the impressive predictive performance of GEC/v2 reported in the initial retrospective studies, subsequent prospective studies assessing the impact of incorporating MT results and appropriateness of surgical intervention ultimately revealed a limited impact on actual practice patterns. For instance, two seminal publications out of a high-volume, tertiary medical center (Johns Hopkins) demonstrated that GEC results changed management strategy in less than 10% of cases, and furthermore led to overtreatment in the majority (72.7%-91%) of the cases where strategy was changed based on MT results. Moreover, these investigations found that over 50% of the patients referred to their practice after MT results had indications for surgical intervention based on clinical assessment alone, suggesting that these tests were being inappropriately ordered for many patients whose recommended treatment was already clear based on standard cytological, radiographical, and physical examination parameters. Another institutional review demonstrated that most lesions *not* designated as "Benign" by GEC ultimately underwent surgical resection, even when the sample was classified as "QNS" (quantity not sufficient) and despite the fact that the GEC is a "rule out" test. Taken together, these investigations have shown that MT results (a) may ultimately influence management in only a subset of patients, (b) do carry a real and significant risk of overdiagnosis and overtreatment, and (c) are often being misused indiscriminately when clinical features alone can dictate appropriate management.

In addition, the overall impact of MT on management decision when compared to that of clinical and radiographic features has been shown to be incremental at best. For instance, a study from Columbia University noted that while supplementing clinical information (history and physical examination) with imaging and cytopathology improves diagnostic accuracy significantly, further incorporation of MT results to these variables leads to only a modest and negligible improvement to overall diagnostic capacity. Similarly, retrospective reviews of single institution series have noted that most patients with clinical indications for surgery (such as compressive symptoms, interval growth of nodules, and presence of secondary nodules) but with "benign" calls in the GEC were in the end managed surgically, with up to a third of these lesions found to harbor malignancy on final pathology.

As such, it is ultimately recommended that decisions regarding when to operate and how much to resect be determined primarily by clinical variables, ultrasound findings, and individual patient preference. One must always ask the question; "What is the likelihood that a MT result would alter the clinical or surgical recommendations?" If the answer is "unlikely" (eg, in the case of a patient with ITN who also has a symptomatic goiter), then MT results should not be routinely or solely pursued to guide management.

E. MT Is Not Cost-Effective at Current Price-Points

One of the postulated benefits of MT is that they can help reduce health-care costs by sparing the need for unnecessary surgeries. Most data regarding cost-effectiveness are derived from modeling studies, and some of these have indicated that MT is indeed not cost-effective. This is due to their current high price-point and the additional costs associated with further workup (neck ultrasound and surgical resection) once these tests determine (often inappropriately) that a lesion may be suspicious. For instance, a modeling study of GEC utilization predicted that while MT could lead to a reduction in the absolute number of patients undergoing surgery by 13%, its use increased *overall cost per nodule* (estimated to be ~$2400 higher compared to no MT over 2 years) because of the need for more frequent repeat biopsies or surveillance imaging of nodules deemed suspicious. The "break-even" price at which molecular tests become cost-effective is estimated to be approximately USD 1000, which is significantly lower than the $3000 to 6000 currently being charged for these tests.

F. Indication for MT in ATC

While the routine use of MT in the context of ITN continues to be debated, the impact of MT on ATC management has been more readily quantifiable and supported by reliable evidence. The 2021 ATA guidelines for ATC, for instance, includes a "strong" recommendation that MT is performed at the time of ATC diagnosis, specifically because the test results can inform which systemic therapy to administer in this aggressive disease. For instance, the presence of $BRAF^{V600E}$ mutation in ATC predicts significant response to combined BRAF + MEK inhibition (discussed further in the section **Targeted Therapies for Thyroid Cancer**), but not in *BRAF* wild-type patients. Similarly, ATC harboring mutations in *ALK* or *NTRK* may be responsive to inhibitors specific to these kinases. Thus, testing for the presence of oncogenic mutations and tailoring inhibitor therapy accordingly is exceedingly important for the management of ATC, and thus underscores the importance of MT in this deadly malignancy.

TARGETED THERAPIES FOR THYROID CANCER

While the incorporation of molecular features into diagnostic testing for thyroid nodules has been fraught with the challenges discussed earlier, it has greatly impacted the development of novel therapeutic agents for TC (Table 24–4). Most of these new therapies are kinase

Table 24–4. List of FDA-approved molecular targeted therapies in thyroid cancer.

Kinase Inhibitor	Molecular Target	Thyroid Cancer Type	Year Approved
Cabozantinib	Multikinase inhibitor, including RET	DTC, MTC	2012 (MTC), 2021 (DTC)
Dabrafenib	RAF	ATC	2018 (in combination with trametinib)
Entrectinib	NTRK	*NTRK*-fusion DTC	2019
Lenvatinib	Multikinase inhibitor	RAI-refractory DTC	2015
Larotrectinib	NTRK	*NTRK*-fusion DTC	2018
Pralsetinib	RET	*RET*-mutant MTC/*RET*-fusion DTC	2020
Selpercatinib	RET	*RET*-mutant MTC/*RET*-fusion DTC	2020
Sorafenib	Multikinase inhibitor	RAI-refractory DTC	2013
Trametinib	MEK	ATC	2018 (in combination with Dabrafenib)
Vandetanib	Multikinase inhibitor, including RET	MTC	2011

inhibitors (KIs) that are administered systemically and play a role in the setting of metastatic, recurrent, or progressive disease where the benefit of surgical intervention is limited. This section summarizes the current approved molecular targeted therapies in TCs. It also includes discussion of investigational use of the molecular targeted therapy, including peptide receptor radionucleotide treatment (PRRT) and immunotherapy for TC.

Metastatic Differentiated Thyroid Cancer

A. Multikinase Inhibitors

As described earlier, constitutive activation of the MAPK and PI3K signaling pathways (either via mutations in specific pathway members such as *BRAF* or activation of upstream receptor tyrosine kinases [RTK]) comprises the majority of actionable mutations in DTC. As such, significant work has been dedicated on developing small molecules that inhibit these oncogenic kinases.

In 2013, sorafenib was the first FDA-approved KI for use in progressive or metastatic radioactive iodine (RAI)-refractory DTC. Sorafenib inhibits the RAF kinases as well as the receptor tyrosine kinases VEGFR1-3, PDGFR, FGFR, KIT, and RET. Cumulatively, inhibition of these targets can lead to downregulation of oncogenic signals via both PI3K and MAPK pathways. Two phase II studies initially demonstrated the efficacy of sorafenib in DTC, which ultimately led to the international, phase III, placebo-controlled randomized DECISION trial in patients with RAI-refractory advanced DTC. In this trial, 417 KI naïve patients were randomized to placebo versus drug treatment, with the latter group demonstrating favorable progression-free survival (PFS) of 10.8 months versus 5.8 months in the placebo group. Response rates were also higher in the sorafenib group at 12.2% (24/196) versus 0.5% (1/201) in the placebo group.

Lenvatinib, another multikinase inhibitor harboring activity against VEGFR1-3, FGFR1-4, PDGFR, KIT, and RET, became FDA-approved for advanced PTC in 2015 after showing superior efficacy in the SELECT trial. In this phase III, multicenter, randomized, placebo-controlled trial in RAI-refractory DTC patients, PFS was six times higher in the drug-treated group at 18.3 months compared to their placebo counterparts. The overall response rate (ORR) was also higher in the lenvatinib group at 64.8%.

Lastly, in September 2021, cabozantinib, a multikinase inhibitor including VEGFR2, was approved for use in RAI-refractory advanced or metastatic DTC based on the outcomes of the COSMIC-311 trial. This was a double-blinded, randomized (2:1), placebo-controlled, multi-institutional trial evaluating 100 patients which revealed a significant increase in median PFS in the cabozantinib treatment group at 11 months compared to 1.9 months in the placebo group. In addition, the treatment group inferred a superior response rate at 18% versus 0% in the cabozantinib and placebo arms, respectively. Thus, single-agent cabozantinib at 60 mg is recommended for appropriate patients until evidence of disease progression or intolerable toxicity is noted.

B. TRK Fusion Inhibitors

Much success has also been demonstrated in targeting *TRK* fusions in TC. Larotrectinib, a highly selective inhibitor of TRKA/B/C, was approved by the FDA in 2018 for treatment of *TRK*-positive solid tumors, including TC, in both the pediatric and adult population. Pooled analysis of phase I/II study protocols containing 55 patients (age range 4 months to 76 years old) with TRK fusion-positive tumors revealed a promising ORR at 75%, with 71% having ongoing responses and 51% remaining progression free at 1 year. Eighty-six percent of patients were continuing treatment or had undergone curative resection at the median follow-up of 9.4 months. Similarly, entrectinib, a TRKA/B/C inhibitor that also demonstrates activity against ALK and ROS1 kinases, was approved by the FDA in 2019. This inhibitor has the added benefit of being able to penetrate the blood-brain barrier, thus being able to potentially target brain metastasis lesions. Pooled data from three trials (STARTRK-1, STARTRK-2, ALK-372-001) on 54 adult patients with TRK fusion-positive tumors of 19 different histologies, comprising four patients with TC, reported an ORR of 57.4%; four patients (7%) with CR, and 27 (50%) had a PR.

C. MEK/ERK Inhibitors in RAI-Refractory DTC

It has been found that downstream activation of the MAPK pathway can contribute to RAI refractoriness in PTC by reducing expression of thyroid-specific genes such as sodium iodide symporter (NIS). Desensitization to RAI occurs due to loss of expression of NIS resulting in the inability of cells to take up and concentrate therapeutic radioactive ^{131}Iodine. Thus, inhibition of this pathway by targeting either RAF or its downstream effectors MEK and ERK kinases has been explored to induce regulation of NIS, thereby promoting the resensitization of RAI therapy. In 2013, a landmark "proof of concept" study investigated the role of pretreatment with selumetinib (MEK1/2 inhibitor) in reversing refractoriness to RAI therapy. Twenty patients with *BRAF* or *NRAS*-mutated RAI-non-avid metastatic DTC were included. Of the 20 patients, selumetinib increased radioactive iodine uptake in 12 patients confirmed by PET/CT. Of the 12 patients, 8 proceeded to complete RAI therapy of which 5 had PR and 3 reported SD. Treatment course was well tolerated, with the majority of patients incurring adverse events of grade 3 or lower. Due to its potential to induce iodine resensitization, trials utilizing pretreatment with selumetinib, other second-generation MEK/ERK inhibitors such as trametinib, as well as BRAF inhibitors are underway in RAI-refractory DTC.

D. BRAF Inhibitors and Other Ongoing Investigative Agents in DTC

Vemurafenib was the first specific BRAF inhibitor to be tested in *BRAF*-mutant thyroid tumors. In a single-agent, multi-institutional, nonrandomized, open-labeled phase II trial, $BRAF^{V600E}$-positive patients were divided into two cohorts based on prior receipt of multikinase inhibitors (including those targeting VEGFRs). Higher response rates were observed in patients with no history of VEGFR inhibitor use; 38.5% experienced PR compared to 27.3% in the comparator arm, as well as a better median PFS at 18.2 months compared to 8.9 months. Likewise, dabrafenib, another selective BRAF inhibitor, had promising results in a phase I trial which led to a multicenter, randomized, open-labeled phase II trial comparing dabrafenib alone to dabrafenib in combination with trametinib (a MEK inhibitor). Overall response rates were 50% in the single-agent arm compared to 54% in the combination arm. Overall, vemurafenib and dabrafenib are currently only FDA-approved for melanoma therapy and not for DTC, although their use continues to be investigated for TC. In addition, ongoing trials are evaluating the use of other TKIs (eg, anlotinib, apatinib, axitinib, cabozantinib, donafenib, dovitinib, nintedanib, pazopanib, sunitinib, vandetinib) in isolation as well as combination for DTC patients as well as patients with PDTC/ATC.

Medullary Thyroid Cancer

A. Multikinase and RET Inhibitors

Cabozantinib and vandetanib (which inhibits VEGFR 2/3, EGFR, KIT, and RET) are multikinase inhibitors that harbor anti-RET kinase activity and are FDA-approved for use in metastatic MTC. A phase III, randomized, double-blinded, placebo-controlled trial using cabozantinib conducted by Elisei and colleagues on 330 locally advanced or metastatic MTC patients revealed a favorable PFS at 11.2 versus 4 months in its placebo arm. Out of these patients, 28% experienced a partial response irrespective of their RET mutation status. A similar phase III randomized placebo-controlled trial (ZETA trial) utilizing vandetanib in 331 patients with unresectable or locally advanced MTC also predicted a median PFS at 30.5 months in the experimental arm versus 19.3 months in the placebo arm with a partial response rate of 45%. Indeed, these two agents, approved in 2012 and 2011 respectively, were some of the earliest targeted therapies approved for TC.

More recently, inhibitors that specifically target mutant RET have been approved for MTC harboring this genetic abnormality. Selpercatinib (LOXO-292) and pralsetinib (BLU-667) demonstrated excellent response in phase I/II trials in patients with advanced metastatic M918T/V804M-positive MTC refractory to prior KI therapy. Selpercatinib's ability to cross the blood-brain barrier provided added benefit to its potential to treat RET-positive brain metastases. Data from subsequent LIBRETTO-001 trial evaluating selpercatinib therapy revealed up to 69% ORR in 55 patients who had previously received kinase-targeted therapy and 73% ORR in 88 treatment naïve patients. In the ARROW trial, pralsetinib demonstrated similar efficacy in the treatment of RET-positive MTCs, yielding an ORR of 60% in patients exposed to prior therapy and 71% in the treatment naïve group. In 2020, both therapies received FDA approval for use in advanced or metastatic RET-mutant MTC.

Anaplastic Thyroid Cancer

A. Multikinase Inhibitors

Given the aggressive nature of this disease, ATC is often diagnosed at an advanced stage and is treated with multimodality therapy that includes chemotherapy and radiation. However, the discovery of BRAF V600E mutation in a subset of ATC led to the exploration of dabrafenib (which inhibits RAF) and trametinib (a MEK inhibitor) for this disease type. This combination ultimately gained approval in 2018 and is now considered the standard of care therapy for ATC with BRAF V600E in both the neoadjuvant setting and in cases of unresectable disease. For ATC without BRAF V600E mutation, the emphasis has been on employing inhibitors that target any other actionable mutation that the tumor may harbor (such as larotrectinib/entrectinib in tumors with *NTRK*-fusions or selpercatinib/pralsetinib for those with *RET* fusions).

Investigational Molecular Targeted Therapeutic Strategies in Thyroid Cancer

A. mTOR Inhibitors

The activation of the PI3K/AKT/mTOR pathway is common on TCs and present in up to 30% to 35% of ATCs. Everolimus, a serine-threonine kinase inhibitor of mTOR, has been studied in multiple trials for the treatment of DTC, MTC, and ATC. The most recent multicenter, phase II trial including 33 patients with DTC, 10 MTC, and 7 patients with ATC revealed a favorable PFS in DTC and MTC at 12.9 months and 13.1 months, respectively but had a relatively low PFS in ATC at 2.2 months. Investigation into combination therapy utilizing everolimus with known KIs is underway.

B. Peptide Receptor Radionuclide Therapy

An exciting molecular therapeutic option for RAI-non-avid metastatic DTC and MTC currently under investigation is PRRT. MTC and a subset of DTC express somatostatin receptors (SSTR) that can be targeted with this therapeutic approach. When administered, PRRT agents like yttrium-90 (^{90}Y)-DOTATOC or lutetium-177 (^{177}Lu)-DOTATATE bind to SSTR and induce cytotoxic effects via lethal radioactivity to the cell, meanwhile sparing adjacent normal cells and thereby limiting systemic effects of therapy. Small pilot studies investigating PRRT have been conducted in Europe. A recent meta-analysis incorporating results from 165 patients revealed an ORR of 8.5% in MTC and 15.6% in DTC, while the DCR were 60% and 54%, respectively. PRRT based on the radioisotope ^{177}Lu was noted to perform better than ^{90}Y.

C. Checkpoint Inhibitors

Modulating the immune landscape of the tumor microenvironment through immune checkpoint blockade has played a significant role in the treatment of metastatic disease. Immune checkpoints such as programmed cell death protein 1 (PD-1) on T cells and its ligand (PDL-1) on tumor cells provide negative feedback to the immune system to prevent excessive activation as in the setting of autoimmunity. Opportunistic tumor cells commandeer this immunosuppressed state to promote proliferation and metastatic disease. PD-1/PDL-1 expression on thyroid tumor cells has been extensively studied. A TCGA analysis of thyroid tumors found higher levels of PDL-1 mRNA expression associated with lymph node metastasis, extrathyroidal invasion, and overall reduced survival. However, while checkpoint inhibitors have received FDA approval for treatment of multiple advanced-staged tumors, metastatic DTC has thus far demonstrated only marginal response to checkpoint blockade therapy. The seminal open-labelled, single-arm, phase Ib trial evaluating pembrolizumab in advanced solid tumors (KEYNOTE-028) included 22 patients with advanced PDL-1 (+) RAI-refractory DTC. Median PFS was 7 months, with 9% (2/22) of patients with PR and 59% (13/22) with SD. This study revealed that although the side effect profile was tolerable, single-agent immunotherapy incurred a favorable response in only a minority of the patients. Given DTC's relatively poor immunogenicity and marginal response to single-agent immunotherapy, clinical trials are underway investigating combination therapy including TKIs and immunotherapy in RAI-refractory DTC.

Unlike DTCs, ATCs have demonstrated high PD-1/PDL-1 expression making immunotherapy an effective agent in the treatment of this disease. A retrospective analysis conducted by MD Anderson of 12 patients with ATC revealed a 42% PR rate, 33% SD rate, and a 25% rate of disease progression in patients treated with combination pembrolizumab and KI therapy. Similarly, MTCs have also been found to have significant T cell infiltration, leading to multiple phase II studies evaluating the checkpoint inhibitors ipilimumab, pembrolizumab, and nivolumab in this disease.

SUGGESTED READING

Alexander EK, Kennedy GC, Baloch ZW, et al. Preoperative diagnosis of benign thyroid nodules with indeterminate cytology. *N Engl J Med*. 2012;367(8):705-715.

Balentine CJ, Vanness DJ, Schneider DF. Cost-effectiveness of lobectomy versus genetic testing (Afirma(R)) for indeterminate thyroid nodules: considering the costs of surveillance. *Surgery*. 2018;163(1):88-96.

Bible KC, Kebebew E, Brierley J, et al. 2021 American Thyroid Association Guidelines for Management of Patients with Anaplastic Thyroid Cancer. *Thyroid*. 2021;31(3):337-386.

Brose MS, Cabanillas ME, Cohen EE, et al. Vemurafenib in patients with BRAFV600E-positive metastatic or unresectable papillary thyroid cancer refractory to radioactive iodine: a non-randomised, multicentre, open-label, phase 2 trial. *Lancet Oncol*. 2016;17(9):1272-1282.

Brose MS, Nutting CM, Jarzab B, et al. Sorafenib in radioactive iodine-refractory, locally advanced or metastatic differentiated thyroid cancer: a randomised, double-blind, phase 3 trial. *Lancet*. 2014;384(9940):319-328.

Brose MS, Robinson B, Sherman SI, et al. Cabozantinib for radioiodine-refractory differentiated thyroid cancer (COSMIC-311): a randomised, double-blind, placebo-controlled, phase 3 trial. *Lancet Oncol*. 2021;22(8):1126-1138.

Cancer Genome Atlas Research Network. Integrated genomic characterization of papillary thyroid carcinoma. *Cell.* 2014; 159(3):676-690.

Chernock RD, Hagemann IS. Molecular pathology of hereditary and sporadic medullary thyroid carcinomas. *Am J Clin Pathol.* 2015;143(6):768-777.

Cibas ES, Ali SZ. The 2017 Bethesda System for Reporting Thyroid Cytopathology. *Thyroid.* 2017;27(11):1341-1346.

Doebele RC, Drilon A, Paz-Ares L, et al. Entrectinib in patients with advanced or metastatic NTRK fusion-positive solid tumours: integrated analysis of three phase 1-2 trials. *Lancet Oncol.* 2020; 21(2):271-282.

Drilon A, Laetsch TW, Kummar S, et al. Efficacy of larotrectinib in TRK fusion-positive cancers in adults and children. *N Engl J Med.* 2018;378(8):731-739.

Drilon A, Siena S, Ou SI, et al. Safety and antitumor activity of the multitargeted Pan-TRK, ROS1, and ALK inhibitor entrectinib: combined results from two phase I trials (ALKA-372-001 and STARTRK-1). *Cancer Discov.* 2017;7(4):400-409.

Elisei R, Schlumberger MJ, Müller SP, et al. Cabozantinib in progressive medullary thyroid cancer [published correction appears in *J Clin Oncol.* 2014;32(17):1864]. *J Clin Oncol.* 2013;31(29):3639-3646.

Endo M, Nabhan F, Porter K, et al. Afirma gene sequencing classifier compared with gene expression classifier in indeterminate thyroid nodules. *Thyroid.* 2019;29(8):1115-1124.

Fagin JA, Wells SA, Jr. Biologic and clinical perspectives on thyroid cancer. *N Engl J Med.* 2016;375(11):1054-1067.

French JD. Immunotherapy for advanced thyroid cancers: rationale, current advances and future strategies. *Nat Rev Endocrinol.* 2020;16(11):629-641.

Hanna GJ, Busaidy NL, Chau NG, et al. Genomic correlates of response to everolimus in aggressive radioiodine-refractory thyroid cancer: a phase II study. *Clin Cancer Res.* 2018;24(7): 1546-1553.

Haugen BR, Alexander EK, Bible KC, et al. 2015 American Thyroid Association Management Guidelines for Adult Patients with Thyroid Nodules and Differentiated Thyroid Cancer: The American Thyroid Association Guidelines Task Force on Thyroid Nodules and Differentiated Thyroid Cancer. *Thyroid.* 2016;26(1):1-133.

Ho AL, Grewal RK, Leboeuf R, et al. Selumetinib-enhanced radioiodine uptake in advanced thyroid cancer. *N Engl J Med.* 2013;368(7):623-632.

Huang BL, Chabot JA, Lee JA, Kuo JH. A stepwise analysis of the diagnostic algorithm for the prediction of malignancy in thyroid nodules. *Surgery.* 2020;167(1):28-33.

Iyer PC, Dadu R, Gule-Monroe M, et al. Salvage pembrolizumab added to kinase inhibitor therapy for the treatment of anaplastic thyroid carcinoma. *J Immunother Cancer.* 2018;6(1):68.

Lee DY, Kim YI. Peptide receptor radionuclide therapy in patients with differentiated thyroid cancer: a meta-analysis. *Clin Nucl Med.* 2020;45(8):604-610.

Lim H, Devesa SS, Sosa JA, Check D, Kitahara CM. Trends in thyroid cancer incidence and mortality in the United States, 1974-2013. *JAMA.* 2017;317(13):1338-1348.

McKelvey BA, Umbricht CB, Zeiger MA. Telomerase reverse transcriptase (TERT) regulation in thyroid cancer: a review. *Front Endocrinol (Lausanne).* 2020;11:485.

Mehnert JM, Varga A, Brose MS, et al. Safety and antitumor activity of the anti-PD-1 antibody pembrolizumab in patients with advanced, PD-L1-positive papillary or follicular thyroid cancer. *BMC Cancer.* 2019;19(1):196.

Nikiforov YE, Carty SE, Chiosea SI, et al. Highly accurate diagnosis of cancer in thyroid nodules with follicular neoplasm/suspicious for a follicular neoplasm cytology by ThyroSeq v2 next-generation sequencing assay. *Cancer.* 2014;120(23): 3627-3634.

Nikiforov YE, Seethala RR, Tallini G, et al. Nomenclature revision for encapsulated follicular variant of papillary thyroid carcinoma: a paradigm shift to reduce overtreatment of indolent tumors. *JAMA Oncol.* 2016;2(8):1023-1029.

Nikiforova MN, Wald AI, Roy S, Durso MB, Nikiforov YE. Targeted next-generation sequencing panel (ThyroSeq) for detection of mutations in thyroid cancer. *J Clin Endocrinol Metab.* 2013;98(11):E1852-E1860.

Noureldine SI, Najafian A, Aragon Han P, et al. Evaluation of the effect of diagnostic molecular testing on the surgical decision-making process for patients with thyroid nodules. *JAMA Otolaryngol Head Neck Surg.* 2016;142(7):676-682.

Noureldine SI, Olson MT, Agrawal N, Prescott JD, Zeiger MA, Tufano RP. Effect of gene expression classifier molecular testing on the surgical decision-making process for patients with thyroid nodules. *JAMA Otolaryngol Head Neck Surg.* 2015;141(12):1082-1088.

Patel KN, Angell TE, Babiarz J, et al. Performance of a genomic sequencing classifier for the preoperative diagnosis of cytologically indeterminate thyroid nodules. *JAMA Surg.* 2018;153(9): 817-824.

Patel KN, Yip L, Lubitz CC, et al. The American Association of Endocrine Surgeons Guidelines for the Definitive Surgical Management of Thyroid Disease in Adults. *Ann Surg.* 2020; 271(3):e21-e93.

Raman P, Koenig RJ. Pax-8-PPAR-gamma fusion protein in thyroid carcinoma. *Nat Rev Endocrinol.* 2014;10(10):616-623.

Sahli ZT, Umbricht CB, Schneider EB, Zeiger MA. Thyroid nodule diagnostic markers in the face of the new NIFTP category: time for a reset? *Thyroid.* 2017;27(11):1393-1399.

Salvatore D, Santoro M, Schlumberger M. The importance of the RET gene in thyroid cancer and therapeutic implications. *Nat Rev Endocrinol.* 2021;17(5):296-306.

Schlumberger M, Jarzab B, Cabanillas ME, et al. A phase II trial of the multitargeted tyrosine kinase inhibitor lenvatinib (e7080) in advanced medullary thyroid cancer. *Clin Cancer Res.* 2016;22(1):44-53.

Schlumberger M, Tahara M, Wirth LJ, et al. Lenvatinib versus placebo in radioiodine-refractory thyroid cancer. *N Engl J Med.* 2015;372(7):621-630.

Silaghi CA, Lozovanu V, Georgescu CE, et al. Thyroseq v3, Afirma GSC, and microRNA panels versus previous molecular tests in the preoperative diagnosis of indeterminate thyroid nodules: a systematic review and meta-analysis. *Front Endocrinol (Lausanne).* 2021;12:649522.

Steward DL, Carty SE, Sippel RS, et al. Performance of a multigene genomic classifier in thyroid nodules with indeterminate cytology: a prospective blinded multicenter study. *JAMA Oncol.* 2019;5(2):204-212.

Subbiah V, Hu MI, Wirth LJ, et al. Pralsetinib for patients with advanced or metastatic RET-altered thyroid cancer (ARROW): a multi-cohort, open-label, registrational, phase 1/2 study [published correction appears in *Lancet Diabetes Endocrinol.* 2021;9(10):e4]. *Lancet Diabetes Endocrinol.* 2021;9(8):491-501.

Subbiah V, Kreitman RJ, Wainberg ZA, et al. Dabrafenib and trametinib treatment in patients with locally advanced or metastatic BRAF V600-mutant anaplastic thyroid cancer. *J Clin Oncol.* 2018;36(1):7-13.

Tahara M, Kiyota N, Yamazaki T, et al. Lenvatinib for anaplastic thyroid cancer. *Front Oncol.* 2017;7:25.

Taye A, Gurciullo D, Miles BA, et al. Clinical performance of a next-generation sequencing assay (ThyroSeq v2) in the evaluation of indeterminate thyroid nodules. *Surgery.* 2018;163(1):97-103.

Valderrabano P, Hallanger-Johnson JE, Thapa R, Wang X, McIver B. Comparison of postmarketing findings vs the initial clinical validation findings of a thyroid nodule gene expression classifier: a systematic review and meta-analysis. *JAMA Otolaryngol Head Neck Surg.* 2019;145(9):783-792.

Wells SA Jr, Robinson BG, Gagel RF, et al. Vandetanib in patients with locally advanced or metastatic medullary thyroid cancer: a randomized, double-blind phase III trial. *J Clin Oncol.* 2012;30(2):134-141.

Wirth LJ, Sherman E, Robinson B, et al. Efficacy of selpercatinib in *RET*-altered thyroid cancers. *N Engl J Med.* 2020;383(9):825-835.

Xing M. Molecular pathogenesis and mechanisms of thyroid cancer. *Nat Rev Cancer.* 2013;13(3):184-199.

Radioactive Iodine Therapy in Thyroid Cancer

25

Kathryn Graham, MB ChB, BSc (Hons)
Ujjal Mallick, MBBS, MS
Nick Reed, MBBS, MRCP (UK)

HISTORY & DEVELOPMENT OF RADIOACTIVE IODINE

Iodine-131 (^{131}I), a radioisotope of iodine, was discovered in 1938. It is a major fission product of uranium and plutonium, significantly contributing to environmental hazards arising from atomic bomb testing in the 1950s and nuclear reactor crises, such as Chernobyl in the 1980s. However, due to favorable physical and chemical properties, controlled use of ^{131}I has been adapted for both imaging and medicinal purposes; ^{131}I now constitutes one of the most important radionuclides in nuclear medicine and is the first example of targeted radiotherapy.

^{131}I Properties

The radioactive half-life decay of ^{131}I is 8.02 days. The isotope emits 90% beta (β) radiation (short range, 192 keV) and 10% gamma (γ) radiation (long range, 383 keV). Therapeutic effects of ^{131}I are derived from β-emission, resulting in DNA damage and cell death, but the short range means that penetration into absorbed tissue is only a few millimeters. While β-rays are essentially invisible, the longer range γ-rays can be detected by nuclear medicine imaging techniques (gamma camera) and facilitate dosimetry. Additional radioisotopes of iodine, for example, ^{123}I and ^{124}I, are also utilized for diagnostic purposes, but ^{131}I is unique, possessing the dual advantage of therapy and imaging applications simultaneously. It can also be generated at relatively low cost from neutron bombardment of tellurium in a nuclear reactor, unlike other isotopes that rely on cyclotron production.

^{131}I Therapeutic Use

Therapeutic use of ^{131}I is possible due to a unique membrane-bound protein, sodium iodide symporter (NIS), present in normal thyroid cells as well as differentiated thyroid cancer (DTC) cells. NIS selectively mediates the active transport of iodine (or isotopes of iodine) inside the cell from the basolateral membrane to the thyroidal colloid. Although the NIS gene was only cloned in 1996,[1] radionuclide therapy with ^{131}I, or radioactive iodine (RAI), has been practiced for 80 years. It was first utilized in a cohort of patients with thyrotoxicosis[2] to render them biochemically and clinically euthyroid (or hypothyroid), based on the understanding of thyroid physiology at that time, as it was already established that iodine was requisite in the biosynthesis of thyroxine (T4) and triiodothyronine (T3). Speculation that ^{131}I could be internalized by DTC cells, and therefore potentially advantageous as a means of cancer therapy, led to successful experimentation in a series of patients in the United States,[3-5] shortly followed in the United Kingdom,[6] often in those with advanced disease who had no other treatment options. NIS expression is not exclusive to the thyroid and has been reported in other tissues, including salivary and lacrimal glands, choroidal plexus, gastric mucosa, and the mammary gland.[7] Extrathyroidal uptake of ^{131}I is known to contribute to acute and late toxicity of RAI, but fortuitously ^{131}I is preferentially concentrated in cells of thyroid origin.

Gradually, RAI was adopted extensively in DTC but due to significant variation in protocols, prescribed activity of ^{131}I, and degree of surgical resection, it was several decades before the full impact of RAI in optimizing the management of DTC was recognized; specifically, the ability to exert a survival benefit in advanced/metastatic disease, reduce recurrence rates in patients with high-risk features, and enable accurate follow-up across the entire spectrum of DTC.[8,9] This early work, performed over many years and often retrospective in methodology, although pivotal, highlighted the importance of good quality evidence in DTC and was instrumental in the design of randomized clinical trials that now define and are continuing to enrich the utilization of RAI in DTC management.

ESTABLISHMENT OF RAI AS STANDARD OF CARE

Surgery is the cornerstone of therapy in differentiated thyroid cancer (DTC), even in the context of metastatic disease, but RAI remains a universally accepted practice in the management of the post-thyroidectomy patients. It can be utilized with ablative, adjuvant, and therapeutic intent. First, it is important to separate ablation from adjuvant treatment. Ablation refers to destruction of the normal thyroid remnant; the main aim of this approach is to facilitate accurate radionuclide imaging and biochemical follow-up, as serum thyroglobulin (Tg) levels should be low or undetectable. Adjuvant RAI additionally sterilizes any residual cancer cells and theoretically minimizes the risk of relapse. Both terms are often used interchangeably, although the principle is different. Therapeutic RAI is the utilization of ^{131}I to achieve tumor control (or eradication) in advanced locoregional disease and/or metastatic disease.

Historically, RAI was considered in all patients with DTC following thyroidectomy (with the exception of solitary microcarcinomas), but in the past 15 years there has been a move to apply evidence-based management to avoid potentially overtreating patients with lower-risk DTC. Just as evolving paradigms promote a more conservative surgical approach, such as hemithyroidectomy rather than total thyroidectomy for small low-risk tumors, clinicians have questioned whether the use of RAI should be similarly constrained. This has led to the development of randomized phase III trials that have investigated de-escalation of ^{131}I activity[10,11] and, more recently, whether RAI can be safely omitted altogether in certain patient cohorts.[12,13]

Traditional Indications for RAI

Over the past few decades, RAI has been shown to improve survival and reduce relapse in specific clinical scenarios, for instance T4 tumors and metastatic disease,[14,15] although the evidence is based on multicenter case series and systematic analyses as opposed to randomized trials. Data on the value of RAI in the absence of these very high-risk features is less robust, but it is well recognized that the following clinical and pathological features can adversely affect outcome in DTC: age; primary tumor size; aggressive histological subtype; regional lymph node involvement; and presence of lymphovascular invasion.[16,17] Age has long been an important prognostic factor in DTC and, in contrast to many other tumor types, it is actually incorporated into various staging systems. Previously, more than 45 years was highlighted as the threshold, above which outcomes are reportedly poorer, but following reanalysis more than 55 years was replaced as the cutoff.[18]

Various international bodies have developed guidelines to direct practice, notably the American Thyroid Association (ATA, 2015),[19] British Thyroid Association (BTA, 2014),[20] European Association of Nuclear Medicine (EANM, 2008),[21] European Society of Medical Oncology (ESMO, 2019),[22] and National Cancer Comprehensive Network (NCCN, 2021) (https://www.nccn.org/), but there is no single overarching protocol. Current recommendations generally concur that RAI is not endorsed in DTC less than 1 cm (ie, T1a N0/Nx). Conversely, RAI is invariably indicated in T4 tumors, especially if there is residual macroscopic disease, and/or in the presence of metastatic disease. In T1b-T3 (or T1a N1) DTC, it is less clear whether adjuvant RAI is advantageous in terms of recurrence and/or survival outcomes. For example, primary tumor more than 4 cm (T3) does not feature in the ATA 2015 guidelines,[19] but still merits adjuvant RAI in both the BTA 2014 guidelines[20] and the recently published NCCN 2021 recommendation (https://www.nccn.org/). An overview of current guidelines is illustrated in Table 25–1.

Risk Stratification in the Modern Era

The most commonly applied staging systems in DTC are the joint American Joint Committee on Cancer-Tumor Node Metastasis (AJCC-TNM, 8th edition, 2018), and Metastases, Age, Completeness of Resection, Invasion, Size (MACIS, https://www.thyroid.org/professionals/calculators/). Both classification schemes use a combination of age, tumor size, extrathyroidal spread, and locoregional and distant metastases to stratify patients, but were derived to predict the risk of cancer-specific mortality from DTC. A recent update modified the age threshold to 55 years, and decreased the unfavorable prognostic significance attributed to certain findings, for example, small-volume cervical lymph node metastases[23] and microscopic extrathyroidal extension as opposed to macroscopic extrathyroidal extension.[24,25] Nonetheless, there is still a wide variation in outcomes across individual stage and it is important to note that survival does not necessarily reflect recurrence rates as many patients with DTC will be cured at relapse. For that reason, it is essential to consider the risk of recurrence as well as the risk of cancer-related death.

The ATA 2015 guidelines provided a detailed breakdown of the likelihood of persistent or structural disease recurrence and not only stratified patients into a specific risk group (low/intermediate/high), but also presented this risk on a continuum that ranges from less than 1% to more than 50%.[19] See Table 25–2. For the first time, "high-risk" included patients with factors other than gross extrathyroidal extension, residual macroscopic disease, and presence of metastases (or postoperative Tg level suggestive of distant metastases), specifically large-volume lymph node involvement (including any metastatic lymph node >3 cm) and/or extranodal extension, and extensive vascular invasion (described as ≥4 foci) in follicular thyroid cancer (FTC). Conversely, minimally invasive (or encapsulated) FTC with less than 4 foci of vascular invasion is deemed

Table 25–1. Overview of indications for RAI based on international guidelines.

	No Indications	Uncertain	Definite Indications
ATA 2015	Low risk* As per ATA	Intermediate risk As per ATA	High risk As per ATA
BTA 2014	If any present: ≤1 cm PTC (unifocal or multifocal†) MI FTC with no VI	If any or all present: Large tumor size Extrathyroidal extension Unfavorable histology Widely invasive histology Nodal involvement: Multiple nodes Large size of involved nodes, high ratio of positive to negative nodes extracapsular nodal involvement	If any present: Tumor >4 cm Gross extrathyroidal extension Distant metastases
EANM 2008	RAI non-avid metastases	RAI-avid metastases (following resection) Nonresectable bone metastases Suspected metastatic DTC (Tg increasing but RAI avidity unknown) Poorly differentiated thyroid cancer with detectable Tg and symptomatic disease	Unresectable RA-avid lymph node metastases RAI-avid lung micrometastases Nonresectable RAI-avid lung metastases Nonresectable soft tissue metastases
ESMO 2019	T1a N0/Nx	Low/Intermediate risk As per ATA	High risk As per ATA
NCCN 2021	If all present: Classical PTC <2 cm Intrathyroidal Unifocal or multifocal (all foci ≤1 cm) No detectable anti-Tg antibodies Postop unstimulated Tg <1 ng/mL†† Negative postoperative USS (if done)	If any or all present: Detectable anti-Tg antibodies†† Largest primary tumor 2-4 cm High-risk histology Lymphovascular invasion Cervical lymph nodes Postop unstimulated Tg <10 ng/mL†† Macroscopic multifocality (focus >1 cm) Microscopic positive margin	If any present: Tumor >4 cm Gross extrathyroidal extension Postop unstimulated Tg >10 ng/mL†† Bulky or >5 positive lymph nodes

*Individual patient factors to be taken into consideration.
†Classical papillary/encapsulated follicular variant papillary thyroid cancer (EFVPTC)/minimally invasive follicular thyroid cancer (MI FTC).
††Tg 6–12 weeks postop.
ATA, American Thyroid Association; BTA, British Thyroid Association; EANM, European Association of Nuclear Medicine; ESMO, European Society of Medical Oncology; FTC, follicular thyroid cancer; NCCN, National Cancer Comprehensive Network; PTC, papillary thyroid cancer; Tg, thyroglobulin; USS, ultrasound scan.

lowrisk as several studies (but not all) purport an excellent clinical outcome.[26-30] Of note, molecular prognostication was introduced in ATA 2015,[19] but not adopted by the most recent guideline published over 5 years later by NCCN (https://www.nccn.org/), and will be discussed in more detail later.

As expected, RAI is recommended in the ATA high-risk group,[19] but RAI is considered optional in the intermediate group and the ATA proposed withholding RAI altogether in the lowest-risk patients.[19] The omission of RAI in the absence of high-risk features has raised controversy[31] and it has been argued that RAI still has a valuable ablative role, especially if there is limited access to essential follow-up techniques such as experienced sonography and/or good quality Tg assay. Since the recent publication of the French ESTIMABL2 trial, however, there is now randomized evidence supporting thyroidectomy alone in T1a(m)/T1b N0/Nx DTC as the 3-year composite structural, functional, and biological outcomes were noninferior to RAI.[12] In addition, emerging data from IoN (Is ablative radioiodine Necessary for low risk differentiated thyroid cancer patients?) suggest that it may be appropriate to withhold RAI in an even wider population of DTC (T1-T3 N0/Nx/N1a).[13] Ultimately, until there is a unified internationally agreed consensus that incorporates the collective findings of these two important randomized trials, the decision whether to proceed with RAI in low-to-intermediate risk DTC will reflect the local and national policies that take

Table 25–2. Postoperative risk stratification.

PTC	FTC	Risk Group
Distant metastases, 100% Postoperative Tg suggestive of distant metastases, 100% Incomplete tumor resection (R2), 100% Concomitant BRAF V600E and TERT mutation, >40% Extranodal extension, 40% Nodal metastases >3 cm, 30% Gross extrathyroidal extension, 30%-40%	Widely invasive, 30%-60% OR Extensive vascular invasion (≥4 foci), 30%-60%	High risk >20%
Clinical N1 disease, 20% Pathological N1 (>5 LNs, all <3 cm), 20% Multifocal mPTC + ETE + BRAF V600E, 20% Vascular invasion, 15%-30% Aggressive histology, up to 15% pT2, BRAF V600E mutated, 10%		Intermediate risk 5%-20%
Clinical N0, <5% Pathological N1 (<5 micrometastases, all < 0.2 cm), <5%	No vascular invasion, >5% OR Minimal vascular invasion (<4 foci), <5%	Low risk <5%

ATA, American Thyroid Association; FTC, follicular thyroid cancer; LN, lymph node; PTC, papillary thyroid cancer; Tg, thyroglobulin; R, resection margin.
Source: Adapted from ATA 2015 Risk Stratification Staging System.

precedence in the treating institution, taking into account individual risk factors, as well as patient choice. Indeed, the BTA advocates "personalized decision-making" between patient and clinician.[20]

Molecular Prognostic/Predictive Factors

More than 10 pathological subtypes of papillary thyroid cancer (PTC) have been documented, of which the most adverse variants are tall cell, columnar, and hobnail. These subtypes have been associated with various mutations, including BRAF V600E.[32] The role of BRAF V600E as an independent prognostic indicator remains contentious. It has been linked with lymph node metastases, and extrathyroidal extension, as well as aggressive histology,[33-35] but the presence of BRAFV600E alone has a limited positive predictive value for recurrence.[36] Therefore, it is difficult to determine the attributable proportional risk. Despite this, BRAF V600E mutational status is included in ATA 2015,[37] although it is emphasized that it is not a prerequisite for initial stratification profiling and should be considered in combination with additional risk factors. More convincing data have highlighted that TERT mutation is an independent predictor of disease-free survival and mortality;[38] as such, TERT is also included in ATA 2015 within the high-risk category.[19] TERT and BRAF V600E appear to have a synergistic effect and dual mutation is associated with a significant preponderance for structural disease recurrence.[39] Many questions still remain over the precise role of molecular prognostication, and many centers do not yet perform next-generation sequencing as standard in DTC, which explains the omission of this technique in NCCN 2021 (https://www.nccn.org/). It is likely that in the future comprehensive genomic analysis incorporating BRAF V600E, TERT, and possibly additional drivers of oncogenesis such as RAS may influence risk stratification, especially as novel gene fusions and deletions (notably RET and NTRK) have been identified and are influencing therapeutic options in the advanced DTC setting.[40,41]

Use of Thyroglobulin (Tg) to Stratify

Serial Tg measurements form the foundation of contemporary DTC monitoring in the long-term follow-up setting. However, Tg is now being investigated as a tool in postoperative risk assessment. The predictive value of Tg will depend on the residual amount of thyroid tissue (and/or thyroid cancer), TSH level at time of Tg measurement, functional sensitivity of the assay, and time elapsed since total thyroidectomy. As the half-life of Tg is 1 to 3 days, the nadir should be reached by 3 to 4 weeks. Several studies have shown that postoperative stimulated or unstimulated Tg (measured at 6-12 weeks after total thyroidectomy), with or without a corresponding neck ultrasound, can be used to predict the likelihood of identifying RAI-avid metastatic thyroid cancer on the post-treatment uptake scan at time of ablation,[42-45] and/or risk of recurrence.[42,46-55] Adverse outcomes generally increase as basal Tg rises above 5 to 10 ng/mL, but there is no agreed cutoff. Even a low or undetectable Tg level cannot completely eliminate the possibility of ^{131}I uptake outside the thyroid bed, especially in higher-risk patients.

However, a recent prospective trial in low-to-intermediate risk DTC with minimum 5-year follow-up suggests that pre-ablation unstimulated highly sensitive Tg (hsTg) less than 0.1 ng/mL (equivalent to stimulated Tg <1 ng/mL) is predictive of cure.[56] In most studies, patients proceeded to ablation regardless of Tg level, but there is increasing interest in potentially withholding RAI based on Tg +/− USS findings despite the lack of phase III or long-term follow-up data to support this. Mature results from the Ion and ESTIMABL2 trials may answer this question in the future. On balance, there is uncertainty over the specific level of stimulated or unstimulated Tg that mandates whether RAI is indicated or not. Based on the available evidence at present, postoperative Tg is more valuable in identifying patients who may benefit from RAI ablation rather than those who do not, with the possible exception of patients who meet only low-risk criteria and have stimulated Tg less than 1 ng/mL or unstimulated hsTg less than 0.1 ng/mL (https://www.nccn.org/).

Activity of RAI

Traditionally, an empirical activity of 3.7 gigabecquerel (GBq) was utilized as standard practice for ablation and/or adjuvant treatment (approximately equivalent to 100 millicurie [mCi]). Following the results of two multicenter randomized phase III trials, HiLo[10] and ESTIMABL1,[11] de-escalation of RAI to an activity of 1.1 GBq (30 mCi) was proven to be noninferior to 3.7 GBq (100 mCi) in terms of successful ablation at 6 to 10 months for patients with T1-T3, N0/Nx/N1 DTC (all had R0 resection). A meta-analysis also reported no difference in efficacy between 1.1 GBq (30 mCi) and 3.7 GBq (100 mCi).[57] Lower activity has the advantage of a shorter in-hospital admission, a briefer period of radiation restrictions post-treatment, and less toxicity. There was a discrepancy over inclusion criteria between the two studies; HiLo permitted patients with T3 and/or N1 DTC,[10] comprising 20% to 25% and 15% to 20% of all trial subjects, respectively, whereas ESTIMABL1 excluded T3 DTC and N1 was restricted to patients with T1/N1 DTC only.[11] 1.1 GBq (30 mCi) has largely replaced the higher activity for T1-T2, N0, R0, DTC, but some centers were reluctant to adopt 1.1 GBq (30 mCi) for T3 DTC, especially in the context of positive nodes. Now that 5-year outcomes have been reported, indicating recurrence rates of up to 2% to 3%, regardless of RAI activity, with no difference in T3 and N1 patients,[58,59] there may be more impetus for utilizing 1.1 GBq (30 mCi) in tumors more than 4 cm and/or those with small volume lymphadenopathy. On a cautionary note, time to recurrence was a secondary endpoint of HiLo and the study was only adequately powered for comparison of proportions rather than hazard ratios. It is unclear precisely how many patients had intermediate risk DTC based on both T3 and N1, leading to a degree of uncertainty over the use of low dose RAI in those with larger tumors and positive nodes. For more advanced DTC (especially T4/R2 and/or metastatic disease), 3.7 GBq (100 mCi) is the activity of choice to achieve ablation as a minimum, followed by additional therapeutic doses as indicated by disease burden and response to ^{131}I (see section Management of Metastatic Disease). In all remaining patients, the decision to proceed with 1.1 GBq (30 mCi) or 3.7 GBq (100 mCi) is based on a careful risk/benefit analysis and the clinician must take into account all of the clinical and pathological factors.

In summary, until a decade ago, 3.7 GBq RAI (100 mCi) was standard practice in virtually all patients with DTC. Contemporary postoperative management is now increasingly complex. There is the option of no RAI or 1.1 GBq (30 mCi) for low-risk DTC, 3.7 GBq (100 mCi) for high-risk DTC, and either no RAI, 1.1 GBq (30 mCi), or 3.7 GBq (100 mCi) for intermediate-risk DTC. A flowchart proposing an algorithm for selection of RAI and/or recommended activity is depicted in Figure 25–1.

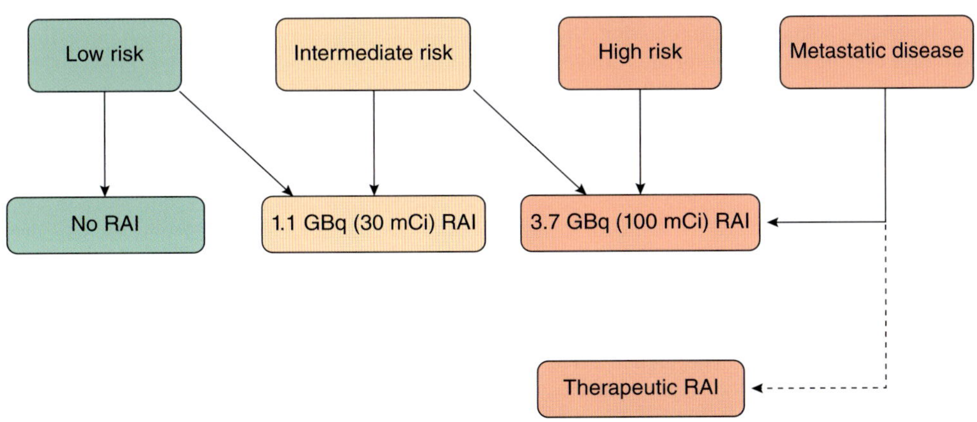

Figure 25–1. Selection of radioactive iodine (RAI) ablation/adjuvant activity.

PREPARATION FOR TREATMENT WITH RAI

Success of RAI treatment is largely dependent on two factors: first, a high TSH level (>30 IU/mL) such that ^{131}I will be driven into thyrocytes and/or DTC cells; and, second, relative deficiency of iodine. The traditional approach is withdrawal of thyroid replacement hormone (levothyroxine for up to 4-5 weeks or liothyronine for 2 weeks) combined with restricting iodine intake for up to 3 weeks prior to treatment. It is well recognized that thyroid hormone withdrawal leads to temporary impairment in quality of life and may exacerbate underlying medical and psychiatric conditions. This has prompted an alternative method, which is now feasible following the development of recombinant human TSH (rhTSH) or Thyrogen®.

Thyroid Hormonal Withdrawal Versus Recombinant TSH (rhTSH)

rhTSH is administered as an intramuscular injection (0.9 mg) 48 hours and 24 hours prior to RAI. The HiLo and ESTIMABL1 trials demonstrated that rhTSH led to equivalent rates of successful ablation (almost 90%) in patients with low/intermediate-risk disease compared with standard withdrawal of thyroid replacement.[10,11] As a result, the ATA[19] and BTA[20] guidelines recommend rhTSH in T1-T3, N0/Nx/N1 DTC (N1a only is specified in ATA as surgery in both trials was generally restricted to the central compartment[19]). However, the use of rhTSH is now becoming standard of care even in patients with high-risk and metastatic disease, although this practice is out with the current licensed indications for Thyrogen® Thyrogen (sanofi.ca). Multiple retrospective analyses support this trend,[60-64] and rhTSH has the additional advantage of more rapid clearance of iodine,[65] potentially resulting in shorter hospital isolation and reduced period of restrictions. While the toxicity from rhTSH is generally minor (headache, nausea, and fatigue), and quality of life superior, at least in the short term,[10,11,66] it is important to be mindful of a potential disadvantage of rhTSH; tumor flare is a small but distinct possibility and in the context of airway compromise or impending spinal cord compression, thyroid hormone withdrawal may be more appropriate. Conversely, the latter is contraindicated in situations where the patient will fail to stimulate TSH on withdrawal of thyroid hormone supplementation, namely hypopituitarism and rare cases where there is exogenous production of thyroxine.

Low Iodine Diet

The recommended adult daily intake of iodine, as indicated by the World Health Organization, is 150 μg (Iodine - Consumer [nih.gov]. A low iodine diet (LID) aims for a daily consumption of less than 50 to 100 μg/day.[67] The highest levels of dietary iodine stem from fish, seafood, dairy, and canned goods; therefore, LID protocols recommend exclusion or limitation of these foods. Iodine may also be ingested from iodized salt and medication/supplements (thyroid hormone replacement itself is a significant source of iodine). As LID is more relevant in areas of the world where nutritional intake is high in iodine and there are no randomized data on the value of LID, some centers have ceased instructing patients on dietary restrictions.[68] Given geographical movement of patients and changing patterns in diet, LID may still have some value, but an extended period of 3 weeks or more is probably unnecessary. Up to 2 weeks is likely more than sufficient.

Pre-ablation Uptake Scan

RAI ablation is typically administered on established empirical activities, specifically 1.1 GBq (30 mCi) and 3.7 GBq (100 mCi), based on clinical and pathological risk factors, as previously discussed. Additional information may be acquired by pre-ablation diagnostic whole-body scintigraphy (DxWBS). This can influence the selection of RAI versus no RAI, as well as activity of RAI, and/or guide personalized dosimetry; the latter will be discussed in more detail in section Personalized Dosimetry & Radiation Protection. DxWBS is performed by using diagnostic activities of ^{131}I, or the alternative isotopes ^{123}I and ^{124}I. It has been suggested that ^{123}I and ^{124}I are preferable as they avoid "stunning," a potential complication of ^{131}I[69] but, providing the activity is well below 400 MBq, diagnostic doses of ^{131}I do not appear to be detrimental in the pre-ablation setting (*Administration of Radioactive Substances Advisory Committee - GOV.UK (www.gov.uk)*). Historically, DxWBS was utilized most commonly to determine the size of the residual thyroid tissue, as a large remnant may have necessitated multiple treatments, or further surgery prior to ablation. This is less relevant nowadays as surgery is increasingly performed by high-volume specialized surgeons. Moreover, the therapeutic and prognostic consequences of a large thyroid remnant are debatable.[70] DxWBS may have a role in patients with nodal or suspected nodal disease. However, one of the limitations of DxWBS is that it does not necessarily differentiate between remnant and lymph node metastases, largely because the resolution of planar scintigraphy is low, although integrated single photon emission computed tomography (SPECT-CT) may augment this.[71] Detection of distant metastases on DxWBS in the absence of any intermediate- to high-risk features and/or Tg level less than 1 ng/mL is unlikely and in the order of 1% to 3%.[11] As DxWBS has no proven role in risk stratification and treatment optimization, pre-ablation scanning is not routinely recommended, but may be selectively applied in centers that have significant experience in interpreting the images. The future of this technique may ultimately depend on its value in personalized dosimetry.

Delay to RAI Due to Recent Contrast Imaging

Significant iodide load from contrast-enhanced CT may compromise ^{131}I uptake in a thyroid remnant or in thyroid metastases. Although most of the iodine from the contrast agent is strongly bound to organic compounds, and is not accessible for uptake by the thyroid, the amount of free iodide is much higher than the quantity of iodine ingested in a regular diet. A minimum interval of 8 weeks is recommended between contrast-enhanced radiological investigations and ^{131}I administration,[19,20] although in younger patients with adequate renal function a shorter time frame may be acceptable,[72] especially in the context of aggressive disease. The timing of contrast-enhanced radiological investigations must be taken into account if requested post-thyroidectomy for staging purposes, particularly as postablation uptake scan, may provide valuable information on the presence or absence of nodal and/or distant metastases.

FOLLOW-UP

One of the main advantages of RAI ablation is that it facilitates long-term monitoring of Tg levels. Biochemical remission is reassuring for both patient and clinician and has formed the backbone of follow-up for many years. Previously, DxWBS was performed in tandem with an unstimulated Tg level at 6 to 12 months postablation. Providing remnant uptake was less than 0.2% and Tg level was below the threshold for detection on the assay of choice, typically 1 to 2 ng/mL, ablation was considered successful. However, this method of evaluation neither provided evidence of a complete radiological response nor estimated the potential risk of recurrence. It has become clearer over the past 10 years that substituting DxWBS with detailed ultrasound neck imaging is a far more robust means of response assessment, especially when combined with a stimulated Tg or nonstimulated hsTg level. Modern analyzers can now detect Tg to a sensitivity of 0.1 ng/mL, obviating the need for stimulation with thyroid hormone withdrawal or rhTSH. Together, these two modalities can be utilized to predict likelihood of recurrence and direct intensity of follow-up as well as documenting whether there has been complete or incomplete response to treatment.

Dynamic Risk Stratification

The introduction of dynamic risk stratification (DRS) means that a static risk estimate, based on clinic-pathological factors following surgery, can be modified and recalculated based on individual response to ablation (or ^{131}I therapy in the context of recurrent/metastatic disease). The results of a neck ultrasound and Tg level assessed after a reasonable time interval postablation are used to categorize patients into the following groups: excellent response; indeterminate response; and incomplete response (either biochemical or radiological). See Table 25–3. The standard interval is 9 to 12 months, but a minimum of 6 months and a maximum of 18 months are considered appropriate.[73]

The majority of patients with DTC have an excellent response following thyroidectomy and RAI ablation. The risk of relapse is low at less than 5% and the incidence of DTC-specific death is even lower at less than 1%.[74] Intensive follow-up is not required; Tg level should be measured on a 12 to 24 monthly basis, and intermittent neck ultrasound is optional. Conversely, the smallest proportion are classified as high risk on DRS. Active regular surveillance may be an option depending on the site and rate of growth of disease,

Table 25–3. Dynamic risk stratification (DRS) groups and proposed TSH level.

Response	Excellent	Indeterminate	Incomplete (Biochemical)	Incomplete (Radiological)
Imaging	Negative	Nonspecific findings OR Faint uptake in thyroid bed on DxWBS	Negative	Structural disease
Tg	Suppressed Tg <0.2 ng/mL OR Stimulated Tg <1 ng/mL	Suppressed Tg ≥0.2 to <1 ng/mL OR Stimulated Tg ≥1 to <10 ng/mL OR Stable/declining Tg Ab level	Suppressed Tg ≥1 ng/mL OR Stimulated Tg ≥10 ng/mL OR Rising Tg Ab level	Any Tg or Tg Ab level
Risk	Low	Intermediate	Intermediate	High
TSH	0.5*-2.0 mU/L OR 0.1-0.5* mU/L (if high risk at diagnosis)	0.1-0.5* mU/L	0.1-0.5* mU/L	<0.1 mU/L

*Lower limit of reference range may be 0.3-0.5 depending on specific assay.
DxWBS, diagnostic whole body scan; Tg, thyroglobulin; Tg Ab, thyroglobulin antibody; TSH, thyroid-stimulating hormone.

but additional therapy is often warranted. Despite further intervention, over 50% of patients will continue to have evidence of persistent DTC[75] and disease-specific mortality ranges from 10% for loco-regional metastases to 50% for distant metastatic spread.[74] The remaining patients with an intermediate propensity for recurrence (approximately 20%) have the most unpredictable outcome, but rates of DTC-specific death are similar to the excellent responders.[74] At least 30% of cases with a biochemical incomplete response spontaneously resolve,[76] with some reports suggesting that the level may be over 70%.[77] Declining Tg level is therefore reassuring. There is no clear protocol on frequency of assessment in this group, particularly in view of heterogeneity of cases, but Tg level should be evaluated at least 6 monthly, in conjunction with interval neck ultrasound every 6 to 12 months. Increasing Tg or Tg Ab levels should prompt additional investigations, such as axial contrast-enhanced CT neck/thorax, DxWBS, and/or fluorodeoxyglucose positron emission tomography (FDG PET-CT).

TSH Suppression

Maintaining complete TSH suppression (<0.1 mU/L) has long been an integral element in the management of DTC, even in low-risk disease. However, observational studies indicate that long-term super-suppression is associated with increased incidence of cardiac and mineral metabolism complications, most notably, atrial arrhythmia and osteoporosis, respectively. Also, it is now recognized that strict manipulation of TSH levels is probably unnecessary in the majority of cases, especially in the context of complete structural and biochemical response. Indeed, another advantage of DRS is the associated framework for guiding TSH level post-treatment[19] (see Table 25–3). Excellent responders no longer need to achieve complete suppression; aiming for a TSH level in the low-to-mid normal range (0.5-2.0 mU/L) is now advocated, minimizing the risk of late sequelae of prolonged over-replacement. The exception to this rule is the presence of high-risk features at initial diagnosis; a more conservative approach of 0.1 to 0.5 mU/L has been suggested as there are conflicting reports of relapse rates in this group varying from less than 5% to 15%.[19,74,78] Mild suppression (0.1-0.5 mU/L) is also advised if there is an indeterminate or biochemical incomplete response at DRS, but can be relaxed further if the patient converts to a complete response (or intensified if Tg level starts to rise/structural disease develops). Full suppression (<0.1 mU/L) is still recommended indefinitely for those at highest risk of progression or relapse, that is, the structural incomplete group.

Clinical judgment should be exercised in patients who are susceptible to complications relating to super-suppression. In the presence of certain risk factors, notably advanced age, postmenopausal status, underlying osteopenia/osteoporosis, and preexisting atrial fibrillation, the level of TSH suppression may need to be adjusted accordingly. Adjunctive therapies such as calcium/vitamin D supplementation, and antiarrhythmic agents are often prescribed to mitigate the endocrine and cardiac risks, but it is important to strike a balance between control of DTC and accepted clinical morbidity of supraphysiological levothyroxine replacement.

Thyroglobulin Antibody (Tg Ab) Monitoring

In the presence of Tg Ab, the results of Tg assay are difficult to interpret. False negative or (less frequently) false positive results are a potential limitation. This can be circumvented with mass spectrometry but is an approach largely restricted to academic settings and not routine clinical practice. On a positive note, monitoring Tg Ab titers over time (preferably, using the same assay) can provide surrogate information on treatment response and recurrence; persistently rising titers should be viewed as suspicious of relapse, whereas declining titers are usually associated with response or remission. To that end, patients with indeterminate response or biochemical incomplete response based on the presence of Tg Ab can be followed up as per other patients within these DRS categories, but regular imaging is often recommended until Tg Ab titer has diminished.

Length of Follow-Up Protocol

Traditionally, follow-up subsequent to thyroidectomy and RAI ablation for DTC has been lifelong, and in many centers this continues to be common practice. Indeed, the BTA guidelines recommend lifetime monitoring,[20] although this is currently being reevaluated. The main reason for ongoing review is that DTC may recur for years, and even decades, after initial treatment. However, more contemporary series indicate that over 80% of recurrences are identified within 5 years of diagnosis.[79] In low-risk patients with an excellent response on DRS, risk of relapse between 5 and 10 years is extremely low at less than 0.5%.[80] The evolution of relapse patterns likely reflects earlier detection of small-volume persistent disease as a result of increasingly sensitive diagnostic tools. As such, the cost-effectiveness and clinical burden of not discharging patients is being called into question.[81] It may be that the lower-risk groups (excellent and perhaps even intermediate response) can safely be discharged to primary care for annual TSH monitoring after up to 5 up to 10 years of follow-up with robust guidance for re-referral back to specialist services, if indicated.

Non-PTC Histotypes

The DRS system was devised based on data pertaining to patients with PTC. Applying the principles of DRS to non-PTC pathological subtypes must take into account the natural history of the underlying disease process. For example, lymph node metastases are more common in Hurthle cell carcinoma (HCC), compared with FTC; therefore, neck ultrasound is a more valuable diagnostic tool in the former compared with the latter. In poorly differentiated thyroid cancer (PDTC), Tg levels may be low, or undetectable, even in the presence of metastatic disease. Hence, radiological assessment may be more reliable than biochemistry; in particular, FDG PET-CT is reportedly more sensitive in PDTC compared to well-differentiated DTC.[82] Follow-up in patients with non-PTC histotypes should be individualized and supervised by the specialist multidisciplinary team.

MANAGEMENT OF METASTATIC DISEASE

RAI has a major role in the treatment of relapsed or newly diagnosed metastatic DTC. In the context of the latter, thyroidectomy is performed to facilitate ^{131}I therapy; otherwise most of the radionuclide will be absorbed by the primary as opposed to the secondary deposits. Fixed activities of 3.7 GBq (100 mCi), 5.5 GBq (150 mCi), or 7.4 GBq (200 mCi) are typically delivered every 6 to 12 months, providing there is ongoing radiological or biochemical response. There is interest in exploiting personalized dosimetry to enable individualization of treatment activity and dose escalation (see section Personalized Dosimetry & Radiation Protection), but this approach remains at a preliminary research level.

Lung and bone metastases are the most common sites of systemic disease. In the case of lung involvement, micronodular or miliary metastases are more likely to respond favorably to ^{131}I therapy, but even with repeated treatments, disease control is usually the aim (with the exception of children and younger adults). For solitary bone metastases, aggressive intervention such as surgical resection or high-dose external beam radiotherapy is warranted, as a cure is achievable. If there is more extensive or widespread bony disease, as shown in Figure 25-2, RAI may be effective in reducing symptom burden, but bisphosphonates or denosumab therapy is also recommended to minimize adverse skeletal-related events. DTC may present at additional or alternative sites, for instance, liver or brain. In selected cases with solitary or oligometastatic deposits, local therapies such as metastasectomy, stereotactic radiotherapy, radiofrequency ablation, or embolization, can be considered in addition to RAI.

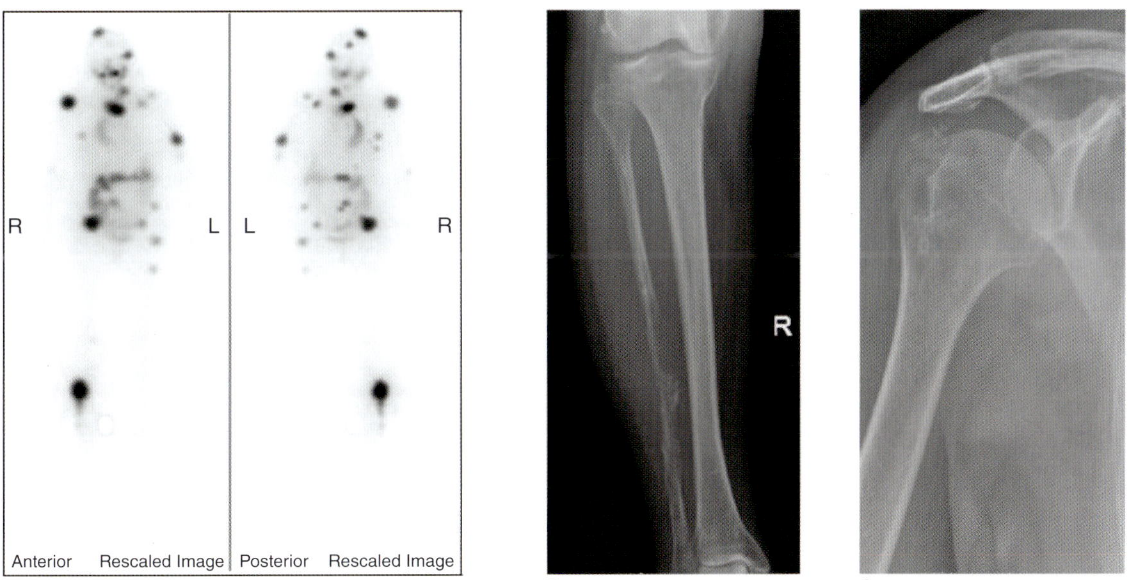

A B C

Figure 25–2. ^{131}I uptake in multiple bone metastases. A 63-year-old female presented with atraumatic left arm pain and underwent intramedullary pinning of a pathological fracture in the shaft of the left humerus. Histology of bone reamings indicated metastatic follicular thyroid cancer. Diffuse involvement of the axial skeleton was noted on CT scan. Following thyroidectomy, the patient received 3.7 GBq (100 mCi) ^{131}I, demonstrating uptake at multiple bony sites, notably the sternum, right hemipelvis, right fibula, and right humeral head **(A)**. Corresponding plain X-rays of right fibula **(B)** and right humerus **(C)** are also shown. The patient proceeded to further therapeutic ^{131}I in addition to palliative external beam radiotherapy for symptom control.

RADIOIODINE REFRACTORY THYROID CANCER & RESENSITIZATION

Up to 10% of patients with DTC will develop advanced disease that is not amenable to complete surgical resection, approximately two-thirds of whom will develop radioiodine-refractory thyroid cancer (RIR-TC). Median survival at this point is less than 5 years. Tyrosine kinase inhibitors (TKI) such as sorafenib[83] and lenvatinib[84] are now established in clinical practice, and novel agents such as highly specific RET inhibitors and NTRK antagonists are also emerging for selected patients with the corresponding mutation.[40,41] As yet, there is no proven overall survival benefit from targeted treatments. In addition, reduced therapeutic efficacy will almost certainly occur as a result of either primary or acquired resistance, or withdrawal may be necessary due to adverse toxicity. The concept of redifferentiation or resensitization has, therefore, emerged to overcome resistance to RAI and initiate durable responses, and perhaps even long-term remission or cure, by facilitating further effective ^{131}I therapy.

Definition of Radioiodine Refractory Thyroid Cancer

The definition of radioiodine refractory thyroid cancer (RIR-TC) has evolved from documented absence of uptake on DxWBS, or more commonly post-therapy uptake scan, to include radiological progression on conventional imaging, based on response evaluation criteria in solid tumors (RECIST 1.1[85]), within a defined time frame (usually between 6 and 18 months). There is debate over precise criteria[31,86] but essentially RIR-TC can be characterized as follows:

- Lesion(s) fail(s) to concentrate therapeutic RAI at outset
- Lesion(s) gradually lose(s) ability to concentrate RAI
- Mixed RAI uptake across multiple lesions
- Radiological progression of lesion(s) despite substantial concentration of RAI

Evidently, some patients have primary refractory disease at diagnosis, whereas others develop insensitivity to ^{131}I over time, although the precise biological explanation for this variation is unclear. Persisting with further therapeutic activities of RAI is usually inappropriate, with the exception of a limited proportion of patients who exhibit a mixed response, depending on the precise site and/or burden of sensitive versus refractory deposits.[86] It has also been suggested that failure to induce remission following 20-22 GBq of RAI (600 mCi) could be added to the inclusion criteria,[31] as complete responses have not been reported above this threshold.[87] Cure is extremely unlikely but patients may continue to respond to further RAI; careful risk/benefit analysis is essential on a case-by-case basis[19,21,86] due to the potential burden of cumulative toxicity from repeated RAI therapy, including hematological sequelae and second malignancy.[87-89]

Mechanism of Radioiodine Refractoriness

NIS plays an essential role in the transmembrane transport of ^{131}I in follicular cells of the thyroid. The level of NIS decreases during dedifferentiation and is instrumental in the development of RIR-TC.[90] In a smaller proportion of cases, there is defective membrane binding of NIS, which lies free in the cytosol thereby reducing intracellular transport.[91] Age-related effects on NIS expression and function have also been reported[92] which may partly explain why older patients have a poorer outcome compared with their younger counterparts, but most of the evidence to date suggests that cell signaling pathways play a key role in downregulation of NIS, most notably mitogen-activated protein kinase (MAPK) and phosphoinositide 3-kinase (PI3K). Additional epigenetic alterations and downstream signaling pathways have been reported to modulate NIS expression and function including histone deacetylation (HDAC) and transforming growth factor (β)/Smad3 (TGF-β/SMAD3) (reviewed by[93]). (See Figure 25–3.)

Predicting RIR-TC

Latterly, Tg doubling time was often utilized to predict RIR-TC in the clinic but is not entirely reliable; although this method has a high sensitivity, the specificity is low. Therefore, Tg monitoring has limited value as a marker of progression and should not be viewed as a surrogate for radiological assessment but may act as a guide and trigger for radiological investigations to look for sites of relapse. The role of FDG PET-CT in DTC is under increasing scrutiny as most studies to date illustrate an association between FDG avidity and disease progression and/or compromised survival.[94] Primarily, this mode of imaging is restricted to detection of lesions responsible for elevated Tg in the context of a negative WBS as an inverse relationship between RAI and FDG uptake has been observed.[95] In patients with metastatic DTC, this so-called flip-flop phenomenon correlates with reduced disease-specific survival.[95] There is also interest in exploiting data from FDG PET-CT at earlier points in the treatment pathway, for example, in the perioperative setting, to predict sensitivity or refractoriness prior to ^{131}I exposure.[96,97] Due to confounding factors relating to patient heterogeneity and variation in imaging parameters, as well as resource issues, routine FDG PET-CT at diagnosis is not standard practice and there is insufficient evidence that the findings should alter immediate management, although follow-up is likely to be more rigorous in PET-positive patients. Similarly, speculation is increasing over the potential application of molecular markers as predictive indicators of RIR-TC. The presence of BRAF V600E, TERT, and NRAS mutations has been shown to inversely correlate with NIS expression,[98] and the specific combination of BRAF V600E and TERT is most robustly linked with loss of RAI avidity in recurrent and/or metastatic DTC.[99] At present, neither FDG PET-CT uptake

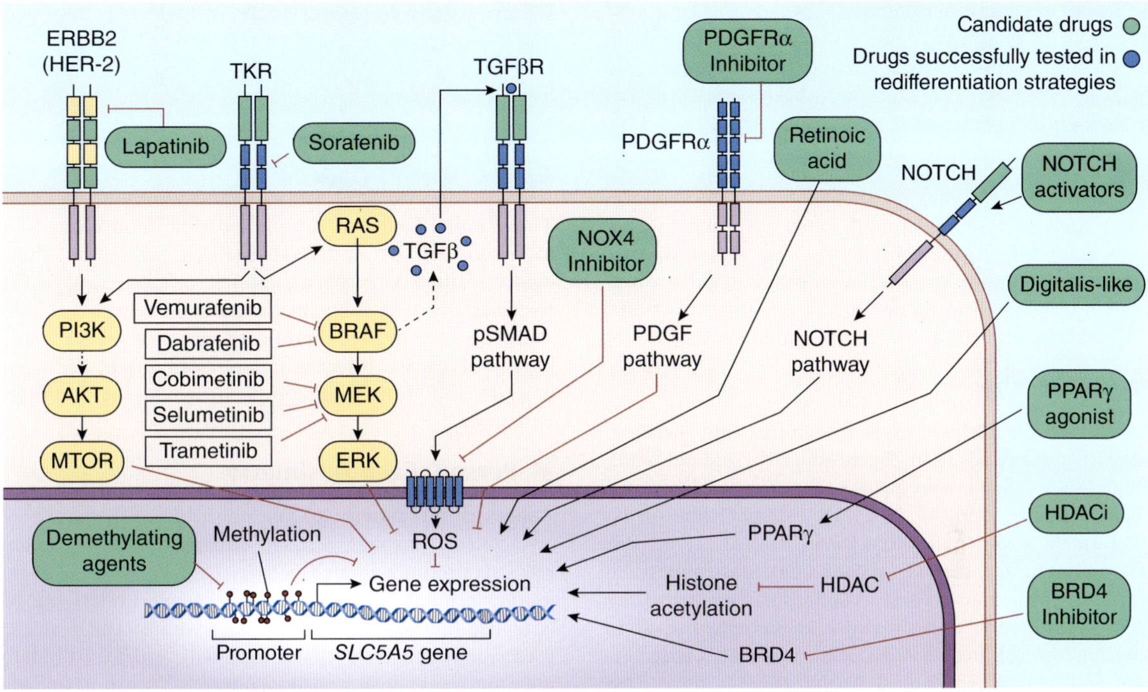

Figure 25–3. Molecular mechanism controlling NIS expression and potential targets to reverse RIR-TC. The most effective means of resensitizing radioiodine refractory thyroid cancer is by inhibiting the mitogen-activated protein kinase (MAPK) pathway, predominantly targeting BRAF and/or MEK. Alternative mechanisms that have yet to be explored in clinical trials include disrupting transcription, post-translational modification, or the TGF-β/Smad3 pathway. (Reproduced with permission from Buffet C, Wassermann J, Hecht F, et al. Redifferentiation of radioiodine-refractory thyroid cancers. *Endocr Relat Cancer*. 2020;27(5):R113-R132.)

nor molecular signature should be considered a deterrent from the administration of adjuvant or therapeutic ^{131}I, but careful monitoring is recommended to detect early relapse and RIR-TC. In the future, treatment intensification and/or alternative pathways may be indicated for patients who are unlikely to derive any advantage from RAI following appropriate interventional studies.

Strategies to Reverse Refractoriness

Attempting to reverse refractoriness is not an entirely new phenomenon. In the 1970s, it was recognized that the mood stabilizer lithium increased thyroidal retention of ^{131}I in patients with thyrotoxicosis.[100] This led to exploratory studies in DTC, and despite increased uptake of ^{131}I with concomitant use of lithium,[101] there has been limited success in terms of treatment outcomes.[102] Contemporary strategies are aimed at specific components of NIS synthesis and function: transcription; post-transcriptional regulation; NIS trafficking to plasma membrane; and modulation of downstream signaling pathways. See Figure 25–3. Thus far, the most studied tactic is the latter, by targeting the MAPK pathway, specifically MAPK/ERK kinase (MEK), which is a substrate of both BRAF and RAS, the most common driver mutations in PTC and FTC, respectively. Selumetinib is an oral agent that selectively inhibits MEK, and has demonstrated promising results in the laboratory that has translated to the clinical setting; 4 weeks treatment with Selumetinib can reestablish uptake of ^{131}I in patients with confirmed RIR-TC.[103] The UK-based SELIMETRY phase II trial (EudraCT No 2015-002269-47) aimed to further explore the resensitizing potential of Selumetinib in tandem with molecular genotyping while simultaneously establishing accurate and reproducible ^{131}I dosimetry across multiple centers. Unfortunately, recruitment was closed early, but several other phase II trials are currently underway (NCT03244956, NCT04619316, NCT04554680). Again, the focus is largely on MEK, albeit with trametinib as opposed to selumetinib, either alone (NCT03244956) or in combination with the BRAF inhibitor dabrafenib (NCT04619316, NCT04554680), which can induce ^{131}I reuptake in BRAF V600E mutant RIR-TC.[104] Dual therapy with vemurafenib (BRAF inhibitor) and cobimetinib

(MEK inhibitor) is another putative approach.[105] Mandatory genetic profiling is stipulated in the inclusion criteria and, in some studies, patients are stratified and treated according to BRAF wild-type, BRAF V600E, and/or RAS status, potentially paving the way for molecular radiotherapy.

CONSEQUENCES & LATE EFFECTS

RAI is a well-tolerated treatment, often resulting in very minimal symptoms in the short term. With repeated high-dose treatments, however, there may be cumulative dose-dependent toxicity leading to effects on quality of life, fertility, and predisposition for second malignancy.

Acute Toxicity

Immediate effects include neck discomfort and swelling, relating to uptake of ^{131}I in the residual thyroid remnant, although this is much less frequent in the era of high-volume specialist surgery. Additional toxicity stems from physiological uptake at other sites that absorb and/or excrete ^{131}I, notably the salivary glands (sialadenitis), gastrointestinal system (dysgeusia, nausea, gastritis), and urinary tract (cystitis).[88,106] Preventative measures such as adequate hydration and antiemetics can negate most of the associated gastrointestinal and urinary symptoms. As yet, there is no proven radioprotective role for amifostine[107] or nonpharmacological methods[108] in limiting salivary gland uptake, especially in high-dose RAI treatments.[107]

Late Effects

Reported late adverse effects associated with RAI include xerostomia, lacrimal gland impairment, gonadal dysfunction (discussed in section Pregnancy & Fertility), hematological sequelae, and risk of second primary malignancy.[106] Pulmonary fibrosis can also occur in patients with diffuse lung involvement and may be a dose-limiting toxicity if multiple therapeutic doses of ^{131}I are required.[109] In such cases, reducing empirical therapy activity and/or utilizing dosimetry should be considered to minimize respiratory compromise. The most common consequence of RAI treatment is xerostomia, affecting up to 30% of patients,[110] but the most potentially devastating sequelae is second primary malignancy. The precise incidence is unclear as the data is conflicting, and in some studies an additional cancer may predate the diagnosis of DTC.[111] RAI has been most strongly associated with hematological disorders, particularly acute myeloid leukemia (AML).[112] Ten-year cumulative AML risk of 0.08% following surgery for DTC compared with 0.12% in patients treated with surgery and RAI was described in a large SEER analysis, but the methodology has been questioned[113-115] and there are likely to be confounding factors such as genetic predisposition and external beam radiotherapy.[114] Overall, the risk of hematological malignancy from a single treatment of RAI is anticipated to be extremely small. Even in DTC patients with aggressive and/or metastatic disease, who may be at higher risk due to repeated ^{131}I therapy,[87,116] the beneficial effect of RAI usually outweighs the low risk of second malignancy.

PERSONALIZED DOSIMETRY & RADIATION PROTECTION

The demand for personalized medicine in oncology is ever-increasing. HiLo[10] and ESTIMABL1[11] highlighted that de-escalation of RAI activity is feasible in lower-risk DTC, but fixed activity of ^{131}I remains the norm for relapsed and metastatic disease, despite significant variation in pattern and burden of disease. It has, therefore, been questioned whether a more individualized approach would yield enhanced outcomes.

Personalized Dosimetry

Adapting ^{131}I activity to optimize tumor response relies on accurate dosimetry, based either on dose to organs at risk, maximum tolerated activity (MTA), or dose to target lesion, lesional dosimetry. The principle underlying MTA is to use the bone marrow as a constraint and restrict the prescribed activity to that which will lead to a predefined maximum safe dose, usually 2 Gy.[117] MTA can be calculated using a tracer of ^{131}I, or an alternative isotope such as ^{124}I, and obtaining radioactivity counts and blood samples at determined time points following administration. While this strategy limits the hematological toxicity of RAI, the dose concentrated in the tumor is unknown and the therapeutic effect is indeterminate.

Lesional dosimetry, on the other hand, reflects the philosophy of external beam radiotherapy and is designed to deliver a precise dose of radiation to the target. Similarly, a tracer activity of ^{131}I (or ^{124}I) is required, and gamma-camera images are captured at regular intervals, to determine the amount of radioactivity absorbed and the effective half-life of the isotope within the lesion(s). A formula is then applied to identify the activity of RAI that will achieve the desired dose (in Gy) to the target, but this may be affected by tumor vascularity, ^{131}I avidity, and TSH stimulation. Observational series comparing empirical with dosimetrically determined activities indicates that doses in excess of 80 Gy may be achieved in the latter group, resulting in higher rates of disease stability and response,[118] although improved survival has not been proven.[119,120] It is unclear whether inconsistent preparation and follow-up protocols may have negatively influenced the outcome of studies to date, emphasizing the need for prospective randomized trials.

Radiation Protection

The use of unsealed radioisotopes must be carefully controlled to minimize risk to patients, carriers, and medical staff. Prior to treatment, a thorough risk assessment should be undertaken to ensure that the patient has adequate swallowing and cognitive function, mobility, and is continent of both urine and feces. To prevent spillages and accidental exposure, ^{131}I oral capsule is preferable to liquid formulation. A period of in-patient isolation is invariably required, usually for 1 to 2 days, but may be longer for a therapeutic activity and/or in the event of delayed ^{131}I excretion, for instance, due to renal impairment. Discharge is permitted when radioactivity levels fall to an acceptable level; this will vary depending on local and nationally agreed guidelines (eg, in the United Kingdom, residual activity <800 MBq or external dose-rate <40 microSv hr^{-1} at 1 m is considered acceptable *IPEM > Scientific Journals & Publications > Medical and Dental Guidance Notes*). Out-patient ablation with 1.1 GBq (30 mCi) is now performed at some centers with suitable facilities.

It is good practice to provide written information for the patient advising on appropriate restrictions that must be followed for a specific period of time. This time frame is typically based empirically on the activity administered; again, subject to the regulatory framework in place, local rules will vary from 1 week to 4 weeks. During this interval, the aim is to keep any dose to the general public (including family members) "as low as reasonably practicable" (ALARP), by applying the three main principles of radiation safety (time, distance, and shielding), but not to unnecessarily mandate long periods of isolation. The patient will be instructed to sleep in a separate bedroom, avoid contact with pregnant women and children aged ≤5 years, refrain from work outside the home, and limit journeys on public transport. Alternative accommodation may need to be arranged temporarily, depending on social circumstances, and should be identified at pretreatment risk assessment. If there is concern about an individual's ability to comply with restrictions then it may be necessary to extend the in-patient stay. To minimize disruption to employment and family life, some centers now perform serial measurements of external dose rate or residual activity not only to confirm discharge but also to aid individualized radiation protection advice and permit earlier easing of restrictions.

PREGNANCY & FERTILITY

DTC is one of the most common malignancies in adolescents and young adults. Females are significantly more likely to be affected than males, and up to 10% of thyroid cancers occurring during the reproductive years are detected during pregnancy. Hence, reproductive issues are paramount and must be taken into account when planning treatment, particularly RAI.

DTC in Pregnancy & Postpartum Period

There is no unequivocal evidence to suggest that pregnancy is a poor prognostic factor. Thus, management of newly diagnosed DTC during pregnancy usually consists of observation, and surgery is delayed until the postpartum period. Termination of pregnancy to facilitate immediate treatment, especially in low-to-intermediate risk DTC, is not advised. In the uncommon situation where more urgent therapy is indicated, surgery can be performed, ideally in the second trimester as maternal and fetal complication rates are lower. There is no evidence for or against suppression of TSH if surgery is electively deferred. If pregnancy occurs following previous treatment for DTC, frequent monitoring of thyroid function is required as T4 requirements generally increase by 20% to 30%. Women can be reviewed in a specialist joint antenatal/endocrine clinic to optimize management.

Pregnancy is an absolute contraindication to RAI. It is also imperative that breastfeeding be discontinued at least 8 weeks before ^{131}I to avoid breast irradiation and ensuing risk of malignancy, as RAI is significantly concentrated in lactating breast tissue.[121] If there is an ongoing concern, DxWBS can be performed to ensure the absence of breast uptake. A dopamine agonist, such as cabergoline, is occasionally administered to suppress lactation, but in most cases RAI ablation can be safely delayed for a number of months, especially in low-risk DTC.[122,123] Breastfeeding should not be resumed until after a subsequent pregnancy.

Female Fertility

Younger women may understandably have concerns about the impact of RAI on future fertility, but little data exist to accurately counsel patients about reproductive outcomes. It is recognized that RAI can precipitate alterations in gonadal function, as reflected by transient changes in serum gonadotrophins (specifically, elevated FSH and LH) and menstrual function; amenorrhea for up to 1 year has previously been reported in up to 30% women.[124] In a US Cancer Registry survey, birth rates were similar between women who did or did not receive RAI following a diagnosis of DTC between the age of 15 and 39 years, suggesting minimal impact of RAI on subsequent fertility.[125] However, subgroup analysis of another US population-based survey indicated that RAI was associated with 29% reduction in birth rate among women aged 35 to 39 years.[126] It is unclear if this finding is due to patient choice or the requisite delay before attempting to conceive rather than a direct biological effect on ovarian function. Nonetheless, anti-Mullerian hormone (AMH), a surrogate for ovarian reserve, has also been noted to fall more rapidly in women more than 35 years who received at least one dose of ^{131}I.[127] Conversely, female survivors of DTC who received RAI in childhood do not appear to be at any higher risk of ovarian dysfunction.[128] Based on current literature, RAI should not be routinely withheld in women over 35 years who are planning a pregnancy, but careful discussion with the patient is required, taking into account risk factors for recurrence and future fertility wishes; another prime example of "personalized decision-making." In women who successfully conceive, pregnancy outcomes and child development are similar to the general population,[129] but due to potential risk of miscarriage,[130] most guidelines strongly recommend delaying a pregnancy for 6 to 12 months post RAI.[17,18,129]

Male Fertility

The testes are more sensitive to ^{131}I compared with ovarian tissue, and temporary reduction in sperm count is well observed.[131,132] A single ablative or adjuvant dose is unlikely to induce permanent male infertility, but there may be cumulative damage with repeated treatments. A reliable means of contraception is strongly advocated for 3 to 4 months following RAI to allow one full sperm cycle, and sperm banking is generally recommended if at least two high-dose treatments (15 GBq or 400 mCi) are anticipated.[19,20,133]

FUTURE DIRECTIONS

Clinicians involved in treating thyroid cancer over the last few decades have observed a remarkable transformation in the management of DTC. From the uniform adoption of empirical RAI across all stages and subtypes, high-level randomized evidence now advocates a more conservative approach for patients with lower-risk disease by omitting RAI or limiting the prescribed activity and subsequently minimizing toxicity (without adversely affecting relapse rates). Looking to the future, personalized medicine will inevitably play an increasing role in the decision to proceed with RAI and also in the selection of RAI activity in both the postoperative and advanced disease settings. Standard activity of 3.7 GBq (100 mCi) will be restricted to adjuvant patients exhibiting more adverse risk features, with the possibility of escalated dose beyond the traditional fixed activities of 5.5 to 7.4 GBq (150–200 mCi) for those with locoregional recurrence/metastatic disease, dependent on the results of well-designed prospective trials incorporating individual dosimetry with appropriate quality assurance. Genetic profiling has yet to enter routine clinical practice, but preliminary indications suggest that molecular signature may influence prognosis, response to RAI and targeted therapies, and the development of resistance to RAI. Risk stratification and treatment pathways are likely to be underpinned by comprehensive genomic analysis, although many questions remain regarding optimal integration of this information into the current model. Interventional studies incorporating molecular biology will be key in addressing this issue.

In conclusion, RAI is well established as a fundamental component in the management of DTC and will almost certainly continue to shape the treatment landscape. RAI represents the first example of targeted radiotherapy in its most basic form but is now in prime position to evolve and deliver advanced molecular radiotherapy to selected patients who are most likely to benefit.

REFERENCES

1. Dai G, Levy O, Carrasco N. Cloning and characterization of the thyroid iodide transporter. *Nature*. 1996;379(6564):458-460.
2. Hertz S, Roberts A. Radioactive iodine in the study of thyroid physiology: the use of radioactive iodine therapy in Graves' disease. *West J Surg Obstet Gynecol*. 1946;54(12):474-486.
3. Leiter L, Seidlin SM, et al. Adenocarcinoma of the thyroid with hyperthyroidism and functional metastases: studies with thiouracil and radioiodine. *J Clin Endocrinol Metab*. 1946;6:247-261.
4. Seidlin SM, Rossman I, et al. Radioiodine therapy of metastases from carcinoma of the thyroid: a 6-year progress report. *J Clin Endocrinol Metab*. 1949;9(11):1122-1137, illust.
5. Siegel E. The beginnings of radioiodine therapy of metastatic thyroid carcinoma: a memoir of Samuel M. Seidlin, M. D. (1895-1955) and his celebrated patient. *Cancer Biother Radiopharm*. 1999;14(2):71-79.
6. Smithers DW. Some varied applications of radioactive isotopes to the localisation and treatment of tumours. *Acta Radiologica*. 1951;35(1):49-61.
7. Vayre L, Sabourin JC, Caillou B, et al. Immunohistochemical analysis of Na^+/I^- symporter distribution in human extrathyroidal tissues. *Eur J Endocrinol*. 1999;141(4):382-386.
8. Mazzaferri EL, Jhiang SM. Differentiated thyroid cancer long-term impact of initial therapy. *Transactions of the American Clinical and Climatological Association*. 1995;106:151-170.
9. DeGroot LJ, Kaplan EL, McCormick M, et al. Natural history, treatment, and course of papillary thyroid carcinoma. *J Clin Endocrinol Metab*. 1990;71(2):414-424.
10. Mallick U, Harmer C, Yap B, et al. Ablation with low-dose radioiodine and thyrotropin alfa in thyroid cancer. *N Engl J Med*. 2012;366(18):1674-1685.
11. Schlumberger M, Catargi B, Borget I, et al. Strategies of radioiodine ablation in patients with low-risk thyroid cancer. *N Engl J Med*. 2012;366(18):1663-1673.
12. Leboulleux S, Bournaud C, Chougnet CN, et al. Thyroidectomy without radioiodine in patients with low-risk thyroid cancer. *N Engl J Med*. 2022;386(10):923-932.
13. Hackshaw A, Newbold N, Beasley M, et al. Major secondary outcomes in the multicentre noninferiority randomised trial IoN: is ablative radioiodine necessary for low-risk differentiated thyroid cancer patients? *Annals of Oncology*. 2023;34(S2):S1145 (abs 2212).
14. Mazzaferri EL, Jhiang SM. Long-term impact of initial surgical and medical therapy on papillary and follicular thyroid cancer. *Am J Med*. 1994;97(5):418-428.
15. Sawka AM, Thephamongkhol K, Brouwers M, et al. Clinical review 170: a systematic review and metaanalysis of the effectiveness of radioactive iodine remnant ablation for well-differentiated thyroid cancer. *J Clin Endocrinol Metab*. 2004;89(8):3668-3676.
16. Guo K, Wang Z. Risk factors influencing the recurrence of papillary thyroid carcinoma: a systematic review and meta-analysis. *Int J Clin Exp Pathol*. 2014;7(9):5393-5403.
17. Gronlund MP, Jensen JS, Hahn CH, et al. Risk factors for recurrence of follicular thyroid cancer: a systematic review. *Thyroid*. 2021;31(10):1523-1530.
18. Nixon IJ, Kuk D, Wreesmann V, et al. Defining a valid age cutoff in staging of well-differentiated thyroid cancer. *Ann Surg Oncol*. 2016;23(2):410-415.
19. Haugen BR, Alexander EK, Bible KC, et al. 2015 American Thyroid Association Management Guidelines for Adult

Patients with Thyroid Nodules and Differentiated Thyroid Cancer: The American Thyroid Association Guidelines Task Force on Thyroid Nodules and Differentiated Thyroid Cancer. *Thyroid*. 2016;26(1):1-133.
20. Perros P, Boelaert K, Colley S, et al. Guidelines for the management of thyroid cancer. *Clinical Endocrinology*. 2014;81(s1):1-122.
21. Luster M, Clarke SE, Dietlein M, et al. Guidelines for radioiodine therapy of differentiated thyroid cancer. *Eur J Nucl Med Mol Imaging*. 2008;35(10):1941-1959.
22. Filetti S, Durante C, Hartl D, et al. Thyroid cancer: ESMO Clinical Practice Guidelines for diagnosis, treatment and follow-up. *Annals of Oncology*. 2019;30(12):1856-1883.
23. Randolph GW, Duh QY, Heller KS, et al. The prognostic significance of nodal metastases from papillary thyroid carcinoma can be stratified based on the size and number of metastatic lymph nodes, as well as the presence of extranodal extension. *Thyroid*. 2012;22(11):1144-1152.
24. Sanabria A, Rojas A, Arevalo J, et al. Microscopically positive surgical margins and local recurrence in thyroid cancer. A meta-analysis. *Eur J Surg Oncol*. 2019;45(8):1310-1316.
25. Back K, Kim SK, Chai YJ, et al. Does microscopic positive tumor margin in papillary thyroid cancer really matter? *Surgery*. 2019;166(6):1160-1167.
26. Sugino K, Ito K, Nagahama M, et al. Prognosis and prognostic factors for distant metastases and tumor mortality in follicular thyroid carcinoma. *Thyroid*. 2011;21(7):751-757.
27. Sugino K, Kameyama K, Ito K, et al. Outcomes and prognostic factors of 251 patients with minimally invasive follicular thyroid carcinoma. *Thyroid*. 2012;22(8):798-804.
28. Ghossein RA, Hiltzik DH, Carlson DL, et al. Prognostic factors of recurrence in encapsulated Hurthle cell carcinoma of the thyroid gland: a clinicopathologic study of 50 cases. *Cancer*. 2006;106(8):1669-1676.
29. Huang CC, Hsueh C, Liu FH, et al. Diagnostic and therapeutic strategies for minimally and widely invasive follicular thyroid carcinomas. *Surg Oncol*. 2011;20(1):1-6.
30. Lo CY, Chan WF, Lam KY, et al. Follicular thyroid carcinoma: the role of histology and staging systems in predicting survival. *Ann Surg*. 2005;242(5):708-715.
31. Tuttle RM, Ahuja S, Avram AM, et al. Controversies, consensus, and collaboration in the use of ^{131}I therapy in differentiated thyroid cancer: a joint statement from the American Thyroid Association, the European Association of Nuclear Medicine, the Society of Nuclear Medicine and Molecular Imaging, and the European Thyroid Association. *Thyroid*. 2019;29(4):461-470.
32. Morandi L, Righi A, Maletta F, et al. Somatic mutation profiling of hobnail variant of papillary thyroid carcinoma. *Endocrine-Related Cancer*. 2017;24(2):107-117.
33. Howell GM, Nikiforova MN, Carty SE, et al. BRAF V600E mutation independently predicts central compartment lymph node metastasis in patients with papillary thyroid cancer. *Ann Surg Oncol*. 2013;20(1):47-52.
34. Xing M, Alzahrani AS, Carson KA, et al. Association between BRAF V600E mutation and mortality in patients with papillary thyroid cancer. *JAMA*. 2013;309(14):1493-1501.
35. Kim TH, Park YJ, Lim JA, et al. The association of the BRAF(V600E) mutation with prognostic factors and poor clinical outcome in papillary thyroid cancer: a meta-analysis. *Cancer*. 2012;118(7):1764-1773.
36. Xing M. Prognostic utility of BRAF mutation in papillary thyroid cancer. *Mol Cell Endocrinol*. 2010;321(1):86-93.
37. Haugen BR. 2015 American Thyroid Association Management Guidelines for Adult Patients with Thyroid Nodules and Differentiated Thyroid Cancer: what is new and what has changed? *Cancer*. 2017;123(3):372-381.
38. Melo M, da Rocha AG, Vinagre J, et al. TERT promoter mutations are a major indicator of poor outcome in differentiated thyroid carcinomas. *J Clin Endocrinol Metab*. 2014;99(5):E754-765.
39. Xing M, Liu R, Liu X, et al. BRAF V600E and TERT promoter mutations cooperatively identify the most aggressive papillary thyroid cancer with highest recurrence. *J Clin Oncol*. 2014;32(25):2718-2726.
40. Drilon A, Laetsch TW, Kummar S, et al. Efficacy of larotrectinib in TRK fusion-positive cancers in adults and children. *N Engl J Med*. 2018;378(8):731-739.
41. Wirth LJ, Sherman E, Robinson B, et al. Efficacy of selpercatinib in RET-altered thyroid cancers. *N Engl J Med*. 2020; 383(9):825-835.
42. Giovanella L, Ceriani L, Ghelfo A, et al. Thyroglobulin assay 4 weeks after thyroidectomy predicts outcome in low-risk papillary thyroid carcinoma. *Clin Chem Lab Med*. 2005;43(8):843-847.
43. Robenshtok E, Grewal RK, Fish S, et al. A low postoperative nonstimulated serum thyroglobulin level does not exclude the presence of radioactive iodine avid metastatic foci in intermediate-risk differentiated thyroid cancer patients. *Thyroid*. 2013;23(4):436-442.
44. de Rosario PW, Guimaraes VC, Maia FF, et al. Thyroglobulin before ablation and correlation with posttreatment scanning. *Laryngoscope*. 2005;115(2):264-267.
45. Oyen WJ, Verhagen C, Saris E, et al. Follow-up regimen of differentiated thyroid carcinoma in thyroidectomized patients after thyroid hormone withdrawal. *J Nucl Med*. 2000; 41(4):643-646.
46. Giovanella L, Ceriani L, Suriano S, et al. Thyroglobulin measurement before rhTSH-aided ^{131}I ablation in detecting metastases from differentiated thyroid carcinoma. *Clin Endocrinol (Oxf)*. 2008;69(4):659-663.
47. Matrone A, Gambale C, Piaggi P, et al. Postoperative thyroglobulin and neck ultrasound in the risk restratification and decision to perform ^{131}I ablation. *J Clin Endocrinol Metab*. 2017;102(3):893-902.
48. Phan HT, Jager PL, van der Wal JE, et al. The follow-up of patients with differentiated thyroid cancer and undetectable thyroglobulin (Tg) and Tg antibodies during ablation. *Eur J Endocrinol*. 2008;158(1):77-83.
49. Vaisman A, Orlov S, Yip J, et al. Application of post-surgical stimulated thyroglobulin for radioiodine remnant ablation selection in low-risk papillary thyroid carcinoma. *Head Neck*. 2010;32(6):689-698.
50. Kim TY, Kim WB, Kim ES, et al. Serum thyroglobulin levels at the time of ^{131}I remnant ablation just after thyroidectomy are useful for early prediction of clinical recurrence in low-risk patients with differentiated thyroid carcinoma. *J Clin Endocrinol Metab*. 2005;90(3):1440-1445.
51. Toubeau M, Touzery C, Arveux P, et al. Predictive value for disease progression of serum thyroglobulin levels measured in the postoperative period and after ^{131}I ablation therapy in patients with differentiated thyroid cancer. *J Nucl Med*. 2004;45(6):988-994.
52. Piccardo A, Arecco F, Puntoni M, et al. Focus on high-risk DTC patients: high postoperative serum thyroglobulin level is a strong predictor of disease persistence and is associated to progression-free survival and overall survival. *Clin Nucl Med*. 2013;38(1):18-24.

53. Polachek A, Hirsch D, Tzvetov G, et al. Prognostic value of post-thyroidectomy thyroglobulin levels in patients with differentiated thyroid cancer. *J Endocrinol Invest.* 2011;34(11): 855-860.
54. Campenni A, Ruggeri RM, Siracusa M, et al. Early preablation rhTSH-stimulated thyroglobulin predicts outcome of differentiated thyroid cancer (DTC) patients. *Eur J Nucl Med Mol Imaging.* 2021;48(8):2466-2475.
55. Tian T, Xu Y, Zhang X, et al. Prognostic implications of preablation stimulated Tg: a retrospective analysis of 2500 thyroid cancer patients. *J Clin Endocrinol Metab.* 2021;106(11): e4688-e4697.
56. Jammah AA, Masood A, Akkielah LA, et al. Utility of stimulated thyroglobulin in reclassifying low risk thyroid cancer patients' following thyroidectomy and radioactive iodine ablation: a 7-year prospective trial. *Front Endocrinol (Lausanne).* 2020;11:603432.
57. Cheng W, Ma C, Fu H, et al. Low- or high-dose radioiodine remnant ablation for differentiated thyroid carcinoma: a meta-analysis. *J Clin Endocrinol Metab.* 2013;98(4):1353-1360.
58. Dehbi HM, Mallick U, Wadsley J, et al. Recurrence after low-dose radioiodine ablation and recombinant human thyroid-stimulating hormone for differentiated thyroid cancer (HiLo): long-term results of an open-label, non-inferiority randomised controlled trial. *Lancet Diabetes Endocrinol.* 2019; 7(1):44-51.
59. Schlumberger M, Leboulleux S, Catargi B, et al. Outcome after ablation in patients with low-risk thyroid cancer (ESTIMABL1): 5-year follow-up results of a randomised, phase 3, equivalence trial. *Lancet Diabetes Endocrinol.* 2018; 6(8):618-626.
60. Pitoia F, Marlowe RJ, Abelleira E, et al. Radioiodine thyroid remnant ablation after recombinant human thyrotropin or thyroid hormone withdrawal in patients with high-risk differentiated thyroid cancer. *J Thyroid Res.* 2012;2012:481568.
61. Sabra MM, Tuttle RM. Recombinant human thyroid-stimulating hormone to stimulate 131-I uptake for remnant ablation and adjuvant therapy. *Endocr Pract.* 2013;19(1):149-156.
62. Klubo-Gwiezdzinska J, Burman KD, Van Nostrand D, et al. Potential use of recombinant human thyrotropin in the treatment of distant metastases in patients with differentiated thyroid cancer. *Endocr Pract.* 2013;19(1):139-148.
63. Bartenstein P, Calabuig EC, Maini CL, et al. High-risk patients with differentiated thyroid cancer T4 primary tumors achieve remnant ablation equally well using rhTSH or thyroid hormone withdrawal. *Thyroid.* 2014;24(3):480-487.
64. Tala H, Robbins R, Fagin JA, et al. Five-year survival is similar in thyroid cancer patients with distant metastases prepared for radioactive iodine therapy with either thyroid hormone withdrawal or recombinant human TSH. *J Clin Endocrinol Metab.* 2011;96(7):2105-2111.
65. Taieb D, Sebag F, Farman-Ara B, et al. Iodine biokinetics and radioiodine exposure after recombinant human thyrotropin-assisted remnant ablation in comparison with thyroid hormone withdrawal. *J Clin Endocrinol Metab.* 2010;95(7): 3283-3290.
66. Tu J, Wang S, Huo Z, et al. Recombinant human thyrotropin-aided versus thyroid hormone withdrawal-aided radioiodine treatment for differentiated thyroid cancer after total thyroidectomy: a meta-analysis. *Radiother Oncol.* 2014;110(1):25-30.
67. Li JH, He ZH, Bansal V, et al. Low iodine diet in differentiated thyroid cancer: a review. *Clin Endocrinol (Oxf).* 2016;84(1):3-12.
68. England CY, Moss L, Beasley M, et al. A survey of UK centres on low iodine diet recommendations prior to radioiodine ablation therapy for differentiated thyroid cancer. *Eur Thyroid J.* 2020;9(3):132-138.
69. McMenemin RM, Hilditch TE, Dempsey MF, et al. Thyroid stunning after ^{131}I diagnostic whole-body scanning. *J Nucl Med.* 2001;42(6):986-987.
70. Leblanc G, Tabah R, Liberman M, et al. Large remnant 131I ablation as an alternative to completion/total thyroidectomy in the treatment of well-differentiated thyroid cancer. *Surgery.* 2004;136(6):1275-1280.
71. Barwick TD, Dhawan RT, Lewington V. Role of SPECT/CT in differentiated thyroid cancer. *Nucl Med Commun.* 2012;33(8):787-798.
72. Padovani RP, Kasamatsu TS, Nakabashi CC, et al. One month is sufficient for urinary iodine to return to its baseline value after the use of water-soluble iodinated contrast agents in post-thyroidectomy patients requiring radioiodine therapy. *Thyroid.* 2012;22(9):926-930.
73. Lamartina L, Grani G, Durante C, et al. Follow-up of differentiated thyroid cancer: what should (and what should not) be done. *Nat Rev Endocrinol.* 2018;14(9):538-551.
74. Tuttle RM, Tala H, Shah J, et al. Estimating risk of recurrence in differentiated thyroid cancer after total thyroidectomy and radioactive iodine remnant ablation: using response to therapy variables to modify the initial risk estimates predicted by the new American Thyroid Association staging system. *Thyroid.* 2010;20(12):1341-1349.
75. Al-Saif O, Farrar WB, Bloomston M, et al. Long-term efficacy of lymph node reoperation for persistent papillary thyroid cancer. *J Clin Endocrinol Metab.* 2010;95(5): 2187-2194.
76. Vaisman F, Momesso D, Bulzico DA, et al. Spontaneous remission in thyroid cancer patients after biochemical incomplete response to initial therapy. *Clin Endocrinol (Oxf).* 2012; 77(1):132-138.
77. Lamartina L, Montesano T, Trulli F, et al. Papillary thyroid carcinomas with biochemical incomplete or indeterminate responses to initial treatment: repeat stimulated thyroglobulin assay to identify disease-free patients. *Endocrine.* 2016;54(2): 467-475.
78. Verburg FA, Stokkel MP, Duren C, et al. No survival difference after successful (131)I ablation between patients with initially low-risk and high-risk differentiated thyroid cancer. *Eur J Nucl Med Mol Imaging.* 2010;37(2):276-283.
79. Durante C, Montesano T, Torlontano M, et al. Papillary thyroid cancer: time course of recurrences during post-surgery surveillance. *J Clin Endocrinol Metab.* 2013;98(2): 636-642.
80. Seejore K, Gerrard GE, Gill VM, et al. Can we discharge dynamically risk-stratified low-risk (excellent response to treatment) thyroid cancer patients after 5 years of follow-up? *Clin Oncol (R Coll Radiol).* 2019;31(4):219-224.
81. Lubitz CC, Kong CY, McMahon PM, et al. Annual financial impact of well-differentiated thyroid cancer care in the United States. *Cancer.* 2014;120(9):1345-1352.
82. Yadav D, Shah K, Naidoo K, et al. PET/computed tomography in thyroid cancer. *Neuroimaging Clin N Am.* 2021; 31(3):345-357.
83. Brose MS, Nutting CM, Jarzab B, et al. Sorafenib in radioactive iodine-refractory, locally advanced or metastatic differentiated thyroid cancer: a randomised, double-blind, phase 3 trial. *Lancet.* 2014;384(9940):319-328.

84. Schlumberger M, Tahara M, Wirth LJ, et al. Lenvatinib versus placebo in radioiodine-refractory thyroid cancer. *N Engl J Med*. 2015;372(7):621-630.
85. Schwartz LH, Litiere S, de Vries E, et al. RECIST 1.1-Update and clarification: from the RECIST committee. *Eur J Cancer*. 2016;62:132-137.
86. Fugazzola L, Elisei R, Fuhrer D, et al. 2019 European Thyroid Association Guidelines for the Treatment and Follow-Up of Advanced Radioiodine-Refractory Thyroid Cancer. *Eur Thyroid J*. 2019;8(5):227-245.
87. Durante C, Haddy N, Baudin E, et al. Long-term outcome of 444 patients with distant metastases from papillary and follicular thyroid carcinoma: benefits and limits of radioiodine therapy. *J Clin Endocrinol Metab*. 2006;91(8):2892-2899.
88. Hyer SL, Newbold K, and Harmer CL. Early and late toxicity of radioiodine therapy: detection and management. *Endocr Pract*. 2010;16(6):1064-1070.
89. Sawka AM, Thabane L, Parlea L, et al. Second primary malignancy risk after radioactive iodine treatment for thyroid cancer: a systematic review and meta-analysis. *Thyroid*. 2009;19(5):451-457.
90. Ravera S, Reyna-Neyra A, Ferrandino G, et al. The sodium/iodide symporter (NIS): molecular physiology and preclinical and clinical applications. *Annu Rev Physiol*. 2017;79:261-289.
91. Dohán O, Baloch Z, Bánrévi Z, et al. Rapid communication: predominant intracellular overexpression of the NA^+/I^- symporter (NIS) in a large sampling of thyroid cancer cases. *J Clin Endocrinol Metabol*. 2001;86(6):2697-2700.
92. Faggiano A, Coulot J, Bellon N, et al. Age-dependent variation of follicular size and expression of iodine transporters in human thyroid tissue. *J Nucl Med*. 2004;45(2):232-237.
93. Buffet C, Wassermann J, Hecht F, et al. Redifferentiation of radioiodine-refractory thyroid cancers. *Endocr Relat Cancer*. 2020;27(5):R113-R132.
94. Wang H, Dai H, Li Q, et al. Investigating (18)F-FDG PET/CT parameters as prognostic markers for differentiated thyroid cancer: a systematic review. *Front oncol*. 2021;11:648658-648658.
95. Hong CM, Ahn BC, Jeong SY, et al. Distant metastatic lesions in patients with differentiated thyroid carcinoma. Clinical implications of radioiodine and FDG uptake. *Nuklearmedizin*. 2013;52(4):121-129.
96. Kwon SY, Choi EK, Kong EJ, et al. Prognostic value of preoperative 18F-FDG PET/CT in papillary thyroid cancer patients with a high metastatic lymph node ratio: a multicenter retrospective cohort study. *Nucl Med Commun*. 2017;38(5):402-406.
97. Pace L, Klain M, Salvatore B, et al. Prognostic role of 18F-FDG PET/CT in the postoperative evaluation of differentiated thyroid cancer patients. *Clin Nucl Med*. 2015;40(2):111-115.
98. Tavares C, Coelho MJ, Eloy C, et al. NIS expression in thyroid tumors, relation with prognosis clinicopathological and molecular features. *Endocr Connect*. 2018;7(1):78-90.
99. Liu J, Liu R, Shen X, et al. The genetic duet of BRAF V600E and TERT promoter mutations robustly predicts loss of radioiodine avidity in recurrent papillary thyroid cancer. *J Nucl Med*. 2020;61(2):177-182.
100. Turner JG, Brownlie BE, Rogers TG. Lithium as an adjunct to radioiodine therapy for thyrotoxicosis. *Lancet*. 1976;1(7960):614-615.
101. Koong SS, Reynolds JC, Movius EG, et al. Lithium as a potential adjuvant to 131I therapy of metastatic, well differentiated thyroid carcinoma. *J Clin Endocrinol Metab*. 1999;84(3):912-916.
102. Luo H, Tobey A, Auh S, et al. The effect of lithium on the progression-free and overall survival in patients with metastatic differentiated thyroid cancer undergoing radioactive iodine therapy. *Clin Endocrinol (Oxf)*. 2018;89(4):481-488.
103. Ho AL, Grewal RK, Leboeuf R, et al. Selumetinib-enhanced radioiodine uptake in advanced thyroid cancer. *N Engl J Med*. 2013;368(7):623-632.
104. Rothenberg SM, McFadden DG, Palmer EL, et al. Redifferentiation of iodine-refractory BRAF V600E-mutant metastatic papillary thyroid cancer with dabrafenib. *Clin Cancer Res*. 2015;21(5):1028-1035.
105. Iravani A, Solomon B, Pattison DA, et al. Mitogen-activated protein kinase pathway inhibition for redifferentiation of radioiodine refractory differentiated thyroid cancer: an evolving protocol. *Thyroid*. 2019;29(11):1634-1645.
106. Clement SC, Peeters RP, Ronckers CM, et al. Intermediate and long-term adverse effects of radioiodine therapy for differentiated thyroid carcinoma—a systematic review. *Cancer Treat Rev*. 2015;41(10):925-934.
107. Ma C, Xie J, Chen Q, et al. Amifostine for salivary glands in high-dose radioactive iodine treated differentiated thyroid cancer. *Cochrane database Syst Rev*. 2009;2009(4):CD007956-CD007956.
108. Haghighatafshar M, Nowshad R, Etemadi Z, et al. The effect of chewing-gum on dose rate of salivary gland in differentiated thyroid carcinoma patients treated with radioiodine. *Q J Nucl Med Mol Imaging*. 2020;64(3):321-325.
109. Chen L, Shen Y, Luo Q, et al. Pulmonary fibrosis following radioiodine therapy of pulmonary metastases from differentiated thyroid carcinoma. *Thyroid*. 2010;20(3):337-340.
110. Chow KY, Kurumety S, Helenowski IB, et al. Association between quality of life and patient-reported complications from surgery and radioiodine in early-stage thyroid cancer survivors: a matched-pair analysis. *Surgery*. 2021;170(2):462-468.
111. Sandeep TC, Strachan MW, Reynolds RM, et al. Second primary cancers in thyroid cancer patients: a multinational record linkage study. *J Clin Endocrinol Metab*. 2006;91(5):1819-1825.
112. Molenaar RJ, Sidana S, Radivoyevitch T, et al. Risk of hematologic malignancies after radioiodine treatment of well-differentiated thyroid cancer. *J Clin Oncol*. 2018;36(18):1831-1839.
113. Fisher R. Questionable relevance of leukemia risk after radioiodine ablation of thyroid cancer. *J Clin Oncol*. 2018;36(18):1885.
114. Hindié E, Récher C, Zerdoud S, et al. Risk of hematologic malignancies after radioactive iodine treatment of thyroid cancer: an unjustified warning. *J Clin Oncol*. 2018;36(18):1881-1882.
115. Verburg FA, Hoffmann M, Iakovou I, et al. Errare humanum est, sed in errare perseverare diabolicum: methodological errors in the assessment of the relationship between I-131 therapy and possible increases in the incidence of malignancies. *Eur J Nuclear Med Mol Imaging*. 2020;47(3):519-522.
116. Teng CJ, Hu YW, Chen SC, et al. Use of radioactive iodine for thyroid cancer and risk of second primary malignancy: a nationwide population-based study. *J Natl Cancer Inst*. 2016;108(2).
117. Benua RS, Cicale NR, Sonenberg M, et al. The relation of radioiodine dosimetry to results and complications in the treatment of metastatic thyroid cancer. *Am J Roentgenol Radium Ther Nucl Med*. 1962;87:171-182.

118. Klubo-Gwiezdzinska J, Van Nostrand D, Atkins F, et al. Efficacy of dosimetric versus empiric prescribed activity of 131I for therapy of differentiated thyroid cancer. *J Clin Endocrinol Metab*. 2011;96(10):3217-3225.
119. Deandreis D, Rubino C, Tala H, et al. Comparison of empiric versus whole-body/-blood clearance dosimetry-based approach to radioactive iodine treatment in patients with metastases from differentiated thyroid cancer. *J Nucl Med*. 2017;58(5):717-722.
120. Finessi M, Liberini V, Deandreis D. Major limits of dosimetrically determined activities in advanced differentiated thyroid carcinoma. *Q J Nucl Med Mol Imaging*. 2019;63(3):258-266.
121. Bakheet SM, Powe J, Hammami MM. Unilateral radioiodine breast uptake. *Clin Nucl Med*. 1998;23(3):170-171.
122. Ahn J, Jin M, Song E, et al. Clinical outcomes after early and delayed radioiodine remnant ablation in patients with low-risk papillary thyroid carcinoma: propensity score matching analysis. *Endocrinol Metab (Seoul)*. 2020;35(4):830-837.
123. Tsirona S, Vlassopoulou V, Tzanela M, et al. Impact of early vs late postoperative radioiodine remnant ablation on final outcome in patients with low-risk well-differentiated thyroid cancer. *Clin Endocrinol (Oxf)*. 2014;80(3):459-463.
124. Sawka AM, Lakra DC, Lea J, et al. A systematic review examining the effects of therapeutic radioactive iodine on ovarian function and future pregnancy in female thyroid cancer survivors. *Clin Endocrinol*. 2008;69(3):479-490.
125. Anderson C, Engel SM, Weaver MA, et al. Birth rates after radioactive iodine treatment for differentiated thyroid cancer. *Int J Cancer*. 2017;141(11):2291-2295.
126. Wu JX, Young S, Ro K, et al. Reproductive outcomes and nononcologic complications after radioactive iodine ablation for well-differentiated thyroid cancer. *Thyroid*. 2015;25(1):133-138.
127. van Velsen EFS, Visser WE, van den Berg SAA, et al. Longitudinal analysis of the effect of radioiodine therapy on ovarian reserve in females with differentiated thyroid cancer. *Thyroid*. 2020;30(4):580-587.
128. Nies M, Cantineau AEP, Arts E, et al. Long-term effects of radioiodine treatment on female fertility in survivors of childhood differentiated thyroid carcinoma. *Thyroid*. 2020;30(8):1169-1176.
129. Cho GJ, Kim SY, Lee HC, et al. Risk of adverse obstetric outcomes and the abnormal growth of offspring in women with a history of thyroid cancer. *Thyroid*. 2019;29(6):879-885.
130. Schlumberger M, De Vathaire F, Ceccarelli C, et al. Exposure to radioactive iodine-131 for scintigraphy or therapy does not preclude pregnancy in thyroid cancer patients. *J Nucl Med*. 1996;37(4):606-612.
131. Wichers M, Benz E, Palmedo H, et al. Testicular function after radioiodine therapy for thyroid carcinoma. *Eur J Nucl Med*. 2000;27(5):503-507.
132. Hyer S, Vini L, O'Connell M, et al. Testicular dose and fertility in men following I(131) therapy for thyroid cancer. *Clin Endocrinol (Oxf)*. 2002;56(6):755-758.
133. Zhang L, Huang Y, Zheng Y, et al. The effect of I-131 therapy on pregnancy outcomes after thyroidectomy in patients with differentiated thyroid carcinoma: a meta-analysis. *Endocrine*. 2021;73(2):301-307.

Percutaneous Ethanol Injection of Thyroid Nodules, Thyroid Cancer, & Cervical Lymph Node Metastasis From Thyroid Cancer

26

Vishnu Sundaresh, MD, MSCI
Dev Abraham, MD, MRCP (UK)

INTRODUCTION

Thyroid nodules and cancers are widely prevalent subclinical disorders of the thyroid gland in humans. These tumors are commonly diagnosed incidentally during imaging performed for other unrelated conditions. There has been an apparent increase in the incidence of thyroid cancer ever since the introduction of medical imaging.[1] Surgical resection is the first-line treatment offered in the United States, especially for malignancy and for large benign goiters. Surgery has a 2% to 10% risk of intra- and postoperative complications, despite being performed by high-volume surgeons.[2] The wide availability of high-resolution ultrasound (US) equipment coupled with increased interventional training has opened a new avenue for office-based US-guided percutaneous interventional procedures, especially the percutaneous ethanol injection (PEI) and radiofrequency ablation (RFA).[3,4] As compared to other procedures, such as RFA or LASER therapy, PEI is cost-effective and also, the equipment requirements are minimal and less expensive. Despite extensive published data regarding the comparative effectiveness of PEI across the globe, it has not become the initial therapy of choice in the United States.[5] In this chapter, ideal patient selection for PEI, its techniques, efficacy, and adverse effects for benign and malignant thyroid nodules and associated cervical lymph node metastasis (CLNM) will be reviewed.

GENERAL PRINCIPLES OF US-GUIDED PERCUTANEOUS ETHANOL INJECTION

The general principles that are common to any percutaneous procedure such as preprocedure patient counseling, adherence to meticulous asepsis, and the administration of local anesthesia also apply to PEI. Prior to the infiltration of local anesthesia, explaining the anticipated sequence of the procedure in a reassuring manner can improve success and patient tolerance. Allowing the patient to speak, swallow, and breathe normally during the intervention does not adversely affect the procedure. Detailed preprocedure neck mapping of blood vessels and a mental "stock-taking" of the typical location of vital structures are very important to avoid complications. During PEI, if a patient encounters unusual pain, voice change (suggestive of recurrent laryngeal nerve-RLN or vagus nerve injury), breathing difficulty, or if there is unsureness about patient safety from the operator's standpoint, the procedure should be terminated immediately.

ULTRASOUND IMAGING ANATOMY OF HEAD & NECK

A comprehensive understanding of the US imaging-specific human neck anatomy (sono-anatomy) is an absolute prerequisite for a successful PEI. Only the most relevant sono-anatomical correlation for PEI is described in this chapter.

The thyroid gland has a ground glass echo appearance and is located anterior to the larynx, posterior to the strap muscles, and flanked bilaterally by the great vessels of the neck. The location of the great vessels along with the RLN, vagus nerve, and sympathetic trunk is depicted in Figure 26–1. The cervical portion of the vagus nerve is commonly located within the carotid sheath, postero-lateral to the common carotid artery (CCA) in 80% of the subjects. Less commonly it can be located anterolateral to the CCA. It appears on the neck US as a hypoechoic 2 to 3 mm thick, linear, avascular structure with echogenic striation. The location can be altered by the presence of metastatic lymph node or a large, laterally protruding nodular goiter. The respective vagus nerve gives off the right and left RLN branches

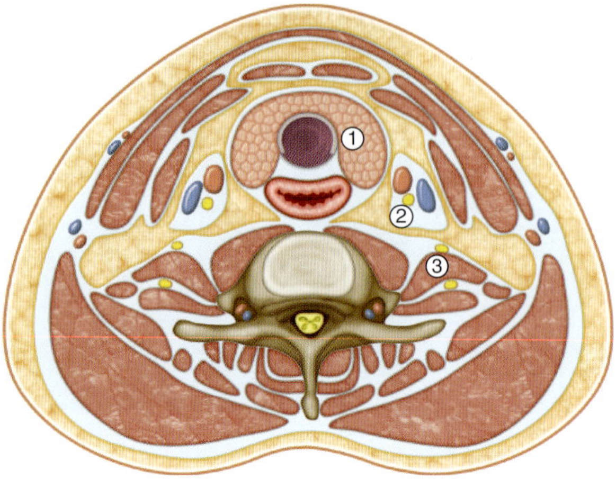

▲ **Figure 26–1.** Cross section at the level of C7 vertebra area 1, 2, and 3 correspond to recurrent laryngeal nerve, vagus nerve, and the sympathetic trunk respectively. (Reproduced with permission from Nikita Abraham, MPH, Department of Public Health, University of Utah.)

caudally in the neck. These nerves travel cranially into the larynx and are situated within the tracheoesophageal (TE) grooves at the level of the thyroid gland. RLNs cannot be reliably visualized with the currently available US technology. PEI performed on thyroid nodules and cysts located within the posteromedial aspect of the thyroid lobes, and medially located central compartment recurrent thyroid cancer carry the risk of injury to the RLN nerves. Attempted PEI of CLNM in the lateral compartment poses the risk of injury to vagus nerves, sympathetic ganglia, and complications from accidental intravascular injection.[6]

Sclerosing Agents Used

Several organic and inorganic chemicals have been used as sclerosing agents in clinical practice to induce tissue destruction and fibrosis. Although ethyl alcohol (ethanol), polidocanol, talc, tetracycline and bleomycin, acetic and hydrochloric acids, and attenuated strains of bacteria have been used, ethanol has become the mainstay for percutaneous injection sclerotherapy.[5,7-10] At higher concentrations (>95%), ethanol effectively induces tissue destruction and sclerosis. Since ethanol is not tissue specific in its destructive ability, whenever possible, only the minimal amount of ethanol required for therapeutic success is recommended to be administered using the thinnest gauge needle for any given tumor. Large-volume ethanol injection in any one sitting is not recommended as it increases the risk of diffusion causing surrounding tissue damage. High concentrations of ethanol destroy any type of tissue, given sufficient duration of contact. Therefore, a clear understanding of the cervical anatomy along with procedural technique will assist in accurate needle placement with US guidance which is crucial to avoid adjacent tissue destruction.[6] Ethanol-mediated tissue destruction is attributed to several mechanisms: (a) The *main effect* is due to acute arteriolar and small vessel coagulation resulting in *gradual* necrosis and fibrosis. (b) A *secondary* effect with *immediate* functional impairment results from acute tissue dehydration and protein denaturation.[7] Ethanol injection into recurrent cystic lesions destroys the epithelial lining and promotes inflammatory obliteration of the cavity. This results in elimination of the dead space and hence reduces recurrences.

Blood ethanol level is known to elevate transiently and drop within 1 hour after the procedure. Signs and symptoms of ethanol toxicity are encountered if the injected volume approaches or exceeds 100 mL in a single sitting.[7] The volume required for PEI of neck tumors is much lower than this limit; therefore, ethanol toxicity is not seen during PEI of thyroid cysts or nodules.

RISKS & SIDE EFFECTS OF PERCUTANEOUS ETHANOL INJECTION

Pain and bruising are the most common side effects of PEI.[11-17] The nontissue discriminative property is the cause for side effects unique to ethanol, which is mostly due to extravasation. Misdirected injections result in tissue necrosis and nerve injury.

Risk Factors for Ethanol Extravasation

1. Use of large bore needle, mostly to drain thick cyst fluid, increases the risk of leak following the injection.
2. Large volume injection of ethanol (>5 mL) into solid nodules.
3. Injection under pressure into thick-walled, non-collapsible cysts or solid nodules.
4. Accidental puncture of posterior capsule resulting in injection outside of the nodule or cyst.

Since solid nodules and lymph nodes require a small volume of ethanol (<1 mL), the risk of extravasation may be lower as compared to cysts. The most common cause of pain, especially in solid lesions is due to capsular stretching during the injection. Intentionally avoiding injections into critical areas (danger areas) especially near the TE groove (RLN) and near the carotid vessel (vagus nerve and sympathetic ganglia) reduces complications.

Strategies to Reduce Risk of Ethanol Extravasation

1. Avoiding large volume injections. Typical volumes include about 30% to 50% of the cyst volume, 1 to 2 mL for TA, and 0.1 to 1 mL for CLNM.
2. Needle tip position awareness during the procedure to avoid capsular damage.

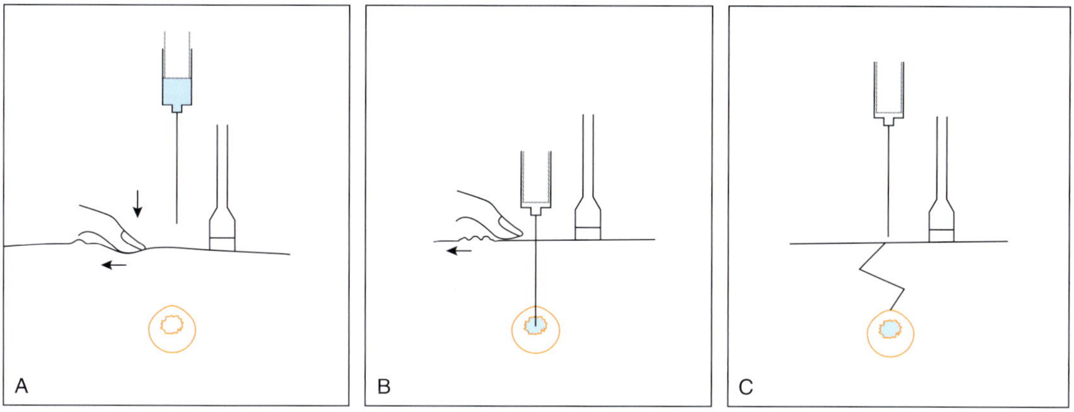

▲ **Figure 26–2.** **(A-C)** Z-track technique. (Reproduced with permission from Nikita Abraham, MPH, Department of Public Health, University of Utah.)

3. Avoiding injection or planned under treatment of lesions located in the danger areas of the neck.
4. Terminating procedure for unusually severe pain or visible extravasation by US.
5. Using the smallest gauge needle possible for successful aspiration and injection.
6. Utilizing the "Z" track technique (Figure 26–2).

Intracavitary bleeding is another complication during PEI for cystic lesions, avoidance of which is crucial for a successful outcome. If bleeding is induced during the procedure, it is very difficult to control it with direct pressure. Once bleeding occurs, the cyst can rapidly fill with blood until spontaneous tamponade ensues. PEI under pressure into tensely cystic recently bled nodule is best avoided due to the risk of extravasation. Immediate aspiration of the blood is almost always unsuccessful. The risk of intracavitary bleeding can be reduced by observing the following two principles. One is to aspirate slowly and the other is to reposition the needle to avoid injury to the posterior capsule of the cyst. If intracystic bleeding is anticipated due to the presence of a vascular mural component, then the use of an intravenous cannula may reduce injury and subsequent bleeding. Fine-bore cannulas tend to kink, and therefore, this should also be taken into consideration. Some cannulas are not sufficiently echogenic and are difficult to visualize. Great care needs to be taken to avoid displacement of the tip of the cannula from the cavity during the injection.

PROCEDURE SUITE SAFETY POLICIES, COMPLICATION RECOGNITION AND RISK MITIGATION STRATEGIES

A small amount of ethanol leakage is inevitable without significant consequence. Extravasation of large volume of ethanol into the soft tissues of neck leading to skin and cartilage necrosis is the most morbid reported complication.[18] Reasons include (a) inadequate expertise and/or skill, and (b) confusion between ethanol and lidocaine, especially after being loaded into the syringe, since both are colorless. This may be prevented by (a) using vials of different sizes, (b) operator self-preloading syringes just prior to procedure, (c) using syringes with different colored hubs, and (d) proper labeling of the syringes. The author practices and recommends pre- and postprocedure US-guided vocal cord function assessment as described by Cheng et al.[19]

PEI for the following etiologies will be discussed in this chapter:

1. Cystic thyroid nodules and thyroglossal cysts
2. Toxic thyroid adenomas and nonfunctional benign thyroid nodules
3. Cervical lymph node metastasis from thyroid cancer

A. Cystic Thyroid Nodules and Thyroglossal Cysts

About 15% to 25% of the thyroid nodules are cystic or predominantly cystic.[20] Most thyroid cysts in adults result from (a) an *acute* spontaneous degeneration of solid nodules or (b) a *gradual* development of simple cysts. The cyst cavity formed after an acute cystic generation are "pseudo cysts" which lack an epithelial lining. Large simple colloid cysts that arise in the thyroid are most likely to have an epithelial lining. The risk of recurrence following aspiration PEI in cysts with a lining epithelium as compared to cysts without, has not been systematically studied with histological correlation. In a surgical series of 71 patients with thyroid cysts, 82% were degenerating adenomas, 4% were simple cysts, and the remaining 14% were papillary cancers.[21] Since there is selection bias in surgical series, cancer risk in thyroid cysts can be estimated to be 2% to 4%.[21,22] Therefore, all cyst aspirates should undergo cytological assessment to evaluate for malignancy prior to PEI. All complex cystic nodules containing mural solid components require fine-needle aspiration (FNA) prior to PEI. The above principle also applies to thyroglossal cysts in adults.

THE PROCEDURE OF PEI IN CYSTIC THYROID NODULES & THYROGLOSSAL CYSTS

Percutaneous ethanol injection is the most effective method to treat simple and complex thyroid cysts.[20,23] The main goal of PEI is to effectively aspirate the contents completely without injury to the posterior or lateral wall of the cyst capsule and introduce ethanol prior to withdrawing the needle (Figure 26–3a, b). The volume of ethanol injection is variable and is dependent on the completeness of aspiration and the absence of mural component. In general, 30% to 50% of the aspirated volume is replaced with 95% ethanol.

The ideal cystic nodule for PEI includes pure or simple cyst, and cysts with contents that can be aspirated easily using smaller gauge needles. Cystic nodules that collapse easily with floppy capsule respond well to PEI. Cysts with vascular mural masses, thick-walled cyst, or those cysts that appear to "re-form" a remnant nodule following aspiration respond less well to PEI. Cysts that contain very thick contents may be impossible to empty and inject in one sitting even with large-bore needles. These cysts may require a second procedure once the content becomes less viscid several days or weeks following the initial injection. If ethanol is injected into the thick viscid content to liquify for subsequent more complete aspiration, then the volume should be reduced appropriately to minimize the risk of extravasation.

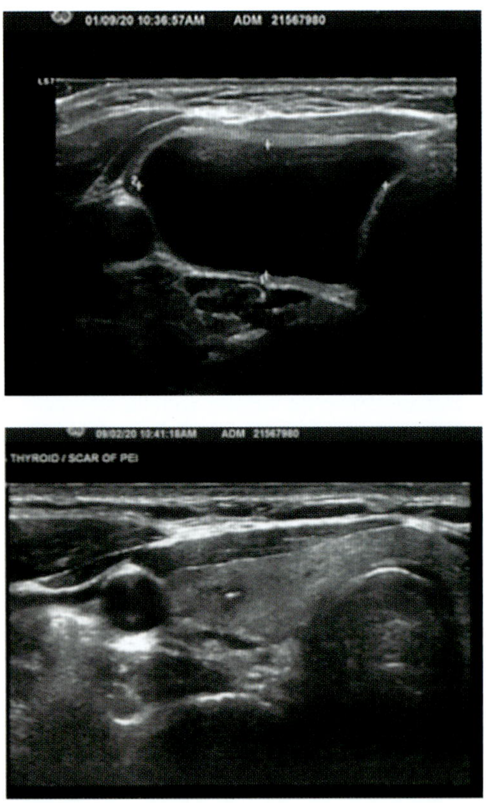

▲ **Figure 26–3.** Cyst aspiration pre- and postimages: Complete resolution of cyst 9 months post-PEI.

Outcomes of PEI in Cystic & Predominantly Cystic Nodules

Percutaneous ethanol injection is feasible in nodules that are more than 50% to 90% cystic in consistency. Since 1989, several publications have reported short- and long-term patient outcomes, which have universally confirmed the effectiveness of PEI.[12,23-27] All cysts do not require PEI, since only a certain percentage of them recur after initial aspiration.

In 2004, Valcavi et al. conducted a controlled randomized study on 281 patients comparing PEI and simple evacuation in which 86% and 7% cyst volume reductions were seen in the respective arms.[23] One among 135 patients involving 218 injections experienced a serious side effect of reduced ipsilateral vocal cord mobility with spontaneous resolution in 2 months. In 2004, Bennedbaek et al. conducted a randomized double-blind controlled trial on 66 patients comparing ethanol and saline injections (placebo) for recurrent cysts.[27] The superiority of PEI over saline was documented with cyst volume reduction by 100% (64% success after first injection) without any serious side effects. Interestingly, 68% reduction in cyst volume was observed with saline injection in the placebo arm. Although the exact reason is not well understood, this further supports the evidence that all cysts do not recur after initial aspiration.

While the above trials have evaluated the effectiveness of PEI wherein the injected ethanol is left inside the cyst permanently after the procedure, a few studies have evaluated the effectiveness of PEI after draining the injected ethanol following a contact time of 2 to 10 minutes with the cyst wall.[12,28] In 2005, Kim et al. examined the effect of PEI with and without aspiration of ethanol in 60 patients (30 in each group).[29] After a mean follow-up of 4.5 months, they reported no difference in outcomes. Pain was the most commonly reported side effect, without a significant difference in the two groups. The re-aspiration group had a significantly higher incidence of intracystic bleeding, more pain and discomfort due to multiple attempts, and twofold procedural time increase as compared to the no re-aspiration group. Hence, the authors concluded that aspiration of the injected ethanol is redundant, not time effective, and has more side effects.

The effectiveness of allowing a certain time of contact between the cyst wall and ethanol with subsequent removal of the instilled ethanol was addressed in 2012 by Kim et al.[28] This retrospective study included 217 patients (127 cystic, 90 predominantly cystic nodules) with a mean follow-up period of 6 months where PEI was performed and ethanol was aspirated after a contact time of 2, 5, and 10 minutes. The success rates were 96% in cystic and 82% in predominantly cystic nodules. The cysts that retained ethanol for 10 minutes were significantly greater in size than those that retained ethanol for 2 and 5 minutes, but there was no significant difference among the three groups in the mean volume reduction rate at last follow-up. With this technique, no major complications were reported.

One of the challenges encountered during attempted PEI of cysts is the unpredictable viscosity of the cyst contents which prevents complete aspiration. To circumvent this challenge, Zieleznik et al. in 2005 reported that the initial introduction of a small amount of ethanol facilitates liquefaction of the contents, enabling a more complete aspiration and introduction of larger amounts of ethanol at a later date for improved success.[30]

In 2021, Yang et al. published a systematic review and meta-analysis to assess the efficacy and safety of PEI for benign thyroid cystic nodules, as compared to other nonsurgical options (simple aspiration with or without saline flush, polidocanol, RFA).[20] This study included 1514 subjects from 4 RCTs and 15 nonrandomized studies which had low-moderate risk of bias. PEI had a higher volume reduction rate compared to other nonsurgical treatment options and was reported to be more effective for thyroid cysts than predominantly cystic thyroid nodules. Although RFA had comparable effectiveness, higher cost and technical complexity are limitations. Also, overall side effects for PEI are mild, with lower risk of major complication (self-limiting dysphonia 0.5% with PEI as compared to 1% with RFA). In summary, this meta-analysis provides evidence that PEI is a highly effective first-line nonsurgical treatment option for symptomatic cystic thyroid nodules with a favorable safety profile and lower cost.

Percutaneous ethanol injection is also a therapeutic option for patients with thyroglossal duct cysts (TGDC). In 2021, Karatay et al. evaluated the efficacy of a single-sitting PEI among 28 patients with TGDC.[31] After 12 months follow-up, 95% decrease in mean volume and 85% decrease in mean diameter were observed. This study demonstrated that PEI is a safe and effective treatment option for TGDC and can be offered as an alternative to surgery.

Predictors of Successful PEI

Based on several studies, the predictors for cyst recurrence are (a) cyst size greater than 10 mL, (b) presence of a mural mass,[28] and (c) vascularity within the mural mass. Blood flow-dependent dilution of the injected ethanol and intracystic bleeding are common reasons for recurrence. Needle-induced injury of the mural mass can cause intracystic bleeding which results in failure of the procedure. Therefore, the use of an intravenous soft-tip cannula instead of hypodermic needles may be used to reduce the risk of intracystic bleeding in nodules with vascular mural mass (Figure 26–4).[32] The use of an extension tube facilitates the aspiration and injection.

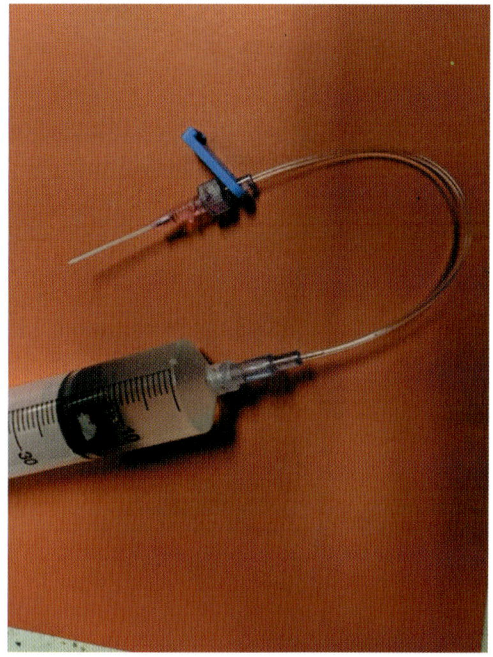

Figure 26–4. Cannula-based PEI set-up.

Cost-Effectiveness of PEI

In 2009, Raggiunti et al. from Italy published a study that not only evaluated the efficacy of PEI, but also performed a cost analysis.[33] They concluded that the cost of PEI was considerably lower than that of surgery and cost saving was about €200,000 for the 110 patients in the study (€1818 per patient).

A. Toxic Thyroid Adenomas and Nonfunctional Benign Thyroid Nodules

Percutaneous ethanol injection has been proven to be beneficial for both functional and nonfunctional thyroid nodules. About 5% to 10% of thyroid nodules are toxic adenomas (TA)[34] and are particularly amenable to PEI because the (a) incidence of malignancy is very low, (b) thyroid-stimulating hormone (TSH) trend allows biochemical monitoring, and (c) normalization of TSH indicates procedural success. Documentation of volume reduction of the nodule by neck US is also a useful parameter for both functional and nonfunctional nodules after PEI. Autoimmune thyroid disease predisposes to postprocedural hypothyroidism, but the risk is negligible in the absence of autoimmunity. PEI of TA leads to a "volume reduction" of the functional nodule, in that, patients with overt hyperthyroidism will improve to subclinical hyperthyroidism but complete destruction of the TA is rarely possible. Therefore, long-term biochemical and nuclear medicine monitoring is recommended to detect recurrences. For this reason, some experts recommend radioactive iodine (RAI) therapy, especially for large TAs.[3]

THE PROCEDURE OF PEI IN TOXIC THYROID ADENOMAS & NONFUNCTIONAL BENIGN THYROID NODULES

Percutaneous ethanol injection can be utilized for percutaneous destruction of benign thyroid nodules and toxic thyroid adenomas. It is particularly useful as an alternative therapy when RAI or surgery is not desired by the patient or if the patient is considered high risk for surgery. The availability of RFA holds promise, although head-to-head comparison studies between the two modalities have not been conducted. PEI for solid nodules is presumed to be cumbersome than RFA since multiple injections are required. Vascularity targeting during PEI is an effective improvisation yielding higher success rates. A detailed power doppler (PD) interrogation is performed on the entire nodule to map its vascularity.[35] Using the Z-track technique, under US guidance, the needle is inserted as close to or into the largest feeding blood vessel inside the capsule of the nodule and ethanol is injected gradually. Toggling between PD and B mode is useful for optimizing needle placement. When vascularity-targeted injection is performed optimally, the injected ethanol will diffuse into the blood vessel and give the appearance of a vasculogram of the nodule (Figure 26–5a). This is followed by the disappearance of blood flow in subsequent doppler interrogation after the injection (Figure 26–5b). Re-establishment of blood flow after transient reduction of flow is because of vascular spasm. If blood flow spontaneously resumes within 5 to 10 minutes after the initial injections, repeat injection can be performed. Vascular TAs can have multiple feeding vessels and may need injection into different blood vessels which can be achieved in the same sitting. There are two intraprocedural predictors for a successful outcome; appearance of (a) intranodular edema and (b) echogenic areas and related acute coagulative changes associated with reduced blood flow.[35]

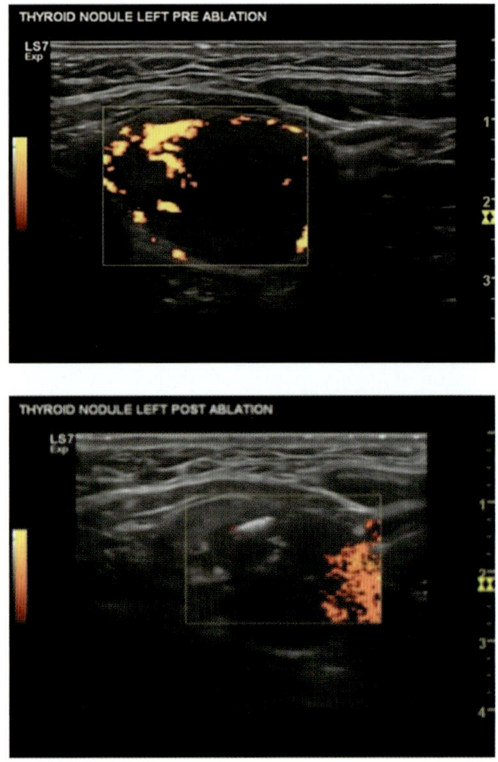

▲ **Figure 26–5.** Pre- and postvascularity targeted PEI depicted using power Doppler.

Outcomes of PEI for Toxic & Pretoxic Adenomas

Goletti and Livraghi initially published outcomes of PEI in the 1990s which was followed by larger studies performed by Papini and others.[3,13-16]

In 1996, Lippi et al. conducted a multicenter study of 429 patients to evaluate the efficacy and feasibility of PEI.[17] It was observed that 242 patients (56%) had TA while the rest had pretoxic adenomas (PTA). Multiple interventionists at different sites were involved in conducting the procedures. Patients underwent 2 to 12 sessions of PEI under US guidance with a median injection of four sessions. The volume of ethanol injected was 1.5 mL/mL of nodule volume with 1 to 8 mL of ethanol injected per session. The total volume of ethanol injected was 2 to 50 mL, followed by biochemical and image monitoring every 3, 6, and 12 months after PEI. Treatment success was higher for PTA (83%) as compared to TA (66.5%) at 12 months. Nodules <15 mL had better outcomes as compared to those >15 mL, with the least favorable outcomes seen for >30 mL. No correlation with success was observed with respect to the number of ethanol injections or methimazole pretreatment. The procedure was generally well tolerated with minor complications of burning and radiating pain in 90% of the patients. Transient hyperpyrexia was seen in 8%, hematoma in 4%, and thrombosis of IJV in 1 patient, with subsequent self-resolution without permanent sequela in any of the patients. Based on these observations, the authors concluded that PEI is safe and feasible in smaller nodules and alternatives such as RAI therapy or surgery are reserved for larger nodules.

In 2003, Monzani et al. published a study of 117 patients with TAs and toxic multinodular goiters (MNG) to report a 5-year outcome after PEI.[16] In this study which included 26 males and 91 females, 60 patients had solitary TAs, 40 pretoxic solitary adenomas (PTA), and 17 had toxic MNGs.

PTA patients had a 100% success rate, whereas it was 78% in those with TA (partial cure in 9%, failure in 13%). Effectiveness was similar irrespective of the number of nodules (1 vs >1) and nodule size (>40 mL vs <40 mL). A significant shrinkage of nodule volume was seen in all patients with no reported recurrence of hyperthyroidism. Methimazole and/or propranolol use did not affect PEI outcomes. Subclinical hypothyroidism developed 3 years after PEI in one patient who had documented high thyroid autoantibody levels.

The efficacy of ethanol has also been compared to suppressive doses of levothyroxine to reduce the volume of nonfunctioning solid nodules. In 1998, Bennedbaek et al. conducted a randomized clinical trial of 50 euthyroid patients with a solitary solid cold nodule where 25 patients were administered 1 ethanol injection and 25 patients were treated with suppressive doses of levothyroxine.[36] Twelve-month follow-up reported a 47% volume reduction in the PEI group as compared to 9% in the levothyroxine group, thus sealing the superiority of ethanol over LT4.

In summary, available evidence from literature suggests that PTAs respond best to PEI. Larger TAs require more ethanol volume higher number of injections to control biochemical hyperthyroidism and carry a higher risk for recurrence. Hence, surgery or RAI therapy is ideal for larger TA. The author published a novel vascularity-targeted approach wherein initial doppler interrogation is conducted to map the intranodular blood vessels that are targeted for injection.[35] A successful outcome of normalization of TSH, lower volume of injected ethanol, and fewer sessions are the advantages of this approach. The universal drawback of PEI akin to RFA is the intentional undertreating of TA near the critical areas (TE groove, carotid, and jugular vessels) that results in recurrence of the residual functional tissue and eventual hyperthyroidism.

Cost-effectiveness of PEI

In the United States, the estimated average Medicare cost for lobectomy is $20,200[37] while the cost of RFA is estimated to be about 30% to 50% of lobectomy.[38]

In 2020, Sharma et al. published the first cohort study in the United States proving the efficacy of TAs with the vascular targeted technique.[35] They reported the cost of first PEI at $508 and subsequent PEI to be $245 at their institution, thus making PEI cost-effective.

A. Cervical Lymph Node Metastasis in Thyroid Cancer

The incidence of thyroid cancer has been increasing over the last few decades, most of which is exclusively due to papillary thyroid carcinoma (PTC).[39] Despite an annual 3% increase in the incidence of PTC from 1975 to 2012 that is mostly attributed to increased detection of smaller tumors fortuitously and mortality remains low.[40] The incidence of cervical lymph node metastasis (CLNM) at diagnosis is different from preoperative imaging as compared to postoperative histological evaluation of the pathology specimen. A 2019 meta-analysis by Zhao et al. reported the incidence of central CLNM of PTC to be 48% on neck US, dropping to 36% after neck dissection, while the incidence of lateral CLNM was 59% and 47%, respectively.[41] Preoperative detection is dependent on the quality of the US machine and expertise of the sonographer, while postoperative incidence depends on the extent of neck dissection and surgical expertise. Timely detection of CLNM is important since treatment has an impact on survival. PTC with CLNM has a significantly lower all-cause survival at 14 years as compared to PTC without CLNM (79% vs 82%).[42]

Continued postoperative surveillance with imaging is indicated for detection of residual and/or recurrent disease, the incidence being 20% to 40%.[43,44] Wide availability of highly sensitive thyroglobulin assays along with increasing quality and expertise with neck US has resulted in the detection of small loco-regional disease. Although surgery is an option for clinically significant low-volume metastatic disease (eg, central CLNM >0.8 cm; lateral CLNM >1.5-2 cm), overall survival is not improved. Since majority of low-risk PTC with small-scale CLNM remains stable without worsening morbidity,[45,46] a risk-benefit analysis should be undertaken regarding management decisions. Although watchful waiting for select patients is an option, most patients are not comfortable "living with cancer" once the diagnosis is confirmed. A low-risk nonsurgical option, such as PEI, may be utilized in select patients. The survival advantage of this approach remains unproven.

THE PROCEDURE OF PEI IN CLNM

The technique is similar to that of solid thyroid nodules. Smaller volumes of ethanol, as little as 0.1 to 0.25 mL, may be sufficient depending on the size of the lymph node.[47,48] The posterior aspect of the lymph node is injected first followed by anterior areas.[47] This approach will not impair needle visualization by the freshly formed echogenic coagulation areas. Similarly, caudal to cranial approach of injection may be practiced based on the positioning of the patient in relation to the operator. Patients often described pain during injection likely due to capsular stretching, and slower injection reduces pain. Disappearance of vascularity and hyperechoic opacification of the lymph nodes predict successful ablation.

Outcomes of PEI in Cervical Lymph Node Metastasis

In 2002, Lewis et al. conducted a prospective study to evaluate the technique, efficacy, and side effect profile of PEI for limited CLNM from PTC.[47] All 14 patients had undergone thyroidectomy and radioactive iodine therapy and presented with recurrent nodal disease. Twenty-nine lymph nodes were injected and mean follow-up was for 18 months. All injected CLNM reduced in volume from a mean volume of 492 mm^3 to a mean volume of 76 mm^3 at 1 year and 20 mm^3 at 2 years. All patients experienced control of CLNM for the duration of follow-up and no major complications were reported.

In 2011, Heilo et al. published the largest retrospective study to date involving 69 patients who had been treated with thyroidectomy for PTC and presenting with recurrent CLNM.[48] The criteria used for successful treatment were (a) complete disappearance of lymph node, (b) reduction of the anteroposterior lymph node diameter to 4 mm or less without visible vascularization, (c) normalization of lymph node size and appearance, and in some nodes scar formation, and (d) no detectable malignant cells in the FNA specimens and no detectable thyroglobulin in needle washouts. PEI was conducted in 63 patients for 109 lymph nodes with 84% success. The authors concluded that PEI is an excellent alternative to surgery in patients with limited CLNM and PEI could replace "berry picking."

Several other studies have confirmed the efficacy and safety of PEI for CLNM from PTC.[49-52] In 2015, Fontenot et al. published a systematic review and pooled analysis evaluating the efficacy and complications comparing PEI to reoperation for the management of locally recurrent PTC.[53] This study included 1617 subjects from 27 studies (mostly retrospective, some prospective) where 168 (11.4%) were treated with PEI and 1449 (88.6%) were treated with reoperation with mean US follow-up of 33 and 31 months, respectively. None of the studies published direct comparison between the two interventions. Reoperation had a significantly higher success rate (95%) as compared to PEI (87.5%) with no difference in recurrence rates. Postprocedural thyroglobulin level median decline was not significantly different for PEI (28%-97%) versus reoperation (31%-98%). Pooled risk of complications was significantly higher with reoperation (3.5%) as compared to PEI (1.2%). A limitation noteworthy of mention is that PEI was mainly used to treat lateral CLNM, wherein the risk of RLN injury is minimal. Also, while most studies discussed RLN injury, only a few included a discussion on routine pre- and post-treatment laryngoscopy to determine vocal cord dysfunction. Hence, information regarding RLN injury is skewed in favor of PEI. In summary, pooled analysis of these observational studies suggests that PEI is less efficacious as compared to reoperation. But, the lower side effect profile, cost-effectiveness, and elimination of surgical risks are all advantages of PEI which should be discussed during shared decision-making. Based on the available evidence, the 2015 American Thyroid Association guidelines recommend formal neck dissection as first-line treatment. PEI is a second-line treatment and may have a limited role in local disease control in patients with medical comorbidities and for palliation.

Indications for PEI

1. Proven small-scale or isolated "left-over" CLNM in patients who have undergone initial surgery and radioactive iodine therapy with a curative intent
2. Patients who refuse further surgery
3. CLNM <2 cm in maximal dimensions
4. Elderly patients or those with comorbidities that increase risk for surgery
5. Palliation in patients who are anxious due to visible or palpable CLNM

Scenarios Where PEI Is Not an Ideal Option or Is Considered High Risk

1. Multi-level disease by neck US
2. Primary therapy for biopsy-proven CLNM
3. Bilateral CLNM in young patients
4. CLNM >2 cm (less responsive to PEI)
5. Patients with distant metastasis proven by imaging (exception when PEI is performed for palliation)
6. Injection of ipsilateral level VI lymph node or thyroid bed disease in patients who have had prior contralateral RLN injury

Cost-effectiveness of PEI in CLNM

Cost of PEI compared to surgery is an important factor in decision-making. Hay et al. in 2013 published data involving 25 patients with recurrent PTC stage III or IVA disease who underwent PEI.[49] Analysis indicated that the 25 patients avoided 40 future neck explorations and saved an average United States $61,440.

SUMMARY & CONCLUSIONS

PEI has been proven to be a safe and effective outpatient procedure. When performed accurately by experienced and skilled interventionists, it yields favorable results and is also cost effective in the management of cystic and solid thyroid nodules. With judicious case selection, PEI is also an effective adjunctive therapy for recurrent CLNM. US-guided PEI requires expert mentorship and continuous practice for a successful outcome. Currently, in the United States, most interventionists are self-trained and training is limited to workshops conducted by professional societies. The incorporation of procedural training into fellowship programs will empower physicians with the necessary interventional skill set and likely achieve improved patient acceptance and outcomes.

ACKNOWLEDGMENT

Images and sketches illustrated by Ms. Nikita Abraham, MPH, Department of Public Health, University of Utah.

REFERENCES

1. Jin J, McHenry CR. Thyroid incidentaloma. *Best Pract Res Clin Endocrinol Metab*. 2012;26(1):83-96.
2. Bergenfelz A, Jansson S, Kristofersson A, et al. Complications to thyroid surgery: results as reported in a database from a multicenter audit comprising 3,660 patients. *Langenbecks Arch Surg*. 2008;393:667-673.
3. Papini E, Pacella CM, Hegedus L. Diagnosis of endocrine disease: thyroid ultrasound (US) and US-assisted procedures: from the shadows into an array of applications. *Eur J Endocrinol*. 2014;170(4):R133-R146.
4. Gharib H, Hegedus L, Pacella CM, et al. Nonsurgical, image-guided minimally invasive therapy for thyroid nodules. *J Clin Endo Metab*. 2013;98(10):3949-3957.
5. Nixon IJ, Angelos P, Shaha AR, et al. Image-guided chemical and thermal ablation for thyroid disease: review of efficacy and complications. *Head Neck*. 2018;40:2103-2115.
6. Ha EJ, Baek JH, Lee JH. Ultrasonography-based thyroidal and perithyroidal anatomy and its clinical significance. *Korean J Radiol*. 2015;16(4)749-766.
7. Cheng D, Amin P, Ha TV. Percutaneous sclerotherapy of cystic lesions. *Semin Intervent Radiol*. 2012;29:295-300.
8. Livraghi T, Paracchi A, Ferrari C, et al. Treatment of autonomous thyroid nodules with percutaneous ethanol injection. *Radiology*. 1990;175:827-829.
9. Hegedus L, Hansen JM, Karstrup S, et al. Tetracycline for sclerosis of thyroid cysts. *Arch Intern Med*. 1988;148:116-1118.
10. Chang HS, Yoon JH, Chung WY, et al. Sclerotherapy with OK-432 for recurrent cystic thyroid nodule. *Yonsei Med J*. 1988; 39:367-371.
11. Zingrillo M, Collura D, Ghiggi MR, et al. Treatment of large cold benign thyroid nodules not eligible for surgery with percutaneous ethanol Injection. *J Clin Endocrinol Metab*. 1998;83:3905-3907.
12. Monzani F, Lippi F, Goletti O, et al. Percutaneous aspiration and ethanol sclerotherapy for thyroid cysts. *J Clin Endocrinol Metab*. 1994;78(3):800-802.
13. Goletti O, Monzani F, Caraccio N, et al. Percutaneous ethanol injection treatment of autonomously functioning single nodule: optimization of treatment and short term outcome. *World J Surg*. 1992;16:784-790.
14. Livraghi T, Paracchi A, Ferrari C, et al. Treatment of autonomous thyroid nodules with percutaneous ethanol injection: Preliminary results. *Radiology*. 1990;175(3):827-829.
15. Papini E, Panunzi C, Pacella CM, et al. Percutaneous US guided ethanol injection: a new treatment of toxic autonomous functioning thyroid nodule? *J Clin Endocrinol Metab*. 76:411-416.
16. Monzani F, Caraccio N, Goetti O, et al. Five year follow-up of percutaneous ethanol injection for the treatment of hyperfunctioning thyroid nodules: a study of 117 patients. *Clin Endocrinol (Oxf)*. 1997;46:9-15.
17. Lippi F, Ferrari C, Manetti L, et al. Treatment of solitary autonomous thyroid nodules by percutaneous ethanol injection: results of an Italian multicenter study. *J Clin Endocrinol Metab*. 1996;81(9):3261-3264.
18. Maz PS, Maasen MM, Braun G, et al. How safe is percutaneous ethanol injection for treatment of thyroid nodule? Report of a case of severe toxic necrosis of the larynx and adjacent skin. *Acta Otolaryngology*. 2004;124(10):1226-1230.
19. Cheng SP, Lee JJ, Liu TP, et al. Preoperative ultrasonography assessment of vocal cord movement during thyroid and parathyroid surgery. *World J Surg*. 2012;36:2509-2515.
20. Yang C, Sgu Y, Liou J. Efficacy of ethanol ablation for benign thyroid cysts and predominantly cystic nodules: a systematic review and meta-analysis. *Endocrinol Metab (Seoul)*. 2021;36(1):81-95.
21. De los Santos ET, Keyhani-Rofagha S, Cunningham JJ, et al. Cystic thyroid nodules: the dilemma of malignant lesions. *Arch Intern Med*. 1990;150(7):1422-1427.
22. Crile G Jr. Treatment of thyroid cysts by aspiration. *Surgery*. 1966;59(2):210-212.
23. Valcavi R, Frasoldati A. Ultrasound guided percutaneous ethanol therapy in thyroid cystic nodules. *Endocr Pract*. 2004; 10(3):269-275.
24. Verde G, Papini E, Pacella CM, et al. Ultrasound guided percutaneous ethanol injection in the treatment of cystic thyroid nodules. *Clin Endocrinol (Oxf)*. 1994;41:719-724.
25. Zingrillo M, Torlontano MD, Ghaggi MR, et al. Percutaneous ethanol injection of larger thyroid cystic nodules. *Thyroid*. 1996;6:403-408.
26. Shu CH, Baek JH, Ha EJ, et al. Ethanol ablation of predominantly cystic thyroid nodules: evaluation of recurrence rate and factors related to recurrence. *Clin Radiol*. 2015;70:42-47.
27. Bennedbaek FN, Hegedus L. Treatment of recurrent thyroid cysts with ethanol: a randomized double-blind controlled trial. *J Clin Endocrinol Metab*. 2003;88;5773-5777.
28. Kim YJ, Baek JH, Ja EJ, et al. Cystic versus predominantly cystic thyroid nodules: efficacy of ethanol ablation and analysis of related factors. *Eur Radiol*. 2012;22:1573-1578.
29. Kim DW, Rho MH, Kim HJ, et al. Percutaneous ethanol injection for benign cystic thyroid nodules: is aspiration of ethanol-mixed fluid advantageous? *Am J Neuroradiol*. 2005; 26(8):2122-2127.
30. Zieleznik W, Kawczyk-Krupka A, Barlik MP, et al. Modified percutaneous ethanol injection in the treatment of viscous cystic nodules. *Thyroid*. 2005;15:683-686.
31. Karatay E, Javadov M. The effectiveness of ethanol ablation in the treatment of thyroglossal duct cysts in adult cases and evaluation with cosmetic scoring. *Jpn J Radiol*. 2021;39(10):994-999.
32. Sundaresh V, Bakian A, Abraham D. Percutaneous Ethanol Injection of Thyroid Cysts using Intravenous Soft Tip Catheter and Z Track Technique: Proof of Concept Study Performed in USA; November 2019, Chicago, IL. American Thyroid Association Annual Meeting.
33. Raggiunti B, Fiore G, Mongia A. A 7-year follow-up of patients with thyroid cysts and pseudocysts treated with percutaneous ethanol injection: volume change and cost analysis. *J Ultrasound*. 2009;12(3):107-111.
34. Hegedus L, Bonnema SJ, Bennedbaek FN. Management of simple nodular goiter: current status and future perspectives. *Endocr Rev*. 2003;24:102-132.
35. Sharma A, Abraham D. Vascularity-targeted percutaneous ethanol injection of toxic thyroid adenomas: outcomes of a feasibility study performed in the USA. *Endocr Pract*. 2020;26(1):22-29.
36. Bennedbaek FN, Nielsen LK, Hegedüs L. Effect of percutaneous ethanol injection therapy versus suppressive doses of L-thyroxine on benign solitary solid cold thyroid nodules: a randomized trial. *J Clin Endocrinol Metab*. 1998;83(3):830-835.
37. Rivas AM, Nassur A, Zhang J, et al. ThyroSeq® V2.0 molecular testing: a cost-effective approach for the evaluation of indeterminate thyroid nodules. *Endocr Pract*. 2018;24(9):780-788.
38. Hamidi O, Callstrom MR, Lee RA, et al. Outcomes of radiofrequency ablation therapy for large benign thyroid nodules: A Mayo Clinic Case Series. *Mayo Clin Proc*. 2018; 93(8):1018-1025.

39. Morris LGT, Tuttle R, Davies L. Changing trends in the incidence of thyroid cancer in the United States. *JAMA Otolaryngol Head Neck Surg*. 2016;142(7):709-711.
40. Noone AM, Howlader N, Krapcho M, et al. SEER Cancer Statistics Review, 1975-2015, National Cancer Institute. Bethesda, MD, https://seer.cancer.gov/csr/1975_2015/. April 2018.
41. Zhao H, Li H. Meta-analysis of ultrasound for cervical lymph nodes in papillary thyroid cancer: diagnosis of central and lateral compartment nodal metastases. *Eur J Radiol.* 2019;112:14-21.
42. Haugen BR, Alexander EK, Bible KC, et al. 2015 American Thyroid Association Management Guidelines for Adult Patients with Thyroid Nodules and Differentiated Thyroid Cancer: The American Thyroid Association Guidelines Task Force on Thyroid Nodules and Differentiated Thyroid Cancer. *Thyroid.* 2016;26(1):1-133.
43. Grebe SKG, Hay ID. Thyroid cancer nodal metastases: biological significance and therapeutic considerations. *Surg Clin North Am*. 1996;5:43-63.
44. Shaha AR, Loree TR, Shah JP. Prognostic factors and risk group analysis in follicular carcinoma of the thyroid. *Surgery.* 1995;118:118-1131-8.
45. Robenshtok E, Fish S, Bach A, et al. Suspicious cervical lymph nodes detected after thyroidectomy for papillary thyroid cancer usually remain stable over years in properly selected patients. *J Clin Endocrinol Metab*. 2012;97:2706-2713.
46. Rondeau G, Fish S, Hann LE, et al. Ultrasonographically detected small thyroid bed nodules identified after total thyroidectomy for differentiated thyroid cancer seldom show clinically significant structural progression. *Thyroid.* 2011;21:845-853.
47. Lewis BD, Hay ID, Charboneau JW, et al. 2002 Percutaneous ethanol injection for treatment of cervical lymph node metastases in patients with papillary thyroid carcinoma. *AJR Am J Roentgenol*. 2002;178:699-704.
48. Heilo A, Sigstad E, Fagerlid KH, et al. Efficacy of ultrasound-guided percutaneous ethanol injection treatment in patients with a limited number of metastatic cervical lymph nodes from papillary thyroid carcinoma. *J Clin Endocrinol Metab.* 2011;96(9):2750-2755.
49. Hay ID, Lee RA, Davidge-Pitts C, et al. Long-term outcome of ultrasound-guided percutaneous ethanol ablation of selected "recurrent" neck nodal metastases in 25 patients with TNM stages III or IVA papillary thyroid carcinoma previously treated by surgery and 131I therapy. *Surgery*. 2013;154(6): 1448-1455.
50. Jin XL, Moley JF. Surgery for lymph node metastasis of medullary thyroid carcinoma: a review. *Cancer*. 2016;122(3): 358-366.
51. Lim CY, Yun JS, Lee J, et al. Percutaneous ethanol injection therapy for locally recurrent papillary thyroid carcinoma. *Thyroid*. 2007;17:347-350.
52. Kim BM, Kim MJ, Kim EK, et al. Controlling recurrent papillary thyroid carcinoma in the neck by ultrasonography-guided percutaneous ethanol injection. *Eur Radiol*. 2008; 18:835-842.
53. Fontenot TE, Deniwar A, Bhatia P, et al. Percutaneous ethanol injection vs reoperation for locally recurrent papillary thyroid cancer: a systematic review and pooled analysis. *JAMA Otolaryngol Head Neck Surg*. 2015;141(6):512-518.

RFA & Ethanol Ablation of Thyroid Nodules, Thyroid Cancer, & Lymph Node Metastases

27

Pia Pace-Asciak, MASc, MD
Ralph P. Tufano, MD, MBA
Alexander Shifrin, MD, FACS
Dev Abraham, MD, MRCP (UK)

GENERAL CONSIDERATIONS

Epidemiology of Benign & Malignant Thyroid Nodules

Thyroid nodules are exceedingly common, particularly among older patients, women, and those with a history of iodine deficiency or exposure to ionizing radiation.[1] Physical exam detects only 4% to 7% of nodules, whereas high-resolution ultrasound detects up to 70%.[1] Most of the time, thyroid nodules are benign; however, malignancy occurs in 7% to 15% of cases depending on age, sex, radiation exposure history, family history, and other factors.[1-3]

Approximately 5% to 10% of nodules degenerate with age whereby they undergo changes to become autonomously functioning thyroid nodules (AFTNs) and secrete an abnormally high amount of thyroid hormone.[4] Determining whether there are multiple nodules, or a single secreting nodule is present helps to determine the likelihood of success in achieving a euthyroid state.

Thyroid cancer is the fastest-growing endocrine malignancy worldwide, with a 300% increase in incidence over the past 3 decades.[5,6] Under the umbrella of differentiated thyroid cancer, papillary thyroid cancer (PTC) is the most common histological subtype of thyroid cancer, accounting for 90% of new cases and with an overall estimated 5-year survival rate of 98.1%: 99.9% for localized disease and 55.5% for distant disease.[7]

Approximately 35% of patients presenting with PTC have clinically positive lymph node metastases, with the most common site being the central neck compartment, and less frequently, the lateral compartments of the neck.[8,9] At the time of surgery, microscopically positive lymph nodes may be present in up to 80% of patients, with clinically N0 disease, but generally, only macroscopic disease requires surgical removal.[1,8,9] Even for patients having what has been deemed appropriate initial treatment, up to 30% of patients suffer persistent disease or recurrence, localized mostly to the cervical lymph nodes.[10] In up to 18% of patients with PTC, more commonly seen with superior pole tumors, skip metastases to the lateral neck can occur even though the central compartment of the neck is negative.[8]

History of Radiofrequency Ablation

Image-guided thyroid ablation procedures can be performed using either thermal energy such as radiofrequency ablation (RFA), laser ablation (LA), high-intensity focused ultrasound (HIFU), and microwave ablation (MA), or with chemical agents such as ethanol.[1-3,5-9,11,12] All thermally ablative techniques cause coagulation necrosis to the desired nodule; however, each technique differs in the type of energy applied and how the tissue is targeted. At the time of writing this chapter, RFA is the most frequently chosen technique and the most studied approach for treating thyroid disease.[13]

RFA is relatively novel for the treatment of thyroid gland pathology in North America but has been offered to patients internationally for decades to treat primary and metastatic tumors of the liver, lung, bone, and kidney and to ablate aberrant conduction pathways in the heart.[14-19] RFA is appealing because it is typically an outpatient procedure that is done in real time, under ultrasound guidance, with the use of a local anesthetic. It avoids the need for a general anesthetic, prolonged recovery time, and the costs associated with surgery. Other morbidities of surgery are avoided with RFA such as a need for an incision or removal of the thyroid gland, and it is much less likely to result in the need for thyroid hormone replacement making it an ideal minimally invasive treatment for patients in whom surgery is inappropriate, contraindicated, or refused.

CLINICAL FINDINGS

Symptoms & Signs for When RFA Is Indicated

Various international societies in Korea, Italy, the United Kingdom, and Austria have established their own clinical practice guidelines, opinion statements, or recommendations for RFA.[20-25] They include the Korean Society of Thyroid Radiology, the Italian Working Group on Minimally Invasive Treatments of the Thyroid, the United Kingdom's National Institute for Health and Clinical Excellence (NICE), the Austrian Thyroid Association, as well as the European Thyroid Association Guidelines. The American Head and Neck Society has initiated a global collaborative consensus guideline which has recently been published.[26]

A. Benign Thyroid Nodules (Nonfunctioning Thyroid Nodules)

Most benign nodules are asymptomatic; however, larger nodules that cause symptoms of compression, globus, dysphagia, throat discomfort, pain, cough, or concern for disfigurement due to a bulging thyroid have been successfully treated with RFA.[11,20,22-25,27,28] A recent systematic review demonstrated a volume reduction ratio (VRR) during long-term follow-up that ranged between 66.9% and 97.9% after 3 years post-RFA.[29] Regrowth was observed in 4.1% to 24.1% of nodules.[29] The consensus among the different society guidelines recommends RFA for patients with benign thyroid nodules with symptoms of compression, dysphagia, throat discomfort, foreign body sensation, pain, or cough as well as cosmetic concerns for those who do not wish to have surgery.[20-25,27] Subtle nuances exist between each society's recommendations regarding the size of the nodule, whether the nodule is autonomously functioning or nonfunctioning, and when to offer a second ablative treatment.[27]

For cytologically benign nodules, the Italian scientific societies recommend RFA for large symptomatic nodules (volume greater than 20 mL) when surgery is contraindicated or declined, whereas the European guidelines recommend RFA if the nodule is growing, the patient is symptomatic, and the nodule is more than 3 cm in size.[21,22,25] The Korean guidelines share a similar approach and recommend offering patients RFA for growing nodules that are greater than 2 cm and causing symptoms.[20] Neither the NICE nor Austrian societies provide a size cutoff for treatment.[23,24]

B. Autonomously Functioning Thyroid Nodules

Thermal ablation remains somewhat controversial for AFTN given the variability in TSH normalization post-treatment.[30] Thus, each society differs in their recommendations for the treatment of AFTN. All societies except the NICE recommend RFA as a therapeutic option for a solitary AFTN but not for Graves' disease and patients with a toxic multinodular goiter. The European Thyroid Association guidelines as well as the Italian society recommend against thermal ablation as first-line treatment for large AFTN (greater than 20 mL) due to the variable rate of therapeutic success for normalizing TSH. They recommend that RFA can be reserved for patients who decline or are not candidates for radioactive iodine (RAI) therapy or surgery[21,22,25] or can be used in combination with RAI to allow for a reduction in the dose of RAI received.[22] Similarly, the revised Korean guidelines and the recommendations from the Asian Task Force agree that RFA is an option for patients who refuse or cannot undergo traditional treatment for AFTN such as RAI or surgery.[20,31]

After careful consideration, patients with smaller single AFTN may be offered thermal ablation, whereas such treatment should be avoided in those with Graves' disease or a toxic multinodular goiter for which antithyroidal medications (ATD) are the cornerstone of therapy. Each society makes slightly different recommendations for the suitability based on the size of the functioning nodule. This notion is supported by Cesareo et al., where comparison was made between the reduction in medium-sized nodules (18 mL) versus smaller-sized nodules (5 mL). Euthyroidism was achieved in 86% of small nodules versus 45% in medium-size nodules.[32] For larger nodules (greater than 15 mL) or multifocal AFTN, the Austrian societies do not recommend RFA. The Italian societies share similar recommendation and tend to treat with RAI for large AFTN (greater than 20 mL), a practice that is more common in Europe than in North America.[13]

In certain circumstances, when a large symptomatic AFTN (volume >20 mL) is present, combined RFA and RAI treatment may be offered (weak evidence and not universally accepted strategy) to induce faster and greater improvement in local symptoms as well as a reduced dose of RAI.[21,33] The Austrian societies do not recommend RFA for larger (>15 mL) or multifocal AFTNs.[23] However, as newer data emerge the recommendations continue to evolve. A recent meta-analysis showed that thermal ablation of AFTN is an option regardless of nodule size.[34] The treatment response rate for TSH normalization was similar for nodules less than 18 mL and those greater than 18 mL (73.6% vs 67% $p = 0.53$).[34] Thus, the Asian task force agrees that RFA may be indicated for AFTNs regardless of nodule size.[31] Although the data show that RFA for smaller AFTNs has a greater success rate, this may be due to the associated initial learning curve combined with the fact that larger nodules have greater volume and are more likely to require repeat treatment.

C. Primary Thyroid Cancer

For patients with primary well-differentiated thyroid carcinoma, the standard of care is surgery or active surveillance for low-risk papillary thyroid cancer patients who do not wish to undergo surgery after having had counsel with a surgeon. RFA has emerged as an alternative therapy for patients who refuse or are ineligible for surgery but is not offered as the first line. The indications for RFA in primary thyroid cancer continue to evolve as new evidence emerges which demonstrates a similar efficacy and lower rate of complications than surgery for low-risk disease.[35-38] It is imperative that an initial evaluation is done by an experienced multidisciplinary team that is well versed in the traditional approaches as well as the novel minimally invasive techniques to allow a patient to make a fully informed value-based decision as to what's best for them.

When RFA is employed for curative intent, the literature supports the efficacy and safety of treating low-risk thyroid carcinoma such as T1aN0M0 or T1bN0M0.[35-37,39-47] The American Joint Committee on Cancer (AJCC) TNM system classifies the T1 category (T1: ≤2 cm) into T1a: ≤1 cm and T1b: ≤2 cm.[48] The main indications for treating low-risk papillary thyroid cancer with RFA include:

(a) pathologically confirmed papillary thyroid carcinoma (PTC) (classical variant) without cytological aggressiveness (such as tall cell, insular, or columnar cell)
(b) single PTC without extrathyroidal extension
(c) no metastatic tumors at the time of treatment
(d) ineligibility for surgery or refuse surgery
(e) refuse active surveillance

Surgery should be offered over RFA if capsular invasion is present at the posterior or medial margin, the tumor is located posteriorly at the tracheoesophageal groove, the presence of lymph node metastases is seen on ultrasonography, or aggressive cytopathology is present on the initial workup.[38,49] In addition, the identification of worrisome molecular patterns such as the detection of TERT promoter and TP53 mutation is a contraindication to minimally invasive thermal techniques, whereby such patients would be better served by surgical removal.[49] Furthermore, other considerations for surgery over RFA might be in patients of a young age, with no comorbidities, or if a familial form of thyroid cancer is present.

The evidence is strong for treating primary low-risk thyroid cancer with RFA. In a systematic review and meta-analysis of 715 patients, Choi et al. demonstrated pooled proportions of complete disappearance and recurrence of thermally ablated PTMC of 57.6% (95% confidence interval (CI): 35.4-79.8) and 0.4% (95% CI: 0-1.1). In a subgroup analysis, RFA showed the highest mean volume reduction rate (99.3%) compared with other treatment modalities such as microwave ablation (95.3%) and laser ablation (88.6%) ($p < 0.001$).[37] Furthermore, when the oncological effectiveness of surgery compared with RFA for PTMC was compared over a 5-year follow-up, similar outcomes were observed.[35] However, when surgery was compared with RFA, the surgery group took longer, required longer hospitalization, was costlier (all $p < 0.001$), and had a higher complication rate compared to the RFA group ($p = 0.095$).[35]

RFA treatment for follicular neoplasm is more controversial than PTC mainly because surgical resection is required to exclude the presence of vascular or capsular invasion for diagnosing whether the thyroid nodule is a follicular adenoma compared with a carcinoma. Thus, the various international societies share the opinion that follicular neoplasm is best treated surgically, as malignancy is assessed by histopathology after surgical resection.[1] Smaller-scale studies, such as one by Ha et al., demonstrated a significant reduction in the volume of RFA-treated follicular thyroid neoplasm (less than 2 cm) with complete disappearance after single treatment and no evidence of recurrence or distant metastases in follow-up (range: 60-76 months).[50] However, further larger-scale studies are required to confirm oncological effectiveness.

For more aggressive cancers such as medullary thyroid cancer (MTC), surgery remains the treatment of choice for curative intent. Few case reports have demonstrated RFA to be a safe and effective option for early MTC in patients ineligible for surgery[51] or for patients with regional recurrence after surgical resection of their MTC.[52] However, the data are somewhat limited for MTC and remains controversial. Similarly, for inoperable poorly differentiated tumors such as anaplastic carcinoma, RFA has a questionable clinical effect unless it is used for temporary relief/palliation.[42]

D. Recurrent Thyroid Cancer and Lymph Node Metastases

Most well-differentiated thyroid cancer is effectively treated by surgery, followed by RAI if deemed necessary.[1] However, local recurrences can occur in the thyroid bed and/or as nodal metastases in the central neck compartment or the lateral neck. The cornerstone of treating recurrent thyroid cancer is surgery, followed by RAI therapy for those that demonstrate iodine avidity and suppressive thyroid hormone replacement treatment, and/or external beam radiotherapy and chemotherapy depending on the extent of recurrent disease.[1] Patients with a malignant diagnosis should be evaluated by a multidisciplinary team before proceeding with alternative therapies such as RFA to ensure that the most effective therapy is offered first. Recurrent disease can be challenging to remove in a previously resected tissue bed making identification of the RLN, parathyroid glands, and other important neurovascular structures difficult potentially leading to a decrease in their quality of life. On the other end of the spectrum, patients reluctant to have surgery can undergo active surveillance for primary low-risk PTC, and serial monitoring for slow-growing, recurrent thyroid cancer, or neck metastases with a diameter less than 10 mm, but this requires close clinical follow-up.[1,35] RFA can be reserved as an alternative treatment for curative or palliative intent in patients deemed to be high surgical risk or for those refusing to undergo repeat surgery but for those who clinically require treatment. Factors that deem patients to be at high risk for reoperative surgery include previous thyroid or neck surgery, poor lung function, poor systemic condition, severe cardiovascular disease, or old age.[20]

When counselling patients to undertake RFA for curative purposes, the most effective outcomes are for locally recurrent small thyroid cancers where disease beyond the neck is absent.[20,49] Recent studies have demonstrated favorable outcomes when the number of locally recurrent well-differentiated papillary thyroid tumors are less than 3 or 4 per patient and the greatest tumor diameter is smaller than 2 cm.[38,53,54] Kim et al. demonstrated a complete disappearance rate of 86.1% (31 of 36 ablation zones) and a low recurrence rate of 11.5% (3 of 26 treated patients) after approximately 3 years of follow-up post-RFA in locally recurrent tumors (central or lateral neck) less than 2 cm in size.[38] When RFA was compared to the surgery group, the 1- and 3-year recurrence-free survival rates were comparable ($p = 0.681$) for RFA (96% and 92.6%, respectively) and reoperation groups (92.2% and 92.2%, respectively).[38]

In a trial where surgery was compared to RFA for small localized recurrent thyroid cancer, Choi et al. showed comparable recurrence-free survival rates between the RFA and surgery groups ($p = 0.2$) with no significant differences in mean serum thyroglobulin levels and their mean decrease after treatment between the groups ($p = 0.891$ and $p = 0.963$).[55] This is further supported by two systematic reviews and a meta-analysis which show a significant improvement in the pooled proportions in reduction of serum level of thyroglobulin, volume reduction, and disappearance of tumor post-RFA treatment for locally recurrent cancers within the neck.[56,57] A subgroup analysis may have been helpful to decipher whether a significant difference is noted when treatment is employed in the central neck compared with the lateral neck.

For patients with unresectable primary or recurrent thyroid cancer (DTC, medullary, or anaplastic), RFA can be used in select cases to rapidly decrease the tumor burden and improve local symptoms, when applied in the context of multimodality treatment.[20,49,58] Studies have shown that RFA can palliate symptoms of dysphagia, hoarseness, dyspnea, or cosmetic concerns for a protruding neck mass in patients with recurrent cancers at the thyroid bed and cervical lymph nodes that are deemed too risky to remove surgically or who refuse surgery.[20,49,58] Patients with progressive RAI refractory cervical recurrences may also benefit from RFA if surgical neck dissection is not a possible option. In this scenario, for symptom relief, RFA can be considered in patients with extensive lymph node involvement, central recurrences, or clinical and histological factors suggesting an aggressive disease.[20,49,58]

An important factor to consider when deciding whether a patient is a candidate for RFA for palliation of symptoms is to assess the degree of tracheal abutment of the tumor. Chung et al. demonstrated a mean volume reduction rate of 81.2% ± 55.7% in 172 recurrent tumors (central compartment after total thyroidectomy), with 72.1% (124 tumors) completely disappearing after a mean follow-up of 4 years depending on the proximity of the tumor to the trachea.[59] Other considerations for palliation of inoperable tumors or recurrences depend on the degree of calcification of the tumor and the severity of tumor vascular encasement which can lend to ineffective ablation.[58] The international societies share similar opinions regarding RFA for the treatment of high surgical-risk patients with local recurrences of their iodine-refractory well-differentiated thyroid carcinoma.[20-25] Furthermore, in select patients with distant RAI refractory metastases from DTC, RFA may be used as a multimodal treatment approach to palliate symptoms associated with bone metastases.[60,61] Thus, recognized indications for RFA include unresectable thyroid cancer, neck lymph-node recurrences of DTC, and even distant metastases.[20,49]

LABORATORY TESTS

Before and after RFA treatments, baseline thyroid function testing (thyroid-stimulating hormone, triiodothyronine, and free thyroxine) are standard tests. In select patients with benign nonfunctioning thyroid nodules and all patients with AFTNs, serum autoantibodies (antithyroid peroxidase antibody and antithyroglobulin antibody) are evaluated after RFA and can be an important blood test for evaluating treatment outcomes specifically for AFTN.[27,62]

As with any preprocedural checklist, the patient's bleeding tendency should be considered with a CBC, and coagulation testing (bleeding time, prothrombin time, and activated partial thromboplastin time). According to the Korean Society guidelines and the Austrian reports, patients taking anticoagulants should discontinue aspirin or clopidogrel 7 to 10 days prior to RFA, 3 to 5 days prior for warfarin, and 4 to 6 hours prior for heparin to avoid risk of hematoma formation.[27] Post-RFA procedure, heparin may be resumed in 2 to 6 hours, the night after RFA for warfarin, and the day after RFA for aspirin or clopidogrel.[27]

Pregnancy status should be evaluated before RFA treatment, as well as the presence of a pacemaker, which is a contraindication to the use of a monopolar electrode.

IMAGING STUDIES

Ultrasound evaluation is the gold standard for evaluating thyroid nodules prior to treatment with RFA.[1] This helps for mapping a treatment plan, ensuring safety for treating a nodule in proximity to critical structures and allowing the operator to ensure that benign biopsy results are consistent with benign sonographic features of the nodule. This congruency between the FNAB result and ultrasound findings for a benign process is especially important since the treatment strategy for the benign nodule is volume reduction and not complete ablation. All societies recommend characterizing the nodule size, composition, and vascularity, as well as the presence or absence of cervical lymph nodes as well as making note of the proximity to surrounding structures such as the trachea, carotid, and "danger triangle" where the recurrent laryngeal nerve sits.[20-25] Suspicious features for papillary thyroid cancer include the presence of microcalcifications, nodule hypoechogenicity, irregular margins (defined as either infiltrative, microlobulated, or spiculated), and a shape taller than wide measured on a transverse view compared with more benign spongiform and cystic features.[1] Different sonographic thyroid nodule assessment protocols exist for categorizing nodules based on the degree of suspicion for malignancy, namely the ACR TIRADS and the ATA guidelines.[1,63] If a patient presents with a large thyroid nodule and has suspected intrathoracic extension, other imaging modalities such as a computed tomography (CT scan) or magnetic resonance (MRI) of the neck and chest with contrast can delineate the extent of disease in relation to the major vasculature for surgical planning.

Mounting evidence demonstrates the importance of documenting pretreatment nodule volume for increasing uniformity of reporting and predicting outcomes when counselling patients.[12] To calculate the nodule volume (mL), the standardized method is to use the ellipsoid volume formula (length × width × depth × 0.524).[12] Nodules should be identified as small (less than 10 mL), medium (11-30 mL), or large (greater than 30 mL) to be able to counsel patients regarding the likelihood of requiring further procedures.[12] Furthermore, since thermal ablation is an area of active research, to track outcomes, a detailed description of the percentage of cystic to solid structure is recommended (eg, solid [less than 10% fluid present], predominantly solid [11%-50% fluid present], mixed solid and cystic, predominantly cystic [51%-90% fluid present], cystic [more than 90% fluid present], spongiform [multiple small cysts less than 5 mm interspersed within solid tissue for nearly all the volume]).[12] It is also key to note the vascularity of the nodule and the main vessels that feed into the nodule since this is a potential site of recurrence and can be addressed by various advanced techniques (described in the treatment section).[64]

As part of the workup of a nodule suspected to be autonomously functioning, usually guided by the TSH value, additional imaging to ultrasound should include a thyroid scan (^{99m}Tc pertechnetate or ^{123}I thyroid scan).[20-25,27] Following RFA treatment of AFTN, TSH should be repeated to evaluate treatment outcomes.

SPECIAL TESTS (FINE-NEEDLE ASPIRATION OR CORE BIOPSY)

Fine-needle aspiration (FNA) is a cost-effective, minimally invasive, readily available test for determining whether a nodule has features of malignancy requiring surgery for therapeutic or diagnostic purposes. The Bethesda classification for cytopathology is the standard system used at most institutions.

Prior to RFA of a benign nonfunctioning nodule, confirmation of at least two benign biopsy results is recommended by the societies (either FNA or core biopsy).[20-25,27] For AFTN, the societies differ slightly in their recommendations, but generally one FNA result can suffice if the ultrasound features are consistent with a benign sonographic appearance (spongiform, cystic, encapsulated, no evidence of extrathyroidal extension or lymphadenopathy).[20-25,27] Any discrepancy between the biopsy results and the ultrasound features can be resolved with repeat FNA or potentially a diagnostic lobectomy. At this point, the use of molecular markers to predict a Bethesda 3 or 4 category as benign and eligible for RFA has not been recommended.[1,49]

SPECIAL EXAMINATION

Flexible laryngoscopy is standard of care to confirm normal vocal cord function for all patients before and after RFA.[25] Ultrasound evaluation may also be used but may not be useful in some patients, especially men who may have an ossified thyroid cartilage.

Pre- and postprocedural symptom score profiles are filled out by patients using a 10 cm visual analog scale (grade 0-10). In addition, a cosmetic score is measured by a physician according to the following grades: 1, no palpable mass; 2, a palpable mass without cosmetic problems; 3, a cosmetic problem.[65]

TREATMENT: HOW RADIOFREQUENCY ABLATION TECHNIQUE WORKS

Patients are brought to the outpatient clinic, prepped in a sterile fashion and positioned supine with mild hyperextension of the neck. Once the nodule of interest has been mapped by ultrasound, including careful note of vital structures in proximity to the area of interest, the first step is to anesthetize the skin puncture site and the thyroid capsule where the sensory nerves exist. One of the key advantages of RFA is that it avoids the costs and risks of surgery; thus, the various societies recommend local anesthetic rather than a general anesthetic for pain control.[20-25] Generally, sedation is avoided since it can delay the detection of complications; however, debate exists among the societies regarding this practice. Using ultrasound guidance, 1% or 2% lidocaine (10-20 mL) is infiltrated in the midline of the neck, and toward the sternothyroid muscle to achieve pericapsular thyroid anesthesia. Once lidocaine is injected, it has a sonographic appearance of an anechoic band separating the thyroid gland from the strap muscle. For nodules that are close in proximity to vital structures, hydrodissection is achieved by injecting 5% dextrose solution (D5W), an iso-osmolar solution, between the thyroid capsule and critical structures to create a thermal barrier.[64,66] Saline is avoided for providing a buffer between critical structures since it is anionic and can potentially conduct electricity or a current that can cause damage from frictional heat.[64]

The RFA probe is generally a monopolar device that is thyroid-use dedicated with an internally cooled electrode.[64] A bipolar electrode is available and can be used for patients with electrical devices such as a pacemaker. Different active electrode tips exist (5 mm, 7 mm, and 10 mm) to precisely target small nodules or cancers near critical areas, but typically the workhorse tips are 7 or 10 mm. The RFA probe is introduced into the midline of the anterior neck at the level of the isthmus (called the trans-isthmic approach) while using ultrasound guidance to monitor the needle tip continuously. The nodule is targeted along the long axis in a medial to lateral direction using the "moving shot technique" where the operator moves the applicator back and forth in the nodule to cause coagulation necrosis of the tissue.[12,19,64,67] The heat from the electrode tip causes tissue necrosis and fibrosis by introducing a high-frequency alternating current, which raises tissue temperatures from 60°C to 100°C. The operator looks for sonographic changes at the tip of the RFA probe to suggest likely successful coagulation of the nodule, such as hyperechoic signals, "micro-bubbling" as well as an increase in the generator impedance as the tissue stiffens.[64,67,68] The operator approaches the nodule "unit by unit," so every part of the nodule is reached systematically starting from the deepest part and going to the most superficial portion of the nodule.[64] Care is taken to avoid extending the probe beyond the posterior or lateral thyroid capsule to avoid injury to nearby structures, particularly within the "danger triangle" where the recurrent laryngeal nerve is tethered to the trachea close to the posterior-medial aspect of the thyroid.[64] Immediate shrinkage of the nodule as well as continued progressive shrinkage over a period of months to a year is appreciated. In benign nodules, the volume of the nodule is thought to decrease between 50% and 90% for most patients which can be both operator and tumor dependent.[67,69-73]

The optimal energy settings are described by Baek et al., where usually 30 W of power is initiated, and then adjusted in increments of 5 W depending on whether a hyperechoic zone appears in the nodule adjacent to the electrode tip.[67] If the patient experiences pain during the procedure, the power can be lowered to 20 to 25 W or managed with further lidocaine injection.[67] Pain during the procedure can be suggestive of thermal propagation outside of the thyroid gland and should be addressed immediately.[64]

Advanced techniques such as artery-first ablation and marginal venous ablation have been introduced for hypervascular tumors to avoid recurrent growth at the margins of the nodule.[64] When a target nodule is in close proximity to a blood vessel (>3 mm in diameter), the flowing blood has a cooling effect, thereby reducing the ability to achieve a volume reduction in that area known as the *heat sink effect*.[64] One approach for mitigating this effect, in addition to limiting hemorrhage during the procedure is to use the "artery first" ablation technique by ablating the main feeding artery into the nodule. Pretreatment, doppler ultrasound is used to identify the nodule's main arterial supply and can be used to confirm successful ablation of the feeding artery post-technique as well. Visual feedback that can be noted by the operator include intranodular linear echogenicities that spread to the periphery of the target nodule and/or wedge-shaped hypoechoic changes which represent infarction in the area supplied by the feeding artery of interest.[64]

The marginal venous ablation technique is a second technique that is useful for ablating the more anterior draining veins which are found along the margin of thyroid nodules. Employing this technique addresses the *heat sink effect* as well as the potential for recurrence along the margin of the thyroid capsule which tends to be more common after ablation of hyperfunctioning thyroid nodules.[64,74] To address this issue, the marginal vein is identified on ultrasound, and using the electrode tip, the vein is punctured. Once the vein is ablated, air bubbles are noted to fill the marginal vein of the nodule, and rapidly flow along the marginal vein until the venous flow gradually decreases. Once the air bubbles remain stagnant inside the vein, complete ablation is accomplished.[64]

POSTPROCEDURAL EVALUATION

Generally, a postprocedural checklist to determine the treatment efficacy consists of bloodwork (TSH for all patients and autoantibodies in select patients) and ultrasound. Efficacy is measured by the volume reduction rate (VRR) on ultrasound as well as the changes in the symptom and cosmetic scores for benign nodules.[20-22] The VRR is equal to: (Initial volume − Final volume × 100/Initial volume). More than a 50% VRR is considered successful, whereas a VRR less than 50% typically requires additional treatment.[20-22] For AFTN, a therapeutic response is measured by the change in the pre- and post-RFA thyroid function tests and reduced uptake of the treated nodule in a thyroid scan. For malignant thyroid nodules, the VRR is a key marker for determining therapeutic success of ablation.

COMPLICATIONS

Although multiple studies have shown that RFA has an excellent safety profile, there are some minor associated complications worth mentioning. In a meta-analysis of 12 studies including RFA-treated benign nodules with follow-up for more than 3 years, Cho et al. found an overall complication rate of 4.6% and a major complication rate of 1.3% in the RFA group.[73] Complications tend to be higher when treating recurrent malignant nodules (10.98%) compared with benign nodules (2.11%) as demonstrated in a systematic review that looked at 2786 nodules (24 studies including both benign and recurrent thyroid cancers).[72]

One of the most common minor complications include pain with an incidence that ranges from 2.6% to 17.5% in a systematic review that included 32 studies with 3409 patients.[75] Chung et al. found transient voice change as one of the common minor complication noted after RFA, with an overall incidence of voice change (transient or permanent) 1.44% (35/2421) demonstrated in their systematic review.[72] The incidence of voice change was 0.94%, 21/2245 for benign nodules compared with 7.95%, 14/176 for recurrent cancer.[72] Benign thyroid nodules have a lower rate of voice change compared with recurrent thyroid cancers likely due to preservation of the thyroid capsule which can be protective against recurrent laryngeal nerve injury and parenchymal involvement and also the intended goal of volume reduction instead of complete ablation for cancer. Other transient minor complications include hematoma, vomiting, skin burn, and transient thyroiditis.[72]

Major complications such as permanent recurrent laryngeal nerve injury, nodule rupture, hematoma requiring surgical drainage, Horner syndrome or injury to the adjacent esophagus, or trachea are rare.[72]

RFA has fewer complications than surgery, particularly for benign thyroid nodules, making nonsurgical treatment a sound option for patients wishing to undergo treatment. One of the important complications that RFA avoids post-treatment compared with surgery is hypothyroidism. Surgery has up to a 30% risk of hypothyroidism post-thyroid lobectomy with some reports demonstrating up to 49%.[76] Total thyroidectomy requires a lifetime of thyroid hormone replacement therapy. The literature demonstrated that RFA has minimal effect on thyroid function mainly because the thyroid nodule is targeted leaving the surrounding normal parenchyma intact.[28]

REFERENCES

1. Haugen BR, Alexander EK, Bible KC, et al. 20215 American Thyroid Association Guidelines for adult patients with thyroid nodules and differentiated thyroid cancer. *Thyroid.* 2016;26(1):1-133.
2. Hegedus L. Clinical practice. The thyroid nodule. *N Engl J Med.* 2004;351:1764-1771.
3. Mandel SJ. A 64-year-old woman with a thyroid nodule. *JAMA.* 2004;292:2632-2642.
4. Ross DS, Burch HB, Cooper DS, et al. 2016 American Thyroid Association Guidelines for diagnosis and management of hyperthyroidism and other causes of thyrotoxicosis. *Thyroid* 2016;26(10):1343-1421.
5. Kilfoy BA, Zheng T, Holford TR, et al. International patterns and trends in thyroid cancer incidence, 1973–2002. *Cancer Causes Control.* 2009;20(5):525-531.
6. Seib CD, Sosa JA. Evolving understanding of the epidemiology of thyroid cancer. *Endocrinol Metab Clinc N Am.* 2019;48:23-35.
7. Surveillance Research Program NCI. Fast stats: an interactive tool for access to SEER cancer statistics. Available at: https://seer.cancer.gov/faststats. Accessed August 21, 2018.
8. Agrawal N, Evasovich MR, Kandil E, et al. Indications and extent of central neck dissection for papillary thyroid cancer: an American Head and Neck Society Consensus Statement. *Head & Neck.* 2017;39:1269-1279.
9. Stack BC, Ferris RL, Goldenberg D, et al. American Thyroid Association consensus review and statement regarding the anatomy, terminology, and rationale for lateral neck dissection in differentiated thyroid cancer. *Thyroid.* 2012;22(5):501-508.
10. Schuff KG. Management of recurrent/persistent papillary thyroid carcinoma: efficacy of the surgical option. *J Clin Endocrinol Metab.* 2011;96(7):2038-2039.
11. Papini E, Gugliemi R, Pacella CM. Laser, radiofrequency, and ethanol ablation for the management of thyroid nodules. *Curr Opin Endocrinol Diabetes Obes.* 2016;23(5):400-406.
12. Mauri G, Pacella CM, Papini E, et al. Image-guided thyroid ablation: proposal for standardization of terminology and reporting criteria. *Thyroid.* 2019;29(5):611-618.
13. Hegedus L, Frasoldati A, Negro R, Papini E. European Thyroid Association Survey on use of minimally invasive techniques for thyroid nodules. *Eur Thyr J.* 2020;9:194-204.
14. Hall WH, McGahan JP, Link DP, deVere White RW. Combined embolization and percutaneous radiofrequency ablation of a solid renal tumor. *Am J Roentgenol.* 2000;174:3.
15. Steinke K. Radiofrequency ablation of pulmonary tumours: current status. *Cancer Imaging.* 2008;8:27-35.
16. McGahan JP, Browning PD, Brock JM, Tesluk H. Hepatic ablation using radiofrequency electrocautery. *Invest Radiol.* 1990;25(3):267-270.
17. Rosenthal DJ, Hornicek FJ, Wolfe MW, Jennings LC, Gebhardt MC, Mankin HJ. Percutaneous radiofrequency coagulation of osteoid osteoma compared with operative treatment. *J Bone Joint Surg.* 1998;80(6):815-821.
18. Sousa J, el-Atassi R, Rosenheck S, Calkins H, Langberg J, Morady F. Radiofrequency catheter ablation of the atrioventricular junction from the left ventricle. *Circulation.* 1991;84(2):567-571.
19. Ha EJ, Baek JH, Lee JH. Moving-shot versus fixed electrode techniques for radiofrequency ablation: comparison in an ex-vivo bovine liver tissue model. *Korean J Radiol.* 2014;15:836-843.
20. Kim JH, Baek JH, Lim HK, et al. 2017 Thyroid radiofrequency ablation guideline: Korean Society of Thyroid Radiology. *Korean J Radiol.* 2018;19:632-655.
21. Papini E, Pacella CM, Solbiati LA, et al. Minimally-invasive treatments for benign thyroid nodules: a Delphi-based consensus statement from the Italian minimally invasive treatments of the thyroid (MITT) group. *Int J Hyperthermia.* 2019;36: 376-382.
22. Garberoglio R, Aliberti C, Appetecchia M, et al. Radiofrequency ablation for thyroid nodules: which indications? The first Italian opinion statement. *J Ultrasound.* 2015;18:423-430.
23. Dobnig H, Zechmann W, Hermann M, et al. Radiofrequency ablation of thyroid nodules: "Good Clinical Practice Recommendations" for Austria: an interdisciplinary statement from the following professional associations: Austrian Thyroid Association (OSDG), Austrian Society for Nuclear Medicine and Molecular Imaging (OGNMB), Austrian Society for Endocrinology and Metabolism (OGES), Surgical Endocrinology Working Group (ACE) of the Austrian Surgical Society (OEGCH). *Wien Med Wochenschr.* 2020;170:6-14.
24. National Institute for Health and Care Excellence. Ultrasound guided percutaneous radiofrequency ablation for benign thyroid nodules [Internet]. London: National Institute for Health and Care Excellence, 2016 [cited 2020 Jul 24]. Available from: https://www.nice.org.uk/guidance/ipg562.

25. Papini E, Monpeyssen H, Frasoldati A, Hegedus L. European Thyroid Association Clinical Guideline for the use of image-guided ablation in benign thyroid nodules. *Eur Thyroid J*. 2020;9:172-185.
26. Orloff L, Noel JE, Stack BC Jr, et al. Radiofrequency ablation and related ultrasound-guided ablation technologies for treatment of benign and malignant thyroid disease: an international multidisciplinary consensus statement of the American Head and Neck Society Endocrine Surgery Section with the Asia Pacific Society of Thyroid Surgery, Associazione Medici Endocrinologi, British Association of Endocrine and Thyroid Surgeons, European Thyroid Association, Italian Society of Endocrine Surgery Units, Korean Society of Thyroid Radiology, Latin American Thyroid Society, and Thyroid Nodules Therapies Association. *Head and Neck*. 2021;1-28.
27. Lee MK, Baek JH, Suh CH, et al. Clinical practice guidelines for radiofrequency ablation of benign thyroid nodules: a systematic review. *Ultrasonography*. 2021;40:256-264.
28. Deandrea M, Sung JY, Limone P, et al. Efficacy and safety of radiofrequency ablation versus observation of nonfunctioning benign thyroid nodules: randomized controlled international collaborative trial. *Thyroid*. 2015;25(8):890-896.
29. Bernardi S, Palmero A, Grasso RF, Fabris B, Stacul F. Current status and challenges of US-guided radiofrequency ablation of thyroid nodules in the long term: systematic review. *Cancers*. 2021;13:2746.
30. Cesareo R, Palermo A, Benvenuto D, et al. Efficacy of radiofrequency ablation in autonomous functioning thyroid nodules. a systematic review and meta-analysis. *Rev Endocr Metab Disord*. 2019;20(1):37-44.
31. Ha EJ, Baek JH, Che Y, et al. Radiofrequency ablation of benign thyroid nodules: recommendations from the Asian Conference on Tumor Ablation Task Force. *Ultrasonography*. 2021;40:75-82.
32. Cesareo R, Naciu AM, Iozzino M, et al. Nodule size as predictive factor of efficacy of radiofrequency ablation in treating autonomously functioning thyroid nodules. *Int J Hyperthermia*. 2018;34:617-623.
33. Mader A, Mader OM, Groner D, et al. Minimally invasive local ablative therapies in combination with radioiodine therapy in benign thyroid disease: preparation, feasibility and efficiency—preliminary results. *Int J Hyperthermia*. 2017;33(8):895-904.
34. Kim HJ, Cho SJ, Baek JH, Suh CH. Efficacy and safety of thermal ablation for autonomously functioning thyroid nodules: a systematic review and meta-analysis. *Eur Radiol*. 2021;31(2):605-615.
35. Zhang M, Tufano RP, Russell JO, et al. Ultrasound-guided radiofrequency ablation versus surgery for low-risk papillary thyroid microcarcinoma: results of over 5 years' follow-up. *Thyroid*. 2020;30(3):408-417.
36. Kim JH, Baek JH, Sung JY, et al. Radiofrequency ablation of low-risk small papillary thyroid carcinoma: preliminary results for patients ineligible for surgery. *Int J Hyperthermia*. 2017;33:212-219.
37. Choi Y, Jung SL. Efficacy and safety of thermal ablation techniques for the treatment of primary papillary thyroid microcarcinoma: a systematic review and meta-analysis. *Thyroid*. 2020;5:720-731.
38. Kim JH, Yoo WS, Park YJ, et al. Efficacy and safety of radiofrequency ablation for treatment of locally recurrent thyroid cancers smaller than 2 cm. *Radiology*. 2015;276:909-918.
39. Ding M, Tang X, Cui D, et al. Clinical outcomes of ultrasound-guided radiofrequency ablation for the treatment of primary papillary thyroid microcarcinoma. *Clinical Radiology*. 2019;74:712-717.
40. Zhang M, Luo Y, Zhang Y, Tang J. Efficacy and safety of ultrasound-guided radiofrequency ablation for treating low-risk papillary thyroid microcarcinoma: a prospective study. *Thyroid*. 2016;26(11):1581-1587.
41. Papini E, Guglielmi R, Hosseim G, et al. Ultrasound-guided laser ablation of incidental papillary thyroid microcarcinoma: a potential therapeutic approach in patients at surgical risk. *Thyroid*. 2011;21(8):917-920.
42. Jeong SY, Baek JH, Choi YJ, et al. Radiofrequency ablation of primary thyroid carcinoma: efficacy according to the types of thyroid carcinoma. *Int J Hyperthermia*. 2018;34:611-616.
43. Teng D, Sui G, Liu C, et al. Long-term efficacy of ultrasound-guided low power microwave ablation for the treatment of primary papillary thyroid microcarcinoma: a 3 year follow up study. *J Cancer Res Clin Oncol*. 2018;144(4):771-779.
44. Yue W, Wang S, Yu S, Wang B. Ultrasound-guided percutaneous microwave ablation of solitary T1N0M0 papillary thyroid microcarcinoma: initial experience. *Int J Hyperthermia*. 2014;30:150-157.
45. Zhang L, Zhou W, Zhan W, Peng Y, Jiang S, Xu S. Percutaneous laser ablation of unifocal papillary thyroid microcarcinoma: utility of conventional ultrasound and contrast-enhanced ultrasound in assessing local therapeutic response. *World J Surg*. 2018;42:2476-2484.
46. Xiao J, Zhang Y, Zhang M, et al. Ultrasonography-guided radiofrequency ablation vs. surgery for the treatment of solitary T1bN0M0 papillary thyroid carcinoma: a comparative study. *Clinical Endocrinology*. 2020;00:1-8.
47. Yan L, Lan Y, Xiao J, Lin L, Jiang B, Luo Y. Long-term outcomes of radiofrequency ablation for unifocal low-risk papillary thyroid microcarcinoma: a large cohort study of 414 patients. *Eur Radiol*. 2021, 31:685-694.
48. Tuttle RM, Haugen B, Perrier ND. Updated American Joint Committee on Cancer/Tumor-Node-Metastasis Staging System for Differentiated and Anaplastic Thyroid Cancer (Eighth Edition): what changed and why? *Thyroid*. 2017;27(6):751-756.
49. Mauri G, Hegedus L, Bandula S, et al. European Thyroid Association and Cardiovascular and Interventional Radiological Society of Europe 2021 Clinical Practice Guideline for the Use of Minimally Invasive Treatments in Malignant Thyroid Lesions. *Eur Thyroid J*. 2021;10:185-197.
50. Ha SM, Sung JY, Baek JH, et al. Radiofrequency ablation of small follicular neoplasms: initial clinical outcomes. *Int J Hyperthermia*. 2017;33(8):931-937.
51. Biamonte E, Solbiati L, Ierace T, et al. Medullary thyroid carcinoma treated with percutaneous ultrasound-guided radiofrequency ablation. *Endocrine*. 2019;65(3):515-519.
52. Tong MY, Li HS, Che Y. Recurrent medullary thyroid carcinoma treated with percutaneous ultrasound-guided radiofrequency ablation: a case report. *World J Clin Cases*. 2021;9(4):864-870.
53. Baek JH, Kim YS, Sung JY, Choi H, Lee JH. Locoregional control of metastatic well-differentiated thyroid cancer by ultrasound-guided radiofrequency ablation. *AJR Am J Roentgenol*. 2011;197:W331-W336.
54. Lim HK, Baek JH, Lee JH, et al. Efficacy and safety of radiofrequency ablation for treating locoregional recurrence from papillary thyroid cancer. *Eur Radiol*. 2015;25:163-170.
55. Choi Y, Jung SL, Bae JS, et al. Comparison of efficacy and complications between radiofrequency ablation and repeat surgery in the treatment of locally recurrent thyroid cancers: a

single-center propensity score matching study. *Int J Hyperthermia*. 2019;36(1):359-367.
56. Zhao Q, Tian G, Kong D, Jiang T. Meta-analysis of radiofrequency ablation for treating the local recurrence of thyroid cancers. *J Endocrinol Invest*. 2016;39:909-916.
57. Suh CH, Baek JH, Choi YJ, Lee JH. Efficacy and safety of radiofrequency and ethanol ablation for treating locally recurrent thyroid cancer: a systematic review and meta-analysis. *Thyroid*. 2016;26:420-428.
58. Park KW, Shin JH, Han BK, Ko EY, Chung JH. Inoperable symptomatic recurrent thyroid cancers: preliminary result of radiofrequency ablation. *Ann Surg Oncol*. 2011;18(9):2564-2568.
59. Chung SR, Baek JH, Choi YJ, et al. Efficacy of radiofrequency ablation for recurrent thyroid cancer invading the airways. *Eur Radiol*. 2021;31(4):2153-2160.
60. Cazzato RL, Bonichon F, Buy X, et al. Over ten years of single-institution experience in percutaneous image-guided treatment of bone metastases from differentiated thyroid cancer. *Eur J Surg Oncol*. 2015;41(9):1247-1255.
61. Bonichon F, Buy X, Godbert Y, et al. Local treatment of metastases from differentiated thyroid cancer. *Ann Endocrinol*. 2015;76(1 Suppl 1):1S40-1S46.
62. Baek JH, Lee JH, Sung JY, et al. Complications encountered in the treatment of benign thyroid nodules with US-guided radiofrequency ablation: a multicenter study. *Radiology*. 2012;262:335-342.
63. Tessler FN, Middleton WD, Grant EG, et al. ACR Thyroid Imaging, Reporting and Data System (TI-RADS): White Paper of the ACR TI-RADS Committee. *J Am Coll Radiol*. 2017;14: 587-595.
64. Park HS, Baek JH, Park AW, Chung SR, Choi YJ, Lee JH. Thyroid radiofrequency ablation: updates on innovative devices and techniques. *Korean J Radiol*. 2017;18(4):615-623.
65. Baek JH, Kim YS, Lee D, Huh JY, Lee JH. Benign predominantly solid thyroid nodules: prospective study of efficacy of sonographically guided radiofrequency ablation versus control condition. *AJR Am J Roentgenol*. 2010;194:1137-1142.
66. Chung SR, Baek JH, Choi YJ, Lee JH. Management strategy for nerve damage during radiofrequency ablation of thyroid nodules. *Int J Hyperthermia*. 2019;36:204-210.
67. Jeong WK, Baek JH, Rhim H, et al. Radiofrequency ablation of benign thyroid nodules: safety and imaging follow-up in 236 patients. *Eur Radiol*. 2008;18(6):1244-1250.
68. Deandra M, Garino F, Alberto M, et al. Radiofrequency ablation for benign thyroid nodules according to different ultrasound features: an Italian multicenter prospective. *Eur J Endocrinol*. 2019;180:79-87.
69. Bernardi S, Giudici F, Cesareo R, et al. Five-year results of radiofrequency and laser ablation of benign thyroid nodules: a multicenter study from the Italian minimally invasive treatments of the thyroid group. *Thyroid*. 2020;30(12):1759-1770.
70. Jung SL, Baek JH, Lee JH, et al. Efficacy and safety of radiofrequency ablation for benign thyroid nodules: a prospective multicenter study. *Korean J Radiol*. 2018;19(1):167-174.
71. Trimboli P, Castellana M, Sconfienza LM, et al. Efficacy of thermal ablation in benign non-functioning solid thyroid nodule: a systematic review and meta-analysis. *Endocrine*. 2020;67:35-43.
72. Chung SR, Suh CH, Baek JH, et al. Safety of radiofrequency ablation of benign thyroid nodules and recurrent thyroid cancers: a systematic review and meta-analysis. *Int J Hyperthermia*. 2017;33:920-930.
73. Cho SJ, Baek JH, Chung SR, Young JC, Lee JH. Long term results of thermal ablation of benign thyroid nodules: a systematic review and meta-analysis. *Endocrinology and Metabolism*. 2020;35:339-350.
74. Baek JH, Moon WJ, Kim YS, Lee JH, Lee D. Radiofrequency ablation for the treatment of autonomously functioning thyroid nodules. *World J Surg*. 2009;33:1971-1977.
75. Wang JF, Wu T, Hu KP, et al. Complications following radiofrequency ablation of benign thyroid nodules: a systematic review. *Chin Med J (Engl)*. 2017;130(11):1361-1370.
76. Stoll SJ, Pitt SC, Liu J, Schaefer S, Sippel RS, Chen H. Thyroid hormone replacement after thyroid lobectomy. *Surgery*. 2009;146(4): 554-558. discussion 558-560.

28 TKI in Treatment of Thyroid Cancer

Loredana Lorusso, MD, PhD
Virginia Cappagli, MD, PhD
Rossella Elisei, MD

INTRODUCTION

Thyroid cancer (TC) corresponds approximately to 2.9% of all new cancer cases in the United States each year,[1] and it remains the most common endocrine neoplasia. Although in the last three decades, an increased detection rate of both tumors less than 1 cm and larger tumors were identified, TC-related death remains uncommon and mainly due to metastases that occur outside the neck.[2,3]

Advanced Differentiated/Poorly Differentiated Thyroid Cancer

Differentiated TC (DTC) derives from follicular cells and the three main subtypes are papillary (PTC), follicular (FTC), and Hürthle cell carcinoma (HTC). DTC is the most frequent tumor type and represents more than 90% of all TC.[4] Poorly differentiated TC (PDTC) is a heterogeneous TC group including those TCs that, after they lose the typical papillary nuclear features, have a solid, insular, or trabecular growth pattern with an increased number of mitoses and necrosis (according to the Turin classification).[5]

Total or near-total thyroidectomy is the gold standard for DTC and PDTC, and, if cervical lymphadenopathies are identified before surgery, their surgical removal simultaneously with the thyroid is recommended. After the initial surgical treatment, radioiodine (^{131}I) therapy and thyroid-stimulating hormone (TSH) suppressive therapy with levothyroxine should be offered to those patients defined at intermediate or high risk of recurrent disease or with known distant metastases.[6]

The overall survival (OS) rate of DTC is about 98.3% at 5 years, but local recurrence in the neck (both thyroid bed or lymph nodes) occurs in about 20% of patients, while distant metastases in less than 10% of cases (lungs in 50% followed by bone in 25%).[4] In this last group, half of metastases are present at diagnosis, while in many other patients they are diagnosed after a median follow-up of 3 to 4 years.[7] When metastatic lesions lose the ability to take up ^{131}I (RAI-refractory DTC) (in up to one-third of advanced DTC), the OS rate drops to less than 10% at 10 years.[7]

A higher risk of persistence/recurrence both in the neck and at distant localization (lung, liver, bone, and brain) and a higher mortality were reported for PDTC with respect to other DTCs.[8]

Anaplastic Thyroid Cancer

The most aggressive TC is anaplastic thyroid carcinoma (ATC), representing about 1% of all TC. Since it is unable to take up ^{131}I with no chance of cure, it accounts for the majority of all TC mortality,[9,10] mainly due to a rapid disease progression, particularly at the local level. In fact, up to 40% of patients have locoregional secondary lesions and/or vocal cord palsy at diagnosis, and up to 70% present a local tissue invasion, including the trachea, larynx, esophagus, and neck muscles. When an initial aggressive local treatment is performed, distant metastases (lungs [50%–80%], bone, skin, and brain [6%–12%]) may appear. Median survival time in these patients is approximately 5 to 6 months, and they rarely survive more than 2 years after diagnosis.[11,12] Only stage IV is assigned to cases of ATC by TNM classification of the American Joint Committee on Cancer, due to the fatal outcome associated nearly universally with ATC, and this underlines the importance of aggressive treatment, including systemic treatment, as soon as possible.

After the initial assessment of airways' stability to identify the urgent need for an immediate intervention, surgery should be the first choice of treatment if a full resection of tumor is possible, and usually when no distant metastases are present.[13] After a total or near-total surgical resection of the primary tumor, standard fractionation radiation therapy, no later than 6 weeks after surgery, with concurrent systemic therapy, should be offered to those patients with both a good performance status and no evidence of metastatic disease.[13]

It has recently become evident (and reported in the most recent guidelines) that once a diagnosis of ATC is confirmed, immunohistochemical and/or molecular assessment for a BRAFV600E mutation should be expeditiously performed, since the molecular profiling of ATC is an important determinant in deciding whether the use of targeted therapies is appropriate, especially after the approval of mutation-specific target therapies by the FDA.[13]

Advanced Medullary Thyroid Cancer

Medullary thyroid carcinoma (MTC) derives from neuroendocrine C cells and represents 5% to 8% of all TC.[14] It has a more aggressive behavior compared to DTC. The most important predicting factor for disease cure is the extent of the disease at diagnosis. In fact, the ability to achieve complete remission of MTC is only 20% in patients with lymph node metastases.[14] Also, distant metastases can be observed at presentation in 7% to 23% of MTC patients, and they represent the main cause of death in MTC patients, with a 10-year survival rate of approximately 10%. The management of advanced MTC can be based both on local (ie, surgery, external-beam radiotherapy, chemoembolization, radionuclide treatments) and on systemic treatments (ie, cytotoxic chemotherapy, TKIs) according to the disease burden and the presence of life-threatening metastases.[15]

RATIONALE TO USE TKI TREATMENTS IN TC

Over the past couple of decades, the Cancer Genome Atlas (TCGA) and several other studies examining the molecular pathogenesis of TC identified mutations affecting the mitogen-activated protein kinase (MAPK) and the phosphatidylinositol-3 kinase (PI3K) pathways as key drivers of TC.[16] These signaling pathways become constitutively activated when a mutation, derived both from somatic or germline genetic alteration, at any level of these pathways, occurs, leading to an unregulated cell replication, loss of cell differentiation, and reduction of cell apoptosis. As shown in Figure 28–1, both transmembrane receptors or a central mediator of the above-mentioned pathways may be involved in tumorigenesis and, particularly in TC the most common genetic alterations are mutations in central mediators such as BRAF, RAS, PTEN, AKT, and PI3KCA.[16,17] NTRK fusions, usually mutually exclusive with other oncogenic driver mutations (see related Molecular Testing in Thyroid Nodules and Thyroid Cancer chapter), are more rare, but detected in several solid tumors including PTC, PDTC, and ATC.

The increasing knowledge of the mechanisms underlying TC tumorigenesis and the importance of tyrosine kinase receptors (TKR) and tyrosine kinases (TK) in general led to the development of tyrosine kinase inhibitor drugs that are specific small oral molecules able to inhibit TK and TKR. The term multikinase inhibitors (MKI) identified a first generation of these drugs that inhibited not only specific oncogene alterations, but also several other tyrosine kinase inhibitors (TKIs). The activity of a TKI on oncogene alterations results in a cytostatic effect on tumoral cells, causing the shrinkage of tumoral mass in very short time, but the activity of these MKI against other receptors may be in some cases very strong, and this "off-target" activity led to the appearance of side effects/adverse events (AEs).

Because of the occurrence of several and severe AEs with first-generation TKIs, recently, a second generation of drugs has been developed. These new TKIs have a higher specificity only for an altered oncogene and fewer "off-target"

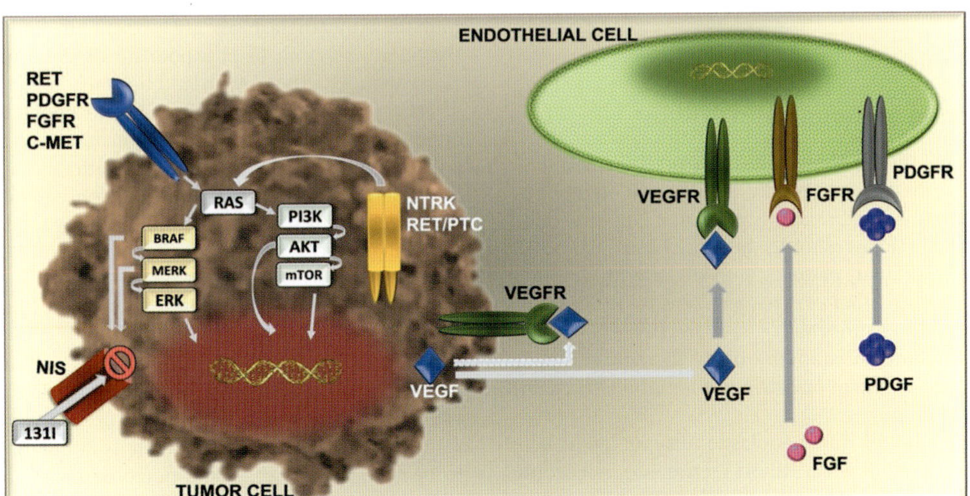

Figure 28–1. Mitogen-activated protein kinase (MAPK) and the phosphatidylinositol-3 kinase (PI3K) pathways signaling.

activities. A greater tolerability and a much smaller number of AEs were witnessed with the second generation of TKIs.

MECHANISM OF ACTION OF TYROSINE KINASE INHIBITORS

Most TKIs compete with adenosine triphosphate (ATP), which consists of adenosine made by an adenine ring and a ribose sugar and three phosphate groups. When ATP binds to a kinase the formation of hydrogen bonds from the adenine ring to the ATP-binding cleft of the kinase takes place.

Kinase inhibitors can target the ATP-binding site of a kinase, through different mechanisms of action. Type I kinase inhibitors recognize the active conformation of a kinase by mimicking the hydrogen bonds normally formed by ATP.[18] On the contrary, type II kinase inhibitors are noncompetitive antagonists of ATP; they recognize the inactive conformation of a kinase, and occupy the hydrophobic pocket directly adjacent to the ATP-binding site, known as allosteric site, modulating kinase activity in an allosteric way.[19] Type III kinase inhibitors, also known as "covalent" inhibitors, covalently and irreversibly bind to cysteine residues at specific sites of the kinase, thanks to the interaction between sulfur, present in the cysteine residue, and an electrophilic group of the inhibitor. This allows the inhibitor to block binding of ATP to the kinase and prevents the kinase's activation.[20]

WHEN TO START TKI TREATMENT IN TC

The decision of when it is appropriate to initiate TKI therapy is still a critical and debated point and the state of the TC, the anticipated duration of therapy itself, possible AEs impairing the patient's quality of life, the performance status of the patient, the drug-resistance problem, and the cost of therapy must all be taken into consideration. These considerations are discussed in following sections.

Progression of Neoplastic Disease

According to the most recent guidelines on TC treatment, patients with a metastatic, rapidly progressive, symptomatic, and/or imminently threatening disease not controlled using other approaches should be considered for TKI therapy.[6,21] In particular, patients with disease progression in less than 6 months that is expected to require intervention and/or to produce morbidity or mortality (eg, pulmonary lesions or lymphadenopathy likely to rapidly invade airways, produce dyspnea, or cause bronchial obstruction) should be treated.

The progression of the neoplastic disease is usually established using radiological RECIST criteria.[22] According to these criteria, after the baseline assessment of diameters of target lesions (defined as any lesion >1 cm for visceral lesions, >1.5 cm short axis for nodal metastases, not considering more than two lesions per disease site/organ) with cross-sectional imaging (computed tomography and/or magnetic resonance imaging), subsequent measurements of the same lesions have to be assessed and compared during follow-up.

Progression of the disease can be defined as an increase in sum of longest diameters of target lesions of at least 20% and/or when a new lesion(s) is identified. Usually, rapid progression is defined when progression according to RECIST occurs within 12 to 14 months of the last restaging of the disease.

In some studies, the assessment of tumor progression by considering the tumor volume instead of the sum of the largest diameters of target lesions used for RECIST seems to have a better clinical utility. Since metastatic nodules have an ellipsoid shape, calculation of tumor volume by using all three dimensions and the doubling time of this volume has demonstrated to be more helpful to identify progression and the time to start systemic therapy.[23]

Diffuse disease progression is another major criterion to start TKI separate from focal progression (eg, in multiple lung metastases, as opposed to a few growing lesions) that may be controlled with local treatment. In fact, before starting systemic treatment with TKI, local treatment modalities, other than surgery, should be used, especially when metastatic lesions are symptomatic or at high risk of local complications as could happen for brain, liver, and bone metastases.

Unfortunately, TKIs appear to be less effective in controlling metastatic disease to bone compared to other metastatic sites (ie, lungs and lymph nodes), and for this reason, progression of bone metastases during TKI treatment commonly occurs despite benefits with respect to disease at other metastatic sites. For this reason, when diffuse and/or symptomatic bone metastases are present, in addition to local treatment, starting bisphosphonate or denosumab therapy, along with TKI therapy, should be considered.

The presence of symptoms due to neoplastic disease is another criterion that has to be considered in advanced TC patients. In fact, since TKIs are very effective antiangiogenic drugs, a rapid devascularization and consequent shrinkage of tumor lesions is expected, leading to a significant and positive impact on symptoms due to the pressure or infiltration of organs.

The doubling time of thyroglobulin and increasing titer trend of thyroglobulin antibodies in DTC, as well as calcitonin and CEA doubling time in MTC, are well-recognized predictors of progression of neoplastic disease and their values correlate to tumor burden.[24,25] Recently, another serum marker, Ca 19.9, along with its doubling time, seemed to be able to predict a fatal outcome in MTC patients.[26,27] Although the usefulness in clinical practice of the above-mentioned serum markers has been well established over the past couple of decades, at the moment no guidelines recommend their use to define disease progression and to decide to start systemic treatment.

Radioiodine Refractory DTC/PDTC

RAI therapy is the gold standard therapy for DTC/PDTC metastatic patients and this treatment should be given to all those patients with so-called RAI-avid metastatic lesions. On the contrary, when a patient with DTC/PDTC is classified as RAI refractory, there is no indication for further treatments.[6]

This condition, known as RAI refractoriness, is another condition that must be present before initiating TKI treatment in DTC patients. As reported in current TC guidelines,[6] in patients with appropriate TSH stimulation and iodine diet preparation, RAI refractoriness can be defined in four different situations (Figure 28–2): (1) the malignant/metastatic tissue does not concentrate RAI since the first therapeutic WBS (Panels A and B), (2) the tumor tissue loses the ability to concentrate RAI after previous evidence of RAI uptake (Panels C and D), (3) RAI is concentrated in some lesions but not in others (Panels E and F); and (4) metastatic disease progresses despite significant RAI uptake (Panels G and H).

According to several evidence, the mean cumulative activity of ^{131}I that is associated with cure of metastases in DTC patients is 22 GBq (600 mCi). In fact, according to some authors, RAI-refractoriness can also be defined when a total activity of 600 mCi is administered without achieving

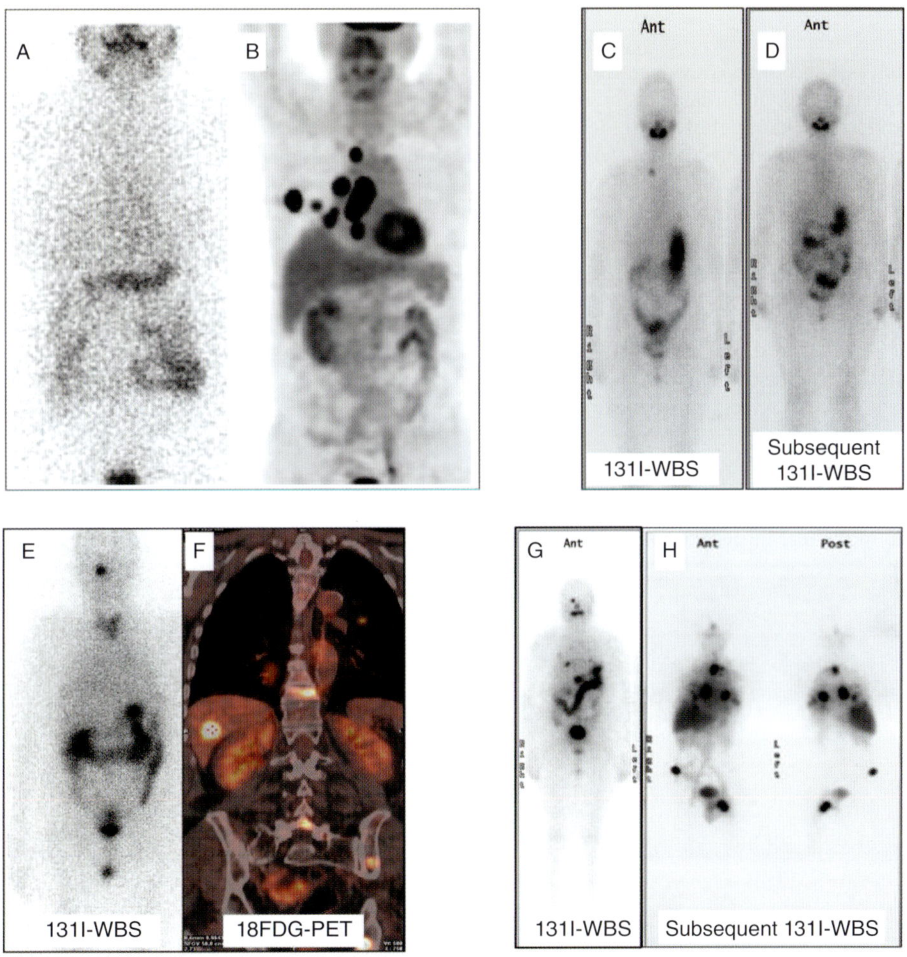

Figure 28–2. Example of radioiodine (RAI) refractoriness: (1) the malignant/metastatic tissue does not concentrate RAI since the first therapeutic WBS (**Panels A** and **B**), (2) the tumor tissue loses the ability to concentrate RAI after previous evidence of RAI uptake (**Panels C** and **D**), (3) RAI is concentrated in some lesions but not in others (**Panels E** and **F**); and (4) metastatic disease progresses despite significant RAI uptake (**Panels G** and **H**).

a disease cure, since these patients will likely never be cured by ^{131}I. On the contrary, other experts are convinced that the evidence of "stable disease" under ^{131}I repeated treatments (every 12-18 months) should not be considered as RAI refractoriness, and they should be continued to be treated with ^{131}I as long as there is evidence of clinical benefit, including stable disease.

Good Clinical Condition

A good performance status should always be present in patients who are being considered for TKI treatment. This is evaluated by the ECOG scale of performance status (ECOG-PS) which is the most utilized method to assess a patient's functional status, and patients are given a score from 0 to 5, representing a fully active patient to a dead patient, respectively.

In addition, as reported in current TC guidelines, some comorbidities, such as active or recently diagnosed intestinal conditions (eg, diverticulitis, inflammatory bowel disease, recent bowel resection), including those with bleeding, liver disease, or coagulopathy, as well as recent cardiovascular event(s), including prolonged QTc interval/history of significant arrhythmia, uncontrolled hypertension, and cachexia/low weight/poor nutrition are considered factors that should discourage the initiation of a TKI until the patient is medically stabilized prior to starting the therapy. Also, untreated brain metastases are considered a controversial contraindication to start of TKI due to the risk of bleeding. In these cases, a stabilization of the metastasis, usually with external radiotherapy, should be obtained before starting systemic treatment.

AVAILABLE SYSTEMIC THERAPIES FOR THE TREATMENT OF ADVANCED & MULTIMETASTATIC THYROID CANCER

Systemic Treatment in DTC & PDTC: Multikinase Inhibitor Approved Drugs

The only two MKI approved by both the Food and Drug Administration (FDA) and the European Medical Agency (EMA) as first-line treatment of advanced RAI-refractory DTC are lenvatinib and sorafenib.

Sorafenib is a small oral molecule with strong anti-angiogenic activity, inhibiting VEGF1-3, PDGF, FGF, KIT, RET receptors and, weakly, RAF (Table 28–1). Based on the results of two different phase 2 clinical trials[28,29] demonstrating the efficacy of sorafenib in DTC patients, a randomized, double-blinded, placebo-controlled phase 3 clinical trial (DECISION study)[30] was conducted, leading to the approval of this drug for advanced DTC treatment. In this study, 417 TKI naïve patients were enrolled (207 assigned to the drug arm receiving an initial dose of 400 mg/daily of sorafenib, and 209 assigned to placebo arm). A significantly longer progression-free survival (PFS) ($p < 0.0001$) was observed in sorafenib group (10.8 months) than in placebo group (5.8 months), with a response rate of 12.2% and 0.5%, respectively. On the contrary, no difference in OS was observed in the two groups, probably due to the permitted crossover phase from placebo to sorafenib when progression of the disease was established.

Lenvatinib is an oral drug, as is sorafenib, with strong anti-angiogenic activity, through the inhibition of VEGF1-3, FGF1-4, PDGF, KIT, and RET receptors (Table 28–1). After

Table 28–1. Main molecular targets of the approved multityrosine kinase inhibitors.

Molecular Target	Lenvatinib (Schlumberger et al.)	Sorafenib (Brose et al)	Vandetanib (Wells et al.)	Cabozantinib (Elisei et al.)
VEGFR-1	+	–	–	–
VEGFR-2	+	+	+	+
VEGFR-3	+	+	–	–
c-KIT	+	+	+	+
RET	+	+	+	+
PDGFR	+	+	–	–
FGFR	+	–	–	–
EGFR	–	–	+	–
Others	RET-KIF5B rearrangements	Raf, FLT3	RET-KIF5B rearrangements	MET, RET-KIF5B rearrangements

EGFR, epidermal growth factor receptor; FGFR, fibroblast growth factor receptor; FLT3, Fms-like tyrosine kinase 3; KIT, v-kit Hardy-Zuckerman 4 feline sarcoma viral oncogene; MET, hepatocyte growth factor receptor; PDGFR, platelet-derived growth factor receptor; Raf, v-raf murine sarcoma viral oncogene homolog; RET, RE arranged during Transfection receptor; TRK, tropomyosin receptor kinase; VEGFR, vascular endothelial growth factor receptor.

phase 2 studies,[31,32] establishing the efficacy of lenvatinib in both DTC and MTC, and a multicentric, randomized, placebo-controlled phase 3 study (SELECT study),[33] the drug was finally approved as treatment for advanced RAI-refractory DTC. In this trial, 392 patients were enrolled (261 randomized to the lenvatinib arm starting with 24 mg/day of drug, and 131 to the placebo arm). A significantly longer PFS ($p < 0.001$) was observed in the lenvatinib group (18.3 months) compared to placebo (3.6 months), with four complete responses (CR) in the drug group. Although again OS was not different between the two groups, a subsequent subanalysis stratifying patients by age showed an OS advantage in patients older than 65 years.

In Table 28–2, the main differences between the DECISION and SELECT studies are delineated.

Another oral molecule, cabozantinib, is also available for the treatment of RAI-refractory, metastatic and progressive DTC/PDTC, but only when standard of care, sorafenib or lenvatinib, fails in controlling neoplastic disease.[34]

Systemic Treatment in MTC: Multikinase Inhibitor Approved Drugs

At this point several TKIs have been studied for the treatment of MTC but only two have been approved by the FDA and EMA and are now available in clinical practice.

Vandetanib (Caprelsa®; Sanofi Genzyme, Cambridge, MA) was the first drug approved by both FDA (2011) and EMA (2013) for the treatment of MTC patients with symptomatic, unresectable, locally advanced or metastatic disease, thanks to the results of the ZETA trial.[35] In this multicenter phase III clinical trial, a longer PFS was observed in patients treated with vandetanib (30.5 months) compared to those on placebo (19.3 months) as well as a higher overall response rate (45% vs 13%).[35] The drug was also approved for the treatment of advanced hereditary MTC in children, thanks to the results obtained in a phase 2 clinical trial.[36] The drug is a multi-target drug able to inhibit VEGFR-2, VEGFR3, EGFR, KIT, and RET as shown in Table 28–1. Its approved recommended starting dose is 300 mg/day in healthy patients, while it is 200 mg/day in case of renal impairment. In case of toxicity during the treatment, the dose can be decreased to 200 mg/day and then to 100 mg/day, maintaining the same stable disease control as demonstrated in the phase IV trial comparing the safety and efficacy of two starting doses of 300 and 150 mg/day.[37] The starting dose could be increased or decreased respectively in case of concomitant use of strong CYP3A4 inducers or inhibitors.[38]

Subsequent to vandetanib, cabozantinib (Cometriq®; Exelixis, South San Francisco, CA) was approved first by the FDA in 2012 and then by EMA in 2014, based on the EXAM trial results. In this randomized, multicentric, phase III trial patients treated with cabozantinb showed a significantly longer median PFS compared to those treated with placebo (11.2 vs 4.0 months) as well as a significantly different overall response (28% vs 0%).[39] Cabozantinib is able to inhibit three main tyrosine kinase receptors: MET, VEGFR2, and RET as shown in Table 28–1. The recommended starting dose is 140 mg/daily or 80 mg/day in case of mild-to-moderate liver impairment. As for vandetanib, during treatment the dose can be reduced to 100 mg/day, 80 mg/day, and 60 mg/day but a phase IV trial was conducted to evaluate the efficacy of 140 mg/day versus 60 mg/day starting dose (NTC01896479) and preliminary data were presented to the last American Thyroid Association Congress.

The efficacy of these drugs cannot be directly compared since some differences exist in the study design of the two trials. In the EXAM trial, documented radiological progression of disease according to RECIST criteria was a mandatory inclusion criterion, while in the ZETA study tumor progression was not required and patients were enrolled by disease-related symptoms and calcitonin levels. This difference in eligibility criteria could explain the difference

Table 28–2. Main differences between sorafenib and lenvatinib based on phase III trials.

Drug	Dose of Drug	PFS (months; drug vs placebo)	PR (%)	CR (%)	SD (%)	Dose Reduced Due to Adverse Events (%)	Dose Interrupted Due to Adverse Events (%)	Most Frequent Adverse Event
Sorafenib	400 mg, twice daily	10.8 vs 5.8	12.2	0	42	77.8	18.8	Hand and foot skin reaction, diarrhea, alopecia, rash, desquamation
Lenvatinib	24 mg, once daily	18.3 vs 3.6	63.2	1.5	NR	78.5	14.2	Hypertension, diarrhea, decreased appetite, weight loss

CR, complete response; PFS, progression-free survival; PR, partial response; SD, stable disease.

in median PFS, since in the EXAM trial more aggressive disease was present.[35,39] Furthermore, in contrast to the ZETA trial, in the EXAM trial crossover to the drug was not allowed, leading to a more consistent evaluation of the drug effect on OS.[35,39]

Although the use of both drugs is recommended by the most important MTC clinical guidelines,[14,15] the choice of which TKI should be used first is still under debate and unclear. No guidelines are available, but several considerations taken from the trial's results could guide clinicians. The safety profile of each drug could facilitate the choice. Since vandetanib could lead to QT elongation, it should be avoided in patients with arrhythmias, heart failure, or unstable electrolyte disorders; instead cabozantinib is associated with a higher risk of intestinal perforation and hemorrhage and should be used carefully in patients with diverticulitis, chronic gastrointestinal disease, active peptic ulcer, or previous irradiation to the neck or mediastinum.[41]

The specific somatic RET gene mutation might also be useful since the subgroup of M918T-RET somatic mutated patients showed a significant increase in OS (median survival 44.3 months) compared to wild type and/or with other gene mutations (median survival 18.9 months).[42] Moreover, cabozantinib has also been demonstrated to be effective as a second-line therapy; in fact, differently from the ZETA trial where patients had to be TKI-naïve, in the EXAM trial patients previously treated with other TKIs were included, and no differences for PFS were observed between the subgroups of naïve and previously treated MTC patients.[39] Finally, the different pharmacokinetic profile and drug interactions could be useful in deciding which drug to recommend upfront. The main differences between the two drugs are summarized in Table 28–3.

Specific Inhibitors of NTRK-Fusions for the Treatment of DTC, PDTC, & ATC

As mentioned earlier, although rare, NTRK fusions can be found in several types of thyroid carcinomas, including PTC, PDTC, and ATC. To date, larotrectinib and entrectinib are the only available specific inhibitors of NTRK fusion-driven TC.

Larotrectinib is a tropomyosin receptor kinase (TRK) A, B, and C selective inhibitor and was approved by the FDA and EMA for the treatment of all solid cancers harboring NTRK fusions, in both adult and pediatric patients. A primary analysis[43] reported the results of two phase 1 trials and one phase 2 trial evaluating the efficacy of larotrectinib. A follow-up paper with 67 supplemental patients treated with the same drug was also published.[44] According to the follow-up paper, about 14% of TC patients showed a CR, while about 47% showed a partial response (PR) after larotrectinib treatment. Moreover, in patients with TRK fusion cancer, and in various tumor types treated with larotrectinib, an objective response rate (ORR) of 79% and a median duration of response of 35.2 months was observed.[44]

Additional data confirmed the efficacy and safety of larotrectinib in adult and pediatric patients with TRK fusion TC.[45] In the study, including 19 PTC, 7 ATC, and 2 FTC with TRK fusion (43% NTRK1 fusion and 57% NTRK3 fusion), the ORR was 75%, including 29% for patients with ATC, and the response duration was from 1.9 to 41.0 months. Median PFS was not reached and the 12-month PFS rate was 81%.

Entrectinib is a selective inhibitor of TRKA, TRKB, and TRKC, but it is also able to inhibit ALK and ROS1. An integrated analysis of three phase 1-2 trials of entrectinib in patients with advanced or metastatic NTRK fusion-positive

Table 28–3. Vandetanib and cabozantinib differences based on phase III trials.

	Vandetanib*	Cabozantinib†
Drug starting dose	300 mg/daily	140 mg/daily
Half-life	19 days	55 hours
Median PFS of drug vs placebo (*p*-value)	Not reached vs 19.3 months ($p < 0.001$)	11.2 vs 4 months ($p < 0.001$)
Objective response rate drug vs placebo (%)	45 vs 13 ($p < 0.001$)	28 vs 0 ($p < 0.001$)
Calcitonin biochemical response rate drug vs placebo (%)	69 vs 3 ($p < 0.001$)	−45.2 vs +57.35 ($p < 0.001$)
Dose reduction due to adverse events	35%	79%
Dose interruption due to adverse events	12%	16%
Most frequent adverse events	Diarrhea, rash, nausea, hypertension	Diarrhea, PPE, decrease appetite, weight loss, nausea, fatigue

*Wells SA Jr, Robinson BG, Gagel RF, et al. Vandetanib in patients with locally advanced or metastatic medullary thyroid cancer: a randomized, double-blind phase III trial. *J Clin Oncol*. 2012;30(2):134-141.

†Elisei R, Schlumberger MJ, Müller SP, et al. Cabozantinib in progressive medullary thyroid cancer. *J Clin Oncol*. 2013;31(29):3639-3646.

solid tumors[46] showed a 7% CR and 50% PR, with a manageable safety profile. Due to its capability to penetrate the blood-brain barrier, entrectinib also showed a very high ORR (50%) when patients with brain metastases were considered, regardless of prior brain radiotherapy.[47]

Larotrectinib has been approved by FDA and EMA as agnostic drug for all human tumors with NTRK fusion as first line and entrectinib was approved by EMA and FDA for the treatment of NTRK-mutant solid tumors and ROS-1 mutant non-small-cell lung cancer. According to the most recent guidelines on the management of ATC,[13] both larotrectinib and entrectinib should be considered for the treatment of NTRK fusion-positive ATC patients with stage IVC disease.

Specific Inhibitors of RET Oncogene for the Treatment of DTC, PDTC, ATC, & MTC Alterations

Selpercatinib (RETEVMO®, Eli Lilly and Company) belongs to a second generation of TKI and shows a high potency to inhibit both RET point mutations and RET fusions, including the V804M one, related to some TKI resistance.[48] In contrast to the previous TKI generation, its activity against other TKI receptors, such as VEGFRs, is very low with a consequent reduction in toxicity. This compound, known also as LOXO-292, with a half-life of 32 hours, was approved by the FDA on 8 May 2020[49] and by EMA on 10 December 2020[50] for the treatment of subgroups of advanced TC—particularly for the treatment of adult and pediatric patients, ≥12 years of age and older, with advanced or metastatic *RET*-mutant MTC or metastatic *RET* fusion-positive RAI-refractory TC who are candidates for systemic therapy.[51] The approved dose was 160 mg twice daily for patients with body weight ≥50 kg, and 120 mg twice daily for patients with a lower body weight.[51]

A phase 1/2 single-arm, multicenter, open-label, multicohort clinical trial (LIBRETTO-001 trial, NCT03157128), conducted in 65 centers in 12 countries, demonstrated the efficacy of selpercatinib in RET-mutated TC.[52] A total of 143 MTC patients were treated across different groups: 55 MTC-RET mutated patients were previously treated with vandetanib or cabozantinib or both, while another 88 patients were naïve. In both cohorts selpercatinib showed a considerable and durable antitumor activity: the ORR was 69% (95% CI, 55-81) in the first cohort, independently from the number of previous multitargeted treatments administered, and 73% (95% CI, 62-82) in the second one. Responses were observed for all RET mutations, including the drug-resistant mutation RET V804.[48] Also, 27 *RET* fusion-positive TC patients (13 PTC, 2 PDTC, 1 HTC, and 2 ATC) were included in the study.[52] In *RET* fusion-positive DTC/PDTC, the overall response rate was 79% in 19 patients previously treated with other TKIs, and 100% in 8 naïve patients.[52] Drug-related AEs led to selpercatinib discontinuation in only 2% of all patients.

An interventional phase 3 multicenter, randomized, open-label study comparing selpercatinib to physician's choice of cabozantinib or vandetanib in patients with progressive, advanced, kinase inhibitor naïve, RET-mutant MTC (LIBRETTO-531 trial, NCT04211337) has been completed and published.[53] In this study, patients were randomized into two different arms, with a 2:1 ratio. In particular, selpercatinib was administered to patients in arm A, while, based on physician decision, cabozantinib or vandetanib was available for arm B patients, with the possibility of crossover to selpercatinib when progression of the disease was identified. On the basis of the results of this study, selpercatinib has been approved as both second and first line for the treatment of advanced and progressive MTC.[54]

Another highly selective *RET* inhibitor targeting oncogenic RET alterations is pralsetinib, known also as BLU-667. After initial in vitro studies,[55] a phase 1/2 open-label multicenter trial (the ARROW study, NCT03037385) was conducted in 11 countries in *RET*-mutated TC and other solid-tumor patients. Positive results were observed and published in 2021[56]: In the 142 *RET* mutation-positive MTC patients an overall response rate of 65% (51 of 79) was observed, in particular 71% in treatment-naïve patients and 60% in those previously treated with cabozantinib or vandetanib. Median duration of response and median progression-free survival was not reached, but the estimated probability of ongoing response at 12 months was 84% in naïve group (95% CI 63-100) and 92% (95% CI 82-100) in the previously treated group, with an estimated 1-year progression-free survival rate of 81% (95% CI 63-98) and 75% (95% CI 63-86), respectively. Responses occurred regardless of *RET* genotypes. Pralsetinib was also highly effective in patients with *RET* fusion TCs showing an ORR of 75% with a median duration of response of 14.5 months. Based on these results, pralsetinib (Gavreto®, Roche) was approved by the FDA in 2020.[55] The recommended dose is 400 mg orally once daily. As with selpercatinib, the drug was well tolerated and only 4% of all patients definitively discontinued the treatment due to AEs.

Specific Inhibitors of BRAFV600E Mutation for the Treatment of DTC, PDTC, & ATC

The T1799A nucleotide transversion in the *BRAF* gene is a prominent oncogenic mutation in PTC, occurring on average in 45% of cases,[57] and causing a valine-to-glutamic acid change in codon 600 of the BRAF protein, (BRAFV600E). *BRAFV600E* has elevated serine/threonine protein kinase activities and constitutively activates the mitogen-activated protein kinase signaling pathway in human cancer, leading to more aggressive clinicopathological characteristics of PTC, including lymph node metastases, extrathyroidal invasion, loss of radioiodine avidity, and, hence, failure of radioiodine treatment and disease recurrence.[58,59] Similar to PTC, somatic alterations of *BRAF* are found in 40% to 70%, depending on series of ATC.[60,61]

To date, dabrafenib in combination with trametinib, an inhibitor of MEK1-2 kinase, is the only drug approved by the FDA for the treatment of ATC, melanoma, and NSCLC, harboring the *BRAFV600E* mutation. The results of a phase 2 study published in 2018[62] led to the approval of these two drugs for ATC treatment. In this study, 16 patients with *BRAFV600E*-mutated ATC were evaluable, after they had received prior radiation treatment and/or surgery, and six had received prior systemic therapy. The ORR was 69% with seven ongoing responses at the end of the study. The median PFS was 60 weeks, and the median OS was 86 weeks.[63]

Dabrafenib alone and dabrafenib in combination with trametinib were also evaluated in *BRAFV600E*-mutated RAI-refractory PTC with evidence of disease progression within 13 months prior to randomization.[64] PR occurred in 38% of patients treated with dabrafenib alone ($N = 26$) and in 33% of patients treated with dabrafenib and trametinib ($N = 27$), while an ORR, defined as a 20% to 29% decrease in the sum of targeted lesions, was 50% and 54%, respectively.

Vemurafenib is another oncogenic BRAF kinase inhibitor actually approved for BRAF-positive melanoma with a clinical benefit in three patients with BRAFV600E-positive PTC in a phase 1 trial. The results of an open-label, nonrandomized, phase 2 multicentric trial confirmed the efficacy and safety of vemurafenib in patients with histologically confirmed recurrent or metastatic RAI-refractory PTC who were positive for the *BRAFV600E* mutation.[65] On the contrary, efficacy of vemurafenib in ATC was not well established since only seven ATC patients were evaluated in a phase 2 study.[66] To date, no phase 3 study has been designed for vemurafenib in TC.

Redifferentiation Treatment in DTC

As mentioned before, RAI remains the gold standard therapy for patients with metastatic TC of follicular origin, but, when metastases no longer concentrate RAI, the 10-year survival rate drops from 60% (RAI-avid metastases) to 10% (RAI-refractory disease). This was the reason why strategies to "re-differentiate" metastatic TCs and render them responsive to RAI have been assessed. Among them can be mentioned retinoids and lithium, but only a very modest clinical benefit was obtained from their use.[67,68]

On the contrary, for redifferentiation in DTC, MEK and BRAF inhibitors have shown some positive results. Selumetinib is a MEK1/2 inhibitor and it was demonstrated to enhance RAI uptake in DTC.[69] However, a recent phase 3 study,[70] evaluating the CR rate for selumetinib in the setting of adjuvant treatment with RAI, demonstrated that selumetinib combined with RAI did not improve CR rate in patients with high risk of primary treatment failure, and the possibility of using selumetinib in clinical practice is still under evaluation.

Vemurafenib is another oncogenic BRAF kinase inhibitor tested in a pilot study aimed at evaluating the proportion of patients in whom vemurafenib increased RAI incorporation.[71] Tumor regression was observed 6 months after the RAI treatment, and, interestingly, analysis of tumor biopsies demonstrated that vemurafenib inhibition of the MAPK pathway was associated with increased thyroid gene expression and RAI uptake.

Dabrafenib is another selective BRAF inhibitor tested to determine whether it is able to "re-differentiate" BRAFV600E mutated, unresectable, or metastatic RAI-refractory PTC.[72] Even though the group of patients examined included only 10 patients, the results were very promising, since 60% of patients demonstrated sites of RAI uptake. Moreover, when standard radiographic restaging at 3 months was performed, a clinical benefit, either PR or SD, was observed in all patients, and 4/6 patients also showed a decreasing serum thyroglobulin.

Interestingly, larotrectinib also seems to be able to restore RAI uptake. Although no preclinical *in vitro* thyroid model to assess the capacity of this NTRK inhibitor to promote redifferentiation is present, a case report was published showing that larotrectinib may inhibit signaling pathways activated by EML4-NTRK3 in a manner similar to the action of MAPK pathway inhibitors.[73]

Although there are very promising results obtained with some TKI in restoring RAI uptake, to date none of them have achieved proven clinical benefits to recommend their use in routine clinical practice.

MOST FREQUENT ADVERSE EVENTS OF TKI & THEIR MANAGEMENT

TKIs are usually associated with several toxicities, shared by all types of molecules, with different percentage and severity grades. Toxicity is unfortunately the consequence of the broad-spectrum of off-target effects of these drugs. There are some general and practical considerations to consider independent of the specific drug.

First, the clinical evaluation and grading of AEs is standardized by the use of the Common Terminology Criteria for Adverse Events (CTCAE) in its last available version 5.0,[74] which is a list of descriptive terminology for each grade of a certain AE, used also in clinical trials. Second, since TKIs are chronic and long-term treatments, the AEs' management is a crucial step in order both to optimize patients' compliance and to avoid potentially life-threatening consequences and should be tailored to each patient. The AEs' management is based on the treatment of all preexisting comorbid conditions, on AEs prevention, when feasible, and on drugs' dose interruption/reductions. Moreover, it is important to avoid drug-drug interaction, which could increase or decrease the plasma concentration of TKIs and consequently their potential toxicity, by reviewing all patients' medications and substituting for potentially the interfering ones if possible. Finally, in most cases, grade 1-2 AE can be easily managed with supporting and/or preventive therapies and measures, while most grade 3-4 AE require dose interruption and dose

Table 28–4. Most frequent adverse events related to the treatment with tyrosine kinase inhibitors in TC patients.

	Main Adverse Events (all grades)									
	Hypertension (%)	Diarrhea (%)	Skin Rash (%)	Anorexia (%)	Fatigue (%)	Nausea (%)	Weight Loss (%)	QT Prolongation (%)	Hand and Foot Syndrome (%)	Weight Gain (%)
Lenvatinib (Schlumberger et al.)	67.8	59.4	16.1	50.2	59	41	46.4	8	31.8	NR
Sorafenib (Brose et al.)	40.6	68.6	50.2	31.9	49.8	20.8	46.9	NR	76.3	NR
Vandetanib (Wells et al.)	32.7	56	45	21	24	33	10	14	NR	NR
Cabozantinib (Elisei et al.)	33	63.1	19.2	45.8	40.1	43	47.7	NR	50	NR
Selpercatinib* (Wirth et al.)	30	17	8	NR	25	15	NR	13	NR	5
Pralsetinib (Kim et al.)	40	34	24°	15	38	17	NR	NR	NR	NR

NR, not reported; TC, thyroid cancer.
Rash includes dermatitis, dermatitis acneiform, eczema, palmar-plantar, erythrodysesthesia syndrome, rash, rash erythematous, rash macular, rash maculopapular, rash papular, rash pustular.
*Considering only AEs related to the treatment.

modification. In some grade 4 AEs, the drug must be discontinued. The more frequent AEs of TKIs are described in detail in the following discussion and reported in Table 28–4.

Dermatological Adverse Events

Dermatological toxicity is very frequent and represented by different clinical manifestations as rash, erythema, pruritus, acneiform rash, paronychia, telangiectasia, alopecia, changes in hair growth or pigmentation, skin discoloration, xerosis (dryness), and hand and foot syndrome (HFSR). The most common are represented by rash and HFSR. The clinical presentation of rash is characterized by widespread and painless erythema, which could be localized or cover the entire body, and have papular, nodular, or blistering shapes and may be pruritic[75] (Figure 28–3). On the contrary, HFSR appears as

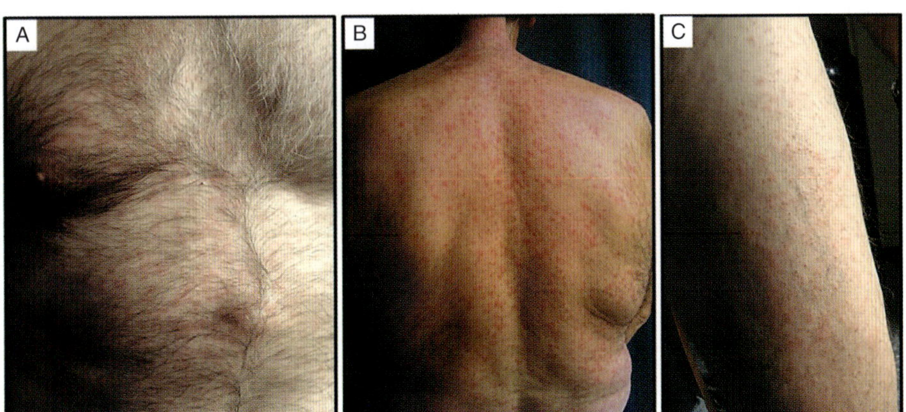

Figure 28–3. Example of cutaneous rash occurred during treatment with TKI.

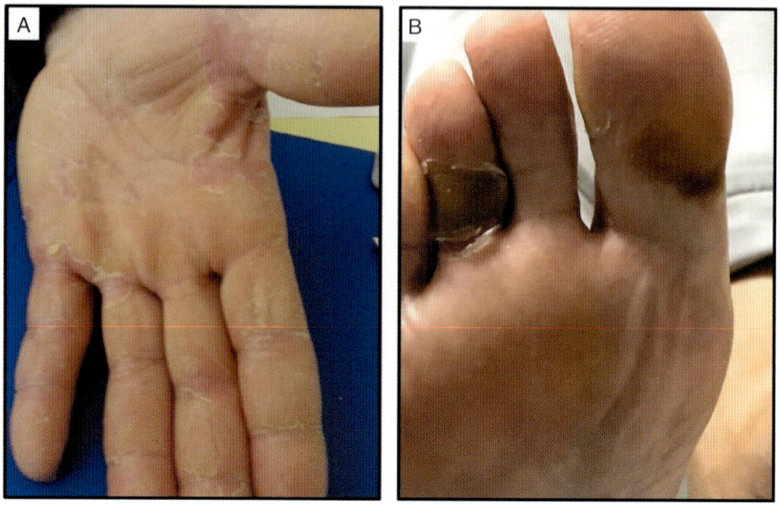

Figure 28–4. Example of hand and foot syndrome occurred during treatment with sorafenib **(A)** and cabozantinib **(B)**.

minimal skin changes or dermatitis of the hands and feet with evolving hyperkeratosis, desquamation, and ulceration of the palmar surfaces of hands or plantar surface of feet, with significant impairment of patient's quality of life, and in some cases bleeding and/or pain[75] (Figure 28–4).

The EGFR is considered the most important mediator in the molecular mechanism underlying TKI toxicity, particularly of rash. In fact, its inhibition in basal keratinocytes is able to induce several alterations in keratinocyte survival, proliferation, differentiation, migration, and attachment as well as an inflammatory reaction.[76] The combined inhibition of VEGFR and PDGFR is instead the suggested pathogenetic mechanism for the HFSR, since it impairs the vascular repair mechanisms in high-pressure areas in the body.[76]

The reported incidence of skin toxicity is different according to the TKI considered. It was the most reported AE in the vemurafenib and sorafenib trial, while it appeared less frequently than other AEs in the lenvatinib, cabozantinib, and vandetanib trials. In particular, patients receiving vandetanib experienced rash (45%), acne (20%), dry skin (15%), and dermatitis acneiform (15%), mainly of grade 1-2,[35] while during cabozantinib treatment HFSR (50%), hair color changes (34%), and rash (19%) were reported in descending order.[39] On the contrary, patients treated with sorafenib experienced mainly HFSR (76.3%), rash (50.2%), and dry skin (14.5%) which are similar to those seen with lenvatinib (HFSR 31.8% and rash 16.1%).[30,33]

No international guidelines for the management of skin toxicity are available, but some recommendations and treatments can be learned from the clinical trial reports. For HFSR, preventive measures include the removal of hyperkeratotic areas in the hands and feet before starting therapy, the application of keratolytic urea creams to aid exfoliation of calluses, and maintaining skin hydration by using fragrance-free and hypoallergenic creams and oily moisturizers.[40,75] In addition, patient education to protect pressure points and tender areas of the feet with comfortable shoes and socks is mandatory, as is education in the recognition and management of cutaneous toxicities. In the case of unresponsive pain, glucocorticoid and anti-inflammatory therapy can be used.[40] The prophylactic use of sunscreen protection cream is the only preventive advice for rash.[75] Topical therapy for symptomatic relief with glucocorticoid cream and/or analgesic cream can be suggested. In the case of acneiform rash, topical corticosteroids and antibiotics may be used.

A rare toxicity that has been reported only during treatment with Raf and BRAF inhibitors, such as sorafenib and vemurafenib, is the development of premalignant or malignant skin lesions such as keratoacanthoma-type squamous cell carcinoma. These appear as solitary or multiple lesions and have been reported to occur after few weeks or months after the initiation of the TKI. In general, these have not been reported to metastasize. Surgical removal is recommended and retreatment with a TKI doesn't appear to increase the risk of secondary skin cancer development.[77]

Gastrointestinal Adverse Events

Gastrointestinal toxicity, represented by a mucositis of the upper and/or lower gastrointestinal tract and presenting as diarrhea, nausea, stomatitis, dysgeusia, or anorexia, occurred in almost all clinical trials with TKIs and is seen in clinical practice. The mechanism of this toxicity remains unclear, but it has been demonstrated that the molecular targets of these drugs, mainly VEGF and VEGFR, play a role in the physiological process of normal proliferation and reparation of gastrointestinal cells.[78,79]

Diarrhea is the most common gastrointestinal AE with all TKIs. In fact, it occurred in 56% of patients treated with vandetanib,[35] 63.1% with cabozantinib,[39] 59.4% with lenvatinib,[33] 68.6% with sorafenib,[30] 17% with selpercatinib,[52] and 34% with pralsetinib.[55] In general, it is an early AE, occurring within the first weeks/months of treatment. Its management includes dietary measures, probiotics, and drugs, and in unresponsive or grade 3-4 cases results in drug interruption and/or dose reduction. Patients have to be educated to avoid food or drinks that may enhance bowel motility, such as spicy foods, fiber, and caffeine, and to adopt a bland diet including things like bananas, rice, and potatoes.[80] Probiotics can also be useful in preventing bowel inflammation. In the majority of patients, drugs are also needed to control this AE: Antidiarrheal/antimotility agents such as loperamide and diphenoxylate/atropine are the most commonly used.[40,80] The use of octreotide, approved for the treatment of diarrhea secondary to VIP-secreting tumors, may be considered in refractory cases.[80] Since diarrhea can lead to dehydration, it is very important to monitor serum electrolyte levels and ECG, and in severe cases, to hospitalize patients to provide intravenous therapy.[40]

Oral and gastrointestinal mucositis is another frequent and early AE during TKI therapy, with clinical manifestation as dysgeusia, oral burning/pain, and pharyngodinia, with or without visible signs of inflammation. Stomatitis occurred in 29% of patients treated with cabozantinib,[39] 35.6% with lenvatinib,[33] 23.2% with sorafenib,[30] while it was not reported with vandetanib[35] and selpercatinib.[52] Pain control and nutritional support are the two main goals of the management of this toxicity. Preventive strategies include the avoidance of spicy foods and appropriate oral care. Supportive measures include daily mouthwashes with sodium bicarbonate and water, or the use of local lidocaine-containing oral rinses that can be useful as symptomatic relief.

Liver transaminase increases are frequent and generally asymptomatic, low grade, and do not require any therapy or dose interruption/modifications.[75] Finally, gastrointestinal perforation and fistula development is a very rare but potentially life-threatening AE that can occur during antiangiogenetic therapy. Fever and abdominal pain are the main suggestive symptoms. Risk factors include the history of surgery/irradiation, diverticulitis, and infiltration or invasion of organs from tumoral disease. If perforation occurs, TKI treatment should be discontinued.

Cardiovascular Adverse Events

Cardiovascular AEs are common and include mainly left ventricular dysfunction, hypertension, conduction abnormalities, and thromboembolism. Drug inhibition by several of the kinases, including VEGF, HIF, PDGF, and KIT, directly impairs physiological compensatory mechanisms in the heart, such as repairing cardiac myocyte necrosis, compensatory hypertrophy, and stem-cell differentiation into cardiomyocytes.[80] In addition, TKI-induced thyroid dysfunction can lead to and/or promote cardiovascular toxicity,[80] as well as TKI-induced electrolyte abnormalities.

The most frequent cardiovascular side effect is hypertension: The reported incidence of all grades is 40.6% with sorafenib,[30] 32.7% with vandetanib,[35] 67.8% with lenvatinib,[33] 33% with cabozantinib,[39] and 30% with selpercatinib.[52] It is a dose-dependent and on-target AE, due to VEGF inhibition, particularly VEGF2 inhibition, resulting in an impairment in the nitric oxide-mediated vasodilatation.[79] The onset of TKI-induced hypertension is variable and there are no clear and specific guidelines for its management, but the Angiogenesis Task Force of the National Cancer Institute Investigational Drug Steering Committee proposed some recommendations.[81] First, it is important to check preexisting high blood pressure and correct potential risk factors (ie, obesity, smoking, etc.); second, it is recommended to monitor blood pressure status throughout TKI therapy, especially during first cycles, both by the clinicians in clinic and by the patient at home.[81] The accepted thresholds of blood pressure are less than 140/90 mmHg for most patients and in case of values above this goal pharmacological therapy must be started. Angiotensin-converting enzyme (ACE) inhibitors, angiotensin II receptor blockers (ARBs), and nondihydropyridine calcium channel blockers are first-line therapies and the treatment strategy should be individualized according to each patient's comorbidities, time available to reach the goal, and drug interactions.[75,81] Since it is a reversible AE, temporary discontinuation and/or dose reduction can also contribute to blood pressure control, especially in urgent cases.

Among conduction abnormalities, the most frequent is QT prolongation, resulting from TKI interactions with the myocardial potassium ion channel involved in cardiac repolarization. It is defined as an increase in the QT interval more than 60 ms from baseline or a QT interval more than 500 ms. It is potentially life-threatening since it can lead to ventricular arrythmias such as torsades de pointes. It has been reported mainly with vandetanib (14% of all grades and 8% of grades 3-4), lenvatinib (8% all grades), and selpercatinib (13% of all grades and 2% of grades 3-4) and not reported for other TKIs. A pretreatment assessment of previous arrhythmias and or cardiac comorbidities, electrolyte disturbances, and a pharmacological history and an electrocardiogram should be done, and subsequently repeated at 7 to 15 days after TKI initiation, monthly during the first 3 months and then periodically.[40,75] Preexisting hypocalcemia, hypomagnesemia, and hypokalemia should be corrected while QT-prolonging drugs, available at https://www.crediblemeds.org should be avoided if possible.[40,75] Drug discontinuation is mandatory if QTc prolongation is above 500 ms.

Renal Adverse Events

The most frequent renal AE is proteinuria, which is related to the specific VEGF signaling inhibition resulting in the loss of integrity of the glomerular filtration barrier. It occurred in 31% of lenvatinib-treated[82] and 1.9% of cabozantinib-treated[39] patients while no cases were reported for vandetanib, selpercatinib,[52] and sorafenib.[30,35] Preexisting renal risk factors and age do not seem to impact the incidence of this AE, while on the contrary preexisting nephrotoxic treatment may be contributory.[83] It is recommended to evaluate both standard urine analysis and protein-to-creatinine ratio or 24-hour urine protein collection both at baseline and then subsequently during TKI treatment. If the 24-hour urine protein collection is more than 1 g/24 h, treatment should be started, generally with ACE or ARB inhibitors, while if it is more than 2 g/24 h it is recommended to withhold TKI treatment and restart at a reduced dose.[75,84]

Endocrine Side Effects

Endocrine side effects of TKI include alterations in thyroid function, bone metabolism, linear growth, gonadal function, fetal development, glucose metabolism, and adrenal function.

Hypothyroidism is the most frequent endocrine alteration. It can be classified into recurrent hypothyroidism, occurring in patients already on levothyroxine therapy, and de novo hypothyroidism. Recurrent hypothyroidism is seen in TC patients who have already had a thyroidectomy during TKI treatment and is thought to be primarily due to lower absorption of thyroid hormone replacement due to gastrointestinal drug-related AEs. Several mechanisms have been proposed for the development of de novo hypothyroidism including accelerated clearance of thyroid hormone through its inactivating pathways, primarily increased activity of type 3 deiodinase, which inactivates both T3 and T4, regression of thyroid capillaries and antibody production.[75] New-onset hypothyroidism occurred in 61.5%, 33.3%, 57%, 49%, and 7%, respectively, of patients treated with lenvatinib, sorafenib, cabozantinib, vandetanib, and selpercatinib.[30,33,35,39,52] Thyroid testing is recommended both before and during TKI therapy and dose adjustment of levothyroxine treatment is the only therapy necessary for this AE.

Primary adrenal insufficiency is a quite frequent but less well-known AE that occurs during TKI treatment whose incidence is not reported in registrative trials of TKIs. Based on animal studies, proposed mechanisms include adrenal cortical hemorrhage or necrosis related to the reduced density of capillary networks during administration of anti-VEGF compounds. The clinical presentation is mainly asymptomatic or pauci-symptomatic with fatigue as the main characteristic symptom,[85,86] which is usually multifactorial in these patients. Also, the time of presentation can be very different among patients since it can be seen early (<12 months) or late (>36 months) after TKI treatment initiation.[86] Since it may represent a life-threatening condition under stress, it is recommended to perform adrenal function testing including serum-free cortisol and ACTH measurement, the ACTH stimulation test and electrolyte levels, both before and during TKI therapy.[85,87] Cortisone acetate replacement therapy must be started in case of adrenal insufficiency to improve related symptoms and avoid TKI discontinuation.

Constitutional Side Effects

Fatigue or asthenia is a very common AE during treatment with all TKIs and occurred in 24% patients treated with vandetanib,[35] 41% with cabozantinib,[39] 59% with lenvatinib,[33] 49.8% with sorafenib,[30] and 25% with selpercatinib.[52] It has been defined as "a subjective state of overwhelming but sustained exhaustion and decreased capacity for physical and mental work that is not relieved by rest."[88] No clear mechanisms have been identified but many factors could contribute to this AE, both cancer and drug related. Among cancer-related mechanisms there is depression syndrome which is frequently described in cancer patients and strongly correlated with fatigue;[89] moreover, pro-inflammatory cytokines, which are responsible for cancer progression, have been also related to the development of fatigue.[80] Many drug-related AEs may also contribute to fatigue: hypothyroidism, hypophosphatemia, malnutrition due to anorexia, diarrhea, and vomiting are frequently clinically associated with fatigue and muscle weakness.[80] Fatigue generally leads to drug discontinuation in a low percentage of patients, but unfortunately, no effective therapies are available to mitigate fatigue. The National Comprehensive Cancer Network (NCC) proposed some practical guidelines for screening and treating this AE.[90] Screening is based on the use of internationally approved questionaries such as the Brief Fatigue Inventory (BFI) and Quality of Life Questionnaire (QLQ-C30), evaluating respectively severe fatigue and patient's quality of life globally.[91,92] Moreover, patients must be evaluated for any concomitant factors known to contribute to fatigue. Intervention is based on both nonpharmacological and pharmacological strategies. An adequate and moderate physical exercise program together with psychoeducation therapy was found to effectively improve fatigue.[90] Pharmacological interventions should include: (1) treatment of any correctable cause of fatigue such as hypothyroidism, anemia, electrolyte disorders, etc.;[90] (2) change in the timing of the daily schedule of TKI, preferring the evening to minimize daytime fatigue;[40] (3) use of medications for emotional distress and sleep dysfunctions as antidepressive and psychostimulants.[90]

Loss of appetite is another frequent, multifactorial, and difficult to manage AE. It occurred in 45.8% of patients on cabozantinib treatment,[39] 21% on vandetanib,[35] 50.2% on lenvatinib,[33] and in 31.9% on sorafenib[30,52] but was not reported in selpercatinib trial. Many drug-related side effects can be responsible for this AE such as nausea, vomiting, dyspepsia, dysgeusia, and stomatitis, and it is important to promptly recognize and treat these side effects.

The anorexia-cachexia syndrome is another complex AE occurring during TKI treatment. It is defined as a metabolic, paraneoplastic syndrome characterized by decreased food intake, with or without involuntary weight loss, and loss of fat and muscle.[93] It has been related to the interaction between cytokines, tumor products inducing lipolysis and protein degradation, and neuropeptides.[94] How these factors are influenced by VEGF inhibitors is not yet established. Medroxyprogesterone acetate and megestrol acetate are the two most common drugs used in clinical practice to treat this AE and the only ones for which there is enough evidence to suggest their use in cancer patients, even though their optimal dose and duration are unknown.[95]

Miscellaneous

Recently, a strong association between TKI treatment and osteonecrosis of the jaw was observed in TC patients. This AE is defined as the presence of exposed bone in the maxillofacial region persisting after 8 weeks from the initial identification,[96] with the degree of severity classified in three stages. Even if this AE is not reported in registrative clinical trials, several case reports have been reported for sorafenib,[97] lenvatinib,[98] and cabozantinib.[99,100] Moreover, for lenvatinib a pharmacovigilance study was also conducted after an FDA warning.[101] In general, the occurrence of this AE is more frequent in patients treated both with TKI and bisphosphonates or denosumab for bone metastases due to the combined inhibition of these drugs respectively on bone vascularization and bone turnover. The prevention strategy is based on dental examination, both before and during these therapies, looking for minimal bone exposure and potential sites of infection and on the treatment of caries and periodontal disease.[102] More aggressive treatment is dependent on the disease stage, varying from antibiotic and microbial therapy to bone resection and subsequent reconstruction. Figure 28–5 is an explicative case of osteonecrosis of the jaw that occurred during TKI and bisphosphonates treatments.

EFFICACY EVALUATION DURING TKI THERAPY & ESCAPE PHENOMENON

During TKI treatment, tumor cells are not killed but are made quiescent and nonproliferative as these drugs act as cytostatic and not cytotoxic agents. This partially explains why, in the above-mentioned studies, CRs were seen in only a small number of patients. The cytostatic action, along with antiangiogenic activity, is responsible for the shrinkage of the tumoral mass, leading to the clinical benefit of TKIs. Unfortunately, cytostatic action also represents a limitation of TKI treatment because, once started, TKIs should be continued indefinitely until evidence of tumoral progression or the appearance of severe side effects occurs, and it seems that, once TKI treatment is stopped, progression of the disease can accelerate.

It is accepted that progression of disease must be established before starting TKI treatment, and RECIST criteria can be used to objectively assess the effects of systemic therapy on tumor dimension/size. A CR is defined as the disappearance of all target lesions; PR is defined when there is at least a 30% reduction in the lesional sum confirmed at least once at a ≥4-week interval once observed; PD is a 20% or greater increase in lesional sum from baseline or nadir, or the appearance of new lesion(s) or a clinically significant increasing of nontarget lesion(s), while SD refers to tumors not reaching criteria for either PR or PD. Examples of some radiological responses are shown in Figure 28–6.

Resistance to TKIs can be either "primary," intrinsic to the tumor cells and present before the TKI treatment has been started or "secondary" when it appears after a variable period of time from the beginning of TKI treatment and cancer cells start to grow again after a period of quiescence. An example of primary resistance in MTCs is represented by the V804M-RET mutation that confers resistance to vandetanib treatment *in vitro* by preventing the binding of the drug to the receptor.[48]

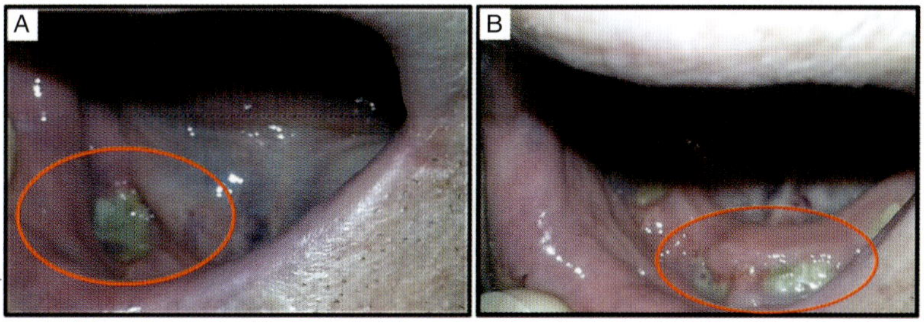

Figure 28–5. Explicative case of osteonecrosis of the jaw occurred during TKI and bisphosphonates treatments in combination.

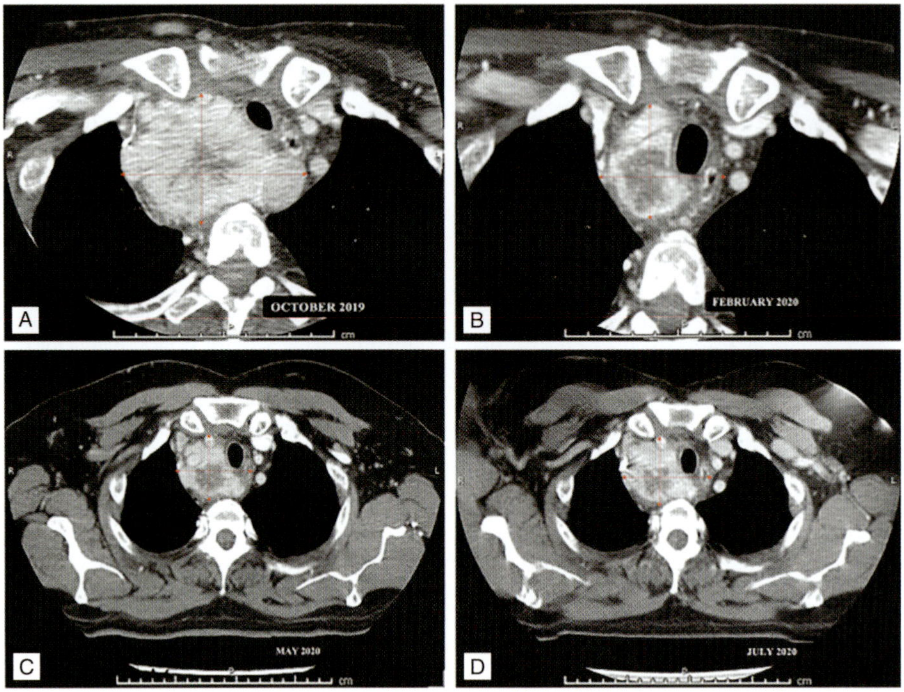

▲ **Figure 28–6.** Radiological response of right paratracheal lesions defined as partial response according to RECIST. **(A)** Before starting TKI treatment the lesion measured 70 × 60 cm and caused dislocation and compression of the trachea. **(B)** After 12 weeks of therapy the lesion decreased to 60 × 39 cm, with improvement in tracheal dislocation and diameter. In the center of the lesion the classical devascularized aspect due the drug-induced necrosis. **(C** and **D)** after 24 and 36 weeks of therapy the lesion was stable.

"Secondary" resistance is likely due to the development of an escape mechanism, independent of the type of TKI or the type of tumor.[103,104] It seems to be due to the appearance of other mutations that occur during TKI therapy. Usually, these mutations are located downstream from the TKI target or in parallel pathways, and they lead to a mechanism to bypass the action of the drug. Similar mechanisms have been demonstrated in lung adenocarcinoma cells treated with TKIs,[105] in chronic myeloid leukemia treated with imatinib,[106] and in TC.[107] Once the efficacy of the TKI is lost, the identification of the new mutations/alterations occurring during TKI treatment and causing TKI resistance could lead to initiation of another drug specifically targeting the new alterations. For this reason, collection of tissue samples both before the start of TKI treatment and when an escape phenomenon is identified can be very useful.[108]

CONCLUSIONS

The vast majority of TC can be cured with "standard" treatments—total thyroidectomy plus/minus lymphadenectomy followed by, when appropriate, RAI treatment. However, a subgroup of multimetastatic, poorly differentiated, and anaplastic tumors require other therapies varying from local treatment—always preferred when the disease is oligometastatic or multimetastatic with only one specific lesion that is growing—to systemic therapy.

Although improvement in OS is not well established, TKI therapy has been demonstrated to improve the outcome of advanced metastatic TC patients, prolonging PFS, and this therapy should be considered in those patients with metastatic, rapidly progressive, symptomatic, and/or imminently threatening disease not otherwise amenable to local control using other approaches.

TKIs are generally not considered curative, and continued treatment is needed to maintain disease response. Thus, consideration must be given to potential side effects that can occur—especially with MKIs, prior to initiating therapy. Once started, side effects that lead to a decreased quality of life can result in drug discontinuation with potential important consequences for disease recurrence/progression. Despite the fact that the new generation of selective TKIs better balances efficacy and AEs in patients with advanced, metastatic, and progressive TC, new therapeutic approaches are still needed.

REFERENCES

1. National Cancer Institute. Surveillance Epidemiology and End Results Program: SEER Stat Facts: Thyroid Cancer. Available from: https://seer.cancer.gov/statfacts/html/thyro.html 2020.
2. Pellegriti G, Frasca F, Regalbuto C, Squatrito S, Vigneri, R. Worldwide increasing incidence of thyroid cancer: update on epidemiology and risk factors. *J Cancer Epidemiol.* 2013;2013.
3. Kitamura Y, Shimizu K, Nagahama M, et al. Immediate causes of death in thyroid carcinoma: clinicopathological analysis of 161 fatal cases. *J Clin Endocrinol Metab.* 1999;84:4043-4049.
4. Dunlap Q, Davies L. Differentiated thyroid cancer incidence. *Surgery of the Thyroid and Parathyroid Glands*; 2021: 174-180.e2.
5. Volante M, Collini P, Nikiforov YE, et al. Poorly differentiated thyroid carcinoma: the Turin proposal for the use of uniform diagnostic criteria and an algorithmic diagnostic approach. *Am J Surg Pathol.* 2007;31:1256-1264.
6. Haugen BR, Alexander EK, Bible KC, et al. 2015 American Thyroid Association Management Guidelines for Adult Patients with Thyroid Nodules and Differentiated Thyroid Cancer: The American Thyroid Association Guidelines Task Force on Thyroid Nodules and Differentiated Thyroid Cancer. *Thyroid.* 2016;26(1):1-133.
7. Durante C, Haddy N, Baudin E, et al. Long-term outcome of 444 patients with distant metastases from papillary and follicular thyroid carcinoma: benefits and limits of radioiodine therapy. *J Clin Endocrinol Metab.* 2006;91:2892-2899.
8. Ibrahimpasic T, Ghossein R, Carlson DL, et al. Poorly differentiated thyroid carcinoma presenting with gross extrathyroidal extension: 1986-2009 memorial Sloan-Kettering cancer center experience. *Thyroid.* 2013;23:997-1002.
9. Molinaro E, Romei C, Biagini A, et al. Anaplastic thyroid carcinoma: from clinicopathology to genetics and advanced therapies. *Nat Rev Endocrinol.* 2017;13: 644-660.
10. Chiacchio S, Lorenzoni A, Boni G; Rubello D, Elisei R, Mariani G. Anaplastic thyroid cancer: prevalence, diagnosis and treatment. *Minerva Endocrinol.* 2008;33:341-357.
11. Neff RL, Farrar WB, Kloos RT, Burman KD. Anaplastic thyroid cancer. *Endocrinol Metab Clin North Am.* 2008;37:525-538.
12. Smallridge RC, Marlow LA, Copland JA. Anaplastic thyroid cancer: molecular pathogenesis and emerging therapies. *Endocr Relat Cancer.* 2009;16:17-44.
13. Bible KC, Kebebew E, Brierley J, et al. 2021 American Thyroid Association Guidelines for management of patients with anaplastic thyroid cancer. *Thyroid.* 2021;31:337-386.
14. Filetti S, Durante C, Hartl D, et al. Thyroid cancer: ESMO Clinical Practice Guidelines for diagnosis, treatment and follow-up. *Ann Oncol.* 2019;*30*:1856-1883.
15. Wells SA, Asa SL, Dralle H, et al. Revised American thyroid association guidelines for the management of medullary thyroid carcinoma. *Thyroid.* 2015;*25*:567-610.
16. Prete A, Borges de Souza P, Censi S, Muzza M, Nucci N, Sponziello M. Update on fundamental mechanisms of thyroid cancer. *Front Endocrinol (Lausanne).* 2020;11:102.
17. Elisei R, Ugolini C, Viola D, et al. BRAFV600E mutation and outcome of patients with papillary thyroid carcinoma: a 15-year median follow-up study. *J Clin Endocrinol Metab.* 2008;93:3943-3949.
18. Zhang J, Yang PL, Gray NS. Targeting cancer with small molecule kinase inhibitors. *Nat Rev Cancer.* 2009;9:28-39.
19. Liu Y, Gray NS. Rational design of inhibitors that bind to inactive kinase conformations. *Nat Chem Biol.* 2006;2:358-364.
20. Kwak EL, Sordella R, Bell DW, et al. Irreversible inhibitors of the EGF receptor may circumvent acquired resistance to gefitinib. *Proc Natl Acad Sci USA.* 2005;102:7665-7670.
21. Kloos RT, Eng C, Evans DB, et al. Medullary thyroid cancer: management guidelines of the American Thyroid Association. *Thyroid.* 2009;19:565-612.
22. Eisenhauer EA, Therasse P, Bogaerts J, et al. New response evaluation criteria in solid tumours: revised RECIST guideline (version 1.1). *Eur J Cancer.* 2009;45:228-247.
23. Sabra MM, Sherman EJ, Tuttle RM. Tumor volume doubling time of pulmonary metastases predicts overall survival and can guide the initiation of multikinase inhibitor therapy in patients with metastatic, follicular cell-derived thyroid carcinoma. *Cancer.* 2017;123:2955-2964.
24. Zhang X, Higuchi T, Tomonaga H, et al. Early detection of progressive disease using thyroglobulin doubling-time in metastatic differentiated thyroid carcinoma treated with radioactive iodine. *Nucl Med Commun.* 2020;350-355.
25. Barbet J, Campion L, Kraeber-Bodéré F, Chatal JF. Prognostic impact of serum calcitonin and carcinoembryonic antigen doubling-times in patients with medullary thyroid carcinoma. *J Clin Endocrinol Metab.* 2005;90:6077-6084.
26. Elisei R, Lorusso L, Piaggi P, et al. Elevated level of serum carbohydrate antigen 19.9 as predictor of mortality in patients with advanced medullary thyroid cancer. *Eur J Endocrinol.* 2015;173:297-304.
27. Elisei R, Lorusso L, Romei C, et al. Medullary thyroid cancer secreting carbohydrate antigen 19-9 (Ca 19-9): A fatal case report. *J Clin Endocrinol Metab.* 2013;98:3550-3554.
28. Gupta-Abramson V, Troxel AB, Nellore A, et al. Phase II trial of sorafenib in advanced thyroid cancer. *J Clin Oncol.* 2008;26:4714-4719.
29. Shah MH, Kloos RT, Ringel MD, et al. Phase II trial of sorafenib in metastatic thyroid cancer. *J Clin Oncol.* 2009;*27*: 1675-1684.
30. Brose MS, Nutting CM, Jarzab B, et al. Sorafenib in radioactive iodine-refractory, locally advanced or metastatic diff erentiated thyroid cancer: a randomised, double-blind, phase 3 trial. *Lancet.* 2014;384:319-328.
31. Schlumberger M, Jarzab B, Cabanillas ME, et al. A phase II trial of the multitargeted tyrosine kinase inhibitor lenvatinib (E7080) in advanced medullary thyroid cancer. *Clin Cancer Res.* 2016;22:44-53.
32. Takahashi S, Kiyota N, Yamazaki T, et al. Phase II study of lenvatinib in patients with differentiated, medullary, and anaplastic thyroid cancer: final analysis results. *J Clin Oncol.* 2016;34:6088-6088.
33. Schlumberger M, Tahara M, Wirth LJ, et al. Lenvatinib versus placebo in radioiodine-refractory thyroid cancer. *N Engl J Med.* 2015;372:621-630.
34. Brose MS, Robinson B, Sherman SI, et al. Cabozantinib for radioiodine-refractory differentiated thyroid cancer (COSMIC-311): a randomised, double-blind, placebo-controlled, phase 3 trial. *Lancet Oncol.* 2021 Aug;22(8):1126-1138. Epub 2021 Jul 5.
35. Wells SA, Robinson BG, Gagel RF, et al. Vandetanib in patients with locally advanced or metastatic medullary thyroid cancer: a randomized, double-blind phase III trial. *J Clin Oncol.* 2012; 30:134-141.
36. Fox E, Widemann BC, Chuk MK, et al. Vandetanib in children and adolescents with multiple endocrine neoplasia type 2b associated medullary thyroid carcinoma. *Clin Cancer Res.* 2013;19:4239-4248.

37. Hu MI, Elisei R, Dedecjus M, et al. Safety and efficacy of two starting doses of vandetanib in advanced medullary thyroid cancer. *Endocr Relat Cancer*. 2019;26:241-250.
38. Cambridge M.S.G. *CAPRELSA® (vandetanib) tablets for oral use [prescribing information]*. 2016.
39. Elisei R, Schlumberger MJ, Müller SP, et al. Cabozantinib in progressive medullary thyroid cancer. *J Clin Oncol*. 2013; 31:3639-3646.
40. Brose MS, Bible KC, Chow LQM, et al. Management of treatment-related toxicities in advanced medullary thyroid cancer. *Cancer Treat Rev*. 2018;66:64-73.
41. Cabanillas ME, Hu MI, Jimenez C. Medullary thyroid cancer in the era of tyrosine kinase inhibitors: to treat or not to treat–and with which drug—those are the questions. *J Clin Endocrinol Metab*. 2014;99:4390-4396.
42. Schlumberger M, Elisei R, Müller S, et al. Overall survival analysis of EXAM, a phase III trial of cabozantinib in patients with radiographically progressive medullary thyroid carcinoma. *Ann Oncol*. 2017;28:2813-2819.
43. Drilon A, Laetsch TW, Kummar S, et al. Efficacy of larotrectinib in TRK fusion-positive cancers in adults and children. *N Engl J Med*. 2018;378:731-739.
44. Hong DS, DuBois SG, Kummar S, et al. Larotrectinib in patients with TRK fusion-positive solid tumours: a pooled analysis of three phase 1/2 clinical trials. *Lancet Oncol*. 2020;21:531-540.
45. Cabanillas ME, Drilon A, Farago AF, et al. 1916P Larotrectinib treatment of advanced TRK fusion thyroid cancer. *Ann Oncol*. 2020;31:S1086.
46. Doebele RC, Drilon A, Paz-Ares L, et al. Entrectinib in patients with advanced or metastatic NTRK fusion-positive solid tumours: integrated analysis of three phase 1–2 trials. *Lancet Oncol*. 2020;21:271-282.
47. John T, Chiu C-H, Cho BC, et al. 364O Intracranial efficacy of entrectinib in patients with NTRK fusion-positive solid tumours and baseline CNS metastases. *Ann Oncol*. 2020;31: S397-S398.
48. Carlomagno F, Guida T, Anaganti S, et al. Disease associated mutations at valine 804 in the RET receptor tyrosine kinase confer resistance to selective kinase inhibitors. *Oncogene*. 2004;23:6056-6063.
49. FDA. FDA approves first RET inhibitor. *Nat Biotechnol*. 2020;38:662.
50. EMA European Medicines Agency Meeting highlights from the Committee for Medicinal Products for Human Use (CHMP) 7-10 December 2020.
51. Bradford D, Larkins E, Mushti SL, et al. FDA approval summary: selpercatinib for the treatment of lung and thyroid cancers with RET gene mutations or fusions. *Clin Cancer Res*. 2021;27(8):2130-2135.
52. Wirth LJ, Sherman E, Robinson B, et al. Efficacy of selpercatinib in RET-altered thyroid cancers. *N Engl J Med*. 2020; 383(9):825-835.
53. Hadoux J, Elisei R, Brose MS, et al. LIBRETTO-531 Trial Investigators. Phase 3 trial of selpercatinib in advanced *RET*-mutant medullary thyroid cancer. *N Engl J Med*. 2023 Nov 16; 389(20):1851-1861. Epub 2023 Oct 21.
54. Hernando J, Tarasova V, Hu MI, et al. 1927TiP LIBRETTO-531: selpercatinib in patients with treatment (Tx)-naïve RET-mutant medullary thyroid cancer (MTC). *Ann Oncol*. 2020; 31:S1091.
55. Kim J, Bradford D, Larkins E, et al. FDA approval summary: pralsetinib for the treatment of lung and thyroid cancers with *RET* gene mutations or fusions. *Clin Cancer Res*. 2021 Oct 15; 27(20):5452-5456. Epub 2021 May 27.
56. Subbiah V, Hu MI, Wirth LJ, et al. Pralsetinib for patients with advanced or metastatic RET-altered thyroid cancer (ARROW): a multi-cohort, open-label, registrational, phase 1/2 study. *Lancet Diabetes Endocrinol*. 2021;9:491-501.
57. Xing M. BRAF mutation in thyroid cancer. *Endocr Relat Cancer*. 2005;12:245-262.
58. Davies H, Bignell GR, Cox C, et al. Mutations of the BRAF gene in human cancer. *Nature*. 2002;417:949-954.
59. Kim TH, Park YJ, Lim JA, et al. The association of the BRAFV600E mutation with prognostic factors and poor clinical outcome in papillary thyroid cancer: a meta-analysis. *Cancer*. 2012;118:1764-1773.
60. Landa I, Ibrahimpasic T, Boucai L, et al. Genomic and transcriptomic hallmarks of poorly differentiated and anaplastic thyroid cancers. *J Clin Invest*. 2016;126:1052-1066.
61. Deeken-Draisey A, Yang GY, Gao J, Alexiev BA. Anaplastic thyroid carcinoma: an epidemiologic, histologic, immunohistochemical, and molecular single-institution study. *Hum Pathol*. 2018;82:140-148.
62. Subbiah V, Cabanillas ME, Kreitman RJ, et al. Dabrafenib and trametinib treatment in patients with locally advanced or metastatic BRAF V600–mutant anaplastic thyroid cancer. *J Clin Oncol*. 2018;36:7-13.
63. Keam B, Kreitman RJ, Wainberg ZA, et al. Updated efficacy and safety data of dabrafenib (D) and trametinib (T) in patients (pts) with BRAF V600E–mutated anaplastic thyroid cancer (ATC). *Ann Oncol*. 2018;29:viii645-viii646.
64. Shah MH, Wei L, Wirth LJ, et al. Results of randomized phase II trial of dabrafenib versus dabrafenib plus trametinib in BRAF-mutated papillary thyroid carcinoma. *J Clin Oncol*. 2017;35:6022-6022.
65. Brose MS, Cabanillas ME, Cohen EE, et al. Vemurafenib in patients with $BRAF^{V600E}$-positive metastatic or unresectable papillary thyroid cancer refractory to radioactive iodine: a non-randomised, multicentre, open-label, phase 2 trial. *Lancet Oncol*. 2016;17(9):1272-1282.
66. Hyman DM, Puzanov I, Subbiah V, et al. Vemurafenib in multiple nonmelanoma cancers with BRAF V600 mutations. *N Engl J Med*. 2015;373:726-736.
67. Handkiewicz-Junak D, Roskosz J, Hasse-Lazar K, et al. 13-Cis-retinoic acid re-differentiation therapy and recombinant human thyrotropin-aided radioiodine treatment of non-functional metastatic thyroid cancer: a single-center, 53-patient phase 2 study. *Thyroid Res*. 2009;2:8.
68. Liu YY, Van Der Pluijm G, Karperien M, et al. Lithium as adjuvant to radioiodine therapy in differentiated thyroid carcinoma: clinical and in vitro studies. *Clin Endocrinol*. 2006;64:617-624.
69. Ho AL, Grewal RK, Leboeuf R, et al. Selumetinib-enhanced radioiodine uptake in advanced thyroid cancer. *N Engl J Med*. 2013;368:623-632.
70. Ho A, Dedecjus M, Wirth LJ, et al. ASTRA: a phase III, randomized, placebo-controlled study evaluating complete remission rate (CRR) with short-course selumetinib plus adjuvant radioactive iodine (RAI) in patients (pts) with differentiated thyroid cancer (DTC). *Proc. 88th Annu. Meet. Am. Thyroid Assoc. 3–7 Oct. 2018;* Washington, DC. *Abstr. short call oral 8.* 2018.
71. Dunn LA, Sherman EJ, Baxi SS, et al. Vemurafenib redifferentiation of BRAF mutant, RAI-refractory thyroid cancers. *J Clin Endocrinol Metab*. 2019;104:1417-1428.

72. Rothenberg SM, McFadden DG, Palmer EL, Daniels GH, Wirth LJ. Redifferentiation of iodine-refractory BRAF V600E-mutant metastatic papillary thyroid cancer with dabrafenib. *Clin Cancer Res*. 2015;21:1028-1035.
73. Groussin L, Clerc J, Huillard O. Larotrectinib-enhanced radioactive iodine uptake in advanced thyroid cancer. *N Engl J Med*. 2020;383:1686-1687.
74. National Institute of Health National Cancer Institute Common Terminology Criteria for Adverse Events (CTCAE) version 5.0.
75. Resteghini C, Cavalieri S, Galbiati D, et al. Management of tyrosine kinase inhibitors (TKI) side effects in differentiated and medullary thyroid cancer patients. *Best Pract Res Clin Endocrinol Metab*. 2017;31:349-361.
76. Lacouture ME, Ciccolini K, Kloos RT, Agulnik, M. Overview and management of dermatologic events associated with targeted therapies for medullary thyroid cancer. *Thyroid*. 2014;24:1329-1340.
77. Brose MS, Cabanillas ME, Cohen EEW, et al. Vemurafenib in patients with BRAFV600E-positive metastatic or unresectable papillary thyroid cancer refractory to radioactive iodine: a non-randomised, multicentre, open-label, phase 2 trial. *Lancet Oncol*. 2016;17:1272-1282.
78. Van Cruijsen H, Van Der Veldt A, Hoekman K. Tyrosine kinase inhibitors of VEGF receptors: clinical issues and remaining questions. *Front Biosci*. 2009;14:2248-2268.
79. Dy GK, Adjei AA. Understanding, recognizing, and managing toxicities of targeted anticancer therapies. *CA Cancer J Clin*. 2013;63:249-279.
80. Schmidinger M. Understanding and managing toxicities of vascular endothelial growth factor (VEGF) inhibitors. *EJC Suppl*. 2013;11(2):172-191.
81. Maitland ML, Bakris GL, Black HR, et al. Initial assessment, surveillance, and management of blood pressure in patients receiving vascular endothelial growth factor signaling pathway inhibitors. *J Natl Cancer Inst*. 2010;102:596-604.
82. Berdelou A, Borget I, Godbert Y, et al. Lenvatinib for the treatment of radioiodine-refractory thyroid cancer in real-life practice. *Thyroid*. 2018;28:72-78.
83. Cappagli V, Moriconi D, Bonadio AG, et al. Proteinuria is a late-onset adverse event in patients treated with cabozantinib. *J Endocrinol Invest*. 2021;44:95-103.
84. Cabanillas ME, Hu MI, Durand JB, Busaidy NL. Challenges associated with tyrosine kinase inhibitor therapy for metastatic thyroid cancer. *J Thyroid Res*. 2011;2011:985780.
85. Colombo C, De Leo S, Di Stefano M, Vannucchi G, Persani L, Fugazzola L. Primary adrenal insufficiency during lenvatinib or vandetanib and improvement of fatigue after cortisone acetate therapy. *J Clin Endocrinol Metab*. 2018;104:779-784.
86. Valerio L, Matrone A, Agate L, et al. MON-537 primary adrenal insufficiency during tyrosine kinase inhibitors treatment in advanced thyroid cancer patients. *J Endocr Soc*. 2020;4:MON-537.
87. Valerio L, Bottici V, Matrone A, et al. Medullary thyroid cancer treated with vandetanib: predictors of a longer and durable response. *Endocr Relat Cancer*. 2020;27:97-110.
88. Cella D, Peterman A, Passik S, Jacobsen P, Breitbart W. Progress toward guidelines for the management of fatigue. *Oncology (Williston Park)*. 1998;12:369-377.
89. Jacobsen PB, Donovan KA, Weitzner MA. Distinguishing fatigue and depression in patients with cancer. *Semin Clin Neuropsychiatry*. 2003;8:229-240.
90. Mock V, Atkinson A, Barsevick A, et al. NCCN practice guidelines for cancer-related fatigue. *Oncology (Williston Park)*. 2000;14:151-161.
91. Mendoza TR, Wang XS, Cleeland CS, et al. The rapid assessment of fatigue severity in cancer patients. *Cancer*. 1999;85:1186-1196.
92. Aaronson NK, Ahmedzai S, Bergman B, et al. The European organization for research and treatment of cancer QLQ-C30: a quality-of-life instrument for use in international clinical trials in oncology. *J Natl Cancer Inst*. 1993;85:365-376.
93. Zhang F, Shen A, Jin Y, Qiang W. The management strategies of cancer-associated anorexia: a critical appraisal of systematic reviews. *BMC Complement Altern Med*. 2018;18:236.
94. Tisdale MJ. Molecular pathways leading to cancer cachexia. *Physiology*. 2005;20:340-348.
95. Yavuzsen T, Davis MP, Walsh D, LeGrand S, Lagman R. Systematic review of the treatment of cancer-associated anorexia and weight loss. *J Clin Oncol*. 2005;23:8500-8511.
96. Khan AA, Morrison A, Hanley DA, et al. Diagnosis and management of osteonecrosis of the jaw: a systematic review and international consensus. *J Bone Miner Res*. 2015;30:3-23.
97. Lorusso L, Pieruzzi L, Gabriele M, et al. Osteonecrosis of the jaw: a rare but possible side effect in thyroid cancer patients treated with tyrosine-kinase inhibitors and bisphosphonates. *J Endocrinol Invest*. 2021;44:2557-2566.
98. Mauceri R, Panzarella V, Morreale I, Campisi G. Medication-related osteonecrosis of the jaw in a cancer patient receiving lenvatinib. *Int J Oral Maxillofac Surg*. 2019;48:1530-1532.
99. Marino R, Orlandi F, Arecco F, Gandolfo S, Pentenero M. Osteonecrosis of the jaw in a patient receiving cabozantinib. *Aust Dent J*. 2015;60:528-531.
100. Bennardo F, Buffone C, Muraca D, Antonelli A, Giudice A. Medication-related osteonecrosis of the jaw with spontaneous hemimaxilla exfoliation: report of a case in metastatic renal cancer patient under multidrug therapy. *Case Rep Med*. 2020;2020:8093293.
101. Lu W, Guo Q, Ma Z, Liu L, Zhao Z. Lenvatinib and osteonecrosis of the jaw: a pharmacovigilance study. *Eur J Cancer*. 2021;150:211-213.
102. Ruggiero SL, Dodson TB, Fantasia J, et al. American association of oral and maxillofacial surgeons position paper on medication-related osteonecrosis of the jaw–2014 update. *J Oral Maxillofac Surg*. 2014;72:1938-1956.
103. Finke J, Ko J, Rini B, Rayman P, Ireland J, Cohen P. MDSC as a mechanism of tumor escape from sunitinib mediated anti-angiogenic therapy. *Int Immunopharmacol*. 2011;11: 856-861.
104. Arao T, Matsumoto K, Furuta K, et al. Acquired drug resistance to vascular endothelial growth factor receptor 2 tyrosine kinase inhibitor in human vascular endothelial cells. *Anticancer Res*. 2011;31:2787-2796.
105. Ohashi K, Sequist LV, Arcila ME, et al. Lung cancers with acquired resistance to EGFR inhibitors occasionally harbor BRAF gene mutations but lack mutations in KRAS, NRAS, or MEK1. *Proc Natl Acad Sci USA*. 2012;109:E2127-E2133.
106. Amsberg GK, Koschmieder S. Profile of bosutinib and its clinical potential in the treatment of chronic myeloid leukemia. *Onco Targets Ther*. 2013;6:99-106.
107. Isham CR, Netzel BC, Bossou AR, et al. Development and characterization of a differentiated thyroid cancer cell line resistant to VEGFR-targeted kinase inhibitors. *J Clin Endocrinol Metab*. 2014;99:E936-E943.
108. Bible KC, Cote GJ, Demeure MJ, Elisei R, Jhiang S, Ringel MD. Correlative studies in clinical trials: a position statement from the international thyroid oncology group. *J Clin Endocrinol Metab*. 2015;100:4387-4395.

29 External Beam Radiation Therapy in the Management of Thyroid Cancer

Jelena Lukovic, MD, FRCPC
James D. Brierley, BSc, MB

OUTLINE

As discussed in earlier chapters, surgery is the primary treatment for thyroid cancer. When there is a high risk of local recurrence, external beam radiotherapy (EBRT) may be considered. In this chapter, the role of EBRT and the identification of patients who may benefit from EBRT for differentiated thyroid cancer (DTC), medullary thyroid cancer (MTC), and anaplastic thyroid cancer are discussed. The role of EBRT in palliation of unresectable and metastatic thyroid cancer is also discussed.

GENERAL CONSIDERATIONS

Surgery is the definitive treatment for almost all forms of thyroid cancer, except for primary lymphoma of the thyroid, in which the role of surgery is limited to diagnosis. Following surgical resection there is a role for additional treatment in certain situations to reduce the risk of recurrence. Postoperative radioactive iodine (RAI) is used in patients with intermediate-risk and high-risk differentiated thyroid cancer (DTC) to reduce the risk of recurrence in the neck and diagnose and treat local and distant disease; this is discussed in Chapter 26. The role of EBRT is limited to certain high-risk situations and will be discussed here. In other circumstances (eg, medullary thyroid cancer [MTC] and anaplastic thyroid cancer [ATC]), RAI is considered to be ineffective and EBRT may be recommended to improve local control or to control unresected disease. EBRT also has an important role in the palliation of symptomatic metastases. Finally, the possibility of long-term control of metastases with stereotactic body radiation therapy (SBRT) is being increasingly explored in selected cases.

GENERAL PRINCIPLES

Unlike RAI, which is a systemic therapy, EBRT is a localized treatment directed at the thyroid bed and adjacent nodal regions. EBRT may be considered in situations where there is a high risk of local relapse after surgical excision and when relapse is unlikely to be controlled with further surgery or in situations where surgery is not possible. The specific indications for EBRT vary by tumor type and are discussed in the subsequent sections in further detail. For DTC and MTC, the extent of extrathyroidal extension (ETE) is important—minimal versus extensive ETE and the presence of invasion of local structures are all essential considerations; invasion of the strap muscles, which can readily be resected with negative margins, is different from posterior extension into the tracheoesophageal grove with involvement of the esophagus, trachea, or larynx, which would require extensive surgery to resect with negative margins. As described in the subsequent section, the situation with ATC is quite different. Palliative radiotherapy should be considered in all forms of thyroid cancer to improve symptoms of metastatic disease.

Differentiated Thyroid Cancer

Surgery is a crucial component of the management of DTC with postoperative RAI used in intermediate-risk and high-risk patients. The role of EBRT, however, is less well-established. EBRT may be considered in two distinct scenarios: (1) in addition to postoperative RAI, to reduce the risk of local-regional (LR) recurrence in high-risk patients; (2) in the definitive treatment of unresectable DTC (eg, due to local extent or patient comorbidities precluding surgery/patient refusal of surgery).

A. Postoperative EBRT to Reduce the Risk of Local-Regional Recurrence

EBRT may be considered in patients with DTC to reduce the risk of LR, which can cause a plethora of severe symptoms including laryngeal, tracheal, and esophageal obstruction, skin ulceration and necrosis, and carotid artery rupture. The 2015 version of the American Thyroid Association (ATA) clinical practice guidelines states that there is no role for routine adjuvant EBRT but that it may be considered in select patients with gross residual disease after surgery and in patients after repeat surgeries for recurrent nodal involvement, especially if the risks of further repeat surgery are high.[1] The United Kingdom National Multidisciplinary Guidelines recommend consideration of EBRT in addition to RAI in patients where there is gross residual disease after surgery.[2] Similarly, the American Head and Neck Society recommends EBRT for patients with gross residual or unresectable locoregional disease; a notable exception is patients less than 45 years of age with limited gross disease that is RAI avid.[3] After complete resection, EBRT may be considered in select patients over the age of 45 years with high likelihood of microscopic residual disease and low likelihood of RAI response.[3] These consensus recommendations are primarily based on single-institution retrospective studies. There is only one randomized trial that attempted to evaluate the role of adjuvant EBRT in DTC. Unfortunately, only 45 out of a planned 311 patients were accrued, the local failure rate in the observation alone group was 3%, and no benefit to EBRT was observed. It is important to note, however, that a large proportion of patients who were included would not be considered at high risk of LR.

Several retrospective series have reported improved local control rates with the addition of EBRT in the setting of gross residual disease, especially in older patients.[4-9] A retrospective review from the Princess Margaret Cancer Centre described the outcomes of 729 patients with papillary or follicular thyroid cancer treated with surgery +/− RAI +/− EBRT between 1958 and 1998.[5] For patients over the age of 60 years with gross ETE but no gross residual disease after surgery, there was a cause-specific survival (CSS) benefit (81.0% vs 64.6%; $p = 0.04$) and local control benefit with EBRT (95.9% vs 85.4%; $p = 0.01$) at 10 years.[5] Similar outcomes were reported by an earlier German study of 874 patients with DTC and ETE with or without invasion of local structures (T3b or T4 in the current classification system).[4] Treatment included thyroidectomy, followed by RAI and TSH suppression. The addition of EBRT was a predictive factor for improvement in time to local regional recurrence ($p < 0.004$) and time to distant failure ($p < 0.001$). A retrospective review of 842 patients with DTC treated with surgery +/− RAI +/− EBRT similarly demonstrated that EBRT improved locoregional control at 10 years in patients with gross residual disease (56% vs 24%; $p < 0.01$).[5]

A French review of 254 patients from 18 centers developed a scoring system to define a cohort of patients who would benefit from EBRT.[6] Two points were awarded for the following high-risk characteristics: age over 60, ETE, and microscopic residual disease—EBRT was recommended for any patient with a score of 6 or more points as there was an improvement in local control. There are two additional meta-analyses worth mentioning.[10,11] A 2014 meta-analysis of 2388 patients from eight studies demonstrated a lower rate of local recurrence for patients receiving EBRT, regardless of stage or residual disease status (8% vs 25%, $p = 0.03$). Conversely, a more recent meta-analysis that included nine studies concluded that although LR was improved by EBRT, the benefit was small and there was no benefit in OS, CSS, or progression-free survival (PFS). The meta-analysis was assessed by a review panel on behalf of the Italian Association of Radiotherapy and Clinical Oncology who judged the harm/benefit balance was uncertain.

A modern retrospective review may help to more clearly identify patients who benefit from EBRT as it includes detailed information on the extent of ETE and includes patients who were treated at high-volume centers, by experienced surgeons, and who received EBRT with modern techniques.[12] Patients in this cohort ($n = 88$) had T4a disease (extent of ETE was classified by the extent of tracheal involvement, esophageal involvement, recurrent laryngeal nerve [RLN] involvement, and extent of resection). They were treated with thyroidectomy followed by RAI; in total, 44 patients received EBRT. Patients who received RAI alone had a lower disease-free survival than those who had RAI and EBRT at 4 years (43% vs 57%).[12] On subgroup analysis, this effect was not seen in patients with only RLN involvement but persisted in patients with minimal tracheal perichondrium or esophageal muscularis involvement.[12] Age and esophageal involvement were additionally significant poor prognostic factors.

In summary, EBRT appears to benefit patients at high risk of LR and may be considered for patients with gross ETE with T4a disease over the age of 55 (excluding patients with RLN involvement). EBRT may also be considered for patients with gross residual disease, unless they are young, the extent of disease is minimal, and there appears to be adequate RAI uptake in the area of concern.

B. Definitive EBRT for Unresectable Differentiated Thyroid Cancer

There is a subgroup of patients with DTC who present with locally advanced disease invading the prevertebral fascia, encasing the carotid artery, and/or encasing the mediastinal vessels rendering their disease unresectable (T4b disease). Patients may also present with extensive disease such that a gross total resection would require extended surgery (eg, laryngopharyngectomy) with significant morbidity or surgery may not be an option due to patient comorbidities. Definitive EBRT may be considered for this subgroup of patients with DTC.

The role of EBRT has been reviewed in a number of retrospective case series, with the earliest publication in 1966 describing a cohort of patients treated between 1935 and 1964.[13] Since then, a number of retrospective series have described improved local-regional control with the use of EBRT in patients with either gross residual or unresectable DTC.[14-17] A study from Hong Kong described the outcomes of 217 patients with DTC and reported improved local relapse free rate (LRFR) survival with EBRT versus no

EBRT (63% vs 24%; $p < 0.001$).[15] A Princess Margaret Cancer Centre review similarly reported a 5-year LRFR of 62% in 33 patients with DTC and gross residual/unresectable disease.[14] A review from the Christie Hospital included 19 patients with DTC and macroscopic residual disease, defined as visible or palpable tumor after surgery. These patients received EBRT with field-based techniques and the local control was 69.2% at 5 years with CSS 58.3%. Finally, a 2009 publication from the MD Anderson Cancer Centre included 15 patients with gross disease from DTC treated with EBRT (63-66 Gy).[17] In this small group of patients, the 4-year LRFR survival was 22%, DSS was 32%, and OS was 32%.[17]

The American Head and Neck Society consensus statement recommends EBRT for patients with DTC and gross residual or unresectable local-regional disease.[3] In general, radiation doses exceeding 60 Gy are recommended as they result in a higher likelihood of long-term control. A phase II study from the Memorial Sloan Kettering Cancer Center is evaluating the role of EBRT in the management of unresectable nonmedullary and nonanaplastic thyroid cancer.[18] Patients are treated with intensity-modulated radiation therapy (IMRT) to a total dose of 70 Gy and receive concurrent low-dose radiosensitizing doxorubicin chemotherapy. The primary outcome is local-regional progression-free survival and secondary outcome measures include overall survival, rates of acute toxicities, and rates of late toxicities (eg, dysphagia, dry mouth, etc.). The estimated study completion date is in 2022 and the results are eagerly anticipated.

Medullary Thyroid Cancer

Given the relative rarity of MTC it is not surprising that data regarding the role of EBRT in MTC are limited and come mainly from small single institution series. Most of these studies include patients who were treated prior to the era of extensive nodal resection. Most series report an improvement in LR in selected patients considered at high risk of local-regional relapse, usually indicated by extensive nodal involvement, ETE, and residual disease (both microscopic and macroscopic.[19-21] The definition of extensive nodal disease is inconsistent and has been defined with as few as four involved nodes; the caveat is that surgical techniques have changed significantly over time and more extensive nodal resections are performed in the modern era. Nevertheless, in one recent systemic review EBRT resulted in improved LR rate by at least 38% with a complete response (CR) rate of 21%.[19] There was no benefit in terms of OS, however, which is not surprising given the natural history of MTC and propensity for distant relapse. In a surveillance, epidemiology, and end results (SEER) analysis of 2046 patients with MTC without metastases at presentation, 152 received EBRT.[20] There was no difference in OS or DSS. In addition, the SEER database does not have data on patterns of relapse (local, regional, or distant). Patients who received EBRT had more advanced disease (T3 and T4, and nodal involvement) and were older; resultantly, a benefit from EBRT in improving local control could not be demonstrated.[20]

Despite the poor quality of data on EBRT in MTC, the 2015 ATA guidelines recommended that EBRT should be considered in patients with incompletely resected MTC or those at high risk for LR to prevent the significant complications of recurrent MTC in the neck.[22] They additionally noted that the potential benefits must be weighed against the probable acute and chronic toxicity associated with the therapy and that a multidisciplinary discussion was essential to ensure that surgical salvage was not an option in the future.[22] The British Thyroid Association guidelines are similar and state that "EBRT should be considered only once optimal surgery has been performed and if there is significant risk of local recurrence." This includes situations where there is macroscopic residual disease or microscopic residual disease in the background of large-volume disease. The guidelines additionally state that "EBRT should not be used to consolidate inadequate surgery," which is true for all tumor sites.

The ATA guideline philosophy outlined above was followed by a group from Memorial Sloane Kettering (New York, United States) and University Medical Centre (Groningen, Netherlands). They reported on a cohort of 297 patients with MTC, 46 of whom received EBRT. Patients who received EBRT had more poor prognostic factors (older age, ETE, residual disease, and nodal involvement). The 10-year LR failure rate was 30.2% (no EBRT) versus 16.9% (EBRT); most patients in the EBRT group relapsed in the mediastinum. The survival was greater at 10 years for patients who did not receive EBRT (76% vs 38%), confirming that local-regional control rather than survival in these high-risk groups is the more relevant outcome given the risk of distant relapse.

It seems appropriate to follow the ATA guidelines and recommend EBRT to patients at high risk of recurrence in the neck. This must be done in consultation with an experienced thyroid surgeon. Recurrence in regional nodes should usually be managed by surgical resection. However, similar to the philosophy used in patients with DTC, if there is extensive ETE and surgical resection of recurrent disease would result in significant morbidity, EBRT should be considered with the proviso that there remains a high risk of distant relapse and risk of long-term side effects of EBRT. In patients with gross residual disease that cannot be resected, given the high likelihood of distant metastases, primary treatment with targeted therapy (eg, vandetanib) may be considered first, reserving EBRT for subsequent recurrent or persistent disease (Figure 29–1) demonstrates a case example of a patient with MTC who was treated with surgery followed by external beam radiation therapy.

Anaplastic Thyroid Cancer

Given the poor prognosis of patients with ATC the TNM staging is somewhat unusual in that all patients are stage IV regardless of initial disease extent. This section will focus on the management of stage IVA (eg, patients without distant

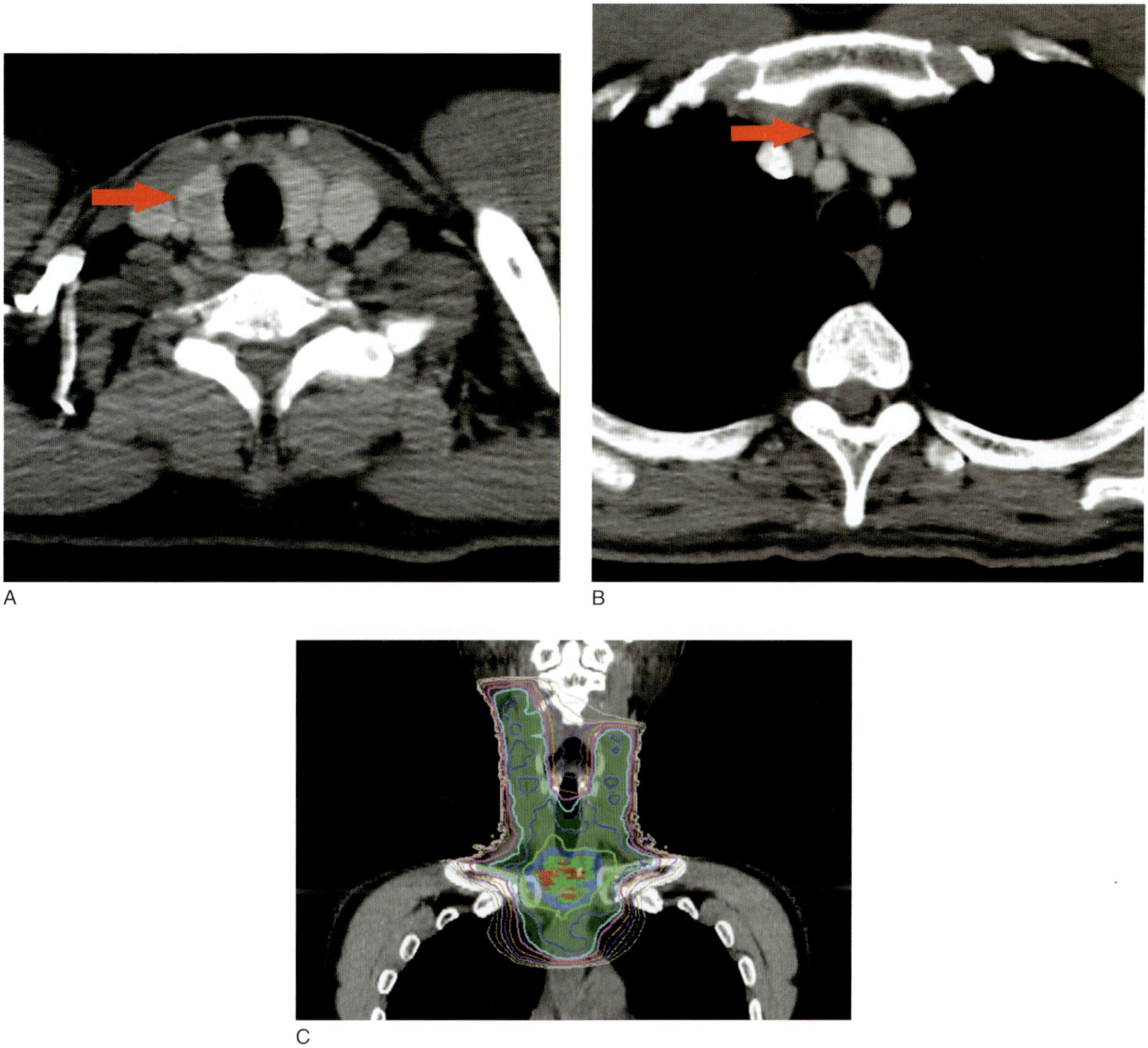

▲ **Figure 29–1.** **(A)** Axial CT image demonstrating the primary thyroid cancer (red arrow). **(B)** Axial CT image demonstrating the enlarged mediastinal node (red arrow). **(C)** Coronal view of the radiation treatment plan. 60 Gy was delivered to the microscopic residual disease in the upper mediastinum and 54 Gy to the resected neck volumes without presumed microscopic residual disease. Note the radiation volume extends more superiorly on the ipsilateral neck as there was more extensive nodal involvement on that side at the time of original surgery.

metastases [DM]) and IVB disease. Given the poor prognosis of patients with ATC, the ATA guidelines strongly recommend five principles that should be followed in determining a treatment approach:[23]

1. The wishes/directives of the patients
2. The fitness of the patient (performance status, comorbidities)
3. The availability of treatment approaches
4. The existence of an experienced treatment team
5. Detailed discussions of the patient's willingness to accept the risks, toxicities, and demands of an aggressive therapeutic treatment

Prior to the introduction of dabrafenib and trametinib (D&T) for patients with *BRAF*V600E (BRAF)-mutated ATC, treatment options were limited. Surgery was reserved for patients with localized resectable disease and EBRT for patients with unresectable disease confined to the neck. The response rate to D&T in patients with BRAF-mutated ATC has changed the treatment paradigm. The ATA guidelines for the management of ATC are based on the resectability of the tumor, presence of a BRAF mutation, and availability of treatment with D&T (which, depending on location, may not be available).

A. Patients With Anaplastic Thyroid Cancer, Stage IVA

Patients with stage IVA tumors often have ATC diagnosed as an incidental finding on pathological assessment of a DTC. If the ATC is incidental and confined to the thyroid, the prognosis is significantly better than for other patients with ATC. The role of additional treatment after resection is controversial. The original ATA guidelines reached a consensus (with one dissenter) that there was no evidence to support further treatment. The 2021 updated guidelines, however, recommend that patients with incidental stage IVA ATC should be managed the same way as others with an R0 resection.[23] Despite that, if there is no ETE and surgical margins are negative, it can be argued that distant relapse is a greater risk than LR and that these patients can forgo EBRT. The NCCN guidelines suggest that this decision can be individualized and highlight the importance of considering patient wishes, fitness for treatment, and particular risk factors. In any discussion of the management of ATC, it is essential that the patients are fully informed of the risks and potential benefits of any treatment, given the generally poor prognosis of these patients and the importance of maintaining a good quality of life. If EBRT is recommended, the treatment would be similar to treatment for IVB disease as described in the following section.

B. Patients With Anaplastic Thyroid Cancer, Stage IVB

The management of patients with stage IVB ATC depends on two factors: (a) tumor resectability and (b) BRAF status. There are no data to support a preoperative approach in resectable tumors with standard chemoradiation, and if an experienced thyroid or head and neck surgeon determines that the tumor is resectable then the patient should have surgery, as discussed in Chapter 18. Assuming that there is no gross residual disease there is strong evidence from both single institutional studies and national database analyses that multimodality treatment results in better outcomes. The most cited approach is surgery followed by postoperative radiotherapy. The 2021 ATA guidelines recommend triple modality with concurrent chemotherapy and radiation after surgery.[23]

Neoadjuvant D&T has been used in *BRAF*V600E-mutated ATC patients, prior to surgical resection. In a recently published case series, six patients with unresectable disease were treated in this manner: four achieved an R0 resection and two an R1 resection. Five of the six patients received postoperative chemoradiation.[28] This study concluded that for patients with unresectable stage IVB ATC and BRAF mutation initial therapy with D&T may be considered.[24] If BRAF is wild-type, however, or D&T is not available, an aggressive approach including EBRT (either hyperfractionated or with concurrent chemotherapy) is recommended.[25-28]

The ATA guideline cites many small institutional series showing a benefit to multimodality treatment; the most intriguing data, however, come from the Mayo Clinic. In 10 consecutively treated IVA and IVB patients with ATC, Foote et al. reported a median OS of 60 months after surgery and postoperative chemoradiotherapy.[24] In a report on 48 patients with ATC, 30 of whom received multimodality therapy (27 had surgery), the median OS was 21 months. In the 18 patients treated with palliative intent, however, the median survival was only 3.9 months.[29] For patients with stage IVB disease, treated with multimodality therapy, the median OS was 22.4 months suggesting that multimodality treatment (eg, surgery combined with chemoradiation) may be optimal for this subgroup. Of note, a variety of different chemotherapy regimens were used and carboplatin plus paclitaxel was the most administered.

There is a paucity of data comparing surgery and radiation to surgery and chemoradiotherapy. Similarly, there is little evidence on accelerated altered fractionation schedules, which have been used to reduce the overall treatment time and try to overcome the risk of tumor repopulation in a rapidly growing tumor with some reported success. The ATA guidelines state that "cytotoxic chemotherapy involving a taxane (paclitaxel or docetaxel), administered with or without anthracyclines (doxorubicin) or platin (cisplatin or carboplatin), is recommended in patients treated with definitive-intention radiation." It is important to note that the Mayo Clinic multimodality treatment was not without toxicity—60% of patients required hospitalization, most frequently for mucositis, dehydration, and failure to thrive. This is an important consideration when discussing patients who may have a short life expectancy given their diagnosis. Figure 29–2 describes a patient with ATC who received EBRT as part of their overall management.

C. Patients With Anaplastic Thyroid Cancer, Stage IVC

Intensive treatment with a high risk of hospitalization may not be appropriate in patients with stage IVC disease or those with a poor performance status. EBRT alone may be of benefit by controlling local symptoms of pain and bleeding and/or palliating obstructive symptoms. Juror et al. reported a 40% CR rate with an overall response rate (RR) of 82% in terms of symptoms, demonstrating a response to palliative radiotherapy using modest doses. Analyses of NCDB data have suggested a survival benefit from higher doses of EBRT,

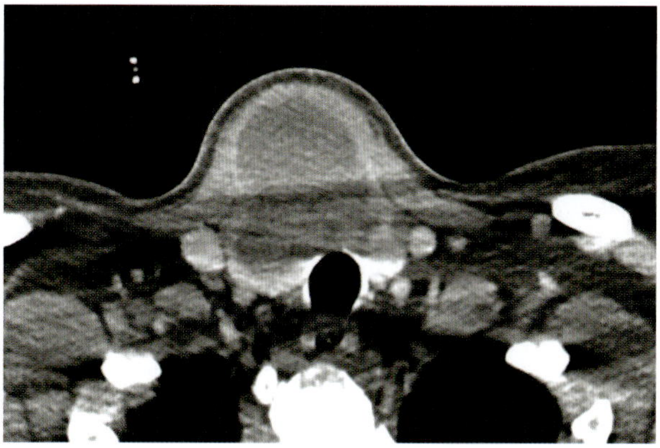

▲ **Figure 29–2.** This figure shows an axial CT slice through the tumor prior to surgery.

exceeding 45 Gy. Unfortunately, response rates and symptom control were not reported, so lower doses that may be well tolerated may have had a good palliative effect as suggested by Juror et al. There is a paucity of data on quality of life in ATC. We recommend palliative radiation in symptomatic patients with poor performance status using doses such as 40 Gy in 10 fractions given as a split course; 2- to 4-week pause after first 20 Gy in five fractions, which if performance status is adequate and no evidence of progression, can be repeated. An alternate regimen to consider is 30 Gy in 10 fractions over 2 weeks.

Palliative External Beam Radiation

A SEER database analysis (1975-2016) identified DM in 2% of DTC thyroid patients at initial diagnosis. The most common metastatic sites were lungs (53.4%), followed by bone (28.1%), liver (8.3%), and brain (4.7%). In patients with MTC and ATC, DM is much more frequently seen. The following section discusses the symptomatic management of metastatic disease with EBRT specifically. The use of RAI and other systemic therapies is discussed elsewhere.

C. Brain Metastases

Brain metastases are rare in patients with thyroid cancers. Historically, the standard treatment has been surgical resection in the presence of a single resectable metastasis or whole brain radiation if widespread disease. The introduction of SBRT, however, has changed the paradigm of management of patients with brain metastases.[30] These patients should be discussed with a multidisciplinary specialized team to determine the most appropriate treatment. The results of SBRT in a multinational consortium identified 42 patients with thyroid cancer brain metastases treated by SBRT—there were no adverse effects and 33% had stable disease, 26% a complete response, and 24% a partial response.

B. Bone Metastases

Compared with lung metastases, bone metastases are less common—it has been estimated that they occur in approximately 4% of thyroid cancer cases at some time in a patient's trajectory. They are more common in ATC and MTC than DTC. There is little evidence to support multifraction radiation over single fraction and the most recent American Society of Therapeutic Radiation Oncology (ASTRO) guidelines support the use of single-fraction radiation for pain relief.[31] EBRT is also recommended after surgery for spinal decompression and after surgery for stabilizing long bone metastases. It is important to remember that thyroid cancer bone metastases are frequently osteolytic and so technetium-99 bone scans are often ineffective in detecting bone metastases.

A. Lung Metastases

Given that lung metastases often have a widespread distribution throughout the lung, the role of EBRT is limited. However, as with metastases from other tumor sites, EBRT can be of benefit in controlling symptoms such as hemoptysis, cough, chest pain, obstructive pneumonia, and dysphagia. There is evidence that higher doses of palliative RT may result in better long-term control but at the expense of more toxicity, such as esophagitis.[32] Doses such as 8 Gy in one fraction, 20 Gy in five fractions, and 30 Gy in 10 fractions are most commonly used for palliation. Higher doses such as 40 Gy in 16 fractions may be used in patients with limited disease and good performance status.

TREATMENT—RADIATION TECHNIQUE

Treatment Planning for EBRT

The goal of EBRT in the treatment of thyroid cancer is to optimize local-regional control while limiting toxicity. Thus, it is important that careful radiation treatment planning is performed, and the potential risk of significant toxicity kept to a minimum, which is aided using modern radiation treatment planning with intensity modulated radiation therapy (IMRT). Radiation planning should be done with simulation including immobilization with a thermoplastic mask to immobilize the head and shoulders. Where available, a preoperative CT with intravenous contrast may aid in radiation treatment planning.

The gross tumor volume (GTV) includes any residual disease; the clinical target volume (CTV) is a 5 mm expansion excluding barriers to spread (eg, bone, air). Our institutional dose is 66 Gy in 33 fractions. The lower risk CTV includes bilateral jugular and posterior cervical lymph nodes from the hyoid to the aortic arch including levels 3, 4, 6, and partial level 5, and receives 56 Gy in 33 fractions. For patients receiving adjuvant EBRT for microscopic residual disease our institutional dose prescriptions are 60 Gy in 30 fractions to the surgical bed and 54 Gy in 30 fractions to the low-risk CTV. Finally, patients with poor performance status who are unable to tolerate 66 Gy can be treated with a dose of 50 Gy in 20 fractions or 40 Gy in 16 fractions.

COMPLICATIONS

Acute & Late Complications of EBRT

Acute and late complications of EBRT are dependent on the volume irradiated and unfortunately, the most significant acute and possible late toxicities to the esophagus, pharynx, larynx, and trachea cannot be avoided as these structures are invariably in the greatest area of concern for recurrence and therefore receive high-dose radiation.[33,34] Other structures of concern where radiation may lead to clinically important radiation toxicity include the mandible (osteoradionecrosis), parotids (xerostomia), and pharyngeal constrictors (dysphagia). The toxicities can potentially be reduced by restricting the volume being irradiated—our institutional treatment volumes are described earlier. An additional consideration is the risk of secondary malignancy, although to our knowledge there are no reports describing this risk following EBRT for thyroid cancer. These are all important considerations when counseling patients about the risks of EBRT. A cross-sectional analysis of 34 patients demonstrated a measurable decrease in head and neck specific quality of life for patients receiving EBRT in addition to thyroidectomy +/− RAI—specifically patients reported decreases in scores for chewing, swallowing, and appetite as wells increased pain.[33] The use of IMRT may help to mitigate some of these toxicities and should be used wherever possible.

Stereotactic Radiation Therapy or Radiosurgery

Stereotactic radiation therapy (SRT) refers to highly conformal or focused radiation that allows either a small number of large fractions (single treatments) of radiation or a single very large fraction of radiation therapy.[35-37] There are a number of different types or names used; these include:

- **Stereotactic radiosurgery (SRS).** SRS usually refers to SRT or radiosurgery to a brain metastases. This may be given by Gamma Knife© radiation.
- **Stereotactic body radiosurgery (SBRS).** SBRS usually refers to radiosurgery to parts of the body other than to the brain (eg, CyberKnife©, X-Knife©).
- **Stereotactic body radiotherapy (SBRT).** SBRT usually refers to highly conformal radiotherapy given in 3 to 10 fractions given by linear accelerator.

SRT has been increasingly used in many cancer types in the setting of a limited number of metastases. In some tumor sites such as limited liver metastases (eg, "oligometastases") from colorectal cancer, ablative treatment with SRT can be curative. Oligometastatic disease, however, is generally not the usual natural history of any of the histological types of thyroid cancer. In most patients in whom widespread metastatic disease is present, such highly focused and high-dose radiation therapy is probably inappropriate given the risk of systemic failure. Conversely, it may have a role in a limited number of thyroid cancer patients with oligometastatic disease. An exception may also be when growth of a very limited number of metastases occurs in the background of widespread metastases (eg, "oligoprogression"). Treating the growing metastases may delay the initiation of or change in systemic therapy. However, there is limited prospective data.

WHEN TO REFER

Given that EBRT is a local therapy, the main aim of treatment is to control local disease. In DTC refer patients for consideration of EBRT if the cancer is unresectable or if the patient has gross residual disease. Refer a patient for consideration of adjuvant RT in older patients (over 55 years) who have gross ETE (especially posteriorly in whom recurrence in that area would not be resectable or would be debilitating). The criteria for referral in MTC are similar; however, given the high risk of metastatic disease in these patients the absolute benefit of EBRT may be less. Finally, all ATC patients should be discussed in a multidisciplinary environment that includes radiation oncology.

For patients with metastatic disease, consider referral of all patients with brain metastases (unless they are being assessed in a dedicated multidisciplinary brain metastasis clinic). Refer symptomatic bone and lung metastases. Finally, consider referral for patients with oligoprogressive disease to delay the start of or change systemic therapy and asymptomatic patients who may shortly become symptomatic with further progression of the metastases.

Case Example—Medullary Thyroid Cancer (Figure 29–1)

A 42-year-old man presents with a mass in his thyroid and biopsy shows MTC. He undergoes a thyroidectomy as well as central and bilateral neck dissection at a high-volume thyroid center. His calcitonin falls but remains high. Further imaging shows an enlarged node in his upper mediastinum but no evidence of other metastases. He has a sternotomy and is found to have an enlarged node invading the thymus and adherent to the innominate vein. The node is subsequently dissected off the vein with presumed residual microscopic residual disease. His case is discussed at a multidisciplinary case conference and radiation is recommended to prevent relapse. He receives 60 Gy in 30 fractions to the region of the mediastinal node and 54 Gy in 30 fractions to the thyroid bed and nodal regions. Nine years later, this patient remains disease free but his calcitonin remains mildly elevated at 24 pmol/L.

Case Example—Anaplastic Thyroid Cancer (Figure 29–2)

A 54-year-old man presented with a rapidly growing thyroid mass, FNA-suggested papillary thyroid carcinoma. At surgery there was evidence of gross extrathyroid extension and invasion of strap muscles. Final pathology showed a mixed thyroid cancer that was primarily anaplastic (85%) with a smaller differentiated component (15%). Further investigations including a PET scan showed no evidence of residual or distant disease. On discussion with the patient, he declined chemotherapy and received EBRT alone. He remains well with no evidence of locally recurrent or distant metastatic disease 18 months after his surgery.

Case Example—Palliative Radiation (Figure 29–3)

Approximately 12 years ago, a 69-year-old man had a total thyroidectomy for a 2.2 cm oncocytic (Hürthle cell) follicular carcinoma with multiple nodes involved. Postoperatively, he received 150 mCi RAI-131. His stimulated thyroglobulin was 65 µg/L with negative antibodies. Post-RAI scan demonstrated uptake in the lumbar spine and faint uptake near his right acetabulum. MRI and CT confirmed the spine lesion but there were no abnormalities noted in the acetabulum. He remained on follow-up and 1 year later, received a further 200 mCi RAI; again, uptake was seen in both the spine and acetabulum. Another year later, an MRI suggested mild progression in the lumbar spine and so he was treated with EBRT (30 Gy in 10 fractions). He remained well for several years but then developed right hip pain; his thyroglobulin rose to 1300. Imaging showed stability of his lumbar spine but now there was an obvious lytic and soft tissue lesion in his acetabulum. He was considered for SBRT but as 30 Gy in 10 fractions had controlled his spinal disease 10 years prior, he was given 30 Gy in 10 fractions to the acetabular lesion as well. Three years later he is pain free and his thyroglobulin has fallen to 300.

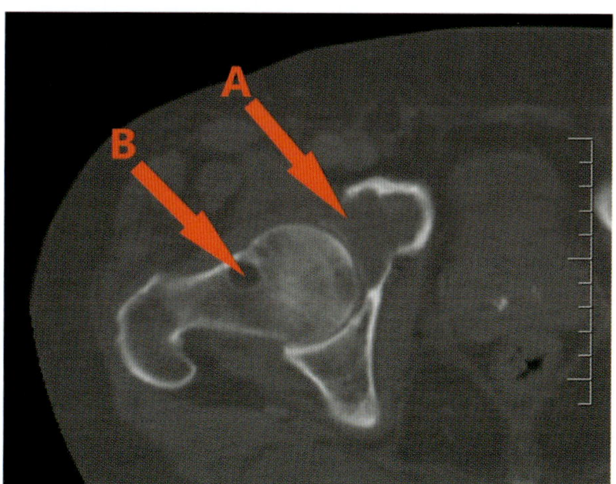

Figure 29–3. Red arrow shows lytic lesion with soft tissue involvement, second arrow shows incidental additional lytic lesion in femoral neck.

REFERENCES

1. Haugen BR, Alexander EK, Bible KC, et al. 2015 American Thyroid Association Management Guidelines for Adult Patients with Thyroid Nodules and Differentiated Thyroid Cancer: The American Thyroid Association Guidelines Task Force on Thyroid Nodules and Differentiated Thyroid Cancer. *Thyroid*. 2016;26:1-133.
2. Mitchell AL, Gandhi A, Scott-Coombes D, Perros P. Management of thyroid cancer: United Kingdom National Multidisciplinary Guidelines. *J Laryngol Otolog*. 2016;130:S150-S160.
3. Kiess AP, Agrawal N, Brierley JD, et al. External-beam radiotherapy for differentiated thyroid cancer locoregional control: a statement of the American Head and Neck Society. *Head Neck*. 2016;38:493-498.
4. Biermann M, Pixberg M, Riemann B, et al. Clinical outcomes of adjuvant external-beam radiotherapy for differentiated thyroid cancer: results after 874 patient-years of follow-up in the MSDS-trial. *Nuklearmedizin*. 2009;48:89-98; quiz N15.
5. Brierley J, Tsang R, Panzarella T, Bana N. Prognostic factors and the effect of treatment with radioactive iodine and external beam radiation on patients with differentiated thyroid cancer seen at a single institution over 40 years. *Clin Endocrinol*. 2005;63:418-427.
6. Farahati J, Reiners C, Stuschke M, et al. Differentiated thyroid cancer. Impact of adjuvant external radiotherapy in patients with perithyroidal tumor infiltration (stage pT4). *Cancer*. 1996;77:172-180.
7. Chow SM, Law SC, Mendenhall WM, et al. Papillary thyroid carcinoma: prognostic factors and the role of radioiodine and external radiotherapy. *Int J Radiat Oncol Biol Phys*. 2002;52:784-795.
8. Sun XS, Sun SR, Guevara N, et al. Indications of external beam radiation therapy in non-anaplastic thyroid cancer and impact of innovative radiation techniques. *Crit Rev Oncol Hematol*. 2013;86:52-68.
9. Servagi Vernat S, Khalifa J, Sun XS, et al. 10-Year locoregional control with postoperative external beam radiotherapy in patients with locally advanced high-risk non-anaplastic thyroid carcinoma de novo or at relapse, a propensity score analysis. *Cancers*. 2019;11(6):849.
10. Fussey JM, Crunkhorn R, Tedla M, Weickert MO, Mehanna H. External beam radiotherapy in differentiated thyroid carcinoma: a systematic review. *Head Neck*. 2016;38(Suppl 1): E2297-E2305.
11. Dicuonzo S, Pedretti S, Mangoni M, et al. Adjuvant radiotherapy and radioiodine treatment for locally advanced differentiated thyroid cancer: systematic review and meta-analysis. *Tumori*. 2021:107:489-497.
12. Tam S, Amit M, Boonsripitayanon M, et al. Adjuvant external beam radiotherapy in locally advanced differentiated thyroid cancer. *JAMA Otolaryngol Head Neck Surg*. 2017;143:1244-1251.
13. Sheline GE, Galante M, Lindsay S. Radiation therapy in the control of persistent thyroid cancer. *Am J Roentgenol Radium Ther Nucl Med*. 1966;97:923-930.
14. Brierley JD, Tsang RW. External radiation therapy in the treatment of thyroid malignancy. *Endocrinol Metab Clin North Am*. 1996;25:141-157.
15. Chow SM, Yau S, Kwan CK, Poon PC, Law SC. Local and regional control in patients with papillary thyroid carcinoma: specific indications of external radiotherapy and radioactive iodine according to T and N categories in AJCC 6th edition. *Endocr Relat Cancer*. 2006;13:1159-1172.

16. Azrif M, Slevin NJ, Sykes AJ, Swindell R, Yap BK. Patterns of relapse following radiotherapy for differentiated thyroid cancer: implication for target volume delineation. *Radiother Oncol.* 2008; 89:105-113.
17. Schwartz DL, Lobo MJ, Ang KK, et al. Postoperative external beam radiotherapy for differentiated thyroid cancer: outcomes and morbidity with conformal treatment. *Int J Radiat Oncol Biol Phys.* 2009;74:1083-1091.
18. Rosenbluth BD, Serrano V, Happersett L, et al. Intensity-modulated radiation therapy for the treatment of nonanaplastic thyroid cancer. *Int J Radiat Oncol Biol Phys.* 2005;63: 1419-1426.
19. Groen AH, Beckham TH, Links TP, et al.; other Group/Consortium Members. Outcomes of surgery and postoperative radiation therapy in managing medullary thyroid carcinoma. *J Surg Oncol.* 2019:10.1002.
20. Jin M, Megwalu UC, Noel JE. External beam radiotherapy for medullary thyroid cancer following total or near-total thyroidectomy. *Otolaryngol Head Neck Surg.* 2021;164(1): 97-103.
21. Rowell NP. The role of external beam radiotherapy in the management of medullary carcinoma of the thyroid: a systematic review. *Radiother Oncol.* 2019;136:113-120.
22. Wells SA Jr, Asa SL, Dralle H, et al. Revised American Thyroid Association guidelines for the management of medullary thyroid carcinoma. *Thyroid.* 2015;25(6):567-610.
23. Bible KC, Kebebew E, Brierley J, et al. 2021 American Thyroid Association Guidelines for management of patients with anaplastic thyroid cancer. *Thyroid.* 2021;31(3):337-386.
24. Foote RL, Molina JR, Kasperbauer JL, et al. Enhanced survival in locoregionally confined anaplastic thyroid carcinoma: a single-institution experience using aggressive multimodal therapy. *Thyroid.* 2011;21(1):25-30.
25. Junor EJ, Paul J, Reed NS. Anaplastic thyroid carcinoma: 91 patients treated by surgery and radiotherapy. *Eur J Surg Oncol.* 1992;18(2):83-88.
26. Prasongsook N, Kumar A, Chintakuntlawar AV, et al. Survival in response to multimodal therapy in anaplastic thyroid cancer. *J Clin Endocrinol Metab.* 2017;102(12):4506-4514.
27. Subbiah V, Kreitman RJ, Wainberg ZA, et al. Dabrafenib and trametinib treatment in patients with locally advanced or metastatic BRAF V600-mutant anaplastic thyroid cancer. *J Clin Oncol.* 2018;36(1):7-13.
28. Wang JR, Zafereo ME, Dadu R, et al. Complete surgical resection following neoadjuvant dabrafenib plus trametinib in BRAF(V600E)-mutated anaplastic thyroid carcinoma. *Thyroid.* 2019;29(8):1036-1043.
29. Wang Y, Tsang R, Asa S, Dickson B, Arenovich T, Brierley J. Clinical outcome of anaplastic thyroid carcinoma treated with radiotherapy of once- and twice-daily fractionation regimens. *Cancer.* 2006;107(8):1786-1792.
30. Bunevicius A, Fribance S, Pikis S, et al. Stereotactic radiosurgery for differentiated thyroid cancer brain metastases: an international, multicenter study. *Thyroid.* 2021;31(8):1244-1252.
31. Lutz S, Balboni T, Jones J, et al. Palliative radiation therapy for bone metastases: update of an ASTRO Evidence-Based Guideline. *Pract Radiat Oncol.* 2017;7(1):4-12.
32. Rodrigues G, Videtic GM, Sur R, et al. Palliative thoracic radiotherapy in lung cancer: an American Society for Radiation Oncology evidence-based clinical practice guideline. *Pract Radiat Oncol.* 2011;1(2):60-71.
33. Gal TJ, Streeter M, Burris J, et al. Quality of life impact of external beam radiotherapy for advanced thyroid carcinoma. *Thyroid.* 2013;23(1):64-69.
34. Schwartz DL, Lobo MJ, Ang KK, et al. Postoperative external beam radiotherapy for differentiated thyroid cancer: outcomes and morbidity with conformal treatment. *Int J Radiat Oncol Biol Phys.* 2009;74(4):1083-1091.
35. Chan M, Palma D, Barry A, et al. Practical considerations for the implementation of a stereotactic body radiation therapy program for oligo-metastases. *Adv Radiat Oncol.* 2020;6(1):100499.
36. Cheung P. Stereotactic body radiotherapy for oligoprogressive cancer. *Br J Radiol.* 2016;89:1066.
37. Palma DA, Olson R, Harrow S, et al. Stereotactic ablative radiotherapy for the comprehensive treatment of oligometastatic cancers: long-term results of the SABR-COMET Phase II randomized trial. *J Clin Oncol.* 2020;38(25):2830-2838.

Recurrent Laryngeal Nerve, External Branch of the Superior Laryngeal Nerve, Vagus Nerve, & Intraoperative Nerve Monitoring

30

Whitney Liddy, MD
Justin M. Soffer, MD
Lauren Williams, MD
Amr H. Abdelhamid Ahmed, MBBCH, MMSc
Gregory W. Randolph, MD, FACS

GENERAL CONSIDERATIONS

Thyroid and parathyroid surgeries are thought to be safe with low rates of postoperative complications.[1] However, one of the most significant contributors to postoperative patient morbidity is vocal fold dysfunction, with vocal fold paresis or paralysis (VFP) caused by intraoperative recurrent laryngeal nerve (RLN) injury and more subtle dysfunction caused by injury to the external branch of the superior laryngeal nerve (EBSLN). The overall rate of RLN injury after thyroid surgery has been reported up to 10% but may range as high as 20% in cases of cancer, Graves' disease, and revision thyroidectomy.[2,3] Given its significant potential burden on patient quality of life, RLN injury resulting in VFP remains the leading cause of medicolegal action after thyroid surgery.[4]

Surgical standards for RLN management include comprehensive knowledge of neural anatomy, adequate cervical exposure, and routine intraoperative visualization of nerves at risk along with preoperative and postoperative laryngoscopy.[3,5] The addition of intraoperative neural monitoring (IONM) as a practical tool for neural mapping, detection of neural anatomic variations, identification of mechanisms of neural injury, and predictions of postoperative vocal fold function has gained widespread acceptance in thyroid and parathyroid surgery.[6-12] This chapter represents a comprehensive review of current knowledge in IONM as it relates to thyroid and parathyroid surgery to provide the surgeon with the tools to utilize IONM for safe and effective RLN and EBSLN management.

NEURAL ANATOMY, ANATOMICAL VARIATIONS, & SURGICAL LANDMARKS

To utilize IONM safely and effectively, a comprehensive understanding of expected neural anatomy, potential anatomic variations, and surgical technique for safe dissection of the vagus, EBSLN, and RLN is essential and will be discussed briefly in this section.

Vagus Nerve

The vagus, or tenth cranial nerve, contains a robust array of nerve fibers with various general, visceral, and special sensory functions as well as autonomic and voluntary motor functions throughout the body. Of importance in thyroid and parathyroid surgery, the vagus nerve carries motor and sensory fibers within its terminal branches to striated muscles of the upper aerodigestive tract, including the laryngeal muscles. The vagus descends in the neck within the carotid sheath and is typically located deep to the common carotid artery (CCA) medially and the internal jugular vein (IJV) laterally.

External Branch of the Superior Laryngeal Nerve

The superior laryngeal nerve (SLN) branches from the vagus at the level of the inferior ganglion just below the jugular foramen. It descends posteromedially in relation to the carotid sheath and divides into internal and external branches roughly 2 cm above the superior pole of the thyroid. The more often encountered EBSLN provides motor control to the cricothyroid to tense the vocal folds, which plays an important role in vocal projection and pitch.

The EBSLN courses inferomedially toward the superior thyroid pole just deep to the superior thyroid vessels and terminates on the cricothyroid muscle fibers. The nerve typically crosses the superior thyroid vessels well above the superior pole; however, its course can be variable. Multiple classification systems have been devised to depict the variable relationship of the EBSLN to the superior thyroid pole, with perhaps the most commonly cited being the Cernea classification system (Figure 30–1).[8,13,14] Type 1 nerves, which cross 1 cm or more above the superior thyroid pole, occur in roughly 60% of cases and confer the lowest surgical risk. Conversely, type 2a nerves (crossing <1 cm above the superior pole) are at higher risk, and type 2b nerves (crossing below the superior pole) are at highest risk of injury during superior pole dissection and ligation of the superior thyroid vessels during thyroidectomy.[15]

Techniques for superior pole dissection reported in the literature include (1) ligation of individual branches of the superior thyroid vessels along the thyroid capsule without attempts to identify the nerve,[16] (2) visual identification of the nerve prior to ligation of the superior pole vessels,[17] and (3) the use of IONM for mapping and confirmation of EBSLN identification and function before and after superior pole dissection.[8] As would be expected, type 2b nerves are at particularly high risk during dissection, especially if the EBSLN is not identified.

Recurrent Laryngeal Nerve

As the left and right vagus nerves descend from the neck into the thoracic cavity, they pass anteriorly to the great vessels, where they give off the RLN. The right RLN courses posteriorly around the right subclavian artery and ascends along the floor of the neck at a more oblique angle compared to the left RLN as it tracks in a superomedial direction toward the tracheoesophageal groove. For this reason, the right RLN has a greater variability in trajectory in comparison with the left RLN. The left RLN branches underneath the aortic arch just lateral to the ligamentum arteriosum, where it then ascends in a more vertical 2D course in closer proximity to the tracheoesophageal groove compared to the right RLN. Distally, as the nerve courses toward its laryngeal nerve entry site at the cricothyroid joint, there is significant neural anatomic variation in relation to the intersecting inferior thyroid artery (ITA) and its branches, in addition to the posterior ligament of Berry (LOB). Extralaryngeal branching of the RLN is very common, with anterior branches most commonly containing the motor fibers to the intrinsic laryngeal muscles (except for the cricothyroid), and posterior branches most commonly providing sensation to the glottic and subglottic mucosa. Extralaryngeal branching of the RLN can be missed during surgery, which can result in neural injury.

Terminology for surgical RLN anatomic variation is in accordance with the International RLN Anatomic Classification System (Figure 30–2),[18] which encompasses both expected anatomical trajectories and embryologic/acquired

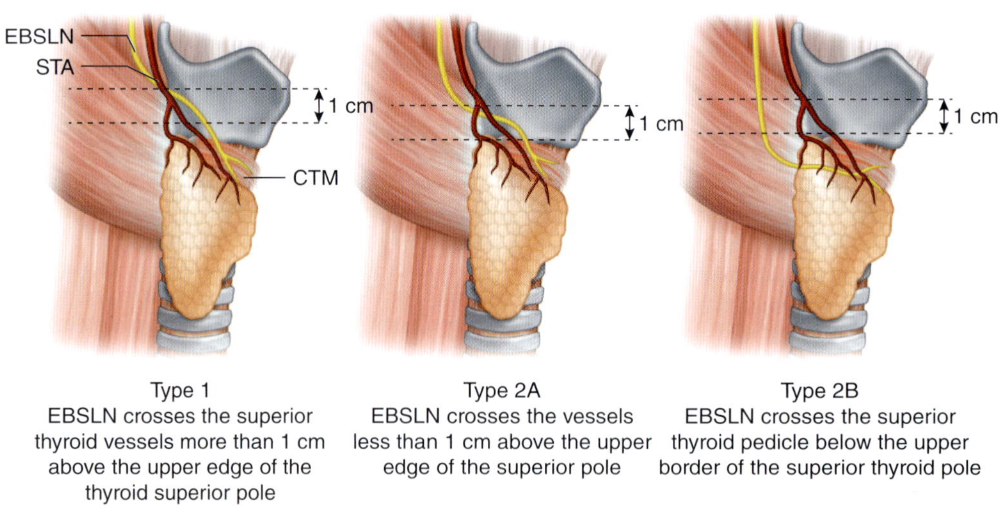

Figure 30–1. Cernea classification of the external branch of the superior laryngeal nerve (EBSLN).[8] (Reproduced with permission from Barczyński M, Randolph GW, Cernea CR, et al. External branch of the superior laryngeal nerve monitoring during thyroid and parathyroid surgery: International Neural Monitoring Study Group standards guideline statement. *Laryngoscope*. 2013;123(Suppl 4):S1-S14.)

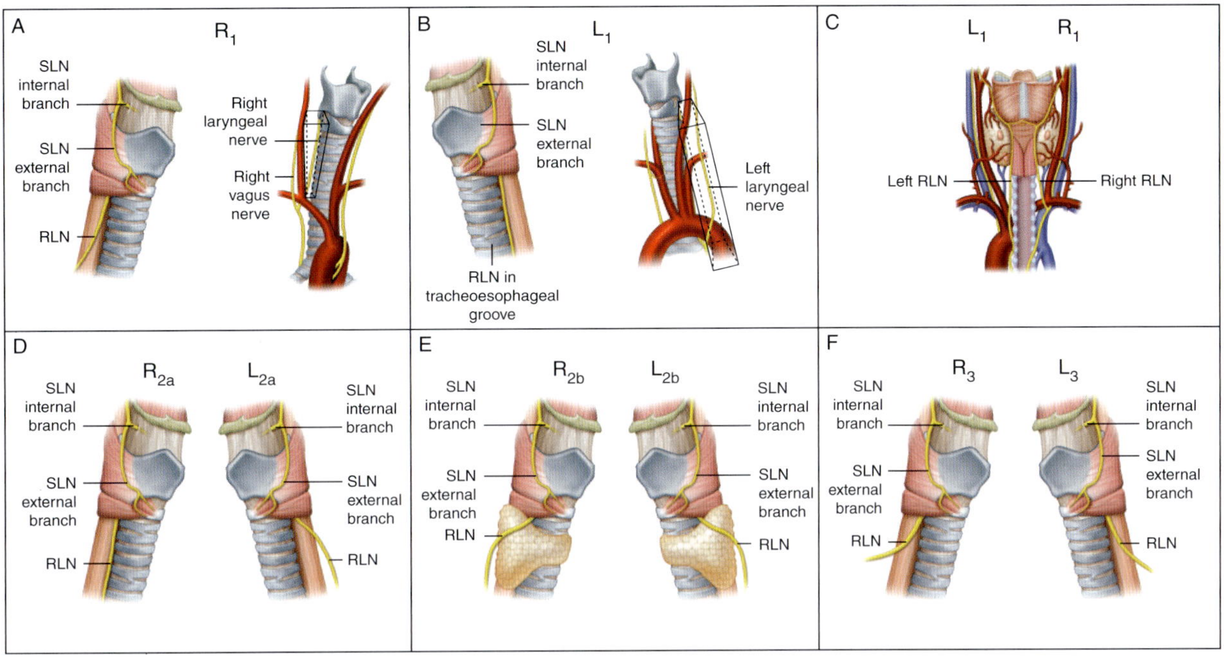

Normal trajectory - L_1: The left RLN travels parallel or at an angle less than 30 degrees relative to the tracheoesophageal groove (TEG); R_1: The right RLN travels at an angle between 15 and 45 degrees relative to the TEG. *Acquired variation* - L_{2a} (lateral nerve displacement): The left RLN travels at an angle greater than 30 degrees relative to the TEG; R_{2a} (medial nerve displacement): The right RLN travels at an angle less than 15 degrees relative to the TEG; L_{2b} (ventral nerve displacement): Ventral displacement of the left RLN; R_{2b} (ventral nerve displacement): Ventral displacement of the right RLN. *Embryologic variation* - L_3: Nonrecurrent left RLN; R_3: Nonrecurrent right RLN.

▲ **Figure 30–2.** The International RLN Anatomic Classification System.[18] (Reproduced with permission from Randolph GW, Wu CW, Dionigi G, et al. The international RLN anatomic classification system. Chapter 12. In: Randolph GW, ed. *The Recurrent and Superior Laryngeal Nerves*. Springer; 2016.)

sources of. Nerves are characterized based on trajectory as well as clinically important neural features. Our current understanding of the estimated prevalence of RLN anatomical variation is based on several multicenter international registry studies. The surgical anatomy of the RLN (SAR) study conducted through the INMSG, for example, included neural anatomical mapping, electromyography (EMG) and loss of signal (LOS) data, mechanisms of neural injury, and postoperative outcomes data related to 1000 RLNs at risk during thyroidectomy in 574 patients across 17 centers.[19]

- Characterization of RLN variants based on trajectory: Trajectory of the RLN can be along the expected “normal” course (L1/R1) or can be described as abnormal-acquired (either ventrally, medially, or laterally displaced by thyroid disease) or abnormal embryologic (ie, nonrecurrent). Normal RLN trajectory is present in 77% of RLNs at risk, as reported in the SAR study.[19] The most common variant trajectories encountered are abnormal-acquired left RLNs that are laterally displaced (L2a) and medially displaced right RLNs (R2a), which can be seen in the setting of large goiters or paratracheal nodal disease.[18,19] Abnormal RLN trajectory has been identified as a significant risk factor for RLN injury.[19]
- Characterization of RLN variants based on neural features: The nerve can be fixed, splayed, or entrapped by the thyroid capsule or associated vessels, directly invaded by tumor, or entrapped by the LOB. In addition, there can be extralaryngeal branching or thin neural caliber (<1 mm). Dynamic elements such as loss of intraoperative EMG signal and extensive intraoperative nerve dissection are also included in the classification scheme due to their functional significance.[18]

There are several useful landmarks for RLN identification that may help in cases of embryologic or acquired variation. The RLN can be found within Simon’s triangle, which refers to the anatomic space bordered by the esophagus medially, the CCA laterally, and the ITA superiorly. Within this space, the nerve will ultimately intersect the ITA either medial/posterior (75.6%), lateral/anterior (17.4%), or between branches of the ITA near the vessel’s trunk (7%).[20]

In 93% of cases, the RLN can be found medial to the tubercle of Zuckerkandl.[21] In addition, the RLN may be identified within 3 mm of the LOB, which is also the most common location for extralaryngeal branching.[22,23] If identification of the RLN using the typical landmarks proves challenging, a nonrecurrent laryngeal nerve should be suspected.

NEURAL INJURY

Epidemiology & Clinical Presentation

Iatrogenic injury to the RLN resulting in postoperative VFP is one of the most feared complications of thyroid surgery and represents the leading cause of medicolegal action following the procedure.[24,25] A review of 27 articles and 25,000 patients who underwent thyroidectomy showed that the average incidence of temporary postoperative VFP was 9.8% and the incidence of permanent VFP was 2.3%.[26] However, high-risk thyroidectomy cases such as Graves' disease, cancer resection, and revision surgery have been associated with a rate of RLN injury of up to 20%.[2,3] Unilateral RLN palsy may cause postoperative voice changes such as a hoarse or breathy voice, vocal fatigue, dysphagia, and aspiration, as the degree of symptoms depends on the resting position of the vocal fold. Laryngoscopy and videostroboscopy findings reveal weakness or immobility of the affected vocal fold and incomplete glottic closure on phonation due to lateralized position of the vocal fold (Figure 30–3).[27,28] Bilateral VFP is an exceedingly rare but potentially life-threatening complication due to airway compromise,[29] and patients typically present shortly after extubation with stridor, persistent tachypnea, and progressive hypoxia. Many of these patients will require urgent airway intervention such as tracheostomy shortly after extubation.[30]

The rate of EBSLN injury after thyroidectomy is highly variable as reported in the literature, reaching as high as 58% of patients.[31] It is considered to be an extremely underestimated complication of thyroidectomy given that many individuals with EBSLN paralysis have minimal symptoms. However, female patients and voice professionals may experience symptomatic voice changes such as vocal fatigue, difficulty to phonate at high-frequency tones, and overall lowered vocal pitch.[13] Laryngoscopy and videostroboscopy findings are very subtle, which further makes the diagnosis challenging by physical exam. Generally, the most noticeable finding is an asymmetric mucosal wave, although clinicians may also detect bowing of the affected vocal fold, posterior glottic rotation toward the side of paralysis, and inferior vocal fold displacement.[32]

Laryngeal EMG is the gold standard to determine the integrity of either the RLN or EBSLN, as well as to differentiate VFP from cricoarytenoid joint injury if the etiology is unclear. However, this procedure is more invasive and less frequently performed.

Risk Factors, Pathophysiology, & Mechanisms of Neural Injury

A thorough understanding of the risk factors for nerve injury as well as the underlying pathophysiology associated with different degrees and mechanisms of nerve injury is important for the surgeon to minimize the risk of harm to the laryngeal nerves during surgery. IONM is an important adjunctive technique to assist the surgeon in a better understanding of some of these key principles.

A. Risk Factors for Nerve Injury

Preoperative risk factors of nerve injury are important to identify for safe and effective intraoperative RLN and EBSLN management. Some examples that have been suggested in the literature include age more than 70 years, diabetes, goiter, previous thyroidectomy, or anterior neck surgery; other risk factors related to operative extent include larger resections and longer operative times.[33-36] Anatomical risk factors that cannot be identified preoperatively also contribute to the risk of nerve injury, which supports the routine use of IONM. Among injured RLNs identified with IONM, there have been higher rates of abnormal trajectory, fixation along the

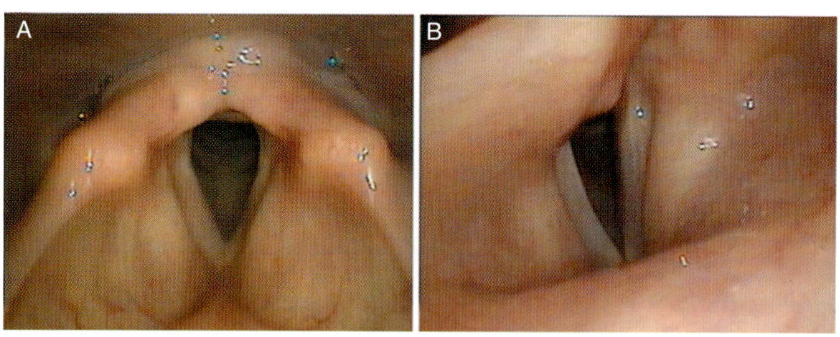

Figure 30–3. Flexible laryngoscopy. **(A)** Symmetric abduction of the vocal folds. **(B)** Unilateral paralysis of the right true vocal fold, demonstrating vocal fold bowing and foreshortening as well as arytenoid medial prolapse.[27] (Reproduced with permission from *The Recurrent and Superior Laryngeal Nerves*, Chapter 2, Randolph GW, Ed, copyright © Springer Nature, Sinclair 2016.)

thyroid capsule and entrapment at the LOB. More extensive neural dissection and invasion of the nerve by cancer also increase the risk nerve injury.[19]

B. Pathophysiology of Neural Injury

Injury to the nerve axon results in a disturbance in electrical conduction at the site of injury. From about 24 hours until 3 to 4 days after injury, Wallerian degeneration occurs in which the myelin sheath is degraded and macrophages infiltrate around the nerve fibers to facilitate nerve regeneration. Because this process has not yet begun immediately following intraoperative nerve injury, electrical stimulation distal to the site of injury will elicit an EMG signal, whereas stimulation proximal to the injury site (ie, away from the larynx) will not. IONM takes advantage of this phenomenon for injury site localization in the setting of segmental (focal) nerve injuries.[10,37,38]

The degree of nerve injury is typically classified by microscopic and electromyographic changes using a system that was first introduced by Dr. Sydney Sunderland in 1951.[39] First-degree injury, or neuropraxia, is defined as a block in electrical conduction due to local myelin damage but without injury to the axon itself. This type of injury is typically caused by traction to the nerve and results in temporary nerve dysfunction with good recovery. However, second- through fifth-degree injuries, which involve injury to the axon sheath components (ie, endoneurium, perineurium, epineurium, or complete transection), are more likely to result in permanent neural dysfunction.[40]

C. Mechanisms of Neural Injury

The most common mechanism of injury resulting in intraoperative LOS in thyroid and parathyroid surgery is traction, which ranges from 63% to 93% of all RLN injuries.[10,19,40,41] This most commonly occurs during RLN dissection distally near the LOB.[40,42] Schneider et al. showed that almost all patients with RLN traction injuries have recovery of vocal fold mobility in 2 to 3 months, while Liddy et al. demonstrated (in a smaller number of injured nerves) that 82% with LOS from traction experienced postoperative VFP with only 61% having recovery of VF function by 12 months.[19,43] Brooks & Ahmed et al. reported that in the cases of RLNs invaded by thyroid carcinomas, segmental LOS (type 1) was documented in 90% compared to 10% for global LOS (type 2).[44] Other mechanisms of neural injury include thermal injury, nerve compression or "crush injury," clamping, ligature entrapment, suction-related injury, and rare transection injuries. Transection rates are likely much higher in the case of the EBSLN, where surgeons less frequently visualize the nerve as part of routine superior pole dissection. In cases of neural injury without a clear mechanism or injury, and often in cases of "global" injury where a focal site of injury cannot be identified, vascular compromise of the nerve may play a role. Though ischemia as an etiology is difficult to confirm, it is thought that circumferentially skeletonizing a nerve may contribute.[18]

Treatment Options

When a nerve injury is identified intraoperatively, immediate maneuvers to mitigate the source of injury should be performed, if able, such as the release of tension on the nerve or removal of a clip or ligature. In the rare case of complete transection of the nerve intraoperatively, tension-free direct nerve anastomosis using microsurgical technique should be considered. If this cannot be achieved, alternative options for repair include most commonly ansa cervicalis-to-RLN anastomosis but also free nerve grafting to fill the defect (ansa cervicalis or supraclavicular, transverse cervical, or greater auricular nerves) and vagus-to-RLN anastomosis, which can yield similar results to that of direct neurorrhaphy.[45,46]

Management of unilateral postoperative VFP can be treated with voice therapy as an initial conservative management approach and/or vocal fold augmentation via injection laryngoplasty with fat, collagen, or calcium hydroxyapatite, which serves to medialize the true vocal fold and close the glottic gap.[9,47] A more permanent alteration of the laryngeal framework is open medialization laryngoplasty, or type I thyroplasty, which involves placement of a Silastic implant or Gore-tex lateral to the vocal fold via a window cut into the thyroid cartilage. This procedure can be accompanied by adduction arytenopexy if there is a large gap or vertical height discrepancy between the immobile and mobile fold.[48]

In the acute setting of postoperative bilateral VFP, some authors advocate for a 24 to 36 hour period of intubation with intravenous corticosteroids followed by a repeat trial of extubation.[49] Should the patient decompensate, tracheostomy is required. Long-term therapies for bilateral VFP include laryngeal framework procedures such as vocal cordotomy; however, these typically lead to poor voice outcomes.[50] Reinnervation procedures are an emerging technique for treating bilateral VFP, although outcomes are variable and are frequently complicated by laryngeal synkinesis.[51]

INTERMITTENT INTRAOPERATIVE NERVE MONITORING

Historical Perspective

While routine use of IONM in thyroid surgery has only recently become widespread in practice, the principles of nerve identification, preservation, and electrical monitoring have been around for much longer. The foundation of electrophysiology and neuromonitoring stems from Luigi Galvani's discovery of the role of bioelectricity in muscular function in 1782.[52] His work was carried on by Emil Du Bois-Reymond in 1848 with the first recording and accurate description of an action potential.[53] The primitive peripheral nerve stimulators used by Guillaume-Benjamin Duchenne and Wilhelm Erb to diagnose Erb-Duchenne palsy, isolate the muscles of facial expression, and identify Erb's point actually resemble modern techniques of nerve stimulation during head and neck surgery.[54-56]

Perioperative nerve assessment using bipolar electrical stimulation was first documented in 1963 by Sir Terence Cawthorne, who demonstrated a relationship between the electrical conduction of the facial nerve following acoustic neuroma surgery with postoperative recovery of nerve function.[57] However, the first intraoperative use of neuromonitoring in history is considered to be by Wilder Penfield, who mapped a patient's cerebral cortex during epilepsy surgery.[58] Since the advent of modern IONM technology, its use has expanded tremendously across surgical fields.

Dr. Frank Lahey (Boston) and Dr. Victor Riddell (London) are credited as the earliest major advocates for routine identification of the RLN during thyroid surgery. They demonstrated a significant decrease in the rate of RLN injury and resultant VFP with intraoperative visual identification of the nerve.[59,60] The use of neuromonitoring to aid in RLN identification did not emerge until much later in the 20th century. One early method of nerve assessment used an endotracheal (ET) tube with a balloon connected to a pressure-recording system, which showed changes upon electrical stimulation.[61] Despite the various methods of RLN monitoring developed and reported in the literature (ie, laryngeal palpation, glottic observation, glottic pressure monitoring, endoscopically placed intramuscular vocal cord electrodes, postcricoid surface electrodes),[7] the use of an ET tube-based system with surface electrodes in conjunction with a monopolar nerve stimulator probe is by far the most widely accepted modality. This is because it can be incorporated into thyroid surgical procedures with relative ease and without additional invasive instrumentation.

Basic Electrophysiology

The general concept of all methods of IONM is to provide electrical stimulation to a nerve and observe whether a response is generated by the target muscle. A nerve of interest may either be stimulated intermittently by a handheld electrode probe, or at certain temporal increments, as will be discussed later in this chapter with continuous IONM. When electricity is applied directly to the nerve, it generates an impulse that is transmitted to the target muscle, thereby producing a myoelectric signal which can be detected with EMG.[62]

The biphasic waveform produced with EMG is characterized by three metrics: amplitude, latency, and threshold. Amplitude, defined as the height of the waves, is dependent on the number of activated muscle fibers. Latency, defined as the time between stimulation to EMG waveform detection, is affected by nerve conduction velocity as well as distance from the point of stimulus to the target muscle (ie, thyroarytenoid-vocalis muscle complex). Threshold is defined as the current in milli-amperes (mA) that will first trigger a recognizable EMG waveform when applied to a nerve. Figure 30–4[63] shows an example of how an evoked EMG waveform of the RLN appears on the neuromonitoring display. There are normative amplitudes, latencies, and thresholds for right and left RLN, EBSLN, and vagus nerves, which can be helpful in distinguishing where an EMG waveform is coming from.

General Setup

The vast majority of neuromonitoring systems utilize an ET tube-based recording system that detects EMG activity from the thyroarytenoid-vocalis muscle complex, in conjunction with intermittent electrical stimulation. A visual schematic of the recording/stimulating components is demonstrated in Figure 30–5.[7] Components of the stimulating end include a handheld stimulator probe, a grounding electrode, and connections to the interface box. The recording components consist of an ET tube with surface electrodes, ground electrodes, connections to the interface box, and an audiovisual monitor. Monitoring systems are broadly categorized into audio only or audio and visual systems. An advantage of audio and visual systems is the ability to monitor the evoked EMG waveform for changes in amplitude, latency, and threshold, which can help distinguish LOS from artifact.

While there is significant variability with respect to the type of recording electrodes used in neuromonitoring systems, the most commonly used are ET tube-based surface electrodes. The confirmation of proper ET tube positioning, which can be aided by the use of a GlideScope or fiber-optic scope at the time of intubation, is critical to ensure that the surface electrodes embedded on the ET tube surface are in contact with both vocal folds. Selection of the properly sized tube, which is typically the largest ET tube tolerated, will also improve electrode-to-glottis contact and impedance.[64] The optimal ET tube positioning is depicted in Figure 30–6.[63] After patient positioning with the neck in final surgical extension, it is important to verify the integrity of the neuromonitoring unit as movement can displace the ET tube sufficiently to lose contact between the electrodes and glottis. Adjunctive tests to help confirm positioning include identification of adequate respiratory variation of the baseline EMG (presence of small waveforms typically 30–70 μV with the patient in a light plane of anesthesia) or the less accurate "tap test" (whereby the thyroid cartilage is tapped on either side with a finger to elicit an EMG response).[65]

Preparing the monitor begins with ensuring that impedance values are less than 5 kΩ per electrode, suggesting good electrode contact with the patient. If impedance is high, the tube may be either slightly displaced or rotated. The threshold is typically set to 1.0 mA but can be set to 2.0 mA if needed—both levels safely above the observed thresholds

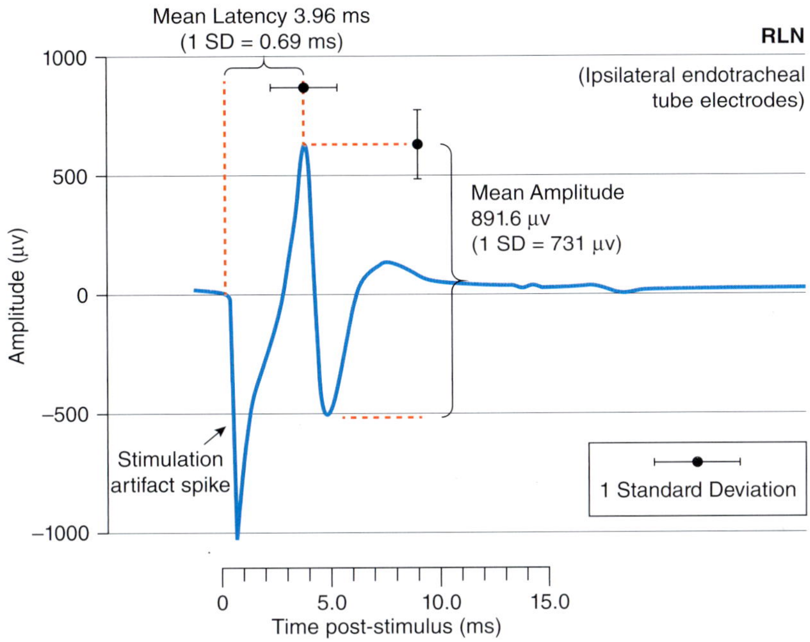

▲ **Figure 30–4.** Depiction of an evoked EMG waveform of the RLN with labeled parameters.[63] (Reproduced with permission from Sritharan N, Chase M, Kamani D, Randolph M, Randolph GW. The vagus nerve, recurrent laryngeal nerve, and external branch of the superior laryngeal nerve have unique latencies allowing for intraoperative documentation of intact neural function during thyroid surgery. *Laryngoscope*. 2015;125[2]:E84-E89.)

for nerve stimulation. One can also choose to set event triggers or thresholds at a certain microvolts (μV) to minimize false-positives; however, caution should be exercised when monitoring the EBSLN as amplitudes can be as low as 100 μV.

Electrical interference can create excessive background noise or artifact that is not only bothersome to the surgeon but may also limit the effectiveness of IONM. It is advised to maintain electrocautery units a minimum distance of 10 feet away from the neural monitoring unit as well as ensure cables/wires are apart and untangled. Cardiac pacemakers do not affect the activity of the EMG monitor.

Anesthetic Considerations

Anesthetic agents can affect various IONM modalities through multiple mechanisms: alteration in synaptic transmission, dampening of cortical and spinal neural processing, and blockade of the lower motor neuron's effect on the neuromuscular junction. Most relevant to IONM of the head and neck is the use of neuromuscular blockade (NMB) and its effect on EMG.

Nondepolarizing agents, which act competitively with acetylcholine for receptor binding, have a duration of action of roughly 1 to 2 hours.[66] For IONM to work correctly, reversal of NMB is required. This can be done with anticholinesterases such as neostigmine, which block the degradation of acetylcholine allowing for increased concentration in the synaptic cleft with more competition with NMB agents, or with Sugammadex, which irreversibly binds to the nondepolarizing NMB agent, thereby removing it from the synaptic cleft.[67-69] Sugammadex is preferred because agents like neostigmine have a poor side effect profile.[68,69]

Conversely, the depolarizing agent succinylcholine, which results in sustained depolarization causing brief fasciculations, has a rapid onset of action and a recovery time of 7 to 12 minutes due to its degradation by plasma cholinesterase.[70] It should be noted that certain genetic mutations of the cholinesterase may prolong the effect of succinylcholine blockade for up to 6 hours.[66]

Standard Procedure

As nerve monitoring becomes increasingly implemented in endocrine and head and neck surgery, along with continued advances in monitoring equipment and increasing literature supporting its use, it is essential that IONM techniques and management protocols are uniform and standardized. The following six steps have been recommended by the 2011 INMSG guidelines as standard operating procedure for the use of IONM in thyroid surgery: (1) preoperative laryngoscopy (L1) to assess vocal cord function before surgery; (2) vagal stimulation before surgical dissection

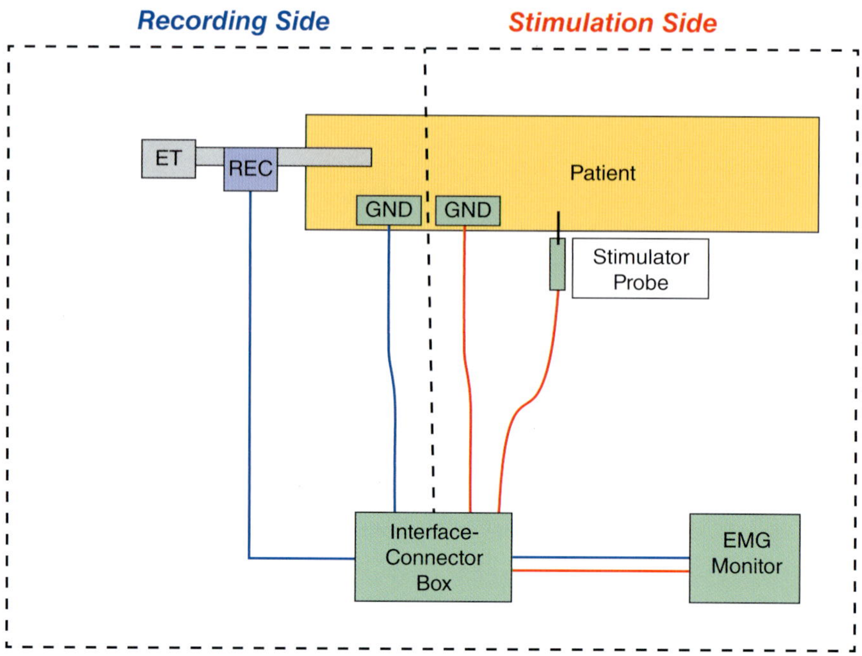

Figure 30–5. Visual schematic of the basic recording/stimulating components of monitoring equipment. EMG = electromyography; ET = endotracheal tube; GND = grounding electrodes; REC = recording electrodes.[7] (Reproduced with permission from Randolph GW, Dralle H, Abdullah H, et al. Electrophysiologic recurrent laryngeal nerve monitoring during thyroid and parathyroid surgery: international standards guideline statement. *Laryngoscope*. 2011;121(1):S1-16.)

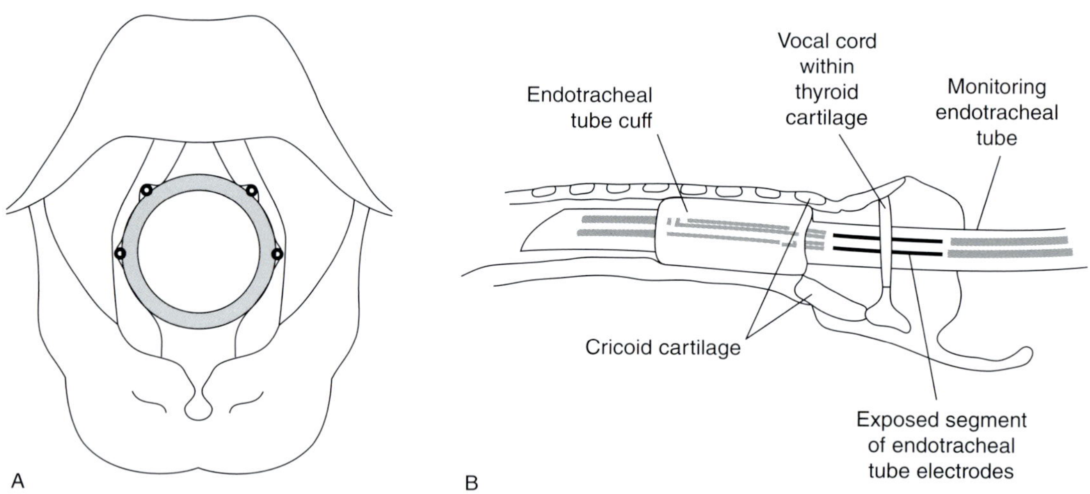

Figure 30–6. **(A)** Endoscopic and **(B)** sagittal cut views of correct endotracheal tube positioning. Note that the parallel lines, representing the surface electrodes, are in contact with the glottis with the endotracheal tube cuff positioned in the subglottis.[63] (Reproduced with permission from Randolph GW, Kamani D, Wu CW, Schneider R. Surgical Anatomy and Monitoring of the Recurrent Laryngeal Nerve. Chapter 36. In: Randolph GW, eds. *Surgery of the Thyroid and Parathyroid Glands*. 3rd ed. Elsevier Saunders; 2021.)

(V1); (3) RLN stimulation at initial identification (R1); (4) RLN stimulation after completion of thyroid dissection and hemostasis (R2); (5) vagal stimulation after completion of thyroidectomy; and (6) postoperative laryngoscopy (L2) to assess vocal fold function after surgery.[7] Of note, vagal stimulation following RLN dissection (V2) was found to be a more reliable predictor of postoperative glottic function than RLN stimulation (R2).[7,71] Vagal stimulation can be done without dissection and direct exposure of the vagal nerve, as stimulation of the carotid sheath between the jugular vein and carotid artery is sufficient.[12]

Contrary to RLN monitoring, IONM of the EBSLN is based not only upon EMG glottic response identified by ET tube-based surface electrodes but also on evaluation of the cricothyroid muscle (CTM) twitch. In fact, while CTM twitch is present in all patients, an electromyographic response is only identified in 70% to 80% of patients when using standard EMG tubes.[8] This improves to essentially 100% of patients with use of ET tubes with more anterior-based electrodes.[72] While the principles of IONM of the RLN described in the International Standards Guideline Statement can be applied to EBSLN stimulation, there are a few modifications.[7,8] The INMSG proposes that the EBSLN should be stimulated both cranial and caudal to the superior pole pedicle prior to ligation of the superior pole vessels with either a positive EMG response or CTM visual twitch. They also recommend stimulation of the pedicle that is to be divided to confirm absence of neural tissue.[8]

Loss of Signal

A. Definitions

The basic criteria for LOS according to the 2011 INMSG guidelines are (1) an EMG change from an initially satisfactory EMG, (2) absence of response or low response to stimulation with a 1 to 2 mA current on a dry field, and (3) absence of laryngeal or glottic twitch.[7] To correctly interpret and diagnose nerve injury, an accurate baseline V1/R1 amplitude reading is essential. More recently, the 2018 INMSG guidelines provided an optimal normative V1/R1 amplitude of greater than 500 μV under a stimulation current of 1 to 2 mA to be obtained prior to thyroid dissection. This is considered a prerequisite for accurate verification of preoperative VFP, intraoperative LOS evaluation, and confirmation of intact RLN integrity following thyroidectomy.[9]

There are five distinct types of events that may be observed following stimulation at each step (ie, V1, R1, R2, V2): stable signal, weak/incomplete LOS, false LOS, LOS type 1, and LOS type 2.[73] Stable signal is defined as improved or unchanged amplitude of R2 and V2 compared to R1 and V1, respectively, indicating normal intraoperative RLN function. Weak or incomplete LOS is defined as a visually intact nerve with a "significant" amplitude reduction, whereby the amplitude at the site of RLN stimulation is still ≥100 μV. Incomplete LOS may indicate a partial or impending nerve injury that may recover intraoperatively; however, it is more commonly identified using continuous methods of IONM, which will be discussed later in this chapter. Of note, significant variability exists among patients with respect to the degree of EMG amplitude reduction and its correlation with postoperative vocal fold function; however, a reduction of 50% or more should increase suspicion for potential postoperative VFP.[74,75] True complete LOS has been more recently accepted by the INMSG as a loss of a normal, biphasic waveform of the RLN at supramaximal stimulation with an amplitude of less than 100 μV, when the initial amplitude was at least 500 μV. False LOS, LOS type 1, and LOS type 2 are discussed in further detail in following sections.

B. False Loss of Signal

The case of absent or significantly reduced EMG amplitude in the presence of normal RLN function is considered false LOS. Suspicion of false LOS is confirmed if there is either no EMG response detected upon contralateral vagal stimulation, or laryngeal/glottic twitch is still present on ipsilateral stimulation.[7] There are several possible etiologies of false LOS:

1. ET tube malposition: Vertical or rotatory displacement during surgical or airway manipulation may result in poor contact between the surface electrodes and vocal cords. This is the most common cause of false LOS and can be corrected with simple readjustment of the ET tube until the vagus can be successfully stimulated again.[7] Confirmation of the presence of laryngeal/glottic twitch using fiberoptic laryngoscopy may be necessary in certain cases.[37]
2. Prolonged effect or repeated use of neuromuscular blockade (NMB): Proper anesthetic planning with respect to choice and timing of NMB is crucial, and in the event of LOS, the surgeon should inquire whether NMB agents are still in effect from the anesthesia team. Should this happen, rapid NMB reversal may be necessary.[76]
3. Equipment malfunction: Verifying correct configuration of the grounding electrodes, recording/stimulating electrodes, and their connections with the interface connector box and monitor should be performed. Electrocautery near cables resulting in damaged fuses should also be considered.

C. True Loss of Signal

True LOS is defined as an evoked EMG amplitude of less than 100 μV obtained under a current of 1 to 2 mA after excluding false LOS (ie, no laryngeal/glottic twitch, positive contralateral vagus stimulation). This should be interpreted as true LOS resulting in a likely ipsilateral nerve injury.[7,9] There are two subtypes of LOS and RLN injury based on electrophysiological parameters. Type 1 indicates a segmental or localized injury of the nerve, whereby proximal RLN stimulation (ie, away from the larynx) exhibits a waveform of less than 100 μV in the presence of normal distal RLN stimulation (ie, toward the larynx). Type 2 indicates a global/diffuse nerve injury, with absence of conduction along the entire course of the RLN and vagus nerve. Possible etiologies of this type of nerve dysfunction are either intralaryngeal traction or nerve ischemia.[7,10,37,77] The reported prevalence of LOS type 1 versus type 2 varies greatly in the literature, and as such, controversy exists as to which type is more common.[10,71,74] Brooks & Ahmed et al. reported that LOS type 1 was documented in 90% of cases of RLNs invaded by thyroid carcinomas.[44]

D. Loss of Signal Troubleshooting

Adherence to the INSMG troubleshooting algorithm for LOS is highly recommended (Figure 30–7),[7] and separates decision-making into recording and stimulating side problems based on whether criteria for false LOS have been met.[7] If true LOS is established, with absence of laryngeal (posterior

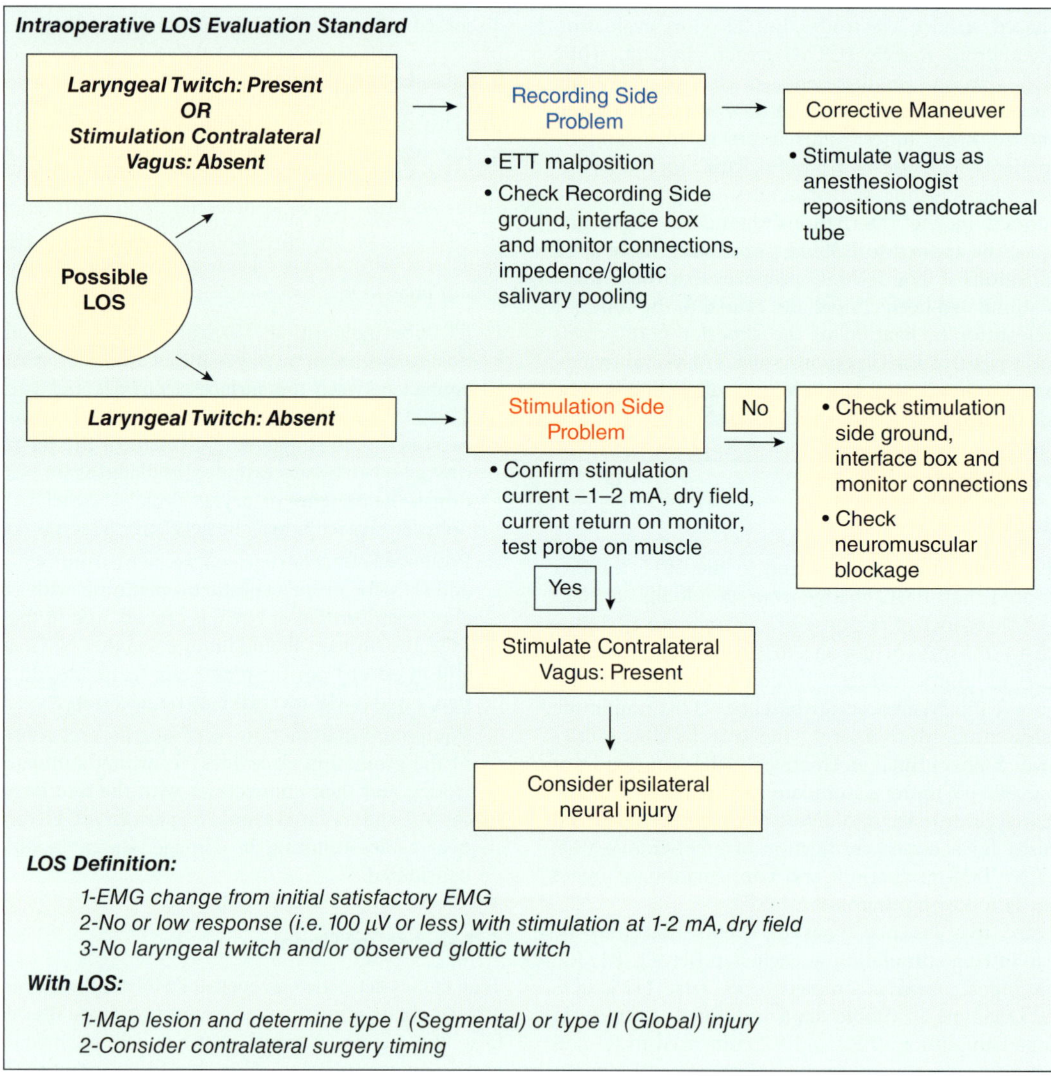

Figure 30–7. Troubleshooting of intraoperative loss of signal.[7] (Reproduced with permission from Randolph GW, Dralle H, Abdullah H, et al. Electrophysiologic recurrent laryngeal nerve monitoring during thyroid and parathyroid surgery: international standards guideline statement. *Laryngoscope*. 2011;121(1):S1-S16.)

cricoarytenoid) twitch on finger palpation, management strategies differ based on the etiology. It is important to determine whether the LOS is segmental (focal) or global (nonlocalizing) and to perform mapping of the lesion, when possible. In some cases, the nerve may manifest ultratransient dysfunction with spontaneous intraoperative recovery; thus, it would be reasonable to wait for a short period of time (ie, 15–30 minutes) to see if the nerve recovers on its own.[78] However, if the signal does not reach at least 50% of baseline amplitude, aborting the contralateral portion of the case to do a staged procedure at a later date is recommended to be considered. Elucidation of the exact mechanism of injury is also essential to determining the timing of a staged contralateral procedure. For example, the majority of traction injuries result in only temporary nerve dysfunction with recovery within 3 to 12 months.[19,43]

In the event of excessive noise or a continuous train of signaling, a separate troubleshooting algorithm is offered by the Iowa Head and Neck Protocols.[79] First, patient and surgical-related factors (ie, depth of anesthesia, metal-on-metal contact, presence of nerve stretch, drying, or cold irrigation) should be explored while having operating room staff verify the correct NIM setup (ie, event threshold ~100 μV, impedance <5 kΩ, muting detector applied, monitoring unit at least 10 feet from electrocautery unit) and electrode positioning (ie, ground and return electrodes in skin 5 cm apart, electrocautery wires looped through the muting detector, no crossing of stimulation and recording electrode wires). If the continuous train of signal persists, proceed with additional troubleshooting by checking the NIM ET-tube setup (ie, correctly sized ET tube with appropriate depth and absence of rotation) and replacing the NIM ET tube, if necessary.

Benefits, Indications, & Applications of RLN Monitoring

A. Evidence-Based Analysis & Benefits of RLN Monitoring

In the most recent decade, IONM has gained popularity among endocrine and head and neck surgeons as a practical tool to assist the surgeon in mapping of the RLN, identifying anatomical variants, evaluating nerve integrity, elucidating mechanisms of injury, and prognosticating vocal fold function.[6-12,40,71,80,81] This section discusses the indications, clinically useful applications, and benefits of intermittent RLN monitoring.

The use of RLN monitoring during thyroid/parathyroid surgery is generally nonrestrictive without specific contraindications. Because it is impossible to reliably predict which cases will prove difficult with respect to RLN identification and risk of injury based on preoperative factors alone, some authors suggest its routine use.[82] Of note, its benefits have been studied extensively with various studies failing to demonstrate statistical significance of the impact of IONM use on the rate of RLN injury;[33,71,83-85] however, there are several limitations to this interpretation. First, there exists significant heterogeneity across studies with respect to factors that affect the rate of RLN injury (ie, surgeon expertise, type of surgical procedure and pathology, use of potentially harmful surgical maneuvers).[26,86-94] Second, the incidence of RLN injury is rare and under-reported; and therefore, studies with sufficient power to show significant differences in RLN injury rate would need to have incredibly large sample sizes (9 million and 40 million patients per arm for benign goiter and malignancy, respectively).[33,71,95-98]

In a study of 850 patients undergoing revision thyroidectomy by Barczyński et al., the use of IONM was shown to reduce the incidence of transient but not permanent RLN injury.[99] These findings have been corroborated by several meta-analyses.[86,94] For example, Zheng et al., who analyzed five prospective randomized studies and 12 comparative nonrandomized studies with a total sample of more than 36,000 nerves at risk, showed a statistical reduction in the rate of transient RLN paralysis with IONM but not with permanent paralysis.[94] In particular, the effect of IONM on the rate of postoperative RLN paralysis is most significant in higher-risk cases such as revision surgery, invasive malignancy, and retrosternal goiter.[100,101]

Along with a potential reduction in RLN injury rates, IONM is also thought to improve the speed of RLN identification with less nerve dissection required. In a recent study by Liddy et al., RLN neural identification was shown to precede visual identification in nearly 35% of cases, suggesting greater surgical efficiency.[102] Moreover, the use of IONM independently predicted shorter time-to-RLN identification in a prospective study of 409 nerves at risk during thyroidectomy.[103]

B. Recommendations for RLN Monitoring

Both the 2018 INMSG Guidelines and the German Association of Endocrine Surgery Guidelines recommend neural monitoring in all cases of thyroid and parathyroid surgery,[7-10,80,104] whereas the American Academy of Otolaryngology–Head and Neck Surgery (AAOHNS) Clinical Practice Guideline: Improving Voice Outcomes After Thyroid Surgery recommends the use of IONM in total thyroidectomy, revision surgery for thyroid malignancy, and surgery on patients with only a single functioning nerve.[105] Other society publications that include specific nerve monitoring indications or highlight the need for IONM to confirm intact neural function at the end of surgery include the 2015 American Thyroid Association (ATA) Thyroid Nodules and Differentiated Thyroid Cancer guidelines, the ATA Surgical Affairs Committee Consensus Statement on Outpatient Thyroid Surgery, and the Evidence-Based American Head and Neck Society (AHNS) Consensus Statement on the Management of Locally Invasive Well-Differentiated Thyroid Cancer.[106-109]

C. Applications of RLN Monitoring

The clinically significant applications and benefits of IONM outlined in the 2018 INMSG Guidelines include:[9]

- RLN mapping to facilitate safe and efficient visual identification to avoid injury[110]
- Identification of RLN anatomical variants that portend greater risk of iatrogenic injury
- Prognostication of RLN function with the effect of reducing the rate of tracheostomy after total thyroidectomy[105,111]
- Correction of harmful surgical maneuvers in cases where impending neural injury is detected[112,113]
- Identification and preservation of the EBSLN[8,14]
- Improvement in overall outcomes with less-experienced thyroid surgeons[114]
- Identification of nonrecurrent laryngeal nerve variation[115]

The capability of IONM to prognosticate vocal fold function postoperatively is another clinically significant application of recent interest. The recently published SAR study showed that an absence of LOS on stimulation of the RLN/vagus following complete thyroid dissection (ie, positive R2 and V2) predicted an absence of postoperative vocal cord paresis or paralysis (VCP) with a negative predictive value (NPV) of 99.8%; positive predictive value was 74.3%.[19] Similarly, a study of 1381 RLNs by Randolph et al. demonstrated an NPV of 99.6%.[116] Given the often-bilateral nature of thyroid surgery, it is essential to appreciate that a visually intact nerve at the end of a unilateral dissection may not always be a functional nerve. With nerve monitoring, the decision to safely proceed to contralateral dissection can be substantiated based on its prognostic ability. In a retrospective study of 1333 patients undergoing total thyroidectomy with IONM, the occurrence of LOS on the first side of dissection resulted in a change in surgical strategy in 100% of cases, which prevented bilateral RLN injury. Conversely, in the group that did not utilize IONM, bilateral VFP occurred in 17% of cases.[111]

Benefits, Indications, & Applications of EBSLN Monitoring

Dissection of the superior thyroid pole with EBSLN identification can be challenging even for highly experienced surgeons, with many tending to avoid rather than readily expose and identify the nerve during thyroidectomy. The nerve runs deep to the fascia of the inferior constrictor in up to 20% of patients, is thin in caliber, and has a varied course through the neck (ie, types 1, 2A, and 2B).[8,117] EBSLN injury is believed by many to be an extremely underestimated cause of morbidity following thyroid surgery. A recent meta-analysis showed that EBSLN injury may occur in as many as 58% of patients undergoing thyroidectomy.[118] Type 2a and 2b nerves according to the Cernea classification are at greater than two and three times higher risk of injury, respectively, compared to type 1 nerves.[119] The use of IONM during superior thyroid pole dissection has been suggested by many authors as a tool for EBSLN mapping of normal and variant courses to minimize the rate of injury.[118,120-123] In a randomized trial comparing thyroidectomy patients with and without EBSLN monitoring, not only was nerve identification more than twice as frequent with IONM (83.8% vs 34.5%) but the rate of nerve injury was also significantly lower (1% vs 5%, $p = 0.02\%$).[121] In a similar comparative study, Uludag et al. demonstrated a reduction in EBSLN injury from 8.6% to 0.9% when EBSLN mapping was performed.[120]

Based on the abundance of literature supporting the use of EBSLN IONM, the 2011 INMSG guidelines provided recommendations to include the routine neurophysiological assessment of the EBSLN before and after superior thyroid pole dissection (S1 and S2).[7]

Prevalence of Neuromonitoring Usage

IONM technology has been available in its most primitive form since the mid-to-late 20th century and was introduced for RLN monitoring almost 30 years ago. Despite this, it is still not the standard of care in most countries, with the exception of Germany.[7,61,82,124] However, more widespread use of IONM is now being seen secondary to technological advancements allowing for more noninvasive, precise, user-friendly, and cost-effective modalities.[125-128]

A shift in surgeon attitudes is now occurring as a result of the publication of prospective trials showing its safe and effective use, society guidelines defining standards for RLN and EBSLN monitoring, and structured training programs for surgical residents.[7,37,105,129-131] The first prevalence study on RLN monitoring among US head and neck surgeons showed in 2007 that while 81% of respondents performed thyroidectomy, only 28% used IONM. Surgeons were 3.14 times more likely to use nerve monitoring if it was used in their training, and those who did report its routine use were 41% less likely to report permanent RLN injury.[126] In 2009, a formal usage pattern study conducted by the American Association of Endocrine Surgeons (AAES) showed that 23% of surgeons reported IONM use for select cases of thyroidectomy, and 13% reported regular IONM use for all thyroidectomies. Nonusers were older, reported a lower case volume, had less familiarity with newer surgical technologies, and had less access to equipment.[127] Since these original surveys, the prevalence of IONM use in the United States appears to be increasing. Based on US surveys concerning practice patterns published in 2012 and 2013, the estimated prevalence of IONM was reported to be 80% for thyroid surgeries performed by OHNS surgeons and 65% for those performed by general surgeons.[128,132] Interestingly, more recently the use of IONM was reported greatest among high-volume surgeons.[133] Medicolegal issues are one of the most cited reasons for use of IONM, likely to mitigate bilateral RLN injury and liability with documented evoked EMG signals at the end of the case.[126,134,135] Residency training programs are now required to include curricula on IONM by the ACGME. A survey of endocrine surgery fellows showed that IONM was utilized over 95% of the time in some or all of thyroid/parathyroid cases.[127] Taken together, these prevalence studies suggest that regular use of IONM during thyroidectomy is becoming an increasingly common practice in the United States.

Limitations of Intermittent IONM

Despite the widespread use of intermittent IONM, there are several potential limitations. With all forms of IONM that use ET tube-based surface electrodes, adequate contact between the electrodes and glottis needs to be maintained to obtain a high-quality recording.[7] With respect to intermittent IONM, since nerve integrity can only be assessed at the time of electrical stimulation, it is limited in its ability to detect nerve injury as it is occurring in real-time. Aside from complete transection injury with immediate LOS, the more common mechanisms of traction, thermal, and clamping forces can result in a more gradual insult to the nerve that is difficult to capture using intermittent stimulation.[62] In addition, user error can occur if the surgeon is not fully familiar with IONM protocols and LOS troubleshooting. A good example is the risk of a false negative IONM signal if the surgeon stimulates the nerve distal to the site of nerve injury (ie, closer to the larynx).[134] To address these potential limitations, a technique was developed employing near-constant assessment of the functional integrity of the entire vagal-RLN axis, known as continuous IONM (C-IONM), which will be discussed in the subsequent section.

CONTINUOUS INTRAOPERATIVE NERVE MONITORING

Introduction

The principal methodologic limitation of intermittent IONM (I-IONM) is that RLN loss of signal (LOS) is most often detected *after* the nerve injury has occurred. This puts the nerve at risk of unmonitored dissection intervals, leaving the surgeon without real-time feedback on potentially harmful surgical maneuvers that cause gradual neural insult. While unable to prevent sudden transection injuries, a more continuous method of IONM could help identification and rectification of those more gradual neural insults such as can be seen with the more common thermal, traction, and clamping injuries.[10]

C-IONM was developed in 2007 as a tool to overcome the limitations of I-IONM by providing near-constant assessment of the functional integrity of the entire vagal-RLN axis to better predict imminent nerve injury.[136,137] With electrode placement around the vagus allowing periodic stimulation at short intervals for ongoing assessment of vagal EMG amplitude and latency, C-IONM is able to provide real-time alerts in response to surgical maneuvers that threaten the RLN and EBSLN, thereby enabling quick corrective action, improving risk management, and facilitating intraoperative decision-making.[113,137] The vagus nerve is chosen because of its location out of the surgical field and for its proximal positioning along the vagus-RLN axis, allowing for the prevention of inadvertent electrode displacement and complete incorporation of all points of potential neural injury. The vagus can also withstand greater surgical manipulation due to its larger caliber compared to the RLN, and it can be readily identified within the carotid sheath with minimal anatomic variability.[138]

C-IONM is a more recent technology that requires a certain amount of experience to gain expertise and has yet to become widespread amongst thyroid surgeons. The introduction of C-IONM was reported in five academic centers in Italy in 2014 (three general surgery and two otolaryngology),[125] and its prevalence continues to increase anecdotally, though more recent prevalence studies are not readily available.

General Setup & Electrophysiology

General setup and equipment used for C-IONM is similar to that of I-IONM with the addition of 360-degree surgical exposure of the vagus and placement of an automatic periodic stimulation (APS) electrode on the nerve at the level of the cricoid cartilage (Figure 30–8). The carotid sheath may be opened from either a medial approach, by making an incision between the left and right sternohyoid muscles, or from a lateral approach, by incising between the lateral border of the sternohyoid muscle and the medial border of the ipsilateral sternocleidomastoid muscle. The preferred approach is the lateral approach, which enables the electrode and connections to be away from the field of thyroid dissection.[139-141] The use of a 1 mA current is recommended for vagal stimulation. The most common stimulation frequency is 1 Hz with a pulse lasting 100 to 200 μs, which is chosen to enable near-continuous stimulation. The IONM system is calibrated to the patient's baseline nerve amplitude of at least 500 μV at the beginning of the procedure.[142] In the event of an initial amplitude less than 500 μV, tube repositioning should be performed. Use of a monopolar or bipolar handheld probe for RLN mapping during dissection is still recommended as with I-IONM.[7]

Impending Nerve Injury & Reversibility

Isolated events, which are defined as periods of increased or decreased amplitude or latency alone, are unrelated to surgical manipulation and can be interpreted as EMG artifact or noise resulting from tube displacement or tracheal shifting

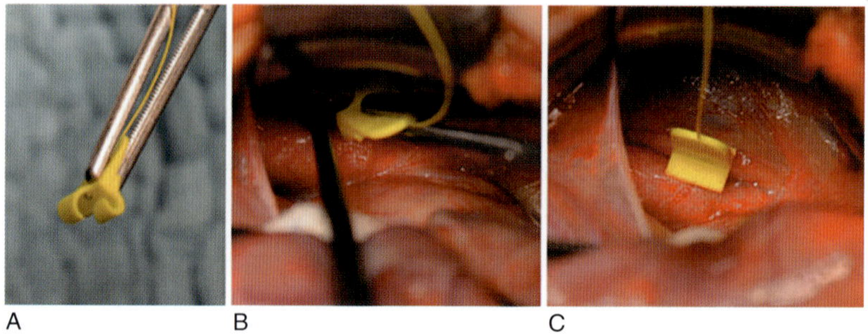

Figure 30–8. Intraoperative placement of the Automatic Periodic Stimulation (APS)® electrode. **(A)** APS electrode prior to vagus nerve placement. **(B)** Placement of the APS electrode on the partially dissected vagus nerve. **(C)** APS electrode resting on the vagus nerve.[140] (Reproduced with permission from Schneider R, Lorenz K, Machens A, Nguyen-Thanh P, Randolph GW, Dralle H. Continuous intraoperative neuromonitoring (CIONM) of the recurrent laryngeal nerve. Chapter 15. In: Randolph GW, ed. *The Recurrent and Superior Laryngeal Nerves*. Springer; 2016:169-183.)

from thyroid manipulation.[142] Conversely, direct traction, pressure or heat applied to the RLN results in a characteristic, reproducible change in both EMG amplitude *and* latency. These adverse EMG events, which have been termed "combined events," are defined as a simultaneous reduction in EMG waveform amplitude of at least 50% from baseline and an increase in latency at least 10% from baseline. EMG changes typically begin with amplitude depression followed by latency elevation with further amplitude depression (Figure 30–9).[140,143]

Combined events have been found to precede imminent RLN injury with high specificity[142,144] and are reversible in 68% to 80% of cases after halting the causative surgical maneuver.[112,145,146] In cases of combined events lasting 40 seconds or more, the risk of VFP increases dramatically.[145,147] Thus, while standard LOS troubleshooting

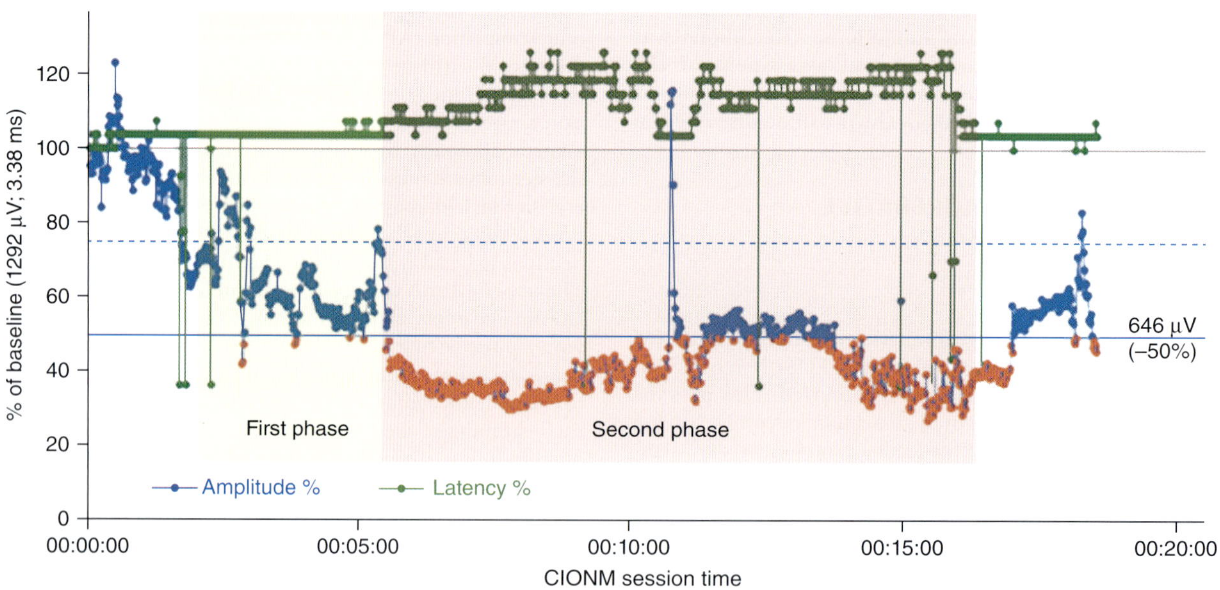

Figure 30–9. Sequential electrophysiologic changes observed during impending nerve injury. Note the decrease in amplitude (first phase) followed by an increase in latency and further amplitude reduction.[140] (Reproduced with permission from Schneider R, Lorenz K, Machens A, Nguyen-Thanh P, Randolph GW, Dralle H. Continuous intraoperative neuromonitoring (CIONM) of the recurrent laryngeal nerve. Chapter 15. In: Randolph GW, ed. *The Recurrent and Superior Laryngeal Nerves*. Springer; 2016.)

algorithms should be followed in accordance with the 2011 INMSG Guidelines,[7] C-IONM offers a window of potential signal reversibility for which the surgeon can make quick corrective action.

Signal recovery of ≥50% of the baseline amplitude during surgery reliably signifies normal postoperative vocal fold function according to a study of 785 patients with 1291 nerves at risk.[74] Segmental LOS typically resolves within 8 minutes and global injury within 16 minutes. Thus, an injured nerve should be observed for a minimum of 20 minutes to evaluate for recovery ≥50% of baseline amplitude before deciding to move forward with contralateral dissection or to stage the procedure.[43,74] A persistent LOS on the first side warrants postponing the contralateral thyroidectomy, since 70% and 95% of patients with segmental and global LOS, respectively, will experience return of VF function postoperatively.[9,43,74]

Comparative Performance

C-IONM is an advanced tool to improve RLN/EBSLN management during thyroidectomy with several advantages over I-IONM. Schneider et al. tested the comparative performance of I-IONM and C-IONM with respect to predictive ability for postoperative VFP in 1526 patients and 2279 nerves at risk.[148] The authors found that the C-IONM group had a lower rate of permanent VFP compared to I-IONM (0% vs 0.4%, $p = 0.019$). Additionally, they estimated how many unnecessary two-staged procedures were avoided in I-IONM versus C-IONM and found that unnecessary two-staged procedures would have been performed in 23% of patients after I-IONM but only 12% of C-IONM patients. More recently, Schneider et al. found in a multivariable analysis of 6029 patients and 10,232 nerves at risk that, in comparison to I-IONM, C-IONM was associated with a 1.8-fold reduction in early postoperative VFP and a 29.4-fold reduction in permanent VFP.[149]

While both modalities are able to identify LOS and RLN injury and predict postoperative VCP with high accuracy, the advantage of C-IONM becomes apparent in technically demanding cases. The ability to recognize impending damage in real time enables the surgeon to take corrective action immediately, giving the nerve a chance to recover before the damage is irreversible. Thus, C-IONM's superior recognition of impending injury to facilitate potential recovery of signal overcomes the principal limitation of I-IONM.

Safety & Limitations

The low-current, short-duration vagal stimulation employed in C-IONM is safe according to a multitude of animal and human studies.[150-157] The major limitation of the continuous method is that it requires surgical exposure and manipulation of the vagus for electrode placement, which takes time and additional dissection and may place the nerve at small risk of injury.[158] Another previously reported adverse event of repeated or continuous stimulation of the vagus is potential cardiovascular side effects such as arrhythmias and hemodynamic changes as a result of disturbances in autonomic parasympathetic resting tone.[158,159] However, chronic vagal nerve stimulation has been used in a variety of other neurologic conditions without evidence of harmful cardiac or pulmonary effects.[153,160,161] The safety of this technique lies in the fact that the current of 1 to 2 mA used in C-IONM does not activate the C-fibers within the vagus nerve, which are the fibers predominantly responsible for autonomic sequelae.[85,151,153,154]

REFERENCES

1. Bergenfelz A, Jansson S, Kristoffersson A, et al. Complications to thyroid surgery: results as reported in a database from a multicenter audit comprising 3,660 patients. *Langenbecks Arch Surg*. 2008;393(5):667-673.
2. Gharib H, Papini E, Paschke R, et al. American Association of Clinical Endocrinologists, Associazione Medici Endocrinologi, and EuropeanThyroid Association Medical Guidelines for Clinical Practice for the Diagnosis and Management of Thyroid Nodules. *Endocr Pract*. 2010;16(Suppl 1):1-43.
3. Bliss RD, Gauger PG, Delbridge LW. Surgeon's approach to the thyroid gland: surgical anatomy and the importance of technique. *World J Surg*. 2000;24(8):891-897.
4. Swonke ML, Shakibai N, Chaaban MR. Medical malpractice trends in thyroidectomies among general surgeons and otolaryngologists. *OTO Open*. 2020;4(2):2473974X20921141.
5. Randolph GW. The importance of pre- and postoperative laryngeal examination for thyroid surgery. *Thyroid*. 2010;20(5):453-458.
6. Wu CW, Wang MH, Chen CC, et al. Loss of signal in recurrent nerve neuromonitoring: causes and management. *Gland Surg*. 2015;4(1):19-26.
7. Randolph GW, Dralle H, Abdullah H, et al. Electrophysiologic recurrent laryngeal nerve monitoring during thyroid and parathyroid surgery: international standards guideline statement. *Laryngoscope*. 2011;121(Suppl 1):S1-S16.
8. Barczyński M, Randolph GW, Cernea CR, et al. External branch of the superior laryngeal nerve monitoring during thyroid and parathyroid surgery: International Neural Monitoring Study Group standards guideline statement. *Laryngoscope*. 2013;123(Suppl 4):S1-S14.
9. Schneider R, Randolph GW, Dionigi G, et al. International neural monitoring study group guideline 2018 part I: staging bilateral thyroid surgery with monitoring loss of signal. *Laryngoscope*. 2018;128(Suppl 3):S1-S17.
10. Chiang FY, Lu IC, Kuo WR, Lee KW, Chang NC, Wu CW. The mechanism of recurrent laryngeal nerve injury during thyroid surgery—the application of intraoperative neuromonitoring. *Surgery*. 2008;143(6):743-749.
11. Chiang FY, Lu IC, Tsai CJ, Hsiao PJ, Lee KW, Wu CW. Detecting and identifying nonrecurrent laryngeal nerve with the application of intraoperative neuromonitoring during thyroid and parathyroid operation. *Am J Otolaryngol*. 2012;33(1):1-5.
12. Wu CW, Dionigi G, Chen HC, et al. Vagal nerve stimulation without dissecting the carotid sheath during intraoperative neuromonitoring of the recurrent laryngeal nerve in thyroid surgery. *Head Neck*. 2013;35(10):1443-1447.
13. Cernea CR. Monitoring of the Superior Laryngeal Nerve. In: Scharpf J, Randolph GW, eds. *Intraoperative Cranial Nerve Monitoring in Otolaryngology-Head and Neck Surgery*. Springer; 2022:83-88.

14. Cernea CR, Ferraz AR, Furlani J, et al. Identification of the external branch of the superior laryngeal nerve during thyroidectomy. *Am J Surg*. 1992;164(6):634-639.
15. Iwata AJ, Liddy W, Barczyński M, et al. Superior laryngeal nerve signal attenuation influences voice outcomes in thyroid surgery. *Laryngoscope*. 2021;131(6):1436-1442.
16. Bellantone R, Boscherini M, Lombardi CP, et al. Is the identification of the external branch of the superior laryngeal nerve mandatory in thyroid operation? Results of a prospective randomized study. *Surgery*. 2001;130(6):1055-1059.
17. Adour KK, Schneider GD, Hilsinger RLJ. Acute superior laryngeal nerve palsy: analysis of 78 cases. *Otolaryngol Head Neck Surg*. 1980;88(4):418-424.
18. Randolph GW, Wu CW, Dionigi G, et al. The international RLN anatomic classification system. In: Randolph GW, ed. *The Recurrent and Superior Laryngeal Nerves*. Springer International Publishing; 2016:125-138.
19. Liddy W, Wu CW, Dionigi G, et al. Varied recurrent laryngeal nerve course is associated with increased risk of nerve dysfunction during thyroidectomy: results of the surgical anatomy of the recurrent laryngeal nerve in thyroid surgery study, an International Multicenter Prospective Anatomic and Electrophysiologic Study of 1000 Monitored Nerves at Risk from the International Neural Monitoring Study Group. *Thyroid*. 2021;31(11):1730-1740.
20. Simon MM. Recurrent laryngeal nerve in thyroid surgery: triangle for its recognition and protection. *Am J Surg*. 1943;60(2):212-220.
21. Gauger PG, Delbridge LW, Thompson NW, Crummer P, Reeve TS. Incidence and importance of the tubercle of Zuckerkandl in thyroid surgery. *Eur J Surg*. 2001;167(4):249-254.
22. Armstrong WG, Hinton JW. Multiple divisions of the recurrent laryngeal nerve. An anatomic study. *AMA Arch Surg*. 1951;62(4):532-539.
23. Sasou S, Nakamura S, Kurihara H. Suspensory ligament of Berry: its relationship to recurrent laryngeal nerve and anatomic examination of 24 autopsies. *Head Neck*. 1998;20(8):695-698.
24. Kern KA. Medicolegal analysis of errors in diagnosis and treatment of surgical endocrine disease. *Surgery*. 1993;114(6):1167-1173; discussion 1173-1174.
25. Rosenthal LHS, Benninger MS, Deeb RH. Vocal fold immobility: a longitudinal analysis of etiology over 20 years. *Laryngoscope*. 2007;117(10):1864-1870.
26. Jeannon JP, Orabi AA, Bruch GA, Abdalsalam HA, Simo R. Diagnosis of recurrent laryngeal nerve palsy after thyroidectomy: a systematic review. *Int J Clin Pract*. 2009;63(4):624-629.
27. Sinclair CF, Duke W, Barbu A, Randolph G. Laryngeal exam indications and techniques. In: Randolph GW, ed. *The Recurrent and Superior Laryngeal Nerves*. Vol 39. Springer; 2016:17-29.
28. Song PC, Hussain I, Bruch J, Franco RA Jr, Randolph GW. Postoperative management of unilateral RLN paralysis. In: *The Recurrent and Superior Laryngeal Nerves*. Springer International Publishing; 2016:125-138.
29. Rosato L, Avenia N, Bernante P, et al. Complications of thyroid surgery: analysis of a multicentric study on 14,934 patients operated on in Italy over 5 years. *World J Surg*. 2004;28(3):271-276.
30. Schneider R, Randolph G, Dionigi G, et al. Prospective study of vocal fold function after loss of the neuromonitoring signal in thyroid surgery: The International Neural Monitoring Study Group's POLT study. *Laryngoscope*. 2016;126(5):1260-1266.
31. Jansson S, Tisell LE, Hagne I, Sanner E, Stenborg R, Svensson P. Partial superior laryngeal nerve (SLN) lesions before and after thyroid surgery. *World J Surg*. 1988;12(4):522-527.
32. Teitelbaum BJ, Wenig BL. Superior laryngeal nerve injury from thyroid surgery. *Head Neck*. 1995;17(1):36-40.
33. Dralle H, Sekulla C, Haerting J, et al. Risk factors of paralysis and functional outcome after recurrent laryngeal nerve monitoring in thyroid surgery. *Surgery*. 2004;136(6):1310-1322.
34. Yuan X, Gao Z, Jiang H, et al. Predictors of facial palsy after surgery for benign parotid disease: multivariate analysis of 626 operations. *Head Neck*. 2009;31(12):1588-1592.
35. Erbil Y, Barbaros U, Işsever H, et al. Predictive factors for recurrent laryngeal nerve palsy and hypoparathyroidism after thyroid surgery. *Clin Otolaryngol*. 2007;32(1):32-37.
36. Dulguerov P, Marchal F, Lehmann W. Postparotidectomy facial nerve paralysis: possible etiologic factors and results with routine facial nerve monitoring. *Laryngoscope*. 1999;109(5):754-762.
37. Chiang FY, Lee KW, Chen HC, et al. Standardization of intraoperative neuromonitoring of recurrent laryngeal nerve in thyroid operation. *World J Surg*. 2010;34(2):223-229.
38. Dionigi G, Wu CW, Kim HY, Rausei S, Boni L, Chiang FY. Severity of recurrent laryngeal nerve injuries in thyroid surgery. *World J Surg*. 2016;40(6):1373-1381.
39. Sunderland S. A classification of peripheral nerve injuries producing loss of function. *Brain*. 1951;74(4):491-516.
40. Snyder SK, Lairmore TC, Hendricks JC, Roberts JW. Elucidating mechanisms of recurrent laryngeal nerve injury during thyroidectomy and parathyroidectomy. *J Am Coll Surg*. 2008;206(1):123-130.
41. Dionigi G, Alesina PF, Barczynski M, et al. Recurrent laryngeal nerve injury in video-assisted thyroidectomy: lessons learned from neuromonitoring. *Surg Endosc*. 2012;26(9):2601-2608.
42. Liu N, Chen B, Li L, et al. Mechanisms of recurrent laryngeal nerve injury near the nerve entry point during thyroid surgery: a retrospective cohort study. *Int J Surg*. 2020;83:125-130.
43. Schneider R, Randolph G, Dionigi G, et al. Prediction of postoperative vocal fold function after intraoperative recovery of loss of signal. *Laryngoscope*. 2019;129(2):525-531.
44. Brooks JA, Abdelhamid Ahmed AH, Al-Qurayshi Z, et al. Recurrent laryngeal nerve invasion by thyroid cancer: laryngeal function and survival outcomes. *Laryngoscope*. 2022;132(11):2285-2292.
45. Miyauchi A, Inoue H, Tomoda C, et al. Improvement in phonation after reconstruction of the recurrent laryngeal nerve in patients with thyroid cancer invading the nerve. *Surgery*. 2009;146(6):1056-1062.
46. Miyauchi A, Matsusaka K, Kihara M, et al. The role of ansa-to-recurrent-laryngeal nerve anastomosis in operations for thyroid cancer. *Eur J Surg*. 1998;164(12):927-933.
47. Laccourreye O, Papon JF, Kania R, Crevier-Buchman L, Brasnu D, Hans S. Intracordal injection of autologous fat in patients with unilateral laryngeal nerve paralysis: long-term results from the patient's perspective. *Laryngoscope*. 2003;113(3):541-545.
48. Franco RA Jr. Adduction arytenopexy, hypopharyngoplasty, medialization laryngoplasty, and cricothyroid subluxation for the treatment of paralytic dysphonia and dysphagia. *Oper Tech Otolayngol Head Neck Surg*. 2012;23(3):164-172.
49. Gelbard A, Netterville JL. Postoperative management of bilateral vocal cord paralysis. In: Randolph GW, ed. *The Recurrent and Superior Laryngeal Nerves*. Springer; 2016:285-293.

50. Bosley B, Rosen CA, Simpson CB, McMullin BT, Gartner-Schmidt JL. Medial arytenoidectomy versus transverse cordotomy as a treatment for bilateral vocal fold paralysis. *Ann Otol Rhinol Laryngol.* 2005;114(12):922-926.
51. Paniello RC. Laryngeal reinnervation. *Otolaryngol Clin North Am.* 2004;37(1):161-181, vii-viii.
52. Galvani L. De viribus electricitatis in motu musculari. Commentarius. In: *De Bonoiensi Scientiarum et Artium Intituo Atque Academie Commentarii.* Vol 7th. Typographia Instituti Scientiarum; 1791:363-418.
53. Schuetze SM. The discovery of the action potential. *Trends Neurosci.* 1983;6:164-168.
54. Erb W. *Handbuch der Elektrotherapie.* (Vogel FCW, ed.). Leipzig; 1882. https://archive.org/details/handbuchderelekt1882erbw.
55. Duchenne GB. *De l'électrisation localisée et de son application à la physiologie, à la pathologie et à la thérapeutique.* 2nd ed.; 1861.
56. Duchenne GB. *Mécanisme de la physionomie humaine: où, Analyse électro-physiologique de l'expression des passions.* Ve Jules Renouard, libraire; 1862.
57. Cawthorne T, Wilson T. Indications for intratemporal facial nerve surgery. *Arch Otolaryngol.* 1963;78:429-434.
58. Penfield W, Boldrey E. Somatic motor and sensory representation in the cerebral cortex of man as studied by electrical stimulation. *Brain.* 1937;60(4):389-443.
59. Riddell VH. Injury to recurrent laryngeal nerves during thyroidectomy: a comparison between the results of identification and non-identification in 1022 nerves exposed to risk. *Lancet.* 1956;271(6944):638-641.
60. Lahey FH, Hoover WB. Injuries to the recurrent laryngeal nerve in thyroid operations: their management and avoidance. *Ann Surg.* 1938;108(4):545-562.
61. Shedd DP, Durham C. Electrical identification of the recurrent laryngeal nerve. I. Response of the canine larynx to electrical stimulation of the recurrent laryngeal nerve. *Ann Surg.* 1966;163(1):47-50.
62. Chen BY, Stack BC. Methods of recurrent laryngeal nerve monitoring. In: Scharpf J, Randolph GW, eds. *Intraoperative Cranial Nerve Monitoring in Otolaryngology-Head and Neck Surgery.* Springer; 2022:73-82.
63. Randolph GW, Kamani D, Wu CW, Schneider R. Surgical anatomy and monitoring of the recurrent laryngeal nerve. In: Randolph GW, ed. *Surgery of the Thyroid and Parathyroid Glands.* Elsevier; 2021:326-359.
64. Noble AR, Bonilla-Velez J. Anesthetic considerations and setup for cranial nerve monitoring. In: Scharpf J, Randolph GW, eds. *Intraoperative Cranial Nerve Monitoring in Otolaryngology-Head and Neck Surgery.* Springer International Publishing; 2022:25-42.
65. Chambers KJ, Pearse A, Coveney J, et al. Respiratory variation predicts optimal endotracheal tube placement for intraoperative nerve monitoring in thyroid and parathyroid surgery. *World J Surg.* 2015;39(2):393-399.
66. Sloan TB. Muscle relaxant use during intraoperative neurophysiologic monitoring. *J Clin Monit Comput.* 2013;27(1):35-46.
67. Carron M, Zarantonello F, Tellaroli P, Ori C. Efficacy and safety of sugammadex compared to neostigmine for reversal of neuromuscular blockade: a meta-analysis of randomized controlled trials. *J Clin Anesth.* 2016;35:1-12.
68. Bevan DR, Donati F, Kopman AF. Reversal of neuromuscular blockade. *Anesthesiology.* 1992;77(4):785-805.
69. Suy K, Morias K, Cammu G, et al. Effective reversal of moderate rocuronium- or vecuronium-induced neuromuscular block with sugammadex, a selective relaxant binding agent. *Anesthesiology.* 2007;106(2):283-288.
70. *Monitoring Neuromuscular Function.* Vol 378; 2018.
71. Dralle H, Sekulla C, Lorenz K, Brauckhoff M, Machens A. Intraoperative monitoring of the recurrent laryngeal nerve in thyroid surgery. *World J Surg.* 2008;32(7):1358-1366.
72. Darr EA, Tufano RP, Ozdemir S, Kamani D, Hurwitz S, Randolph G. Superior laryngeal nerve quantitative intraoperative monitoring is possible in all thyroid surgeries. *Laryngoscope.* 2014;124(4):1035-1041.
73. Wu CW, Chiang FY, Karcioglu AS, Iwata AJ, Abdelhamid Ahmed AH, Randolph GW. Rationale and indications for vagus/recurrent laryngeal nerve monitoring. In: Scharpf J, Randolph GW, eds. *Intraoperative Cranial Nerve Monitoring in Otolaryngology-Head and Neck Surgery.* Springer International Publishing; 2022:57-72.
74. Schneider R, Sekulla C, Machens A, Lorenz K, Thanh PN, Dralle H. Dynamics of loss and recovery of the nerve monitoring signal during thyroidectomy predict early postoperative vocal fold function. *Head Neck.* 2016;38(Suppl 1):E1144-E1151.
75. Wu CW, Hao M, Tian M, et al. Recurrent laryngeal nerve injury with incomplete loss of electromyography signal during monitored thyroidectomy-evaluation and outcome. *Langenbecks Arch Surg.* 2017;402(4):691-699.
76. Lu IC, Wu SH, Chang PY, et al. Precision neuromuscular block management for neural monitoring during thyroid surgery. *J Invest Surg.* 2021;34(12):1389-1396.
77. Dionigi G, Snyder SK, Chiang FY, Liddy W, Kamani D, Kyriazidis N. Mechanism of injury. In: Randolph GW, ed. *The Recurrent and Superior Laryngeal Nerves.* Springer; 2016:222-237.
78. Sitges-Serra A, Gallego-Otaegui L, Fontané J, Trillo L, Lorente-Poch L, Sancho J. Contralateral surgery in patients scheduled for total thyroidectomy with initial loss or absence of signal during neural monitoring. *Br J Surg.* 2019;106(4):404-411.
79. Hoffman HT. Thyroidectomy and thyroid lobectomy. Iowa Head and Neck Protocols. Published 2020. Accessed January 18, 2024. https://medicine.uiowa.edu/iowaprotocols/thyroidectomy-and-thyroid-lobectomy.
80. Wu CW, Dionigi G, Barczynski M, et al. International neuromonitoring study group guidelines 2018: Part II: optimal recurrent laryngeal nerve management for invasive thyroid cancer-incorporation of surgical, laryngeal, and neural electrophysiologic data. *Laryngoscope.* 2018;128(Suppl 3):S18-S27.
81. Chiang FY, Lu IC, Chen HC, et al. Anatomical variations of recurrent laryngeal nerve during thyroid surgery: how to identify and handle the variations with intraoperative neuromonitoring. *Kaohsiung J Med Sci.* 2010;26(11):575-583.
82. Dionigi G, Dralle H, Liddy W, Kamani D, Kyriazidis N, Randolph GW. Intraoperative nerve monitoring of the recurrent laryngeal nerve. In: Randolph GW, ed. *The Recurrent and Superior Laryngeal Nerves.* Springer; 2016:147-168.
83. Dionigi G, Van Slycke S, Boni L, Rausei S, Mangano A. Limits of neuromonitoring in thyroid surgery. *Ann Surg.* 2013;258(1):e1-e2.
84. Yarbrough DE, Thompson GB, Kasperbauer JL, Harper CM, Grant CS. Intraoperative electromyographic monitoring of the recurrent laryngeal nerve in reoperative thyroid and parathyroid surgery. *Surgery.* 2004;136(6):1107-1115.
85. Ulmer C, Friedrich C, Kohler A, et al. Impact of continuous intraoperative neuromonitoring on autonomic nervous system during thyroid surgery. *Head Neck.* 2011;33(7):976-984.

86. Pisanu A, Porceddu G, Podda M, Cois A, Uccheddu A. Systematic review with meta-analysis of studies comparing intraoperative neuromonitoring of recurrent laryngeal nerves versus visualization alone during thyroidectomy. *J Surg Res.* 2014;188(1):152-161.
87. Kunath M, Hussock J, Marusch F, Horschig P, Gastinger I. [Identifying the recurrent laryngeal nerve by intraoperative neuromonitoring]. *Zentralbl Chir.* 1999;124(7):641-645.
88. Lamadé W, Renz K, Willeke F, Klar E, Herfarth C. Effect of training on the incidence of nerve damage in thyroid surgery. *Br J Surg.* 1999;86(3):388-391.
89. Thomusch O, Machens A, Sekulla C, et al. Multivariate analysis of risk factors for postoperative complications in benign goiter surgery: prospective multicenter study in Germany. *World J Surg.* 2000;24(11):1335-1341.
90. Hermann M, Alk G, Roka R, Glaser K, Freissmuth M. Laryngeal recurrent nerve injury in surgery for benign thyroid diseases: effect of nerve dissection and impact of individual surgeo n in more than 27,000 nerves at risk. *Ann Surg.* 2002;235(2):261-268.
91. Chiang FY, Wang LF, Huang YF, Lee KW, Kuo WR. Recurrent laryngeal nerve palsy after thyroidectomy with routine identification of the recurrent laryngeal nerve. *Surgery.* 2005;137(3):342-347.
92. Barczyński M, Konturek A, Cichoń S. Randomized clinical trial of visualization versus neuromonitoring of recurrent laryngeal nerves during thyroidectomy. *Br J Surg.* 2009;96(3):240-246.
93. Dionigi G, Chiang FY, Dralle H, et al. Safety of neural monitoring in thyroid surgery. *Int J Surg.* 2013;11(Suppl 1):S120-S126.
94. Zheng S, Xu Z, Wei Y, Zeng M, He J. Effect of intraoperative neuromonitoring on recurrent laryngeal nerve palsy rates after thyroid surgery—a meta-analysis. *J Formos Med Assoc.* 2013;112(8):463-472.
95. Rulli F, Ambrogi V, Dionigi G, et al. Meta-analysis of recurrent laryngeal nerve injury in thyroid surgery with or without intraoperative nerve monitoring. *Acta Otorhinolaryngol Ital.* 2014;34(4):223-229.
96. Cernea CR, Brandão LG, Hojaij FC, et al. How to minimize complications in thyroid surgery? *Auris Nasus Larynx.* 2010;37(1):1-5.
97. Cernea CR, Brandão LG, Brandão J. Neuromonitoring in thyroid surgery. *Curr Opin Otolaryngol Head Neck Surg.* 2012;20(2):125-129.
98. Mangano A, Wu CW, Lianos GD, et al. Evidence-based analysis on the clinical impact of intraoperative neuromonitoring in thyroid surgery: state of the art and future perspectives. *Surg Technol Int.* 2014;25:91-96.
99. Barczyński M, Konturek A, Pragacz K, Papier A, Stopa M, Nowak W. Intraoperative nerve monitoring can reduce prevalence of recurrent laryngeal nerve injury in thyroid reoperations: results of a retrospective cohort study. *World J Surg.* 2014;38(3):599-606.
100. Wong KP, Mak KL, Wong CKH, Lang BHH. Systematic review and meta-analysis on intra-operative neuro-monitoring in high-risk thyroidectomy. *Int J Surg.* 2017;38:21-30.
101. Chuang YC, Huang SM. Protective effect of intraoperative nerve monitoring against recurrent laryngeal nerve injury during re-exploration of the thyroid. *World J Surg Oncol.* 2013;11:94.
102. Liddy W, Lawson BR, Barber SR, et al. Anterior laryngeal electrodes for recurrent laryngeal nerve monitoring during thyroid and parathyroid surgery: new expanded options for neural monitoring. *Laryngoscope.* 2018;128(12):2910-2915.
103. Sarı S, Erbil Y, Sümer A, et al. Evaluation of recurrent laryngeal nerve monitoring in thyroid surgery. *Int J Surg.* 2010;8(6):474-478.
104. Musholt TJ, Clerici T, Dralle H, et al. German Association of Endocrine Surgeons practice guidelines for the surgical treatment of benign thyroid disease. *Langenbecks Arch Surg.* 2011;396(5):639-649.
105. Chandrasekhar SS, Randolph GW, Seidman MD, et al. Clinical practice guideline: improving voice outcomes after thyroid surgery. *Otolaryngol Head Neck Surg.* 2013;148 (6 Suppl):S1-S37.
106. Haugen BR, Alexander EK, Bible KC, et al. 2015 American Thyroid Association Management Guidelines for Adult Patients with Thyroid Nodules and Differentiated Thyroid Cancer: The American Thyroid Association Guidelines Task Force on Thyroid Nodules and Differentiated Thyroid Cancer. *Thyroid.* 2016;26(1):1-133.
107. Terris DJ, Snyder S, Carneiro-Pla D, et al. American Thyroid Association statement on outpatient thyroidectomy. *Thyroid.* 2013;23(10):1193-1202.
108. Chen AY, Bernet VJ, Carty SE, et al. American Thyroid Association statement on optimal surgical management of goiter. *Thyroid.* 2014;24(2):181-189.
109. Shindo ML, Caruana SM, Kandil E, et al. Management of invasive well-differentiated thyroid cancer: an American Head and Neck Society consensus statement. AHNS consensus statement. *Head Neck.* 2014;36(10):1379-1390.
110. Chiang FY, Lu IC, Chen HC, et al. Intraoperative neuromonitoring for early localization and identification of recurrent laryngeal nerve during thyroid surgery. *Kaohsiung J Med Sci.* 2010;26(12):633-639.
111. Goretzki PE, Schwarz K, Brinkmann J, Wirowski D, Lammers BJ. The impact of intraoperative neuromonitoring (IONM) on surgical strategy in bilateral thyroid diseases: is it worth the effort? *World J Surg.* 2010;34(6):1274-1284.
112. Phelan E, Schneider R, Lorenz K, et al. Continuous vagal IONM prevents recurrent laryngeal nerve paralysis by revealing initial EMG changes of impending neuropraxic injury: a prospective, multicenter study. *Laryngoscope.* 2014;124(6):1498-1505.
113. Schneider R, Lamade W, Hermann M, et al. [Continuous intraoperative neuromonitoring of the recurrent laryngeal nerve in thyroid surgery (CIONM)—where are we now? An update to the European Symposium of Continuous Neuromonitoring in Thyroid Surgery]. *Zentralbl Chir.* 2012;137(1):88-90.
114. Alesina PF, Hinrichs J, Meier B, Cho EY, Bolli M, Walz MK. Intraoperative neuromonitoring for surgical training in thyroid surgery: its routine use allows a safe operation instead of lack of experienced mentoring. *World J Surg.* 2014;38(3):592-598.
115. Kamani D, Potenza AS, Cernea CR, Kamani YV, Randolph GW. The nonrecurrent laryngeal nerve: anatomic and electrophysiologic algorithm for reliable identification. *Laryngoscope.* 2015;125(2):503-508.
116. Randolph GW, Kamani D. Intraoperative electrophysiologic monitoring of the recurrent laryngeal nerve during thyroid and parathyroid surgery: experience with 1,381 nerves at risk. *Laryngoscope.* 2017;127(1):280-286.
117. Lennquist S, Cahlin C, Smeds S. The superior laryngeal nerve in thyroid surgery. *Surgery.* 1987;102(6):999-1008.
118. Naytah M, Ibrahim I, da Silva S. Importance of incorporating intraoperative neuromonitoring of the external branch of the superior laryngeal nerve in thyroidectomy: a review and meta-analysis study. *Head Neck.* 2019;41(6):2034-2041.

119. Cernea CR, Brandão LG, Hisham AN. Surgical anatomy of the superior laryngeal nerve. In: Randolph GW, ed. *Surgery of the Thyroid and Parathyroid Glands*. Elsevier; 2018:316-325.
120. Uludag M, Aygun N, Kartal K, et al. Contribution of intraoperative neural monitoring to preservation of the external branch of the superior laryngeal nerve: a randomized prospective clinical trial. *Langenbecks Arch Surg*. 2017;402(6):965-976.
121. Barczyński M, Konturek A, Stopa M, Honowska A, Nowak W. Randomized controlled trial of visualization versus neuromonitoring of the external branch of the superior laryngeal nerve during thyroidectomy. *World J Surg*. 2012;36(6):1340-1347.
122. Dionigi G, Kim HY, Randolph GW, et al. Prospective validation study of Cernea classification for predicting EMG alterations of the external branch of the superior laryngeal nerve. *Surg Today*. 2016;46(7):785-791.
123. Lee J, Fraser S, Glover A, Sidhu S. Prospective evaluation of the utility of routine neuromonitoring for an established thyroid surgical practice. *ANZ J Surg*. 2017;87(10):E138-E142.
124. Lamadé W, Meyding-Lamadé U, Hund E, Senninger N, Herfarth C. [Transtracheal monitoring of the recurrent laryngeal nerve. Prototype of a new tube]. *Chirurg*. 1997;68(2):193-195.
125. Dionigi G, Lombardi D, Lombardi CP, et al. Intraoperative neuromonitoring in thyroid surgery: a point prevalence survey on utilization, management, and documentation in Italy. *Updates Surg*. 2014;66(4):269-276.
126. Horne SK, Gal TJ, Brennan JA. Prevalence and patterns of intraoperative nerve monitoring for thyroidectomy. *Otolaryngol Head Neck Surg*. 2007;136(6):952-956.
127. Sturgeon C, Sturgeon T, Angelos P. Neuromonitoring in thyroid surgery: attitudes, usage patterns, and predictors of use among endocrine surgeons. *World J Surg*. 2009;33(3):417-425.
128. Ho Y, Carr MM, Goldenberg D. Trends in intraoperative neural monitoring for thyroid and parathyroid surgery amongst otolaryngologists and general surgeons. *Eur Arch Otorhinolaryngol*. 2013;270(9):2525-2530.
129. Dionigi G, Bacuzzi A, Barczynski M, et al. Implementation of systematic neuromonitoring training for thyroid surgery. *Updates Surg*. 2011;63(3):201-207.
130. Lamade W, Fogel W, Rieke K, Senninger N, Herfarth C. [Intraoperative monitoring of the recurrent laryngeal nerve. A new method]. *Chirurg*. 1996;67(4):451-454.
131. Dionigi G, Barczynski M, Chiang FY, et al. Why monitor the recurrent laryngeal nerve in thyroid surgery? *J Endocrinol Invest*. 2010;33(11):819-822.
132. Singer MC, Rosenfeld RM, Sundaram K. Laryngeal nerve monitoring: current utilization among head and neck surgeons. *Otolaryngol Head Neck Surg*. 2012;146(6):895-899.
133. Marti JL, Holm T, Randolph G. Universal use of intraoperative nerve monitoring by recently fellowship-trained thyroid surgeons is common, associated with higher surgical volume, and impacts intraoperative decision-making. *World J Surg*. 2016;40(2):337-343.
134. Dionigi G, Wu CW, Lombardi D, et al. The current state of recurrent laryngeal nerve monitoring for thyroid surgery. *Curr Otorhinolaryngol Rep*. 2014;2(1):44-54.
135. Dralle H, Sekulla C, Lorenz K, Nguyen Thanh P, Schneider R, Machens A. Loss of the nerve monitoring signal during bilateral thyroid surgery. *Br J Surg*. 2012;99(8):1089-1095.
136. Ulmer C, Koch KP, Seimer A, et al. Real-time monitoring of the recurrent laryngeal nerve: an observational clinical trial. *Surgery*. 2008;143(3):359-365.
137. Lamadé W, Ulmer C, Seimer A, et al. A new system for continuous recurrent laryngeal nerve monitoring. *Minim Invasive Ther Allied Technol*. 2007;16(3):149-154.
138. Singer MC. Safety and feasibility of a novel recurrent laryngeal nerve monitoring technique. *Laryngoscope*. 2018;128(Suppl 4):S1-S8.
139. Schneider R, Rangel L, Bertelli A. Intraoperative cranial nerve monitoring in otolaryngology-head and neck surgery. In: Scharpf J, Randolph GW, eds. *Intraoperative Cranial Nerve Monitoring in Otolaryngology-Head and Neck Surgery*. Springer; 2022:89-98.
140. Schneider R, Lorenz K, Machens A, Thanh PN, Randolph GW, Dralle H. Continuous intraoperative neuromonitoring (CIONM) of the recurrent laryngeal nerve. In: Randolph GW, ed. *The Recurrent and Superior Laryngeal Nerves*. Springer International Publishing; 2016:169-183.
141. Schneider R, Machens A, Lorenz K, Dralle H. Intraoperative nerve monitoring in thyroid surgery-shifting current paradigms. *Gland Surg*. 2020;9(Suppl 2):S120-S128.
142. Schneider R, Randolph GW, Sekulla C, et al. Continuous intraoperative vagus nerve stimulation for identification of imminent recurrent laryngeal nerve injury. *Head Neck*. 2013;35(11):1591-1598.
143. Schneider R, Machens A, Randolph G, et al. Evolution and progress of continuous intraoperative neural monitoring. *Ann Thyroid*. 2018;3:29-29.
144. Kandil E, Mohsin K, Murcy MA, Randolph GW. Continuous vagal monitoring value in prevention of vocal cord paralysis following thyroid surgery. *Laryngoscope*. 2018;128(10):2429-2432.
145. Marin Arteaga A, Peloni G, Leuchter I, et al. Modification of the surgical strategy for the dissection of the recurrent laryngeal nerve using continuous intraoperative nerve monitoring. *World J Surg*. 2018;42(2):444-450.
146. Schneider R, Lorenz K, Sekulla C, Machens A, Nguyen-Thanh P, Dralle H. [Surgical strategy during intended total thyroidectomy after loss of EMG signal on the first side of resection]. *Chirurg*. 2015;86(2):154-163.
147. Phelan E, Potenza A, Slough C, Zurakowski D, Kamani D, Randolph G. Recurrent laryngeal nerve monitoring during thyroid surgery: normative vagal and recurrent laryngeal nerve electrophysiological data. *Otolaryngol Head Neck Surg*. 2012;147(4):640-646.
148. Schneider R, Sekulla C, Machens A, Lorenz K, Nguyen Thanh P, Dralle H. Postoperative vocal fold palsy in patients undergoing thyroid surgery with continuous or intermittent nerve monitoring. *Br J Surg*. 2015;102(11):1380-1387.
149. Schneider R, Machens A, Sekulla C, Lorenz K, Elwerr M, Dralle H. Superiority of continuous over intermittent intraoperative nerve monitoring in preventing vocal cord palsy. *Br J Surg*. 2021;108(5):566-573.
150. Wu CW, Lu IC, Randolph GW, et al. Investigation of optimal intensity and safety of electrical nerve stimulation during intraoperative neuromonitoring of the recurrent laryngeal nerve: a prospective porcine model. *Head Neck*. 2010;32(10):1295-1301.
151. Schneider R, Przybyl J, Pliquett U, et al. A new vagal anchor electrode for real-time monitoring of the recurrent laryngeal nerve. *Am J Surg*. 2010;199(4):507-514.
152. Castoro MA, Yoo PB, Hincapie JG, et al. Excitation properties of the right cervical vagus nerve in adult dogs. *Exp Neurol*. 2011;227(1):62-68.
153. Groves DA, Brown VJ. Vagal nerve stimulation: a review of its applications and potential mechanisms that mediate its clinical effects. *Neurosci Biobehav Rev*. 2005;29(3):493-500.

154. Yoo PB, Lubock NB, Hincapie JG, Ruble SB, Hamann JJ, Grill WM. High-resolution measurement of electrically-evoked vagus nerve activity in the anesthetized dog. *J Neural Eng.* 2013;10(2):026003.
155. Ben-Menachem E. Vagus-nerve stimulation for the treatment of epilepsy. *Lancet Neurol.* 2002;1(8):477-482.
156. Ben-Menachem E, Revesz D, Simon BJ, Silberstein S. Surgically implanted and non-invasive vagus nerve stimulation: a review of efficacy, safety and tolerability. *Eur J Neurol.* 2015;22(9):1260-1268.
157. Cohen-Gadol AA, Britton JW, Wetjen NM, Marsh WR, Meyer FB, Raffel C. Neurostimulation therapy for epilepsy: current modalities and future directions. *Mayo Clin Proc.* 2003;78(2):238-248.
158. Terris DJ, Chaung K, Duke WS. Continuous vagal nerve monitoring is dangerous and should not routinely be done during thyroid surgery. *World J Surg.* 2015;39(10): 2471-2476.
159. Choi SY, Son YI. Intraoperative neuromonitoring for thyroid surgery: the proven benefits and limitations. *Clin Exp Otorhinolaryngol.* 2019;12(4):335-336.
160. Hatton KW, McLarney JT, Pittman T, Fahy BG. Vagal nerve stimulation: overview and implications for anesthesiologists. *Anesth Analg.* 2006;103(5):1241-1249.
161. Agnew WF, McCreery DB. Considerations for safety with chronically implanted nerve electrodes. *Epilepsia.* 1990;31 (Suppl 2):S27-S32.

Voice Evaluation & Flexible Laryngoscopy

31

Defne Altan, AB
Rajshri M. Gartland, MD, MPH
Richard A. Hodin, MD

INTRODUCTION

Voice quality is an important outcome after thyroidectomy. Thyroidectomy involves a risk of recurrent laryngeal nerve (RLN) injury and subsequent temporary or permanent vocal fold dysfunction.[1] Overall rates of RLN injury are low when thyroidectomy is performed by high-volume surgeons.[2,3] An annual volume of over 50 cases has been shown to be protective, and over 100 cases even more so.[4,5] Very rarely (<0.1%), direct trauma from endotracheal intubation can also cause vocal fold dysfunction.[6] Postoperative voice changes unrelated to nerve injury are common after thyroidectomy and usually resolve with time.[7-10]

Flexible laryngoscopy can be used to investigate suspected damage to the RLN both pre- and postoperatively. Unilateral RLN injury affects vocal fold position and can cause voice hoarseness, difficulty swallowing, and aspiration.[5,11] Bilateral RLN injury compromises the airway by limiting bilateral vocal fold abduction on inspiration and can necessitate tracheostomy.[12] Bilateral injury can considerably impair patient quality of life[13-15] as well as increase economic burden,[16] and it is associated with plaintiff payout in thyroidectomy-related malpractice cases.[17] Recommendations from the American Association of Endocrine Surgeons on voice assessment pre- and postoperatively are shown in Table 31–1, and are centered around patient history and physical exam, surgical indication, and intraoperative events and findings.[18] In this chapter, we discuss perioperative voice evaluation and flexible laryngoscopy.

PREOPERATIVE EVALUATION & INDICATIONS FOR LARYNGOSCOPY

A careful history and physical exam should be used to screen patients before thyroidectomy. While some societies advocate for routine preoperative screening with flexible laryngoscopy, many endocrine surgeons safely screen only patients at risk for prior nerve injury and/or current vocal fold dysfunction.[19-22] As a general guideline, flexible laryngoscopy should be performed for the following listed indications.[21,22]

1. *Persistent hoarseness or change in voice quality noted by the patient or surgeon:* Questionnaires assessing voice quality can be used to screen patients, but none have been standardized. Pain or difficulty with swallowing, voice huskiness or hoarseness, and difficulty speaking loudly, singing, or producing high pitch correspond to items on the Thyroidectomy Related Voice Questionnaire (TRVQ) and can indicate the need for flexible laryngoscopy.[23,24]
2. *History of prior surgery in which the recurrent laryngeal or vagus nerves might have been at risk:* Examples include prior thyroid/parathyroid operations, cervical spine procedures involving an anterior approach, carotid endarterectomies, and certain cardiac and thoracic surgery procedures.
3. *Suspicion of locally advanced cancer based on physical exam or imaging findings:* For example, a posteriorly situated thyroid cancer, loss of normal anatomic planes between the thyroid and adjacent structures, or direct invasion into adjacent organs may be indications for flexible laryngoscopy.[25] Knowledge of vocal fold dysfunction in the setting of locally advanced cancer could change surgical management. For instance, a multidisciplinary team may consider neoadjuvant treatment in this setting. In some cases, a decision is made to limit the operation to one side of the neck, that is, the side that already has the vocal cord paralysis. At the time of surgery, a surgeon may decide to use intraoperative nerve monitoring to help assess function of both the involved and uninvolved nerves. Information garnered from flexible laryngoscopy can also help guide preoperative patient counseling and expectations.[14]

Table 31–1. Recommendations from the American Association of Endocrine Surgeons for pre- and postoperative voice assessment.

47	In preoperative discussion of thyroidectomy, the surgeon should disclose to the patient the possibility, likelihood, and implications of permanent vocal fold dysfunction (moderate-quality evidence)
48	Prior to thyroidectomy, laryngeal examination should be performed in patients determined to have vocal abnormalities as assessed by the surgeon, preexisting laryngeal disorders, prior at-risk surgery, or locally advanced thyroid cancer (low-quality evidence)
49	Voice assessment should be performed at the postoperative visit (low-quality evidence)
50	After thyroidectomy, laryngeal examination should be performed in patients with known or suspected new RLN dysfunction or aspiration (moderate-quality evidence)
51	If vocal fold motion impairment is suspected or identified, early referral of the patient to a laryngologist is recommended (moderate-quality evidence)

Source: Reproduced with permission from Patel KN, Yip L, Lubitz CC, et al. The American Association of Endocrine Surgeons Guidelines for the definitive surgical management of thyroid disease in adults. *Ann Surg*. 2020;271(3):e21-e93.

4. *A thyroid gland with anatomic features suggesting that laryngeal nerves may be at higher risk than normal during the operation:* For example, a large multinodular goiter may obscure normal anatomy secondary to displacement of the trachea and/or nerve and a retrosternal goiter may predispose to stretch injury during thyroid retraction.

INTRAOPERATIVE CAUSES OF VOCAL FOLD DYSFUNCTION & ANATOMIC CONSIDERATIONS

Intraoperatively, vocal fold dysfunction can be caused by intubation, thermal or traction-related nerve trauma, or nerve transection. Injury to the RLN can be avoided by visually identifying and avoiding injury to the nerve on the operative side along the entire field of dissection.[26,27] Some surgeons use intraoperative nerve monitoring routinely while others may use it selectively depending on the clinical situation. While nerve monitoring has not been shown in large, randomized control trials to significantly decrease rates of permanent nerve palsy,[28,29] a unilateral loss of signal may alert the surgeon to delay operating on the contralateral side to avoid the small but morbid risk of bilateral laryngeal paralysis.[5]

Many different parts of the larynx and surrounding structures contribute to voice and can affect postoperative function.[5,30] The RLN supplies all extrinsic muscles of the larynx except the cricothyroid muscle.[5] During thyroidectomy, injury to the RLN can lead to an immobile vocal fold that does not close adequately leading to suboptimal speaking and/or swallowing.[5] The external branch of the superior laryngeal nerve (EBSLN), and the cricothyroid muscle it innervates, is important for producing higher pitch as well as forceful speech, and thus injury to these structures can lead to altered pitch, limited projection, and tiring of the voice (Figure 31–1).[26,31,32] Traumatic intubation, while rare, can cause laceration, hematoma, edema, or rupture of the vocal folds, with or without chronic granulation or polyp formation, and rarely can result in arytenoid dislocation.[15] Other intraoperative occurrences, such as mild soft tissue injury to the structures surrounding the larynx or postoperative local edema, have an unknown impact on postoperative voice.[33] Sternothyroid muscle division, which is occasionally deployed during thyroidectomy to gain access to the superior pole, has not been shown to lead to adverse voice outcomes.[34,35]

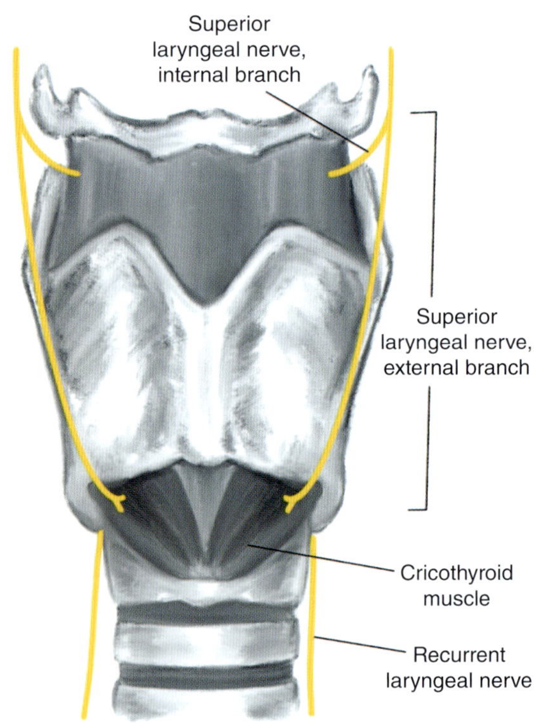

▲ **Figure 31–1.** Laryngeal anatomy.

POSTOPERATIVE EVALUATION & INDICATIONS FOR LARYNGOSCOPY

Voice changes are common after thyroid surgery and are usually transient.[36] Postoperative symptoms can include hoarseness, voice fatigue, and reduction in vocal range. Subjective voice changes after surgery are common, occurring in up to one-third of patients postoperatively.[37,38] The overall incidence of RLN injury after thyroidectomy is low among high-volume surgeons (<6%),[4] though the true percentage is difficult to assess without routine laryngoscopy and thus likely an underestimate, especially given that postoperative symptoms do not reliably indicate intraoperative nerve injury.[5]

Postoperatively, when the primary goal is to optimize patient voice outcomes and quality of life, auditory assessment of voice is adequate in most cases.[39] Voice symptoms may prompt assessment with flexible laryngoscopy, as well as other adjuncts such as laryngeal stroboscopy, transcutaneous laryngeal ultrasound, CT, MRI, and laryngeal electromyography.[11,14] While not used routinely, some centers will also administer pre- and postoperative surveys to assess voice outcomes, such as the Voice Handicap Index (VHI), which can assess voice symptoms and their impact on quality of life.[40,41]

The following indications can be considered for evaluation with laryngoscopy:[22]

1. *Voice symptoms or hoarseness that is significantly bothersome to the patient:* In this situation, laryngoscopy should be performed even if full recovery of the voice is anticipated and the surgeon is certain that the RLNs are intact.
2. *Significant hoarseness persisting more than 2 to 8 weeks postsurgery:* Postanesthetic voice changes can last up to 2 weeks; hoarseness persisting after 2 weeks warrants investigation.[15] Performing a laryngoscopy after 8 weeks postoperatively diminishes the benefit a patient with vocal fold dysfunction might receive from treatment.[15]
3. *Known nerve injury or loss of signal observed during thyroidectomy with postoperative symptoms:* While voice symptoms often improve over several months after thyroidectomy, early intervention and referral to a laryngologist have been consistently associated with better outcomes.[15] Treatment options for acute vocal fold paralysis include temporary vocal fold medialization via cord injection[42] as well as nimodipine, a calcium channel blocker shown in limited studies to improve nerve reinnervation and voice outcomes.[43] Once referred to a laryngologist, patients may work with a speech-language pathologist on voice and swallowing optimization and potentially pursue medialization via cord injection or arytenoid adduction.[11,42] Vocal fold augmentation produces the best patient outcomes when performed less than 3 months after thyroidectomy.[15,44] In the case of bilateral vocal fold dysfunction, therapies such as cordotomy and arytenoidectomy prioritize ventilatory function, though voice outcomes (in addition to ventilation) may be improved with newer reinnervation and laryngeal pacing techniques.[12,45,46]

GUIDELINES FOR PRACTICAL USE OF FLEXIBLE LARYNGOSCOPY

Flexible laryngoscopy can easily be performed in an office setting. A laryngoscope with a flexible fiberoptic camera is used to evaluate the nasopharynx, oropharynx, and laryngopharynx. The main equipment for flexible laryngoscopy includes:[47]

- flexible laryngoscope with light source
- gloves and protective eyewear
- nasal speculum and lubricant
- topical vasoconstrictor or anesthetic with cotton swabs or pledgets for any nonspray topical vasoconstrictor/anesthetics[47]

The patient should sit upright and lean forward, chin up and out, and legs should not be crossed. To apply topical anesthetic, the speculum is inserted so its handle is parallel to the floor, and its tongs open vertically. The nares can be held open and the topical anesthetic applied several minutes before the procedure. If using spray, it should be directed posteriorly toward the floor of the nasopharynx.

After the anesthetic has taken effect, the lubricated laryngoscope tip is inserted into the nose and advanced parallel to the floor of the nasopharynx below the inferior turbinate (Figure 31–2). The laryngoscope tip should be tilted slightly upward. In cases of septal deviation or large inferior turbinates, the path of the laryngoscope tip can also be directed above the inferior turbinate. Care should be taken not to touch the mucosa, especially the septum, to minimize irritation.[32] In the back of the nasopharynx, the laryngoscope tip should be flexed using the thumb control to go down past the palate, then straightened to avoid curling forward into the uvula.[47] Once the vocal folds come into view, they are assessed for masses or mucosal abnormalities. Arytenoid mobility is assessed as well as mucosal wave and completeness of glottic closure.[48] The patient can be asked to say "eeee" and sniff in through their nose to visualize vocal fold adduction and abduction, respectively.[49] After evaluation is complete, the laryngoscope can be gently withdrawn. Potential complications include nasal irritation and bleeding as well as gagging, coughing, or vomiting. The procedure is typically well tolerated with minimal risk to patients.[50] After the procedure, the patient should not eat or drink for 20 minutes to avoid aspiration in the setting of residual

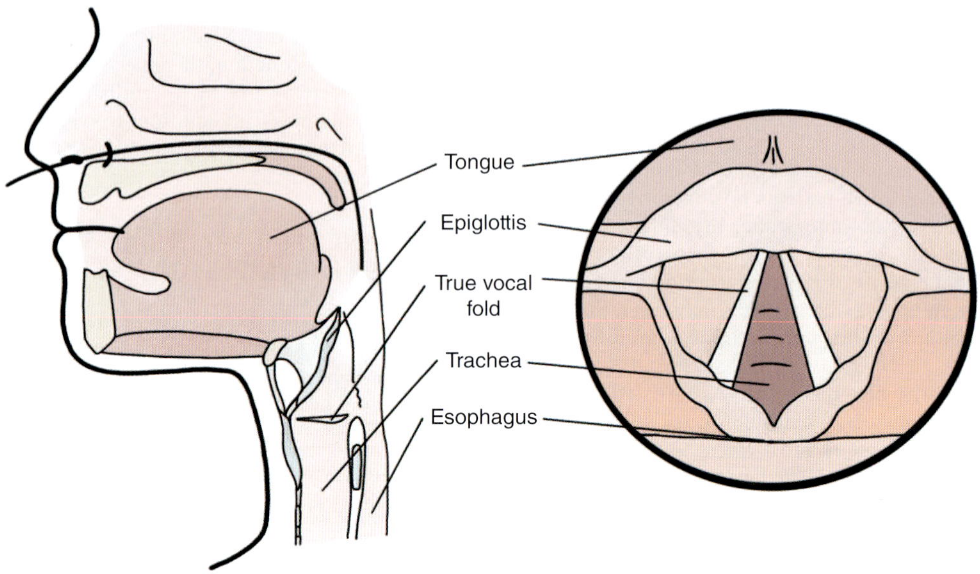

Figure 31–2. View of vocal cords during flexible laryngoscopy.

anesthesia.[49] Tips and tricks for the procedure are summarized in Table 31–2.

CONCLUSIONS

Voice and quality of life are important outcomes after thyroidectomy. A key priority for thyroid surgeons is to avoid preventable voice issues and recognize vocal cord dysfunction when it does occur. Transient or permanent postoperative voice changes can occur due to a number of etiologies, including RLN, EBSLN, or cricothyroid muscle damage as well as intubation trauma. Flexible laryngoscopy is a high-yield, accessible, and well-tolerated procedure to assess vocal fold function before and after thyroidectomy as needed.

Table 31–2. Tips and tricks when performing flexible laryngoscopy.

- Before the procedure, give the patient a tissue as tearing may occur.
- The initial positioning can be described to the patient similar to leaning forward to smell a flower, or a turtle sticking their head out of its shell.
- Some patients may hold their breath during the procedure—remind them to breathe.
- Ask the patient to swallow as needed during the procedure to clear the scope.
- Common errors include: not using enough vasoconstrictor, inserting the scope too forcefully, and losing situational awareness of the scope tip.

REFERENCES

1. Schneider M, Dahm V, Passler C, et al. Complete and incomplete recurrent laryngeal nerve injury after thyroid and parathyroid surgery: characterizing paralysis and paresis. *Surgery*. 2019;166(3):369-374.
2. Adam MA, Thomas S, Youngwirth L, et al. Is there a minimum number of thyroidectomies a surgeon should perform to optimize patient outcomes? *Ann Surg*. 2017;265(2):402-407.
3. Bedi HK, Jedrzejko N, Nguyen A, Aspinall SR, Wiseman SM. Thyroid and parathyroid surgeon case volume influences patient outcomes: a systematic review. *Surg Oncol*. 2021;38:101550.
4. Aspinall S, Oweis D, Chadwick D. Effect of surgeons' annual operative volume on the risk of permanent hypoparathyroidism, recurrent laryngeal nerve palsy and haematoma following thyroidectomy: analysis of United Kingdom registry of endocrine and thyroid surgery (UKRETS). *Langenbeck's Arch Surg*. 2019;404:421-430.
5. Tolley N, Witterick I, Randolph GW. *Laryngeal Examination in Thyroid and Parathyroid Surgery. In: Randolph GW, eds. Surgery of the Thyroid and Parathyroid Glands*. 3rd ed. Philadelphia, PA: Elsevier; 2021:156-162.
6. Kikura M, Suzuki K, Itagaki T, Takada T, Sato S. Age and comorbidity as risk factors for vocal cord paralysis associated with tracheal intubation. *Br J Anaesth*. 2007;98(4):524-530.
7. Tedla M, Chakrabarti S, Suchankova M, Weickert MO. Voice outcomes after thyroidectomy without superior and recurrent laryngeal nerve injury: VoiSS questionnaire and GRBAS tool assessment. *Eur Arch Oto-Rhino-L*. 2016;273:4543-4547.
8. Sinagra DL, Montesinos MR, Tacchi VA, et al. Voice changes after thyroidectomy without recurrent laryngeal nerve injury. *J Am Coll Surg*. 2004;199(4):556-560.
9. Maeda T, Saito M, Otsuki N, et al. Voice quality after surgical treatment for thyroid cancer. *Thyroid*. 2013;23(7):847-853.

10. Kuhn, MA, Gary B, David M. Patient perspectives on dysphonia after thyroidectomy for thyroid cancer. *J Voice*. 2013;27(1):111-114.
11. Culp JM, Patel G. Recurrent Laryngeal Nerve Injury. [Updated 2023 May 22]. In: StatPearls [Internet]. Treasure Island (FL): StatPearls Publishing; 2024 Jan-. Available from: https://www.ncbi.nlm.nih.gov/books/NBK560832/
12. Czesak MA, Osuch-Wójcikiewicz E, Niemczyk K. Methods of surgical treatment of bilateral vocal fold paralysis. *Endokrynologia Polska*. 2020;71(4):350.
13. Gardner GM, Smith MM, Yaremchuk KL, Peterson EL. The cost of vocal fold paralysis after thyroidectomy. *Laryngoscope*. 2013;123(6):1455-1463.
14. Dhillon VK, Randolph GW, Stack Jr BC, et al. Immediate and partial neural dysfunction after thyroid and parathyroid surgery: need for recognition, laryngeal exam, and early treatment. *Head & Neck*. 2020;42(12):3779-3794.
15. Chandrasekhar SS, Randolph GW, Seidman MD, et al. Clinical practice guideline: improving voice outcomes after thyroid surgery. *Otolaryngol Head Neck Surg*. 2013;148(6_suppl):S1-S37.
16. Cohen SM, Kim J, Roy N, Asche C, Courey M. Direct health care costs of laryngeal diseases and disorders. *Laryngoscope*. 2012 Jul;122(7):1582-1588.
17. Gartland RM, Bloom JP, Parangi S, et al. A long, unnerving road: malpractice claims involving the surgical management of thyroid and parathyroid disease. *World J Surg*. 2019;43(11):2850-2855.
18. Patel KN, Yip L, Lubitz CC, et al. The American Association of Endocrine Surgeons Guidelines for the definitive surgical management of thyroid disease in adults. *Ann Surg*. 2020;271(3):e21-e93.
19. Maher DI, Goare S, Forrest E, Grodski S, Serpell JW, Lee JC. Routine preoperative laryngoscopy for thyroid surgery is not necessary without risk factors. *Thyroid*. 2019;29(11):1646-1652.
20. Black KA, Wilkinson DS. Selective laryngoscopy before thyroidectomy: a risk assessment. *ANZ J Surg*. 2022;92(6):1423-1427.
21. Franch-Arcas G, González-Sánchez C, Aguilera-Molina YY, Rozo-Coronel O, Estévez-Alonso JS, Muñoz-Herrera Á. Is there a case for selective, rather than routine, preoperative laryngoscopy in thyroid surgery? *Gland Surg*. 2015;4(1):8-18.
22. Hodin R, Clark O, Doherty G, Grant C, Heller K, Weigel R. Voice issues and laryngoscopy in thyroid surgery patients. *Surgery*. 2013;154(1):46-47.
23. Hwang YS, Shim MR, Kim GJ, et al. Development and validation of the thyroidectomy-related voice and symptom questionnaire (TVSQ). *J Voice* 32022:6(1):145.e15-145.e22.
24. Nam IC, Bae JS, Shim MR, Hwang YS, Kim MS, Sun DI. The importance of preoperative laryngeal examination before thyroidectomy and the usefulness of a voice questionnaire in screening. *World J Surg*. 2012 Feb;36(2):303-309.
25. Haugen BR, Alexander EK, Bible KC et al. 2015 American Thyroid Association management guidelines for adult patients with thyroid nodules and differentiated thyroid cancer: the American Thyroid Association guidelines task force on thyroid nodules and differentiated thyroid cancer. *Thyroid*. 2016 Jan 1; 26(1):1-33.
26. Varaldo E, Ansaldo GL, Mascherini M, Cafiero F, Minuto MN. Neurological complications in thyroid surgery: a surgical point of view on laryngeal nerves. *Front Endocrinol*. 2014 Jul 15;5:108.
27. Hermann M, Alk G, Roka R, Glaser K, Freissmuth M. Laryngeal recurrent nerve injury in surgery for benign thyroid diseases: effect of nerve dissection and impact of individual surgeon in more than 27,000 nerves at risk. *Ann Surg*. 2002;235(2):261-268.
28. Pisanu A, Porceddu G, Podda M, Cois A, Uccheddu A. Systematic review with meta-analysis of studies comparing intraoperative neuromonitoring of recurrent laryngeal nerves versus visualization alone during thyroidectomy. *J Surg Res*. 2014 May 1;188(1):152-161.
29. Davey MG, Cleere EF, Lowery AJ, Kerin MJ. Intraoperative recurrent laryngeal nerve monitoring versus visualisation alone: a systematic review and meta-analysis of randomized controlled trials. *Am J Surg*. 2022 Sep 1;224(3):836-841.
30. Sung ES, Kim KY, Yun BR, et al. Long-term functional voice outcomes after thyroidectomy, and effect of endotracheal intubation on voice. *Eur Arch Otorhinolaryngol*. 2018;275(12):3049-3058.
31. Potenza AS, Araujo Filho VJF, Cernea CR. Injury of the external branch of the superior laryngeal nerve in thyroid surgery. *Gland Surg*. 2017 Oct;6(5):552-562.
32. Sinclair CF, Bumpous JM, Haugen BR, et al. Laryngeal examination in thyroid and parathyroid surgery: an American Head and Neck Society consensus statement: AHNS consensus statement. *Head Neck*. 2016;38(6):811-819.
33. Maeda T, Saito M, Otsuki N, et al. Voice quality after surgical treatment for thyroid cancer. *Thyroid*. 2013 Jul;23(7):847-853.
34. Henry LR, Solomon NP, Howard R, et al. The functional impact on voice of sternothyroid muscle division during thyroidectomy. *Ann Surg Oncol*. 2008;15(7):2027-2033.
35. Barron C, Hamberis A, Gold B, Yun J, Chai RL. Impact of sternothyroid muscle division on patient-reported voice outcomes after thyroid surgery: a prospective study. *Otolaryngol Head Neck Surg*. 2023;169(6):1550-1555.
36. Kwon HK, Cheon YI, Shin SC, et al. Clinical significance of the preoperative thyroidectomy-related voice questionnaire score in thyroid surgery. *J Voice*. 2022;36(1):145-e7.
37. de Pedro NI, Fae A, Vartanian JG, et al. Voice and vocal self-assessment after thyroidectomy. *Head Neck*. 2006;28(12):1106-1114.
38. Li C, Lopez B, Fligor S, et al. Long-term voice changes after thyroidectomy: results from a validated survey. *Surgery*. 2021 Dec;170(6):1687-1691.
39. Heikkinen M, Penttilä E, Qvarnström M, Mäkinen K, Löppönen H, Kärkkäinen JM. Perceptual assessment and acoustic voice analysis as screening tests for vocal fold paresis after thyroid or parathyroid surgery. *World J Surg*. 2021;45(3):765-773.
40. Solomon NP, Helou LB, Henry LR, et al. Utility of the voice handicap index as an indicator of postthyroidectomy voice dysfunction. *J Voice*. 2013;27(3):348-354.
41. Rosen CA, Lee AS, Osborne J, Zullo T, Murry T. Development and validation of the voice handicap index-10. *Laryngoscope*. 2004;114(9):1549-1556.
42. Joliat GR, Guarnero V, Demartines N, Schweizer V, Matter M. Recurrent laryngeal nerve injury after thyroid and parathyroid surgery: incidence and postoperative evolution assessment. Medicine (Baltimore). 2017 Apr;96(17):e6674.
43. Lin RJ, Klein-Fedyshin M, Rosen CA. Nimodipine improves vocal fold and facial motion recovery after injury: a systematic review and meta-analysis. *Laryngoscope*. 2019 Apr;129(4):943-951.
44. Alghonaim Y, Roskies M, Kost K, Young J. Evaluating the timing of injection laryngoplasty for vocal fold paralysis in an attempt to avoid future type 1 thyroplasty. *J Otolaryngol Head Neck Surg*. 2013;42(1):24. Published 2013 Mar 19.

45. Powell ME, Zealear DL, Li Y, Garrett CG, Von Wahlde K, Netterville J. Unilateral and bilateral laryngeal pacing for bilateral vocal fold paralysis. Current otorhinolaryngology reports. 2020 Dec;8:395-401.
46. Prades JM, Lelonge Y, Dubois MD, et al. Dual laryngeal reinnervation in bilateral vocal fold paralysis: anatomical pitfalls. *Surg Radiol Anat*. 2021:43:1745-1751.
47. Mehta V. How to Do Flexible Laryngoscopy. MSD Manual Professional Edition, MSD Manuals, Sept. 2020, www.msdmanuals.com/professional/ear,-nose,-and-throat-disorders/how-to-do-throat-procedures/how-to-do-flexible-laryngoscopy. Accessed August 14, 2021.
48. Sinclair CF, Bumpous JM, Haugen BR, et al. Laryngeal examination in thyroid and parathyroid surgery: an American Head and Neck Society consensus statement. *Head Neck*. 2016;38:811-819.
49. Khaja S, Hoffman H. Flexile Fiberoptic Laryngoscopy (written instruction). Iowa Head and Neck Protocols, University of Iowa Health Care. Nov. 2023, https://medicine.uiowa.edu/iowaprotocols/flexible-fiberoptic-laryngoscopy-written-instruction. Accessed February 7th, 2024.
50. Paul BC, Rafii B, Achlatis S, Amin MR, Branski RC. Morbidity and patient perception of flexible laryngoscopy. *Ann Otol Rhinol Laryngol*. 2012 Nov;121(11):708-713.

Parathyroid Anatomy

32

Rajshri M. Gartland, MD, MPH
Sean Wrenn, MD
Matthew A. Nehs, MD

INTRODUCTION

The parathyroid gland was first identified in an Indian rhinoceros in 1849 by Sir Richard Owen and was first identified in a human by Swedish medical student Ivar Sandstrom in 1880.[1] Since this time, our knowledge of the parathyroid embryologic origin, typical and atypical locations, blood supply, and relation to other structures has grown tremendously. This knowledge is paramount for performing safe and effective thyroid and parathyroid surgery. This chapter outlines the anatomy of the parathyroid glands and their neurovascular relations.

EMBRYOLOGY

The superior parathyroid glands develop from the dorsal wing of the fourth pharyngeal pouch between the fifth and twelfth weeks of gestation.[2] The superior parathyroid gland shares a common origin with the lateral thyroid which develops from the vestigial fifth pharyngeal pouch and is ultimately incorporated in the fourth pharyngeal pouch.[2,3] Because of their limited embryologic migration, the superior parathyroid glands are typically more predictable in location when compared to the inferior glands.[4]

The inferior parathyroid glands and thymus develop from the third pharyngeal pouch during the same time period.[4] The parathyroid and thymus complex have a relatively long descent before reaching their final anatomic position.[4] The pathway of descent of the thymus extends from the angle of the mandible to the pericardium and accordingly inferior parathyroid glands are more likely to be variably located, asymmetric, or ectopic.[2,5]

LOCATION & BLOOD SUPPLY

Blood Supply

Both the superior and inferior parathyroid glands receive blood supply from the inferior thyroid artery (ITA) in the vast majority of cases.[6] Given the shared blood supply with the thyroid gland, an important risk of total thyroidectomy is parathyroid devascularization resulting in transient or permanent hypocalcemia. To avoid this, ligating and dividing the most distal branches of the ITA on the thyroid capsule is recommended during thyroidectomy.[7] Parathyroid glands often have a distinct polar vessel that comes off the ITA; acknowledgment of this anatomy can provide operative guidance if identified preoperatively on imaging. If the feeding vessel is embedded in the thyroid capsule, the thyroid capsule itself carrying the vessel should be preserved if possible.[7] In terms of venous drainage, similar to the thyroid, the parathyroid glands are drained by the superior, middle, and inferior thyroid veins.

Superior Parathyroid Gland Location & Variants

In approximately 80% of cases, the superior parathyroid glands are located posterior to the thyroid lobe near the cricothyroid junction at the intersection of the ITA and recurrent laryngeal nerve (RLN).[2,3,8] Given the more posterior location of the superior parathyroid gland, starting one's exploration with dissection down to the level of the prevertebral fascia can facilitate efficient identification. The superior glands often have a "halo" of surrounding fat and are freely mobile from the thyroid capsule but can occasionally be adhered to the thyroid capsule.[2] Superior parathyroid glands are almost always located posterior to the plane of the ipsilateral RLN. In about 15% of cases, the superior parathyroid gland can be located on the posterior lateral surface of the superior thyroid pole, and in less than 1% of cases, it may be located higher above the superior pole.[2] The superior gland can also be located more caudally (ie, descended, sometimes posterior to the inferior thyroid pole) or can be found in the retropharyngeal or retroesophageal space, though this is more common for pathologically enlarged glands.[2]

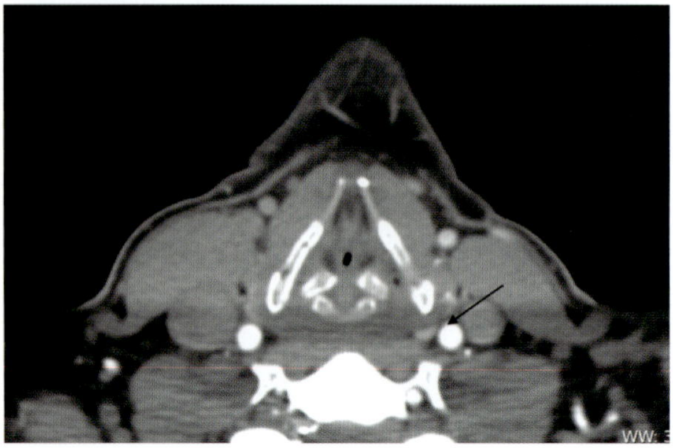

▲ **Figure 32–1.** Left retropharyngeal superior parathyroid adenoma seen on 4D CT (black arrow).

(Figure 32–1). Major ectopic locations for superior glands are rare but may include position adjacent to the common carotid artery or an intrathyroidal position.[2,3,8]

Inferior Parathyroid Gland Location & Variants

Compared to superior parathyroid glands, inferior glands are more widely distributed and more likely to be ectopic given their longer embryologic migration.[2,5] In about half of cases, inferior glands are located at the level of the inferior thyroid pole on the anterior, lateral, or posterior aspect, and typically are anterior to a plane drawn along the course of the RLN (Figure 32–2).[2] They are often located in a fat lobule

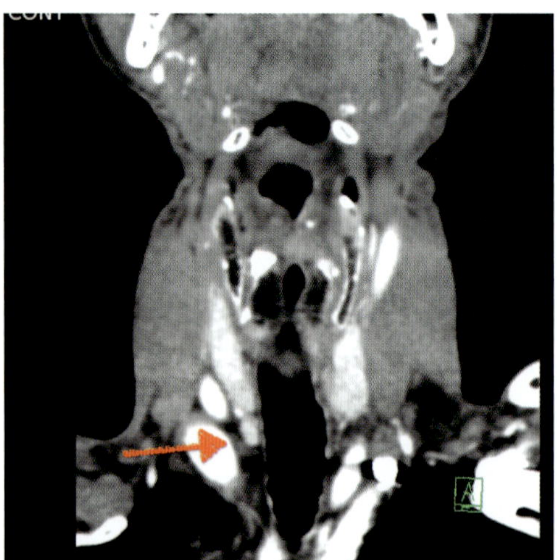

▲ **Figure 32–2.** 4D CT demonstrating most common location of an inferior parathyroid gland adjacent to the inferior thyroid pole (red arrow).

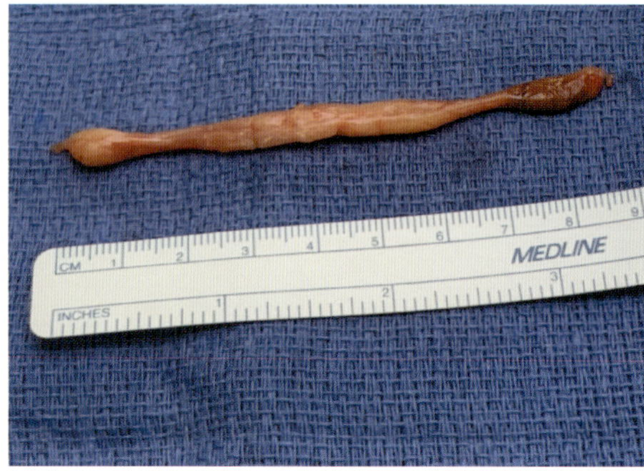

▲ **Figure 32–3.** Intrathymic abnormal inferior parathyroid gland.

near the inferior pole but can also be adhered to the posterior aspect of the thyroid capsule. In about 25% of cases, the inferior gland is located in the thyrothymic ligament or in the cervical portion of the thymus (Figure 32–3).[8] When separation from the thymus is delayed during embryology, an inferior parathyroid gland may get pulled down with the thymus and 4% to 5% of inferior glands are located in the chest.[2] In this situation, potential locations for the inferior glands include within or posterior to the retrosternal thymus or along the great mediastinal vessels such as the left innominate vein and ascending aorta. Such glands can develop an ectopic blood supply from the internal mammary artery, a thymic artery, or a direct branch from the aorta. In 1% to 3% of cases, the inferior parathyroid gland is truly intrathyroidal, a phenomenon deemed more common in inferior glands compared to superior glands (Figure 32–4).[3,6,8] Rarely, when the parathyroid-thymic complex fails to fully descend, it may be located high in the neck in areas such as the carotid bifurcation or elsewhere along the carotid sheath, adjacent to the angle of the mandible, or even near the hyoid bone.[2] In these situations, the inferior parathyroid glands may obtain blood supply from the superior thyroid artery.[2]

Symmetry

Symmetry of the superior parathyroid glands is reported in ~80% of cases, whereas symmetry of the inferior glands is reported in ~70% of cases. Symmetry of all four glands is reported in ~60% of cases.[8] These percentages fall when a gland is located at an uncommon site, and the most common asymmetric site is when one of the inferior glands is located in the thymus. Because the descent of the superior gland is crossed by that of the inferior glands during embryology, it is also possible to see both glands located in close proximity to

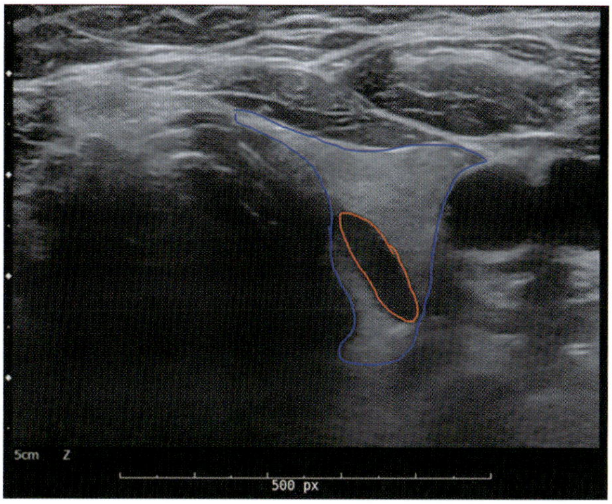

▲ **Figure 32–4.** Ultrasound demonstrating left intrathyroidal adenoma.

the crossing of the ITA and RLN.[4,8] Very rarely these glands can appear fused in a condition called "kissing pairs."[3] This can be distinguished from a bilobed gland given that a kissing pair will have two distinct vascular pedicles.[2]

GROSS ANATOMY & SUPERNUMERARY GLANDS

The average weight of a normal parathyroid gland is 35 to 50 mg and the average size is 5 × 3 × 1 mm.[3] The average weight of an enlarged parathyroid gland is 1000 mg, though this value can range from 50 mg to 20,000 mg. Figure 32–5 demonstrates a large right superior parathyroid adenoma found in a 56-year-old woman with primary hyperparathyroidism. The color of the parathyroid gland depends on the amount of fatty tissue and degree of vascularity, but generally ranges from yellowish-tan for most normal glands to reddish-brown for adenomatous or hyperplastic glands.[3] Glands may appear paler yellow, similar to the color of fat, in patients with malnutrition, chronic illness, or interstitial edema. The parathyroid glands are generally soft and can assume several different shapes and contours secondary to their intrinsic inelasticity (Figure 32–6).[3] Their pliable nature leads them to be molded by adjacent tissue; when the gland is subcapsular it may appear flattened like a pancake, whereas when located in the cricothyroidal or intrathymic position, it may appear more like a bean or teardrop.[3] Its soft consistency helps distinguish it from lymph nodes and thyroid tissue which are generally more firm and elastic.[3] In addition, parathyroid tissue can be distinguished from fat in that it will sink rather than float in normal saline solution.[3] On sectioning, parathyroid tissue is generally finely granular in texture.

While most individuals have four parathyroid glands, supernumerary glands have been reported in up to 2.5% to 15% of individuals, ranging from 5 to 8 in number.[2,3,8] Most supernumerary glands are small and rudimentary and can be found inferior to the lower pole of the thyroid associated with the thyrothymic ligament or thymus. In the setting of persistent hyperparathyroidism, supernumerary glands may be the cause of persistent hyperparathyroidism after surgery, especially in patients with secondary hyperparathyroidism or hyperparathyroidism in the setting of a genetic syndrome.[3,5]

PRACTICAL CONSIDERATIONS

When a surgeon is unable to locate a parathyroid gland during surgery for hyperparathyroidism, despite investigating the most common ectopic positions listed above, there may be benefit in obtaining more imaging prior to further exploration. Such modalities include neck ultrasound, 99mTc Sestamibi scan, 4D CT, selective venous sampling, and newer modalities such as 18F-fluorocholine PET.[5] Fine-needle aspiration or biopsy of a candidate parathyroid

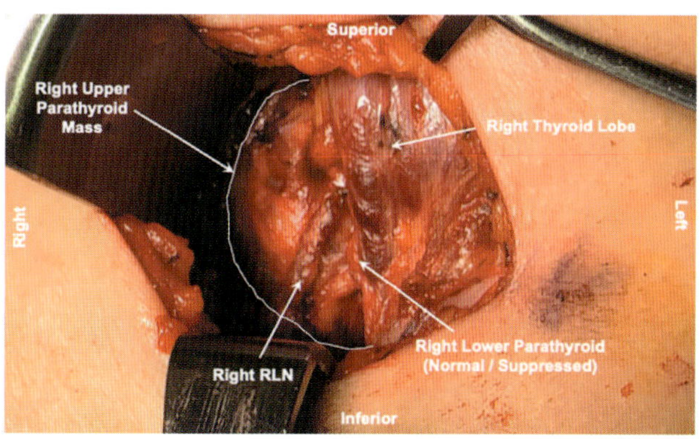

▲ **Figure 32–5.** Large right superior parathyroid adenoma in patient with primary hyperparathyroidism.

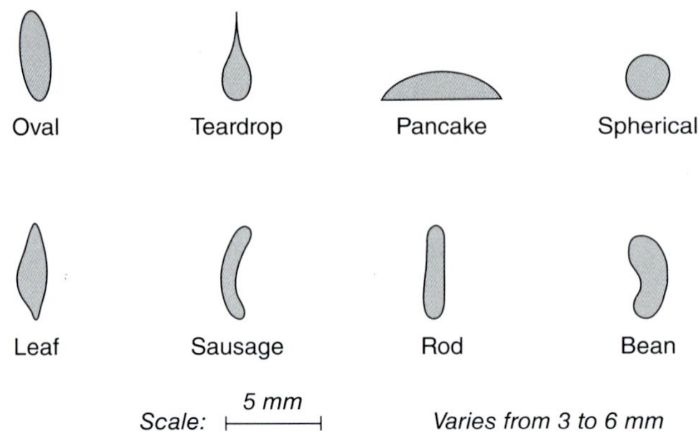

Figure 32–6. Variations in shape of normal parathyroid glands. (Reproduced with permission from Wang C. The anatomic basis of parathyroid surgery. *Ann Surg*. 1976;183(3):271-275.)

lesion should not be performed routinely preoperatively but can be a useful adjunct intraoperatively or postoperatively after a negative exploration.[5] At the time of reoperation, expert knowledge of normal and aberrant parathyroid anatomy is critical for success, and deductive reasoning based on the embryologic origin of target glands can help elucidate their location.

REFERENCES

1. Udelsman R, Citino SB, Prasad M, Donovan PI, Fredholm DV. Parathyroid, thyroid and recurrent laryngeal nerve anatomy in the Indian Rhinoceros (Rhinoceros unicornis). *World J Surg*. 2018;42:514-520.
2. Pradhan R, Agarwal A, Lombardi CP, Raffaelli M. Applied embryology of the thyroid and parathyroid glands. In: Randolph GW, eds. *Surgery of the Thyroid and Parathyroid Glands*. 3rd ed. Philadelphia, PA: McGraw-Hill; 2021:15-25.
3. Wang C. The anatomic basis of parathyroid surgery. *Ann Surg*. 1976;183:271-275.
4. Fancy T, Gallagher D, Hornig JD. Surgical anatomy of the thyroid and parathyroid glands. *Otolaryngol Clin N Am*. 2010;43:221-227.
5. Noussios G, Anagnostis P, Natsis K. Ectopic parathyroid glands and their anatomical, clinical and surgical implications. *Exp Clin Endocrinol Diabetes*. 2012;120:604-610.
6. Mohebati A, Shaha AR. Anatomy of thyroid and parathyroid glands and neurovascular relations. *Clin Anat*. 2012;25:19-31.
7. Park I, Rhu J, Woo JW, Choi JH, Kim JS, Kim JH. Preserving parathyroid gland vasculature to reduce post-thyroidectomy hypocalcemia. *Would J Surg*. 2016;40:1382-1389.
8. Akerstrom G, Malmaeus J, Bergstrom R. Surgical anatomy of human parathyroid glands. *Surgery*. 1984;95:14-21.

Parathyroid Physiology

Richard C. Maduka, MD
Jennifer B. Ogilvie, MD, FACS

33

INTRODUCTION

The balance of calcium within our bodies is carefully regulated by hormonal feedback from cells found within both the parathyroid glands and the thyroid gland. The chief cells (originating within the parathyroid glands) synthesize, store, and release parathyroid hormone (PTH) in response to low serum calcium levels detected by the calcium-sensing receptors (CaSR) on chief cell surfaces. When released, activated PTH circulates in the blood before it is removed rapidly (within minutes) by the kidney and liver. Conversely, the parafollicular C cells (originating within the thyroid gland) release calcitonin in response to elevated serum calcium levels. These two hormones competitively modulate fluctuations in plasma levels of ionized calcium.

There are three primary mechanisms by which PTH raises serum calcium levels. PTH will indirectly stimulate osteoclast cells within the bone to cause resorption, with release of both calcium and phosphate into the blood. In the kidneys, circulating PTH will increase reabsorption of calcium via the renal tubules (both in the ascending loop of Henle, and the distal convoluted tubule), while decreasing the reabsorption of phosphate (by the proximal convoluted tubule) allowing excretion into the urine. In addition, PTH works to convert the inactive form of vitamin D (25-hydroxycholecalciferol) to the active form of vitamin D (1,25-dihydroxycholecalciferol) via enzymatic conversion within the proximal convoluted tubule. Active vitamin D will in turn increase calcium absorption within the small intestine. The overall effect of PTH in patients with normal functioning kidneys is an increase in serum calcium and a decrease in serum phosphate. Notably, this effect is magnified in hyperparathyroidism.

Parathyroid Hormone Release & Receptor Activation

The CaSR complex is located on the surface of the cells in the PTH-producing cells in the parathyroid glands and is extremely sensitive to small changes in serum calcium ion concentration. A decrease in serum ionized calcium activates the process of exocytosis of PTH from secretory vesicles into the extracellular fluid. This process occurs within seconds to minutes, increasing the serum concentration of PTH to allow for distant organ manipulation to increase serum calcium levels. In addition, as the CaSR continues to detect low calcium ion levels, PTH degradation is slowed, and transcription of the PTH gene is upregulated. An increase in serum ionized calcium has the opposite effect, resulting in cessation of vesicle secretion of PTH, rapid degradation of intact hormone, and decreased transcription.[1]

Action of Parathyroid Hormone in the Skeletal System

PTH has two predominant effects within bone. First is the mobilization of free calcium in equilibrium with the bone and extracellular fluid that is rapidly available. The second effect is to increase bone resorption. PTH works at the cellular level by indirectly stimulating osteoclasts to resorb or break down bone. Osteoclasts (multinucleated cells originally derived from monocytes) will liberate minerals such as calcium phosphate during bone remodeling. Notably, however, PTH will first bind to cell receptors on premature osteoblasts, cells whose primary function is bone formation. This binding will stimulate the release of cytokines such as receptor activator of nuclear factor kappa B ligand (RANKL).

RANKL then binds to its receptor on osteoclast precursors, stimulating them to fuse into mature osteoclasts.[1] Chronic PTH exposure indirectly stimulates an increased maturation of osteoclasts, as well as upregulation of their activity to increase calcium resorption from bone. The overall effect is an increased release of calcium and phosphate ions into the serum.[2,3]

Action of Parathyroid Hormone in the Gastrointestinal System

Dietary calcium absorption occurs throughout the small intestines both passively (paracellular diffusion through tight junctions) and actively (energy-dependent transcellular absorption), with 70% to 80% being absorbed in the ileum. PTH has no direct effects on calcium absorption in the small intestine; however, the hormone is a vital component of vitamin D metabolism. Vitamin D is first introduced into the body from the diet or via dermal synthesis through the exposure of 7-dehydrocholesterol within the skin to ultraviolet sunlight. It is then transported to the liver where the hepatic enzyme 25-hydroxylase converts dietary and synthesized vitamin D to 25-hydroxyvitamin D. Following the first enzymatic conversion, vitamin D will then travel to the kidney for further processing.[2,3]

PTH stimulates the synthesis of the enzyme 1-α hydroxylase within the proximal tubules of the kidney, which in turn converts 25-hydroxyvitamin D to its most active form 1,25-dihydroxyvitamin D prior to traveling to the intestine. Once bound to receptors along the intestinal epithelium, active vitamin D or calcitriol affects the process of active transcellular calcium transport by increasing transcription and translation of calcium transport proteins in the epithelium, including transient receptor potential vanilloid type 6 (TRPV6), calbindin, and ATP-dependent calcium pumps. Following the initial calcium influx, translocation of calcium through the interior of the intestinal enterocyte occurs through the apical calcium channel TRPV6, and basolateral extrusion of calcium occurs via the intestinal plasma membrane pump. Notably, some studies have shown an effect of calcitriol on paracellular diffusion of calcium as well. Active vitamin D also increases the intestinal absorption of dietary phosphorus but to a much lesser extent than dietary calcium. The overall effect is an increased absorption of calcium and phosphate ions into the serum.[2,3]

Action of Parathyroid Hormone in the Renal System

PTH has two main roles in the kidney. The first is to increase the absorption of calcium filtered from serum within the nephron, and the second is to inhibit the absorption of phosphorus so that it is excreted in the urine. PTH works in the cortical thick ascending limb of the loop of Henle (LoH) and distal convoluted tubule (DCT) to increase transcellular absorption of calcium ion by upregulating transcription and translation of calcium transport proteins on the tubular epithelium such as transient receptor potential vanilloid type 5 (TRPV5). PTH also regulates sodium-phosphate cotransporters in the proximal convolute tubule via both protein kinase A and protein kinase C-dependent pathways. This blocks phosphate reabsorption and increases urinary phosphate excretion Therefore, the net effect of PTH is to increase calcium absorption and increase phosphate excretion in the urine.[2,3]

Note: Parathyroid hormone-related peptide (PTHrP) is associated with paraneoplastic syndromes and can cause humoral hypercalcemia of malignancy (most common in squamous cell carcinoma of the lung). Although PTHrP and PTH share the same end organ receptors, there are differences in presentation. Patients suffering from PTHrP syndromes will have suppressed bone formation, metabolic alkalosis, and decreased levels of active vitamin D.

REFERENCES

1. Lofrese JJ, Basit H, Lappin SL. StatPearls [Internet]. StatPearls Publishing; Treasure Island (FL): Jul 22, 2021. Physiology, Parathyroid.
2. Christakos S, Dhawan P, Porta A, Mady LJ, Seth T. Vitamin D and intestinal calcium absorption. *Mol Cell Endocrinol.* 2011;347(1-2):25-29.
3. Gesek FA, Friedman PA. On the mechanism of parathyroid hormone stimulation of calcium uptake by mouse distal convoluted tubule cells. *J Clin Invest.* 1992;90(3):749-758.

34 Parathyroid Imaging

Paladino Nunzia Cinzia, MD, PhD
Taïeb David, MD, PhD
Sebag Frédéric, MD

INTRODUCTION

The treatment of primary hyperparathyroidism (pHPT) is surgical and consists of removal of hyperfunctioning parathyroid glands.[1] From the first parathyroidectomy, performed by Mandl in 1925, bilateral cervical neck exploration with identification of all glands was the standard treatment.[2-4] The development of parathyroid imaging has revolutionized the surgical approach to pHPT allowing for the development of focused exploration and minimally invasive surgery. Though still controversial, today a focused exploration with confirmation by intraoperative PTH measurement (IOPTH) is the preferred option by some surgeons for 80% to 85% of patients. However, the classical bilateral cervical exploration with four gland identification remains necessary in 15% to 20% of patients with multiple abnormal glands.[1,5] For surgeons who wish to pursue a focused exploration, parathyroid imaging is critical before deciding on the surgical approach.[6] Most common first-line imaging strategies include parathyroid ultrasound and parathyroid scintigraphy (PS)[1] and have a reported sensitivity of 73% to 90% and 78% to 90%, respectively, and a positive predictive value (PPV) of 86% to 93% and 83% to 94%.[7-9]

FIRST-LINE IMAGING

Ultrasonography

Parathyroid ultrasonography (US) is performed with a high-resolution linear probe from 5 to 15 Mhz.

It has the advantage of low cost, is noninvasive, and does not expose the patient to any radiation. US is also widely available and provides important information about the thyroid gland.[10]

Only hyperfunctioning parathyroid glands are detectable by US as a result of their size and echogenicity. Enlarged parathyroid glands are usually hypoechoic, oval in shape, and can be delineated from the thyroid gland by hyperechoic connective tissue (Figures 34–1 and 34–2). Rarely cystic degeneration can be found, and the gland may present as an anechoic nodule.[6] However, the quality of US is largely dependent on the radiologist's experience and the patient's body habitus.[11] The limitations of US are low sensitivity in identifying mediastinal ectopic glands, small glands, or multiglandular disease. False negative results can occur in presence of intrathyroidal location (Figure 34–3). In this case, it is possible to perform fine-needle aspiration cytology with measurement of the PTH, if deemed necessary.[6] Schenk et al. reported US sensitivity of 64% to 89%.[12] According to a recent meta-analysis by Cheung et al. the overall sensitivity is 76.1% with a PPV of 93.2% in the preoperative localization of abnormal glands. The overall accuracy of parathyroid US increases with radionuclide imaging, and thus ultrasound should be used in combination with scintigraphy or another cross-sectional imaging technique.[6,13]

Parathyroid Scintigraphy

In the late 1980s, technetium-thallium scintigraphy was a commonly used parathyroid imaging method.[10] Later, technetium-thallium was replaced with ^{99m}Tc-labeled tracers with better physical characteristics. The advantages were provided by shorter physical half-life of the isotope and thus lower radiation exposure, as well as less expense.[6] Today SestaMIBI (methoxyisobutylisonitrile) radiolabeled with technetium-99m (^{99m}Tc-MIBI) is used in virtually all PS protocols. The tracer is taken up not only by the parathyroid glands but also by the thyroid so it is converted into a parathyroid agent in two ways:

1. Delayed acquisition which demonstrates a prolonged retention within hyperfunctioning parathyroid glands (**single tracer-dual-phase protocol**)
2. Subtraction of the thyroid image using thyroid tracers (**dual tracer-subtraction protocol**) (Figure 34–4)

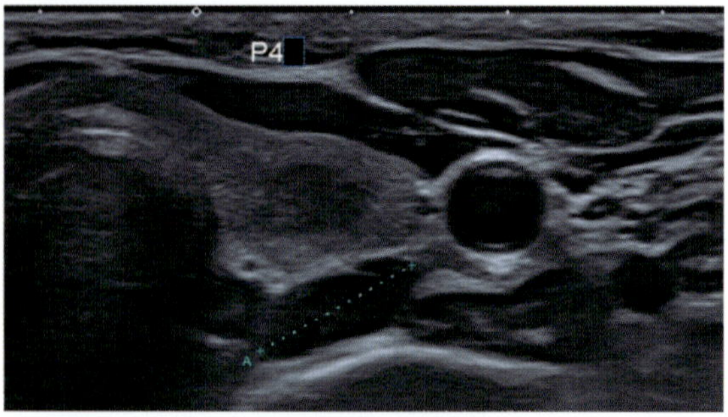

▲ **Figure 34–1.** Left upper parathyroid (P4).

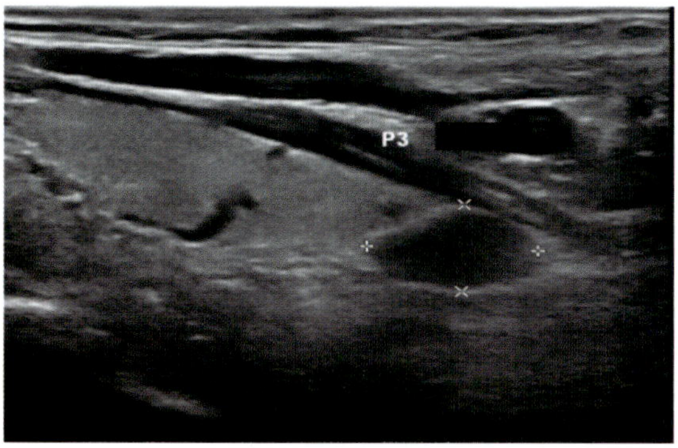

▲ **Figure 34–2.** Left inferior parathyroid (P3).

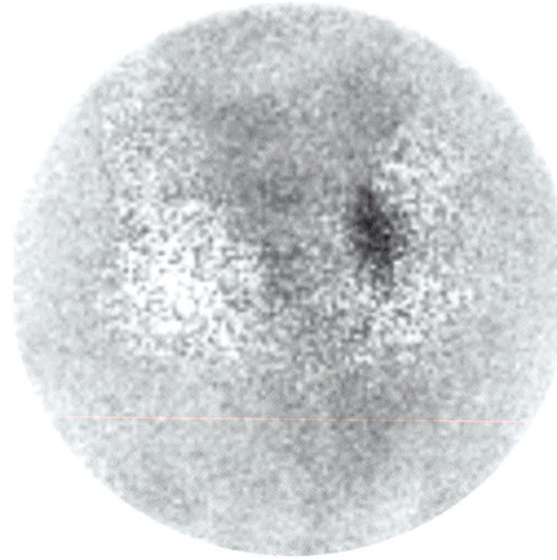

▲ **Figure 34–4.** Subtraction scintigraphy revealing the presence of a left P4 parathyroid.

In the single-tracer protocol, ^{99m}Tc-MIBI tracer retention is prolonged in parathyroid lesions, whereas the tracer washes out at a faster rate in normal thyroid tissue. It is based on the difference of ^{99m}Tc-MIBI retention in thyroid and parathyroid gland.[14]

A limitation of this method is conferred by the presence of thyroid nodules which can lead to false positive results—particularly oncocytic nodules or nodules in the setting of thyroiditis.[10] The original dual-phase protocol requires

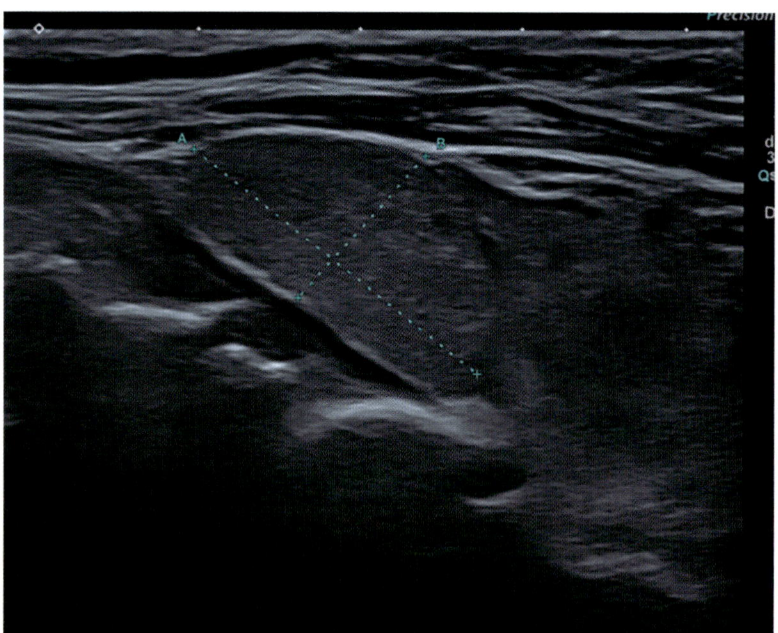

▲ **Figure 34–3.** Ectopic adenoma in intrathyroidal position.

only two planar images, one recorded early (15 minutes) and late (2–3 hours) after ^{99m}Tc-MIBI injection. Enlarged parathyroid glands show increased uptake compared with the thyroid gland. The dual-tracer protocol uses ^{99m}Tc-MIBI (half-life of 6 hours, 140 KeV gamma-ray emission) and iodine-123 (12 hours, 159 Kev). The advantage of using ^{123}I is that thyroid and parathyroid images can be acquired simultaneously. After acquisition, the ^{123}I thyroid image is digitally subtracted from the ^{99m}Tc-MIBI image. The residual activity correlates to the hyperfunctioning parathyroid gland(s) (Figure 34–4). This protocol has optimal sensitivity to detect single or multiple ectopic glands.

Regardless of the protocol used, the entire neck and the chest from the angle of the mandible to the upper part of the myocardium should be included in the field of view considering the wide distribution of ectopic parathyroid glands.[6,14] Therefore, a cervico-mediastinal SPECT/CT (Figure 34–5), should follow pinhole acquisition, preferably with dual-tracer acquisition.[11,14-17] This is less sensitive than the pinhole technique in the thyroid area, but may reveal parathyroid glands that are not seen on planar images and provide a superior anatomic localization of lesions.[6,14]

Numerous studies have shown the superiority of the dual-tracer protocol with an increase of at least 20% in sensitivity, including for the identification of multiglandular disease.[1,7,18] Dual-tracer scintigraphy with subtraction imaging has an excellent performance in the detection of hyperfunctioning parathyroid glands with accuracy in detecting and localizing 94% and 92%, respectively. However, this technique is more expensive and takes longer than a single-tracer method.[6]

Planar scintigraphy or SPECT has higher sensitivity in identifying adenomas than hyperplastic glands, probably due to the fact that hyperplastic glands tend to be smaller than adenomas. During image acquisition, the patient should be calm since the duration of the examination is long.

Before scheduling a patient for scintigraphy it is necessary to inform patients to stop the intake of vitamin D and calcimimetics for at least 2 weeks because they can decrease ^{99m}Tc-MIBI uptake. In addition, calcium channel blockers may reduce uptake of ^{99m}Tc-MIBI.[6] Chen et al. report

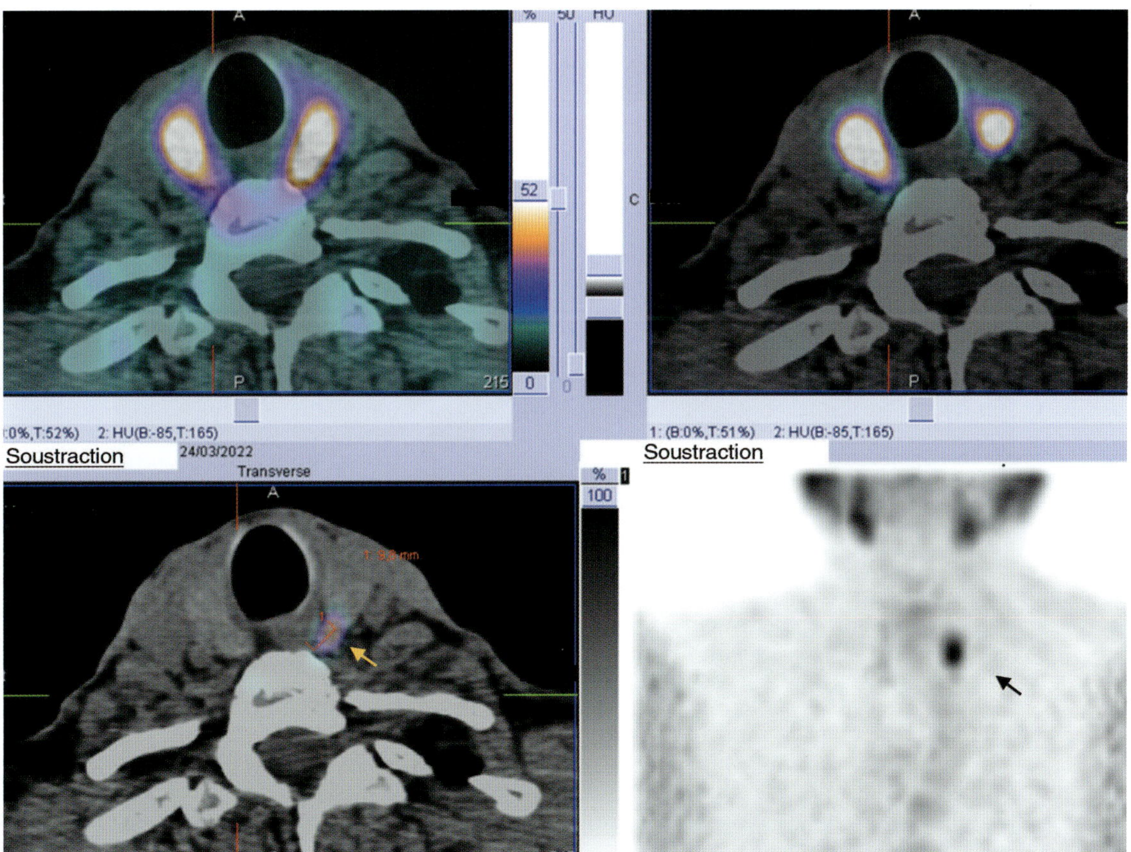

Figure 34–5. SPECT/CT scintigraphy showing a left upper parathyroid gland.

SestaMIBI scintigraphy sensitivity of 62% to 100%.[19] The combination of scintigraphy and cervical US is currently used with a sensitivity of 81% to 95%. The advantage of radionuclide imaging over US is the identification of ectopic glands and posteriorly located upper glands.[6]

In the presence of negative or inconclusive first-line imaging, it is possible to propose a bilateral cervical exploration or a second-line imaging technique such as parathyroid 4D-computed tomography (CT), magnetic resonance imaging (MRI), or ^{18}F-fluorocholine (^{18}F-FCH) PET/CT.[1,6]

If initial imaging identifies the presence of an ectopic gland in the mediastinum, a CT or MRI could be helpful to guide the surgeon toward the more suitable surgical approach—cervical vs thoracic.[7,20]

CT Scan

A CT scan with thin sections can give important information since it can provide precise anatomical localization. Unlike conventional cervical CT scan which reconstructs images with a thickness of 2.5 to 3 mm, the dynamic CT scan provides thin-cut reconstruction of 1.5 mm, using images without injection and multiphase after injection. It is also possible to make 3D reconstructions.[10,21,22] A sensitivity of 60% to 88% is reported.[21,22] It should be noted that CT scans without contrast enhancement have much lower sensitivity and specificity for enlarged parathyroid glands.

CT scans can identify an ectopic adenoma in the thymus or mediastinum with a sensitivity of 40% and specificity of 88%.[10] MIBI scan and CT scan images can be fused to locate the pathological gland and, recently four-dimensional CT (4D-CT) contributes functional information in addition to anatomical data (Figures 34–6 and 34–7). 4D-CT consists of standard CT imaging with three vascular phases (non-enhanced, arterial, and venous), which is the fourth dimension that allows enhancement evaluation over time. Fast uptake and washout of contrast are considered typical for parathyroid adenomas.[6,23] The advantage of 4D-CT is short imaging time and the possibility to detect small and ectopic parathyroid glands, but the disadvantages are irradiation and the need for iodinated contrast.

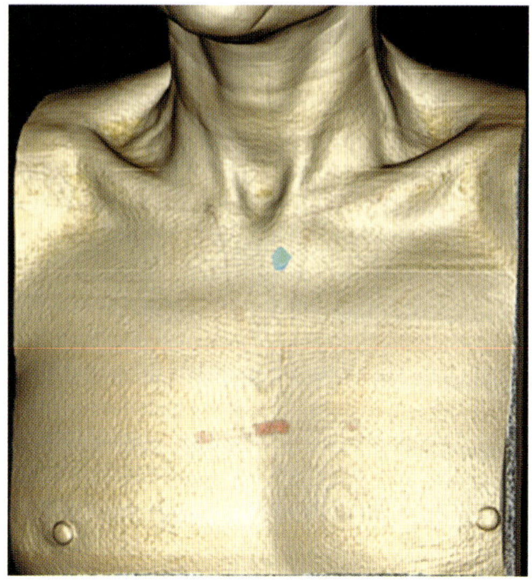

Figure 34–7. 4D-CT with reconstruction finding an ectopic parathyroid adenoma between the brachiocephalic trunk and left primary carotid artery.

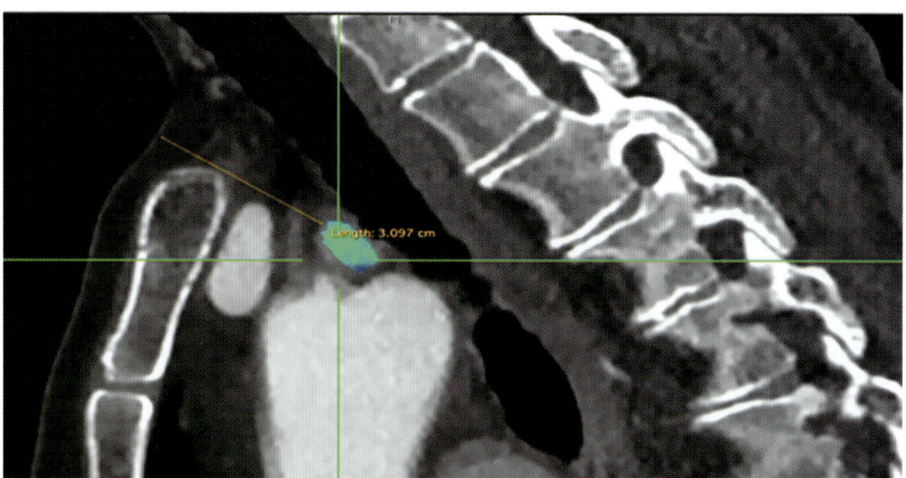

Figure 34–6. 4D-CT with reconstruction finding an ectopic parathyroid adenoma between the brachiocephalic trunk and left primary carotid artery.

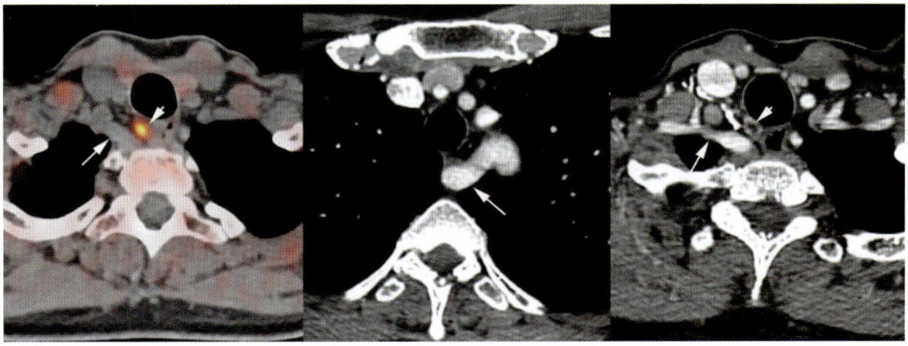

Figure 34–8. ^{18}F-FCH PET/CT. Right P4-derived (ie, superior) parathyroid adenoma located in the tracheoesophageal groove with an aberrant right subclavian artery (ie, arteria lusoria) indicating the presence of a nonrecurrent ILN.

Contrast-enhanced CT scanning can be used in cases of negative previous imaging studies or in persistent pHPT after the unsuccessful initial surgery. The combination of [18F] fluorocholine PET and 4D contrast-enhanced CT can be considered in pHPT with negative or inconclusive first-line imaging.[6] However, the sensitivity of CT for the detection of multiglandular disease is only 32% to 52%.[24]

MRI

Less used, MRI has the advantage of being nonradiating. Parathyroid adenomas are hypointense in T1 phase imaging and hyperintense in T2. Hyperfunctioning parathyroid glands display intense contrast on T1 sequences. The sensitivity reported for this method is 60% to 88% with a false positive rate of 1.6% to 14% and is related to the presence of lymph nodes or thyroid nodules.[6,10] MRI is used as a second-line imaging technique. Its use is limited in patients with kidney failure and implanted medical devices. It also fails to differentiate hyperfunctioning glands from lymph nodes.[6] However, since it is nonirradiating, it can be used for pregnant women though it does have lower sensitivity than 4D-CT.[25]

SECOND-LINE IMAGING

^{18}F-FCH PET/CT

Some PET tracers can be helpful for parathyroid imaging such as ^{11}C-methionine, ^{11}C-choline, and ^{18}F-fluorocholine. In recent years, ^{18}F-FCH PET/CT (Figure 34–8) has demonstrated utility in pHPT with negative or inconclusive findings on initial PS and thus may be a valuable tool as second-line imaging.[1] It is more expensive than scintigraphy.[25] Quak et al. report a high detection rate and suggest that fluorocholine PET is capable of predicting that unilateral cervical neck exploration will be adequate in 75% of patients.[26] Michaud et al. found a sensitivity of 89% for the detection of parathyroid adenoma or hyperplasia.[27] In our recent publication, conducted on 72 patients with pHPT and negative first-line imaging, we found the sensitivity and specificity of ^{18}F-FCH PET/CT to predict uniglandular disease as 92.7% and 46%, respectively. When the data of ^{18}F-FCH PET/CT was combined with first-line imaging data, we were able to complete a minimally invasive surgery in 92% of patients with pHPT.[1]

Selective Venous Sampling

Selective venous sampling consists of obtaining serial blood samples from the superior vena cava, bilateral brachiocephalic, internal jugular, vertebral, thymic, superior, middle, and inferior thyroid veins. The increase in PTH level from the vein drainage sites is compared with a peripheral sample.[6] It is performed only in patients with previous surgery and negative preoperative imaging.[25]

A sensitivity of 75% has been reported.[28]

Selective Arteriography

Selective arteriography can be useful in patients with altered venous drainage due to prior neck surgery,[6] though this is a rarely utilized technique.

CONCLUSION

PS and US are the preferred imaging methods for endocrine surgeons to select candidates for a focused approach.[29] Dual-radiopharmaceutical 123I/99mTc-sestamibi subtraction pinhole imaging followed by SPECT acquisition is more accurate than US for directing a minimally invasive surgery. 123I/99mTc-sestamibi using a pinhole collimator may be sufficient when US is negative in the presence of posterior adenomas, major ectopia, or in cases of previous cervical surgery. This method also facilitates the detection of multiglandular disease in the majority of cases.[11]

In the presence of major ectopia in the mediastinum, CT scan and MRI can be helpful in guiding the surgical approach.[7,20] In recent years, the use of ^{18}F-FCH PET/CT has proven to be a useful diagnostic tool after negative or inconclusive findings on initial PS as second-line imaging.

REFERENCES

1. Goren S, Paladino NC, Laks S, et al. Diagnostic rechallenge with 18F-FCH PET/CT often allows minimally invasive parathyroidectomy while maintaining exceptional cure rates. *World J Surg*. 2022;46(10):2409-2415.
2. Mandl F. Klinisches und Experimenteles zur Frage der lakalisierten und generalisiereten Osteitis Fibrosa. *Arch Klin Chir*. 1926;143:1.
3. Fraser WD. Hyperparathyroidism. *Lancet*. 2009;374(9684):145-158.
4. Delbridge LW, Palazzo FF. First parathyroid surgeon: Sir John Bland-Sutton and the parathyroids. *ANZ J Surg*. 2007;77(12):1058-1061.
5. Paladino NC, Guerin C, Slotema E, Franco IF, Henry JF, Sebag F. Endoscopic parathyroidectomy. In: Lombardi CP, Bellantone R, eds. *Minimally Invasive Therapies for Endocrine Neck Diseases*. Springer; 2016:167-179.
6. Ovčariček PP, Giovanella L, Gasset IC, et al. The EANM practice guidelines for parathyroid imaging. *Eur J Nucl Med Mol Imaging*. 2021;48(9):2801-2822.
7. Guerin C, Paladino NC, Lowery A, Castinetti F, Taieb D, Sebag F. Persistent and recurrent hyperparathyroidism. *Updates Surg*;2017:161-169.
8. Hessman O, Stalberg P, Sundin A, et al. High success rate of parathyroid reoperation may be achieved with improved localization diagnosis. *World J Surg*. 2008;32(5):774-781.
9. Feingold DL, Alexander HR, Chen CC, et al. Ultrasound and sestamibi scan as the only preoperative imaging tests in reoperation for parathyroid adenomas. *Surgery*. 2000;128(6):1103-1110.
10. Lee Js, Carnaille B, Inabnet WB. Chapitre 25, Imagerie preoperatoire. 243-251. Traité de chirurgie endocrinienne, thyroïde, parathyroïdes, néoplasies endocriniennes multiples C Trésallet, F. Menegaux. Volume 1. 2015, Doin Editeurs (Edictions John Libbey Eurotext).
11. Guerin G, Lowery A, Gabriel S, et al. Preoperative imaging for focused parathyroidectomy: making a good strategy even better. *Eur J Endocrinol*. 2015;172(5):519-526.
12. Schenk WG, Hanks JB, Smith FW. Surgeon-performed ultrasound for primary hyperparathyroidism. *Surg*. 2013;79(7):681-685.
13. Cheung K, Wang TS, Farrokhyar F, Roman SA, Sosa JA. A meta-analysis of preoperative localization techniques for patients with primary hyperparathyroidism. *Ann Surg Oncol*. 2012;19(2):577-583.
14. Hindié E, Paladino NC, Meuter L, et al. Primary hyperparathyroidism and renal hyperparathyroidism. In: Taieb D, Pacak K, eds. *Current Diagnostic and Therapeutic Approaches in Nuclear Endocrinology*. Cambridge Scholars Publishing.
15. Lavely WC, Goetze S, Friedman KP, et al. Comparison of SPECT/CT, SPECT, and planar imaging with single- and dual-phase (99m) Tc-sestamibi parathyroid scintigraphy. *J Nucl Med*. 2007;48(7):1084-1089.
16. Tunninen V, Varjo P, Schildt J, et al. Comparison of five parathyroid scintigraphic protocols. *Int J Mol Imaging*. 2013;2013:921260.
17. Klingensmith WC III, Koo PJ, Summerlin A, et al. Parathyroid imaging: the importance of pinhole collimation with both single- and dual-tracer acquisition. *J Nucl Med Technol*. 2013;41:99-104.
18. Hindie E, Melliere D, Jeanguillaume C, et al. Unilateral surgery for primary hyperparathyroidism on the basis of technetium Tc 99m sestamibi and iodine 123 subtraction scanning. *Arch Surg*. 2000;135:1461-1468.
19. Chen CC, Holder LE, Scovill WA, Tehan AM, Gann DS. Comparison of parathyroid imaging with technetium-99m-pertechnetate/sestamibi subtraction, double-phase technetium-99m-sestamibi and technetium-99m-sestamibi SPECT. *J Nucl Med*. 1997;38(6):834-839.
20. Yen TWF, Wang TS, Doffek KM, Krzywda EA, Wilson SD. Reoperative parathyroidectomy: an algorithm for imaging and monitoring of intraoperative parathyroid hormone levels that results in a successful focused approach. *Surgery*. 2008;144(4):611-621.
21. Lumachi F, Tregnaghi A, Zucchetta P, et al. Technetium-99m sestamibi scintigraphy and helical CT together in patients with primary hyperparathyroidism: a prospective clinical study. *Br J Radiol*. 2004;77(914):100-103.
22. Zald FB, Hamilton BE, Larsen ML, Cohen JI. The role of computed tomography for localization of parathyroid adenomas. *Laryngoscope*. 2008;118(8):1405-1410.
23. Hoang JK, Williams K, Gaillard F, Dixon A, Sosa JA. Parathyroid 4D-CT: multi-institutional international survey of use and trends. *Otolaryngol Head Neck Surg*. 2016;155(6):956-960.
24. Sho S, Yuen AD, Yeh MW, Livhits MJ, Sepahdari AR. Factors associated with discordance between preoperative parathyroid 4-dimensional computed tomographic scans and intraoperative findings during parathyroidectomy. *JAMA Surg*. 2017;152(12):1141.
25. Khan AA, Hanley DA, Rizzoli R, et al. Primary hyperparathyroidism: review and recommendations on evaluation, diagnosis, and management. A Canadian and international consensus. *Osteoporos Int*. 2017;28(1):1-19.
26. Quak E, Blanchard D, Houdu B, et al. F18-choline PET/CT guided surgery in primary hyperparathyroidism when ultrasound and MIBI SPECT/CT are negative or inconclusive: the APACH1 study. *Nucl Med Mol Imaging*. 2018;45(4):658-666.
27. Michaud L, Burgess A, Huchet V, et al. Is 18F-fluorocholine-positron emission tomography/computerized tomography a new imaging tool for detecting hyperfunctioning parathyroid glands in primary or secondary hyperparathyroidism? *J Clin Endocrinol Metab*. 2014;99:4531-4536.
28. Witteveen JE, Kievit J, van Erkel AR, Morreau H, Romijn JA, Hamdy NA. The role of selective venous sampling in the management of persistent hyperparathyroidism revisited. *Eur J Endocrinol*. 2010;163:945-952.
29. Greene AB, Butler RS, McIntyre S, et al. National trends in parathyroid surgery from 1998 to 2008: a decade of change. *J Am Coll Surg*. 2009;209:332-343.

Primary Hyperparathyroidism

35

Kimberly M. Ramonell, MD
Sally E. Carty, MD

GENERAL CONSIDERATIONS

Primary hyperparathyroidism (pHPT) is a relatively common disorder that arises from the autonomous overproduction of parathyroid hormone (PTH) by one or more abnormal parathyroid glands. Historically thought to be rare, the prevalence of pHPT is now estimated at 0.3% of the general population. Moreover, this rate likely represents an underestimation due to widespread underdiagnosis in the United States today.[1-3] The diagnosis of pHPT is biochemical and is characterized by repeatedly elevated serum calcium levels with concomitantly elevated or inappropriately normal PTH levels. In a hypercalcemic patient, the finding of a nonsuppressed PTH level should be considered pathognomonic for pHPT and mandates appropriate evaluation and treatment.

The majority of pHPT is due to a single adenomatous gland (80%-85%) and resection of the adenoma is associated with durable cure in more than 90% of patients. The remaining 15% to 20% of pHPT is caused by multigland disease (MGD) including four-gland hyperplasia (15%) and double adenoma or asymmetric hyperplasia (3%-5%). Rarely, parathyroid carcinoma is present (<1%).

Surgery is the only curative treatment for pHPT and remains exceptionally safe and effective in appropriately trained hands. Today, operative failure remains the highest risk of parathyroid surgery. However, a thoughtful and methodical preoperative evaluation contributes integrally to the success of a parathyroid surgeon with high cure rates, low risks, and excellent outcomes.

CLINICAL FINDINGS & DIAGNOSTIC APPROACH

Clinical Evaluation & Symptomatology

The clinical presentation of pHPT is quite heterogeneous and can span from no appreciable symptoms to significant physical and psychological disability. Historically, pHPT was associated with "classic" manifestations of bone, renal, and neuropsychiatry symptoms but as our understanding expands and management evolves, so too does the definition of symptomatic disease. Over the past three decades, the subjective and objective manifestations of pHPT have been recognized to include a variety of neurocognitive, psychiatric, cardiovascular, musculoskeletal, and gastrointestinal symptoms that were previously not considered. At the same time, with the adoption of routine serum calcium testing, the diagnosis of pHPT is being made earlier in the disease process.

Whether or not symptoms are reported at diagnosis, a careful history for target organ involvement should be conducted by the evaluating surgeon. Objective renal involvement now includes not only evidence of clinically overt nephrolithiasis or nephrocalcinosis but also silent nephrolithiasis/nephrocalcinosis identified on renal imaging, hypercalciuria (24-hour urine calcium level >400 mg/dL), or impaired renal function (glomerular filtration rate <60 mL/min). Objective bone involvement now includes evidence of osteoporosis/osteopenia, fragility fracture, or vertebral compression fracture on DXA imaging and successful parathyroid surgery improves BMD in 40% to 67% of osteoporotic and osteopenic patients.[4]

Severe neuro-psychiatric, -cognitive, and -muscular manifestations of pHPT including psychosis, obtundation, and myopathy are rare and mostly of historical interest. However, subjective complaints of fatigue, weakness, altered sleep, depressed mood, anxiety, irritability, memory/concentration impairment, joint pain, arthritis, heartburn, prior "fibromyalgia" diagnosis, or erectile dysfunction are commonly reported and should be queried in all patients undergoing evaluation, along with documentation of the use of diuretics, narcotics, or other medications being used to treat such conditions. Although improvement in subjective symptoms is demonstrated in the majority of patients after parathyroidectomy, the primary reason for parathyroid surgery is to promote and restore renal and bone health.

The clinical assessment should also include a careful history elucidating prior anterior neck surgery, which if present very much influences the preoperative evaluation, surgical indications, and conduct of parathyroidectomy. As such, reoperative parathyroid surgery is discussed later. Other influential history includes previous radioiodine treatment of thyroid disease, external beam radiation exposure to the head, neck or chest, or exceptionally high doses of environmental radiation exposure, as each of these increases the risk of developing pHPT. Moreover, the latter two circumstances are associated with thyroid cancer that may require concurrent management. A personal and family history of hereditary syndromes associated with parathyroid disease should include queries about a history in first-degree relatives of hypercalcemia, neck surgery, nephrolithiasis, pituitary or pancreatic tumors, and peptic ulcer disease.[5]

Biochemical Assessment

The initial biochemical workup of pHPT should include serum total calcium, intact PTH, creatinine, and 25-hydroxyvitamin D levels performed synchronously for accurate interpretation; for best diagnostic value, it is often very helpful to test in the fasting state. In pHPT, patients may have intermittently normal total and/or ionized calcium levels but will be hypercalcemic the majority of the time. Conversely, normocalcemic pHPT (NpHPT) is an uncommon, recently recognized and incompletely understood variant of pHPT that is often confused with unrecognized vitamin D deficiency, renal insufficiency, and/or the use of confounding medications such as thiazide diuretics, potassium citrate, and lithium. Patients with NpHPT have normal serum and ionized calcium levels; therefore, measurement of ionized calcium is necessary to establish the diagnosis of normocalcemic (but not hypercalcemic) pHPT.

In pHPT, PTH levels are high or inappropriately normal (nonsuppressed) for the hypercalcemic state. The threshold to define a nonsuppressed and thus an abnormal PTH level in the setting of hypercalcemia varies as serum PTH levels can be influenced by multiple factors including venous collection site, phlebotomy conditions, sample preparation and handling, and generation/type of assay used. In general, utilization of a threshold of 15 to 25 pg/mL is justified by available literature and this situation represents an uncommon but well-documented variant of pHPT.[6,7] When hypercalcemic patients have PTH levels in the lower range of normal, it is prudent to rule out hypercalcemia of malignancy and a fasting PTHRP should be performed. Very high PTH levels (>500-800 pg/mL) have been associated with parathyroid carcinoma, but modestly elevated PTH levels do not exclude the possibility of parathyroid carcinoma.[8]

The essential role of 25-hydroxyvitamin D in PTH pathophysiology has been well documented. Under normal conditions, vitamin D deficiency and hypocalcemia both will trigger increased production of PTH. Today vitamin D deficiency is endemic in the United States (possibly leading to a skewed "normal" range curve) and deficiency is associated with an increased risk of hypocalcemic symptoms after parathyroid or thyroid surgery.[9] In pHPT, 25-hydroxyvitamin D deficiency has been associated with more significant hypercalcemia, more severe bone disease, and increased parathyroid adenoma weight. Measurement of 25-hydroxyvitamin D is the best available test to assess the adequacy of vitamin D levels and should be obtained in all patients being evaluated for pHPT. In patients with low vitamin D levels, repletion is safe to use preoperatively, should be prescribed in doses sufficient to achieve a robustly normal level, and provides a modality that is quite useful in managing diagnostic ambiguity for pHPT.[10]

A 24-hour total urine calcium and creatinine level can help distinguish pHPT from familial hypocalciuric hypercalcemia (FHH). FHH is an autosomal dominant condition caused by heterogenous mutations in the renal calcium-sensing receptor which result in lifelong hypercalcemia and hypocalciuria that rarely requires treatment but can be a major cause of unnecessary parathyroid surgery when unrecognized.[11] FHH should be considered in patients with urinary calcium levels <100 mg/24 h and can be differentiated from pHPT by a calcium/creatinine clearance ratio (CCCR) <0.01, whereas a CCCR >0.02 is diagnostic of pHPT. In vitamin D–deficient patients with a CCCR <0.01, a repeat urinary calcium level should be obtained after repletion. Mutational analysis for FHH is now 98% effective in diagnosing or excluding the condition.[11]

Parathyroid Imaging & Preoperative Localization Studies

Multiple imaging modalities are available to localize hyperfunctional parathyroids in patients with pHPT, and choice of imaging modality and protocols varies by surgeon and institution. Negative imaging does not preclude a patient from being a candidate for initial surgery but does generally contraindicate reoperation. However, preoperative knowledge of the location of the abnormal gland(s) can simplify the dissection and minimize its risks.

All patients should undergo preoperative neck ultrasound to assess for concomitant thyroid pathology, which is frequent (40%) and may require fine-needle biopsy and/or concurrent thyroid surgery; ultrasound also often helps to localize parathyroid pathology. Localization of abnormal parathyroid gland(s) can also be achieved with functional nuclear medicine techniques performed with or without synchronous computed tomography (CT) by sestamibi imaging (Figure 35–1A) or SPECT-CT (Figure 35–1B), respectively. Other approaches include four-dimensional (4D) CT neck with IV contrast, which characteristically identifies a parathyroid adenoma to have lower attenuation than the

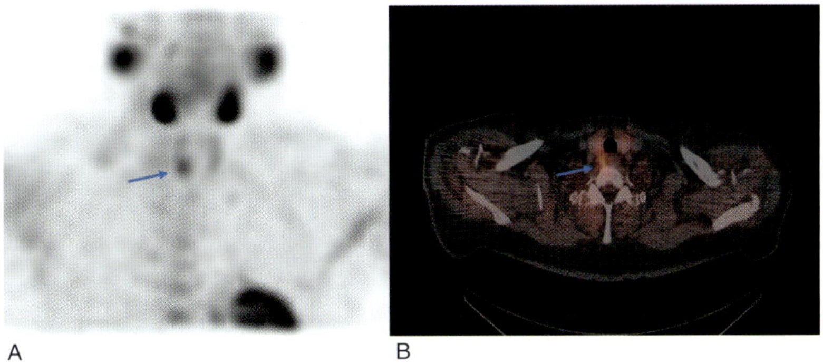

Figure 35–1. Delayed planar sestamibi **(A)** and fused SPECT-CT **(B)** images of a localized right superior parathyroid adenoma (blue arrow.)

surrounding thyroid tissue in the noncontrast phase, peak enhancement greater than that of the thyroid in the arterial phase, and washout of contrast material in the delayed phase. However, 4D CT requires multiple fine cuts with significant radiation exposure for the patient.

To avoid operative failure, expert surgeons utilize multiple approaches to diagnose and manage MGD, which preoperatively is often undiagnosed. In a recent study of 245 patients with sporadic pHPT due to MGD, 30% had imaging findings that were incorrectly concordant for apparent *single* gland disease, and altogether the imaging results indicated MGD in only 36%; conversely, 96% of MGD cases were detected intraoperatively and 5% were diagnosed postoperatively when early or late hypercalcemia was observed.[12] Studies have demonstrated that discordant imaging and intraoperative findings are more common in MGD, with hyperfunctional inferior parathyroids, and with hyperfunctional glands less than 10 mm in greatest dimension. Awareness of these drawbacks and potential limitations allows surgeons to minimize costs and better utilize localization techniques in preoperative planning and intraoperative troubleshooting.[13]

Special Tests & Considerations

The detrimental effects of pHPT on bone mineralization are well documented. Patients diagnosed with pHPT should have their bone density evaluated with dual-energy X-ray absorptiometry (DXA) imaging to assess the lumbar spine, distal radius, and femoral head/neck. Skeletal symptoms can take the form of any combination of fragility fractures, skeletal deformities, and bone pain. In the classic setting, osteitis fibrosa cystica describes the radiographic features of severe pHPT in which brown tumors, lytic lesions, subperiosteal bone resorption of the phalanges, and bone cysts are seen, although these findings are exceedingly rare now.

Genetic counseling should be offered to patients younger than 40 years with pHPT, particularly in the setting of known multigland disease, a strong family history, and syndromic manifestations of known hereditary causes of pHPT (discussed later).

Genetic Syndromes

The majority of pHPT cases are sporadic but in 3% to 5% of patients, pHPT occurs in association with an inherited syndrome.

A. Multiple Endocrine Neoplasia Syndromes

pHPT is associated with MEN syndromes types 1, 2A, and 4; due to founder effects these autosomal dominant conditions have varying regional incidences. Unlike the predominance of single gland adenomatous disease in sporadic pHPT, MEN-associated pHPT is often asymmetrical multigland hyperplasia, in MEN-2, and is always multigland hyperplasia in MEN-1. MEN-1 is characterized by pHPT, pituitary tumors, pancreaticoduodenal neuroendocrine tumors, adrenal adenomas, and thymic carcinoids; pHPT is often (but not always) the first clinical manifestation and generally presents in the second to fourth decade of life, which is generally earlier than sporadic pHPT.[14]

MEN-2A is characterized by medullary thyroid cancer (90%), pheochromocytoma (40%-50%), and pHPT (20%) with such a strong genotype–phenotype relationship that the specific RET mutation can be used to estimate the likelihood of developing pHPT. In patients with a known RET mutation, surveillance for pHPT should be performed annually at the time of screening for pheochromocytoma and should include serum calcium and PTH levels. Patients with RET mutations in high-risk codons 634 and 883 should undergo evaluation by the age 11 versus by age 16 in patients with other "moderate-risk" RET mutations.

MEN-4 is related to an inactivating mutation of the cyclin-dependent kinase (CDK) inhibitor 1b (*CDKN1B*) gene on chromosome 12. Approximately 3% of patients clinically diagnosed with MEN-1 do not have MEN-1 mutations but carry CDKN1B mutations; these patients carry the diagnosis of MEN-4. The clinical manifestations of MEN-4 are similar to those of MEN-1; pHPT and pituitary tumors are common manifestations of MEN-4 but prolactin-producing pituitary tumors are less common. Other tumors, such as gastro-entero-pancreatic endocrine tumors, adrenal tumors, lipomas, meningiomas, and carcinoids, can also be found in patients with MEN-4 but appear to occur less commonly than in MEN-1.[15]

B. Hyperparathyroidism-Jaw Tumor Syndrome

Hyperparathyroidism-jaw tumor syndrome (HPT-JT) is an uncommon autosomal dominant disorder in which a mutation in the tumor suppressor gene *CDC73* that encodes parafibromin causes pHPT, ossifying tumors of the maxilla and mandible, and renal cysts and tumors. The majority of patients develop pHPT and it is often associated with more severe hypercalcemia than in sporadic pHPT. In addition, this syndrome is associated with a significantly higher risk of developing parathyroid cancer, which occurs in 10% to 15% of patients.

C. Familial Isolated Hyperparathyroidism

Familial isolated pHPT (FIHP) is pHPT identified with a clear familial history but without characteristic features of a known familial hyperparathyroid syndrome (MEN, FHH, HPT-JT). The concept and etiology of FIHP has undergone drastic evolution over the past 60 years but a significant deficit in our understanding and characterization of this disease persists. Most recently, an autosomal dominant pathologic mutation in the transcription factor GCM2 has been identified in 17% of FIHP kindreds. The features of FIHP with or without a GCM2 mutation (and without mutation of MEN1, CASR, or CDC73) include adult age at diagnosis, mild hypercalcemia, and predominance of multigland disease—but occasional single adenomas in FIHP have been reported.[16]

DIFFERENTIAL DIAGNOSIS OF HYPERCALCEMIA

Hyperparathyroidism is the most common cause of hypercalcemia in adults, but it is important to consider other non-HPT etiologies during evaluation. While this list is not exhaustive, this most commonly includes malignancy, osteolytic metastases, thiazide and lithium therapy, prolonged immobilization, sarcoidosis, 1-25-dihydroxyvitamin D production or toxicity, and FHH (Table 35–1). Malignancy-related hypercalcemia is driven by tumoral production of parathyroid hormone-related peptide (PTHrP) which stimulates osteoclastic PTH receptors and results in excessive bone resorption and hypercalcemia.

Table 35–1. Causes of hypercalcemia.

Malignancy
PTHrP secreting tumors (small-cell lung, renal)
Metastatic breast cancer
Osteolytic metastases of other primary cancers
Multiple myeloma
Leukemia
Iatrogenic
Thiazide diuretic use
Lithium
Excess vitamin D, vitamin A, or calcium consumption
Endocrinopathy
Hyperparathyroidism
Granulomatous disease
Tuberculosis
Sarcoidosis
Idiopathic diseases and other rare etiologies
Benign familial hypocalciuric hypercalcemia (FHH)
Idiopathic hypercalcemia of infancy
Paget disease
Aluminum toxicity
Prolonged immobilization
Ectopic PTH production

SURGICAL MANAGEMENT OF PRIMARY HYPERPARATHYROIDISM

Parathyroidectomy is the only definitive treatment for pHPT. Compared to surgery, nonoperative approaches including pharmacological therapy or long-term observation are less effective and less cost-effective at reducing serum calcium levels and improving bone demineralization. Therefore, current guidelines recommend that all patients with the diagnosis of pHPT, regardless of symptomatology, be referred to a high-volume parathyroid surgeon for evaluation, and risk-benefit discussion about candidacy for parathyroidectomy.[17]

In several respects, a comprehensive understanding of parathyroid embryology and surgical anatomy (Chapters 33 and 34, respectively) is vital for successful parathyroid surgery. The following concepts serve as the foundation for mastering parathyroid operations:

- First, parathyroid surgery is properly termed "exploration" because parathyroid glands can reside at any site along their embryologic track from the base of the skull to the upper chest resulting in highly variable anatomy and an obligatory understanding of the compartments and contents of the anterior neck.
- Second, the intraoperative skill of estimating gland weight is crucial (discussed later).
- Third, although most patients have four parathyroid glands (85%), and while autopsy series claim there are

patients with only three glands, this occurs quite rarely. Conversely, the situation of >4, that is, supernumerary glands, is surprisingly common. To achieve a cure in patients with supernumerary glands, identification of said glands is necessary but compromised when precursory knowledge of embryologic and anatomic data is applied. The authors have seen several patients with seven parathyroid glands and one patient who had nine.

- Fourth, during dissection, knowing the embryologic origins of the already-identified gland(s) can be very helpful in deducing the identity, and thus the location, of a missing culprit gland. The superior parathyroid glands originate from the fourth branchial pouch and descend with the thyroid to rest near the upper pole of the thyroid gland or drop posteriorly within the tracheoesophageal groove. The inferior parathyroids arise from the third branchial pouch along with the thymus and migrate anteriorly to rest near the inferior pole of the thyroid gland but have notoriously variable locations and 40% are located elsewhere, including within the thymus, carotid sheath, at the carotid bulb, or intrathyroidally.

Operative cure is currently defined by documented normocalcemia at 6 months after parathyroidectomy. Operative failure occurs in two settings: persistent disease and recurrent disease. In persistent pHPT (surgical failure), patients do not achieve normocalcemia within the 6 months after surgery. Broadly speaking, this is due to the insufficient removal of abnormal parathyroid tissue leaving the patient with ongoing disease, and occurs in several scenarios: (1) failure to remove any abnormal parathyroid on exploration; (2) insufficient resection of MGD; (3) false positive intraoperative parathyroid hormone (ioPTH) results (eg, an insufficient ioPTH decline was not recognized/performed, or ioPTH was falsely low due to aberrant venous sampling techniques); or (4) incorrect diagnosis of pHPT.[18]

Recurrent disease occurs when the patient is biochemically cured with normal serum calcium levels at 6 months, but subsequently develops hypercalcemia with elevated or nonsuppressed PTH levels. Long-term recurrence has unknown etiology and with widespread use of electronic medical records is considerably more common than was appreciated years ago—with recurrence rates now estimated at 10.7% up to 17 years after initial surgery.[19] Management of recurrent/persistent disease and reoperative surgery is discussed later.

In the hands of experienced parathyroid surgeons, initial surgical cure rates are greater than 95% and are often 98% to 99% today.

Indications for Surgery

Parathyroid exploration is indicated in all symptomatic patients with biochemically confirmed pHPT, and should be considered for most asymptomatic patients as well; indications for surgery in patients truly considered to be asymptomatic include age <50 years, clinical or biochemical suspicion for parathyroid cancer, and serum calcium level greater than 1 mg/dL above normal range. Patients with severe hypercalcemia should be cautioned to stay well hydrated preoperatively and are at an increased risk for parathyroid carcinoma and thus should be counseled about the possible need for en bloc resection (discussed later).

In symptomatic patients, curative parathyroidectomy has repeatedly been shown to provide benefit in affected bone, renal, and/or neurocognitive systems. Parathyroidectomy markedly reduces future kidney stone formation and attenuates further decline in glomerular filtration in patients with pHPT-related renal disease. On average, bone mineral density (BMD) is expected to improve by 12% to 14% over 10 years, and fracture-free survival is increased by 12% in osteoporotic patients who undergo successful parathyroidectomy.[20] Neuropsychiatric symptoms including depression and anxiety have shown significant improvement after curative parathyroidectomy based on validated patient questionnaire results.[21] The impact of parathyroidectomy on mitigating cardiovascular-disease-specific sequela including hypertension, stroke, and myocardial dysfunction remains equivocal based on limited observational studies and remains an area of ongoing research.

Parathyroid Surgery

In performing parathyroid surgery, there is a substantial risk of unrecognized MGD which occurs anatomically in 15% to 20% of pHPT patients. Two techniques have been validated to date to reliably exclude or identify and manage MGD, and both methods (discussed in following discussion) are widely used today: routine bilateral exploration (BE) and focused dissection with ioPTH monitoring.

Other adjuncts exist, including intraoperative recurrent laryngeal nerve monitoring (IONM) which for initial parathyroid operations can be used at the discretion of the surgeon but has not been demonstrated to provide benefit; it is our institutional practice to use IONM in select high-risk initial operations and frequently in reoperative cases.

During any type of parathyroid operation, care should be taken not to disrupt the capsule of an enlarged parathyroid gland which can cause the complication of parathyromatosis. Moreover, when the surgeon encounters an enlarged firm pale mass, which may be adherent to surrounding structures, this is parathyroid carcinoma until proven otherwise and en bloc resection of adjacent adherent tissues such as fat, thymus, or even the ipsilateral thyroid lobe should be performed to achieve durable cure.

In performing parathyroidectomy it is essential to keep in mind that the surgeon's intraoperative assessment of the parathyroid anatomy does not define or guarantee operative success. At all times the surgeon strives to achieve cure of pHPT while keeping all normal parathyroid tissue intact and leaving the patient with sufficient parathyroid tissue to prevent hypoparathyroidism.

Intraoperative Parathyroid Hormone Monitoring

Intraoperative parathyroid hormone (ioPTH) monitoring is widely accepted for use during initial or reoperative parathyroidectomy for pHPT to guide extent of dissection. Its use provides a functional equivalent to the visual inspection of routine BE. Even with *strongly* positive concordant SPECT/CT and ultrasound findings suggesting a single adenoma, the rate of multigland disease is as high as 3% to 5%, and ioPTH testing has value in detecting and managing these patients at surgery.[22,23] Currently, there are at least seven ioPTH protocols, in which the criteria for operative cure vary based on PTH assay type, local practices and capabilities, timing of ioPTH draw, and the percentage decline or absolute value at which exploration is terminated. Using the dual criteria, a level is drawn prior to the incision to set a baseline value, an ioPTH sample is sent 10-minutes after the surgeon thinks resection is complete, and a drop in ioPTH of at least 50% from baseline plus to within normal range (<65 pg/mL) is considered sufficient to terminate surgery, using further exploration and ioPTH testing if the postresection level does not drop adequately.[24] Alternatively, employing a lower post-excision cutoff of <40 pg/mL may aid further in predicting operative success.[25]

Bilateral Exploration for Hyperparathyroidism

Historically a bilateral neck exploration was the gold standard surgical approach to sporadic pHPT. Advancements in imaging techniques and enthusiastic adoption of minimally invasive options have successfully challenged that dogma over the past two decades. Nonetheless, bilateral four-gland exploration (BE) remains a safe, efficient, and effective approach to pHPT, is the default operation when ioPTH monitoring is unavailable or when intraoperative findings suggest MGD, and should be the planned approach in primary sporadic patients with discordant preoperative imaging. In addition, BE is the planned approach for primary familial, secondary, and tertiary hyperparathyroidism. In addition, some experts also use ioPTH monitoring when performing BE.

In general, BE is a sequential exercise in logical deduction that is performed by the authors with the following approach: as the thyroid lobes are rotated anteriorly with care taken to preserve their capsular integrity as well as the integrity of the RLN, all four of the parathyroids are identified and are delicately preserved on intact vascular pedicles. The surgeon then visually compares the parathyroid sizes to assign an estimated anatomic diagnosis of single or multiple gland disease. A normal parathyroid weighs 20 to 50 mg, measures 5 mm in longest dimension, is typically flat, may be oblong, and histologically is comprised of chief cells. In contrast, a hyperfunctional parathyroid is visibly enlarged and is typically plump and/or round and can also be bilobed. Thus, in resection, the surgeon should be careful not to leave a deeper half behind. A normal parathyroid is too small for intraoperative tissue PTH analysis, but during exploration may undergo a delicate shave biopsy if necessary for tissue and weight documentation.

Based on the surgeon's assessment of the parathyroid anatomy, if during BE one identifies a single enlarged and three small glands, the single adenoma is resected. If two enlarged and two small glands are identified, the double adenomas are resected. If all parathyroids are big, a subtotal (typically 3.5 gland) resection of the four-gland hyperplasia is performed leaving a viable remnant approximated at 40 to 50 mg.

The authors perform subtotal parathyroidectomy by choosing the most normal-looking gland as the planned remnant, placing a clip across it, and transecting the tissue superficial to the clip using a 15-blade knife; because the intended remnant can later become dusky or inadvertently disrupted from its pedicle, it is generally created early to leave the possibility of using another gland as the remnant if necessary. When possible, cryopreservation of parathyroid tissue is performed in subtotal cases in the event postoperative hypoparathyroidism is later diagnosed. All resected glands or parathyroid biopsy specimens should be immediately weighed.

If one cannot find a missing hyperfunctional gland, the approach to identifying ectopically located glands may include: cervical thymectomy, liberal medialization of the thyroid lobe with evaluation of the tracheoesophageal groove and retroesophageal space as far cranially and caudally as can be visualized, opening of the carotid sheaths, and a thorough interrogation of the thyroid lobes. Blind thyroid lobectomy is rarely necessary and with the use of intraoperative ultrasound, probably contraindicated.

Minimally Invasive Parathyroid Surgery

The many heterogenous published studies about techniques for minimally invasive parathyroid surgery all share the intent to provide a focused and unilateral dissection through a short incision. Unfortunately, some studies in the literature coded as "minimally invasive" those operations in which an unplanned BE was performed; in other studies, any operation in which BE was performed was counted as BE. The important point is that during a planned focused initial operation for pHPT, any concern for MGD should prompt conversion to BE because the goal of initial surgery is cure.

Preoperative identification of a target parathyroid gland by one or more imaging modalities allows the surgeon to start with a focused parathyroidectomy. Use of ioPTH monitoring as an intraoperative adjunct provides intraoperative biochemical confirmation of resection adequacy, but failure of ioPTH levels to drop adequately warrants conversion to BE, as does inability to identify the target gland in the expected location; some experts at least attempt to examine the ipsilateral gland as well. In the hands of an experienced parathyroid surgeon, a focused unilateral approach confers equivalent or slightly improved outcomes compared to BE including cure rates, operative times, length of stay, and complication rates.[26] Another distinct advantage of MIP approach is the more liberal use of regional anesthesia compared to general anesthesia for BEs.

Tissue PTH Analysis

An intraoperative adjunct to confirm parathyroid tissue is fine-needle aspiration and washing of an enlarged parathyroid specimen for ioPTH analysis. This can be utilized in lieu of frozen section analysis which can be more expensive and time intensive. To perform it, a 25-gauge needle is used to aspirate the gland multiple times with the purpose of agitation to create a cloudy solution that is sent in a phlebotomy tube for ioPTH analysis similar to a serum specimen. A value >50,000 pg/mL unequivocally confirms parathyroid tissue.

Parathyroid Autotransplantation & Cryopreservation

Permanent hypoparathyroidism is a rare but potentially devastating complication of thyroid and parathyroid surgery. It is functionally defined as persistent hypocalcemia requiring calcium and active vitamin D supplementation (calcitriol) that persists at least 6 months after surgery. It requires lifelong medical therapy that is laborious and reduces quality of life. To avoid hypoparathyroidism, most endocrine surgeons acquire considerable expertise in finding and delicately preserving normal parathyroids in situ. Two further methods of parathyroid tissue salvage and preservation are autotransplantation and cryopreservation.

Parathyroid autotransplantation permits immediate tissue reimplantation during either parathyroid or thyroid surgery; the autografted tissue then takes 6 to 12 weeks to function. However, nonselective use of autotransplantation at least theoretically increases the risk of later hyperparathyroidism at the transplanted site, and if overused demonstrably carries an increased risk of otherwise transient hypoparathyroidism after thyroid surgery.

Parathyroid cryopreservation allows for fresh tissue to be stored in a sterile fashion for potential future reimplantation if hypoparathyroidism is later diagnosed; it avoids unnecessary autotransplantation at the time of the initial surgery but carries a higher rate of graft nonfunction. Cryopreservation is indicated in initial or reoperative surgery for primary hyperparathyroidism when there is a high risk for permanent postoperative hypoparathyroidism such as patients with multigland disease undergoing a subtotal parathyroidectomy.

Reoperative Parathyroid Surgery

Any anterior cervical operation, such as thyroidectomy, parathyroidectomy, anterior cervical disk fusion, thoracic and thoracoscopic surgery, and carotid endarterectomy, generates scar tissue that can impede or prohibit successful parathyroid dissection. Moreover, both these operations and prior cervical or upper thoracic surgery can be associated with RLN dysfunction. With any such history, the preoperative evaluation and intraoperative management of patients undergoing initial surgery for pHPT requires modification which must sometimes be extensive, and which routinely includes preoperative assessment of vocal cord function.

In patients diagnosed specifically with recurrent or persistent pHPT a reoperation may be necessary but is unique in its preoperative diagnostic approach and intraoperative management. As above, any prior operation to the anterior cervical neck or that places a recurrent laryngeal nerve at risk has the potential to devascularize normal parathyroid glands. Because reoperative parathyroid surgery is technically more challenging and has higher risks of failure, RLN injury, and hypoparathyroidism compared to initial parathyroid exploration, the threshold for indication in reoperations is higher and most parathyroid surgeons require significant symptomatology, nephrolithiasis, osteoporosis, hypercalciuria, or a documented decrease in renal function before recommending reoperation for persistent or recurrent pHPT.[17] In asymptomatic patients with recurrent or persistent pHPT a calcium of 12.0 mg/dL or greater is typically used as a biochemical threshold for reintervention. Importantly, in contrast to initial surgery, positive preoperative imaging is essential in planning reoperative parathyroidectomy. Most experienced surgeons require at least one positive imaging study prior to reoperation, and some require two concordantly positive studies as this increases the sensitivity to >90%.[27]

The decision to proceed with re-exploration in a patient with appropriate indications is tailored to each patient scenario and must be carefully weighed against the risks and only after a thorough investigation and review of prior operative findings, pathology reports, vocal cord function, and imaging studies. The managing team needs to realize that just because an abnormal gland is identified on imaging does not mean that it represents the only abnormal parathyroid; if the assessment is inadequately treated MGD, staged unilateral reoperations are occasionally employed. Nonoperative management of persistent or recurrent pHPT can be pursued in patients with mild disease and/or nonlocalizing imaging studies.

Most residual parathyroid disease is accessible by a transcervical approach, but previous surgery may result in dense adhesions between strap muscles and thyroid capsule, making an anterior approach more difficult. In this situation, a lateral approach can be utilized by dissecting in the plane between the sternohyoid and sternocleidomastoid muscles. Even in the setting of a reoperation, mediastinal parathyroid glands are usually accessible from a cervical incision which facilitates a cervical thymectomy to remove parathyroid tissue within the thyrothymic ligament or anterior mediastinum.

Intraoperative adjuncts that are utilized in initial parathyroid explorations are applicable to reoperative cases including ioPTH monitoring and RLN monitoring. Parathyroid autotransplantation and cryopreservation are of particular importance as the reoperative specimen may be the patient's last remaining viable parathyroid tissue. While selective parathyroid jugular venous sampling is generally not utilized for localization in initial operations, it has been demonstrated to be a useful adjunct in otherwise nonlocalizing reoperative cases and should be kept in the parathyroid surgeon's toolbelt.[28]

REFERENCES

1. Duh QY, Suh I, Stoller ML. Underdiagnosis of primary hyperparathyroidism: the need for a system-level fix. *JAMA Surg*. 2020;155(9):868-869.
2. Seib CD, Meng T, Suh I, et al. Undertreatment of primary hyperparathyroidism in a privately insured US population: decreasing utilization of parathyroidectomy despite expanding surgical guidelines. *Surgery*. 2021;169(1):87-93.
3. Griebeler ML, Kearns AE, Ryu E, Hathcock MA, Melton LJ, 3rd, Wermers RA. Secular trends in the incidence of primary hyperparathyroidism over five decades (1965-2010). *Bone*. 2015;73:1-7.
4. Khan R, Martin J, Das G. The impact of observation versus parathyroidectomy on bone mineral density and fracture risk determined by FRAX tool in patients with primary hyperparathyroidism. *J Clin Densitom*. 2021;24(4):571-580.
5. Yip L, Ogilvie JB, Challinor SM, et al. Identification of multiple endocrine neoplasia type 1 in patients with apparent sporadic primary hyperparathyroidism. *Surgery*. 2008;144(6): 1002-1006; discussion 1006-7.
6. Hollenberg AN, Arnold A. Hypercalcemia with low-normal serum intact PTH: a novel presentation of primary hyperparathyroidism. *Am J Med*. 1991;91(5):547-548.
7. Wallace LB, Parikh RT, Ross LV, et al. The phenotype of primary hyperparathyroidism with normal parathyroid hormone levels: how low can parathyroid hormone go? *Surgery*. 2011;150(6):1102-1112.
8. Quaglino F, Manfrino L, Cestino L, et al. Parathyroid carcinoma: an up-to-date retrospective multicentric analysis. *Int J Endocrinol*. 2020;2020:7048185.
9. Tripathi M, Karwasra RK, Parshad S. Effect of preoperative vitamin D deficiency on postoperative hypocalcemia after thyroid surgery. *Thyroid Res*. 2014;7:8.
10. Grubbs EG, Rafeeq S, Jimenez C, et al. Preoperative vitamin D replacement therapy in primary hyperparathyroidism: safe and beneficial? *Surgery*. 2008;144(6):852-858; discussion 858-9.
11. Dershem R, Gorvin CM, Metpally RPR, et al. Familial hypocalciuric hypercalcemia type 1 and autosomal-dominant hypocalcemia type 1: prevalence in a large healthcare population. *Am J Hum Genet*. 2020;106(6):734-747.
12. Shah US, McCoy KL, Kelly ML, Carty SE, Yip L. How and when is multigland disease diagnosed in sporadic primary hyperparathyroidism? *Surgery*. 2022;171(1):36-39.
13. Sho S, Yuen AD, Yeh MW, Livhits MJ, Sepahdari AR. Factors associated with discordance between preoperative parathyroid 4-dimensional computed tomographic scans and intraoperative findings during parathyroidectomy. *JAMA Surg*. 2017;152(12):1141-1147.
14. Nastos C, Papaconstantinou D, Kofopoulos-Lymperis E, et al. Optimal extent of initial parathyroid resection in patients with multiple endocrine neoplasia syndrome type 1: a meta-analysis. *Surgery*. 2021;169(2):302-310.
15. Hu X, Guan J, Wang Y, et al. A narrative review of multiple endocrine neoplasia syndromes: genetics, clinical features, imaging findings, and diagnosis. *Ann Transl Med*. 2021;9(11):944.
16. Marx SJ. New concepts about familial isolated hyperparathyroidism. *J Clin Endocrinol Metab*. 2019;104(9):4058-4066.
17. Wilhelm SM, Wang TS, Ruan DT, et al. The American Association of Endocrine Surgeons Guidelines for Definitive Management of Primary Hyperparathyroidism. *JAMA Surg*. 2016;151(10):959-968.
18. Lee S, Ryu H, Morris LF, et al. Operative failure in minimally invasive parathyroidectomy utilizing an intraoperative parathyroid hormone assay. *Ann Surg Oncol*. 2014;21(6):1878-83.
19. Mallick R, Nicholson KJ, Yip L, Carty SE, McCoy KL. Factors associated with late recurrence after parathyroidectomy for primary hyperparathyroidism. *Surgery*. 2020;167(1):160-165.
20. VanderWalde LH, Liu IL, Haigh PI. Effect of bone mineral density and parathyroidectomy on fracture risk in primary hyperparathyroidism. *World J Surg*. Mar 2009;33(3):406-411.
21. Liu JY, Peine BS, Mlaver E, et al. Neuropsychologic changes in primary hyperparathyroidism after parathyroidectomy from a dual-institution prospective study. *Surgery*. Jan 2021;169(1):114-119.
22. Lu R, Zhao W, Yin L, et al. Efficacy of ultrasonography and Tc-99m MIBI SPECT/CT in preoperative localization of parathyroid adenomas causing primary hyperthyroidism. *BMC Med Imaging*. May 21 2021;21(1):87.
23. Tawfik AI, Kamr WH, Mahmoud W, Abo Shady IA, Mohamed MH. Added value of ultrasonography and Tc-99m MIBI SPECT/CT combined protocol in preoperative evaluation of parathyroid adenoma. *Eur J Radiol Open*. 2019;6:336-342.
24. Wharry LI, Yip L, Armstrong MJ, et al. The final intraoperative parathyroid hormone level: how low should it go? *World J Surg*. Mar 2014;38(3):558-563.
25. Heller KS, Blumberg SN. Relation of final intraoperative parathyroid hormone level and outcome following parathyroidectomy. *Arch Otolaryngol Head Neck Surg*. Nov 2009;135(11):1103-1107.
26. Udelsman R, Lin Z, Donovan P. The superiority of minimally invasive parathyroidectomy based on 1650 consecutive patients with primary hyperparathyroidism. *Ann Surg*. Mar 2011;253(3):585-591.
27. Patel SG, Saunders ND, Jamshed S, Weber CJ, Sharma J. Multimodal preoperative localization improves outcomes in reoperative parathyroidectomy: a 25-year surgical experience. *Am Surg*. 2019;85(9):939-943.
28. Zolin SJ, Crawford K, Rudin AV, et al. Selective parathyroid venous sampling in reoperative parathyroid surgery: a key localization tool when noninvasive tests are unrevealing. *Surgery*. 2021;169(1):126-132.

Secondary Hyperparathyroidism

36

Denise Carneiro-Pla, MD, FACS
Mahsa Javid, MBBChr, DPhil

GENERAL CONSIDERATIONS

Over the years, nephrologists have had a wide range of medical therapies to help manage this disease, such as vitamin D analogues and phosphate binders. However, the introduction of cinacalcet, a calcimimetic, has changed the management of secondary HPT from an often surgically treated disease to a mostly medically managed condition. Since cinacalcet approval in 2004, parathyroidectomy rates decreased worldwide, resulting in a decrease in the United States from 6.8-11.8 to 3.3-5.5/1000 patients per year, depending on the year evaluated.[1] Recently, the use of cinacalcet (oral) and etelcalcetide (parenteral) has been limited, and secondary HPT due to ESRD has become a common surgical disease once again. According to kidney disease: Improving Global Outcomes (KIDGO) guidelines, parathyroid hormone (PTH) levels should be maintained between 2 and 9 times the upper normal limit for the assay.[2] On updates of these guidelines, it has been recommended that the trend of PTH levels long-term is more important than absolute values.[3,4] Parathyroid hormone targets in the dialysis population have varied widely across professional organizations in the absence of high-level evidence: from 60-240 pg/mL (Japanese Society for Dialysis Therapy 2012) to 130-600 pg/mL (KDIGO 2009).[5]

Furthermore, it has been shown that PTH levels >600 pg/mL are associated with a higher risk for all-cause and cardiovascular mortality and cardiovascular hospitalizations.[5] Furthermore, lowering pre-kidney transplantation PTH levels may be of benefit to prevent eventual tertiary HPT following kidney transplantation.[6,7]

In summary, patients with autonomous parathyroid function with unsuppressed serum PTH production or hypercalcemia despite adequate medical treatment can benefit from surgical intervention.

PATHOGENESIS

In conjunction with bone and the parathyroid glands, the kidneys are a fundamental part of calcium and phosphorous hemostasis. Secondary HPT, also known as uremic hyperparathyroidism, is a disorder in which patients with ESRD have excessive secretion of PTH. In these patients, the kidneys cannot adequately hydroxylate the inactive form of vitamin D (25-hydroxyvitamin D) and convert it to its active form (1,25 hydroxyvitamin D). The chronic decrease in vitamin D leads to hypocalcemia and chronic excess secretion of PTH. As a result, the parathyroid glands exist under a constant drive to produce PTH; they become hyperplastic and eventually lose feedback regulation from serum calcium levels. Moreover, phosphorous levels are also increased in patients with ESRD, which stimulates further parathyroid secretion of PTH.

A key modulator of calcium and phosphorous levels is fibroblast growth factor-23 (FGF-23). Physiologically, in the presence of normal renal function, FGF-23 is released from bones in the presence of high serum phosphorous levels and acts on the kidneys to increase phosphorous excretion and decrease 1-alpha-hydroxylation of 25 hydroxyvitamin D to reduce the activation of vitamin D. In patients with ESRD, FGF-23 levels are increased, leading initially to increased renal phosphorous excretion. FGF-23 also directly suppresses PTH gene expression; however, its inhibitory effect on secondary HPT is relatively limited because of decreased klotho expression in parathyroid glands.[8] Eventual resistance of the diseased kidneys and the parathyroid glands to FGF-23 leads to reduced phosphorus excretion with resultant hyperphosphatemia. Subsequently, the parathyroid glands are subjected to continuous stimulation resulting in parathyroid hyperplasia.

Prevention

Most patients with ESRD will develop secondary HPT, and the only true prevention is kidney transplantation prior to the transformation of the parathyroids into autonomous glands that no longer respond to negative feedback. Correcting the biochemical abnormalities causing the parathyroid glands to become hyperplastic and occasionally adenomatous is critical in preventing secondary HPT from becoming a surgical disease. Optimal PTH levels in patients with ESRD are unknown; however, those with progressively rising values should be evaluated for modifiable factors. These include hypocalcemia, hyperphosphatemia, and vitamin D deficiency. Aggressive calcium replacement, during dialysis and orally, use of phosphate binders, and vitamin D replacement are critical to lessening the detrimental effects of secondary HPT. KDIGO guidelines recommend lowering phosphorous levels to the normal range and avoiding hypercalcemia. When the parathyroid glands become autonomous due to chronic stimulation, the efficacy of medical treatment of these biochemical abnormalities is limited and hypercalcemia will develop, often requiring parathyroidectomy.

Clinical Findings

A. Symptoms and Signs

Patients with secondary HPT can present with bone pain, joint pain, intractable pruritus, muscle weakness, pathologic fractures, and occasionally calciphylaxis. The latter presents as painful necrotic skin lesions that carry a poor prognosis.[9]

Renal osteodystrophy can present as adynamic bone disease due to low bone turnover resulting from over suppression of PTH to <100 mg/mL or osteitis fibrosa, a high turnover bone disease that increases the risk of bone fractures. The different forms of renal osteodystrophy are diagnosed by bone biopsy. Subperiosteal erosions, brown tumors, and tissue calcification can be seen radiographically.

Anemia is a common complication in hemodialysis patients. Decreased erythropoietin production, iron deficiency, and increased hemolysis are important contributing factors for anemia. Progressive secondary HPT induces bone marrow resistance and decreases its response to erythropoietin treatment.

B. Laboratory Findings

- Low to high corrected serum calcium depending on the stage of secondary HPT
- Elevated PTH
- Hyperphosphatemia
- Vitamin D deficiency
- Alkaline phosphatase is often high due to bone turnover

C. Imaging Studies

Although some surgeons do not use imaging prior to neck exploration in secondary hyperparathyroidism, since all parathyroid glands need to be identified and evaluated at surgery, many will obtain imaging to help localize the glands preoperatively. Preoperative cervical imaging can be performed, as recommended by the American Association of Endocrine Surgeon guidelines, usually with ultrasonography to evaluate possible thyroid pathology prior to neck exploration.[10]

- Ultrasonography (US): This method is often adequate to visualize enlarged parathyroid glands. Adenomatous glands are usually more hypoechoic and easier to appreciate than hyperplastic glands that contain more fat and are more difficult to identify on US. That being said, an experienced cervical ultrasonographer can often localize all parathyroid glands (Figures 36–1 to 36–6). The parathyroid glands may contain calcifications in patients with secondary HPT (Figure 36–4). When fewer than four glands are visualized on US, another imaging modality can be obtained to rule out intrathoracic and ectopic locations. The accuracy of US in this population is 91% to 97% in localizing all parathyroid glands.[11,12] Furthermore, preoperative US is useful in identifying any thyroid pathology that might need to be managed either prior to surgery or intraoperatively. It is important to understand that the accuracy and usefulness of preoperative ultrasound in localizing parathyroid glands in patients with secondary HPT is based on the sonographer's experience.
- Technitium-99m Sestamibi scan (MIBI scan): The results of MIBI scan in localizing parathyroid glands in secondary HPT are inferior compared with those in primary HPT. This imaging modality has 50% to 56% accuracy, increasing to 78% when SPECT MIBI scan is used to localize all parathyroid glands.[11,12] MIBI scans are helpful to localize mediastinal glands, which cannot be visualized with US. Some suggest combined US and MIBI scan is the best imaging strategy with higher accuracy in localizing all glands.[13] The authors prefer to use MIBI scans selectively following surgeon-performed US.
- Four-dimensional computed tomography (4DCT): This method requires IV contrast, which is more complex in these patients. The scan needs to be coordinated with the patient's dialysis sessions. There are few reports of this modality in this patient population, but for surgeons who do not perform US themselves, this method might be beneficial to localize all parathyroid glands and help identify them preoperatively.

Complications

Patients with ESRD and long-standing secondary HPT will develop nonsuppressible parathyroid gland function,

Figure 36–1 through 36–6. Cervical ultrasonography of a patient with secondary hyperparathyroidism. The images 36-1 through 36-6 show 4 eutopic parathyroid glands, a thyroid nodule and an ectopic parathyroid gland in the lateral neck.

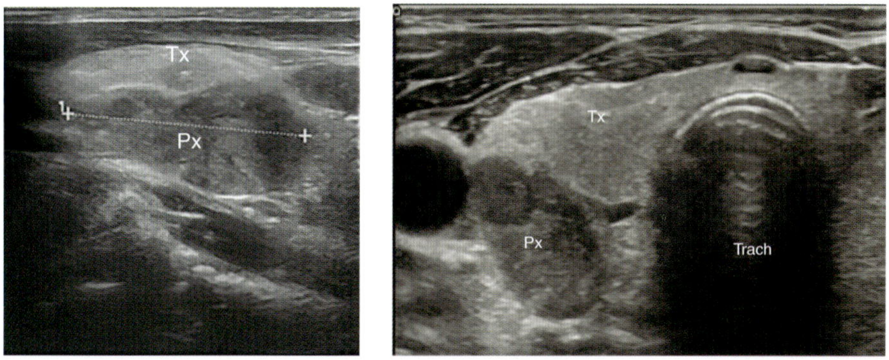

▲ **Figure 36–1.** Longitudinal and transverse views of the superior enlarged parathyroid gland.

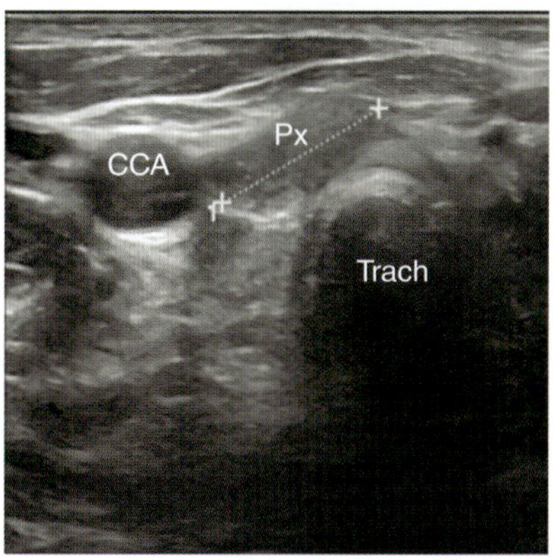

▲ **Figure 36–2.** Transverse view of right inferior enlarged parathyroid gland located inferior to the right thyroid lobe.

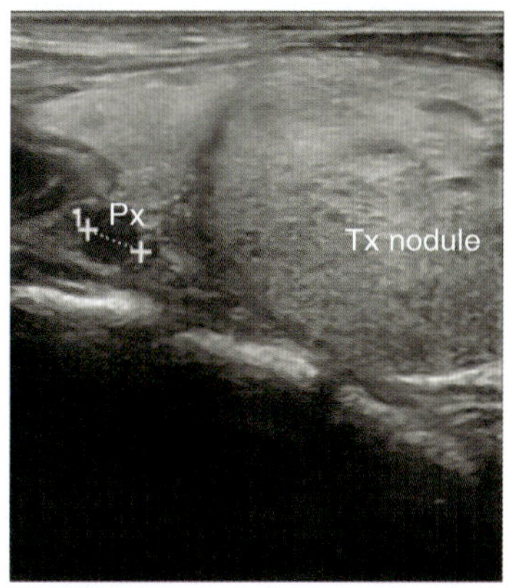

▲ **Figure 36–3.** Longitudinal eutopic left superior parathyroid gland at the level of the superior pole of the thyroid.

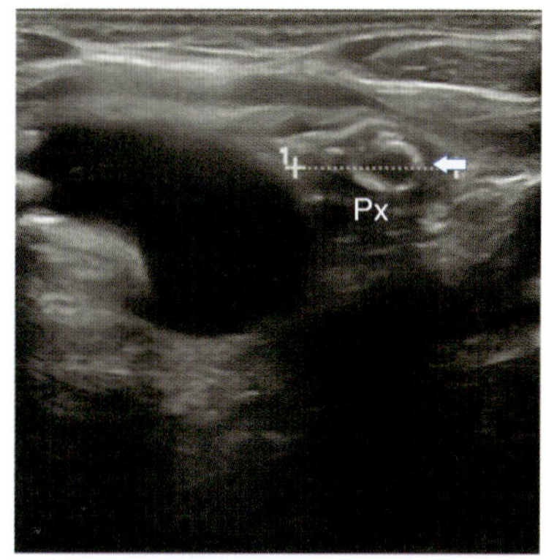

▲ **Figure 36–4.** Transverse view of an enlarged left inferior parathyroid gland with calcifications inferior to the left thyroid lobe. Arrow points to part of the parathyroid with calcification.

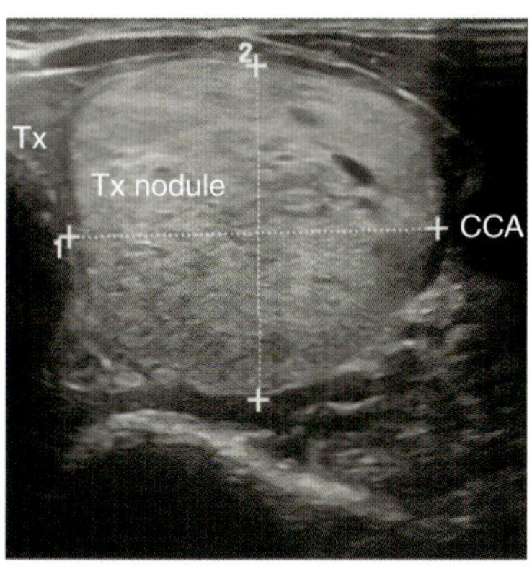

▲ **Figure 36–5.** Transverse view of large biopsy-proven benign left thyroid nodule.

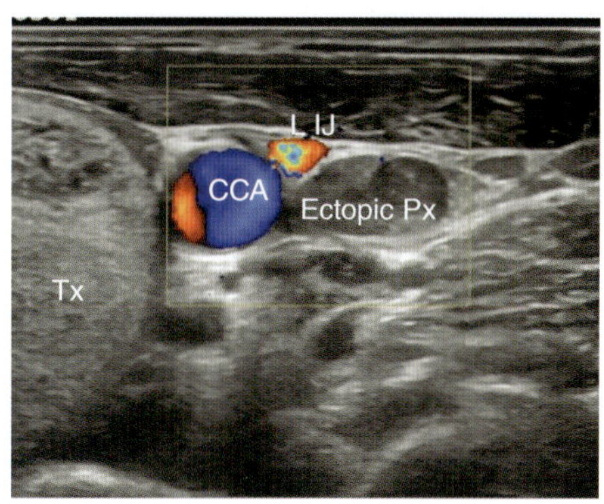

▲ **Figure 36–6.** Transverse view of an enlarged ectopic parathyroid gland in the left lateral neck at level III, diagnosed preoperatively with FNA and PTH washout.

Abbreviations: CCA, common carotid artery; FNA, fine-needle aspiration; L IJ, left internal jugular vein; Px, parathyroid gland; Tx, thyroid; Trach, trachea.

eventually leading to hypercalcemia. Elevated PTH levels outside the recommended range increase mortality and worsen bone disease. Furthermore, one of the most feared complications of secondary HPT is calciphylaxis which has a high mortality rate.[9,14]

Control of PTH levels is important for a successful outcome in patients with secondary HPT requiring kidney transplantation. In these patients, pretransplantation parathyroidectomy is associated with a lower risk of graft failure.[7] In comparison, pretransplantation PTH level ≥6 times the normal range is associated with a higher risk of graft failure.[7] Therefore, PTH levels should be reduced before transplantation to improve outcomes. Parathyroidectomy should be considered prior to transplantation if this level of PTH reduction cannot be achieved by medical treatment. Studies have not determined the optimal level of PTH in kidney transplant candidates. Also, the severity of hyperparathyroidism prior to transplantation in patients with secondary HPT plays a major role in the development of tertiary HPT post-transplantation with higher pretransplantation PTH levels associated with higher rates of tertiary HPT. The level of PTH at the time of and after kidney transplantation may have adverse consequences on the transplanted kidney graft, not only while the tertiary HPT is medically managed but also when this condition requires surgical intervention. Parathyroidectomy for tertiary HPT can decrease graft function if excessive parathyroid glands are resected; therefore, preventing surgical tertiary HPT would benefit these patients.[15,16]

Surgical Treatment

A study showed that 15% and 38% of patients require parathyroidectomy after 10 and 20 years of dialysis, respectively.[17,18] Most patients with secondary HPT can be treated medically; however, parathyroidectomy is indicated when PTH levels can no longer be suppressed despite aggressive medical therapy with calcium, vitamin D replacement, phosphate binders, and calcimimetics. The most recent KDIGO guidelines no longer recommend specific biochemical values to trigger consideration of surgery and state that those with severe hyperparathyroidism, despite medical management, should undergo parathyroidectomy.[4] However, the following metabolic and laboratory changes are generally considered appropriate indications for surgery.

Indications for Parathyroidectomy

- Hypercalcemia
- Intractable hyperphosphatemia
- Calciphylaxis, especially in the presence of hypercalcemia
- Symptoms such as bone and joint pain, pruritus
- PTH levels >800-1000 pg/mL despite medical management; however, intervention in severe hyperparathyroidism with even lower PTH levels has been shown to improve graft function following kidney transplantation[7,19]
- Erythropoietin-resistant anemia despite correction of iron deficiency and after ruling out gastrointestinal bleeding.

When a surgical indication is present, parathyroid localization can be obtained as described above. Surgeon-performed ultrasonography can localize most parathyroid glands and can also identify concomitant thyroid pathology. MIBI scans can be used when not all four glands are visualized on US in an attempt to localize ectopic and mediastinal glands.

Parathyroidectomy aims to decrease PTH, calcium, and phosphorus to target ranges as per KIDGO guidelines.[4] A 3.5 gland excision or total parathyroidectomy with autotransplantation in the upper extremity can be performed to accomplish this goal. Total parathyroidectomy without autotransplantation is an option for patients who are not transplant candidates; however, adynamic bone disease can result from the absence of PTH, therefore often not recommended for patients who are transplant candidates. Overtreating hyperparathyroidism by lowering PTH levels to <200 pg/mL is associated not only with adynamic bone disease but also accelerated vascular calcification and increased fracture risk.[20]

Subtotal Parathyroidectomy

This procedure aims to remove almost all abnormal glands leaving only a small remnant of the most "normal appearing" gland to maintain postoperative PTH levels around 250 to 300 pg/mL, return calcium and phosphorus to normal range, and avoid postoperative permanent hypocalcemia. Through a Kocher incision, the platysma is divided, and the subplatysmal flaps are elevated superiorly and inferiorly. The median raphe is divided with electrocautery. If no localization studies were performed, sequential bilateral exploration of the central neck to visualize all four parathyroid glands is performed. When all parathyroid glands are visualized, subtotal resection of the most "normal appearing" gland is performed. It is transected to leave *in situ* a small remnant, usually around 30 to 60 mg, with good vascularization. It is recommended that the size of the remnant is adjusted according to the expected time the patient will remain on dialysis, balancing the possibility of recurrence versus permanent hypocalcemia and adynamic bone disease. Larger remnants can be left *in situ* in kidney transplant candidates, while smaller remnants should be considered for nontransplant candidates. The remnant gland can be marked with nonabsorbable sutures or large titanium clips to facilitate its localization at reoperation in case of recurrence. It is important to perform the subtotal resection early in the procedure to assess its viability before further parathyroid resection. If the blood supply of the partially resected gland is not ideal, then the next most "normal appearing" gland should be selected for subtotal excision. If this is viable, then the initial remnant should be fully resected. The remaining glands should not be devascularized until a well vascularized half-gland is achieved. When this is accomplished, the remaining glands are removed and passed to the back table and preferably kept on ice for potential autotransplantation in the event that the remnant becomes devascularized during hemostasis. A frozen section of these glands could be obtained to confirm that all four parathyroid glands were identified. Alternatively, each gland can be aspirated *ex vivo* for PTH washout in 1 cc of saline when intraoperative PTH is available. Levels greater than the assay scale confirm that the aspirated tissue is parathyroid. Another approach is to use one of the parathyroid autofluorescence systems to confirm the excised tissue is parathyroid.

When preoperative imaging such as ultrasonography is used, the side with the smallest visualized gland can be explored first. The smaller gland on this side can then be partially excised at the beginning of the procedure. If the subtotal remnant is viable, the remaining three glands can be removed expeditiously.

Total Parathyroidectomy

This operative approach can be performed with or without autotransplantation. Total parathyroidectomy with autotransplantation is preferred as very low PTH levels postoperatively will lead to adynamic bone disease and should be avoided, as previously mentioned. During a total parathyroidectomy, all parathyroid glands are visualized as described above and are excised along with the thymus, which can also be performed during subtotal parathyroidectomy as per the surgeon's preference. All parathyroid glands are excised and kept on ice until autotransplantation is performed. The most "normal appearing" gland is then minced and transplanted into the brachioradialis muscle either in the nondominant upper extremity or the opposite side from the vascular access used for dialysis. This location, rather than one in the neck, is favorable in the event that reoperation becomes necessary, as this can be performed under local anesthesia with low morbidity. Also, if hyperparathyroidism persists or recurs, the source of excess PTH can be identified by collecting blood for PTH from each antecubital vein, differentiating a cervical source from a brachial one due to the transplanted tissue. MIBI scan can also establish the source of recurrent disease. The chosen parathyroid gland is transplanted into the muscle in four to six different pockets and marked with nonabsorbable sutures or titanium clips that will be evident at reoperation in case re-excision is required. It is important to avoid bleeding into the muscle pocket as significant bleeding would prevent revascularization of the autotransplanted tissue. The amount of autotransplanted tissue, the number of pockets in the muscle, and the location of autotransplantation in muscle versus subcutaneous tissue are debated. The authors suggest mincing the parathyroid to the smallest size possible, then transplanting the parathyroid in four to six pockets in the upper extremity.

The results of total parathyroidectomy with autotransplantation are similar to those following subtotal parathyroidectomy; however, until the transplanted parathyroid tissue starts to function following total parathyroidectomy, calcium levels may be more difficult to manage.[21]

Total parathyroidectomy without transplantation is an option for patients who are not candidates for a kidney transplant in whom this approach decreases the chance of recurrence. Low bone turnover is the main downside of this approach, along with permanent hypocalcemia, and the latter is an undesirable outcome for kidney transplantation candidates.

Intraoperative PTH Monitoring

Many surgeons use intraoperative PTH monitoring to guide the extent of parathyroidectomy in patients with primary HPT. The use of this adjunct in secondary HPT is less clear. The authors use intraoperative PTH monitoring to confirm that excision of almost all hyperfunctioning glands was accomplished. An elevated PTH at the end of the dissection might indicate that supernumerary gland(s) is(are) present, and further dissection is necessary. The PTH is expected to drop to around 250-300 pg/mL by 30 minutes after the subtotal parathyroidectomy. This absolute value also depends on the intraoperative PTH assay used. Some surgeons require the PTH level to decline a certain percentage from the baseline value. Determining a percent PTH decline can be challenging, as the baseline PTH level is often far above the assay scale and needs to be diluted to obtain an absolute value.

Furthermore, the PTH decline following sequential gland excision does not necessarily occur in a stepwise manner since the glands have different morphologies, with some being more adenomatous and others more hyperplastic. Also, the vascularization of the remaining parathyroid gland remnant can affect the final PTH value with better-vascularized remnants resulting in higher final PTH levels. An important consideration, and likely the most helpful use of intraoperative PTH, is to ensure that supernumerary parathyroid glands are not left *in situ* as these glands are more common in patients with secondary HPT. An inadequate decrease in PTH levels will lead the surgeon to further explore the neck and superior mediastinum for supernumerary glands and, often, ectopic parathyroid glands. An adequate PTH drop also assures that thymectomy is not needed to achieve operative success. Although having fewer than four glands is uncommon, it can occur in these patients, especially those who have undergone previous cervical and upper mediastinal procedures. In these cases, intraoperative PTH monitoring can signal adequate excision

Table 36–1. Different criteria used to predict intraoperatively, operative success in secondary hyperparathyroidism.

Authors	Intraoperative PTH Criteria to Predict Operative Success in Secondary Hyperparathyroidism
Chou et al.[23]	>60% decrease in rapid PTH levels at 10 minutes after total parathyroidectomy and autotransplantation predicted PTH <60 pg/mL POD1
Zhang et al.[24]	>86.8 and 90.6% PTH in 10 and 20 minutes after total parathyroidectomy and thymectomy predicated PTH <300 pg/mL postoperatively
Chavez et al.[25]	>90% PTH drop 15 minutes after subtotal parathyroidectomy predicted PTH <150 pg/mL on POD1
Ohe et al.[26]	>80% PTH from the 0 minute value, 20 minutes after total parathyroidectomy with autotransplantation predicted the restoration of serum calcium and PTH levels as expected for each renal function stage, throughout the first 6 months after surgery
Barczynski et al.[27]	>60% from pre-excision 10 minutes after subtotal parathyroidectomy
Hiramitsu et al.[28]	>70% PTH drop from the baseline 10 minutes after total parathyroidectomy and thymectomy predicated PTH <60 pg/mL on POD1

POD1, postoperative day 1.

when fewer than four glands are found and possibly indicate that total parathyroid excision has been performed and autotransplantation is required.

A "differential jugular venous sampling" for PTH can be performed to localize the side of the missing hyperfunctioning gland. Aspiration of whole blood from the left and right internal jugular veins, sequentially, is sent for intraoperative PTH levels, and a 10% difference in levels indicates lateralization. This is less helpful for mediastinal lesions and also in cases where the middle thyroid vein was already ligated during the procedure.

Several criteria can be used to predict operative success in secondary HPT, as shown in Table 36–1. Each criterion has an associated accuracy in predicting the desired outcome.

Surgical Outcomes

Parathyroidectomy for secondary HPT presents favorable results in most symptomatic patients with significant improvement in bone pain, joint pain, and pruritus.[22] Parathyroidectomy resulted in BMD increase of 7% to 23% within 6 months following a successful procedure.[19] In addition, improvement of nonvisceral calcification occurs in most patients following parathyroidectomy. Parathyroidectomy is associated with 20% to 57% and 33% to 41% all-cause and cardiovascular mortality, respectively, compared to the matched control group.[8,29] Surgical intervention also improves hypercalcemia, hyperphosphatemia, tissue calcification, bone mineral density, and health-related quality of life.[8]

Operative failure occurs when the hyperfunctioning parathyroid tissue is not all visualized and appropriately resected. This can occur during a subtotal parathyroidectomy where the remnant left *in situ* is too large or by failing to find and resect all or sufficient abnormal glands. Supernumerary glands are present in 5% to 30% of the patients and are often the cause of operative failure.[20,30]

It is quite challenging to define the reported outcomes of different operative approaches due to multiple definitions of operative failure and the heterogenicity of the population in several studies, which often include secondary and tertiary HPT together. Operative failure has been defined as postoperative hypercalcemia, PTH levels outside the expected range by guidelines, or merely PTH above normal limits.[20] In the authors' opinion, a successful parathyroidectomy should achieve a postoperative PTH of 250 to 300 pg/mL and within the expected range based on guidelines. At the same time, calcium and phosphorus levels are controlled with medical management.

Hungry bone syndrome is common following parathyroidectomy in patients with secondary HPT, especially when significant bone disease is present. Severe hypocalcemia, symptomatic or not, requires aggressive treatment following parathyroidectomy in this population. There are several approaches to correct postoperative hypocalcemia, including orally with vitamin D and calcium supplementation and intravenously with calcium gluconate. Coordination with nephrology, to treat with an adequate calcium bath that is available both during the hospital stay and at the patient's regular dialysis clinic, is necessary to control hypocalcemia in a timely fashion.

Ergocalciferol replacement a few weeks prior to parathyroidectomy may help increase absorption of calcium following parathyroidectomy. Although the data about ergocalciferol use in this population is unclear, many specialists will replace vitamin D before surgery to facilitate postoperative calcium management.[8]

When to Refer

Patients with secondary HPT should be referred when PTH levels are greatly elevated despite exhaustive pharmacological treatment, if tolerated, or if hypercalcemia has developed. In addition, patients with or at high risk for calciphylaxis, inadequate phosphorus control, erythropoietin-resistant anemia, and debilitating symptomatology should be considered for parathyroidectomy. Furthermore, in kidney transplant candidates, perhaps PTH >800-1000 pg/mL with or without cinacalcet could be considered an indication for parathyroidectomy in the hope of preventing the development of tertiary hyperparathyroidism.[10,19]

REFERENCES

1. Kim SM, Long J, Montez-Rath ME, Leonard MB, Norton JA, Chertow GM. Rates and outcomes of parathyroidectomy for secondary hyperparathyroidism in the United States. *Clin J Am Soc Nephrol.* 2016;11(7):1260-1267.
2. Kidney Disease: Improving Global Outcomes (KDIGO) CKD-MBD Work Group. KDIGO clinical practice guideline for the diagnosis, evaluation, prevention, and treatment of Chronic Kidney Disease-Mineral and Bone Disorder (CKD-MBD). *Kidney Int Suppl.* 2009;(113):S1-130.
3. Ketteler M, Block GA, Evenepoel P, et al. Executive summary of the 2017 KDIGO Chronic Kidney Disease-Mineral and Bone Disorder (CKD-MBD) Guideline Update: what's changed and why it matters. *Kidney Int.* 2017;92(1):26-36.
4. Kidney disease: improving global outcomes (KDIGO) CKD-MBD Update Work Group. KDIGO 2017 Clinical Practice Guideline Update for the Diagnosis, Evaluation, Prevention, and Treatment of Chronic Kidney Disease-Mineral and Bone Disorder (CKD-MBD). *Kidney Int Suppl* (2011). 2017; 7(1):1-59.
5. Tentori F, Wang M, Bieber BA, et al. Recent changes in therapeutic approaches and association with outcomes among patients with secondary hyperparathyroidism on chronic hemodialysis: the DOPPS study. *Clin J Am Soc Nephrol.* 2015;10(1):98-109.
6. Isakova T, Nickolas TL, Denburg M, et al. KDOQI US Commentary on the 2017 KDIGO Clinical Practice Guideline Update for the Diagnosis, Evaluation, Prevention, and Treatment of Chronic Kidney Disease-Mineral and Bone Disorder (CKD-MBD). *Am J Kidney Dis.* 2017;70(6):737-751.
7. Callender GG, Malinowski J, Javid M, et al. Parathyroidectomy prior to kidney transplant decreases graft failure. *Surgery.* 2017;161(1):44-50.
8. Lau WL, Obi Y, Kalantar-Zadeh K. Parathyroidectomy in the management of secondary hyperparathyroidism. *Clin J Am Soc Nephrol.* 2018;13(6):952-961.
9. Udomkarnjananun S, Kongnatthasate K, Praditpornsilpa K, Eiam-Ong S, Jaber BL, Susantitaphong P. Treatment of calciphylaxis in CKD: a systematic review and meta-analysis. *Kidney Int Rep.* 2019;4(2):231-244.
10. Dream S, Kuo LE, Kuo JH, et al. The American Association of Endocrine Surgeons guidelines for the definitive surgical management of secondary and tertiary renal hyperparathyroidism. *Ann Surg.* 2022 Sep 1;276(3):e141-e176. Epub 2022 Jul 18.
11. Li X, Li J, Li Y, et al. The role of preoperative ultrasound, contrast-enhanced ultrasound, and 99mTc-MIBI scanning with single-photon emission computed tomography/X-ray computed tomography localization in refractory secondary hyperparathyroidism. *Clin Hemorheol Microcirc.* 2020;75(1): 35-46.
12. Lee JB, Kim WY, Lee YM. The role of preoperative ultrasonography, computed tomography, and sestamibi scintigraphy localization in secondary hyperparathyroidism. *Ann Surg Treat Res.* 2015;89(6):300-305.
13. Yuan LL, Kan Y, Ma DQ, Yang JG. Combined application of ultrasound and SPECT/CT has incremental value in detecting parathyroid tissue in SHPT patients. *Diagn Interv Imaging.* 2016;97(2):219-225.
14. McCarthy JT, El-Azhary RA, Patzelt MT, et al. Survival, risk factors, and effect of treatment in 101 patients with calciphylaxis. *Mayo Clin Proc.* 2016;91(10):1384-1394.
15. Lee PP, Schiffmann L, Offermann G, Beige J. Effects of parathyroidectomy on renal allograft survival. *Kidney Blood Press Res.* 2004;27(3):191-196.
16. Schwarz A, Rustien G, Merkel S, Radermacher J, Haller H. Decreased renal transplant function after parathyroidectomy. *Nephrol Dial Transplant.* 2007;22(2):584-591.
17. Shih ML, Duh QY, Hsieh CB, et al. Total parathyroidectomy without autotransplantation for secondary hyperparathyroidism. *World J Surg.* 2009;33(2):248-254.
18. Fassbinder W, Brunner FP, Brynger H, et al. Combined report on regular dialysis and transplantation in Europe, XX, 1989. *Nephrol Dial Transplant.* 1991;6(Suppl 1):5-35.
19. Coyne DW, Delos Santos R. Evaluating the safety and rationale for cinacalcet posttransplant hyperparathyroidism and hypercalcemia. *Am J Transplant.* 2014;14(11):2446-2447.
20. Steinl GK, Kuo JH. Surgical management of secondary hyperparathyroidism. *Kidney Int Rep.* 2021;6(2):254-264.
21. Chen J, Jia X, Kong X, Wang Z, Cui M, Xu D. Total parathyroidectomy with autotransplantation versus subtotal parathyroidectomy for renal hyperparathyroidism: a systematic review and meta-analysis. *Nephrology* (Carlton). 2017;22(5): 388-396.
22. Zhang Y, Lu Y, Feng S, Zhan Z, Shen H. Evaluation of laboratory parameters and symptoms after parathyroidectomy in dialysis patients with secondary hyperparathyroidism. *Ren Fail.* 2019;41(1):921-929.
23. Chou FF, Lee CH, Chen JB, Hsu KT, Sheen-Chen SM. Intraoperative parathyroid hormone measurement in patients with secondary hyperparathyroidism. *Arch Surg.* 2002;137(3): 341-344.
24. Zhang L, Xing C, Shen C, et al. Diagnostic accuracy study of intraoperative and perioperative serum intact PTH level for successful parathyroidectomy in 501 secondary hyperparathyroidism patients. *Sci Rep.* 2016;6:26841.
25. Chavez KV, Marquez-Gonzalez H, Chavez-Tostado M. The usefulness of intraoperative PTH as a predictor for successful parathyroidectomy in secondary hyperparathyroidism. *Front Surg.* 2021;8:696469.
26. Ohe MN, Santos RO, Kunii IS, et al. Intraoperative PTH cutoff definition to predict successful parathyroidectomy in secondary and tertiary hyperparathyroidism. *Braz J Otorhinolaryngol.* 2013;79(4):494-499.

27. Barczynski M, Cichon S, Konturek A, Cichon W. A randomised study on a new cost-effective algorithm of quick intraoperative intact parathyroid hormone assay in secondary hyperparathyroidism. *Langenbecks Arch Surg.* 2005;390(2): 121-127.
28. Hiramitsu T, Tominaga Y, Okada M, Yamamoto T, Kobayashi T. A retrospective study of the impact of intraoperative intact parathyroid hormone monitoring during total parathyroidectomy for secondary hyperparathyroidism: STARD study. *Medicine* (Baltimore). 2015;94(29):e1213.
29. Komaba H, Taniguchi M, Wada A, Iseki K, Tsubakihara Y, Fukagawa M. Parathyroidectomy and survival among Japanese hemodialysis patients with secondary hyperparathyroidism. *Kidney Int.* 2015;88(2):350-359.
30. Schneider R, Waldmann J, Ramaswamy A, Fernandez ED, Bartsch DK, Schlosser K. Frequency of ectopic and supernumerary intrathymic parathyroid glands in patients with renal hyperparathyroidism: analysis of 461 patients undergoing initial parathyroidectomy with bilateral cervical thymectomy. *World J Surg.* 2011;35(6):1260-1265.

Tertiary Hyperparathyroidism

37

Taylor C. St. Amour, MD
Carmen C. Solórzano, MD, FACS

GENERAL CONSIDERATIONS

By definition, tertiary hyperparathyroidism, also referred to as persistent or autonomous hyperparathyroidism, is preceded by a prolonged period of secondary hyperparathyroidism, classically in the setting of chronic kidney disease (CKD). While it is estimated that at least 25% to 30% of patients with CKD will develop secondary hyperparathyroidism, only a small minority (1%-3%) of these patients will go on to develop tertiary parathyroid disease.[1,2] However, tertiary hyperparathyroidism is more prevalent within the subset of patients with end-stage renal disease (ESRD) who ultimately go on to receive renal transplantation, where it is seen in 20% to 30% of cases.[2,3]

While secondary and tertiary hyperparathyroidism most commonly occur in the setting of CKD and ESRD, these conditions can rarely occur in other clinical settings. Specifically, PTH homeostasis can become deranged in cases of chronic decreased calcium absorption, such as in cases of vitamin D deficiency, malabsorption-dependent bariatric surgery, celiac disease, or pancreatic conditions associated with fat malabsorption.[2,3] Similarly, renal calcium losses, such as in cases of idiopathic hypercalciuria or secondary to loop diuretic usage, can also lead to hyperparathyroidism.[4] Finally, hyperparathyroidism can rarely occur secondary to phosphate replacement therapy, such as in the case of genetic disorders including X-linked hypophosphatemic rickets or adult-onset (autosomal dominant) hypophosphatemic rickets, or oncogenic osteomalacia.[5] However, given the rarity of these conditions in comparison to CKD as the impetus for hyperparathyroidism, this chapter will largely focus its discussion of tertiary hyperparathyroidism as it relates to CKD.

Finally, it is important to note that there is a paucity of high-quality data regarding tertiary hyperparathyroidism when compared to primary and secondary forms. Consequently, a recurring challenge in the diagnosis and management of this condition is the lack of consensus regarding diagnostic criteria and treatment. Indeed, a significant proportion of the recommendations that exist regarding the management of tertiary hyperparathyroidism are based on comparatively small retrospective studies and expert opinions or are extrapolated from research in primary and secondary hyperparathyroidism.[2]

PATHOGENESIS

The cellular etiology that guides the progression from secondary to tertiary hyperparathyroidism remains uncertain. Some authors postulate that, as parathyroid hyperplasia progresses in the setting of secondary hyperparathyroidism, the expression of both the calcium-sensing receptor and vitamin D receptor on parathyroid tissue is downregulated. Eventually, polyclonal hyperplasia transitions to a monoclonal expansion of parathyroid cells, in which the sensitivity of the calcium-sensing receptor has been permanently altered such that PTH is continuously produced and excreted irrespective of serum calcium levels, which defines tertiary hyperparathyroidism.[2,3,6] Accordingly, the majority of patients with tertiary hyperparathyroidism are indeed found to have four-gland disease (hyperplasia), though recent data suggest that the rate of single- or double-gland disease (adenoma) may reach as high as 30%.[7-9] Ultimately, however, the molecular trigger that drives this transition remains to be determined.

While a thorough discussion of the pathogenesis of secondary hyperparathyroidism is beyond the scope of this chapter, it is important to note that the majority of these patients do not progress to tertiary parathyroid disease. Rather, it is more common to see PTH levels decline and electrolyte levels normalize following kidney transplantation, often most steeply in the first 3 months post-transplant and then gradually over the remainder of the first year.[2,7-9]

PREVENTION

Unfortunately, few preventive therapies exist to halt the progression from secondary to tertiary hyperparathyroidism in the ESRD population. However, there are several features that have been shown to be predictive of the development of tertiary hyperparathyroidism in the CKD patient population, which can help to identify these patients earlier in their course. Prompt recognition of these factors, when present, and timely intervention can prevent the sequelae of prolonged hyperparathyroidism in renal transplant recipients.[10,11] These features include:

- Severe hypercalcemia
- Markedly elevated PTH levels (≥300 pg/mL)
- Prolonged pretransplant duration of dialysis
- Immediate post-transplant hypercalcemia (<2 weeks)
- Elevated alkaline phosphatase post-transplant
- Pretransplant use of calcimimetics
- Enlarged parathyroid glands detected on imaging prior to renal transplantation

Unfortunately, many of these features are not clearly defined, which can limit their clinical utility. While severe hypercalcemia is generally agreed to be greater than 13 to 14 mg/dL, no consensus currently exists regarding this cutoff.[12,13] Similarly, an exact duration of time that qualifies as prolonged duration of pretransplant dialysis has yet to be adopted. Finally, pretransplant cervical ultrasonography or other imaging is rarely performed in this patient population and, when obtained, has been associated with a very high false negative rate, reported up to 96% in some series.[14-16] Therefore, until a consensus is reached regarding these criteria, physicians are often left to use their own discretion and clinical judgment to identify these patients, leading to considerable variability in their management.

Importantly, as tertiary hyperparathyroidism most commonly occurs in the setting of ESRD, prevention of CKD is critical. Unfortunately, the incidence of CKD continues to rise as several of its major contributors, namely diabetes and hypertension, become increasingly prevalent. Preventative recommendations for these common conditions are well known, though are beyond the scope of this chapter. Ultimately, without successful prevention of these contributing diseases, the incidence of tertiary hyperparathyroidism is likely to similarly increase in the future.

CLINICAL FINDINGS

Symptoms & Signs

The symptom profile of tertiary hyperparathyroidism (Table 37–1) largely overlaps with that of primary and secondary parathyroid disease. These symptoms can range from mild to severe, though symptoms do not always correlate with the degree of PTH or calcium elevation in most instances. Commonly cited symptoms include generalized weakness and fatigue, bone and joint aches, concentration or memory difficulties, and mood disturbances.[3] In many cases, however, patients can also present without any overt symptoms despite marked hormonal or electrolyte abnormalities.

Table 37–1. Symptoms and signs associated with tertiary hyperparathyroidism.

Symptoms	Signs
Asymptomatic	Osteoporosis (*T* score >2.5 SD below mean), pathologic bone fractures
Weakness and/or fatigue	Nephrocalcinosis
Pruritis	Nephrolithiasis
Increased thirst	Calciphylaxis
Bone and/or joint pains	Vascular calcifications
Concentration and/or memory difficulties, "brain fog"	Peptic ulcer disease
Headache	Pancreatitis
Mood changes, such as depression or irritability	

Table created using data from Chandran M, Wong J. Secondary and tertiary hyperparathyroidism in chronic kidney disease: an endocrine and renal perspective. *Indian J Endocrinol Metab.* 2019;23(4):391-399. [PMID: 31741895] and van der Plas WY, Noltes ME, van Ginhoven TM, Kruijff S. Secondary and tertiary hyperparathyroidism: a narrative review. *Scand J Surg.* 2020;109(4):271-278. [PMID: 31364494]

In addition to the similar symptomatology seen among primary, secondary, and tertiary hyperparathyroidism, there are also several signs commonly seen across these conditions. These include osteoporosis and increased risk of pathologic or atraumatic bone fractures, as well as nephrocalcinosis and nephrolithiasis, both of which are often indications for surgical intervention in these conditions.[17,18] While nephrolithiasis can result from calcium oxalate stone formation following calcification within the collecting system, nephrocalcinosis involves calcification of the renal tubules from calcium deposition occurring within the renal parenchyma itself.[18]

Calciphylaxis is most commonly seen in cases of secondary and tertiary hyperparathyroidism and occurs when high levels of phosphate bind with calcium and form intravascular and soft tissue calcifications, causing painful purpuric cutaneous lesions. If left untreated, these lesions can progress to dry gangrene and ulceration, and reported mortality rates are variable but can reach as high as 90%.[19] For this reason, calciphylaxis is often considered a strong indication for surgical intervention, as further outlined below.[20]

Finally, severe vascular calcifications can be seen in cases of tertiary hyperparathyroidism, thought to be the direct result of prolonged hypercalcemia, and is associated with increased risk of cardiovascular morbidity and mortality. Vascular calcification is believed to occur in two ways. First, atherosclerotic intimal plaques can become calcified, most commonly in the coronary arteries, leading to increased cardiovascular events, such as myocardial infarction. In addition, calcification can occur diffusely within the muscular media layer of major vessels, contributing to vascular stiffness and increased pulse pressure seen in these patients.[21]

Laboratory Findings

Tertiary hyperparathyroidism is a biochemical diagnosis that is made based on the patient's elevated PTH and calcium levels in the appropriate clinical context. Notably, no standardized cutoff values have been established for either PTH or calcium in the diagnosis of tertiary hyperparathyroidism. However, according to the 2017 Kidney Disease: Improving Global Outcomes (KDIGO) guideline, an increased serum PTH level greater than two to nine times the upper limit of normal in the setting of an elevated serum calcium and in the context of CKD or ESRD is consistent with the diagnosis of tertiary hyperparathyroidism.[1] It is important to note that total calcium must always be corrected for serum albumin concentration, as patients with CKD and ESRD are often hypoalbuminemic.

Imaging Studies

Several imaging studies are utilized to better characterize the extent of disease in patients with tertiary hyperparathyroidism, though no imaging study is required to establish the diagnosis. Rather, imaging studies are often obtained to identify all parathyroid glands, including possible ectopic or supernumerary glands, during the preoperative planning process.[22] There is currently no consensus regarding the optimal imaging modality, if any, to obtain preoperatively in this patient population. Some surgeons strongly advocate for the role of preoperative imaging to optimize early identification of ectopic parathyroid glands and, thus, reduce the risk of operative failure in these otherwise frail, medically comorbid patients. Conversely, others feel that imaging results are unlikely to affect their surgical management, as bilateral neck exploration with examination of the usual four glands remains the gold standard. The authors always explore all glands in these patients, though we feel that imaging is useful to potentially speed the operation.

When obtained, the most commonly utilized studies include cervical ultrasonography, technetium (Tc-99m) sestamibi scintigraphy, and four-dimensional computed tomography. F-18 fluorocholine positron emission tomography with computed tomography (PET/CT) scan is a newer imaging modality increasingly utilized in primary hyperparathyroidism with preliminary data in tertiary parathyroid disease, though this modality is not widely available in the United States.[23-25]

A. Cervical Ultrasonography

Cervical ultrasonography represents the most commonly utilized preoperative imaging modality, as it allows for simultaneous assessment for both the parathyroids and the thyroid for any abnormalities that would necessitate concomitant surgical intervention. Ultrasonography is often performed by the operating surgeon in clinic and is the most cost-effective imaging modality available. Furthermore, ultrasonography has been shown to have a sensitivity, specificity, and overall accuracy of 62%, 87%, and 65%, respectively, for identification of hyperplastic parathyroid glands in patients with secondary and tertiary hyperparathyroidism.[26] However, it is important to note that this modality is highly operator dependent and is limited in its ability to identify ectopic parathyroid glands. The authors believe that ultrasound should always be performed in patients with any form of surgically treated hyperparathyroidism to assess for thyroid disease and to possibly localize the affected parathyroid(s).

Figures 37-1A and B demonstrate the appearance of enlarged left inferior and right superior parathyroid glands, respectively, on cervical ultrasonography in a patient with tertiary hyperparathyroidism referred for surgical evaluation. When all four parathyroids are not visualized on ultrasound, particularly the inferior glands, the authors prefer to also obtain a sestamibi scan.

B. Sestamibi Scintigraphy

Technetium (Tc-99m) sestamibi scintigraphy offers additional merits in the identification of ectopic, particularly mediastinal, parathyroid glands not detected on cervical ultrasonography. While this modality has been thoroughly investigated in the context of primary hyperparathyroidism, data are conflicting regarding its utility in the context of tertiary parathyroid disease.[27] A recent study by Chen and colleagues cited a sensitivity, specificity, and overall accuracy of 55%, 80%, and 59%, respectively, in the identification of hyperplastic parathyroids in secondary and tertiary hyperparathyroidism, significantly inferior to the 70% to 80% sensitivity seen in primary parathyroid disease.[28] Another group cited an even lower sensitivity (29%) of this modality in the identification of ectopic parathyroid glands in the ESRD patient population. Due to these limitations, recent studies suggest reserving this modality only in the setting of a nonlocalizing ultrasound given its overall poor sensitivity and specificity and comparatively higher cost and exposure to ionizing radiation.[28]

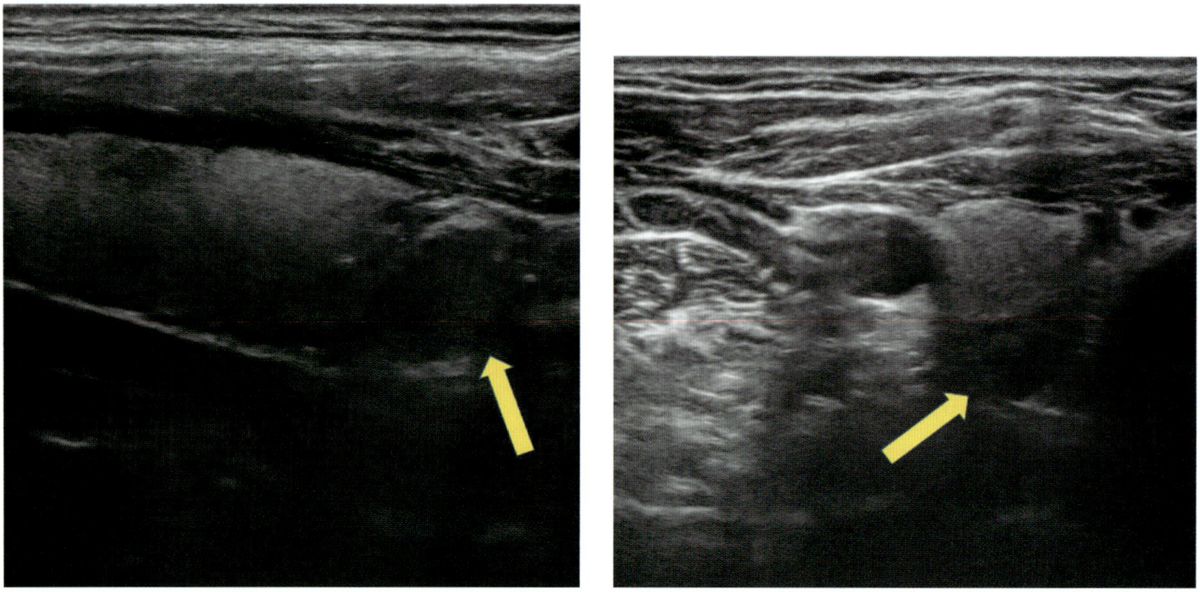

A B

Figure 37–1. Enlarged left inferior **(A)** and right superior **(B)** parathyroid glands on cervical ultrasonography in a patient with tertiary hyperparathyroidism. This patient previously underwent deceased donor kidney transplantation, after which he was found to have persistently elevated calcium (11.1 mg/dL) and PTH (924 pg/mL) levels, consistent with the diagnosis of tertiary hyperparathyroidism. He was initially medically managed with calcitriol and cinacalcet with subsequent improvement in his calcium (8.8 mg/dL) and PTH (399 pg/mL) levels, though he was recently found to have severe osteopenia on DEXA scan, prompting his referral to an endocrine surgeon.

C. Computed Tomography

Four-dimensional computed tomography (4D-CT), also referred to as a parathyroid protocol or multiphase CT, was first described for parathyroid gland localization by Rodgers and colleagues in 2006.[29] This modality combines the standard three-dimensional anatomic CT scan with a fourth dimension of time, which allows for the visualization of differences in perfusion characteristics of the neck soft tissues. Hyperfunctioning parathyroid glands are characterized by increased perfusion, which appears as rapid contrast uptake and washout, and allows them to be readily distinguished from normal parathyroids and other surrounding soft tissues. This functional information, combined with the highly detailed anatomic images of CT, can be easily interpreted by the operating surgeon and may allow for improved operative planning. These scans are protocolized to routinely include the upper mediastinum.

While this imaging modality has not yet been specifically evaluated in cases of secondary or tertiary hyperparathyroidism, numerous studies have demonstrated its improved sensitivity and specificity in primary hyperparathyroidism. In their early study, Rodgers and colleagues found that 4D-CT offered a higher sensitivity in lateralizing and localizing diseased glands to the correct quadrant of the neck (88% and 70%, respectively) compared to ultrasonography (57% and 29%) and sestamibi scintigraphy (65% and 33%).[29] Recent studies have since confirmed the high sensitivity of 4D-CT in identifying hyperfunctioning parathyroid glands, ranging between 73% and 98% for accurate lateralization and 60% and 88% for localization to the correct quadrant of the neck.[30] Even more impressively, these studies have found that the sensitivity of 4D-CT does not decrease in reoperative settings, as is often the case with ultrasonography and sestamibi scintigraphy.[31] Furthermore, 4D-CT has been found to outperform ultrasonography and sestamibi scans in cases of multiglandular disease and double adenomas, both of which are commonly seen in cases of tertiary hyperparathyroidism.[31,32] These qualities make 4D-CT especially useful for preoperative planning in the reoperative setting or when other imaging studies are nonlocalizing. However, the clear advantages of this imaging technique must be weighed against its risks, most notably the increased ionizing radiation exposure and requirement for the use of potentially nephrotoxic contrast.

D. Positron Emission Tomography

F-18 fluorocholine PET/CT has been shown to offer the highest sensitivity, specificity, and overall accuracy for the identification of hyperplastic parathyroids in patients with secondary and tertiary hyperparathyroidism (86%, 93%, and 87%, respectively) compared to ultrasonography and sestamibi scintigraphy.[28] Furthermore, fluorocholine PET/CT has been shown to identify smaller parathyroid glands with improved sensitivity compared to sestamibi scintigraphy. Chen and colleagues found the sensitivity of fluorocholine PET/CT to be >90% for parathyroid glands ≥175 mg and 95% for those ≥200 mg, compared to a sensitivity of 90% for parathyroids ≥300 mg for sestamibi scans.[28] However, this same study also found that the negative predictive value of fluorocholine PET/CT was similarly poor (52%) when compared to ultrasound (27%) and sestamibi (23%), thus limiting its ability to decrease the rate of bilateral neck exploration.[28] Ultimately, the role of PET/CT in the management of tertiary hyperparathyroidism has yet to be clearly defined, though recent studies suggest it may offer a useful complement to cervical ultrasonography, particularly in the reoperative setting. It should be noted that this modality is costly, not always available, and suffers from the same limitations of less costly imaging studies, specifically regarding its poorer sensitivity in multiglandular disease.

DIFFERENTIAL DIAGNOSIS

There are several defining features that allow tertiary hyperparathyroidism to be distinguished from cases of primary and secondary parathyroid disease (Table 37–2). First, while both primary and tertiary hyperparathyroidism are characterized by the inappropriate overproduction and secretion of PTH, tertiary hyperparathyroidism can be easily distinguished, as it occurs in the setting of another chronic condition, such as ESRD or chronic malabsorption. Conversely, there is no such clinical history in the case of primary hyperparathyroidism. Second, while both secondary and tertiary hyperparathyroidism occur in the context of chronic stimulation of PTH secretion as the result of an underlying disorder, the serum calcium level allows one to easily distinguish these two conditions. In particular, the serum calcium concentration is normal or low in cases of secondary hyperparathyroidism, whereas the transition to hypercalcemia is a defining feature of tertiary parathyroid disease. It is important to note that this transition can occur before or after renal transplantation, as pretransplant tertiary hyperparathyroidism is becoming an increasingly recognized disease among ESRD patients.

Table 37–2. Biochemical distinction of primary, secondary, and tertiary hyperparathyroidism.

Hyperparathyroidism	Calcium	PTH
Primary	Normal to high	High
Secondary	Low to normal	High
Tertiary	High	High

Table created using data from Jamal SA, Miller PD. Secondary and tertiary hyperparathyroidism. *J Clin Densitom*. 2013;16(1):64-68. [PMID: 23267748] and Kidney Disease: Improving Global Outcomes (KDIGO) CKD-MBD Update Work Group. KDIGO 2017 Clinical Practice Guideline Update for the Diagnosis, Evaluation, Prevention, and Treatment of Chronic Kidney Disease-Mineral and Bone Disorder (CKD-MBD). *Kidney Int Suppl*. 2017;7:1-59. [PMID: 30675420]

COMPLICATIONS

Recent data suggest that as many as 40% to 64% of patients with tertiary hyperparathyroidism receive no treatment despite the documented long-term complications associated with this condition, many of which can be prevented with treatment.[33,34] While there is significant overlap between the adverse effects of primary, secondary, and tertiary hyperparathyroidism, there are unique complications that arise in this subset of patients following renal transplantation.

Renal Allograft Function

Untreated tertiary hyperparathyroidism in renal transplant recipients has been repeatedly found to be associated with delayed graft function, renal allograft calcifications and dysfunction, and subsequent increased risk of renal allograft loss.[4] In a recent study by Prakobsuk and colleagues, hyperparathyroidism (PTH >90 pg/mL) and increased fractional excretion of phosphate (>20%) were predictive of allograft loss in long-term kidney transplant recipients.[35] While the mechanism underlying graft loss in this disease is not fully understood, it is believed to be associated with increased calcium oxalate levels and nephrocalcinosis in the renal allograft, resulting in papillary or urinary tract damages.[34]

Recently, several studies have found that persistent hyperparathyroidism and hypercalcemia following renal transplantation are associated with worse graft outcomes, whereas patients who underwent parathyroidectomy and, thus, correction of these hormonal and electrolyte derangements, saw improved graft function and long-term outcomes.[4,36-41] In a study by Finnerty and colleagues, the authors found that patients treated with parathyroidectomy experienced lower rates of renal allograft failure when compared to those who received medical management alone with cinacalcet.[42] It is important to note, however, that these data are based on relatively small, retrospective studies, so further work is needed to characterize the effect of tertiary hyperparathyroidism and its medical and surgical treatment more completely on renal allograft function.

Skeletal Manifestations

A. Osteoporosis & Fragility Fractures

Loss of bone mineral density in hyperparathyroidism is thought to occur due to the binding of PTH to its receptor on osteoblasts, which indirectly stimulates osteoclasts and leads to increased bone turnover. As a result, osteopenia (*T* score 1-2.5 SD below mean) and, eventually, osteoporosis (*T* score >2.5 SD below mean) develop in many patients and can lead to an increased risk of fragility fractures. Fragility fractures have been shown to be two to four times more frequent in patients with secondary and tertiary hyperparathyroidism and are associated with increased risk of mortality in this patient population.[42] Some studies have shown an association between PTH levels and fracture risk, particularly when PTH levels are very high (>900 pg/mL). Importantly, however, there is robust evidence that successful treatment can not only halt, but also reverse, this loss of bone mineral density.

B. Osteitis Fibrosa Cystica

Osteitis fibrosa cystica, also referred to as brown tumors, so called due to their abundance of hemosiderin deposition and hypervascularity, is an infrequent complication of hyperparathyroidism. While often previously the presenting sign of hyperparathyroidism, this condition is now much rarer, as hyperparathyroidism is frequently diagnosed earlier and managed more successfully. This complication is most commonly seen in cases of primary hyperparathyroidism (4.5%), though it has also been reported in secondary (1.5%-1.7%) and tertiary parathyroid disease (very rare with unknown prevalence).[42] Treatment is centered on management of the underlying disorder, often with parathyroidectomy, though resection of the bony lesion is sometimes required, particularly if the tumor is symptomatic or impairing essential functions, such as eating, speaking, or breathing.[42]

C. Uremic Leontiasis Ossea

Uremic leontiasis ossea is another rare complication that can occur in cases of secondary and tertiary hyperparathyroidism. This disorder resembles fibrous dysplasia and Paget disease on histopathology but can be distinguished based on the patient's clinical history and laboratory data. This skeletal complication preferentially affects the cranial and facial bones, presenting as diffuse bony expansion, which can ultimately lead to vision loss, exophthalmos, dysphagia, speech impairment, or airway obstruction, depending on the site(s) of involvement. Parathyroidectomy is required to prevent further progression and may eventually lead to improvement of the bony deformities.[42]

Cardiovascular Complications

It is well established that prolonged hyperparathyroidism is associated with several cardiovascular complications, including hypertension, heart failure, arrhythmias, and severe vascular calcifications.[43] However, this risk is not unique to tertiary hyperparathyroidism and has been more thoroughly examined in the context of primary and secondary parathyroid disease. Hyperparathyroidism is believed to contribute to the development of hypertension through alterations in the vasodilatory properties of the endothelium and through still incompletely understood interactions with the renin-angiotensin-aldosterone system. Further, the binding of excess PTH to its receptor on cardiac myocytes leads to increased intracellular calcium and, over time, can lead to the development of left ventricular hypertrophy and, eventually, heart failure. In addition, chronic hypercalcemia can have further deleterious effects, including calcium deposition within blood vessels, cardiac myocytes, and cardiac valves, further perpetuating the risk of myocardial infarction, stroke, and heart failure. Finally, hypercalcemia has also been associated with prolonged cardiac intervals on electrocardiography (particularly PR and QRS), leading to arrhythmias in this population. Together, these cardiovascular changes contribute to the increased cardiac morbidity and mortality seen in patients with hyperparathyroidism, many of which can be halted or reversed with correction of the underlying disorder.[43]

A. Hypercalcemic Crisis

Hypercalcemic crisis is a life-threatening emergency characterized by marked elevation in serum calcium and acute onset of symptoms of hypercalcemia. This condition most commonly occurs in the setting of malignancy and primary hyperparathyroidism, though there have been case reports of hypercalcemic crisis in the setting of tertiary hyperparathyroidism. Presenting symptoms can include constitutional, neurologic, gastrointestinal, and renal manifestations. Treatment is centered on correcting dehydration, lowering serum calcium, and addressing the underlying condition, usually with parathyroidectomy.[44]

TREATMENT

While the 2017 KDIGO and 2022 American Association of Endocrine Surgeons (AAES) guidelines offer the only available recommendations regarding the management of tertiary hyperparathyroidism in the United States, no consensus or standardized guidelines exist for this condition worldwide.[1,2] Given the overall rarity of this disorder, there are comparatively few dedicated studies on this topic, and those that do exist are relatively small and largely retrospective in nature. Based on the most recent 2017 KDIGO and 2022 AAES guidelines, treatment of this condition usually begins by optimizing medical management of hormonal and electrolyte derangements, followed by surgical intervention in severe or refractory cases.[1,2] However, much debate exists regarding the most appropriate therapy for this condition, particularly related to the role and timing of surgical intervention.

Medical Therapies

Current optimal medical management of tertiary hyperparathyroidism includes a multipronged approach with vitamin D supplementation, phosphate-binding agents, and calcimimetics.[1,2]

A. Vitamin D Supplementation

Vitamin D supplementation is often initiated in CKD patients before the development of even secondary hyperparathyroidism, as many of these patients are vitamin D deficient long before initiating dialysis. In this population, vitamin D replacement works to correct hypocalcemia, decrease serum PTH levels, decrease bone turnover, prevent fractures, and reduce proteinuria. Vitamin D is initially replenished with cholecalciferol or ergocalciferol. A monthly dose of 50,000 to 100,000 IU, often administered in daily or weekly increments, is frequently recommended to achieve these benefits.[1-3] It is important to note, however, that vitamin D replacement is discontinued in cases of hyperphosphatemia or hypercalcemia, as its use can further exacerbate these conditions.

In cases of progressive and severe hyperparathyroidism (PTH >2-3 times the upper limit of normal), such as in cases of secondary and tertiary hyperparathyroidism, synthetic vitamin D receptor activators are introduced.[1-3] While calcitriol is one of the most commonly used vitamin D derivatives, other agents including alfacalcidol, doxercalciferol, and paricalcitol are also used. These agents have been shown to reduce and stabilize PTH levels and improve bone histology, though there is an overall paucity of high-quality data regarding their impact on cardiovascular events, quality of life, and overall mortality in the ESRD population. Dosing for these medications begins at 0.25 μg three times weekly and can be increased to up to 1 μg daily to maintain a PTH level <150 pg/mL according to the 2017 KDIGO guideline.[1]

B. Phosphate Binders

Hyperphosphatemia is one of the earliest clinical manifestations of renal excretion failure and the development of secondary hyperparathyroidism, and it has been associated with increased mortality in this population. Thus, the 2017 KDIGO guideline recommends maintaining serum phosphate within the normal range.[1] Given the difficulty associated with strict adherence to a low-phosphorus diet, phosphate binders are frequently initiated at the earliest indication of hyperphosphatemia in most ESRD patients. Phosphate binders can be broadly categorized into calcium-based and calcium-free formulations. While an exhaustive discussion of phosphate binders is beyond the scope of this chapter, the use of calcium-based phosphate binders can exacerbate the hypercalcemia seen in tertiary hyperparathyroidism and, thus, should be considered when managing these patients.[1-3]

C. Calcimimetics

As vitamin D supplementation and phosphate binders alone are seldom able to reestablish normal calcium-phosphate homeostasis amidst failing renal function, the 2017 KDIGO guideline recommends the addition of calcimimetics as first-line therapy in the management of secondary and tertiary hyperparathyroidism.[1] Calcimimetics are allosteric modulators of the calcium-sensing receptor and mimic the binding of calcium to this receptor.[45] In doing so, these compounds also cause a conformational change of the calcium-sensing receptor, further increasing the sensitivity of this receptor to the circulating serum calcium. Through this dual mechanism, calcimimetics reduce PTH production and excretion by the parathyroid glands and, consequently, work to reestablish hormonal and electrolyte homeostasis. Calcimimetics are currently available in an oral formulation (cinacalcet) and an intravenous formulation (etelcalcetide).

Cinacalcet was introduced in the United States in 2004, at which time it was approved for the treatment of secondary hyperparathyroidism and hypercalcemia of malignancy. Notably, it is not approved in the management of tertiary hyperparathyroidism and is used off-label in this population.[2] In a large meta-analysis, cinacalcet was shown to significantly reduce PTH concentrations, calcium levels, and phosphate levels in patients with secondary hyperparathyroidism.[46] However, data have been conflicting regarding the effect of cinacalcet on bone resorption and formation markers, bone mineral density, and fracture risk.[47] Further, several recent studies, including the Evaluation of Cinacalcet Hydrochloride Therapy to Lower Cardiovascular Events (EVOLVE) trial, have failed to demonstrate a significant reduction in cardiovascular and all-cause mortality with the use of calcimimetics.[48] Finally, compliance with cinacalcet remains problematic due to bothersome side effects reported in almost half of patients (most frequently gastrointestinal distress), prohibitive cost, and polypharmacy.[46,48,49]

To address some of these issues associated with cinacalcet and increase drug compliance, etelcalcetide was approved in 2016.[50] This formulation is administered three times weekly as a bolus injection, making it convenient for the dialysis patient. However, there was no difference in its observed side effect profile, and the associated costs are even greater.[50] For these reasons, etelcalcetide remains second-line, reserved for those who are unresponsive or intolerant of cinacalcet. Again, this medication is not approved for the treatment of tertiary hyperparathyroidism and is rarely used in this population.

Importantly, with the development of calcimimetics, there has been a large shift in the approach to the treatment of tertiary hyperparathyroidism. While this was previously considered to be a largely surgical disease, first-line treatment has primarily become medical, and only a small minority (6%-7%) of patients are eventually referred for surgical evaluation in the modern era.[9,24,25] In fact, a retrospective study by van der Plas and colleagues found that, following the introduction of cinacalcet, there has been an average 22-month delay in surgical referral of patients with tertiary hyperparathyroidism despite no significant differences in their baseline characteristics or severity of PTH elevation.[9] Given the frequent comorbidities and frailty of this patient population, it is true that surgery might not be appropriate or feasible for all patients with tertiary hyperparathyroidism. However, several recent studies have questioned the appropriateness of this paradigm shift, especially as it relates to treatment efficacy, outcomes, and cost.

Surgical Intervention

Despite the promise of medical therapies in the management of tertiary hyperparathyroidism, parathyroidectomy remains the only curative treatment for this disease.[2,3,51,52] General surgical approaches include focused, subtotal, or total parathyroidectomy, the last of which can be performed with or without parathyroid autotransplantation. While several studies have attempted to identify the optimal surgical approach in tertiary hyperparathyroidism, results are varied, so this decision ultimately remains at the discretion of the operating surgeon on a case-by-case basis.[2]

A. Focused Parathyroidectomy

Focused, or limited, parathyroidectomy is the approach whereby fewer than four parathyroid glands are intentionally identified, and the surgeon limits their dissection, often removing only one gland. While this technique is commonly employed in cases of primary hyperparathyroidism, particularly when a single adenoma is identified on preoperative imaging, this approach is widely considered insufficient in cases of tertiary hyperparathyroidism. While some authors suggest that the rate of single or double adenomas in tertiary parathyroid disease might reach as high as 30% of cases, this approach has been associated with exceedingly high rates (91%) of persistent or recurrent disease.[1-3,51] The authors do not practice this approach in tertiary hyperparathyroidism, as it is our belief that all glands are affected in this disease, though to a variable degree, and, therefore, warrant intraoperative direct evaluation.

B. Subtotal Parathyroidectomy

Subtotal, or near-total, parathyroidectomy is defined as the reduction of parathyroid tissue mass, often removing three glands completely and a part of the fourth gland, leaving a sufficient size remnant *in situ*. While some groups debate the ideal amount of parathyroid tissue that ought to be left in these cases, it is generally recommended leaving roughly 50 to 100 mg of the most normal-appearing gland.[2] The surgeon must balance the removal of too much versus too little glandular tissue while also ensuring adequate remnant vascularization. The cure rate following subtotal parathyroidectomy has been estimated to be as high as 98.7%, with low rates of recurrent or persistent disease (7.6% and 1.3%, respectively).[2,3,51]

Certain groups strongly prefer subtotal parathyroidectomy to alternative techniques given that the underlying metabolic disorder that incited the patient's hyperparathyroidism has been corrected. Furthermore, studies have demonstrated a lower risk of postoperative hypocalcemia and persistent hypoparathyroidism following subtotal compared to total resection.[51,53] In addition, a recent meta-analysis by Chen and colleagues found no significant difference in rates of persistent or recurrent disease, symptomatic improvement, need for reoperation, readmission, complications, or 30-day mortality in subtotal compared to total parathyroidectomy with autotransplantation.[54] Recent studies have also shown no significant differences in preoperative, intraoperative, or postoperative PTH levels in patients who underwent either of these approaches.[53] Other studies, however, have cited a risk of persistent or recurrent disease following subtotal parathyroidectomy that is significantly greater than those who underwent total parathyroidectomy.[2,3,51]

C. Total Parathyroidectomy With or Without Autotransplantation

Total parathyroidectomy consists of removal of all parathyroid tissue and can be performed with or without parathyroid autotransplantation. In a systematic review by Dulfer and colleagues, the cure rate of total parathyroidectomy with or without autotransplantation was as high as 100%, and recurrent or persistent disease was rare (4% and 0%, respectively).[33] Similarly, in a case series by Casarim and colleagues, cure rate following parathyroidectomy with autotransplantation was high (94.3%) and relapse infrequent (5.7%).[53]

When used, total parathyroidectomy without autotransplantation is often performed in the management of secondary hyperparathyroidism, though its use in cases of tertiary parathyroid disease remains more controversial and ill-defined. Unsurprisingly, this approach is associated with the lowest rates of persistent or recurrent disease and need for reoperation (0%-4%).[51] While it seems logical that this approach would be associated with the highest rates of transient and permanent postoperative hypocalcemia and hypoparathyroidism, this assumption has not been borne out in the current literature. Importantly, however, all available studies comparing total parathyroidectomy with and without autotransplantation in cases of tertiary hyperparathyroidism also include patients with the more prevalent secondary form of parathyroid disease. To date, these studies suggest comparable rates of transient postoperative hypocalcemia (15%-30%) and permanent hypoparathyroidism requiring prolonged calcium and vitamin D supplementation (up to 7%).[53,54] Ultimately, however, total parathyroidectomy without autotransplantation remains controversial and infrequently utilized in cases of tertiary hyperparathyroidism, and total parathyroidectomy with autotransplantation is largely preferred in most centers.

In cases of tertiary hyperparathyroidism, parathyroid autotransplantation is usually performed in the patient's sternocleidomastoid or in the brachioradialis muscle of the forearm, the latter offering easier access to the reimplanted parathyroid tissue in cases of exuberant growth of the autotransplant.

D. Parathyroid Cryopreservation

While parathyroid autotransplantation is most often performed at the time of parathyroidectomy, certain groups have sought to enable delayed heterotopic parathyroid autotransplantation in cases where persistent hypoparathyroidism develops with cryopreservation. However, this technique is almost never used in clinical practice, as it is quite time-consuming and associated with prohibitive costs. In addition, the banked tissue may not be functional after prolonged (>1 year) storage.[55]

E. Transcervical Thymectomy

Recent studies suggest that up to 32% of patients with secondary or tertiary hyperparathyroidism have ectopic parathyroid glands, most frequently located within the thymus. Even more, autopsy studies suggest a prevalence of 13% to 30% of supernumerary parathyroid glands, also often found within the thymus.[51,54] Some researchers suggest that the chronic parathyroid stimulation seen in secondary and tertiary hyperparathyroidism can cause hyperplasia of small, supernumerary parathyroid tissues, contributing to the high rates of recurrence in these patients. Nonetheless, patients who received bilateral prophylactic thymectomy at the time of parathyroidectomy had significantly higher cure rates, so some authors now recommend bilateral prophylactic transcervical thymectomy in all patients undergoing parathyroidectomy for tertiary hyperparathyroidism, regardless of surgical approach.

F. Recurrent Laryngeal Nerve Monitoring

The benefit of recurrent laryngeal nerve monitoring during parathyroidectomy for tertiary hyperparathyroidism is unclear. Studies have largely failed to show a protective benefit with nerve monitoring during thyroid and parathyroid procedures for other reasons, though no studies have examined its utility in cases of tertiary hyperparathyroidism specifically. Therefore, the use of this surgical adjunct is left to the discretion of the operating surgeon. The authors do not use nerve monitoring for parathyroidectomy unless it is in the reoperative setting.

G. Intraoperative PTH Monitoring

While the utility of intraoperative PTH monitoring (IPM) is well established in cases of primary hyperparathyroidism, its role in secondary and tertiary parathyroid disease remains unclear, and the degree to which PTH should decrease intraoperatively is widely contested. Due to the often drastically elevated PTH levels seen in tertiary hyperparathyroidism preoperatively, most authors agree that the PTH level should not necessarily be expected to return to normal, as is often the case with primary hyperparathyroidism. Studies also generally agree that PTH levels should drop by more than 50% of the baseline value intraoperatively to be predictive of cure, similar to the case of primary parathyroid disease. However, several authors advocate for even higher thresholds in tertiary hyperparathyroidism. One recent study by Casarim and colleagues found that an intraoperative drop in PTH level of ≥71.2% at 20 minutes following total parathyroidectomy had a sensitivity of 100%, specificity of 93.9%, and positive predictive value of 100% for probability of cure.[53] These results are similar to a previous study, which found that a PTH drop of ≥80% predicted a 100% cure rate, whereas a drop <70% was associated with surgical failure in 66.6% of cases.[24]

Therefore, given the ongoing debate regarding the most appropriate threshold to predict success in this patient population, IPM is often not routinely utilized in cases of tertiary hyperparathyroidism. However, surgeons who intend to perform focused parathyroidectomy based on imaging studies should likely utilize IPM, as these surgeons are not exploring all of the parathyroids in these cases, and imaging studies often fail to detect multiple gland disease. The authors routinely utilize IPM in cases of tertiary hyperparathyroidism and aim to achieve a PTH decrease of more than 50% of the baseline and into or close to the normal range within 10 to 15 minutes following reduction of parathyroid tissue in patients with normal renal function.

H. Postoperative Care and Complications

The postoperative course and complications following parathyroidectomy for secondary and tertiary hyperparathyroidism appear to be very similar based on current data, though many of the available studies do not distinguish these variants of uremic hyperparathyroidism in their study populations. Notably, some reports indicate that the overall complication rate following parathyroidectomy for secondary or tertiary hyperparathyroidism is slightly higher than for primary parathyroid disease, though the overall complication rate is still low, approximated at 7.9% overall.[24,51]

Recent data suggest that parathyroidectomy for tertiary hyperparathyroidism is associated with slightly higher rates of severe hypocalcemia (15%-23%), hungry bone syndrome (8%-87%), and neck hematoma requiring evacuation (1.5%).[2,3] These patients also experience longer initial postoperative hospitalizations and are more likely to return to the emergency room following discharge (7.5%) and be readmitted (5.1%-23.8%) than those with primary hyperparathyroidism. However, the rates of serious postoperative complications, including recurrent laryngeal nerve injury, permanent hypocalcemia or hypoparathyroidism, pneumonia, prolonged ventilation, cardiovascular events, and mortality are no different than in cases of primary parathyroid disease.[24,51,54]

1. Hungry bone syndrome—Hungry bone syndrome is characterized by the rapid occurrence of severe and prolonged hypocalcemia lasting greater than 4 days following parathyroidectomy and is thought to occur due to the rapid cessation of bone resorption.[42] In this new environment of unchecked bone formation, there is an increased skeletal uptake of calcium and a resulting drop in serum calcium. The prevalence of this complication is estimated to be as high as 13% in secondary and tertiary hyperparathyroidism and is associated with older age, elevated alkaline phosphatase, hypomagnesemia, hypoalbuminemia, and the presence of other skeletal complications at the time of surgery.[42] Treatment is centered on calcium replacement, often requiring doses of 6 to 12 g/day, and can require close monitoring.[42] Some studies suggest that preoperative correction of vitamin D deficiencies or use of bisphosphonates may help to prevent this condition, though this approach is not standardized.

Cost Effectiveness

A recent study estimates the cost associated with cinacalcet to exceed $100,000 per quality-adjusted life year (QALY), and the cost associated with the intravenous etelcalcetide to be even greater.[49,50] This cost is further confounded by the off-label use of calcimimetics in the management of tertiary hyperparathyroidism. Accordingly, several studies have found that parathyroidectomy and its associated postoperative care becomes more cost-effective after only 14 months of treatment with cinacalcet is exceeded, though others cite an even shorter duration of 7 months.[40] Even further, recent data from a large microsimulation study suggests that parathyroidectomy performed prior to kidney transplantation is the most cost-effective strategy of all.[56]

Other Treatment Modalities

While the previously outlined medical and surgical approaches represent the cornerstone of tertiary hyperparathyroidism management, several other techniques have been trialed with variable success and are briefly included here for completeness.

Percutaneous fine-needle ethanol injection was first reported in 1985 and was recommended for the selective destruction of enlarged parathyroid glands with nodular hyperplasia in the revised 2008 Japanese Society of Parathyroid Intervention guideline.[57] Similarly, percutaneous injection of calcitriol was also attempted though with inconsistent results. More recently, Hu and colleagues demonstrated that microwave ablation might offer a safe and effective alternative for patients with tertiary hyperparathyroidism who are ineligible for parathyroidectomy.[58] Ultimately, however, none of these approaches are commonly employed or recommended at this time.

PROGNOSIS

Current medical and surgical therapies for tertiary hyperparathyroidism are highly effective overall, with normocalcemia being achieved in the majority of patients.[2,3,34,51] A retrospective study by Dulfer and colleagues identified an 80.8% rate of normocalcemia with cinacalcet treatment in uremic hyperparathyroidism, though this rate varies widely in the available literature from 28% to 100%.[34] It is important to note that many authors define cure of tertiary hyperparathyroidism differently, likely contributing to this wide range.

In the first of its kind, a recent randomized control trial by Cruzado and colleagues compared the efficacy of cinacalcet and parathyroidectomy in the management of tertiary hyperparathyroidism.[59] In this study, the authors defined cure as normocalcemia at 12 months following initiation of therapy or surgery. Cure rates were high, though statistically greater in the surgery group, where cure was achieved in 100% of patients versus 67% in the cinacalcet group. Furthermore, reduction of PTH level during this same timeframe was also significantly greater in the parathyroidectomy group (67%) compared to no significant reduction in the cinacalcet group. Almost all patients in both groups achieved normophosphatemia, and there were no significant differences between fracture risk, renal allograft function, or mortality.[59] It is important to note that this study is limited by its relatively small sample size ($n = 30$). Other retrospective studies have corroborated these results, citing cure rates ranging from 85% to 100% following parathyroidectomy. In a 5-year follow-up to Cruzado's study, Moreno and colleagues found that both medical and surgical therapies are effective in maintaining normocalcemia at long-term follow-up.[60] However, the reduction in PTH level remained statistically greater in the parathyroidectomy group, and surgical intervention was found to be more cost effective than treatment with cinacalcet.

Other sequelae of tertiary hyperparathyroidism can also be positively impacted with successful treatment. A recent study by See and colleagues found a significant improvement in hyperparathyroidism-associated symptoms following parathyroidectomy based on patients' self-report.[61] These symptoms included bone pains, pruritis, abdominal pain, weakness, fatigue, mood derangements, and memory and cognitive complaints, among others.[61] Similarly, markers of bone turnover, rates of osteoporosis, and fragility fractures have been shown to significantly improve with successful treatment, though several studies have found this trend to be more significant following parathyroidectomy.[62] While the impact of parathyroidectomy timing on renal allograft function remains widely contested, there is a consensus that treatment of tertiary hyperparathyroidism is essential to prevent renal allograft dysfunction and, eventually, loss.[63]

A single retrospective study demonstrated decreased GFR with prolonged cinacalcet treatment, though this finding has not been repeated.[62]

At the writing of this chapter, no studies exist that specifically examine the impact of successful medical or surgical treatment of tertiary hyperparathyroidism on cardiovascular or all-cause morbidity and mortality. However, several studies have identified a positive association between successful management of secondary hyperparathyroidism and these outcomes in dialysis patients.[63-66] In particular, the current literature supports a significantly reduced risk of cardiovascular and all-cause hospitalizations and mortality following successful parathyroidectomy in patients with secondary parathyroid disease. Komaba and colleagues observed a 34% lower risk for all-cause mortality and 41% lower risk for cardiovascular mortality in patients with uncontrolled secondary hyperparathyroidism.[65] While these results appear promising, other studies have failed to demonstrate a similar survival benefit in the ESRD population. Some authors postulate that this survival benefit might be artificially inflated, as patients undergoing parathyroidectomy are often deemed healthier and better able to tolerate an operation.

In summary, the successful treatment of tertiary hyperparathyroidism appears to offer a significant benefit to patients in several ways, including symptomatic improvement and reversal of skeletal and renal complications. However, the impact on cardiovascular and all-cause mortality has yet to be borne out in this population and should be the area of future research.

WHEN TO REFER

Many transplant nephrologists traditionally wait at least 1 year following renal transplantation to monitor for normalization of serum calcium and PTH levels before initiating treatment for tertiary hyperparathyroidism, as these hormonal and electrolyte derangements frequently improve post-transplant. Indeed, studies have demonstrated that calcium and PTH levels significantly and rapidly improve in the first 3 months following transplant and then continue to gradually improve further over this first year.[5,9,24] However, recent studies have suggested that earlier surgical referral could be associated with improved renal allograft function, with some authors suggesting even pretransplant referral for parathyroidectomy.[40,67]

While there is significant overlap between the presentation, pathogenesis, and manifestations of primary and tertiary hyperparathyroidism, the approach to management, especially timing of surgical referral, vary widely between these two diseases.[68] Furthermore, in stark opposition to primary parathyroid disease, the role of PTH level as an indicator for surgery in tertiary hyperparathyroidism is still under debate.[67] In fact, there is no consensus between nephrologists and surgeons regarding the absolute indications for parathyroidectomy in tertiary hyperparathyroidism, though the following are common relative indications for surgical referral:[5,9,24,69]

- Symptomatic disease (severe pruritis, bone pain, etc.)
- Persistent PTH levels >9 times the upper limit of normal despite maximum medical therapy
- Severe or persistent hypercalcemia (>3-12 months post-transplant)
- Nephrocalcinosis or nephrolithiasis
- Osteoporosis or pathologic bone fracture
- Significantly enlarged parathyroid glands on imaging (>500 mg)
- Intolerance or noncompliance with medical therapy
- Patient preference

The 2017 KDIGO guideline recommends that ESRD patients with severe uremic hyperparathyroidism, including both secondary and tertiary forms, who fail medical therapy be referred for surgical evaluation.[1] However, this guideline does not clearly define at what point a patient has failed medical therapy, ultimately leaving the timing of referral to the discretion of the patient's nephrologist in most cases. Recently, the European Society of Endocrine Surgeons (ESES) has defined medical failure in cases of secondary hyperparathyroidism as persistent PTH >85 pmol/L, hypercalcemia, and hyperphosphatemia, though this definition has yet to be widely adopted or applied to cases of tertiary parathyroid disease.

Historically, there has been much debate surrounding the optimal timing of parathyroidectomy for tertiary hyperparathyroidism given concerns regarding its potential impact on renal allograft function. Many have advocated to postpone parathyroidectomy until at least 1 year following renal transplantation, citing that operative intervention within the first year of transplant might jeopardize graft function.[38] Indeed, a recent prospective cohort study by Littbarski and colleagues found that parathyroidectomy within the first year of transplantation is an independent risk factor for permanently impaired allograft function as measured by glomerular filtration rate (GFR), though this effect was only transient if parathyroidectomy was delayed until after the first post-transplant year.[38] However, these findings have not been reproduced in several other recent retrospective studies, in which no long-term decline in graft function or other adverse outcomes were observed regardless of the timing of parathyroidectomy.[67,69-71]

In a recent study by Dream and colleagues, the authors found that most patients with tertiary hyperparathyroidism wait, on average, at least 1 year prior to receiving endocrine surgery referral.[70] However, in this study, earlier referral (<1 year) was associated with improved long-term allograft function. Several other studies have similarly found that parathyroidectomy within the first-year post-transplant, while sometimes associated with a transient decline in graft function, has not been associated with long-term adverse outcomes.[67,69-71] Even more, several studies have found that elevated PTH levels before kidney transplant significantly increase the likelihood of graft failure and, thus, strongly advocate for parathyroidectomy pretransplant in many cases. These studies have similarly demonstrated that parathyroidectomy before kidney transplantation was also associated with the greatest overall life expectancy, least yearly and lifetime risk of graft failure, and overall greater quality of life. However, this practice has not been widely adopted in most centers.

Ultimately, treatment of tertiary hyperparathyroidism is essential, as persistently elevated calcium and PTH levels following renal transplantation are associated with increased morbidity and mortality.[2] While parathyroidectomy has been associated with improved outcomes, surgical intervention is not without risk, and the literature is currently divided regarding the optimal timing of referral for these patients.

REFERENCES

1. Kidney Disease: Improving Global Outcomes (KDIGO) CKD-MBD Update Work Group. KDIGO 2017 Clinical Practice Guideline Update for the Diagnosis, Evaluation, Prevention, and Treatment of Chronic Kidney Disease-Mineral and Bone Disorder (CKD-MBD). *Kidney Int Suppl.* 2017;7:1-59.
2. Dream S, Kuo LE, Kuo JH, et al. The American Association of Endocrine Surgeons Guidelines for the Definitive Surgical Management of Secondary and Tertiary Renal Hyperparathyroidism. *Ann Surg.* 2022 Sep 1;276(3):e141-e176.
3. Chandran M, Wong J. Secondary and tertiary hyperparathyroidism in chronic kidney disease: an endocrine and renal perspective. *Indian J Endocrinol Metab.* 2019;23(4):391-399.
4. Lou I, Schneider DF, Leverson G, Foley D, Sippel R, Chen H. Parathyroidectomy is underused in patients with tertiary hyperparathyroidism after renal transplantation. *Surgery.* 2016; 159(1):172-179.
5. Tang JA, Friedman J, Hwang MS, Salapatas AM, Bonzelaar LB, Friedman M. Parathyroidectomy for tertiary hyperparathyroidism: a systematic review. *Am J Otolaryngol.* 2017;38(5):630-635.
6. DeLellis RA. Parathyroid tumors and related disorders. *Mod Pathol.* 2011;24 (Suppl 2):S78-S93.
7. Jamal SA, Miller PD. Secondary and tertiary hyperparathyroidism. *J Clin Densitom.* 2013;16(1):64-68.
8. Patel A, Lee CY, Sloan DA, Randle RW. Parathyroidectomy for tertiary hyperparathyroidism: a multi-institutional analysis of outcomes. *J Surg Res.* 2021;258:430-434.
9. van der Plas WY, Noltes ME, van Ginhoven TM, Kruijff S. Secondary and tertiary hyperparathyroidism: a narrative review. *Scand J Surg.* 2020;109(4):271-278.
10. Sutton W, Chen X, Patel P, et al. Prevalence and risk factors for tertiary hyperparathyroidism in kidney transplant recipients. *Surgery.* 2021;S0039-6060(21)00536-5.
11. Schlosser K, Zielke A, Rothmund M. Medical and surgical treatment for secondary and tertiary hyperparathyroidism. *Scand J Surg.* 2004;93(4):288-297.
12. Dewberry LC, Tata S, Graves S, Weber CJ, Sharma J. Predictors of tertiary hyperparathyroidism: who will benefit from parathyroidectomy? *Surgery.* 2014;156(6):1631-1637.
13. Cabo J, Gallagher KC, Baregamian N. Challenges and controversies in the surgical management of uremic hyperparathyroidism: a systematic review. *Am J Surg.* 2018;216(4):713-722.
14. McHenry CR, Shi HH. Can parathyroid hyperplasia be predicted preoperatively? *Am J Surg.* 2018;215(3):389-392.
15. Yamamoto T, Tominaga Y, Okada M, et al. Characteristics of persistent hyperparathyroidism after renal transplantation. *World J Surg.* 2016;40(3):600-606.
16. Schlosser K, Endres N, Celik I, Fendrich V, Rothmund M, Fernández ED. Surgical treatment of tertiary hyperparathyroidism: the choice of procedure matters! *World J Surg.* 2007; 31(10):1947-1953.
17. Colares Neto GP, Ide Yamauchi F, Hueb Baroni R, et al. Nephrocalcinosis and nephrolithiasis in X-linked hypophosphatemic rickets: diagnostic imaging and risk factors. *J Endocr Soc.* 2019;3(5):1053-1061.
18. Hruska KA, Mathew S, Lund R, Qiu P, Pratt R. Hyperphosphatemia of chronic kidney disease. *Kidney Int.* 2008;74(2): 148-157.
19. Roy R, Lee JA. Calciphylaxis due to hyperparathyroidism. *Endocr Pract.* 2011;17 (Suppl 1):54-56.
20. Pasieka JL, Parsons LL. A prospective surgical outcome study assessing the impact of parathyroidectomy on symptoms in patients with secondary and tertiary hyperparathyroidism. *Surgery.* 2000;128(4):531-539.
21. van der Plas WY, Dulfer RR, Engelsman AF, et al. Effect of parathyroidectomy and cinacalcet on quality of life in patients with end-stage renal disease-related hyperparathyroidism: a systematic review. *Nephrol Dial Transplant.* 2017;32(11): 1902-1908.
22. Broome DT, Naples R, Bailey R, et al. Use of preoperative imaging in primary hyperparathyroidism. *J Clin Endocrinol Metab.* 2021;106(1):e328-e337.
23. Expert Panel on Neurological Imaging, Zander D, Bunch PM, et al. ACR Appropriateness Criteria® Parathyroid Adenoma. *J Am Coll Radiol.* 2021;18(11S):S406-S422.
24. Pitt SC, Sippel RS, Chen H. Secondary and tertiary hyperparathyroidism, state of the art surgical management. *Surg Clin North Am.* 2009;89(5):1227-1239.
25. Saunders BD. Surgery for secondary hyperparathyroidism. *Oper Tech Otolaryngol Head Neck Surg.* 2016;27(3):136-144.
26. Alkhalili E, Tasci Y, Aksoy E, et al. The utility of neck ultrasound and sestamibi scans in patients with secondary and tertiary hyperparathyroidism. *World J Surg.* 2015;39(3): 701-705.
27. Karipineni F, Sahli Z, Somervell H, et al. Are preoperative sestamibi scans useful for identifying ectopic parathyroid glands in patients with expected multigland parathyroid disease? *Surgery.* 2018;163(1):35-41.
28. Chen YH, Chen HT, Lee MC, et al. Preoperative F-18 fluorocholine PET/CT for the detection of hyperfunctioning parathyroid glands in patients with secondary or tertiary hyperparathyroidism: comparison with Tc-99m sestamibi scan and neck ultrasound. *Ann Nucl Med.* 2020;34(8):527-537.
29. Rodgers SE, Hunter GJ, Hamberg LM, et al. Improved preoperative planning for directed parathyroidectomy with 4-dimensional computed tomography. *Surgery.* 2006;140(6):932-941.
30. Brown SJ, Lee JC, Christie J, et al. Four-dimensional computed tomography for parathyroid localization: a new imaging modality. *ANZ J Surg.* 2015;85(6):483-487.
31. Hamidi M, Sullivan M, Hunter G, et al. 4D-CT is superior to ultrasound and sestamibi for localizing recurrent parathyroid disease. *Ann Surg Oncol.* 2018;25(5):1403-1409.

32. Kedarisetty S, Fundakowski C, Ramakrishnan K, Dadparvar S. Clinical value of Tc99m-MIBI SPECT/CT versus 4D-CT or US in management of patients with hyperparathyroidism. *Ear Nose Throat J.* 2019;98(3):149-157.
33. Dulfer RR, Franssen GJH, Hesselink DA, Hoorn EJ, van Eijck CHJ, van Ginhoven TM. Systematic review of surgical and medical treatment for tertiary hyperparathyroidism. *Br J Surg.* 2017;104(7):804-813.
34. Dulfer RR, Koh EY, van der Plas WY, et al. Parathyroidectomy versus cinacalcet for tertiary hyperparathyroidism; a retrospective analysis. *Langenbecks Arch Surg.* 2019;404(1):71-79.
35. Prakobsuk S, Sirilak S, Vipattawat K, et al. Hyperparathyroidism and increased fractional excretion of phosphate predict allograft loss in long-term kidney transplant recipients. *Clin Exp Nephrol.* 2017;21(5):926-931.
36. Ozdemir FN, Afsar B, Akgul A, Usluoğullari C, Akçay A, Haberal M. Persistent hypercalcemia is a significant risk factor for graft dysfunction in renal transplantation recipients. *Transplant Proc.* 2006;38(2):480-482.
37. Pihlstrøm H, Dahle DO, Mjøen G, et al. Increased risk of all-cause mortality and renal graft loss in stable renal transplant recipients with hyperparathyroidism. *Transplantation.* 2015;99(2):351-359.
38. Littbarski SA, Kaltenborn A, Gwiasda J, et al. Timing of parathyroidectomy in kidney transplant candidates with secondary hyperparathryroidism: effect of pretransplant versus early or late post-transplant parathyroidectomy. *Surgery.* 2018;163(2):373-380.
39. Lou I, Foley D, Odorico SK, et al. How well does renal transplantation cure hyperparathyroidism? *Ann Surg.* 2015;262(4):653-659.
40. McManus C, Oh A, Lee JA, Hur C, Kuo JH. Timing of parathyroidectomy for tertiary hyperparathyroidism with end-stage renal disease: a cost-effectiveness analysis. *Surgery.* 2021;169(1):94-101.
41. Finnerty BM, Chan TW, Jones G, et al. Parathyroidectomy versus cinacalcet in the management of tertiary hyperparathyroidism: surgery improves renal transplant allograft survival. *Surgery.* 2019;165(1):129-134.
42. Bransky N, Iyer NR, Cannon SM, et al. Three rare concurrent complications of tertiary hyperparathyroidism: maxillary brown tumor, uremic leontiasis ossea, and hungry bone syndrome. *J Bone Metab.* 2020;27(3):217-226.
43. Brown SJ, Ruppe MD, Tabatabai LS. The parathyroid gland and heart disease. *Methodist Debakey Cardiovasc J.* 2017;13(2):49-54.
44. Shen Y, Fei P. Refractory hypercalcemia due to an ectopic mediastinal parathyroid gland in a hemodialysis patient: a case report. *BMC Nephrol.* 2019;20(1):165.
45. Palmer SC, Nistor I, Craig JC, et al. Cinacalcet in patients with chronic kidney disease: a cumulative meta-analysis of randomized controlled trials. *PLoS Med.* 2013;10(4):e1001436.
46. Greeviroj P, Kitrungphaiboon T, Katavetin P, et al. Cinacalcet for treatment of chronic kidney disease-mineral and bone disorder: a meta-analysis of randomized controlled trials. *Nephron.* 2018;139(3):197-210.
47. Behets GJ, Spasovski G, Sterling LR, et al. Bone histomorphometry before and after long-term treatment with cinacalcet in dialysis patients with secondary hyperparathyroidism. *Kidney Int.* 2015;87(4):846-856.
48. EVOLVE Trial Investigators, Chertow GM, Block GA, et al. Effect of cinacalcet on cardiovascular disease in patients undergoing dialysis. *N Engl J Med.* 2012;367(26):2482-2494.
49. Belozeroff V, Chertow GM, Graham CN, Dehmel B, Parfrey PS, Briggs AH. Economic evaluation of cinacalcet in the United States: the EVOLVE trial. *Value Health.* 2015;18(8):1079-1087.
50. Martin KJ, Bell G, Pickthorn K, et al. Velcalcetide (AMG 416), a novel peptide agonist of the calcium-sensing receptor, reduces serum parathyroid hormone and FGF23 levels in healthy male subjects. *Nephrol Dial Transplant.* 2014;29(2):385-392.
51. Shindo M, Lee JA, Lubitz CC, et al. The changing landscape of primary, secondary, and tertiary hyperparathyroidism: highlights from the American College of Surgeons Panel, "What's New for the Surgeon Caring for Patients with Hyperparathyroidism." *J Am Coll Surg.* 2016;222(6):1240-1250.
52. Tominaga Y, Matsuoka S, Uno N, Sato T. Parathyroidectomy for secondary hyperparathyroidism in the era of calcimimetics. *Ther Apher Dial.* 2008;12 (Suppl 1):S21-S26.
53. Casarim ALM, Arcadipane FAMC, Martins AS, et al. Pattern of intraoperative parathyroid hormone and calcium in the treatment of tertiary hyperparathyroidism. *Otolaryngol Head Neck Surg.* 2019;161(6):954-959.
54. Chen J, Jia X, Kong X, Wang Z, Cui M, Xu D. Total parathyroidectomy with autotransplantation versus subtotal parathyroidectomy for renal hyperparathyroidism: a systematic review and meta-analysis. *Nephrology (Carlton).* 2017;22(5):388-396.
55. Shepet K, Alhefdhi A, Usedom R, Sippel R, Chen H. Parathyroid cryopreservation after parathyroidectomy: a worthwhile practice? *Ann Surg Oncol.* 2013;20(7):2256-2260.
56. Callender GG, Malinowski J, Javid M, et al. Parathyroidectomy prior to kidney transplant decreases graft failure. *Surgery.* 2017;161(1):44-50.
57. Onoda N, Fukagawa M, Tominaga Y, et al. New clinical guidelines for selective direct injection therapy of the parathyroid glands in chronic dialysis patients. *NDT Plus.* 2008;1(Suppl 3):iii26-iii28.
58. Hu Z, Han E, Chen W, Chen J, Chen W, Guo R. Feasibility and safety of ultrasound-guided percutaneous microwave ablation for tertiary hyperparathyroidism. *Int J Hyperthermia.* 2019;36(1):1129-1136.
59. Cruzado JM, Moreno P, Torregrosa JV, et al. A randomized study comparing parathyroidectomy with cinacalcet for treating hypercalcemia in kidney allograft recipients with hyperparathyroidism. *J Am Soc Nephrol.* 2016;27(8):2487-2494.
60. Moreno P, Coloma A, Torregrosa JV, et al. Long-term results of a randomized study comparing parathyroidectomy with cinacalcet for treating tertiary hyperparathyroidism. *Clin Transplant.* 2020 Aug;34(8):e13988.
61. See A, Lim AEL, Wong J, et al. The effect of parathyroidectomy on patients' symptoms in tertiary hyperparathyroidism. *Head Neck.* 2019;41(8):2748-2755.
62. Tentori F, Wang M, Bieber BA, et al. Recent changes in therapeutic approaches and association with outcomes among patients with secondary hyperparathyroidism on chronic hemodialysis: the DOPPS study. *Clin J Am Soc Nephrol.* 2015;10(1):98-109.
63. Chen L, Wang K, Yu S, et al. Long-term mortality after parathyroidectomy among chronic kidney disease patients with secondary hyperparathyroidism: a systematic review and meta-analysis. *Ren Fail.* 2016;38(7):1050-1058.
64. Ivarsson KM, Akaberi S, Isaksson E, et al. The effect of parathyroidectomy on patient survival in secondary hyperparathyroidism. *Nephrol Dial Transplant.* 2015;30(12):2027-2033.
65. Komaba H, Taniguchi M, Wada A, Iseki K, Tsubakihara Y, Fukagawa M. Parathyroidectomy and survival among Japanese

hemodialysis patients with secondary hyperparathyroidism. *Kidney Int.* 2015;88(2):350-359.
66. El-Husseini A, Wang K, Edon A, et al. Value of intraoperative parathyroid hormone assay during parathyroidectomy in dialysis and renal transplant patients with secondary and tertiary hyperparathyroidism. *Nephron.* 2018;138(2):119-128.
67. Okada M, Hiramitsu T, Ichimori T, et al. Comparison of pre- and post-transplant parathyroidectomy in renal transplant recipients and the impact of parathyroidectomy timing on calcium metabolism and renal allograft function: a retrospective single-center analysis. *World J Surg.* 2020;44(2):498-507.
68. Wilhelm SM, Wang TS, Ruan DT, et al. The American Association of Endocrine Surgeons Guidelines for Definitive Management of Primary Hyperparathyroidism. *JAMA Surg.* 2016;151(10):959-968.
69. Bures C, Seika P, Skachko T, et al. Influence of parathyroidectomy on kidney graft function in secondary and tertiary hyperparathyroidism. *Transplant Proc.* 2020;52(10): 3134-3143.
70. Dream S, Chen H, Lindeman B. Tertiary hyperparathyroidism: why the delay? *Ann Surg.* 2021;273(3):e120-e122.
71. Triponez F, Clark OH, Vanrenthergem Y, Evenepoel P. Surgical treatment of persistent hyperparathyroidism after renal transplantation. *Ann Surg.* 2008;248(1):18-30.

Parathyroid Carcinoma

Oliver J. Fackelmayer, MD, FACS
Avital Harari, MD, MBA

38

GENERAL CONSIDERATIONS

EPIDEMIOLOGY & CLINICALLY HELPFUL BACKGROUND STATEMENTS

Parathyroid carcinoma (PC) is an extremely rare malignancy and accounts for less than 1% of cases of hyperparathyroidism.[1] It typically presents as a severe case of hypercalcemia with markedly elevated parathyroid hormone (PTH), consistent with severe primary hyperparathyroidism (PHPT). It can present with a palpable neck mass in approximately 40% to 70% of cases.[2] There are rare (5%-10%) reported cases of nonfunctional PC that present with a palpable firm neck mass that does not secrete excess PTH and thus the patient remains normocalcemic.[3,4]

Pathogenesis

The vast majority of PC is sporadic with only a small minority associated with genetic syndromes such as hyperparathyroidism-Jaw Tumor Syndrome (HPT-JT) and multiple endocrine neoplasia (MEN) types 1 and 2a syndromes. The molecular pathogenesis of PC is just beginning to be understood, both for sporadic PC and the autosomal dominant HPT-JT. The proposed genetic pathogenesis involves inactivating mutations in the tumor-suppressor gene *HRPT2* (CDC73), causing loss of function of the product parafibromin which seems to regulate gene expression and dampen cell proliferation.[5] Germline mutation in HRPT2, as seen in HPT-JT, will develop PC in approximately 15% of cases.[6] Somatic inactivating mutations in HRPT2 are seen in the majority of sporadic PC, and immunohistochemistry for parafibromin can confirm the diagnosis.[7] Importantly, HRPT2 mutations are not seen in benign parathyroid adenomas (<1%).[8] Additional genetic alterations are still being elucidated but include mutations in the PI3K/AKT/MTOR pathway in 20% of PC[9] and mutations of CCND1 causing amplification of cyclin D1 in 30% of cases.[10] Another gene of interest is the GCM2 parathyroid transcription factor. Missense germline mutations in GCM2 have been implicated in familial isolated hyperparathyroidism and may contribute to more aggressive disease (ie, more difficult to achieve biochemical cure).[11,12] The association, if any, with the development of PC is unclear at this time.

Prevention

Given the rarity of PC, with so little known about pathogenesis, it is difficult to deduce much about preventing this disease. One could argue that earlier detection of PC is possible by attention to serum calcium level on routine metabolic profiles and that an elevated calcium value should be rechecked with an intact PTH level. Evidence to support early diagnosis is limited but there had been a trend toward decreased tumor size and lymph node involvement in the last two decades.[13] It is possible that this could be attributed to increasing awareness and thus earlier diagnosis and management of PHPT.

Differential Diagnosis

By far the most common presentation of patients with PC is severe hypercalcemia with a markedly elevated PTH level, thus limiting the differential to benign PHPT or PC. This excludes those patients with end-stage renal disease who manifest extremely high PTH levels from secondary hyperparathyroidism; these patients will typically have low-normal serum calcium levels. If the presenting sign is a palpable neck mass, the differential is broad and ranges from benign lymphadenopathy to malignancy of many possible origins such as (but not limited to) thyroid carcinoma and esophageal carcinoma.

Clinical Findings

A. Symptoms & Signs
B. Laboratory Findings
    a. Calcium
    b. Parathyroid hormone, intact
C. Imaging Studies
    a. Ultrasound
    b. CT
    c. PET/CT
D. Special Tests
    a. Avoid percutaneous biopsy attempts (FNA)
E. Special Examinations, etc.
    a. Laryngoscopy

Patients with severe hypercalcemia usually present to the emergency department but can be encountered in the ambulatory setting. Signs and symptoms are myriad and include progressive nausea, polyuria, polydipsia, dehydration, altered mental status, coma, and cardiac arrhythmia.

Most patients with PC present in the mid-fifth to mid-sixth decade of life with extremely high serum calcium and PTH levels, and there is roughly equivalent incidence in females and males (up to 1:1.5). PC is also much more commonly seen in the inferior glands (Table 38–1).[14]

Perhaps the single most pivotal point in the consideration of PC is the initial workup. It cannot be overemphasized that the only chance of cure for PC is complete surgical *en bloc* resection at the initial operation. Early consideration of PC allows the surgeon to amend the preoperative workup and discussion of parathyroid disease, including obtaining additional preoperative imaging. Surgeon-performed ultrasound is used in all cases of parathyroid disease to evaluate for parathyroid candidates, assess for invasive features, scrutinize the cervical lymph nodes, and evaluate for concomitant thyroid pathology.[15] In addition to typical parathyroid localization imaging including nuclear medicine Sestimibi study and 4-dimensional CT scan, an FDG-PET/CT can be helpful to evaluate for metastatic disease. Evidence of widely metastatic disease can temper the aggressiveness of the index operation from curative to palliative intention. Fine-needle aspiration (FNA) biopsy of a target lesion should not be entertained as this will not provide a definitive diagnosis and violation of the tumor capsule with spilling of parathyroid cells can predispose to locoregional spread and possible seeding of the biopsy tract. FNA can be performed, however, on metastatic lesions for confirmation. Laryngoscopy is a useful adjunct to examine for recurrent laryngeal nerve involvement, especially in the setting of voice changes.[16]

Given the rarity of this cancer, there was previously no established TNM staging system. The most recent eighth edition of the American Joint Committee on Cancer does include a TNM system for PC. There are still insufficient data to propose anatomic stage and prognostic groups for PC.[17] Tumors are generally categorized as being localized, locally invasive, or metastatic.

Localized disease has histologic characteristics of carcinoma but is confined to the gland. As these tumors do not have invasive features to be classified as malignant, they can be termed atypical adenomas. These tumors generally lack somatic HRPT2 mutations and show low (<10%) biochemical recurrence.[18] Locally invasive disease shows gross or microscopic invasion involving adjacent fat, strap muscle, vessels, esophagus, thyroid, trachea, or recurrent laryngeal nerve (Figure 38–1). Metastatic disease to distant

Table 38–1. Benign primary hyperparathyroidism vs parathyroid carcinoma.[2]

	Primary Hyperparathyroidism	Parathyroid Carcinoma
Age at diagnosis	Sixth-seventh decade	Fifth-sixth decade
Female:male sex distribution	4:1	1:1, possible slight male predilection
Serum calcium (mg/dL)	<13	>14
Intact parathyroid hormone level	>1-3× upper limit of normal	≥4× upper limit of normal
Palpable neck mass	Rarely	70%

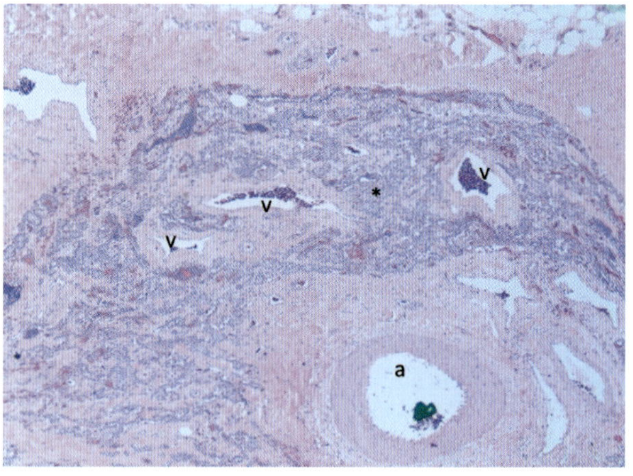

Figure 38–1. Histopathology of parathyroid carcinoma demonstrates extracapsular soft tissue invasion with tumor cells (blue, *) invading around a muscular artery (lower right, a) and several muscular veins (v). (Photo credit: Dr. Jeffery Goldstein, Department of Pathology, UCLA.)

organs outside the neck is most commonly to bone, lung, or liver. Metastatic disease is rare on presentation (1 of 27 cases in one series) but later developed in six patients in that same series.[16]

Treatment

A. Index operation
B. Reoperation
C. Concurrent thyroid lobectomy
D. Lymph node dissection
E. Adjuvant therapies
  a. Cytotoxic chemotherapy
  b. EBRT
  c. Targeted therapies

All of the preoperative data taken in context allows the surgeon to have the most informed and complete preoperative counseling with the patient. The surgeon must be attuned to any suggestion of an invasive process including severely elevated calcium or PTH, voice changes, a palpable neck mass, ultrasound with concern for invasion or abnormal lymph nodes, or other suggestions of malignant process. Consent should include verbiage for a typical parathyroid operation, as well as a more radical resection to potentially include any involved structures such as the ipsilateral thyroid lobe, recurrent laryngeal nerve, lymph nodes in the ipsilateral central compartment, trachea, esophagus, and major vasculature. Hypercalcemia should be medically managed preoperatively.

A complete (R0) resection offers the only change of cure for this disease and as such the surgeon must be attuned to intraoperative findings that suggest malignancy, including but not limited to invasive features and malignant appearing lymphadenopathy. As previously mentioned, surgical *en bloc* resection to negative microscopic margins should include all involved structures. It is not mandatory to remove the ipsilateral thyroid lobe or to perform a compartmental level VI lymph node dissection if not involved by the tumor. In a study identifying 114 cases of PC with lymph nodes assessed at time of operation, only 10.5% showed lymph node metastases, which were associated with tumors >3 cm in size and not correlated with disease-specific survival.[19]

Regarding possible multigland disease in the setting of a PC, one quarter of PCs coexist with other pathologic glands—either benign adenoma or multigland hyperplasia.[20] However, index resection should focus on the malignant side and delay operation of the contralateral side containing benign pathology so as not to seed the contralateral field with malignant cells. Two separate but coexisting malignant parathyroid glands would be exceedingly rare, and although rare still, patients with HPT-JT carrying germline HRPT2 mutations do have the risk of subsequently developing a second metachronous PC in a remaining parathyroid gland following curative resection of an index PC.

Histopathology is not always definitive for the diagnosis of PC. Without suggestive diagnostic findings such as gross local invasion or known metastatic disease, there can be ambiguity in the histopathologic diagnosis of PC. In suspicious cases, including cases categorized as atypical parathyroid adenoma, patients should be followed closely for recurrence and metastasis, which would secure a malignant diagnosis.

Each patient has an average of three neck dissections over the course of their disease. Therefore, surgically resectable, recurrent, and metastatic disease should undergo reoperation balanced by the compounded surgical morbidity.[20] Once a patient's disease is deemed unresectable or associated with unacceptably high surgical morbidity, ethanol, or radiofrequency ablation can be considered, although the malignant target may be difficult to hydrodissect from surrounding structures to allow for safe ablation. The surgical goal in the management of recurrent disease is control of disease burden to allow for mitigation of hypercalcemia causing end-organ damage.

Neoadjuvant therapies are not applicable for PC, as the diagnosis, though suspected, cannot be made preoperatively. Adjuvant therapies include systemic chemotherapy, external beam radiation, and control of hypercalcemia medically and with palliative tumor debulking. Traditional systemic chemotherapy and external beam radiation are generally ineffective at reducing functional tumor burden but several series document external beam radiation administration in up to 70% of cases.[21,22] Hypercalcemia is managed per routine regardless of etiology and includes intravenous fluid resuscitation specifically with normal saline, intravenous bisphosphonates, calcimimetics, and denosumab for refractory cases.

An exciting and evolving area of promising research is the sequencing of tumors and targeted therapies. HRPT2 (CDC73) is a tumor suppressor gene that has undergone somatic inactivating mutation in the majority of cases of sporadic PC (Table 38–2).[7] Germline mutation in HRPT2 is the genetic marker for HPT-JT syndrome as discussed above. Theoretically, gene therapy to transfect an HRPT2-expressing plasmid could be used in the future to downregulate tumorgenesis.[23] Studies have demonstrated the tumor-suppressing activity of HRPT2 and the exogenous HRPT2 attenuated protumorigenic activity.[24] Mutations in PTEN and PIK3CA in the mTOR pathway occur in 24% of cases of PC and offer targets for mTOR inhibitors.[9] Mutations in *KDR* (producing VEGFR-2) occur in 13% of cases of PC and offer targets for tyrosine kinase inhibitors.[25] A high tumor mutation burden, >20 m/Mb, seen in 18.7% of cases, allows for potential use of immune checkpoint inhibitors.[25]

Table 38–2. Theoretic and potential future targeted therapies for PC.

Target	Frequency	Therapeutic Class	Notes/Examples
HRPT2 (CDC73)	77%	Gene therapy	<1% of benign hyperparathyroidism
mTOR (PTEN, PIK2CA)	24%	mTOR inhibitors	Sirolimus, everolimus, temsirolimus
KDR (gene product = VEGFR-2)	13%	Tyrosine kinase inhibitors	Oral bioavailability, antiangiogenic. Sorafenib, sunitinib, lenvatinib
High tumor mutation burden	19%	Immune checkpoint inhibitors	Pembrolizumab

Precision personalized medicine is a promising field for rare diseases such as PC.

Complications

1. Hypercalcemic crisis
2. Perioperative morbidity
    i. Recurrent laryngeal nerve injury/sacrifice
    ii. Esophageal injury
    iii. Tracheal injury
3. Hungry bone syndrome

Untreated PC can present with severe hypercalcemic crisis and should be medically stabilized. Morbidity from parathyroid surgery is well described and usually low risk. However, the invasive nature of PC increases the need to resect involved organs to achieve an *en bloc* resection required for potential cure. Additional morbidity from such resections includes palsy of the recurrent laryngeal nerve (either from injury or sacrifice), esophageal leak, and tracheal fistula.

Following resection of the hypersecreting parathyroid tumor, patients are at risk of developing hungry bone syndrome characterized by refractory and severe hypocalcemia. Patients should be monitored for this occurrence postoperatively and managed accordingly.

Prognosis

Disease onset in the fifth and sixth decade of life is young enough that patients are more likely to enjoy good health and functional status at diagnosis. The option to reoperate on recurrences becomes less palatable with each reoperation and will reach a time when reoperative intervention is no longer possible or comes with excessively high morbidity and risk of mortality. As such, tumor burden will eventually exceed the ability to medically mitigate hypercalcemia. Mortality is usually the result of severe hypercalcemia and not directly from invasive or metastatic disease. Fortunately, given the availability of cinacalcet and other medications that can initially assist in reducing hypercalcemia for noncurable patients, median survival for patients with PC is approximately 15 years with an overall recurrence rate of 39%.[26] Five year survival ranges from 77% to 100% and 10-year survival ranges from 49% to 91%.[27]

When to Refer/When to Admit

Severe hypercalcemia should prompt PC to be included in the differential diagnosis. Patients with markedly elevated calcium usually present to the emergency department with symptoms of dehydration, altered mental status, and cardiac arrhythmia, but can also be encountered in the office setting. The patient should be admitted to the hospital to stabilize the calcium level and workup possible causes. Patients in parathyroid crisis (severe hypercalcemia usually >15 mg/dL) mandate careful resuscitation and advanced supportive care, as most patients have altered sensorium. Consider nephrology consultation as severe hypercalcemia impaires the concentrating capacity in the distal tubule resulting in a nephrogenic diabetes incipidus and renal insufficiency or acute renal failure.

Once PC is suspected, patients should be referred to an experienced endocrine or head and neck surgeon. Most cases of PC will be diagnosed intraoperatively when confronted by an invasive parathyroid tumor or postoperatively by histology. Every effort should be made to clear that side of the neck of disease, being prepared to remove all involved structures without spilling parathyroid cells. Keep in mind that the index operation is the only opportunity to achieve curative R0 resection. Postoperatively, the patient should be referred to a multidisciplinary tumor board with expertise in endocrine oncology. Regular monitoring of calcium and PTH is essential to detect recurrence and should occur every 6 months for the first few years and then yearly indefinitely, as recurrence can manifest after a long disease-free interval —up to 12 years.[26]

The best chance of cure is a thorough and meticulous index operation and should be undertaken by an experienced endocrine/head and neck surgeon who is familiar with the disease, and at an institution with a multidisciplinary team required for the treatment of this rare but fascinating malignancy. Long-term survival is possible with multimodal management of tumor recurrence and hypercalcemia.

REFERENCES

1. Ruda JM, Hollenbeak CS, Stack BC Jr. A systematic review of the diagnosis and treatment of primary hyperparathyroidism from 1995 to 2003. *Otolaryngol Head Neck Surg.* 2005;132(3):359-372.
2. Fingeret AL. Contemporary evaluation and management of parathyroid carcinoma. *JCO Oncol Pract.* 2021;17(1):17-21.
3. Wang L, Han D, Chen W, et al. Non-functional parathyroid carcinoma: a case report and review of the literature. *Cancer Biol Ther.* 2015;16(11):1569-1576.
4. Harari A. Parathyroid Carcinoma. In: Clark OH, ed. *Textbook of Endocrine Surgery*. Jaypee Brothers Medical Publishers; 2016.
5. Cetani F, Pardi E, Borsari S, et al. Genetic analyses of the HRPT2 gene in primary hyperparathyroidism: germline and somatic mutations in familial and sporadic parathyroid tumors. *J Clin Endocrinol Metab.* 2004;89(11):5583-5591.
6. Sharretts JM, Simonds WF. Clinical and molecular genetics of parathyroid neoplasms. *Best Pract Res Clin Endocrinol Metab.* 2010;24(3):491-502.
7. Gill AJ. Understanding the genetic basis of parathyroid carcinoma. *Endocr Pathol.* 2014; 25(1):30-34.
8. Tan MH, Morrison C, Wang P, et al. Loss of parafibromin immunoreactivity is a distinguishing feature of parathyroid carcinoma. *Clin Cancer Res.* 2004;10(19):6629-6637.
9. Pandya C, Uzilov AV, Bellizi J, et al. Genomic profiling reveals mutational landscape in parathyroid carcinomas. *JCI Insight.* 2017;2(6):e92061.
10. Zhao L, Sun L-H, Liu D-M, et al. Copy number variation in CCND1 gene is implicated in the pathogenesis of sporadic parathyroid carcinoma. *World J Surg.* 2014;38(7):1730-1737.
11. El Lakis M, Nockel P, Guan B, et al. Familial isolated primary hyperparathyroidism associated with germline GCM2 mutations is more aggressive and has a lesser rate of biochemical cure. *Surgery.* 2018;163(1):31-34.
12. Song A, Yang Y, Wang Y, et al. Germline GCM2 mutation screening in chinese primary hyperparathyroidism patients. *Endocr Pract.* 2020;26(10):1093-1104.
13. James BC, Kilfoy BA, Cipriyani N, et al. The incidence and survival of rare cancers of the thyroid, parathyroid, adrenal, and pancreas. *Ann Surg Oncol.* 2016;23(2):424-433.
14. Busaidy NL, Jimenez C, Habra MA, et al. Parathyroid carcinoma: a 22-year experience. *Head Neck.* 2004;26(8):716-726.
15. Wilhelm SM, Wang TS, Ruan DT, et al. The American Association of Endocrine Surgeons Guidelines for Definitive Management of Primary Hyperparathyroidism. *JAMA Surg.* 2016;151(10):959-968.
16. Maher DI, Goare S, Forrest E, et al. Routine preoperative laryngoscopy for thyroid surgery is not necessary without risk factors. *Thyroid.* 2019;29(11):1646-1652.
17. Landry C, Wang T, Asare E. Parathyroid. In: Amin M, editor. *AJCC Cancer Staging Manual.* 8th edn. New York, NY: Springer International Publishing; (2017). p. 903.
18. Saponaro F, Pardi E, Mazoni L, et al. Do patients with atypical parathyroid adenoma need close follow-up? *J Clin Endocrinol Metab.* 2021;106(11):e4565-e4579.
19. Hsu KT, Sippel RS, Chen H, Schneider DF. Is central lymph node dissection necessary for parathyroid carcinoma? *Surgery.* 2014;156(6):1336-1341; discussion 1341.
20. Harari A, Waring A, Ranvier GF, et al. Parathyroid carcinoma: a 43-year outcome and survival analysis. *J Clin Endocrinol Metab.* 2011;96(12):3679-3686.
21. Erovic BM, Goldstein DP, Kim D, et al. Parathyroid cancer: outcome analysis of 16 patients treated at the Princess Margaret Hospital. *Head Neck.* 2013;35(1):35-39.
22. Nayyar SS, Thiagrajan S, Chaukar D, et al. Parathyroid carcinoma: an experience of the enigma over 10 years. *Indian J Endocrinol Metab.* 2020;24(2):137-142.
23. Shen DF, Liu X, Yang XF, et al. The roles of parafibromin expression in ovarian epithelial carcinomas: a marker for differentiation and prognosis and a target for gene therapy. *Tumour Biol.* 2016;37(3):2909-2924.
24. Rather MI, Swamy S, Gopinath KS, Kumar A. Transcriptional repression of tumor suppressor CDC73, encoding an RNA polymerase II interactor, by Wilms tumor 1 protein (WT1) promotes cell proliferation: implication for cancer therapeutics. *J Biol Chem.* 2014; 289(2):968-976.
25. Kang H, Pettinga D, Schubert AD, et al. Genomic profiling of parathyroid carcinoma reveals genomic alterations suggesting benefit from therapy. *Oncologist.* 2019;24(6): 791-797.
26. Iihara M, Okamoto T, Suzuki R, et al. Functional parathyroid carcinoma: Long-term treatment outcome and risk factor analysis. *Surgery.* 2007;142(6):936-943; discussion 943 e1.
27. Cetani F, Pardi E, Marcocci C. Parathyroid carcinoma. *Front Horm Res.* 2019;51:63-76.

39 Parathyroidectomy: Indications, Operative Techniques, Intraoperative Parathyroid Hormone Monitoring, Management of Complications

Alexander Shifrin, MD, FACS
Oliver Gimm, MD, FEBS

GENERAL CONSIDERATIONS

Diagnosis of primary hyperparathyroidism (PHPT) is biochemical. Therefore, the following laboratory measurements are essential to establish the diagnosis: serum calcium, parathyroid hormone (PTH), vitamin D, phosphate, creatinine levels, glomerular filtration rate (GFR), alkaline phosphatase activity, 24-hour urine calcium, and at times, ionized calcium levels.[1-3] Bone mineral density (BMD) by DEXA scan is essential to evaluate for osteoporosis in the lumbar spine, femoral hip, and, importantly, at the most common site for PHPT-related osteoporosis, the wrist. Approximately 85% of patients with PHPT will have a single parathyroid adenoma; the rest of the patients will have either double adenoma or hyperplasia. Radiological localization studies are obtained to localize an adenoma and to help plan for a minimally invasive surgical approach, but not to establish the diagnosis of PHPT. When imaging studies do not localize a parathyroid adenoma, but surgical criteria are met, the patient is still a candidate for parathyroid exploration.[2]

Based on the current guidelines for managing PHPT, it is stated that parathyroidectomy is indicated for all symptomatic patients and should be considered for most asymptomatic patients. Parathyroidectomy is more cost-effective than observation or pharmacologic therapy. Parathyroidectomy is recommended regardless of the results of preoperative localizing studies for all patients who have met surgical criteria (see following discussion). Minimally invasive parathyroidectomy can achieve cure in up to 97% to 99% of patients when intraoperative PTH (IOPTH) monitoring is used.[2] Minimally invasive approaches have shown no differences in recurrence compared to more traditional techniques.[4]

Over the last two decades, several new minimally invasive techniques for parathyroidectomy have developed, including mini-open, video-assisted, and totally endoscopic approaches. The benefits include a targeted surgical approach to a parathyroid adenoma and the ability to perform a neck exploration, even with possible thyroid lobectomy, without the need to convert to a standard open procedure. This allows for cosmetically pleasing and curative results.[5,6]

Preoperative localization studies include dedicated parathyroid ultrasound (Figure 39–1A), sestamibi (Figure 39–1B), SPECT CT sestamibi scan (Figure 39–2), and 4D-CT scan (Figure 39–3). Ultrasound is the safest imaging study for preoperative localization of parathyroid adenoma with no risk of radiation exposure. A designated parathyroid ultrasound, not just a neck or a thyroid gland ultrasound, is recommended before a parathyroidectomy for operative planning of all patients with PHPT. The sensitivity of high-resolution ultrasonography has been reported to be between 51% and 89% if a radiologist interpreted the study. Surgeon-performed ultrasonography correctly identified a parathyroid adenoma in 74% to 90% of patients with a sensitivity of 87% and specificity of 88%.[7,8]

Dual-isotope subtraction single-photon emission computed tomography-computed tomography (SPECT-CT) scan is a newer diagnostic technique with superior results to the traditional sestamibi scan (Figure 39–2). A recent study showed that the sensitivity of the SPECT-CT scan was 95%, with a specificity of 89% for detecting and localizing a parathyroid adenoma. The positive predictive value was estimated at 97%, and the negative predictive value was 83%. The accuracy of the technique was reported from 80% to 94% in detecting a parathyroid adenoma and 92% in accurate localization to the appropriate gland and not only

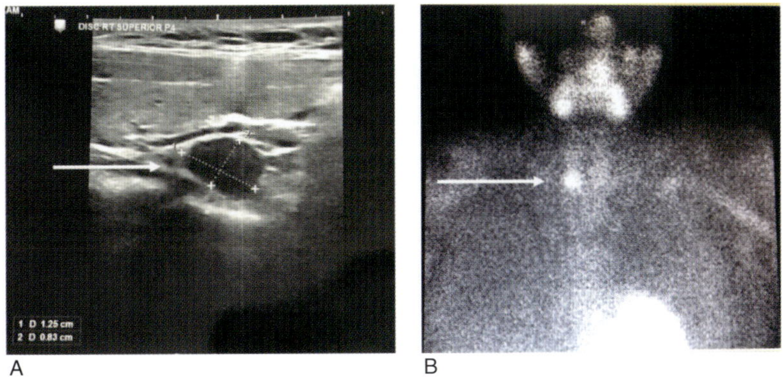

▲ **Figure 39–1.** Right superior parathyroid adenoma. **(A)** A dedicated, surgeon-performed parathyroid ultrasound, transverse view, showing a solid hypoechoic mass located deep and posterior to the middle of the right thyroid lobe consistent with enlarged descended right superior parathyroid gland (adenoma). The arrow is pointing at the parathyroid adenoma. **(B)** Sestamibi scan, 3 (hours delayed image) performed in the same patient; the arrow points to the area of persistent uptake consistent with a hyperfunctioning parathyroid adenoma. By the radiologist's assessment, it was described as the right inferior parathyroid adenoma. In correlation with an ultrasound and subsequent surgical findings, it appeared to be an enlarged, descended right superior parathyroid gland.

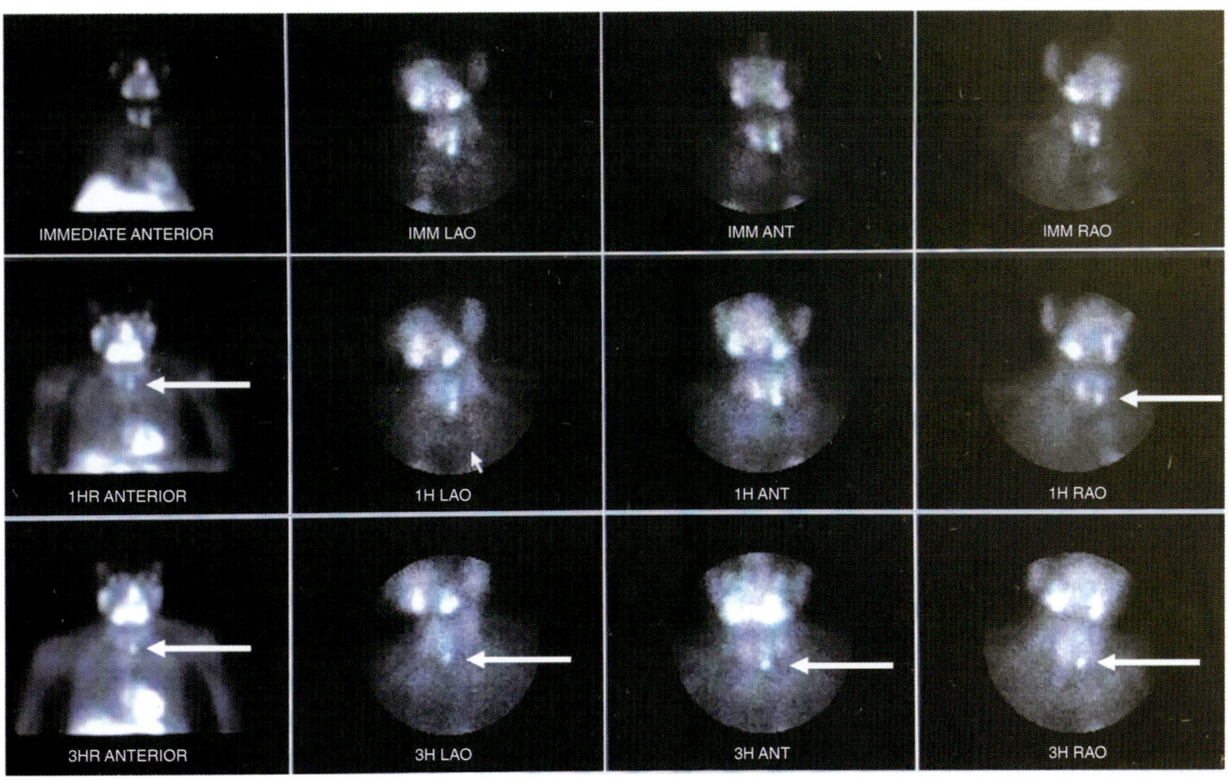

▲ **Figure 39–2.** SPECT CT Sestamibi scan showing persistent uptake at 3 hours consistent with a left inferior parathyroid adenoma (arrows).

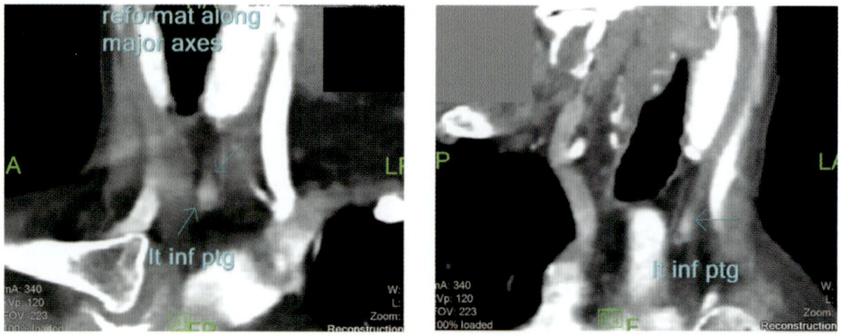

A B

▲ **Figure 39–3.** Dedicated parathyroid 4D-CT scan. An enlarged supernumerary left inferior parathyroid gland (arrows) lies 1.5 cm below the extreme lower pole of the left lobe thyroid, abutting the medial margin of the strap muscle, at and to the left of the midline, 2.2 cm above the suprasternal notch. The enlarged gland is an 11 mm major axis with a calculated weight of 103 mg. (Figure provided with permission by Daniel Neistadt, MD.)

the laterality.[7,9] A minimally invasive parathyroid surgery is a successful parathyroidectomy performed through a small incision, with short duration under anesthesia, minimal postoperative pain, low complication rate, and high long-term success rates.[10,11] If a patient were to develop recurrent disease after first parathyroid surgery, the complication rate has been reported to be increased if the initial surgery performed was a 4-gland neck exploration (44%) versus the minimally invasive approach (15%).[12] There is no difference in long-term recurrence rates between a minimally invasive approach and a bilateral exploration.[4,13] Furthermore, the use of IOPTH monitoring has been associated with cure rates with a minimally invasive parathyroidectomy as high as 97% to 99%.[2]

IOPTH monitoring has become an essential part of performing a parathyroidectomy. The goal of the IOPTH assessment is to achieve an instant intraoperative confirmation of the biochemical cure of hyperparathyroidism. IOPTH assay facilitates a minimally invasive surgical approach by minimizing the extent of surgery, leading to minimal surgical trauma. The goal of the IOPTH assessment is not only to have a 50% drop in PTH levels but also to achieve a final IOPTH value down into the normal range and, in ideal circumstances, to less than 40 pg/mL after the parathyroidectomy.[14-24]

Indications for Parathyroidectomy

Based on the recent guidelines for the management of asymptomatic PHPT from the summary statement of the Fifth International Workshop and the American Association of Endocrine Surgeons (AAES) Guidelines for Definitive Management of Primary Hyperparathyroidism, the following are indications for surgical treatment of PHPT: serum calcium 1.0 mg/dL (0.25 mmol/L) above upper limit of normal; skeletal involvement such as a fracture by vertebral fracture assessment (VFA) or vertebral X-ray, or the presence of osteoporosis defined as BMD by DEXA scan, a T score of less than −2.5 at lumbar spine, total hip, femoral neck, and especially, distal one-third of the radius (Z scores should be used instead of T scores in premenopausal women and men younger than 50 years of age); the presence of nephrolithiasis or nephrocalcinosis by X-ray, ultrasound, or other imaging modality; hypercalciuria defined by the measurements of 24-hour urine calcium above 250 mg/day in women, and above 300 mg/day in men; and individuals less than 50 years of age.[1-3]

Surgical Techniques

The patient is placed in a supine position. Usually, general anesthesia is performed by intubating the patient with an ET tube that has a sensor for intraoperative monitoring (IONM) of the recurrent laryngeal nerve (RLN). However, the procedure can also be performed under local anesthesia with mild sedation with or without a deep cervical block. A shoulder roll is placed to keep the head and the neck in an extended position. A shoulder roll is not required if the procedure is a video-assisted approach. It is important to confirm the position of the ET tube IONM sensor at the vocal cords after placing a shoulder roll by either direct laryngoscopy (by anesthesiologist) or by the surgeon with flexible laryngoscopy. Both arms are tucked at the patient's sides, ensuring pressure points are padded to mitigate the possibility of brachial and ulnar nerve injury. The head is placed in a foam head cradle. The patient is prepped with chlorhexidine or other surgical skin prep, and we recommend draping with sterile paper drape towels and strips of an IOBAN antimicrobial adhesive drape to seal off the paper drapes for a tight seal of the field. This is done to prevent accidental gas leaks from the anesthesia machine from infiltrating the field (to avoid fire hazards from using a bovie cautery in the presence of oxygen) and for sterility of the field.

Preoperative antibiotics are usually not given unless the patient is immunocompromised, has some other source of infection, or has some implantable device. Sequential compression devices are placed on the lower extremities bilaterally for deep venous thrombosis prophylaxis.

Understanding the anatomical location of parathyroid glands is essential to avoid complications. The upper parathyroid glands are most commonly located dorsal to the RLN, while the lower parathyroid glands are most commonly located ventral to the RLN. IONM can help identify the RLN in case of limited visualization during a minimally invasive approach.

Precise and meticulous dissection is crucial in performing a parathyroidectomy. Incidental disruption of the parathyroid adenoma can result in the seeding of parathyroid cells in the surgical field and, subsequently, the development of parathyromatosis. A clean and dry surgical field with good hemostasis is essential for clearly visualizing parathyroid glands and their differentiation from lymph nodes or satellite thyroid nodules. Any blood staining of the surgical field can compromise the view and not only cause frustration to the surgeon due to decreased visualization of the parathyroid glands but also potentially increase the possibility of complications due to injury of the RLN.

A small skin incision is carried out at a natural skin crease using a #15 blade. The platysma muscle is transected with a bovie cautery. Then, subplatysmal flaps are created superiorly and inferiorly with the bovie cautery (Figure 39–4). Strap muscles are separated at the midline along the *linea alba* with a bovie cautery, and the space is created between the

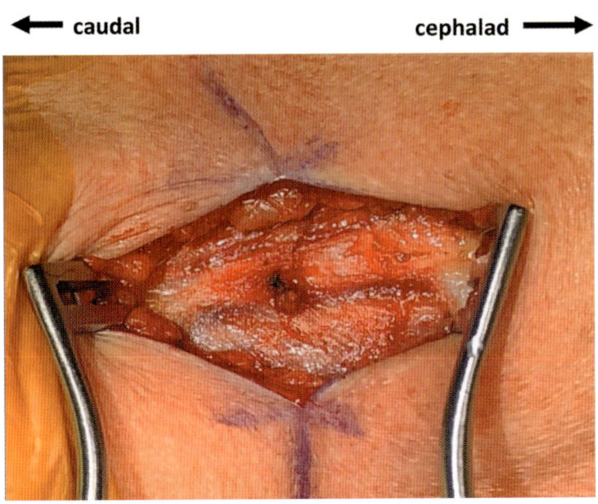

▲ **Figure 39–4.** Parathyroidectomy. Subplatysmal flaps are created superiorly and inferiorly with a bovie cautery. A small Weitlaner surgical retractor is placed to retract the platysma flaps in caudal and cephalad directions and expose the underlying strap muscles.

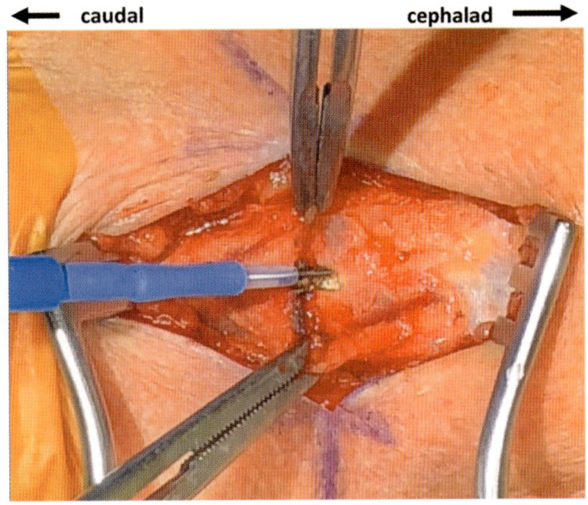

▲ **Figure 39–5.** Parathyroidectomy. Strap muscles are separated at the midline along the *linea alba* with a bovie cautery.

anterior strap muscles and the thyroid lobes (Figure 39–5). The left thyroid lobe is retracted medially and anteriorly with peanuts on Allis hemostatic clamps. The strap muscles are retracted laterally and inferiorly with army-navy retractors. Another Allis clamp is used to develop the space between the thyroid lobe and the carotid artery and to dissect the middle thyroid vein (Figure 39–6). Fibrous tissue overlying a parathyroid adenoma can be picked up with Debakey forceps. Adson hemostatic forceps (or mosquito) are used to spread overlying tissue over and around the parathyroid adenoma to dissect the adenoma circumferentially. IONM may help with localization of the RLN, especially when it is not initially visualized (Figures 39–7 and 39–8). The parathyroid adenoma is gently picked up with the DeBakey forceps at the level of the vascular pedicle. The surgeon must be cautious not to tear off the thin parathyroid capsule and avoid seeding parathyroid cells. The Adson hemostatic forceps (or mosquito) are used to dissect the RLN away from the adenoma (Figure 39–9).

If the location of the parathyroid adenoma corresponds to an inferior parathyroid gland, the following technique is used. Inferior attachments of the parathyroid adenoma to the thymus are mobilized and transected. The parathyroid adenoma is then mobilized medially, laterally, and posteriorly. If a superior parathyroid gland has to be removed, dissection should be handled very carefully since, most of the time, it will be located posterior to the RLN.

A nerve stimulator can be used to locate the position of the RLN if it is not visualized. Once the RLN is located, posterior attachments to the adenoma are transected. The parathyroid adenoma is then held up with Debakey forceps, and the adenoma pedicle with blood vessels is mobilized

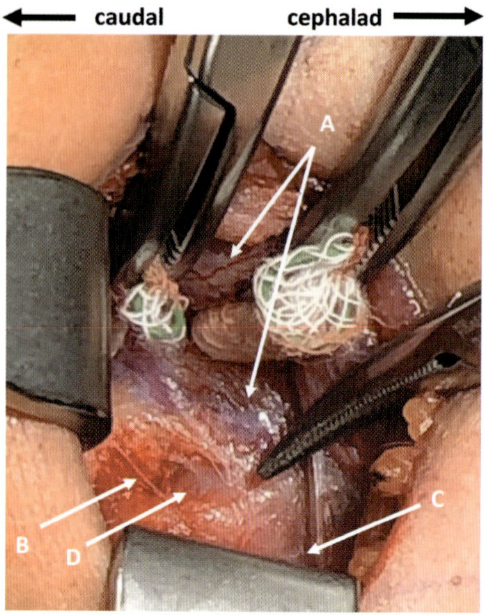

▲ **Figure 39–6.** Parathyroidectomy, excision of a left superior parathyroid adenoma. The left thyroid lobe is retracted medially and anteriorly with peanuts on Allis hemostatic clamps. Strap muscles are retracted laterally and inferiorly with army-navy retractors. An Adson clamp creates the space between the thyroid lobe and the carotid artery and dissects the middle thyroid vein. Parathyroid adenoma is visualized under the fibrous tissues **(A)** left thyroid lobe; **(B)** middle thyroid veins; **(C)** tissues overlying the left carotid artery; **(D)** parathyroid adenoma.

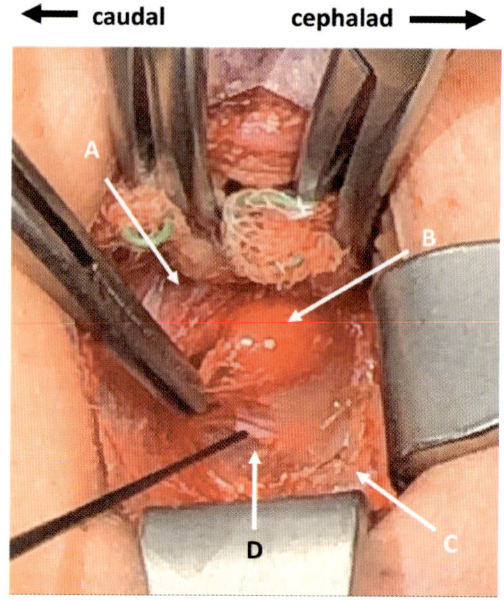

▲ **Figure 39–7.** Parathyroidectomy, excision of a left superior parathyroid adenoma. The DeBakey forceps pick up fibrous tissue overlying the parathyroid adenoma **(B)**. Adson hemostatic forceps (or mosquito) are used to spread overlying tissue over and around the parathyroid adenoma to dissect the adenoma circumferentially. The IONM technique may help with the localization of the RLN, especially when it is not initially visualized. The left superior parathyroid adenoma is located above the recurrent laryngeal nerve (RLN), between the RLN and Berry's ligament. The intraoperative nerve stimulator points at the RLN **(D)**. **(A)** left thyroid lobe; **(B)** left superior parathyroid adenoma; **(C)** fibrous tissue overlying the carotid artery; **(D)**. the RLN.

circumferentially with a mosquito clamp. The parathyroid adenoma can then be reflected anteriorly and caudally away from the RLN. The vascular pedicle is held with the DeBakey forceps, and after confirmation that the RLN is away, the adenoma vascular pedicle is transected using the Harmonic Focus device (Figure 39–10). The adenoma is retrieved (Figure 39–11). The wound is irrigated with saline solution, and a small piece of Fibrillar (absorbable hemostatic agent) may be placed into the remaining space (Figure 39–12). In some patients with suspicion of possible parathyroid hyperplasia or equivocal PTH results, or when IOPTH testing is unavailable, visualization of a normal parathyroid gland on the same side can help with deciding on completing the procedure (Figure 39–13). After that, the strap muscles are reapproximated with absorbable sutures, as is the platysma. Skin closure is carried out with a subcutaneous or intracutaneous running 5-O Monocryl. A Dermabond is placed over the closed skin incision. Monocryl stitch ends are cut at the skin level. IOPTH levels should be measured at baseline (T baseline), during manipulation of the adenoma (T 0), and in 5 (T 5) and 10 (T 10) minutes after dividing the adenoma pedicle. Two measurements, five and 10-minute time points after the removal of the parathyroid adenoma, are used not only to see the drop in the PTH level but also to see the decreasing values trend in the PTH levels. Some patients may have underlying renal dysfunction, and the PTH level will not drop very quickly, but the trend will show a drop; in this instance, we usually add T-20 to see the drop in the PTH level to normal ranges. In addition, if the T-0 (stimulation) level is drastically elevated several times over the T-baseline, then one measurement (5 or 10 min) after removing the parathyroid adenoma will not be enough to confirm that the PTH level is down to normal rangers and still might be several times over the baseline numbers, the trend in decreasing the PTH level may help to determine if the second parathyroid adenoma (or multifocal adenomas) is present. An intraoperative frozen section of the parathyroid gland is recommended to confirm the removal

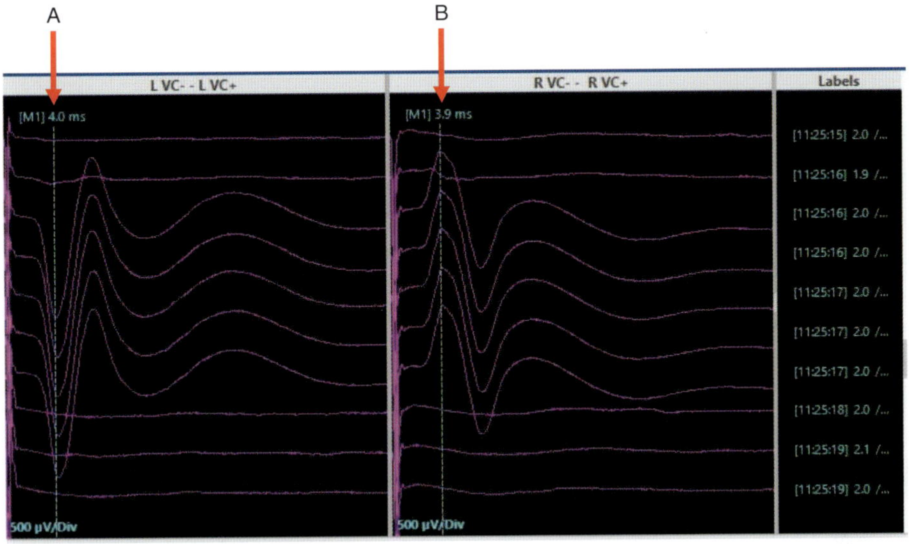

▲ **Figure 39–8.** The IONM technique shows the signal from the stimulation of the RLN (**A** - left RLN, **B** - right RLN).

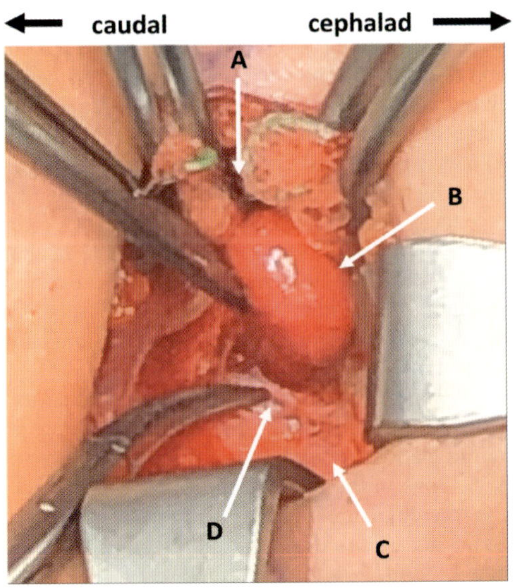

▲ **Figure 39–9.** Parathyroidectomy, excision of a left superior parathyroid adenoma. The parathyroid adenoma is gently picked up with the DeBakey forceps at the level of the vascular pedicle. The surgeon must be cautious not to tear the thin parathyroid capsule to avoid seeding parathyroid cells. The Adson hemostatic forceps (or mosquito) are used to dissect the RLN away from the adenoma. **(A)** left thyroid lobe; **(B)** left superior parathyroid adenoma; **(C)** carotid artery; **(D)** the RLN.

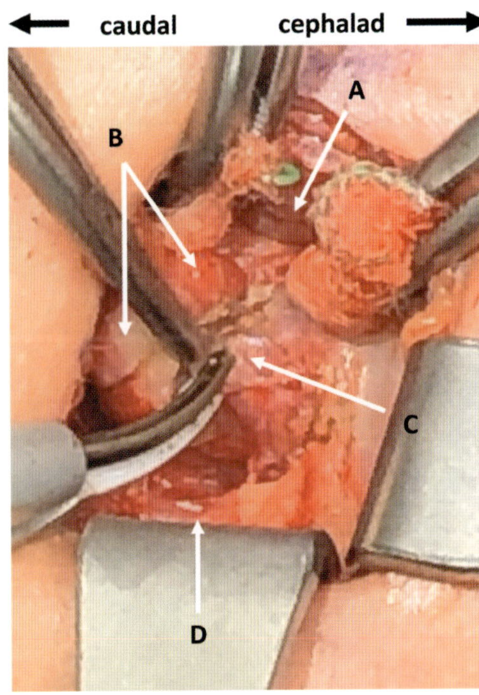

▲ **Figure 39–10.** Parathyroidectomy, excision of a left superior parathyroid adenoma. The parathyroid adenoma is reflected anteriorly and caudally away from the RLN. The DeBakey forceps hold the adenoma vascular pedicle, and, after confirmation that the RLN is away, the adenoma vascular pedicle is transected by using the Harmonic Focus device. **(A)** left thyroid lobe; **(B)** left superior parathyroid adenoma; **(C)** adenoma vascular pedicle; **(D)** the RLN.

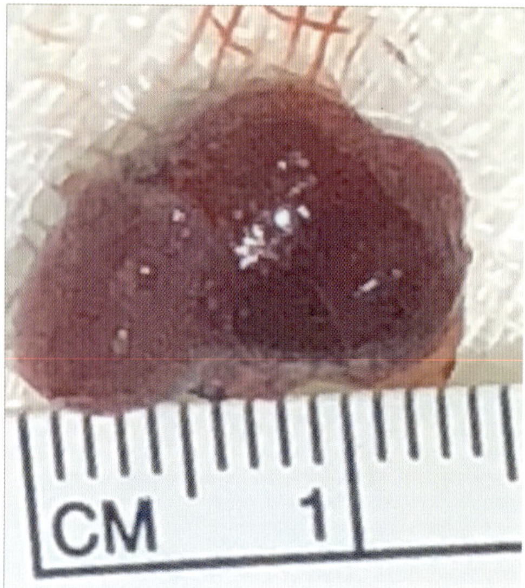

▲ **Figure 39–11.** Parathyroidectomy, excision of a left superior parathyroid adenoma. The left superior parathyroid adenoma.

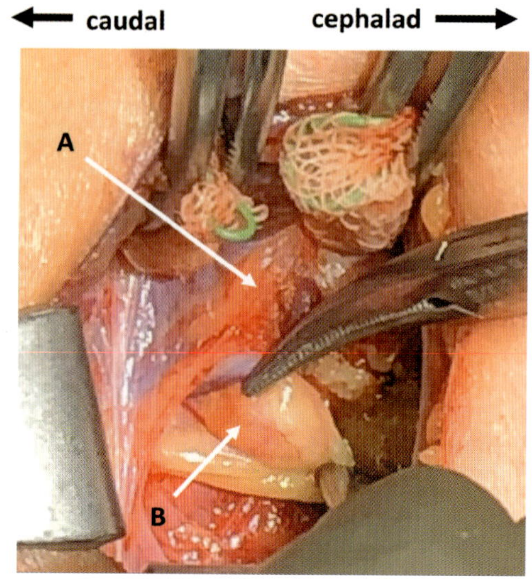

▲ **Figure 39–13.** Normal left inferior parathyroid gland. Adson hemostatic forceps point at the normal left inferior parathyroid gland within the tip of the thymus **(A)**. **(A)** left thyroid lobe, **(B)** normal left inferior parathyroid gland.

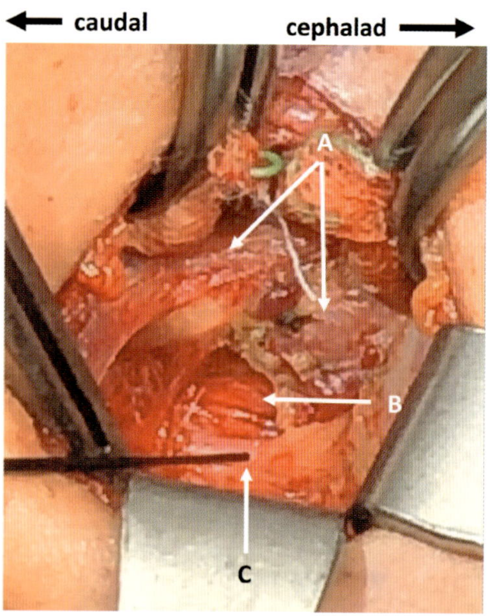

▲ **Figure 39–12.** Parathyroidectomy, excision of a left superior parathyroid adenoma. The space remained after the excision of the left superior parathyroid adenoma. The intraoperative nerve stimulator is used to confirm the integrity of the RLN **(C)**. **(A)** left thyroid lobe; **(B)** the space remained after the removal of the parathyroid adenoma; **(C)** the RLN.

of a hypercellular parathyroid gland. The intraoperative frozen section helps to decide whether the procedure is complete. Based on the intraoperative frozen section assessment of the parathyroid adenoma or gland, the pathologists will give the percentage of hypercellularity. If the percentage is higher than 30%, it is considered hyperplastic parathyroid, gland, or adenoma, which helps with intraoperative planning. Knowing the percentage of hypercellularity may help determine the procedure's completion. On a few occasions, a satellite thyroid nodule or a lymph node may visually appear very similar to a parathyroid adenoma. After 3 hours of observation, the patient is discharged on an empiric dose of calcium carbonate with vitamin D until the postoperative visit.

The following surgical steps can be undertaken to locate a missing parathyroid gland. To locate a missing inferior parathyroid gland, the surgeon can dissect the lower pole of the thyroid lobe in the plane to the RLN, then dissect along and into the thyro-thymic ligament or posterior thymus, looking for intra-thymic parathyroid gland. If a parathyroid adenoma is found within a thymus, cervical thymectomy could be performed. It is important not to miss a subcapsular intrathyroidal parathyroid adenoma at the inferior pole of the thyroid by retracting the thyroid medially with the peanut and carefully evaluating the inferior pole, specifically looking for intracapsular yellowish/brownish color parathyroid gland. Then, the surgeon can open the carotid sheath at the level of the carotid bifurcation and above the bifurcation at the skull base level to look for an undescended lower gland in the skull base.[25] Ectopic superior parathyroid glands can be found between the thyroid gland and the carotid artery or adjacent to the carotid artery. Superior parathyroid glands can also be intrathyroidal but are less likely than inferior glands. The surgical steps that can be undertaken to locate a missing superior parathyroid gland include: mobilization of the superior pole of the thyroid lobe with rotation of the thyroid medially, then looking superiorly, medially, or posteriorly to the upper pole of the thyroid lobe; then dissecting posterior to the tubercle of Zuckerkandl. Occasionally, glands can descend posterior to the RLN along the esophagus toward the posterior mediastinum, and thus dissection inferiorly in the paraesophageal or retroesophageal plane should be pursued. Finally, dissection lateral to the RLN along the medial border of the common carotid artery and into the carotid sheath caudally should be performed if a superior gland is still not identified.[25,26]

A. Intraoperative PTH Monitoring

The serum half-life of PTH is approximately 3 to 4 minutes, while ionized calcium decreases at about 30 minutes after removal of an adenoma. PTH levels nadir about 5 hours after an adenoma removal. PTH levels start to increase again on postoperative day two.[27] IOPTH guides a surgeon's assessment of the completeness of a parathyroid exploration as an adjunct to visual morphologic characteristics used by surgeons in the past.[28] The ability to perform a rapid IOPTH assessment has become possible due to the development of a new generation of PTH assay with two monoclonal antibodies specific for the N- and C-terminal regions of the (1-84)PTH. In contrast, earlier assays were directed to the N-terminal, mid, or C-terminal regions.[29] Although there is still some debate on the timing and the best criteria for interpreting the IOPTH assay, a 50% drop in PTH level at 5 and 10 minutes after the excision of the parathyroid adenoma has become the gold standard for IOPTH criteria. Therefore, the ideal time points for IOPTH measurements are as follows: Tb—at baseline (before the parathyroidectomy); at the T0—during the parathyroid adenoma manipulation; T5—at 5 minutes after the adenoma removal; T10—at 10 minutes after the adenoma removal; T20 can be added if IOPTH levels are decreasing slowly as seen in the case of very high initial preoperative PTH level.

Despite literature debating the optimal criteria, this approach has been utilized by most endocrine and head and neck surgeons who are high-volume parathyroid surgeons.[18-20] It has been shown that IOPTH monitoring accurately predicts operative success or failure in 96% of patients. Some authors also recommend using an additional measurement of IOPTH at 20 minutes after removing a parathyroid adenoma, which was associated with a 97% operative success rate.[30] Earlier data on IOPTH measurements established that the goal of a 50% IOPTH drop was enough to achieve a biochemical cure, even if the final IOPTH level was still above the upper limit of normal.[21] More recent data have shown that in addition to a 50% IOPTH level drop, it must also go down into the normal range. A study of patients with 2-year follow-up after parathyroidectomy has shown that patients with a final IOPTH level less than 40 pg/mL had a lower persistence and recurrence rate than patients with IOPTH levels between 40 and 59 pg/mL. Patients with a final IOPTH level between 41 and 65 pg/mL have a higher likelihood of persistent disease due to a missed hyperplastic gland. Patients with final IOPTH ≥60 pg/mL were reported to have a recurrence rate of 5.9% and a persistence rate of 5.4% as compared to patients with an IOPTH level <40 pg/mL, who had a recurrence rate of 1.3% and a persistence rate of only 0.2%.[22-24] In a retrospective study, Chen et al. showed that an IOPTH level drop greater than 70% was also protective against a recurrence.[13]

Treating patients with normocalcemic or normohormonal PHPT can be challenging, and relying only on the IOPTH levels may not be sufficient. It has been shown that patients who presented with normocalcemic PHPT may have approximately a 12% chance of multigland disease. Patients with normohormonal PHPT may have up to a 58% chance of multiglandular disease (44% of them were reported to have hyperplasia). Therefore, bilateral parathyroid exploration should be considered in perioperative planning of normocalcemic or normohormonal PHPT.[31,32] The primary cause of operative failure of a minimally invasive surgical approach utilizing IOPTH monitoring was not the failure of the IOPTH technique itself but rather the surgeons' misinterpretation of the IOPTH result and the failure to identify all abnormal parathyroid glands.[33]

Management of Complications

A. Development of Hematoma

Development of acute postoperative hematoma during the immediate postoperative period is quite rare but may require urgent exploration in the operating room. If severe stridor develops, the incision should be opened at the bedside, and the hematoma should be drained, followed by immediate re-exploration in the operating room to control the bleeding.

Delayed postoperative hematoma or seroma (several days after the surgery) can usually be managed in an outpatient setting. If drainage is deemed necessary, it can be done either by ultrasound-guided drainage using a sterile technique with a 20G or 18G needle on a 20-cc syringe or by opening the corner of the incision and draining the hematoma and then packing the opening with gauze loosely into the wound. The dressing and the packing gauze must be changed daily until the wound is healed. If the wound has to be opened, prophylactic oral antibiotics can be considered for 1 to 2 weeks (until the wound is healed).

B. Postoperative Hypocalcemia

Development of acute hypocalcemia after a focused exploration and single parathyroid gland removal is infrequent since the three other parathyroid glands were undisturbed, except in the setting of a prior thyroid or parathyroid operation on the contralateral side. Nevertheless, younger patients may develop transient hypocalcemia that can be easily controlled by administering oral calcium carbonate with vitamin D 1000 mg every 6 to 8 hours for 1 to 2 weeks. If a patient has a 3-1/2 gland parathyroidectomy for hyperplasia, severe hypocalcemia can develop during the first 2 to 3 days after the surgery. Measurement of PTH levels after parathyroidectomy can predict the development of hypocalcemia. If the IOPTH level is less than 15 pg/mL, the development of severe hypocalcemia can be predicted, and the patient would benefit by receiving prophylactic calcitriol (Rocatrol) 0.25 to 0.5 μg once or twice a day for 1 to 2 weeks. In severe cases of hypocalcemia refractory to oral supplementation or with severe symptoms, intravenous calcium should be administered as an initial bolus of 1 to 2 g of calcium in 50 mL of 5% dextrose infused over 20 minutes. If symptoms of severe hypocalcemia persist, intravenous calcium infusion of a solution composed of 11 g of calcium gluconate added to normal saline or 5% dextrose water to provide a final volume of 1000 mL is administered at 50 mL/h intravenous infusion rate and adjusted to maintain the calcium level in the low normal range.[34]

C. RLN Injury

Injury to the RLN is a devastating complication of a parathyroidectomy. Consequences of RLN injury are especially pronounced in older patients who, in addition to the severe voice hoarseness, may also develop dysphagia with aspiration, especially of liquids.

1. Transient injury to the RLN—RLN injury can be due to traction of the thyroid that results in neural stretch and temporary paralysis. This usually resolves within days to weeks after surgery.

2. Complete transection of the RLN—If the RLN injury is recognized intraoperatively, several options for immediate repair can be accomplished. If both ends of the RLN are visible and can be approximated, it should be repaired by direct approximation of the RLN ends. If there is a segment of the RLN loss, flipping the end of *ansa cervicalis* to the proximal end of the RLN, the vagus-RLN anastomosis or free nerve grafting can be used. The specific techniques for nerve repair are addressed in another publication.[35]

REFERENCES

1. Bilezikian JP, Khan AA, Silverberg SJ, et al. International Workshop on Primary Hyperparathyroidism. Evaluation and management of primary hyperparathyroidism: summary statement and guidelines from the Fifth International Workshop. *J Bone Miner Res.* 2022 Nov;37(11):2293-2314.
2. Wilhelm SM, Wang TS, Ruan DT, et al. The American Association of Endocrine Surgeons Guidelines for Definitive Management of Primary Hyperparathyroidism. *JAMA Surg.* 2016;151(10):959-968.
3. Udelsman R, Åkerström G, Biagini C, et al. The surgical management of asymptomatic primary hyperparathyroidism: proceedings of the Fourth International Workshop. *J Clin Endocrinol Metab.* 2014;99(10):3595-3606.
4. Schneider D, Mazeh H, Chen H, Sippel R. Predictors of recurrence in primary hyperparathyroidism: an analysis of 1,386 cases. *Ann Surg.* 2014;259(3):563-568.
5. Fouquet T, Germain A, Zarnegar R, et al. Totally endoscopic lateral parathyroidectomy: prospective evaluation of 200 patients. ESES 2010 Vienna presentation. *Langenbecks Arch Surg.* 2010;395(7):935-940.
6. Bakkar S, Matteucci V, Corsini C, Pagliaro S, Miccoli P. Less is more: time to expand the indications for minimally invasive video-assisted parathyroidectomy. *J Endocrinol Invest.* 2017; 40(9):979-983.
7. Arora S, Balash PR, Yoo J, Smith GS, Prinz RA. Benefits of surgeon-performed ultrasound for primary hyperparathyroidism. *Langenbecks Arch Surg.* 2009;394(5):861-867.
8. Deutmeyer C, Weingarten M, Doyle M, Carneiro-Pla D. Case series of targeted parathyroidectomy with surgeon-performed ultrasonography as the only preoperative imaging study. *Surgery.* 2011;150(6):1153-1160.
9. Keidar Z, Solomonov E, Karry R, Frenkel A, Israel O, Mekel M. Preoperative [99mTc]MIBI SPECT/CT interpretation criteria for localization of parathyroid adenomas-correlation with surgical findings. *Mol Imaging Biol.* 2017;19(2):265-270.
10. Henry JF. Minimally invasive thyroid and parathyroid surgery is not a question of length of the incision. *Langenbecks Arch Surg.* 2008;393(5):621-626.
11. Starker LF, Fonseca AL, Carling T, Udelsman R. Minimally invasive parathyroidectomy. *Int J Endocrinol.* 2011;2011:206502.
12. Morris LF, Lee S, Warneke CL, et al. Fewer adverse events after reoperative parathyroidectomy associated with initial minimally invasive parathyroidectomy. *Am J Surg.* 2014;208(5): 850-855.
13. Lou I, Balentine C, Clarkson S, Schneider DF, Sippel RS, Chen H. How long should we follow patients after apparently curative parathyroidectomy? *Surgery.* 2017;161(1):54-61.
14. Irvin GL 3rd, Dembrow VD, Prudhomme DL. Operative monitoring of parathyroid gland hyperfunction. *Am J Surg.* 1991;162(4):299-302.
15. Irvin GL 3rd, Dembrow VD, Prudhomme DL. Operative monitoring of parathyroid gland hyperfunction. *Am J Surg.* 1991;162(4):299-302.
16. Irvin GL 3rd, Deriso GT 3rd. A new, practical intraoperative parathyroid hormone assay. *Am J Surg.* 1994;168(5): 466-468.
17. Carneiro-Pla D. Contemporary and practical uses of intraoperative parathyroid hormone monitoring. *Endocr Pract.* 2011;17 (Suppl 1):44-53.
18. Carneiro DM, Irvin GL 3rd. New point-of-care intraoperative parathyroid hormone assay for intraoperative guidance in parathyroidectomy. *World J Surg.* 2002;26(8):1074-1077.
19. Carneiro-Pla D. Recent findings in the use of intraoperative parathyroid hormone monitoring in parathyroid disease. *Curr Opin Oncol.* 2009;21(1):18-22.
20. Trinh G, Noureldine SI, Russell JO, et al. Characterizing the operative findings and utility of intraoperative parathyroid hormone (IOPTH) monitoring in patients with normal baseline IOPTH and normohormonal primary hyperparathyroidism. *Surgery.* 2017;161(1):78-86.

21. Carneiro-Pla DM, Solorzano CC, Lew JI, Irvin GL 3rd. Long-term outcome of patients with intraoperative parathyroid level remaining above the normal range during parathyroidectomy. *Surgery*. 2008;144(6):989-993; discussion 993-4.
22. Wharry LI, Yip L, Armstrong MJ, et al. The final intraoperative parathyroid hormone level: how low should it go? *World J Surg*. 2014;38(3):5.
23. Rajaei MH, Bentz AM, Schneider DF, Sippel RS, Chen H, Oltmann SC. Justified follow-up: A final ioPTH over 40 pg/mL is associated with an increased risk of persistence and recurrence in primary hyperparathyroidism. *Ann Surg Oncol*. 2015;22(2):454-459.
24. Rajaei MH, Bentz AM, Schneider DF, Sippel RS, Chen H, Oltmann SC. Justified follow-up: a final intraoperative parathyroid hormone (ioPTH) over 40 pg/mL is associated with an increased risk of persistence and recurrence in primary hyperparathyroidism. *Ann Surg Oncol*. 2015;22(2):454-459.
25. Cheatem D, Sturgeon C. Technique of Parathyroidectomy. In: Clark O, Duh Q-Y, Kebebew E, Gosnell J, Shen W., eds. *Textbook of Endocrine Surgery*. 3rd ed. Jaypee, 2016: Chapter 60.
26. Randolph GW. *Surgery of the Thyroid and Parathyroid Glands*. 2nd ed. Saunders; 2012.
27. Maier GW, Kreis ME, Renn W, Pereira PL, Häring HU, Becker HD. Parathyroid hormone after adenectomy for primary hyperparathyroidism. A study of peptide hormone elimination kinetics in humans. *J Clin Endocrinol Metab*. 1998;83(11):3852-3856.
28. Irvin GL 3rd, Dembrow VD, Prudhomme DL. Clinical usefulness of an intraoperative "quick parathyroid hormone" assay. *Surgery*. 1993;114(6):1019-1022; discussion 1022-3.
29. Bieglmayer C, Prager G, Niederle B. Kinetic analyses of parathyroid hormone clearance as measured by three rapid immunoassays during parathyroidectomy. *Clin Chem*. 2002;48(10):1731-1738.
30. Calò PG, Pisano G, Loi G, et al. Intraoperative parathyroid hormone assay during focused parathyroidectomy: the importance of 20 minutes measurement. *BMC Surg*. 2013;13:36.
31. Trinh G, Rettig E, Noureldine SI, et al. Surgical management of normocalcemic primary hyperparathyroidism and the impact of intraoperative parathyroid hormone testing on outcome. *Otolaryngol Head Neck Surg*. 2018;159(4):630-637.
32. Javid M, Callender G, Quinn C, Carling T, Donovan P, Udelsman R. Primary hyperparathyroidism with normal baseline intraoperative parathyroid hormone: a challenging population. *Surgery*. 2017;161(2):493-498.
33. Lee S, Ryu H, Morris LF, et al. Operative failure in minimally invasive parathyroidectomy utilizing an intraoperative parathyroid hormone assay. *Ann Surg Oncol*. 2014;21(6):1878-1883.
34. Stack BC, Bimston DN, Bodenner DL, et al. American Association of Clinical Endocrinologists and American College of Endocrinology Disease State Clinical Review: Postoperative Hypoparathyroidism—Definitions and Management. *Endocr Pract*. 2015;21(No. 6).
35. Ito Y, Miyauchi A. Recurrent laryngeal nerve paralysis—management of recurrent laryngeal nerve injuries. In: Shifrin A, ed. *Endocrine Emergencies*. Elsevier; 2020.

40 Parathyroidectomy: Thoracoscopic/Robotic Approach to Ectopic Parathyroid Adenoma

Roy Oommen, MD Joshua Sonett, MD

GENERAL CONSIDERATIONS

Primary hyperthyroidism is a disease process characterized by the unopposed secretion of parathyroid hormone along with elevated serum concentrations of calcium. It is a common disease that affects approximately 1% of the adult population. The oversecretion of PTH leads to issues with bone absorption and decalcification, affecting not only the bones but the digestive system, nervous system, and urinary system as well.

Approximately 95% of patients with primary hyperparathyroidism are cured after neck exploration. In many of those in whom a cure is not achieved after parathyroidectomy, an ectopic or supernumerary parathyroid is found in a different location. An ectopic mediastinal parathyroid adenoma may be present in as many as 25% of patients with primary hyperparathyroidism, although only about 2% of them are inaccessible through a standard cervical incision and require a thoracic approach. Though previously performed through a median sternotomy, the use of video-assisted thoracic surgery (VATS) for the removal of ectopic mediastinal parathyroid glands has been associated with lower postoperative complications and length of hospital stay.[1-3]

Pathogenesis

The superior parathyroid glands arise from the fourth branchial pouch while the inferior parathyroid glands originate from the dorsal aspect of the third brachial pouch along with the thymus gland. Inferior parathyroid glands travel for a longer distance, in an inferomedial direction, and are thus more variable in location when compared to superior parathyroid glands. Ectopic inferior parathyroid glands are most frequently found in the anterior mediastinum, usually within the thymus gland, while superior ectopic parathyroids are typically found posteriorly and superiorly in the mediastinum. Ectopic glands may be found along the course of the esophagus, the thyrothymic ligament, within the thyroid gland, or the carotid sheath. Less commonly, ectopic parathyroid glands may be found in the aortopulmonary window, pericardium, or right dome of the diaphragm.[4,5]

Clinical Findings

The spectrum of symptoms and signs of primary hyperparathyroidism can range from subtle to severe. Classic symptoms include osteoporosis, renal failure, nephrolithiasis, peptic ulcer disease, pancreatitis, and cardiovascular disease. Nonclassical symptoms may include depression, fatigue, and hypertension. Most of these conditions are reversible with parathyroidectomy. Hyperparathyroidism can also occur as a part of multiple endocrine neoplasia type 1 (MEN1) syndrome, which consists of pancreatic islet cell tumors, pituitary adenoma, and primary hyperparathyroidism.

Ectopic parathyroid adenomas have been reported to be associated with more severe clinical manifestations of primary hyperparathyroidism, presenting with higher calcium levels and more frequently with bone disease. This could be partly due to delayed diagnosis and localization as most of them are diagnosed in patients who present with persistent hypercalcemia after surgery for primary hyperparathyroidism. Rarely, an ectopic parathyroid adenoma may result in thoracic bleeding or cause obstructive symptoms resulting in stridor or vocal cord palsy from its large size or extracapsular hematoma.[6-8]

Differential Diagnosis

Many mediastinal structures can be mistaken for a parathyroid adenoma, including lymph nodes, which are typically differentiated by their location along lymph node chains and the presence of an echogenic fatty hilum with hilar vascularity. If the nodule is located lateral to the common carotid artery, it is very unlikely to be a parathyroid adenoma. Other differential considerations include ectopic thyroid nodules or separate thyroid lobulations most often found along the posterior border of the mid to lower portion of the thyroid due to an anatomic variant known as the tubercle of Zuckerkandl. A fluid-filled esophageal diverticulum or a vascular structure might be mistaken for a very hypoechoic parathyroid adenoma.[9]

On sestamibi scan, a thyroid adenoma can be differentiated from a parathyroid adenoma with a dual-tracer study in which a thyroid adenoma demonstrates uptake of Tc-99m pertechnate of I-123 but a parathyroid adenoma remains photopenic (cold). Other causes of false positive sestamibi uptake in the neck are rare and include malignancies such as lung, breast, and papillary thyroid cancer, in addition to reactive and metastatic lymph nodes.[10]

Treatment

A. Preoperative Imaging Modalities

Preoperative localization studies are necessary before mediastinal exploration for parathyroid adenoma; however, the optimal approach to preoperative localization has not been determined.[11] Parathyroid glands larger than 1.5 cm can be detected by CT scan, but it may be difficult to identify smaller glands. Magnetic resonance imaging is reported to be more sensitive than CT, but not as sensitive as nuclear scanning. Technetium-99 sestamibi scanning (99Tc-MIBI) combined with sestamibi single-photon emission computed tomography (SPECT) has the highest positive predictive value of the available imaging techniques; however, if not available, the combination of chest CT and 99Tc-MIBI imaging should be used. The typical pattern in cases of parathyroid tumor is prolonged retention of 99m Tc-MIBI in the adenoma with rapid washout of the tracer from normal thyroid tissue. Mitochondrial density within a tumor is associated with the retention of 99m-TC sestamibi, and it should be borne in mind that some mitochondrial-rich mediastinal tumors, such as thymoma, can appear false-positive for this reason. As scintigraphy does not provide sufficient anatomic detail to guide the surgical approach, combination with US or CT is necessary to increase the sensitivity. 4D CT as well as 18F-FCH PET are modalities that also demonstrate a high sensitivity for parathyroid adenomas in patients with hyperparathyroidism.[12,13]

Select venous sampling (SVS) may be helpful in patients who have disscordant sestamibi and CT scans; however, SVS has been demonstrated to have a very high sensitivity (95%) and fairly good specificity (86%). In the patient in whom all other localization studies are unrevealing, a positive SVS may be justification for mediastinal exploration, with the caveat that these patients appear to have a lower rate of successful cure of hyperparathyroidism.[14,15]

B. Operative Technique

Once a mediastinal location is determined based on localization studies, the patient is taken to the operating room for VATS or mediastinoscopic exploration.[16] Exploration and resection with conventional mediastinoscopy is used if the parathyroid adenoma appeared localized in the middle mediastinum on preoperative imaging, whereas VATS/RATS is used when the gland is localized in the anterior or part of the middle mediastinum which would be difficult to access with the mediastinoscopy. The decision to perform right-sided versus left-sided VATS/RATS is determined by the location of the parathyroid adenoma on the preoperative CT scan. A left-sided approach is more commonly used as it allows the surgeon to visualize the aorticopulmonary window and to have easier access to the paratracheal region above the innominate vein. The right-sided approach allows the surgeon better visualization of the superior vena cava and the right phrenic vein.

The patient should be intubated with a double-lumen endotracheal tube, placed in a standard lateral decubitus position with three thoracoscopic ports. CO_2 insufflation to 10 or 12 mmHg as tolerated is essential for good visualization. If the adenoma is located in the anterior mediastinum, thymectomy and excision of mediastinal fat tissue are performed with the assistance of the Ligasure TM (Medtronic) instrument. If the parathyroid adenoma is located in a part of the middle mediastinum not easily accessible with mediastinoscopy, a more targeted exploration with VATS is recommended and the thymectomy and resection of mediastinal fat can be omitted. The specimen is removed from the thorax by using a protected bag. Given the ability of an active adenoma to seed if the capsule is violated, great care is taken during dissection not to violate the capsule of the adenoma. The specimen is sent for frozen section to confirm that it is indeed an enlarged parathyroid gland.

Intraoperative PTH values are obtained at baseline, when the specimen is removed (ie, T-0), at 5 and 10 minutes after the removal of the gland, and at the discretion of the surgeon, 20 minutes after removal of the specimen. A value drop of 50% from baseline and into the normal range is considered indicative of removal of the hyperfunctioning parathyroid gland. A PTH drop to less than 15 pg/mL may indicate the possibility of ultimate permanent hypoparathyroidism, and the need to reimplant a fragment of the parathyroid gland to avoid hypoparathyroidism should be considered. The decision to reimplant should be made in conjunction with a dedicated endocrine surgeon, endocrinologist, and the history of previous explorations with removal of normal parathyroid glands. A portion of the excised gland should be kept on ice while the final parathyroid hormone levels are obtained and a decision made regarding the need for reimplantation. Reimplantation is easily performed in a subcutaneous position in the forearm.

After hemostasis is achieved, the lung is re-expanded, evacuation of air from the chest can be performed and chest tube placement omitted. Patients are routinely prescribed supplemental calcium postoperatively for hypocalcemia prophylaxis.

We consider resection for primary hyperparathyroidism successful if we achieved (1) an intraoperative decrease in PTH levels of 50% or greater from the higher of the baseline and T-0 values, (2) pathologic confirmation of removal of parathyroid gland or adenoma from the mediastinum, and (3) postoperative normalization of calcium levels.[1,17] In patients in whom two-point preoperative imaging concur on location of parathyroid adenoma, concurrent CT and sestamibi, CT and venous sampling, minimally invasive resection of the mediastinal parathyroid is 100% effective in successful resection of the pathologic adenoma.[1] However, if only one preoperative imaging study suggests a mediastinal adenoma, the success rate dramatically decreases, and intraoperative localization techniques may be employed to improve the results of explorative surgery. These techniques include intraoperative autofluorescence techniques and intraoperative gamma probe localization.[18,19]

Complications

A uncommon and concerning complication of open parathyroidectomy is hoarseness.

During thoracoscopic resection, recurrent laryngeal nerve injury can occur with dissection at the aortic arch.

It is important to remember that hoarseness due to surgical resection does not require full transection; even intact nerves can be injured due to traction injury. If permanent vocal cord paralysis is suspected, direct laryngoscopy is indicated and the vocal cords can be medialized using autologous fat, or synthetic options such as calcium hydroxyapatite or collagen. Surgical medialization of the injured vocal cord can also be performed by arytenoid adduction.

Other rare complications of thoracoscopic resection include hemorrhage, pneumothorax, and subcutaneous emphysema.

Prognosis

Thoracoscopy (RATS or VASTS) is a safe and successful means of resecting ectopic parathyroid adenomas. Many series report no conversion to sternotomy or thoracotomy with near complete control of hyperparathyroidism in all patients.

Either a right-sided, left-sided, or bilateral approach can be used with significantly less morbidity and length of hospital stay when compared to sternotomy or thoracotomy.

REFERENCES

1. Wei B, Sonett JR, Lee JA, Sonett JR. Optimizing the minimally invasive approach to mediastinal parathyroid adenomas. *Ann Thorac Surg*. 2011;92(3):1012-1017.
2. Alesina PF, Moka D. Thoracoscopic removal of mediastinal hyperfunctioning parathyroid glands: personal experience and review of the literature. *World J Surg*. 2008;32:224-231.
3. Hu J, Ngiam KY. Mediastinal parathyroid adenomas and their surgical implications. *Ann R Coll Surg Engl*. 2015;97(4):259-261.
4. Fancy T, Gallagher D, Hornig JD. Surgical anatomy of the thyroid and parathyroid glands. *Otolaryngol Clin North Am*. 2010;43(2):221-227.
5. LoPinto M, Rubio, Khan ZF, Vaghaiwalla TM, Farra JC, Lew JI. Location of abnormal parathyroid glands: lessons from 810 parathyroidectomies. *J Surg Res*. 2017;20(7):22-26.
6. Sheldon DG, Lee FT. Surgical treatment of hyperparathyroidism improves health-related quality of life. *Arch Surg*. 2002; 137:1022-1028.
7. Wieneke, JA, Smith A. Parathyroid adenoma. *Head Neck Pathol*. 2008;2(4):305-308.
8. Lassen T, Friis-Hansen L. Primary hyperparathyroidism in young people. When should we perform genetic testing for multiple endocrine neoplastia 1 (MEN-1)? *J Clin Endocrinol Metab*. 2014;99(11):3983-3987.
9. Itaki M, Middleton W. Parathyroid imaging. *Radio Clin North Am*. 2020;58(6):1071-1083.
10. Norman JG, Jaffray CE. The false-positive parathyroid sestamibi. *Ann Surg*. 2000; 231(1):31.
11. Cordes M, Coerper S. Ultrasound imaging of cervical anatomic variants. *Curr Med Imaging*. 2021;17(8):966-972.
16. Du H, Shi M. Comparison of video-assisted thoracic surgery with open surgery in the treatment of ectopic mediastinal parathyroid tumors. *J Thorac Dis*. 2017;9(12):5171-5175.
12. Baj J, Sitarz R. Preoperative and intraoperative methods of parathyroid gland localization and the diagnosis of parathyroid adenomas. *Molecules*. 2020;25(7):1724.
13. Kumar A, Kumar S, Aggarwal S, et al. Thoracoscopy: the preferred method for excision of mediastinal parathyroids. *Surg Laparosc Endosc Percutan Tech*. 2002;12(4):295-300.
14. Whitman J, Allen IE. Assessment and comparison of 18F-Flurocholine PET and 99m Tc-Sestamibi scans in identifying parathyroid adenomas: a metaanalysis. *J Nucl Med*. 2021;62(9):1285-1291.
15. Clark O. Mediastinal parathyroid tumors. *Arch Surg*. 1988; 123:1096-1100.
17. Gorobeiko M, Dinets A. Intraoperative detection of parathyroid glands by autofluorescence identification using image-based system: report of 15 cases. *J Med Case Reports*. 2021;15(1):414.
18. Daliakopoulos SI, Chatzoulis G, Lampridis S, et al. Gamma probe-assisted excision of an ectopic parathyroid adenoma located within the thymus: case report and review of the literature. *J Cardiothorac Surg*. 2014;9:62.
19. Karpinski S, Sardi A. Thoracoscopic resection of a mediastinal intrathymic parathyroid adenoma. *Am Surg*. 2005;71(12): 1070-1072.

Adrenal Anatomy

41

Rafael Humberto Pérez-Soto, MSc
David Butrón-Hernández, MD
Miguel F. Herrera, PhD

INTRODUCTION

Since its first description by Bartolomeo Eustachius, the adrenal gland has fascinated the field of endocrinology and endocrine surgery due to its innate complexity regarding the inner structure and metabolic pathways. Although it is considered to be one anatomic gland, embryologically and functionally it is composed of two different structures, the adrenal cortex and the medulla, as described initially by Georges Cuvier in 1805.[1] Both structures play an important role in the organism's short- and long-term response to stress, as well as fluid volume, electrolyte concentrations, and blood pressure homeostasis. Table 41–1 summarizes historical milestones related to the adrenal gland.[1,2]

EMBRYOLOGY

The *adrenal gland cortex* and the kidney are embryologically related, as both emerge from the thoracolumbar mesoderm, known as the urogenital ridge. Around the fourth or fifth week of gestation, the adrenal-gonadal primordium rises in the form of epithelial cells from the celomic cavity, and mesonephric mesenchymal cells start to migrate (Figure 41–1A and B).[3,4] This first wave of migrating cells will form the primitive or fetal cortex. In the seventh week, a second wave of cells migrates to the adrenal-gonadal primordium to give rise to the secondary cortex, which will persist until adult age (adult cortex). This migration event explains the finding of ectopic adrenal cortex tissue around the urogenital system. Finally, connective tissue surrounds this group of cells to give shape to the adrenal gland cortex.[5] The adrenal cortex begins to function between the 24th and 28th gestational week.[6]

Around the seventh week of gestation, neural crest cells (chromaffin cells) from the celiac plexus sympathetic ganglion migrate to the adrenal primordium, becoming the *adrenal medulla*. Under pathologic conditions, tumors rising from remnants of these groups of cells (paraganglioma) may develop in the paraaortic region. This primitive adrenal medulla is progressively encapsulated by the adrenal cortex, a process that is completed by the end of gestation.[3,4]

Near the end of gestation, the adrenal glands develop the following zones: glomerulosa, transitory, and dominant fetal zone. Approximately 6 months after birth, the fetal cortex regresses and the adrenal gland reduces its size by a tenth, shaping the adult adrenal gland. The zona reticularis starts to develop sometime around 4 to 8 years of age and finishes development by 10 to 20 years of age.[6]

GROSS ANATOMY

The adrenal gland is a paired organ located in the retroperitoneal cavity, lateral to the diaphragmatic crura and anterior to the thoracic spine (T11 for the left and T12 for the right gland).[4] Typically, the right adrenal gland has a pyramidal shape, whereas the left is semilunar.[7] Both glands are approximately 5 × 3 × 1 cm in size, with an average weight of 4 to 7 g. Their dark yellowish color, granular surface, consistency, and surrounding connective tissue layer allow for easy identification within the perinephric fat.[4,8]

Relations

Immersed in the retroperitoneal and perirenal fat, the right adrenal gland relates to adjacent organs as follows: the right lobe of the liver and the inferior vena cava in the anterior aspect; posteriorly, the diaphragm and the ipsilateral psoas muscle; the bare area of the liver at the superior surface; and the upper pole of the right kidney inferiorly (Figure 41–2).[4,7] Regarding the left adrenal gland: the stomach, pancreas, and spleen are in contact with the anterior surface of the gland; the posterior surface contacts the left psoas muscle and the diaphragm; the spleen and the dome of the diaphragm are at the superior surface; and inferiorly the upper pole of the left kidney (Figure 41–3).[4,7] The knowledge of these

Table 41–1. Historical milestone regarding the adrenal gland.

1563	Discovery of the adrenal gland by **Eustachius**
1855	Description of Addison disease
1856	Importance of the adrenal gland, adrenalectomy by Brown-Sequard
1912	Adrenal gland atrophy after hypophysectomy (Ascoli and Legnani)
1930-1947	Steroid purification and structures
1960	Dexamethasone suppression test
1962	Nuclear action of steroid hormones
1969	Transcriptional properties of the steroid hormones
1985	Glucocorticoid receptor clonation
1987	Mineralocorticoid receptor clonation

anatomical relationships is important during the mobilization maneuvers needed to have access to the glands during the transabdominal surgical approach. For the retroperitoneoscopic approach, the upper pole of the kidney and the diaphragm are the most important landmarks for adrenal gland identification.

Arterial Supply

As with any endocrine tissue, the adrenal gland receives a generous amount of blood (approximately 5 mL per minute) to fulfill its metabolic needs. These blood volume requirements are supplied by three main arteries.[9] On the right side, the superior adrenal artery (SAA) is a terminal branch of the inferior phrenic artery (Figure 41–4B). On the left side, the SAA can emerge from the lateral margin of the abdominal aorta (AA) or the splenic artery. The middle adrenal artery (MAA) is a terminal branch of the AA, and it is more constant on the left side (Figure 41–4A). Eighteen percent of the time the MAA originates from an accessory renal artery on the right side and 6% on the left. The absence of the right MAA has been described in 29% of autopsy studies. Regarding the inferior adrenal artery (IAA), on the left side it arises 76% of the time from the ipsilateral renal artery, 18% from the gonadal artery, and 6% from the lateral margin of the AA. On the right side, the IAA originates from the ipsilateral renal artery in 59% of the cases, from the gonadal artery in 6%, and in 35% of the cases, it is absent.[10]

Each artery divides into 10 to 50 branches before entering the adrenal gland capsule, shaping the capsular plexus in proximity with the zona glomerulosa. The latter gives multiple straight capillaries that pass through the zona fasciculata, ending abruptly near the zona reticularis where they form a capillary sinusoid. This intraglandular vascular anatomy has two implications. First, the direction of the arterial circulation from the cortex to the medulla allows a biochemical communication between the two structures, an important mechanism for the conversion of norepinephrine to epinephrine in the medulla by glucocorticoid induction of the PMNT (phenyl ethanolamine *N* methyltransferase) enzyme. Second, this abrupt ending of the arterial circulation makes the adrenal gland prone to hemorrhagic necrosis, an event commonly associated with fungal and mycobacterial infectious diseases.[11]

Venous Drainage

The venous drainage of each adrenal gland depends largely on a single vein. Both veins (right and left) rise from a central adrenomedullary vein that forms from the junction of multiple collecting vessels from the gland cortex and medulla. On the right side, the adrenal vein is short (1-5 mm); it emerges from the gland apex and runs transversely to drain directly into the inferior vena cava on the posterolateral face. The length of the right adrenal vein has important implications during adrenal venous sampling (AVS), making the

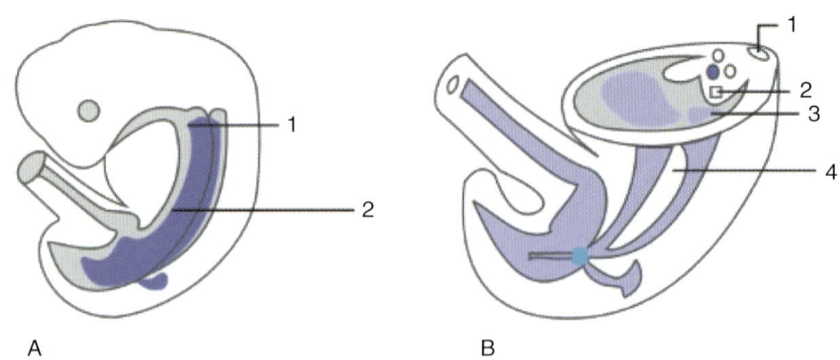

Figure 41–1. **(A)** Embryologic development of the adrenal gland (7th week): 1 mesonephros, 2 gonadal ridges. **(B)** View of an axial plane slide of the embryo: 1 spine, 2 adrenal cortex primordium, 3 urogenital ridge, 4 bowel mesentery.

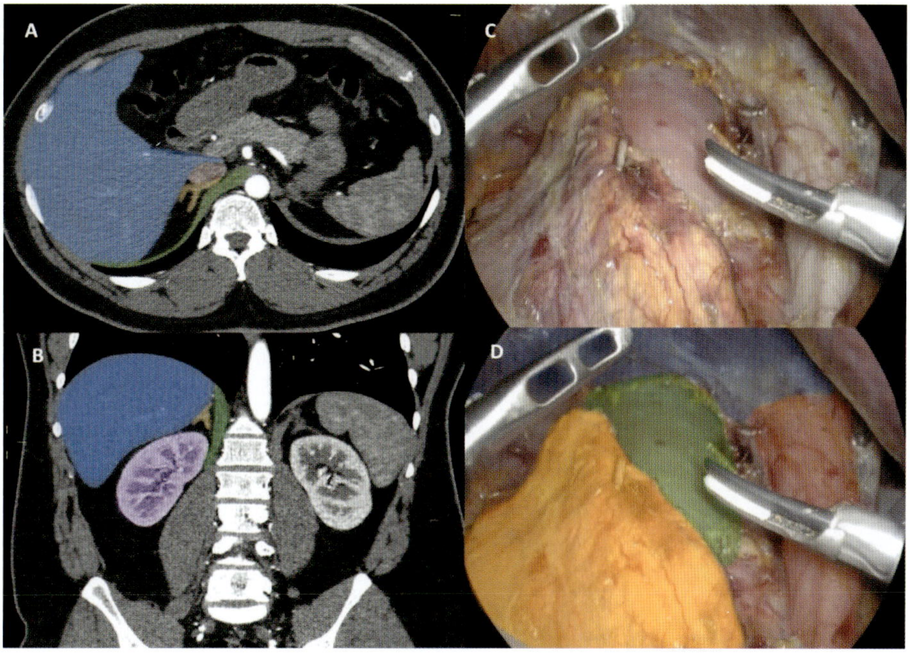

▲ **Figure 41–2.** Anatomic relations of the right adrenal gland. **(A)** CT-scan image on the axial axis plane. **(B)** CT-scan image on the coronal axis plane. **(C)** and **(D)** Laparoscopic view of the right adrenal gland and adjacent viscera. Light blue: right lobe of the liver; light purple: right kidney; light red: inferior vena cava; light green: right diaphragmatic crura and right psoas muscle; and light yellow: right adrenal gland.

canulation process difficult.[12] This anatomical feature also makes vein control challenging at surgery.

As for the left side, the adrenal vein is 2 to 4 cm long and runs posterior to the body of the pancreas to join with the left inferior phrenic vein to finally drain into the left renal vein. In addition, adrenal gland venous drainage also occurs through the small superficial capsular veins and retroperitoneal veins.[12] The latter could explain how adrenal cortical function is maintained after partial adrenalectomy with main adrenal vein ligation, as well as persistent variability of heart rate and blood pressure after adrenal vein ligation in patients who are being surgically treated for unilateral pheochromocytoma.

Despite these classic anatomic descriptions, some variations have been reported as a result of identification of adrenal vein anatomy at laparoscopic adrenalectomy in 546 patients. In 70 (13%) of these patients, an anatomic variation regarding the adrenal vein was found. Of these, 18 lacked a central adrenal vein, 11 had a central adrenal vein and multiple accessory veins, 20 had two adrenal veins, and 14 had more than two adrenal veins. Furthermore, seven patients had variants in relation to the hepatic vein, inferior vena cava, or the inferior phrenic vein. Identification of these variations through cross-sectional imaging could influence AVS and surgical treatment planning.[12]

Lymphatic Drainage

Microscopic studies have shown a total absence of lymphatic vessels in the adrenal cortex and medulla. Nevertheless, these can be found in the capsule and adventitia of the main central vein, draining the cortex but not the medulla. Interestingly, there is a close relationship between lymphatic vessels and large blood vessels. Given this fact, lymphatic drainage follows three pathways. On the right side, these vessels drain into the lateral aortic lymph nodes (passing through the lymph vessels of the right crus of the diaphragm and those proximal to the junction between the left renal vein and the inferior vena cava) and directly into the thoracic duct or the posterior mediastinal nodes. On the left side, two out of the three pathways drain into the left lateral aortic nodes, proximal to the celiac trunk and left renal vein, with the third pathway draining to the thoracic duct and posterior mediastinal nodes after perforating the diaphragm as on the right side.[13]

Innervation

Innervation of the adrenal medulla comes from preganglionic nerve fibers from the intermediolateral cell column of the lateral horn of the spinal cord. These nerves derive from the sympathetic visceral nervous system, which arises from

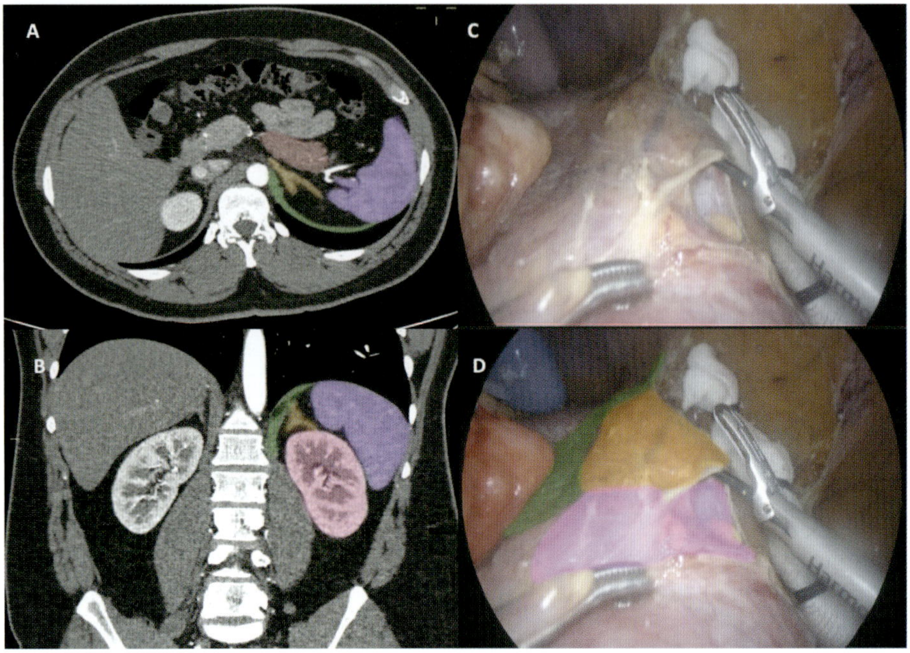

▲ **Figure 41–3.** Anatomic relations of the left adrenal gland. **(A)** CT scan image on the axial axis plane. **(B)** CT scan image on the coronal axis plane. **(C)** and **(D)** Laparoscopic view of the left adrenal gland and adjacent viscera. In light yellow: left adrenal gland; light green: left diaphragmatic crura and left psoas muscle; light red: tail and body of the pancreas; light purple: spleen; and light pink: left kidney.

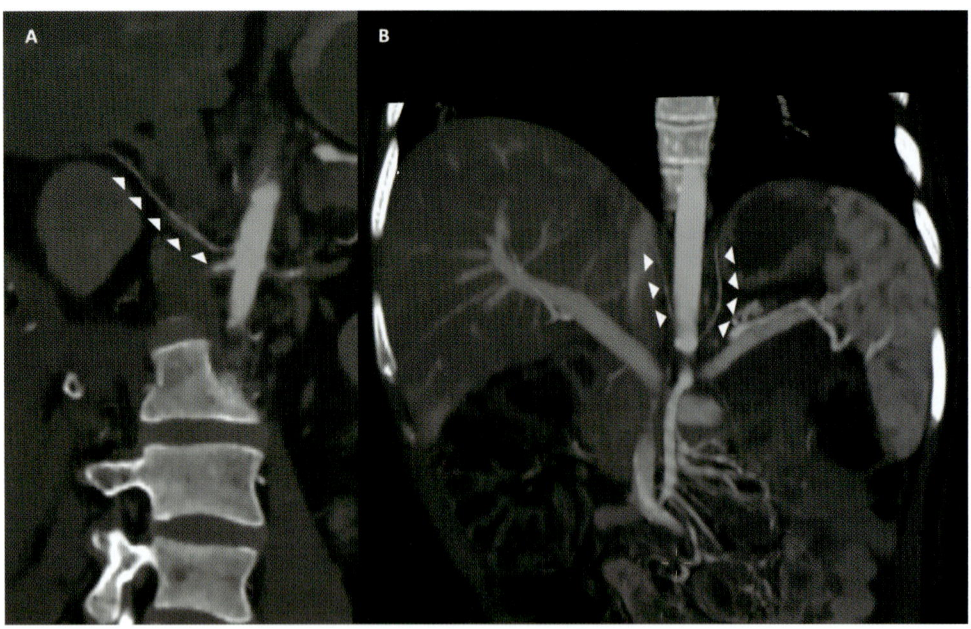

▲ **Figure 41–4.** Contrast-enhanced CT (CECT) arterial phase. **(A)** Multiplanar reconstruction shows adrenal artery arising from the abdominal aorta (white arrowheads). **(B)** MIP coronal CT shows right and left inferior phrenic arteries (white arrowheads) arising from the celiac artery.

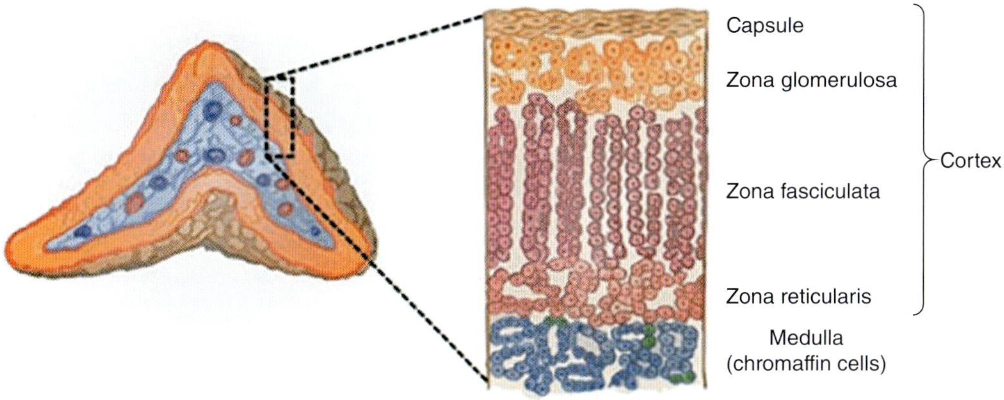

Figure 41–5. Adrenal gland gross and microscopic structure.

the celiac ganglia and connects with the posterior vagus nerve and greater and lesser splanchnic nerves.[4,8,9] From a functional standpoint, we can consider the adrenal medulla as part of the nervous system, working as a presynaptic sympathetic nerve that drives the acute stress response through cholinergic stimulation.

On the other hand, the adrenal cortex's main stimulation comes from a hormonal pathway via adrenocorticotropic hormone (ACTH). This pituitary hormone induces the synthesis of corticosteroids in the different zones of the adrenal cortex.[8]

MICROSCOPIC ANATOMY

Around 80% to 90% of the adrenal volume corresponds to the cortex, and the medulla constitutes the remaining 10% to 20% (Figure 41–5). Although its significance is not well understood, microscopically and functionally the adrenal cortex is organized in three zones: *zona glomerulosa (zG), zona fasciculata (zF), and zona reticularis (zR),* which display clear differences between their cellular structure and organization.[8,9] zG (the outermost layer) represents around 15% of the entire adrenal cortex. Typically, its cells show a central nucleus and a small foamy cytoplasm (lipid-rich) that is arranged in densely packed cellular clusters (glomeruli) surrounded by basement membrane proteins and a capillary network rising from the adrenal capsule. Regarding their ultrastructure, zG cells may show one or two nucleoli, the Golgi system is polarized toward the nearest blood vessel and the junction between cells is mediated through desmosomes and small gap junctions. zG is responsible for mineralocorticoid production and secretion is mediated by the renin-angiotensin-aldosterone system and serum potassium level changes.[14]

Around 80% of the adrenal cortex is represented by the zF. zF cells are organized in a cord-like structure surrounded by fenestrated blood vessels. These cells are larger than zG cells and have a more developed smooth endoplasmic reticulum (40%-50% of the cell volume) with a larger cytoplasm rich in lipid droplets and rounded mitochondria. Glucocorticoid production is the main function of the zone through ACTH stimulation.[14]

The most inner layer (5%-7% of the cortex) is the zR. Cells from zR show a central nucleus and eosinophilic cytoplasm with lipofuscin pigment, lysosomes, and less lipid droplets as compared with zF cells that arrange in large clusters. zR thickness is highly variable, as well as the vacuolation and lipid content of their cells. In addition, zR cells can migrate to the zF and secrete cortisol. Their main function is the synthesis of dehydroepiandrostenedione (DHEA) and the sulfated form of DHEA (DHEA-S) during fetal development and adrenarche.[14]

Regarding the adrenal medulla, its composition comes from rounded clusters of large and polyhedric chromaffin cells in close contact with capillaries and venules, connective tissue, and nerves. These cells are considered modified postganglionic sympathetic neurons that secrete catecholamines. Within this structure, two types of chromaffin cells can be identified using histochemical staining reactions: (a) chromaffin cells with granules storing norepinephrine, and (b) those storing epinephrine (representing 85% of all chromaffin cells). This disparity in epinephrine:norepinephrine cell ratio is due to the high activity of the PMNT enzyme within the adrenal medulla, which is stimulated directly by the high levels of glucocorticoids coming from the zF.[14]

REFERENCES

1. Miller WL. A brief history of adrenal research. *Mol Cell Endocrinol.* 2013;371(1-2):5-14.
2. Miller WL. The hypothalamic-pituitary-adrenal axis: a brief history. *Horm Res Paediatr.* 2018;89(4):212-223.
3. Ross IL, Louw GJ. Embryological and molecular development of the adrenal glands. *Clin Anat.* 2015;28(2):235-242.
4. Avisse C, Marcus C, Patey M, Ladam-Marcus V, Delattre JF, Flament JB. Surgical anatomy and embryology of the adrenal glands. *Surg Clin North Am.* 2000;80(1):403-415.

5. Barwick TD, Malhotra A, Webb JAW, Savage MO, Reznek RH. Embryology of the adrenal glands and its relevance to diagnostic imaging. *Clin Radiol.* 2005;60(9):953-959.
6. Kempná P, Flück CE. Adrenal gland development and defects. *Best Pract Res Clin Endocrinol Metab.* 2008;22(1):77-93.
7. Ritchie JE, Balasubramanian SP. Anatomy of the pituitary, thyroid, parathyroid and adrenal glands. *Surgery.* 2014;32(10):499-503.
8. Megha R, Wehrle CJ, Kashyap S, Leslie SW. Anatomy, abdomen and pelvis, adrenal glands (Suprarenal Glands). In: *StatPearls.* StatPearls Publishing; 2021. http://www.ncbi.nlm.nih.gov/books/NBK482264/. Accessed August 29, 2021.
9. Willenberg HS, Bornstein SR. Adrenal cortex; Development, anatomy, physiology. In: Feingold KR, Anawalt B, Boyce A, et al., eds. *Endotext.* MDText.com, Inc.; 2000. http://www.ncbi.nlm.nih.gov/books/NBK278945/. Accessed August 29, 2021.
10. Dutta S. Suprarenal gland-arterial supply: an embryological basis and applied importance. *Rom J Morphol Embryol.* 2010; 51(1):137-140.
11. Fowler AM, Burda JF, Kim SK. Adrenal artery embolization: anatomy, indications, and technical considerations. *Am J Roentgenol.* 2013;201(1):190-201.
12. Cesmebasi A, Du Plessis M, Iannatuono M, Shah S, Tubbs RS, Loukas M. A review of the anatomy and clinical significance of adrenal veins. *Clin Anat.* 2014;27(8):1253-1263.
13. Merklin RJ. Suprarenal gland lymphatic drainage. *Am J Anat.* 1966;119(3):359-374.
14. Pignatti E, Leng S, Carlone DL, Breault DT. Regulation of zonation and homeostasis in the adrenal cortex. *Mol Cell Endocrinol.* 2017;441:146-155.

Adrenal Physiology

Sara Abou Azar, MD
Courtney E. Gibson, MD, FACS

42

I. ADRENAL ANATOMY AND PHYSIOLOGY

INTRODUCTION

After the first description of adrenal gland anatomy by Bartolomeo Eustachius in the 1500s, many prominent scientists worked to establish its function and vitality, including Thomas Addison and Brown-Sequard.[1,2] Cuvier noted that the gland's outer and inner portions were different, and Nagel in 1836 coined the terms *cortex* and *medulla*.[3] However, it wasn't until 1852 when R.A. Von Kolliker microscopically characterized and defined the structure of the adrenal gland.[4] Embryologically, the adrenogonadal primordium, which is a collection of cells within the urogenital ridge, forms around 28 to 30 days postconception, as a result of increased expression of nuclear factor steroidogenic factor 1 (SF1, NR5A1).[4,5] Other involved pathways include the Hedgehog, Wnt, and ACTH/PKA signaling pathways, where adrenocorticotropin hormone (ACTH) becomes essential after the first trimester in the evolution of the adrenal gland.[4,5] The adrenal gland has dual embryologic origins: the medulla from the neural crest and the cortex from the intermediate mesoderm. The latter eventually encapsulates the medulla and differentiates into three zones: zona glomerulosa, zona fasciculata, and zona reticularis, each with different functions.[6]

ANATOMY

The adrenal gland is pyramidal in shape and usually lies in a suprarenal position. On the left side, it is more posteromedial while on the right, it is more anteromedial to the upper pole of the kidney.[4] The average weight of a normal gland is close to 4-6 g.[7,8] The outer cortex has a higher lipid concentration, and the inner medulla comprises about 15% of the gland.[4]

- Blood supply: Variations are quite common. There are three arteries that supply blood to the adrenal gland: the superior suprarenal artery (from the inferior phrenic artery), the middle suprarenal artery (from the abdominal aorta), and the inferior suprarenal artery (from the renal artery).[1,4] Some variants include arteries branching directly off the aorta, celiac axis, intercostal arteries, and superior mesenteric arteries.[9] As for the venous system, the left adrenal veins drain into the left renal vein, while the right adrenal vein drains directly into the inferior vena cava.[4] Variations also exist in the venous drainage of adrenal glands, such as double left adrenal veins.[10,11]
- Innervation: The adrenal gland has two forms of innervation—synaptic and hormonal. The anterior pituitary gland releases ACTH that acts on the adrenal cortical zones, leading to the activation of biochemical pathways depicted later in this chapter. Splanchnic nerve fibers are also believed to play a role in these pathways.[1] In addition, chromaffin cells in the adrenal medulla, once innervated by splanchnic fibers originating from the intermediolateral cell column of the spinal cord, secrete catecholamines leading to a sympathetic response.[12]

PHYSIOLOGY (FIGURE 42–1)

The adrenal Cortex has three functional zones. The zona glomerulosa (outer zone) is where mineralocorticoids are synthesized, including aldosterone (80-200 μg/day varies per salt consumption). The zona fasciculata (middle zone) is where glucocorticoids, such as cortisol (10-20 mg/day), which plays an important role in feedback for the hypothalamic-pituitary-adrenal (HPA) axis, are made. Finally, the zona reticularis (inner zone) is where androgens are produced, such as dehydroepiandrosterone (DHEA), which is a precursor for sex hormones.[4] The adrenal medulla, as noted previously, is where catecholamines are synthesized. L-tyrosine is enzymatically converted to L-DOPA then to dopamine, which can subsequently be converted to norepinephrine (noradrenaline) via dopamine β-hydroxylase and stored in

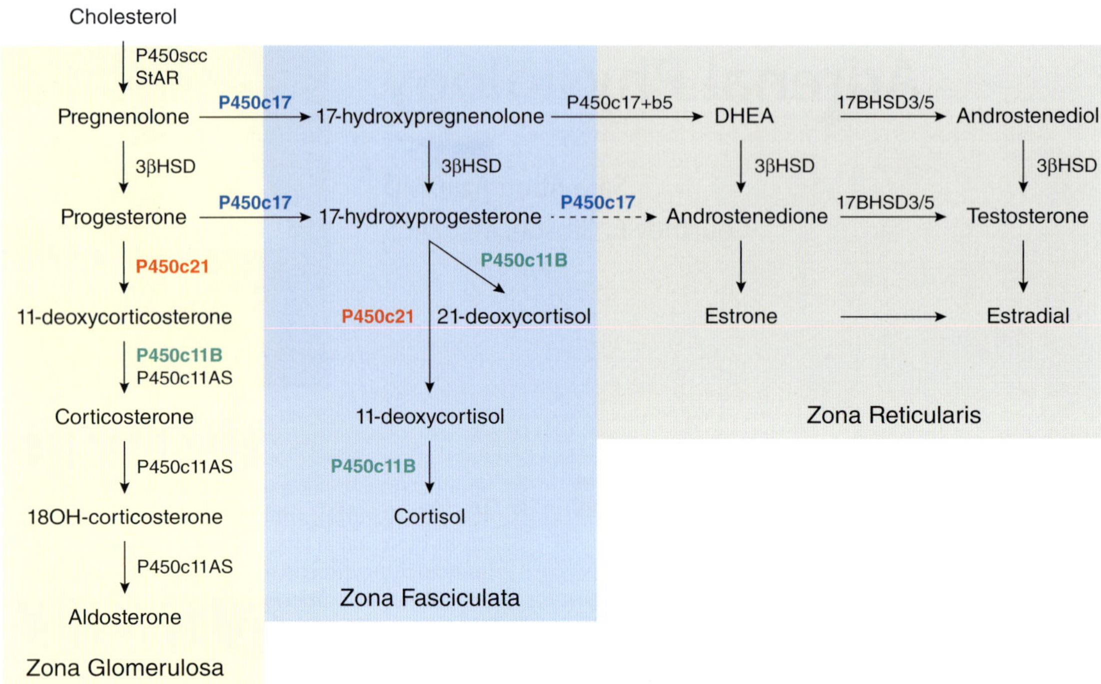

Figure 42–1. Steroidogenesis pathway within the three zones of the adrenal gland (zona glomerulosa, zona fasciculata, and zona reticularis). (Reproduced from Held PK, Bird IM, Heather NL. Newborn screening for congenital adrenal hyperplasia: review of factors affecting screening accuracy. *Int J Neonat Screen*. 2020;6(3):67.)

chromaffin cells. Phenylethanolamine *N*-methyltransferase (PNMT) converts norepinephrine to epinephrine (adrenaline) within the adrenal medulla.[13]

II. ADRENAL INCIDENTALOMA

DEFINITION/OVERVIEW

An adrenal incidentaloma is usually discovered on imaging meant to rule out other nonadrenal pathologies.[14,15] Its prevalence is reported at around 2% to 3% but varies between 1% and 8.7%.[15,16] This increases with age and in the elderly.[4,14] It is rare in young people (<40 years of age) and should prompt investigation to rule out malignancy.[17] There is no major difference in gender distribution and there is a similar distribution in terms of laterality, though some studies report a higher incidence of left-sided incidentalomas compared to right.[18] The frequency of the different types of adrenal incidentalomas can be seen in Table 42–1 below.

Genetic mutations have been implicated in both benign and malignant disease and different syndromes of hormonal excess have been linked to various mutations described in subsequent sections.

DIAGNOSIS/IMAGING

a. History and physical exam should be focused on identifying signs and symptoms of excess adrenal function and any familial disorders.[16] Depending on what part of the adrenal gland is involved and which pathways are functioning, symptoms can range from headaches, skin changes such as abdominal striae, to variations in blood pressure and the body's response to catecholamine surge, as well as an array of psychological disturbances.[19]
b. Laboratory evaluation is aimed at identifying the abnormality to target therapy.
   - In cases of suspected hypercortisolism, a serum ACTH level and a 24-hour urinary-free cortisol or midnight salivary cortisol levels are obtained. Low-dose dexamethasone suppression test can be performed either as a screening or confirmatory test for hypercortisolism. This will be discussed further under Cushing syndrome.[14,15]
   - In hypertensive patients, biochemical evaluation should include plasma aldosterone and renin levels as well as serum potassium levels to rule out primary hyperaldosteronism (though not all patients with this entity will have hypokalemia).[15,16,20] The ratio of plasma aldosterone concentration to plasma renin

Table 42–1. Frequency of the different types of adrenal incidentaloma.

Type	Average, %	Range, %
Clinical studies		
Adenoma	80	33-96
Nonfunctioning	75	71-84
Cortisol secreting	12	1.0-29
Aldosterone secreting	2.5	1.6-3.3
Pheochromocytoma	7.0	1.5-14
Carcinoma	8.0	1.2-11
Metastasis	5.0	0-18
Surgical studies		
Adenoma	55	49-69
Nonfunctioning	69	52-75
Cortisol secreting	10	1.0-15
Aldosterone secreting	6.0	2.0-7.0
Pheochromocytoma	10	11-23
Carcinoma	11	1.2-12
Myelolipoma	8.0	7.0-15
Cyst	5.0	4.0-22
Ganglioneuroma	4.0	0-8.0
Metastasis	7.0	0-21

Source: Reproduced with permission from Lee JM et al. Clinical Guidelines for the Management of Adrenal Incidentaloma. *Endocrinol Metab (Seoul)*. 2017;32(2):200-218.

activity is calculated. In primary hyperaldosteronism, the plasma renin activity is low (<1 ng/mL/h) and the plasma aldosterone concentration is high (>15 ng/dL) with a ratio more than 20.[21]

- Plasma-fractioned metanephrines and/or 24-hour urine-fractionated metanephrines and catecholamines are obtained to rule out pheochromocytoma.[15,22]
- Sex steroid hormonal levels, such as DHEA-S, androstenedione, testosterone, 17-OH-progesterone, and 17-B-estradiol are measured if there are signs of virilization, hirsutism, and other changes in secondary sex characteristics or concerns for carcinoma.[16,17]

c. Radiographic assessment: Computed tomography is usually the first-line imaging modality for assessing the adrenal gland. The mean diameter on CT varies among studies but is roughly 3 cm (0.8-23 cm),[23] with higher incidences of adrenocortical carcinoma in sizes exceeding 4 cm.[14,24] Hounsfield unit (HU) can help differentiate benign versus malignant tumors depending on the attenuation (< 10 for benign). If the Hounsfield unit reading is equal to or above 10, then washout of contrast at 15 minutes when greater than 60% indicates a higher likelihood of the tumor being benign. In addition, MRI with and without contrast can help differentiate benign from malignant tumors.[14,16]

SURVEILLANCE

Per ENSAT guidelines, for patients who have an incidentaloma but no indications for surgical intervention, recommendations include no follow-up for an adrenal mass less than 4 cm with benign features. For indeterminate lesions that do not undergo adrenalectomy, repeat imaging with CT or MRI is warranted at 6 to 12 months to monitor for an increase in size.[17]

III. SYNDROMES OF HORMONAL EXCESS

CUSHING SYNDROME

Definition/Overview

A plethora of clinical signs and symptoms have been described depending on chronicity and level of cortisol secretion, from subclinical to overt disease.[16] Common signs and symptoms in adults include obesity, moon facies, plethora, hirsutism, dorsal fat pad, high blood pressure, glucose intolerance, lethargy, menstrual irregularities, and decreased libido.[14,15] Striae, edema, proximal muscle weakness, skin atrophy, bruising, hyperpigmentation, osteopenia, acne, and female balding can also be seen in Cushing syndrome.[25-27] Increased cardiovascular risks have been documented in patients with Cushing syndrome due to the metabolic sequelae of this disease.[28] Causes include ACTH-independent Cushing syndrome, Cushing disease, ectopic ACTH syndrome, and other rare entities such as ectopic CRH production.[29] Pituitary adenomas are usually evident in Cushing disease, often as microadenomas and up to 10% being macroadenomas.[30,31] An increase in ACTH leads to bilateral adrenocortical hyperplasia and increased cortisol secretion.[32] ACTH-independent Cushing syndrome includes iatrogenic or factitious Cushing syndrome (exogenous corticosteroid use), adrenocortical tumors (functioning unilateral adrenal adenomas or carcinomas), bilateral macronodular adrenal hyperplasia (<2%), and primary pigmented nodular adrenocortical disease (~ 1%, sporadic and familial forms—Carney syndrome/complex).[33-35] Adrenal adenomas are responsible for around 10% to 20% of Cushing syndrome with a bimodal age distribution.[36] In some cases, cortisol hypersecretion is regulated by abnormal expression and activation of adrenal G-protein coupled receptors. Mutations in the G alpha subunit (GNAS) have been observed. Overt Cushing syndrome has been linked to somatic mutations of protein kinase A catalytic subunit (PRKACA).[36]

Laboratory Evaluation of Hypercortisolism

Initial workup can include starting with measurement of late-night salivary cortisol, measurement of 24-hour urinary free cortisol (UFC) excretion, or overnight 1 mg or two-day 2 mg dexamethasone suppression test.[14-16] In the overnight test, a 1 mg dexamethasone dose is given the evening before a fasting morning blood cortisol sample is collected. If no suppression (cortisol > 5 μg/dL) with low ACTH, then Cushing syndrome is confirmed. If incomplete suppression (cortisol 1.9-5 μg/dL) occurs, sub-clinical Cushing is suspected. If this test is positive, high dose dexamethasone suppression test can be used to differentiate between ACTH dependent and independent Cushing syndrome.[33] In the 2-day 2 mg test, the patient is given 0.5 mg of dexamethasone orally every 6 hours over 2 days (8 total doses), followed by serum cortisol measurement 6 hours from the final dose.[32,36] It is imperative to rule out other causes of excess physiologic hypercortisolism, including a pregnancy test, checking for polycystic ovary syndrome, stress, poorly controlled diabetes, or recent surgery/hospitalization.

Treatment

Surgical intervention is the first-line therapy for functioning unilateral adenomas or ectopic sites with resultant Cushing syndrome.[14,27] Medical treatment is usually reserved for bilateral disease and to control chronic cortisol excess, with bilateral adrenalectomy usually performed if medical management fails to control the hypercortisolism.[15,16] Medical treatment may include inhibition of steroidogenesis (ketoconazole, mitotane, metyrapone) or blockade of glucocorticoid receptor (mifepristone).[37]

PHEOCHROMOCYTOMA

Overview

Pheochromocytomas are catecholamine-secreting tumors, and chromaffin cells of the adrenal medulla are the cells of origin for this disease.[22] Catecholamine-secreting paragangliomas refer to a similar entity with its origin in the sympathetic and parasympathetic ganglia, that is, an extra-adrenal pheochromocytoma.[38] These tumors are rare, presenting most commonly in the fourth to fifth decade, with equal distribution between genders.[39] A larger proportion is noted on autopsy and may indicate underdiagnosis.[39] Patients usually present with headache, diaphoresis, and tachycardia. Almost half develop paroxysmal hypertension and rarely can present in crisis, with high-grade fever (> 40° C), altered mental status, labile blood pressure, and organ dysfunction.[39,40] Other rare findings include takotsubo stress-induced cardiomyopathy, orthostasis, visual disturbances, and others.[40] A small percentage may be asymptomatic.

Labs

Biochemical testing is performed to evaluate for abnormal catecholamine secretion. 24-hour urinary fractionated metanephrines and catecholamines and plasma fractionated metanephrines are measured 20 minutes after lying supine.[41] If normal, these labs are repeated while the patient is symptomatic. Levels greater than 3 times the upper limit of normal indicate the presence of a catecholamine-secreting tumor.[16,22]

Imaging

Following biochemical testing, imaging is utilized to localize the lesion. Abdominal CT scan or MRI are the modalities of choice (elevated Hounsfield units HU >10 on CT and enhancement on T2-weight MRI phase).[16,39] FDG or Dotatate PET scans are helpful in metastatic disease with a higher sensitivity than Metaiodobenzylguanidine (I-123 MIBG) scan.[15,22] It is recommended to avoid image-guided biopsy in suspected catecholamine-secreting tumors.[15]

Genetic Testing

Though most lesions are sporadic, hereditary tumors should be suspected in younger adults. Associated familial disorders include Von Hippel-Lindau syndrome (VHL tumor-suppressor gene on chromosome 3p25-26), neurofibromatosis type 1 (NF1), and multiple endocrine neoplasia type 2A and B (RET proto-oncogene on chromosome 10).[19,40] Other germline mutations have been described as well, with SDHB, SDHAF2, SDHC and SDHD variants seen in paragangliomas.[40] As such, all patients with catecholamine-secreting tumors should be monitored for signs of genetic disease and screened, especially in young patients and extra-adrenal pheochromocytomas.[14,16]

Perioperative Management

Per the Endocrine Society Clinical Practice guideline, preoperative alpha-blockers should be initiated 1 to 2 weeks prior to operation.[42] Phenoxybenzamine is usually started at 10 mg once or twice a day and uptitrated to achieve blood pressure control.[16] Selective alpha 1 adrenergic blocking agents such as prazosin, terazosin, or doxazosin can also be used.[40] Beta blockade may need to be added to the regimen if patients remain tachycardic after alpha blockade.[16] Propranolol and metoprolol are usually the agents of choice.[16,40] Metyrosine is a catecholamine synthesis inhibitor and can be used when alpha/beta blockade is not sufficient.[15,16] A high-salt diet and oral hydration to counteract catecholamine-induced volume contraction are a very important part of the preoperative regimen once alpha blockade has been initiated.[15,16,40] The key to success is a multidisciplinary approach and good communication with the anesthesia team preoperatively and intraoperatively.[14,16,39] In the setting of a hypertensive crisis, sodium nitroprusside, phentolamine, or nicardipine are good agents for control. Postoperative cardiac monitoring and glucose levels are encouraged.

A. Follow-up

Urine and plasma metanephrines can be checked at the postoperative follow-up visit (within 2-6 weeks) as well as annual testing to rule out recurrence or metastases in malignant cases.[14,16] For patients with persistently elevated biochemical testing postoperatively or preoperative normal levels, the European Society of Endocrinology recommends repeat imaging 3 months postoperatively.[22] Follow-up is encouraged for at least 10 years postoperatively in high-risk patients; those with familial disease will need lifelong follow-up.[16,22]

HYPERALDOSTERONISM

Overview

Up to 70% of patients with primary hyperaldosteronism have bilateral disease, while the remainder represent unilateral adenomas.[43] Mutations in ATP1A1, ATP2B3, CTNNB1, CYP11B1/CYP11B2 (familial hyperaldosteronism type I), CLCN2 (familial hyperaldosteronism type II), KCNJ5 (familial hyperaldosteronism type III), CACNA1H (familial hyperaldosteronism, type IV), CACNA1D, and ARMC5 can also be found.[43,44] Primary hyperaldosteronism remains underdiagnosed in the setting of hypertension and can be found in up to 20% of patients with resistant hypertension, that is, poorly controlled high blood pressure on three drug therapy.[45,46] The combination of hypertension and low serum potassium was classically described, but hypokalemia may not always be present.[16,21] As such, it is recommended to test for hyperaldosteronism in all patients with incidentalomas and elevated blood pressure.[14] Metabolic alkalosis can also be seen due to hydrogen excretion in the renal tubules in the setting of hypokalemia and hyperaldosteronism. This disease is also associated with an increase in cardiovascular morbidity and mortality.[46]

Labs

Testing should begin by measuring paired plasma renin activity (PRA) and plasma aldosterone concentration (PAC). PRA values of <1 ng/mL/h, PAC >15-20 ng/dL, or PAC/PRA ratio of >20-30 ng/dL per ng/mL/h are considered indicative of disease.[16,21] If PAC is ≥20 ng/dL, with evidence of hypokalemia and undetectable PRA, no further confirmatory tests are needed. Otherwise, a salt-loading test is performed by administering oral sodium chloride and measuring urine aldosterone excretion, or administration of intravenous sodium chloride and measuring PAC levels.[16,21,46]

Imaging & Treatment

Following confirmation of hyperaldosteronism, an adrenal CT scan should be obtained. In younger patients (<35 years of age), if a unilateral nodule is identified >1 cm in size, positive biochemical testing and surgery is desired, one should proceed with surgical resection, while in most other conditions, adrenal venous sampling (AVS) should be performed to lateralize the lesion.[21,46] AVS is a well-tolerated procedure with low risk for complications (estimated at <1%) though it may be technically challenging.[47] If unilateral disease is identified, then the next step is to proceed with unilateral adrenalectomy. If bilateral disease is found, then pharmacologic therapy with mineralocorticoid receptor blockade, such as eplerenone (selective antagonist) or spironolactone (nonselective antagonist with lower cost) is instituted.[21,46]

SEX-HORMONE SYNDROMES

Overview

Androgen and estrogen-secreting adrenal gland tumors are associated with malignancy and are overall rare. The European and American guidelines recommend against screening for sex hormones except if the patient presents with obvious clinical signs and symptoms.[14,16]

Labs

Measurement of serum dehydroepiandrosterone-sulfate (DHEA-S), testosterone, 17-hydroxyprogesterone and androstenedione levels can be performed.[14] Elevated DHEA-S (>700 μg/dL) should alert the presence of adrenal hyperandrogenism.[48]

Imaging and Treatment

As described earlier, CT and MRI are imaging modalities to localize adrenal lesions and differentiate between benign and malignant tumors. Surgery is the first-line therapy for sex-hormone-secreting adrenal tumors.

IV. SURGICAL MANAGEMENT OF ADRENAL DISEASE

MINIMALLY INVASIVE ADRENALECTOMY

Minimally invasive adrenalectomy was first introduced in the early 1990s and has since become the most widely used procedure for adrenal tumor resection. Michel Gagner defined the first laparoscopic adrenalectomy and it was quickly evident that this technique was associated with lower morbidity, as well as shorter hospital stay.[49,50] This was formally demonstrated in multiple studies comparing the open versus laparoscopic approach; for example, Thompson et al. early on showed that the laparoscopic approach was also associated with improved perioperative pain control, decreased length of hospital stay, and quicker recovery.[51] Mortality rates were not significantly different and better outcomes were directly correlated with high-volume centers.[49] Two main techniques have evolved and become widely used: the laparoscopic transabdominal and the posterior retroperitoneoscopic approach (PRA).[50] The transabdominal approach can be performed with the patient in either a supine or lateral position, whereas the patient is positioned either lateral or prone (jackknife) during an PRA.[49] The latter technique usually requires a higher CO_2 pressure on insufflation (~25 mmHg).

Laparoscopic Transabdominal

The lateral approach is the most commonly utilized approach due to improved exposure in the lateral decubitus position.[49] To increase the space between the costal margin and the anterior superior iliac spine, the patient is placed in a flexed position. Three ports are used in general, with a fourth one reserved for liver retraction (for right-sided tumors). On the left, the splenic flexure and spleen are mobilized medially, and the avascular plane lateral to the tail of pancreas and medial to the kidney is dissected to expose the adrenal bed. The adrenal vein is identified, clipped, and ligated. Then, the adrenal gland is dissected out circumferentially, generally using laparoscopic energy devices. On the right side, the right triangular ligament is taken down and the liver is mobilized and retracted for adequate exposure. The lateral edge of the IVC is dissected and the adrenal vein is identified, clipped, and ligated. Then, circumferential dissection of the adrenal gland proceeds, and the specimen is removed. The fully supine anterior approach is not widely used and may require more ports for access and single-port transabdominal adrenalectomies have been described and deemed safe in expert hands.[49]

Robotic Adrenalectomy

This technique gained wide use in the 2000s. Multiple studies have shown the benefit of this approach in obese patients with BMI more than 30 to 35 and in larger tumors, due to the known advantages of greater degree of freedom, ergonomics, and exposure.[49] This approach may be limited by a steep learning curve, longer operative times, and increased cost.

Retroperitoneoscopic Approach

Multiple studies have shown that the PRA approach is safe and comparable to the laparoscopic approach. In 2006, Walz et al. published their study that included 520 PRAs for adrenal disease including Cushing, adenomas, pheochromocytomas, and other tumors, and found there were no significant differences in perioperative major complications and mortality compared to the lateral laparoscopic approach.[52] Evans et al. again confirmed those findings in their cohort of 62 patients.[53] Chiu et al. looked at all adrenalectomies at a single tertiary center over a 7-year period with a total of 237 PRAs. Complication rates were lower than reported in the literature (under 7%), and mortality rates were less than 1% with a short hospital stay.[54] Modification of the conventional retroperitoneoscopic approach using single incision has been described with comparable outcomes.[55] In this chapter, we will describe the PRA approach used in our institution. The patient is placed in the jack-knife position, prone and flexed to increase the space between the 12th rib and the iliac crest. A 10 to 12 mm port is placed below the tip of the 12th rib and introduced into the retroperitoneal space. Blunt finger dissection is used to develop a cavity within that space. Two additional 5 mm ports are placed medially adjacent to the paraspinous muscles and laterally below the 11th rib. CO_2 insufflation to a pressure between 20 and 30 mmHg is established. The diaphragm, superior pole of the kidney, and spleen or liver (depending on side) are clearly identified. Then, a plane along the superior pole of the kidney is developed and dissection of the adrenal gland is undertaken first along the inferior aspect. The adrenal vein is identified coursing either to the IVC or left renal vein. We usually double clip the adrenal vein and divide it. Then, we proceed with circumferential dissection of the adrenal gland and ligate all tributaries of the adrenal arteries using the Harmonic scalpel. Once the entire gland is resected with its surrounding fat pad, a specimen-retrieval bag is used to remove it. Hemostasis is then achieved, the ports removed after de-sufflation, and the fascia is closed.

V. ADRENAL CORTICAL CARCINOMA (ACC)

ACCs are rare with peaks in early childhood and fourth to fifth decades of life, and it is more common in females than males.[56] They can be associated with hereditary syndromes such as Li-Fraumeni, Lynch, MEN 1, familial adenomatous polyposis (FAP), Carney complex, and Beckwith-Wiedemann syndrome.[56,57] Per the SEER database (2012-2018), 5-year relative survival rate for ACC approaches 50%, with poor prognosis in advanced metastatic disease (~38%).[58] It is recommended by multiple local and international guidelines that ACC should be managed in a multidisciplinary setting at a high-volume referral center.

Diagnosis

ACC can be asymptomatic or symptomatic, depending on the size and functional status (~60% present with Cushing syndrome).[57] Tumors measuring >4 cm on imaging with irregular margins and heterogenous consistency raise concern for malignancy.[16,57] On CT, tumors typically measure ≥10 HU, with a washout of <60%.[16,17] Imaging can also reveal adjacent lymphadenopathy, invasion into surrounding tissues/organs and/or intra-abdominal metastases. MRI can help identify locoregional tissue invasion when CT findings are inconclusive and assess resectability.[57] PET scans can be used as an additional workup for distant metastases. FDG PET can be helpful for staging and prognosis. Although less commonly used nowadays, metomidate (11C MTO) PET scan can aid in identifying ACCs due to higher tracer uptake, as it specifically binds to CYP11B enzymes.[56] Preoperative biopsy of ACC is generally not recommended. On pathology, classification systems exist, most notably the Weiss score that includes nine histological criteria, out of which at least three should be present. Markers, such as Ki-67 index and mitotic count, are helpful for prognostication and in deciding who may benefit from adjuvant therapy.[59]

Determinants of Resectability

Tumor staging of ACC follows the ENSAT TNM classification.[60] Prognosis depends on three main factors: staging, resection "R" status, and grade of tumor (Ki-67 and mitotic indices). Stage IV has <30% 5-year overall survival.[60] Achieving complete R0 radical resection is associated with an overall improved prognosis and is the mainstay of therapy when possible.[56,57,60,61] Tumor thrombus in the IVC or renal vein does not obviate resection as complete resection with vascular reconstruction may be feasible depending on extent of the thrombus.[60] If R0 is achieved, adjuvant therapy is dictated by stage and prognostic markers such as Ki-67 index to determine risk of recurrence. If high risk of recurrence or R1/R2/Rx, next step should be adjuvant therapy as indicated, such as mitotane or external beam radiotherapy.[60]

Management of Metastatic Disease

In cases of locoregional unresectable or metastatic disease, surgery can only be performed if able to remove the primary and metastatic lesions in an R0 fashion or in case of symptomatic palliation (debulking).[59] In most ACC patients who are eligible for systemic therapy, mitotane (oral adrenocorticolytic agent) alone or in combination with EDP is often initiated. Other additional therapy may include thermal ablative therapies (radiofrequency/microwave/cryo-ablation), liver-directed therapies, and/or immunotherapy.[60] Treatment with radiation can be considered for more advanced stages or with postoperative high-risk features such as positive margins, although definitive consensus was not reached in the 2018 ENSAT guidelines.[60] These cases should be approached individually and discussed in a multidisciplinary tumor board.

Operative Approach

Laparoscopy in the setting of ACC remains a controversial topic due to concern for local recurrence and poor oncologic outcomes in the past.[16] However, in the hands of experienced surgeons, smaller tumors without evidence of invasion can safely be resected with a minimally invasive approach.[56,60] Open adrenalectomy with complete en bloc resection, however, remains the mainstay approach for resection of ACC, especially for tumors >10 cm in size and radiographic evidence of invasive cancer.[16,59,60] The open anterior approach allows for wide resection, debulking, regional lymphadenectomy, and metastatectomy. Perioperative corticosteroids should be initiated to avoid adrenal insufficiency in functional ACC with hypercortisolism.[60]

Follow-up

This includes imaging and biomarker testing every 3 to 12 months for at least 5 years, then surveillance as indicated.

VI. METASTASIS TO THE ADRENAL GLAND

Metastatic disease to the adrenal glands is rare and often originates from the kidneys, lung, breast, skin (melanomas), lymphomas, and the gastrointestinal tract.[62] In the presence of known primary tumor and imaging findings, the diagnosis is achieved, and image guided biopsy, after ruling out pheochromocytoma biochemically, may be done if clinically indicated to decide on possible targeted treatment.[16] Decision for adrenalectomy is tailored to each patient in a multidisciplinary discussion to assess if this will prolong disease-free survival.[16,63]

REFERENCES

1. Nicolaides, N.C., et al., *Adrenal Cortex: Embryonic Development, Anatomy, Histology and Physiology*, in *Endotext*, K.R. Feingold, et al., Editors. 2000: South Dartmouth (MA).
2. Hiatt, J.R. and N. Hiatt, *The conquest of Addison's disease*. Am J Surg, 1997. **174**(3): p. 280-83.
3. Miller, W.L. and P.C. White, *A brief history of congenital adrenal hyperplasia*. Horm Res Paediatr, 2022. **95**(6): p. 529-45.
4. Sherlock, M., et al., *Adrenal Incidentaloma*. Endocr Rev, 2020. **41**(6): p. 775-820.
5. Kim, J.H. and M.H. Choi, *Embryonic development and adult regeneration of the adrenal gland*. Endocrinol Metab (Seoul), 2020. **35**(4): p. 765-73.
6. Xing, Y., et al., *Development of adrenal cortex zonation*. Endocrinol Metab Clin North Am, 2015. **44**(2): p. 243-74.
7. Studzinski, G.P., D.C. Hay, and T. Symington, *Observations on the weight of the human adrenal gland and the effect of preparations of corticotropin of different purity on the weight and morphology of the human adrenal gland*. J Clin Endocrinol Metab, 1963. **23**: p. 248-54.
8. Lam, K.Y., A.C. Chan, and C.Y. Lo, *Morphological analysis of adrenal glands: a prospective analysis*. Endocr Pathol, 2001. **12**(1): p. 33-8.
9. Priya, A., R.K. Narayan, and S.K. Ghosh, *Prevalence and clinical relevance of the anatomical variations of suprarenal arteries: a review*. Anat Cell Biol, 2022. **55**(4): p. 525-28.
10. Cesmebasi, A., et al., *A review of the anatomy and clinical significance of adrenal veins*. Clin Anat, 2014. **27**(8): p. 1253-63.
11. Scholten, A., et al., *Variant adrenal venous anatomy in 546 laparoscopic adrenalectomies*. JAMA Surg, 2013. **148**(4): p. 378-83.
12. Guerineau, N.C., *Cholinergic and peptidergic neurotransmission in the adrenal medulla: a dynamic control of stimulus-secretion coupling*. IUBMB Life, 2020. **72**(4): p. 553-67.
13. van Berkel, A., J.W. Lenders, and H.J. Timmers, *Diagnosis of endocrine disease: biochemical diagnosis of phaeochromocytoma and paraganglioma*. Eur J Endocrinol, 2014. **170**(3): p. R109-19.

14. Fassnacht, M., et al., *Management of adrenal incidentalomas: European Society of Endocrinology Clinical Practice Guideline in collaboration with the European Network for the Study of Adrenal Tumors*. Eur J Endocrinol, 2016. **175**(2): p. G1-G34.
15. Lee, J.M., et al., *Clinical guidelines for the management of adrenal incidentaloma*. Endocrinol Metab (Seoul), 2017. **32**(2): p. 200-218.
16. Zeiger, M.A., et al., *American Association of Clinical Endocrinologists and American Association of Endocrine Surgeons Medical Guidelines for the Management of Adrenal Incidentalomas: executive summary of recommendations*. Endocr Pract, 2009. **15**(5): p. 450-53.
17. Fassnacht, M., et al., *European Society of Endocrinology clinical practice guidelines on the management of adrenal incidentalomas, in collaboration with the European Network for the Study of Adrenal Tumors*. Eur J Endocrinol, 2023. **189**(1): p. G1-G42.
18. Barzon, L., et al., *Prevalence and natural history of adrenal incidentalomas*. Eur J Endocrinol, 2003. **149**(4): p. 273-85.
19. Farrugia, F.A., et al., *A step by step approach in differential diagnosing of adrenal incidentaloma (epinephroma), (with comments on the new Clinical Practice Guidelines of the European Society of Endocrinology)*. Rom J Intern Med, 2017. **55**(4): p. 188-97.
20. Tezuka, Y., et al., *Recent development toward the next clinical practice of primary aldosteronism: a literature review*. Biomedicines, 2021. **9**(3).
21. Wachtel, H. and D.L. Fraker, *Therapeutic outcomes with surgical and medical management of primary aldosteronism*. Curr Cardiol Rep, 2021. **23**(7): p. 89.
22. Plouin, P.F., et al., *European Society of Endocrinology Clinical Practice Guideline for long-term follow-up of patients operated on for a phaeochromocytoma or a paraganglioma*. Eur J Endocrinol, 2016. **174**(5): p. G1-G10.
23. Shah, A.N., et al., *Adrenal incidentaloma needs thorough biochemical evaluation: an institutional experience*. Indian J Endocrinol Metab, 2022. **26**(1): p. 73-78.
24. Vural, V., et al., *Association between tumor size and malignancy risk in hormonally inactive adrenal incidentalomas*. Cureus, 2020. **12**(1): p. e6574.
25. Lefkowitz, E.G., J.P. Cossman, and J.B. Fournier, *A case report of Cushing's disease presenting as hair loss*. Case Rep Dermatol, 2017. **9**(1): p. 45-50.
26. Sharma, S.T., L.K. Nieman, and R.A. Feelders, *Cushing's syndrome: epidemiology and developments in disease management*. Clin Epidemiol, 2015. **7**: p. 281-93.
27. Nieman, L.K., et al., *The diagnosis of Cushing's syndrome: an Endocrine Society Clinical Practice Guideline*. J Clin Endocrinol Metab, 2008. **93**(5): p. 1526-40.
28. Fleseriu, M., et al., *Consensus on diagnosis and management of Cushing's disease: a guideline update*. Lancet Diabetes Endocrinol, 2021. **9**(12): p. 847-75.
29. Balomenaki, M., et al., *Diagnostic workup of Cushing's syndrome*. J Neuroendocrinol, 2022. **34**(8): p. e13111.
30. Lonser, R.R., L. Nieman, and E.H. Oldfield, *Cushing's disease: pathobiology, diagnosis, and management*. J Neurosurg, 2017. **126**(2): p. 404-417.
31. Hakami, O.A., S. Ahmed, and N. Karavitaki, *Epidemiology and mortality of Cushing's syndrome*. Best Pract Res Clin Endocrinol Metab, 2021. **35**(1): p. 101521.
32. Raff, H. and T. Carroll, *Cushing's syndrome: from physiological principles to diagnosis and clinical care*. J Physiol, 2015. **593**(3): p. 493-506.
33. Newell-Price, J., et al., *The diagnosis and differential diagnosis of Cushing's syndrome and pseudo-Cushing's states*. Endocr Rev, 1998. **19**(5): p. 647-72.
34. Bouys, L., et al., *Update on primary bilateral macronodular adrenal hyperplasia (PBMAH)*. Endocrine, 2021. **71**(3): p. 595-603.
35. Liu, X., et al., *Treatment of primary pigmented nodular adrenocortical disease*. Horm Metab Res, 2022. **54**(11): p. 721-30.
36. Stratakis, C.A., *Cushing syndrome caused by adrenocortical tumors and hyperplasias (corticotropin-independent Cushing syndrome)*. Endocr Dev, 2008. **13**: p. 117-32.
37. Pivonello, R., et al., *The treatment of Cushing's disease*. Endocr Rev, 2015. **36**(4): p. 385-486.
38. Pacak, K., *Phaeochromocytoma: a catecholamine and oxidative stress disorder*. Endocr Regul, 2011. **45**(2): p. 65-90.
39. Farrugia, F.A. and A. Charalampopoulos, *Pheochromocytoma*. Endocr Regul, 2019. **53**(3): p. 191-212.
40. Lenders, J.W.M., et al., *Genetics, diagnosis, management and future directions of research of phaeochromocytoma and paraganglioma: a position statement and consensus of the Working Group on Endocrine Hypertension of the European Society of Hypertension*. J Hypertens, 2020. **38**(8): p. 1443-56.
41. Lenders, J.W., et al., *Biochemical diagnosis of pheochromocytoma: which test is best?* JAMA, 2002. **287**(11): p. 1427-34.
42. Lenders, J.W., et al., *Pheochromocytoma and paraganglioma: an endocrine society clinical practice guideline*. J Clin Endocrinol Metab, 2014. **99**(6): p. 1915-42.
43. Rege, J., A.F. Turcu, and W.E. Rainey, *Primary aldosteronism diagnostics: KCNJ5 mutations and hybrid steroid synthesis in aldosterone-producing adenomas*. Gland Surg, 2020. **9**(1): p. 3-13.
44. Itcho, K., et al., *Update on genetics of primary aldosteronism*. Biomedicines, 2021. **9**(4).
45. Garcia, E.A., et al., *Resistant hypertension and undiagnosed primary hyperaldosteronism detected by use of a computerized database*. J Clin Hypertens (Greenwich), 2011. **13**(7): p. 487-91.
46. Funder, J.W., et al., *The management of primary aldosteronism: case detection, diagnosis, and treatment: an Endocrine Society Clinical Practice Guideline*. J Clin Endocrinol Metab, 2016. **101**(5): p. 1889-916.
47. Quencer, K.B., *Adrenal vein sampling: technique and protocol, a systematic review*. CVIR Endovasc, 2021. **4**(1): p. 38.
48. Sharma, A. and C.K. Welt, *Practical approach to hyperandrogenism in women*. Med Clin North Am, 2021. **105**(6): p. 1099-1116.
49. Stefanidis, D., et al., *SAGES guidelines for minimally invasive treatment of adrenal pathology*. Surg Endosc, 2013. **27**(11): p. 3960-80.
50. Tanaka, M., et al., *Guidelines for urological laparoscopic surgery*. Int J Urol, 2009. **16**(2): p. 115-25.
51. Thompson, G.B., et al., *Laparoscopic versus open posterior adrenalectomy: a case-control study of 100 patients*. Surgery, 1997. **122**(6): p. 1132-36.
52. Walz, M.K., et al., *Posterior retroperitoneoscopic adrenalectomy–results of 560 procedures in 520 patients*. Surgery, 2006. **140**(6): p. 943-48; discussion 948-50.
53. Perrier, N.D., et al., *Posterior retroperitoneoscopic adrenalectomy: preferred technique for removal of benign tumors and isolated metastases*. Ann Surg, 2008. **248**(4): p. 666-74.
54. Chiu, A., et al., *Contemporary experience of posterior retroperitoneoscopic adrenalectomy in the US*. J Am Coll Surg, 2021. **232**(6): p. 815-21.
55. Sho, S., et al., *Single-incision retroperitoneoscopic adrenalectomy: a North American experience*. Surg Endosc, 2017. **31**(7): p. 3014-19.

56. Libe, R., *Adrenocortical carcinoma (ACC): diagnosis, prognosis, and treatment.* Front Cell Dev Biol, 2015. **3**: p. 45.
57. Benassai, G., et al., *Adrenocortical carcinoma: what the surgeon needs to know. Case report and literature review.* Int J Surg, 2014. **12 Suppl 1**: p. S22-8.
58. SEER*Explorer. *An interactive website for SEER cancer statistics [Internet]. Surveillance Research Program, National Cancer Institute.* [cited 2023 February 23]; Available from: https://seer.cancer.gov/explorer/.
59. Gaujoux, S., et al., *European Society of Endocrine Surgeons (ESES) and European Network for the Study of Adrenal Tumours (ENSAT) recommendations for the surgical management of adrenocortical carcinoma.* Br J Surg, 2017. **104**(4): p. 358-76.
60. Fassnacht, M., et al., *European Society of Endocrinology Clinical Practice Guidelines on the management of adrenocortical carcinoma in adults, in collaboration with the European Network for the Study of Adrenal Tumors.* Eur J Endocrinol, 2018. **179**(4): p. G1-G46.
61. Anderson, K.L., Jr., et al., *Impact of Micro- and macroscopically positive surgical margins on survival after Resection of Adrenocortical Carcinoma.* Ann Surg Oncol, 2018. **25**(5): p. 1425-31.
62. Lam, K.Y. and C.Y. Lo, *Metastatic tumours of the adrenal glands: a 30-year experience in a teaching hospital.* Clin Endocrinol (Oxf), 2002. **56**(1): p. 95-101.
63. Yip, L., et al., *American Association of Endocrine Surgeons Guidelines for Adrenalectomy: Executive Summary.* JAMA Surg, 2022. **157**(10): p. 870-77.

43

Adrenal Incidentaloma

Dimitrios A. Linos, MD, PhD

ADRENAL INCIDENTALOMA

Introduction

An adrenal tumor ≥1 cm in diameter discovered incidentally, usually during an imaging procedure (CT, MRI, ultrasound) for symptoms unrelated to adrenal disease (eg, back pain) is called an incidentaloma. Other terms such as "Adrenaloma" or "Clinically inapparent adrenal mass" have been coined but the term adrenal incidentaloma (AI) has prevailed. Adrenal tumors discovered during the evaluation and follow-up for nonadrenal cancers as well as screening and surveillance of hereditary syndromes are not considered incidentalomas. The unexpected discovery of an AI raises two questions. Is this lesion malignant? Is this lesion producing an excess of any of the known adrenal hormones?

Epidemiology

The prevalence of AIs remains around 5% among adults. In autopsy studies, the reported prevalence ranges from 1% to 8.7%. Over the last 20 years, by using a high-resolution modern CT scan equipment, the prevalence of AIs has increased from 1% to 5%. Autopsy and imaging studies have shown that the prevalence of AIs increases with age with a peak incidence in the fifth to seventh decades. An adrenal tumor discovered at a younger age requires prompt evaluation to rule out malignancy or a functioning tumor. Literature has shown that AIs can be bilateral in 10% to 20% of patients.[1]

Pathology

On pathology, most surgically removed AIs are cortical adenomas. Benign masses, such as nodular hyperplasia, adrenal cysts, myelolipomas, ganglioneuromas, hamartomas, hemangiomas, leiomyomas, neurofibromas, teratomas, as well as infection processes (mycobacterial, fungal, parasitic or bacterial), have also been discovered after removal of nonfunctional AIs.[2]

Pheochromocytomas and primary adrenal carcinomas have been reported in up to 10% and 5% of patients, respectively, supporting a thorough investigation of AIs when they are identified (Figure 43–1).[3]

Bilateral adrenal masses can include metastatic disease, congenital adrenal hyperplasia, cortical adenomas, bilateral macronodular hyperplasia, and ACTH-dependent Cushing's. Occasionally, in patients with bilateral disease, one adrenal mass is functioning while the contralateral mass is nonfunctioning. Therefore, all AIs—unilateral and bilateral—should be evaluated for possible subclinical function.[4]

Screening for "Subclinical Cushing Syndrome"

Subclinical Cushing syndrome, described also as minimal autonomous cortisol secretion (MACS), is the most frequent hormonal abnormality discovered in patients with AIs with prevalence rates up to 20%. Despite the absence of the usual symptoms and signs of overt Cushing syndrome, patients with AIs and MACS have been documented to have a higher incidence of hypertension, insulin resistance, type 2 diabetes mellitus, obesity, and metabolic syndrome. More specifically, patients with MACS present with moderate hypertension in 41% to 92% of cases. In addition, they present with a higher prevalence of cardiovascular events compared to patients with nonfunctional AI, and increased rates of cardiovascular morbidity (43% vs 8.8%) and mortality (22.6% vs 2.5%) have been reported with 15 years of follow-up.

Impaired glucose tolerance or diabetes occurs in 10% to 69% of patients with MACS. Interestingly, there have been several studies describing reversal of hypertension and diabetes following surgical treatment of subclinically functioning or even "nonfunctioning" AIs.

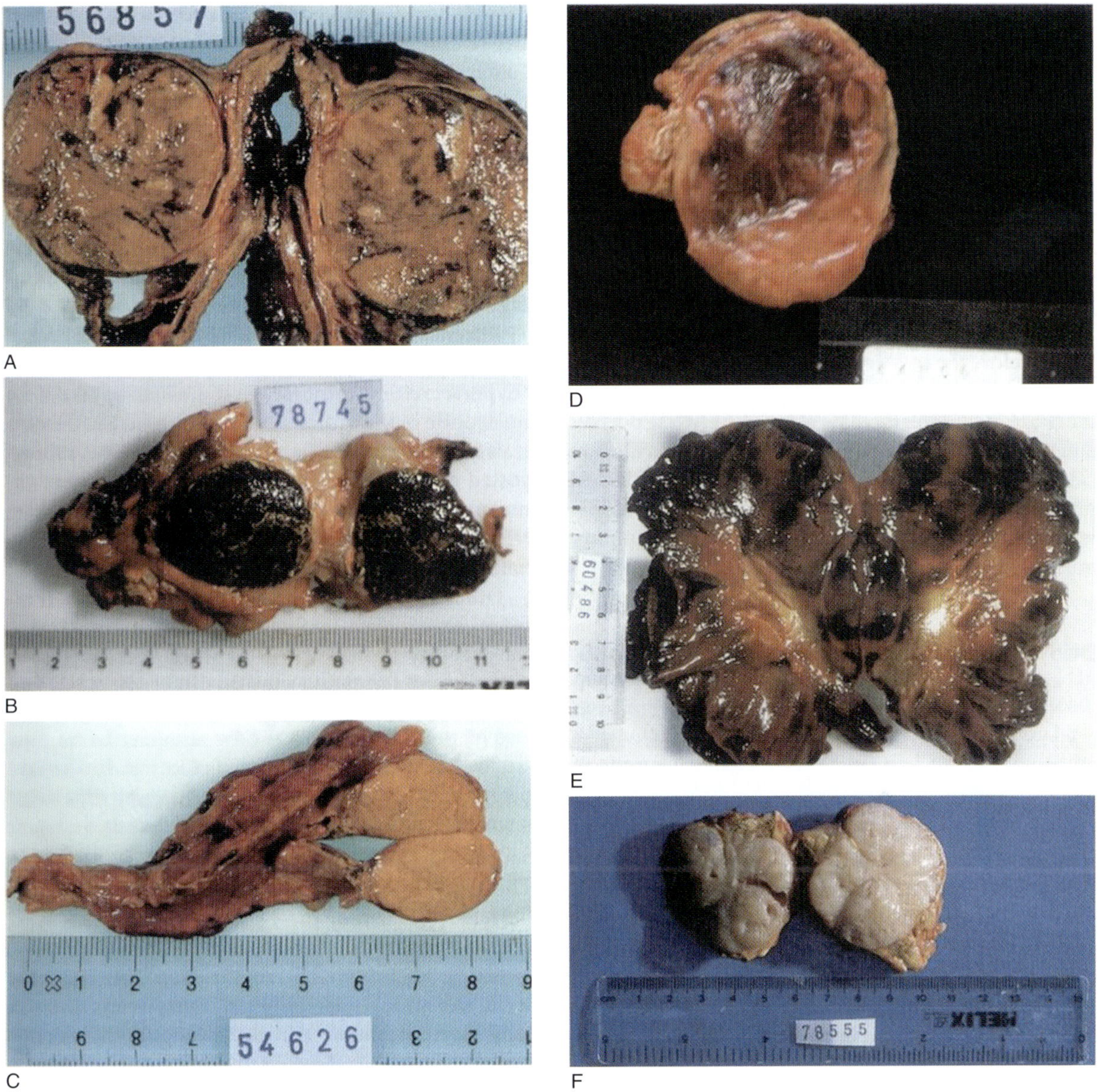

Figure 43–1. Adrenal incidentalomas with different pathology and clinical behavior. **(A)** Cortical adenoma in a 37-year-old female with subclinical Cushing syndrome and metabolic syndrome significantly improved after surgery. **(B)** Cortical adenoma in a 40-year-old male that over 3 years of follow-up turned from "nonfunctioning" to overt Cushing syndrome. **(C)** Aldosteronoma in a 45-year-old hypertensive but normokalemic male followed for years for this 2.5 cm "incidental" mass. **(D)** Pheochromocytoma in a 32-year-old asymptomatic normotensive female. **(E)** "Indolent" myelolipoma that ruptured during its follow-up causing severe intra-abdominal bleeding in a 27-year-old male. **(F)** Solitary metastatic carcinoma, 10 years after hysterectomy for cervical cancer in a 62-year-old female. (Reproduced with permission from Linos DA. *Adrenal Glands: Diagnostic Aspects and Surgical Therapy*. Heidelberg: Springer-Verlag, 2005: 243.)

In patients with subclinical Cushing syndrome, trabecular and cortical bone loss have been described, as well as a higher rate of bone fracture. A meta-analysis reported a prevalence of 63.6% of vertebral fracture in patients with MACS and this risk was independent of age, sex, gonadal status, or bone mineral density.

The best test to rule out autonomous cortisol production from an AI remains the overnight dexamethasone (1 mg) suppression test (the Pavlatos Test). A suppressed morning serum cortisol (<1.8 μγ/dL or <50 nmol/L) excludes MACS. A level of more than 1.8 μg/dL has high sensitivity (95%-100%) but low specificity (60%-80%), whereas a level of more than 5.0 μg per deciliter (>138 nmol/L) has lower sensitivity (86%) but higher specificity (92%-97%). Additional tests may include measurements of morning serum corticotropin and cortisol levels, 24-hour urinary cortisol, late-night salivary cortisol, midnight serum cortisol, and dehydroepiandrosterone sulfate (DHEAS).

Screening for "Subclinical Primary Aldosteronism"

Primary aldosteronism has been found in 1.6% to 5.5% of cases of AIs. These patients typically do not have a classic clinical picture of hypertension and hypokalemia. They can be normotensive and may have spontaneous hypokalemia, or they may have normokalemia with hypertension. A recent multicenter study has estimated that only 9% to 37% of patients with primary aldosteronism were hypokalemic. All patients with AI and a history of hypertension or hypokalemia should undergo measurements of mid-morning plasma aldosterone concentration and plasma renin activity. A ratio of the plasma aldosterone concentration to plasma renin activity that is higher than 20 is considered a positive test for the presence of the disease. If the ratio is high but below 20, further confirmatory tests are needed, such as measurement of 24-hour urinary aldosterone excretion while the patient is receiving a high sodium diet.

It should be noted that primary aldosteronism is associated with an increased risk of stroke, coronary artery disease, atrial fibrillation, heart failure, and mortality compared with matched patients with essential hypertension. Thus, a detailed screening for primary aldosteronism should be performed in all small-size AIs which may be described as "nonfunctioning" lesions on imaging reports.

Screening for "Subclinical Pheochromocytoma"

Among patients with AI, pheochromocytoma is found in 10% of cases ranging in different studies from 1.5% to 40%, though it is likely to be closer to the lower figure. It is known that up to 15% of patients with pheochromocytoma have normal blood pressure at presentation, so the term subclinical pheochromocytoma applies to patients without classical symptoms of paroxysmal sweating, headache, hypertension, and tachycardia. Patients with familial pheochromocytoma may be asymptomatic in 50% of cases.

All patients with AI should have measurements of plasma-free metanephrines and/or a 24-hour urinary fractionated metanephrine levels.

False positive findings may be found in patients who are in distress or have severe illness requiring hospitalization. Medications also may cause false positive test results, such as sympathomimetic drugs or substances that interfere with the hormonal assays such as caffeine or amphetamines. For plasma-free metanephrines, blood should be drawn after resting for at least 30 minutes. For 24-hour urine estimation, the use of acidified containers (to achieve urine pH <4) and storage in the refrigerator is recommended.

Small pheochromocytomas (eg, <1.5 cm) may have normal biochemical testing. Pheochromocytomas need to achieve a critical mass before they become biochemically detectable.

Screening for Adrenal Carcinoma

A primary adrenocortical carcinoma or less often, a primary carcinoma arising from the adrenal medulla or metastatic carcinoma to the adrenal gland, can present as an AI. Studies have reported that 1.2% to 11% of AIs prove to be carcinomas. The size of the incidentaloma and its imaging features are important determinants of the likelihood of cancer and inform subsequent management.

A. Size of Tumor

The risk of adrenocortical carcinoma is less than 2% among patients with incidentalomas smaller than 4 cm in diameter, 6% among those with tumors between 4 cm and 6 cm in diameter, and 25% or higher among those with tumors larger than 6 cm in diameter. In several series, adrenocortical carcinomas with a maximum diameter of 3 cm or less have been described. Similarly, large adrenal tumors that appeared to be suspicious for malignancy on CT scan, turned out to be benign on the final histology (Figure 43–2).

When a cut-off size of 4 cm is used to recommend surgery for an AI one should consider two additional facts. First, the age of the patient. An AI less than 4 cm in a patient who is younger than 40 years of age carries a high probability of cancer. Second, the size of an AI reported by the CT scan is usually less than the real size of the tumor reported on the final pathology. This underestimation of the size ranges from 16% to 47%. The formula "Histologic size = 0.85 + (1.0 + 9 × CT size)" can be used to correct the CT scan size and predict the real histological tumor size. An independent study from Mexico showed that the above-mentioned "Linos formula" is significantly more accurate than the direct radiological measurements in the prediction of the real pathological size of the tumor.

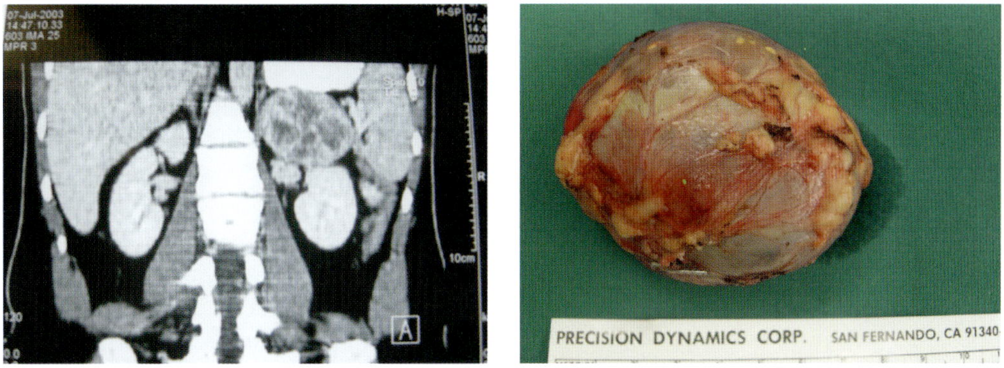

A B

▲ **Figure 43–2.** A larger than 6 cm adrenal incidentaloma was suspicious for malignancy on CT scan **(A)** but histologically proved to be a benign cortical tumor **(B)**. (Reproduced with permission from Linos DA. *Adrenal Glands: Diagnostic Aspects and Surgical Therapy*. Heidelberg: Springer-Verlag, 2005:246.)

Imaging Studies

A. Computed Tomography

The computed tomography (CT) scan not only measures the size of the tumor, but can differentiate a benign lesion from a malignant AI. Features such as irregular tumor margins, heterogeneity, necrosis, vascularity, and calcifications raise suspicion of malignancy. An attenuation of 10 Hounsfield units (HU) or less on unenhanced CT is consistent with a benign lesion. All AIs with an attenuation of >10 HU need to have follow-up imaging including a contrast-enhanced CT scan measuring the percentage of contrast washout at different times.

Features of benign tumors include rapid enhancement and prompt washout of intravenous contrast. Malignant tumors usually enhance rapidly but demonstrate a slower washout of contrast medium. Dual- or multiple-energy CT scan can provide additional specific data about attenuation properties of different materials at different energies.

B. Magnetic Resonance Imaging

Magnetic resonance imaging (MRI) with chemical shift imaging can be used if a CT scan is not desirable, for example during pregnancy, in children, and in patients with allergies to iodinated contrast. Visual analysis and quantitative analysis of adrenal signal intensity index and adrenal-to-spleen ratio have high accuracy for identifying lipid-rich AIs.

C. Positron Emission Tomography—Computed Tomography

A meta-analysis of 29 studies involving 2421 patients showed that FDG PET-CT has a high diagnostic accuracy for characterization of adrenal masses with pooled sensitivity of 91% and specificity of 91%. This technique has the ability to identify malignant adrenal nodules and is able to discriminate metastatic disease from benign masses in patients with known malignancy. Nevertheless, some functional AIs, nonmetastatic pheochromocytomas, and ganglioneuromas can be FDG positive (Figure 43–3).[5]

D. Measurement of Sex Hormones and Steroid Precursors

It has been shown that steroid profiling by gas chromatography mass spectrometry (GC-MS) of 24-hour urine samples has diagnostic value in discriminating benign and malignant adrenal tumors. Because urine collection is more time consuming and prone to sampling errors, the liquid chromatography-tandem mass spectrometry (LC-MS/MS) for measurement of sex steroids and steroid precursors, such as androstenedione, testosterone, DHEA-S, and 17β estradiol, is used more frequently for the evaluation of an AI suspicious for cancer. These hormones can also be used as tumor markers after surgical removal of the tumor when they are positive.

E. Adrenal Biopsy

Biopsy of an AI is not indicated because it has a low accuracy for distinguishing benign from malignant lesions and may lead to tumor seeding if the mass is an adrenocortical carcinoma, or a hypertensive crisis if the mass is a pheochromocytoma. One exception is in the case of a suspected adrenal metastasis from a known extra-adrenal carcinoma.

Screening of Bilateral Adrenal Masses

Ten to 15% of patients with AI have bilateral adrenal masses. These include primary bilateral macronodular adrenal

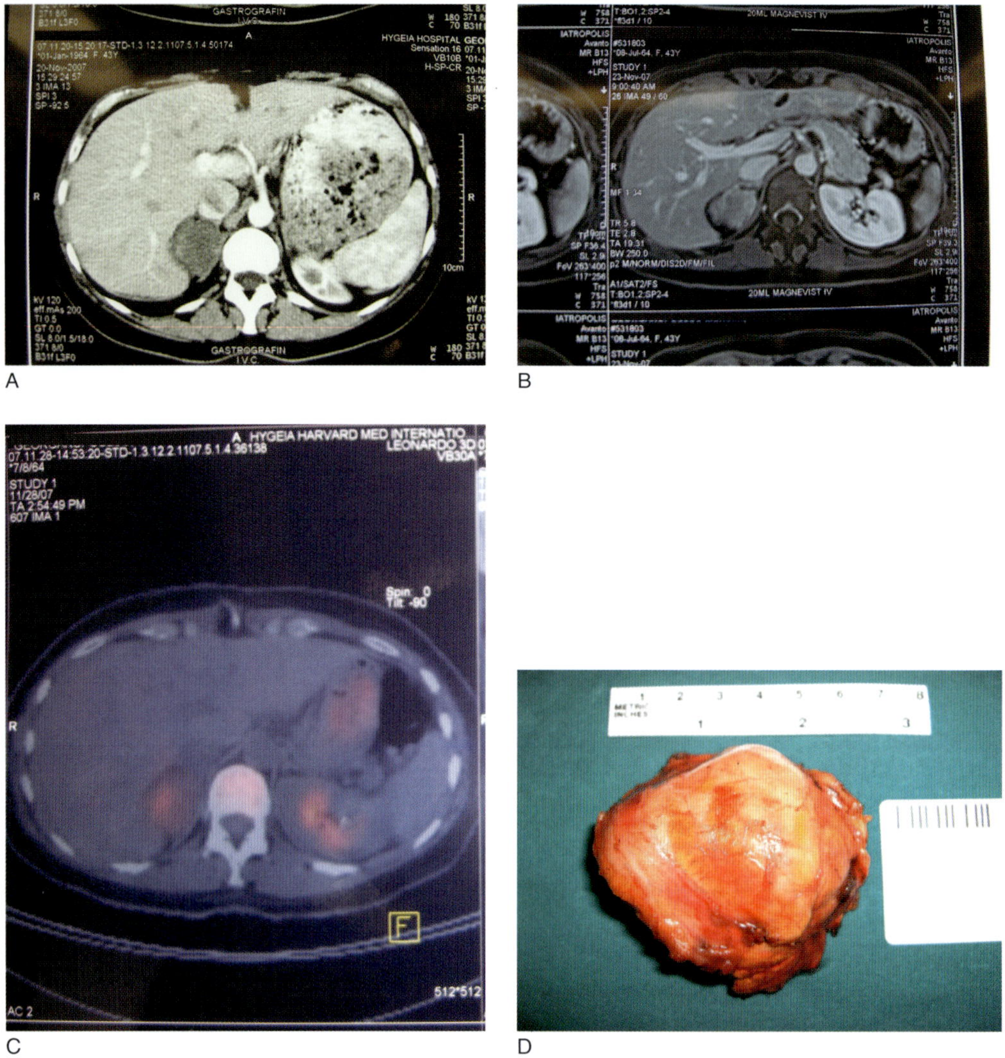

▲ **Figure 43–3.** A 43-year-old female with a history of bilateral mastectomies for extensive in situ lobular breast carcinoma 18 months ago. Currently, a right adrenal incidentaloma is discovered. **(A)** CT scan of a 5 cm right adrenal mass (30 units of Hounsfield). **(B)** MRI appearance of the same lesion. **(C)** 18F-FDG-PET-scan with increased metabolic function (SUV max 4) in the right adrenal indicating metastatic lesion. **(D)** The gross specimen (6.7 × 6.4 cm in diameter) that eventually proved to be a benign ganglioneuroma.

hyperplasia and adenomas, bilateral adrenal hyperplasia due to Cushing disease or ectopic corticotropin secretion, metastases or primary cancer, myelolipomas, infections, hemorrhage, and partial glucocorticoid resistance. The previously described biochemical evaluation of unilateral AIs should be applied when bilateral AIs are encountered as well. In addition, measurement of serum 17-hydroxyprogesterone level is indicated to exclude congenital adrenal hyperplasia.

In patients with bilateral adrenal masses, imaging characteristics of each adrenal lesion should be evaluated independently. This is important to decide the best management approach. In some patients, one adrenal mass can be found to be a nonfunctioning adenoma, while the contralateral adrenal mass can be a hormone-secreting tumor. In addition, if bilateral adrenal masses appear on imaging to be hemorrhagic or infiltrating, the patient should be tested for adrenal insufficiency.

Conservative Management & Follow-up

Patients with nonfunctioning AIs, especially those <4 cm in size and with imaging features suggesting a benign lesion, can be managed conservatively. The age of the patient should also be considered when the decision is made not to operate. The need for follow-up hormonal studies and imaging remains controversial. The American Association of Clinical Endocrinologists recommends repeat imaging for up to 5 years for benign nonfunctioning tumors. However, some studies recommend that no further follow-up imaging is needed if an AI is smaller than 4 cm and is ≤10 HU on CT scan. In a meta-analysis involving 4121 patients with nonfunctioning adrenal lesions, the mean tumor growth was 2 mm over a medium of 52.8 months of follow-up. Tumor enlargement of 1 cm or more was encountered in 2.5% of the patients.

Repeated hormonal evaluation should be considered in patients with minimal autonomous cortisol secretion, if surgery is deferred, to detect progression to overt Cushing syndrome. This possibility is real but occurs in a small percentage of patients.

The most appropriate time interval for repeat hormonal and imaging studies is also unclear. Studies looking at different follow-up strategies for patients with nonfunctioning AI are inconclusive and no consensus recommendations can be made. This is especially true for younger individuals. It is reasonable to consider repeating a serum dehydroepiandrosterone sulfate (DHEAS) and an overnight Dexamethasone Suppress Test (DST) at least once at 1 year when the initial evaluation is negative.[6]

Surgical Management

All patients with subclinical functioning AIs, as well as those with tumors larger than 4 cm in size, are candidates for surgery. More specifically surgery is indicated:

1. In all patients with subclinical Cushing syndrome (MACS) especially those who have comorbidities potentially attributable to autonomous glucocorticoid secretion such as hypertension, diabetes, obesity, and low bone mass. Several studies have documented impressive improvements in hypertension, glycemic control, and normalization of markers of bone turnover following unilateral adrenalectomy in patients with even minimal evidence of autonomous cortisol secretion.[7]
2. In all patients with subclinical primary aldosteronism and pheochromocytoma.
3. Adrenal lipid-poor masses with either suspicious imaging or size larger than 4 cm should be considered for surgical removal because a fraction of them will be adrenocortical carcinomas. The size of the AI does not necessarily predict the clinical severity of the problem (Figure 43–4).

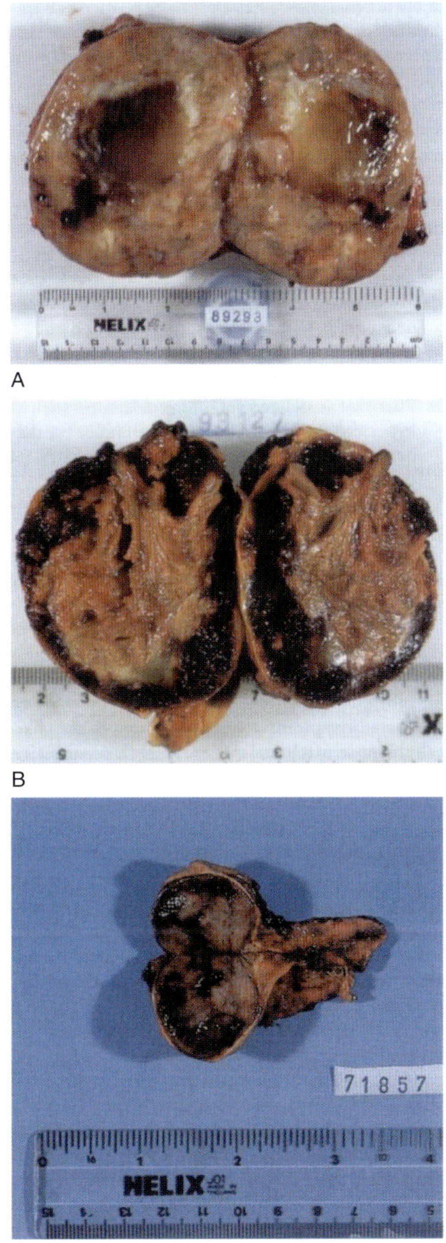

Figure 43–4. The size of the adrenal incidentaloma does not necessarily predict the clinical severity of the problem. **(A)** A 9 cm maximum diameter benign schwannoma. **(B)** A 7 cm maximum diameter benign hemorrhagic cortical adenoma. **(C)** A 2.9 cm potentially dangerous pheochromocytoma. (Reproduced with permission from Linos DA. *Adrenal Glands: Diagnostic Aspects and Surgical Therapy*. Heidelberg: Springer-Verlag, 2005:247.)

4. Adrenal myelolipomas, once considered safe to just follow, can be considered for elective surgery when larger than 6 cm in diameter because of the risk of bleeding and associated local mass-effect symptoms.

Today's endoscopic adrenalectomy techniques, both the laparoscopic anterior adrenalectomy approach and the posterior retroperitoneoscopic approach, offer the opportunity for definitive diagnosis and treatment with a very low morbidity rate. The decision to use an anterior or posterior approach ultimately has to be determined by the operating surgeon, taking into account characteristics of the tumor and the patient. The few patients with AIs suspicious for cancer on imaging, as well as those with lesions larger than 4 cm in size, can still be approached by a minimally invasive surgical technique. The "open" approach can be reserved for large lesions or tumors with definite evidence of malignancy on preoperative imaging. Patients with a solitary metastasis to the adrenal gland can be treated either by a minimally invasive or open approach.[8,9]

Management of Bilateral Adrenal Masses

Bilateral adrenal masses interestingly carry a higher risk of autonomous cortisol secretion and malignancy compared to unilateral adrenal masses. Thus, their management poses diagnostic and therapeutic challenges when surgery is indicated. Because bilateral adrenalectomy carries additional problems related to the need for lifelong glucocorticoid and mineralocorticoid replacement, several authors have suggested only removal of the larger adrenal gland. As might be expected, recurrence can be found in 20% to 70% of cases with 33% of patients ultimately found to undergo contralateral adrenalectomy. Adrenal venous sampling (AVS) can and usually should be utilized to identify the side of dominant cortisol secretion, which can mitigate the need for bilateral adrenalectomy and facilitate the appropriate management of bilateral AIs.

REFERENCES

1. Kebebew E. Adrenal incidentaloma. *N Engl J Med*. 2021;384(16):1542-1551.
2. Sherlock M, Scarsbrook A, Abbas A, et al. Adrenal incidentaloma. *Endocr Rev*. 2020;41(6):775-820.
3. Young WF, Kebebew E. Evaluation and management of the adrenal incidentaloma. July 2021. https://www.uptodate.com/contents/evaluation-and-management-of-the-adrenal-incidentaloma.
4. Bourdeau I, Ghorayeb NE, Gagnon N, et al. Management of endocrine disease: differential diagnosis, investigation and therapy of bilateral adrenal incidentalomas. *Eur J Endocrinol*. 2018;179(2):R57-R67.
5. Kim SJ, Lee SW, Pak K, et al. Diagnostic accuracy of 18 F-FDG PET or PET/CT for the characterization of adrenal masses: a systematic review and meta-analysis. *Br J Radiol*. 2018;91(1086):20170520.
6. Mayo-Smith WW, Song JH, Boland G, et al. Management of incidental adrenal masses: a white paper of the ACR incidental findings committee. *J Am Coll Radiol*. 2017;14(8):1038-1044.
7. Elhassan YS, Alahdab F, Prete A et al. Natural history of adrenal incidentalomas with and without mild autonomous cortisol excess: a systematic review and meta-analysis. *Ann Intern Med*. 2019;171(2):107-116.
8. Gavriilidis P, Camenzuli C, Paspala A, et al. Posterior retroperitoneoscopic versus laparoscopic transperitoneal adrenalectomy: a systematic review by an updated meta-analysis. *World J Surg*. 2021;45(1):168-179.
9. Vrielink OM, Wevers KP, Kist JW, et al. Laparoscopic anterior versus endoscopic posterior approach for adrenalectomy: a shift to a new golden standard? *Langenbecks Arch Surg*. 2017;402(5):767-773.

Cushing Disease & Syndrome

44

Effie Tsomos, MD
Alice C. Levine, MD

GENERAL CONSIDERATIONS

Endogenous Cushing syndrome (CS) is an uncommon disorder with an incidence of 3.2 cases per million population per year. The disease is more prevalent in females with a 3:1 ratio except for CS due to ectopic ACTH, a disorder that is equally common in both sexes. In a Swedish epidemiological study on the incidence of CS, out of the 3.2 cases per million per year of endogenous Cushing's, 48% were attributable to Cushing disease (pituitary ACTH overproduction), 26% were attributable to CS due to ectopic ACTH, 21% to benign adrenal CS, and 6% to adrenocortical carcinoma (ACC). This breakdown differs slightly from prior studies that had lower percentages of CS due to ectopic ACTH. Increased awareness of hypercortisolism in patients with malignant tumors as well as variation in the diagnostic process and management of these patients can potentially explain this discrepancy.

Mild autonomous cortisol secretion (MACS) is the most common secretory syndrome in benign adrenal nodules. Patients with MACS do not exhibit signs and symptoms of overt hypercortisolism. The disease has multiple names in scientific literature. In addition to MACS, this disorder is commonly referred to as Subclinical Cushing's or Mild Autonomous Cortisol Excess (MACE). MACS is reported to be present in up to 30% of all adrenal incidentalomas. There is accumulating evidence, primarily from retrospective studies, that MACS is associated with increased mortality due to cardiovascular disease. In fact, in a recent systematic review of over 4000 patients with nonfunctioning adrenal incidentalomas or adrenal adenomas resulting in MACS, cardiovascular mortality represented 43.2% of all deaths with an incidence of 5% in those with MACS. There has been no consensus to-date about the optimal management of MACS due to benign adenomas.

Pathogenesis

The molecular pathophysiology underlying pituitary ACTH-producing tumors and adrenal causes of CS is beginning to be elucidated. With the advent of rapid whole-exome sequencing, some pituitary corticotroph tumors were found to have mutations in a gene transcribing the mRNA for the peptide ubiquitin-specific protease-8 (USP8). This protein normally decreases the ubiquitination and degradation of EGF-R. The somatic mutation leads to increased activity of USP8, and therefore, decreased ubiquitination and degradation of EGF-R. This single mutational hotspot in the ubiquitin-specific protease 8 (USP8) gene has been demonstrated in almost half of pituitary Cushing disease tumors.

Adrenal CS is primarily due to cortisol-producing adrenal adenomas. Rarely, adrenal CS is due to bilateral micronodular or macronodular hyperplasia. Adrenal cortical carcinomas often have a pattern of disorganized steroidogenesis with the accumulation of cortisol precursors. However, because of their large size and vascularity, they often produce CS in spite of inefficient production of cortisol.

Germline and somatic mutations have been identified as the underlying cause of hypercortisolism due to various adrenal pathologies. In most cases of overt hypercortisolism due to adrenal disease, mutations that lead to increased cAMP-dependent protein kinase A (PKA) signaling (cAMP-PKA-signaling) are involved. Activating mutations in guanine nucleotide binding protein, alpha stimulating (GNAS), a key part of the cAMP-PKA pathway, is the heritable cause of cortisol-producing adrenal tumors in infants with the McCune-Albright syndrome. Mutations in the regulatory subunit type 1 alpha (R1alpha) of PKA cause primary pigmented nodular adrenocortical disease (PPNAD). In addition, inactivating mutations in inhibitors of cAMP-PKA signaling pathways (phosphodiesterases) were demonstrated in patients with adrenal hyperplasia and adenomas. Somatic mutations in the main catalytic subunit of PKA were found in cortisol-producing adenomas. Preclinical and clinical studies indicate that PKA-activating mutations in adrenocortical cells predominantly stimulate steroidogenesis with less effect on proliferation.

In patients with bilateral macronodular adrenal hyperplasia (BMAH), hypercortisolism tends to be milder and develops later in life when nodules are quite large. Analysis of blood and tumor DNA from patients with apparently sporadic BMAH revealed a frequent mutation in the armadillo-repeat containing 5 (*ARMC5*) gene, a putative tumor-suppressor gene. ARMC5 was analyzed in leukocyte DNA in 14 of 18 patients with ARMC5 mutations, and in all 14 tumors both alleles of ARMC5 carried mutations: one germline and the other somatic. The requirement for both a germline mutation and a secondary somatic mutation (Knudson's two-hit hypothesis) may explain why the disease presents later in life. Interestingly, ARMC5 inactivation decreased steroidogenesis *in vitro*, consistent with the observation that very large nodules are required to produce even mild degrees of hypercortisolism. Therefore, in contrast to mutations that activate the PKA pathway, ARMC5-inactivating mutations promote tumor growth rather than steroidogenesis.

Similarly, benign adenomas with MACS were associated with Wnt/beta-catenin (CTNNB1) mutations. CTNNB1 mutations, activating the Wnt/beta-catenin pathway, are also commonly found in adrenal cortical cancers. This mutation, like ARMC5, primarily stimulates adrenal tumorigenesis with less effect on steroidogenesis.

Clinical Findings

A. Symptoms and Signs

There is a wide spectrum of clinical manifestations of Cushing's. Patients with Cushing's often develop features of the metabolic syndrome including hypertension, diabetes, and central obesity. With the increase in the rate of obesity in the general population, however, metabolic effects of hypercortisolism are less specific to CS. Thus, anti-anabolic changes in CS can be more helpful in raising suspicion for the diagnosis. Such effects include osteopenia, thin skin, and ecchymoses. These features are present in patients with Cushing syndrome but not in patients with simple obesity. Patients in whom osteoporosis is diagnosed radiographically are 11 times more likely to have Cushing syndrome than those who do not have osteoporosis.

Patients who have thin skin are also more likely to have Cushing syndrome, with a positive likelihood ratio of 116. The area suggested for such assessment is the skin over the proximal phalanx of the middle finger of the nondominant hand, measured using an electrocardiographic caliper. Finally, patients who have three or more ecchymoses that are larger than 1 cm in diameter and not associated with trauma are more likely to have Cushing syndrome than are patients without such findings, with a positive likelihood ratio of 4.

Other potential features of hypercortisolism include gonadal dysfunction and psychiatric and cognitive dysfunction. Gonadal dysfunction presents as decreased libido, infertility, menstrual irregularity or amenorrhea in women, and erectile dysfunction in men. The psychiatric manifestations include depression, emotional lability, irritability, anxiety, acute psychosis, mania, suicidal ideation, and paranoia.

B. Laboratory Findings

The diagnosis of Cushing's is reliant on the demonstration of hypercortisolism or the loss of negative feedback for cortisol secretion. Cortisol is normally released in a predictable circadian rhythm, peaking in the morning within the first hour of awakening and reaching a nadir in the evening. Therefore, testing for hypercortisolism entails assessment for elevated cortisol secretion with a 24-hour urine-free cortisol excretion (UFC), assessment for elevated evening cortisol levels by testing midnight salivary cortisol levels, and assessment for defects in negative feedback by testing 9 AM cortisol concentrations after an overnight low-dose (1 mg) dexamethasone suppression test (LDDST).

Dexamethasone is chosen for suppression testing because it does not cross-react with the biochemical assays used to assess cortisol. A serum cortisol concentration of >1.8 μg/dL (50 nmol/L) after LDDST is recommended by the American Association of Clinical Endocrinologists as the cutoff of cortisol suppression used to diagnose overt Cushing syndrome. It is important to simultaneously measure a dexamethasone level in serum to ensure that it is high enough for reliable interpretation of the cortisol results.

Determination of ACTH-independence or dependence is ascertained with a serum ACTH level. ACTH-independent Cushing syndrome is the result of autonomous adrenal cortisol production. This is therefore associated with low ACTH levels as a result of feedback inhibition. Of note, in ACTH-dependent Cushing syndrome, the ACTH levels are generally elevated, but may even be in the normal range. In the setting of hypercortisolism, a nonsuppressed ACTH confirms ACTH-dependent disease.

Distinguishing pituitary (eutopic) from ectopic ACTH secretion can be difficult as they both may present with elevated ACTH and cortisol levels. Severe elevations in ACTH and 24-hour urine-free cortisol levels suggest ectopic disease. High-dose dexamethasone suppression testing (HDDST) can also be used to differentiate between eutopic and ectopic ACTH secretion. The test utilizes 8 mg of oral dexamethasone and is performed either as an overnight or two-day test. Cortisol is expected to suppress to <5 μg/dL or is expected to decrease by 50%. The reported sensitivity and specificity of the test varies widely in the scientific literature. Ectopic ACTH-secreting malignant tumors usually do not suppress after HDDST, whereas ectopic ACTH-secreting benign neuroendocrine tumors can partially suppress after HDDST. Therefore, up to 30% of patients with ectopic ACTH may suppress after HDDST. Thus, HDDST is usually performed with a corticotropin-releasing hormone (CRH) stimulation test to enhance the diagnostic accuracy.

Use of dexamethasone suppression testing is ineffectual in conditions resulting in elevated levels of corticosteroid binding globulin (CBG) such as pregnancy or use of oral contraceptives or conditions resulting in reduced levels of CBG such as nephrotic syndrome, liver disease, and malnutrition. This limitation is a result of the cortisol assay as it measures total cortisol which consists of both free and protein-bound cortisol. In such cases, late-night salivary cortisol or 24 h UFC is preferred when testing for hypercortisolism.

C. Imaging Studies

MRI pituitary imaging is warranted when there is suspicion for ACTH-dependent CS as this is the most common etiology of this disease. MRI reveals a pituitary adenoma in 40% to 60% of cases of Cushing disease.

When ectopic ACTH secretion is suspected, contrast-enhanced CT of the chest is recommended as half of corticotropin-secreting solid tumors can be found in the thorax. If the more common intrathoracic source of ectopic ACTH is excluded, a CT or MRI of the abdomen and pelvis should be performed to evaluate for an intra-abdominal source. CT or MRI of thorax and abdomen and scintigraphic studies localize tumors in 70% to 90% of ectopic ACTH cases.

ACTH-independent disease is due to either exogenous steroids or an adrenal source. Once careful history has excluded the use of glucocorticoids, adrenal CT should be performed.

Adrenal tumors that secrete cortisol are generally large and easily detected on routine CT or MRI of the abdomen. If the lesion raises suspicion for ACC based on morphology or size, F-fluorodeoxyglucose (FDG) PET scan and MRI may be needed prior to adrenalectomy.

D. Special Tests

Most ACTH-secreting pituitary tumors are microadenomas less than 1 cm in diameter and therefore may not be identified on MRI imaging. If the clinical suspicion for pituitary Cushing's is high despite an unremarkable or indeterminate pituitary MRI, bilateral inferior petrosal sinus sampling (IPSS) of ACTH is justified. In pituitary Cushing disease, ACTH levels in the venous drainage of the pituitary are anticipated to be higher than ACTH levels of peripheral blood. Use of CRH or vasopressin to directly stimulate pituitary corticotrophs will increase the sensitivity of this test. A positive test that confirms a pituitary source of ACTH overproduction is a pituitary to peripheral ACTH ratio more than 3 with CRH.

Differential Diagnosis

There are several conditions that can mimic CS clinically. ACTH-independent disease is most commonly due to exogenous steroids and a careful history to rule out use of oral, topical, intra-articular, and inhaled steroids must be undertaken. In addition, other medications such as megestrol acetate (Megace) activate the glucocorticoid receptor and can produce all the clinical signs and symptoms of CS. ACTH-dependent hypercortisolism may also be seen in patients with severe depression and/or anorexia, both of which activate the HPA axis. It is important to rule these conditions out before embarking on extensive workup and treatment.

Complications

The cardiovascular, thromboembolic, metabolic, and infectious complications of CS result in increased morbidity and mortality.

A. Cardiovascular

CS is associated with an increased prevalence of hypertension and elevated cardiovascular risk. The mechanism for elevated blood pressure in hypercortisolism is related to an enhanced response to angiotensin II. More significantly, cortisol itself is a potent activator of the mineralocorticoid receptor (MR). Under normal conditions, kidney cells express 11β-hydroxysteroid dehydrogenase isozyme 2 (11BHSD2) that inactivates cortisol via conversion to cortisone. In CS, high cortisol levels exhaust the ability of this enzyme to fully inactivate cortisol and its actions at the MR. This leads to fluid retention and has toxic effects on the heart resulting in left ventricular hypertrophy and heart failure. Medical management of hypertension related to hypercortisolism often requires MR antagonist treatment with spironolactone at doses of 100 to 300 mg daily until the CS can be cured medically or surgically.

B. Thromboembolic

When considering surgical management, one of the more concerning risks in CS is hypercoagulability. In a retrospective trial involving 208 patients undergoing surgical (pituitary, unilateral, and bilateral adrenalectomy) and medical treatment, the risk of thromboembolic events was found to be about 20%. Such thromboembolic events (TEs) included DVT, MI, PE, and CVA. In the study, hypercoagulability persisted even after surgical intervention. Patients who underwent bilateral adrenalectomy (BLA) had the highest probability of TEs with an odds ratio of 3.74, possibly because they had severe hypercortisolism. Of patients with TEs, 40.5% experienced the event within the first 60 days after surgery. Therefore, although the optimal duration of anticoagulation is unknown, it is recommended for AC to be continued for at least 60 days postoperatively.

C. Hypokalemia

Cortisol-mediated activation of the MR in the kidneys results in urinary loss of potassium resulting in hypokalemia. If hypokalemia is severe, patients can experience muscle weakness, rhabdomyolysis, and cardiac arrhythmias such as QT interval prolongation, supraventricular tachyarrhythmias, and life-threatening ventricular arrhythmias. Concomitant hypomagnesemia increases the risk of such arrhythmias. Thus, correction of hypomagnesemia and hypokalemia is imperative to decreasing the risk of such a complication. In addition, MR antagonism with spironolactone is often required.

D. Metabolic

Chronic excess of cortisol leads to metabolic syndrome. Glucocorticoids stimulate enzymes involved in liver gluconeogenesis resulting in increased glucose output and subsequent insulin resistance. Glucocorticoids increase lipid oxidation and lipolysis in adipose and skeletal muscle, and stimulate enzymes involved in fatty acid synthesis, resulting in liver steatosis and insulin insensitivity. Changes in adipocyte differentiation and lipoprotein lipase activity result in visceral rather than subcutaneous storage of fat and increased waist-to-hip circumference.

These changes in glucose metabolism also result in hyperglycemia. An impairment of glucose metabolism has been described in 27% to 87% of patients with CS. In addition, glucose and insulin concentrations are higher in patients with CD compared with sex- and age-matched controls and BMI-matched controls after glucose loading. The prevalence of impaired glucose tolerance or diabetes is higher in patients with pituitary (33%) or adrenal CS (34%) than in BMI-matched controls without difference between sexes. The prevalence of diabetes in patients with ectopic CS is highest at 74%.

Infections

Infections are common in patients with CS because of the immunosuppressive effects of cortisol, leaving patients vulnerable to opportunistic infections like *Pneumocystis jirovecii* (PCP). There is a strong association between the development of PCP and the degree of cortisol excess and is therefore more commonly seen in patients with ectopic CS. Interestingly, it is usually diagnosed after initiation of cortisol-lowering therapy, suggesting that immune reconstitution plays a role in development of the infection. Such infection is associated with a high mortality rate of 60% to 65% and therefore prophylaxis with trimethoprim-sulfamethoxazole should be initiated when cortisol-lowering therapy is initiated.

Treatment

A. Pituitary Tumor-Directed Drugs

Pasireotide is a somatostatin receptor (SSTR) ligand used in pituitary Cushing's as corticotroph tumor cells express somatostatin receptors. Pasireotide is used for treatment of Cushing disease when surgery is not an option. Although effective, the use of pasireotide is limited by the side effect of hyperglycemia due to a decrease in incretin and insulin secretion.

Corticotroph adenomas can also express dopamine receptors that can be targeted with the dopamine receptor agonist, cabergoline. High doses can induce long-term biochemical remission in about 30% of patients, although escape occurs.

B. Steroidogenesis Inhibitors

The most commonly used steroidogenesis inhibitor is ketoconazole, a drug that blocks multiple cytochrome P450 steroidogenic enzymes needed for cortisol synthesis. Generally, doses of 400 to 1600 mg/day are needed depending on the degree of hypercortisolism. The main toxicity of ketoconazole is hepatitis, although several reports have demonstrated that only a minority of patients develop severe transaminitis.

Levoketoconazole is a ketoconazole stereoisomer that is more potent than ketoconazole with less hepatotoxicity and a more favorable pharmacokinetic profile resulting in higher plasma concentration levels. Use of levoketoconazole for treatment of patients with CS leads to sustained improvements in urinary-free cortisol with an acceptable safety and tolerability profile.

Etomidate is an intravenously administered hypnotic drug that inhibits 11β-hydroxylase and also 20, 22 desmolase. It is helpful for severe hypercortisolism as it is very effective with a rapid onset of action, but its use is limited to intensive care units due to its sedative properties.

Metyrapone is a potent inhibitor of 11β-hydroxylase and a partial inhibitor of 18-hydroxylase with a rapid absorption and onset of action. The drug has a short half-life and must be given four times daily in doses ranging from 750 to 4000 mg/day depending on the degree of hypercortisolism. Side effects may include nausea and vomiting, worsening hypokalemia/hypertension due to accumulation of aldosterone precursors with mineralocorticoid action, and hirsutism in women due to increased adrenal androgens.

Another 11β-hydroxylase inhibitor drug, osilodrostat, produces similar results to metyrapone by reducing the synthesis of aldosterone and cortisol. This medication rapidly reduces mean 24-hour UFC and improves clinical signs of hypercortisolism when given in doses of 2 to 30 mg twice daily. Side effects are similar to those reported with metyrapone, namely nausea, headache, fatigue, adrenal insufficiency, hypokalemia, hypertension, and hirsutism.

With either of the 11β-hydroxylase inhibitor drugs, accumulation of 11-deoxycortisol occurs and can falsely elevate cortisol levels measured by immunoassays because of cross-reactivity. Therefore, when monitoring cortisol levels in patients on these drugs, the preferred assay is liquid chromatography/mass spectrometry (LC/MS). Both drugs also cause accumulation of 11-deoxycorticosterone (DOC) which has mineralocorticoid activity and can result in worsening hypertension and hypokalemia, necessitating addition or increased dosing of a mineralocorticoid receptor blocker spironolactone.

Mitotane (OP'-DDD) is an adrenolytic drug that is a mainstay of therapy for adrenal cortical carcinoma. With the higher doses needed for its anticancer activity, mitotane is associated with significant side effects and drug interactions. However, lower doses inhibit steroidogenesis and are better tolerated. Low-dose mitotane has been utilized alone and in combination with other steroidogenesis inhibitors for the long-term medical management of severe hypercortisolism.

C. Glucocorticoid Receptor Antagonist

Mifepristone is a glucocorticoid receptor-blocking agent. It is FDA approved for treatment of CS of any cause if a patient has glucose intolerance and cannot undergo surgery. The efficacy of this drug cannot be tracked using cortisol values and, therefore, response is assessed based on monitoring of clinical features. Because the drug does not block cortisol actions at the MR, it can worsen hypertension and hypokalemia-associated hypercortisolism, necessitating the addition of potassium and spironolactone.

Of note, many of the medications currently in use to treat CS are used off label. The only medications that are FDA approved for CS in the United States are mifepristone, osilodrostat, levoketoconazole, and pasireotide.

D. Surgery

The selection of an appropriate surgical candidate can be challenging as the comorbidities caused by cortisol excess are otherwise prevalent in the general population and may be difficult to distinguish from those induced by hypercortisolism.

A pituitary mass larger than 6 mm in diameter in a patient with ACTH-dependent CS is referred for pituitary surgery. Surgical removal of a pituitary adenoma by transsphenoidal resection is the only definitive cure and is first-line for treatment of pituitary Cushing's. Ideally, the surgery is a selective adenomectomy that preserves pituitary function. If no adenoma is identified, partial or subtotal hypophysectomy can be successful in induction of remission. In the hands of experienced neurosurgeons, the remission rate for microadenomas is 81% to 89% and less than 67% for macroadenomas. The occurrence of hypopituitarism is dependent on the extent of the surgery. The mean frequency of partial hypopituitarism is 6.6% in patients who had undergone selective adenomectomy and 20.2% in those who have undergone partial hypophysectomy.

In regard to hypercortisolism related to adrenal adenomas, European guidelines from 2016 suggest adrenalectomy in patients with higher degrees of biochemical hypercortisolism with a DST >5 μg/dL (140 nmol/L) and the presence of cortisol-related comorbidities like hypertension, diabetes, obesity, or low bone mass.

In critically ill patients with severe hypercortisolism, BLA may be necessary to prevent death as a result of cardiovascular, metabolic, or infectious complications. This is considered in patients with CS when: (1) there is severe life-threatening hypercortisolism necessitating a rapid decline in glucocorticoid levels, (2) the primary tumor cannot be identified, (3) the tumor(s) are deemed unresectable, and (4) medical therapies are unavailable, ineffective, or poorly tolerated. It can also be helpful when attempting to prevent drug interactions in patients with neuroendocrine tumors in whom the efficacy or safety of antineoplastic agents would be affected by cortisol-lowering drugs. An important disadvantage to bear in mind when considering BLA is the danger of primary adrenal insufficiency that can be fatal in 6% of cases. Postoperative glucocorticoid and mineralocorticoid replacement and patient education regarding stress dosing of steroids is imperative to survival given the lack of adrenocortical function.

Prognosis

Effective treatment of CS clearly reduces the morbidity and mortality due to hypercortisolism. However, epidemiologic studies have shown that excess morbidity persists even after successful treatment of CS and CD and this may correlate with the duration of disease prior to therapy. Therefore, it is imperative to identify patients with CS and initiate treatment as early as possible to reduce morbidity and mortality from the disease.

When to Refer/When to Admit

In patients with benign appearing adrenal masses who lack the classic clinical features of overt hypercortisolism, referral to an endocrinologist for workup and management of hormonal hypersecretion is appropriate.

Patients with severe life-threatening hypercortisolism should be admitted to the ICU for acute management of CS and all of its comorbidities. If the primary tumor cannot be identified or is deemed unresectable, urgent BLA should be considered.

SUGGESTED READING

Albani A, Perez-Rivas LG, Reincke M, Theodoropoulou M. Pathogenesis of Cushing disease: an update on the genetics of corticotropinomas. *Endocr Pract*. 2018;24(10):907-914.

Beuschlein F, Fassnacht M, Assié G, et al. Constitutive activation of PKA catalytic subunit in adrenal Cushing's syndrome. *N Engl J Med*. 2014;370(11):1019-1028.

Delivanis DA, Athimulam S, Bancos I. Modern management of mild autonomous cortisol secretion. *Clin Pharmacol Ther.* 2019;106(6):1209-1221.

Elhassan YS, Alahdab F, Prete A, et al. Natural history of adrenal incidentalomas with and without mild autonomous cortisol excess: a systematic review and meta-analysis. *Ann Intern Med.* 2019;171(2):107-116.

Faillot S, Foulonneau T, Néou M, et al. Genomic classification of benign adrenocortical lesions. *Endocr Relat Cancer.* 2021;28(1):79-95.

Feelders RA, Newell-Price J, Pivonello R, Nieman LK, Hofland LJ, Lacroix A. Advances in the medical treatment of Cushing's syndrome. *Lancet Diabetes Endocrinol.* 2019;7(4):300-312.

Fleseriu M, Pivonello R, Elenkova A, et al. Efficacy and safety of levoketoconazole in the treatment of endogenous Cushing's syndrome (SONICS): a phase 3, multicentre, open-label, single-arm trial. *Lancet Diabetes Endocrinol.* 2019;7(11): 855-865.

Groussin L, Jullian E, Perlemoine K, et al. Mutations of the PRKAR1A gene in Cushing's syndrome due to sporadic primary pigmented nodular adrenocortical disease. *J Clin Endocrinol Metab.* 2002;87(9):4324-4329.

Horvath A, Giatzakis C, Robinson-White A, et al. Adrenal hyperplasia and adenomas are associated with inhibition of phosphodiesterase 11A in carriers of PDE11A sequence variants that are frequent in the population. *Cancer Res.* 2006;66(24):11571-11575.

Lacroix A, Feelders RA, Stratakis CA, Nieman LK. Cushing's syndrome. *Lancet.* 2015;386(9996):913-927.

Lamberts SW, van der Lely AJ, de Herder WW. Transsphenoidal selective adenomectomy is the treatment of choice in patients with Cushing's disease. Considerations concerning preoperative medical treatment and the long-term follow-up. *J Clin Endocrinol Metab.* 1995;80(11):3111-3113.

Lodish M, Stratakis CA. A genetic and molecular update on adrenocortical causes of Cushing syndrome. *Nat Rev Endocrinol.* 2016;12(5):255-262.

Lonser RR, Nieman L, Oldfield EH. Cushing's disease: pathobiology, diagnosis, and management. *J Neurosurg.* 2017;126(2):404-417.

Loriaux DL. Diagnosis and differential diagnosis of Cushing's syndrome. *N Engl J Med.* 2017;376(15):1451-1459.

Nieman LK, Biller BM, Findling JW, et al. The diagnosis of Cushing's syndrome: an endocrine society clinical practice guideline. *J Clin Endocrinol Metab.* 2008;93(5):1526-1540.

Ma ZY, Song ZJ, Chen JH, et al. Recurrent gain-of-function USP8 mutations in Cushing's disease. *Cell Res.* 2015;25(3): 306-317.

Papakokkinou E, Olsson DS, Chantzichristos D, et al. Excess morbidity persists in patients with Cushing's disease during long-term remission: a Swedish nationwide study. *J Clin Endocrinol Metab.* 2020;105(8):2616-2624.

Pivonello R, Fleseriu M, Newell-Price J, et al. Efficacy and safety of osilodrostat in patients with Cushing's disease (LINC 3): a multicentre phase III study with a double-blind, randomised withdrawal phase. *Lancet Diabetes Endocrinol.* 2020;8(9):748-761. Erratum in: *Lancet Diabetes Endocrinol.* 2020;8(9):e4.

Pivonello R, Isidori AM, De Martino MC, Newell-Price J, Biller BM, Colao A. Complications of Cushing's syndrome: state of the art. *Lancet Diabetes Endocrinol.* 2016;4(7):611-629.

Reincke M, Sbiera S, Hayakawa A, et al. Mutations in the deubiquitinase gene USP8 cause Cushing's disease. *Nature Genet.* 2015;47(1):31-38.

Sathyakumar S, Paul TV, Asha HS, et al. Ectopic Cushing syndrome: a 10-year experience from a tertiary care center in southern India. *Endocr Pract.* 2017;23(8):907-914.

Sharma ST, Nieman LK, Feelders RA. Cushing's syndrome: epidemiology and developments in disease management. *Clin Epidemiol.* 2015;7:281.

Suarez MG, Stack M, Hinojosa-Amaya JM, et al. Hypercoagulability in Cushing syndrome, prevalence of thrombotic events: a large, single-center, retrospective study. *J Endocr Soc.* 2020;4(2):bvz033.

Terzolo M, Pia A, Reimondo G. Subclinical Cushing's syndrome: definition and management. *Clin Endocrinol.* 2012;76(1):12-18.

van Halem K, Vrolijk L, Pereira AM, de Boer MG. Characteristics and mortality of pneumocystis pneumonia in patients with Cushing's syndrome: a plea for timely initiation of chemoprophylaxis. *Open Forum Infect Dis.* 2017;4(1):ofx002.

Wagner-Bartak NA, Baiomy A, Habra MA, et al. Cushing syndrome: diagnostic workup and imaging features, with clinical and pathologic correlation. *Am J Roentgenol.* 2017;209(1):19-32.

Weinstein LS, Shenker A, Gejman PV, Merino MJ, Friedman E, Spiegel AM. Activating mutations of the stimulatory G protein in the McCune–Albright syndrome. *N Engl J Med.* 1991;325(24):1688-1695.

Wengander S, Trimpou P, Papakokkinou E, Ragnarsson O. The incidence of endogenous Cushing's syndrome in the modern era. *Clin Endocrinol.* 2019;91(2):263-270.

Young J, Haissaguerre M, Viera-Pinto O, Chabre O, Baudin E, Tabarin A. Management of endocrine disease: Cushing's syndrome due to ectopic ACTH secretion: an expert operational opinion. *Eur J Endocrinol.* 2020;182(4):R29-R58.

Primary Aldosteronism

Maheshwaran Sivarajah, MD, MSc
Rasa Zarnegar, MD

45

GENERAL CONSIDERATIONS

Primary aldosteronism (PA) is the most common cause of secondary hypertension that is likely underdiagnosed.[1,2] The autonomous hypersecretion of aldosterone drives a clinical syndrome of hypertension, hypokalemia, and low plasma renin levels in the renin-angiotensin system. PA was originally described by Jerome W. Conn in 1955 who associated an aldosterone-producing tumor of the adrenal gland with its biological actions.[3] He hypothesized that the disease may not only be associated with resistant hypertension but may originate in normotensive patients with normokalemia progressing to a more severe phenotype of hypertension with hypokalemia. He established that hypokalemia was not pathognomonic for the diagnosis of the disease. However, it is now believed that PA may present within a continuum of renin-independent aldosteronism that may be identified in healthy normotensive and moderately hypertensive individuals with an absence of the clinical findings of the disease.[4] These individuals would be at a higher risk for developing hypertension with subtle presumed "normal" or high aldosterone levels described as subclinical or nonclassical PA. Closer to the other end of the spectrum lie individuals with unrecognized yet biochemically overt PA with largely normotension and mild-to-moderate hypertension. This category of patients is followed by individuals with overt PA with an obvious clinical syndrome of hyperaldosteronism and at the highest risks of cardiovascular disease.

Prevalence rates of PA have been described with a range from 3.2% to 7.2% in mild-to-moderate hypertension, more than 15% in moderate-to-severe hypertension, and ≥20% in resistant hypertension and/or sleep apnea.[5] However, inconsistencies in reported studies are largely due to the variations in patient population, diagnostic algorithm, health-care settings, and geographic location.[1,6] Notably, there is no universal "gold standard" diagnostic test for PA, and published prevalence statistics have varied test conditions, medication regimens, and cutoff thresholds. Hypokalemia is present in up to 28% of patients and may also reflect diuretic treatment of essential hypertension, demonstrating that hypokalemia is not a prerequisite for further testing for PA.[7]

It has been proposed that the female sex is a positive predictor of bilateral PA, with underlying bilateral idiopathic hyperaldosteronism, in contrast to their male counterpart.[8] However, younger age is positively associated with unilateral disease in women, whereas younger-aged men have a negative association with unilateral PA. This suggests that sex may have a clinically significant impact on the distribution of subtypes among the generations. The body mass index (BMI) may also play a role in the distribution of PA with obesity being positively associated with a higher plasma aldosterone concentration (PAC) and aldosterone-to-renin ratio (ARR) in hypertensive individuals.[8]

Aldosterone-associated hypertension may be more common in Black patients. In contrast to Caucasians, the phenomenon of increased "salt sensitivity" may be more prominent in the Black population—greater sodium accumulation causing a more intense response of aldosterone release with volume expansion and elevated blood pressure (BP) with inversely correlated renin activity.[9,10] This clinical scenario has been thought to be found in up to 75% of non-Hispanic Black patients and 50% of all patients with hypertension. Salt-sensitive patients with long-standing poorly controlled hypertension are also at an increased risk of developing target organ damage, such as renal failure, cardiac ventricular hypertrophy, and incident cardiovascular events.[11] Treatment approaches that antagonize the actions of aldosterone could have relevance to reducing these complications.

PATHOGENESIS

PA is caused by an excess secretion of the adrenal salt-retaining corticoid hormone, aldosterone, within the renin-angiotensin-aldosterone system (RAAS) (Figure 45–1).

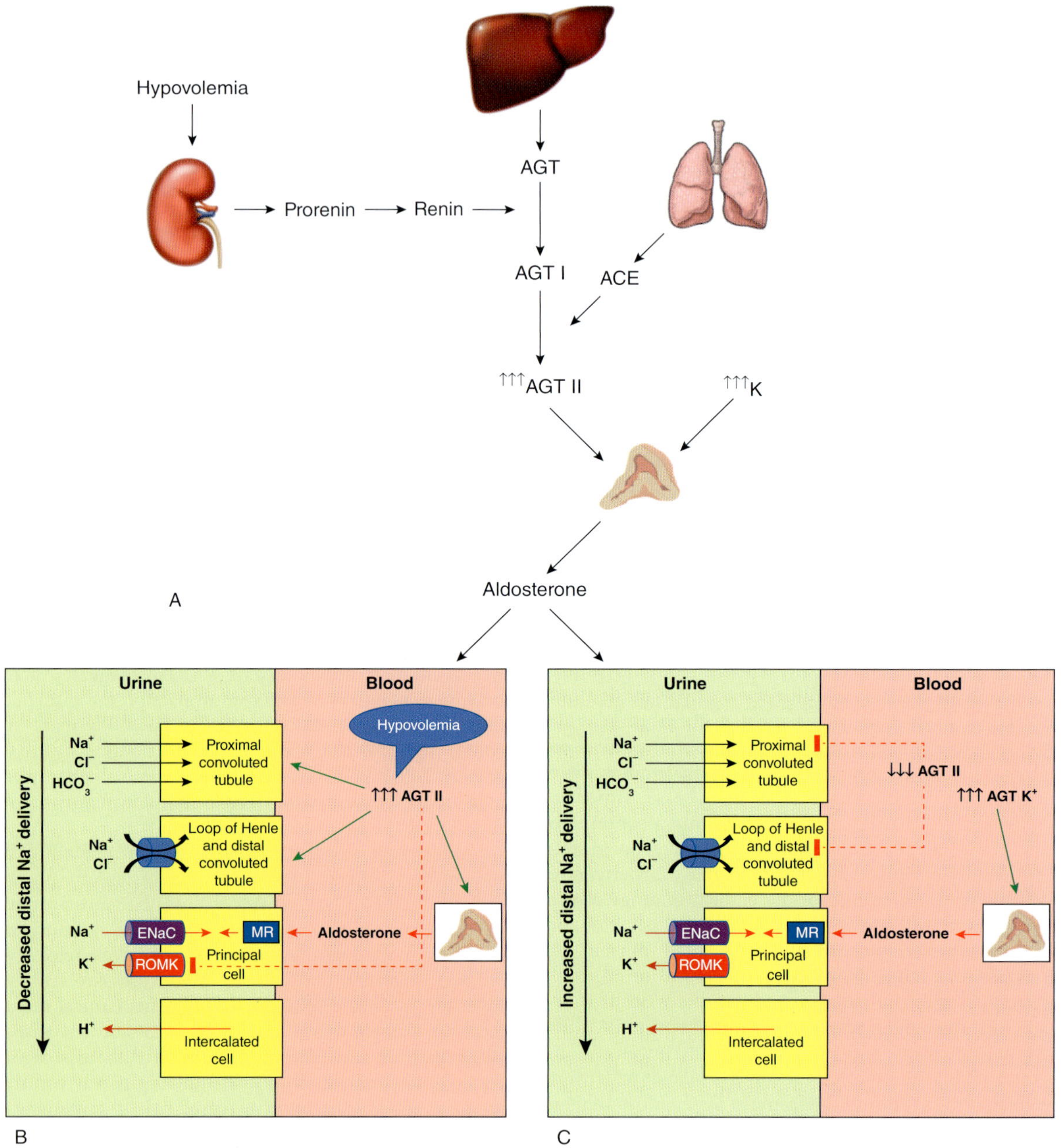

▲ **Figure 45–1.** The renin-angiotensin-aldosterone and physiologic hyperaldosteronism pathways. **(A)** *Aldosterone production*. Activated renin action on AGT leads to downstream effect of aldosterone production. **(B)** *Renin-dependent hyperaldosteronism*. Physiological mechanism to maintain homeostasis. **(C)** *Renin-independent hyperaldosteronism*. Primary aldosteronism is a pathophysiological mechanism with suppression of renin. AGT, angiotensinogen; AGT I, angiotensin I; AGT II, angiotensin II; ACE, angiotensin-converting enzyme; ENaC, epithelial sodium channel; K, potassium; MR, mineralocorticoid receptor.

This system regulates blood volume and systemic vascular resistance through a feedback mechanism triggered by a decrease in renal BP, decrease in salt delivery to the distal convoluted tubule, and/or an increase in sympathetic activity. The primary response of RAAS is to elevate arterial blood volume, pressure, and peripheral arterial tone.

The initiating hormone in RAAS is renin which is secreted by the juxtaglomerular cells as a prohormone within the kidney. The afferent feedback triggers that produce the downstream release and conversion of prorenin to renin are:

a. Reduced delivery of sodium chloride sensed by *macula densa* cells within the early distal renal tubule.
b. Reduced stretch of baroreceptors in the renal afferent arteriolar system with decreased BP.
c. Enhanced sympathetic neural activity and increased levels of catecholamines on β-1-adrenergic receptors within the cardiac and arterial baroreceptors.

The activated hormone, renin, cleaves plasma substrate angiotensinogen (AGT), produced by the liver, into the angiotensin I (AGT I). The angiotensin-converting enzyme (ACE), largely present within pulmonary and renal vascular endothelial cells, converts AGT I to the angiotensin II (AGT II). This messenger binds to AGT II receptors present on a variety of organs and initiates effects that include the following:[12]

a. Stimulate the zona glomerulosa within the adrenal cortex to release aldosterone. This mineralocorticoid hormone acts on mineralocorticoid receptors (MR) within the kidney, heart, and endothelial smooth muscle cells. The effects discussed below are a result of aldosterone binding to the MR.
b. Increase sodium reabsorption in the proximal convoluted tubule, loop of Henle, and distal convoluted tubule of the kidney through sodium-proton exchange. As a result, isotonic fluid shifts into the blood volume, interstitial, and extracellular space, increasing the arterial BP.
c. Arteriolar vasoconstriction occurs when AT II binds to G-protein-coupled receptors in systemic arterioles. This increase in total peripheral resistance causes an increase in BP.
d. Within the brain, AT II in the hypothalamus stimulates the thirst trigger to increase water intake and initiates the release of antidiuretic hormone, or vasopressin, by the posterior pituitary to incorporate aquaporin channels in the renal collecting duct and increase water reabsorption.
e. Inhibit firing of the aortic arch baroreceptors or vagal afferents to impair arterial baroreceptor reflex function and decrease efferent parasympathetic tone to the heart to increase cardiac output.
f. Facilitates norepinephrine release from sympathetic nerve endings and inhibits norepinephrine reuptake, thereby enhancing sympathetic adrenergic transmission.

Aldosterone, a steroid hormone, secreted by the adrenal cortex is under the control of several factors: AT II, potassium, and to a lesser degree, adrenocorticotrophic hormone (ACTH), endothelin 1, estrogens, and urotensin II. AT II is the major stimulus for the secretion of aldosterone. The MR present on the surface of the principal cells, in the distal tubules and collecting ducts of the nephron, is activated by aldosterone to promote sodium retention through an increase in luminal epithelial sodium channels (ENaC) and basolateral Na-K ATPase proteins. This potent electronegative luminal potential induces the efflux of cations from the principal cell, namely potassium and hydrogen ions. Potassium is excreted through the renal outer medullary potassium channels (ROMKs) present in the luminal surface of the principal cell, and hydrogen ions through the neighboring α-intercalated cells. However, AT II directly acts on the principal cells to minimize potassium excretion through the ROMKs and instead, promote hydrogen ion loss through the α-intercalated cells. Through the initiation of this renin-dependent-aldosteronism pathway by low intravascular volume, sodium is reabsorbed leading to an increase in osmolarity and subsequent increase in volume while minimizing the loss of potassium.

Hyperkalemia, however, can also be a trigger for aldosterone release. In the setting of volume expansion and extracellular hyperkalemia, aldosterone is released from the adrenal glands to act on the renal principal cells to excrete the excess potassium ions. Both renin and AT II are suppressed, and proximal tubular sodium reabsorption is decreased as a result of volume expansion in this setting, creating a renin-independent-aldosteronism pathway. The high concentration of sodium delivered to the distal nephron is exchanged for further potassium release.

The renin-dependent and -independent aldosteronism are essential physiological mechanisms that are integrated and can occur concurrently to maintain homeostasis. PA is a pathophysiological state driven primarily by a renin-independent pathway. Aldosterone hypersecretion, from one or both adrenal glands, causes appropriate suppression of renin resulting in an elevated plasma ARR. The production of AT II is reduced which prevents the absorption of sodium in the proximal nephron. The increased sodium delivery to the distal nephron induces aldosterone-mediated sodium reabsorption, together with water, at the expense of potassium resulting in a metabolic alkalosis. The fluid volume expansion creates an increase in arterial BP, which in turn causes a glomerular hyperfiltration. Eventually, the continued sodium reabsorption-driven fluid expansion results in hypertension.

The majority of PA is caused by bilateral adrenal hyperplasia (60%) (BAH) or an aldosterone-producing adrenal adenoma (30%) (APA).[13,14] A less common form of the disease consists of unilateral adrenal hyperplasia (2%) caused by micro- or macronodular hyperplasia of the zona glomerulosa of predominantly one gland. The remaining consists of aldosterone-producing adrenocortical carcinoma (<1%), hereditary familial hyperaldosteronism (<1%), and ectopic aldosterone-producing adenoma or carcinoma (<0.1%). The underlying pathophysiology of APAs involve somatic mutations of the potassium channel KCNJ5, sodium/potassium and calcium ATPases (ATP1A1 and ATP2B3), and the calcium channel CACNA1D.[15-17]

Hereditary familial hyperaldosteronism (FH) is an extremely rare cause of PA and should be considered when individuals are diagnosed with the disease at less than 20 years of age or when it presents in multiple members within a family. FH Type I (FH I) is caused by a chimeric gene where the gene coding for aldosterone synthase—$CYP_{11}B_2$—is under the regulation of the promoter for 11β-hydroxylase—$CYP_{11}B_1$—the enzyme involved in the last step in cortisol biosynthesis.[16,18] Instead of the usual AT II messenger initiating the generation of aldosterone synthase in the zona glomerulosa, the production of the enzyme in FH I is controlled by ACTH and occurs in the zona fasciculata. It is also known as glucocorticoid-remediable aldosteronism (GRA) and can be treated with physiologic doses of glucocorticoid to suppress ACTH secretion.

The germline mutations involved in FH II–IV produce elements that regulate cell membrane potential in the secretion of aldosterone. Individuals with FH II possess a gain-of-function germline mutation of the voltage-gated CLCN2 chloride channel in zona glomerulosa.[16,18] A mutation within the *KCNJ5* gene in FH III, which encodes for a potassium channel, causes a lack of ion selectivity and an inward leak of sodium ions resulting in increased cell depolarization and aldosterone secretion. Similarly, FH IV involves a spectrum of mutations such as the gain-of-function mutation in the *CACNA1H* gene, which encodes the α-subunit of an L-type voltage-gated calcium channel causing increased calcium influx and aldosterone production. Mutations involved in the *CACNA1D* gene encode for the α1D-subunit of the calcium channel. In addition to PA, individuals with this germline mutation present with neurocognitive disorders such as epilepsy and autism.

PREVENTION

The overall treatment goal in patients with PA is to prevent the adverse outcomes associated with excess aldosterone, including hypertension, hypokalemia, progressive chronic kidney disease, and further cardiovascular damage. The early diagnosis of the disease provides the opportunity either to cure hypertension or to direct targeted pharmacotherapy, both of which can prevent end-stage PA. The prevalence of target-organ damage to the heart and kidney is increased in patients with PA in contrast to patients with apparent essential hypertension matched for age, sex, and BP.[19] Patients with suppressed plasma renin activity (PRA) levels treated with mineralocorticoid receptor antagonists (MRAs) still have a higher risk of cardiovascular events than in those with essential hypertension. This is fundamentally due to the inadequate dosing of MRAs which should fully block the adverse consequences of hyperaldosteronism. In addition, PA has also been linked to the progression of insulin resistance, metabolic syndrome, depression, and osteoporotic fractures—all of which are also consistent with the concomitant increase in cortisol.[20-23] Believed to be secreted by adenomas >2 cm, this cortisol cosecretion may indicate why treatment with MRAs alone in patients with an aldosterone-secreting adenoma or idiopathic hyperaldosteronism may not fully mitigate the risk of developing glucocorticoid-dependent metabolic syndrome.[24]

Patients with an underlying APA or BAH have an increased risk of left ventricular hypertrophy, stroke, coronary artery disease, atrial fibrillation, and heart failure.[21] Thus, the early diagnosis of PA provides the opportunity either to cure hypertension or to direct targeted pharmacotherapy with surgery or medical treatment, respectively, both of which can prevent end-stage renal disease and irreversible cardiovascular damage.

Although BP normalization with medical and surgical intervention is essential in the prevention of the morbidity and mortality associated with PA, dietary sodium restriction is effective at lowering BP and may also contribute toward the effects of MRAs.[25] In adopting a sodium-restricted diet, less sodium is delivered to the distal nephron, substantially reducing the fluid expansion, increasing renin, normalizing the ARR, reducing hypokalemia, and help mitigate complications from PA. However, the level to which sodium should be restricted is not known, nor is it practical to implement and adhere to.

CLINICAL FINDINGS

Symptoms & Signs

The classic features of moderate-to-severe hypertension, hypokalemia, and metabolic alkalosis are highly suggestive of hyperaldosteronism. However, there is no consistent and reliable clinical phenotype indicative of patients with underlying PA. The phenotype depends largely on the underlying cause and the degree of hyperaldosteronism, as well as the presence of other comorbidities. Hypertension is the major clinical finding, typically moderate to severe, and may be resistant to several antihypertensive pharmacologic treatments. When compared with essential hypertension, individuals with PA have a higher risk of coronary artery disease, atrial fibrillation, left ventricular hypertrophy, heart failure, metabolic syndrome, diabetes, worsening mean eGFR, decreased bone density and higher rate of fracture, and death even after initiation of medical treatment to control BP and MRAs.[21,26-29]

Historically, hypokalemia has been considered one of the major clinical features of PA. However, it has now been shown to be less synonymous with the disease, thought to be present in up to 57% of patients.[7] The fall in potassium ions is accompanied with metabolic alkalosis largely due to increased urinary hydrogen excretion. It is usually mild with no significant sequelae. Additional electrolyte disturbances, such as hypomagnesemia and hypernatremia, can also be observed, with patients experiencing neuromuscular symptoms including paresthesia or weakness.

Laboratory Findings

There are several clinical practice guidelines published by different countries and international organizations for the screening and management of PA. These include guidelines presented by the *Endocrine Society* (ES), *European Society of Hypertension/European Society of Cardiology*, the *American Association of Clinical Endocrinologists/American Association of Endocrine Surgeons*, the *Canadian Hypertension Education Program* (CHEP), the *Italian Association of Clinical Endocrinologists, American Heart Association*, the *Japan Endocrine Society*, and the *French Endocrinology Society/French Hypertension Society/Francophone Endocrine Surgery Association* (Figure 45–2).[2,30-36] Discrepancies exist at all levels between these guidelines—screening, case confirmation, classification, treatment, and follow-up. This may cause confusion in clinicians regarding the management of the disease. Based on the 2019 Wu et al. systematic literature review of existing guidelines on the management of PA, the 2016 ES and 2016 CHEP publications are regarded as of good methodological quality according to the assessment tools *Appraisal of Guidelines Research and Evaluation* updated 2017 version and *Institute of Medicine* tools for quality assessment.[37]

Screening for PA is made by the PAC/PRA ratio, known as the ARR. Although this investigation is consistently recommended in all published guidelines, the cutoff value varies considerably.[2,38,39] In addition, most guidelines require a washout period for certain antihypertensive medications due to their effects on raising the renin activity level and therefore lowering the ARR value. Although there is consensus in stopping MRAs, β-adrenergic antagonists, epithelial channel inhibitors, and potassium-wasting diuretics prior to measuring ARR in all guidelines, there are inconsistencies in the recommendations of withdrawing other medications such as calcium channel blockers, ACE-inhibitors, renin inhibitors, NSAIDs, and contraceptives.[40] The 2016 ES guidelines state

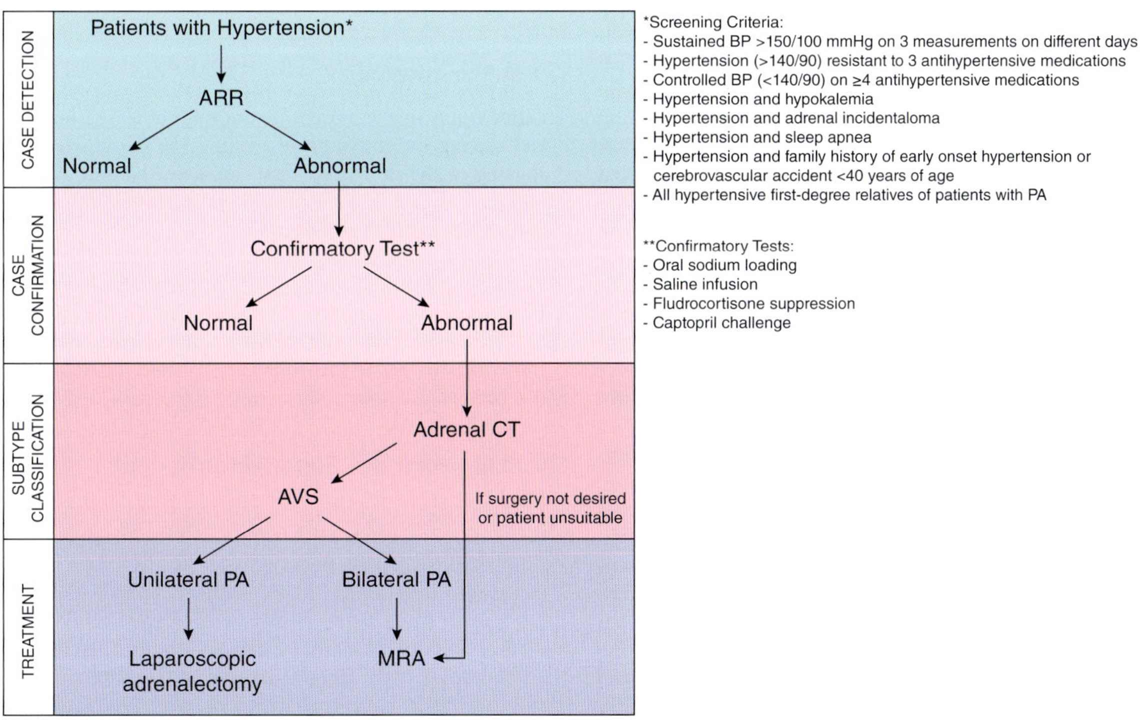

Figure 45–2. Algorithm for screening and management of primary aldosteronism. Flowchart for the diagnostic workup of primary aldosteronism according to the 2016 Endocrine Society Practice Guidelines. ARR, aldosterone-to-renin ratio; CT, computed tomography; AVS, adrenal vein sampling; PA, primary aldosteronism; MRA, mineralocorticoid receptor antagonist.

that the ARR test can still be performed despite continuing all antihypertensive medications, including MRAs, provided the result is clarified with these potential confounding factors.[2] In any case, if the initial ARR is abnormal, difficult to interpret due to suboptimal conditions, or the clinical diagnosis is strongly suspected despite a negative result, the test should be repeated. If still abnormal, the presence of an autonomous hypersecretion of aldosterone should be proven by failure to suppress aldosterone levels through one or more confirmatory tests.

Most guidelines recommend screening for PA in patients at moderate-high risk of the disease, the exception being the practice guidelines developed by the Japan Endocrine Society which advocates screening all hypertensive patients.[35] This practice, however, would not be cost-effective and will likely place an additional burden on primary care physicians. In this setting, prediction tools to reduce the number of patients screened for PA have been developed but hampered by the lack of generalizability of the models. Yamashita et al. developed a scoring system based on specific coefficients obtained from multivariable logistic regression of candidate variables of potential markers of PA in 130 patients—the *pH* of urine, female sex, and low serum K^+ score (*PFK score*).[41] The receiver operating characteristic (ROC) area under curve (AUC) for the model was 0.73 (95% CI: 0.61-0.85). Although a similar result was obtained on external validation, limitations of the PFK score include a small sample size and the derivation from untreated patients with PA. Based on a larger population of patients (420 patients) and enhanced AUC, Kietsiriroje et al. developed the *Predictive Scoring System* (PSS) that used predictive factors age <60 years, BMI <25 kg/m^2, presence of diabetes, ≥3 antihypertensive agents, serum sodium ≥141 mmol/L, and serum potassium <3.5 mmol/L with ROC curve AUC 0.87 (95% CI: 0.83-0.91).[42] Similar to the PFK score, the PSS score was developed from a retrospective design with its inherent biases that may limit the application of the models. Finally, Buffolo et al. have developed two models that have also been validated within an independent external cohort that are promising—a conventional scoring system and a novel machine learning-based model.[43] The *Score To Predict Primary Aldosteronism* (SToP-PA), based on six independent predictors of PA—male sex, systolic BP, antihypertensive treatment, BMI, lowest potassium, and signs of organ damage (left ventricularly hypertrophy, or microalbuminuria and cardiovascular events)—has an optimized sensitivity of 90.7% for PA and 92.3% for unilateral PA; and the machine-learning classifier *Random Forest Regressor* (RFr) has an optimized sensitivity of 96.6% for PA and 100.0% for unilateral PA. By applying the SToP-PA score and RFr-model, the number of patients undergoing PA screening would reduce by 11.6% and 32.7%, respectively. However, it still remains to be determined how best, and at what point in the patient's course, such scoring systems should be incorporated into the routine clinical care of patients with PA.

Patients successfully screened with the ARR test, or to exclude a diagnosis of PA in a borderline case, should undergo one of four confirmatory tests: oral sodium loading, saline infusion, fludrocortisone suppression, or a captopril challenge test. There is no one specific benchmark confirmatory test that should be performed. Instead, the choice of test should be made according to the local expertise, practice, cost, and patient compliance.

A. Oral Sodium Loading

Patients should increase their sodium intake to >200 mmol (~5 g) for 3 days prior to testing. In addition, serum potassium concentration should be normal with the addition of potassium chloride supplements. Urinary aldosterone is measured in the 24-hour collection time starting from the morning of day 3.

Interpretation: Elevated urinary aldosterone excretion, with cutoff values from >10 μg/24h (28 nmol/d) to >14 μg/24 h (>33 nmol/d), indicative of PA.

Problem: Should not perform in patients with uncontrolled HTN, renal insufficiency, cardiac dysrhythmias, or severe hypokalemia.

B. Saline Infusion

Patients stay in recumbent position for at least 1 hour before and during the infusion of 2 L of 0.9% saline over 4 hours starting in the morning. Vitals are assessed and blood samples for PAC, PRA, cortisol, and plasma potassium are drawn at time zero and after 4 hours.

Interpretation: If aldosterone levels <5 ng/dL (140 pmol/L), PA is very unlikely; indeterminate if levels between 5 to 10 ng/dL; and indicative of PA if levels >10 ng/dL (280 nmol/L).

Problem: Should not perform in patients with uncontrolled HTN, renal insufficiency, cardiac dysrhythmias, or severe hypokalemia.

C. Fludrocortisone Suppression

Patients receive 0.1 mg oral fludrocortisone every 6 hours for 4 days, together with slow-release potassium chloride supplements to keep potassium levels close to 4.0 mmol/L (measured four times a day), sodium chloride supplements (30 mmol three times a day with meals), and sufficient dietary salt to maintain a urinary sodium excretion rate ≥3 mmol/kg body weight. On day 4, cortisol is measured at 7 AM; at 10 AM, cortisol, along with PAC and PRA are measured with the patient in a seated position.

Interpretation: Upright aldosterone level >6 ng/dL (170 nmol/L) on day 4 at 10 AM confirms PA provided PRA is <1 ng/mL/h and cortisol concentration is lower than the value obtained at 7 AM (to exclude the confounding effect of ACTH).

Problem: Need for inpatient assessment requiring hospital admission for accurate testing in some institutions.

D. Captopril Challenge

Patients receive 25 to 50 mg captopril orally in the morning after sitting or standing for at least 1 hour. With the patient remaining seated, blood samples are drawn at time zero and at 1 or 2 hours after the challenge measuring PRA and PAC.

Interpretation: Aldosterone is normally suppressed by captopril but remains elevated and PRA remains suppressed in patients with PA.

Problem: False negative or equivocal results.

However, these confirmatory tests can be bypassed in patients with a combination of a high PAC with concomitant sufficient renin suppression and spontaneous hypokalemia, as recommended by the ES guidelines.[2] Wang et al. had shown that, in addition to the optimized and guideline criteria, combining spontaneous hypokalemia, a PAC >20 ng/dL, and plasma renin concentration <2.5 μIU/mL were 100% specific for the diagnosis of PA (CI: 0.97-1.00).[44] This led to bypassing confirmatory tests in 12% of patients with PA in their validation cohort.

Imaging Studies

Computed tomography (CT) or magnetic resonance imaging (MRI) of the adrenal glands should be performed to localize the responsible lesion and to eliminate other aldosterone-producing tumors, such as adrenal carcinoma. A CT of the abdomen with and without contrast per institutional adrenal protocol with 2.5-mm slice thickness, or MRI abdomen with and without contrast should be done in every patient. Imaging features seen in patients with PA can include structurally normal-appearing bilateral adrenal glands, unilateral adenoma, bilateral adenoma, micronodular hyperplasia, bilateral macronodular hyperplasia, or unilateral adrenocortical carcinoma. An adrenal aldosteronoma is usually small (<2 cm in diameter), homogenous, often hypodense, with an attenuation value near that of water; whilst an adrenal carcinoma, producing aldosterone-excess, is usually >4 cm in diameter, irregularly shaped, with an attenuation of >20 Hounsfield units, and characterized by marked biochemical abnormalities and severe hypertension.[45] The specificity and sensitivity of detecting an adrenal adenoma on CT are 98% and 88%, respectively. Although an MRI can accurately detect a lipid-rich adenoma with a sensitivity nearing 100%, it is less discriminate with lipid-poor adenomas.

The accuracy of diagnosis by imaging tests is not always precise as the prevalence of nonfunctioning adrenocortical nodules increases with age and distinguishing the source of aldosterone excess in small adenomas (<10 mm) is often challenging.

Special Tests

Patients confirmed to have PA are recommended to undergo adrenal venous sampling (AVS) in the setting of bilateral abnormal glands, bilateral nodules, bilateral normal glands with biochemical evidence of PA, or assessment of small adenomas (<10 mm). The role of AVS is to differentiate unilateral from bilateral forms of PA. Although recommended in all guidelines and consensus statements, the AVS can be bypassed in a young patient (<35 years old) with spontaneous hypokalemia, marked aldosterone excess (PAC >30 ng/dL), and the presence of a solitary, hypodense, unilateral nodule, with normal contralateral adrenal gland imaging.[2]

It is usually performed by a dedicated interventional radiologist who is adept technically and able to interpret the results proficiently. Apart from the added benefit of obtaining a functional diagnosis in CT-identified nodules, performing the AVS can help locate an APA that is below the threshold of identification via CT-alone. In the largest registry of individual AVS studies performed in major referral centers between 2000 and 2015, the AVIS-2 study had shown that subtyping of PA by AVS was associated with a higher rate of clinical and biochemical successes, and a reduced number of antihypertensive medications for persistently elevated BP after surgery.[46]

The meta-analysis of 38 studies describing adults with PA who underwent CT/MRI and AVS performed by Kempers et al. produced a concordance rate of only 62%.[47] However, a more recent study performed by Thiesmeyer et al. revealed a concordance rate of 100% based on retrospective data from three tertiary medical centers, likely due to improved sensitivities and specificities for lipid-rich adenomas found on CT and MRI.[48] In addition, they had shown that there were no differences in complete chemical and biochemical successes between patients who underwent AVS versus those who proceeded directly to surgery.

The complexity in executing an AVS is confounded mainly by anatomical variations, such as aberrant adrenal venous drainage and cannulation of the inaccurate draining vein of the adenoma. Additional factors include the technical aspects related to the procedure, sampling conditions, a standardized written protocol for diagnosis with wide between-center success rates, appropriate patient selection and preparation, coordinated sample handling, respective cutoff values for laterality index (LI), and the use of cosyntropin.[49] The rationale for cosyntropin-stimulated AVS is to minimize fluctuations in aldosterone secretion caused by stress, amplify the adrenal-to-IVC cortisol gradient, which, in turn, confirm successful sampling of the appropriate draining vein, and to promote the secretion of aldosterone from the suspected adenoma.

Complications from the AVS procedure include adrenal vein rupture, bleeding from the entry site, localized hematoma, dissection of the vein(s), and adrenal hemorrhage or ischemia. Although initially reported up to 10%, complication

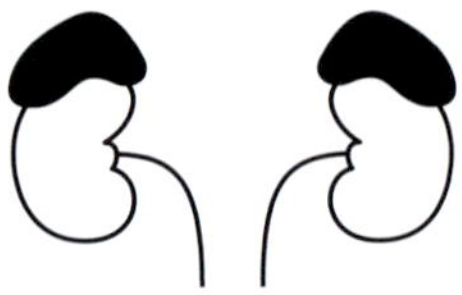

$$\text{Selectivity index} = C_{AV} \div C_{IVC}$$

$$\text{Lateralization index} = A_{DAV}/C_{DAV} \div A_{NDAV}/C_{NDAV}$$

$$\text{Contralateral suppression index} = A_{NDAV}/C_{NDAV} \div A_{IVC}/C_{IVC}$$

Figure 45–3. Adrenal vein sampling indices and definitions. *Selectivity Index* = If greater than cutoff confirm blood sample obtained from adrenal vein. *Lateralization Index* = If greater than cutoff confirm blood sample from lateralized aldosterone excess. *Contralateral Suppression Index* = If lesser than cutoff confirm ipsilateral aldosterone suppression and contralateral excess. A, plasma aldosterone concentration; C, plasma cortisol concentration; AV, adrenal vein; DAV, dominant adrenal vein; NDAV; nondominant adrenal vein; IVC, inferior vena cava.

rates have decreased down to 0.61% likely due to improved procedural skills.[50,51] The procedure is time-consuming, expensive, invasive, technically difficult, requires access to a specialty center, and with success rates ranging between 42% and 99%.[52] Given the complications associated with this approach and the increased sensitivity of CT, selective utilization of the AVS procedure would be prudent.

Clinical prediction scores (CPS) can be used to distinguish between unilateral and bilateral PA since the treatment options are different for the two disorders. It can also be useful before proceeding to an AVS study especially when dealing with a lack of availability, technical procedural performance issues, and when performed at lower volume centers. These score-based algorithms have largely been developed by combining clinical and biochemical parameters along with significant imaging findings. The prediction models include those designed by Küpers, Nanba, Kocjan, Kobayashi, Nagano, Puar, and Burrello.[53-59] Although CPS algorithms may be clinically valid and beneficial within its specific patient cohort, the majority lack external validation, and for those that do, had variable results unlike the high diagnostic performance originally reported.[60,61] In addition, due to differences in lab assays and confirmatory tests, the prediction model may not be applicable in other cohorts.

A percutaneous femoral approach is used in the AVS procedure, and blood, which is assayed for aldosterone and cortisol, is obtained both from adrenal veins and from the external iliac vein (labelled "IVC"). A sample of blood from the common phrenic trunk next to the left adrenal vein is considered as drainage from the left adrenal gland, and its counterpart is obtained from the orifice of the right adrenal vein. The different concentrations of cortisol obtained from the paired glands and IVC are used as confirmation of accurate catheterization. Blood from the inferior phrenic veins into the common phrenic trunk causes a dilutional effect and is corrected by dividing each PAC by its respective cortisol concentrations, the cortisol-corrective ratio, to determine the aldosterone LI (Figure 45–3). An LI of ≤4:1 is the threshold for the diagnosis of a unilateral adrenal gland disease, and a ratio of <3:1 suggests bilateral hypersecretion. Determining a contralateral suppression index (CSI), by dividing the contralateral aldosterone/cortisol ratio by the IVC aldosterone/cortisol ratio, is useful when the LI is in the grey zone (3.0-<4.0) and if the AVS is not successful in determining laterality. A CSI of <0.5 denotes contralateral disease.

Segmental selective AVS (sAVS) is a novel technique, performed in some countries, that has provided the option of performing a partial adrenalectomy.[62] An intra-adrenal gland aldosterone concentration is obtained from each adrenal vein tributary and central vein with the composite producing a gradient map. This specialized study provides the ability to distinguish the location of a single macro- or micro-aldosterone-producing nodule from diffuse hyperplasia, the advantage of preserving sufficient glandular tissue on the affected side, and the surgical treatment for bilateral aldosterone-secreting nodules. Further investigations are required to demonstrate the accuracy of sAVS and to facilitate the development of this new diagnostic strategy.

DIFFERENTIAL DIAGNOSIS

The following are the causes of secondary hypertension that may present with elevated PAC.

Renal Artery Stenosis

Hypertension caused by narrowing of unilateral or bilateral renal arteries with atherosclerosis. Diagnosed by imaging studies of kidney and renal arteries—ultrasound, magnetic resonance arteriogram, computed tomographic angiography. Treatment with medical therapy involving antihypertensive medication and/or renal artery angioplasty with stenting if medical therapy is unsuccessful.

Apparent Mineralocorticoid Excess

Rare form of juvenile hypertension characterized by low birth weight, failure to thrive, hypercalciuria, nephrocalcinosis, and end-organ damage, such as renal failure, due to early onset of hypertension. Accompanied by all findings of PA (hypertension, hypokalemia, metabolic alkalosis, low PRA) except for low PAC. Caused by autosomal recessive trait in mutation of 11-β-hydroxysteroid dehydrogenase enzyme type 2 isoform (11-β-HSD2) that normally converts cortisol to cortisone. Cortisone does not bind to the MR. The build-up of cortisol is approximately 100-fold higher than plasma aldosterone concentration but binds as avidly to the MR creating a marked elevation in net MR activity. Diagnosis confirmed by genetic testing. Treatment includes dexamethasone, amiloride, triamterene, spironolactone, eplerenone; all agents which reduce endogenous cortisol production or block the MRA.

Excessive Licorice Intake

Chronic ingestion induces a rise in BP in normal individuals. Licorice contains glycyrrhetinic acid, a steroid, that inhibits 11-β-HSD2 and produces a syndrome similar to AME. Testing is not necessary and cessation of licorice ingestion results in cure.

Gitelman Syndrome

Rare disorder due to a defective sodium/chloride cotransporter in the distal convoluted tubule. Autosomal recessive genetic disorder with mutations in SLC12A3 that produces less sodium reabsorption in the distal convoluted tubule with increased delivery to the collecting duct. This results in increased potassium and hydrogen excretion causing the similar characteristics of PA—hypokalemia and metabolic alkalosis.

Liddle Syndrome

Rare autosomal dominant mutation on chromosome 16p12 condition with increased sodium reabsorption and potassium secretion due to increase in collecting tubules. This gain-of-function mutation of the ENaC leads to manifestations of mineralocorticoid excess: hypertension, hypokalemia, and metabolic alkalosis. Diagnosed by genetic testing. Management consists of amiloride or triamterene, potassium-sparring diuretics, that directly block the collecting tubule ENaC channels correcting both hypertension and hypokalemia. Spironolactone is ineffective as the syndrome is not mediated by aldosterone.

Pregnancy-Exacerbated Hypertension

Rare autosomal dominant condition due to a mutation in the MR that constitutively activates the receptor, which is also nonspecific and causes activation by progesterone (lack of response to spironolactone). Treated with amiloride. Characterized by early onset low renin/low aldosterone hypertension with hypokalemia. BP levels typically increase during pregnancy.

COMPLICATIONS

The necessity to treat patients with PA is largely due to the deleterious hormonal effects of hyperaldosteronism—increased perivascular inflammation, oxidant stress, interstitial fibrosis, vascular tone dysfunction, with subsequent remodeling. The excessive activation of the MR results in volume expansion, hypertension, hypokalemia, and metabolic alkalosis. The disease manifests in end-organ damage in the cardiovascular, renal, musculoskeletal, endocrine, and systems. This target-organ damage associated with PA can be reversed with appropriate treatment.

Hyperaldosteronism leads to an increased risk for developing coronary artery disease, atrial fibrillation, stroke, left ventricularly hypertrophy, and, ultimately, cardiac failure.[21] These consequences are more commonly observed in patients with hyperaldosteronism than essential HTN—matched individuals. Thus, aldosterone-mediated MR stimulation is pathologic and induces cardiovascular injury, independent of the influence of BP. Contributing factors in hyperaldosteronism include the (1) hypertrophic effect on the myocardium and vascular smooth muscle cells mediated by dose-dependent myosin light-chain phosphorylation; (2) formation of reactive oxygen species resulting in cardiac and vascular fibrosis; (3) direct effects of the hormone on the extracellular matrix leading to cardiovascular dysregulation; and (4) hypokalemia coupled with atrial structural and electrical remodeling.[21] In comparing 385 patients with PA caused by an aldosteronoma-producing adenoma matched with 385 patients with essential hypertension, Wu et al. had shown that patients with hyperaldosteronism had a higher nocturnal systolic (130 ± 16 vs 127 ± 17 mmHg, $p < 0.05$) and diastolic (82 ± 10 vs 79 ± 11 mmHg, $p < 0.01$) BP, a reduced nocturnal BP decline and higher median N-terminal pro-BNP (53.7 vs 33.2 pg/mL, $p < 0.001$) and left ventricular mass index (113 ± 25 vs 102 ± 26 g/m^2, $p < 0.001$).[63]

In the large retrospective cohort study by Hundemer et al., PA patients treated with MR, to achieve similar BPs as age-matched patients with essential hypertension, still had an approximately twofold higher risk for incident cardiovascular outcomes, diabetes, atrial fibrillation, and death, even with comparable cardiovascular risk profiles in both groups.[27] The increased risk was primarily seen in PA patients with persistent renin suppression even on MRA therapy. PA patients treated with higher doses of MRAs with a consequential rise in renin had comparable risks with patients with essential hypertension. This suggests that MRA therapy should be titrated for a concomitant rise in renin levels for effective risk reduction in medical management of patients with PA.

Renal consequences of hyperaldosteronism have been presumptively attributed to mesangial cell proliferation, podocyte injury, and endothelial dysfunction, culminating in albuminuria with decline in glomerular filtration. The vicious cycle of increased sodium reabsorption and volume expansion leads to increased renal perfusion pressure and ultimately glomerular capillary noncompliance and hypertension.[64] Additionally, enhanced excretion of potassium and hydrogen in the distal nephron results in hypokalemia and metabolic alkalosis, increasing the risk of renal damage.

The association between PA and an increased risk of insulin resistance and metabolic syndrome is thought to be based on several observations: (1) hyperaldosteronism impairing insulin sensitivity and differentiation of adipose cells causing it to be more resistant to insulin; (2) reducing the level and expression of an adipocyte-produced peptide in visceral adipose tissue, adiponectin, that has been shown to have insulin-sensitizing, anti-atherogenic, and anti-inflammatory effects; (3) augment hepatic gluconeogenesis and impair pancreatic β-cell function, and (4) decrease expression of insulin receptors in skeletal muscles leading to decreased glucose uptake.[28] The increased metabolic risk may also be accounted for by the significant and consistent increase in cortisol and total glucocorticoid metabolites in patients with PA. Clinically relevant cortisol secretion from an adrenal adenoma is correlated with tumor size, typically with adenomas measuring >2 cm. This glucocorticoid excess has also been shown to cause bone disease and osteoporotic fractures in patients with PA.[23]

Finally, PA may also contribute to obstructive sleep apnea due to the underlying volume overload. This is demonstrated by the fluid shift to the neck structures that occur in a supine state during sleep leading to upper respiratory tract soft tissue oedema with subsequent airflow obstruction. This has major implications resulting in neuropsychiatric dysfunction, cardiovascular and cerebrovascular morbidity, pulmonary hypertension or right heart failure, and metabolic syndrome.[28]

TREATMENT

The primary aim for treatment of PA is to prevent the morbidity and mortality associated with hypertension, kidney disease, and cardiovascular damage. Thus, either curative surgery or medical therapy by antagonizing the MR is essential for the management of the disease. Although, the question of one treatment being more superior than the other is problematic due to the inherent differences and biases in treatment selection. Older patients tend to have bilateral disease, prolonged hypertension, and more medical comorbidities. Thus, they are more ideally suited for MRAs. Younger individuals, who present with more severe hypertension that has developed over a relatively short time, tend to undergo surgical intervention for effective treatment. These patients have been shown to require less follow-up, achieve higher quality of life scores, and are less likely to develop type 2 diabetes than patients treated with MRAs.[65]

Surgery

Management with adrenalectomy should be reserved for unilateral secreting tumors. Surgical adrenalectomy has been shown to cure or, at least, significantly improve the hypertension and hypokalemia associated with PA and even lead to improved quality of life.[65] A unilateral minimally invasive adrenalectomy is the optimal surgical procedure with a transperitoneal or retroperitoneal approach. The latter has the benefit of avoiding the peritoneal cavity especially in patients with previous abdominal surgeries. Preoperative management includes BP control and repletion of hypokalemia, if present. All potassium supplements and MRAs should be discontinued after an adrenalectomy. Patients who are not candidates for surgery, or who prefer a noninvasive approach to management, can be treated with medical pharmacotherapy agents.

Medical

Medical management with MRAs can be used as effective therapy in PA caused by bilateral idiopathic hyperaldosteronism, FH I, and in patients with contraindications to surgery. It is vital to ensure that complete MR blockade is reached, as despite normalization of BP and/or hypokalemia, a rise in renin corresponds to a lower risk of cardiovascular complications, death, and atrial fibrillation, similar to a patient undergoing an adrenalectomy for PA. Persistently low renin, despite starting MRAs, signifies an incomplete response and effects of the medication. In addition to its effects on BP, MRAs also mitigate the adverse cardiovascular and renovascular effects of aldosterone excess.

Spironolactone is a potassium sparing MRA that additionally works as an antagonist of the androgen and agonist of the progesterone receptors. This nonselectivity produces the characteristic adverse side effects of the treatment that include gynecomastia, mastodynia, irregular menses, decreased libido, and erectile dysfunction. Spironolactone is also listed as a pregnancy category C medication due to the nonselectivity of its receptor-binding activity.

On the contrary, the competitive and selective MRA, eplerenone, does not cause these side effects, but demonstrates lower efficacy and comes at a higher cost to the patient. Low doses of eplerenone, a pregnancy category B medication, are relatively safe in pregnant women with severe PA where an adrenalectomy is not an option. The ideal MRA chosen for treatment of PA in any individual should be based on a shared decision-making process with the patient.

Short-acting glucocorticoids, such as hydrocortisone, should be used with the smallest effective dose to treatment PA due to GRA confirmed by germline mutation assessment.

In addition to correcting hypokalemia and reducing hypertension, higher doses may cause Cushing syndrome. Other options for GRA treatment include the MRAs mentioned above.

PROGNOSIS

The excess risk for adverse health outcomes in PA is thought to be independent of BP control but instead due to the direct pathophysiological effects of chronic hyperaldosteronism and continuous stimulation of the MR.[12,28,64] The *Primary Aldosteronism Surgical Outcome* (PASO) study group, comprised of 31 experts from 28 countries worldwide, established consensus criteria for outcomes in the management of PA. The success of treatment can be categorized as biochemical versus clinical.[66]

Biochemical Success

Complete

- Correction of hypokalemia, if present presurgery, and normalization of the ARR; in patients with a raised ARR postsurgery, aldosterone secretion should be suppressed in a confirmatory test.

Partial

- Correction of hypokalemia, if present presurgery, and a raised ARR with one or both of the following (compared with presurgery): ≥50% decrease in baseline PAC or abnormal but improved postsurgery confirmatory test result.

Absent

- Persistent hypokalemia, if present presurgery, or persistent raised ARR, or both, with failure to suppress aldosterone secretion with a postsurgery confirmatory test.

Clinical Success

Complete

- Normal BP without the aid of antihypertensive medication.

Partial

- The same BP before surgery with less antihypertensive medication or a reduction in BP with either the same amount or less antihypertensive medication.

Absent

- Unchanged or increased BP with either the same amount or an increase in antihypertensive medication.

The goals of management are to reduce the hyperaldosteronism-associated comorbidities, improve quality of life, and reduce mortality. Early systematic screening, diagnosis, and initiation of specific treatment for PA may lead to the reversal of cardiovascular risk excess compared with patients with essential hypertension.[67] Where overall medical management aims to normalize the systolic and diastolic BP in accordance with current guidelines, surgery, in selective patients, provides the added benefit of removing the source of aldosterone excess. The immediate effects of eliminating aldosterone overproduction seen in surgery may be the ultimate benefit to the spectrum of improvement, from possibly partial to near complete.[66,68]

The laparoscopic adrenalectomy is the treatment of choice for patients with unilateral PA. Compared to a laparotomy, a minimally invasive adrenalectomy performed by an expert adrenal surgeon is associated with a shorter duration of hospitalization and a lower rate of clinical complications.[69,70] In the PASO study, based on a large worldwide retrospective analysis of 705 patients who underwent an adrenalectomy for PA between 1994 and 2015, complete or partial clinical success was achieved in 37% and 47% patients, respectively; complete biochemical success was seen 94% of the cohort.[66] Continued reliance on medication and persistent hypertension following an adrenalectomy have been correlated with use of ≥2 antihypertensive agents preoperatively, increasing age, male sex, increased serum creatinine level, chronicity of hypertension, higher BMI, and is most likely due to coexistent essential hypertension. Current theories suggest structural vascular remodeling caused by chronic elevations in peripheral vascular resistance with long-term exposure to excess aldosterone as the main instigating factor to an incomplete response to surgery.

The assessment of preoperative factors can be used to help provide individualized objective measures of the potential benefit of an adrenalectomy, predict complete clinical cure, and help support the shared decision-making process between physician and patient. These scoring systems include the *Aldosteronoma Resolution Score* (ARS), *PASO score*, *Nomogram-based Predictive Score*, the *Spanish Primary Aldosteronism Registry Score*, and those proposed by Utsumi, Kaneko, Wachtel, and Morisaki.[71-78] The variable parameters in these scoring systems include BMI, the antihypertensive medication profile, evidence of end-organ damage, nodule size, age, ARR, and coexistent diabetes mellitus, whilst the common factors are sex and chronicity of hypertension. Important limitations in these scoring systems relate to the lack of generalizability, paucity of prospective external validation, and short duration of follow-up. In the retrospective comparative analysis of six of these preoperative scoring systems in a single tertiary referral center performed by O'Toole et al., although each scoring system had demonstrated significance within the defined population it was based on, there was no overall single best system.[79] The PASO and Utsumi scoring systems demonstrated more universal relevance and stronger predictive performances than the rest with similar prediction accuracy and result concordance up to 70% and 90%, respectively.[79]

The PASO scoring system was derived to classify postsurgical clinical outcomes from 380 patients who underwent adrenalectomy for unilateral PA. Six variables from the algorithm, confirmed as independent predictors, were selected to develop a 25-point predictive score with an optimal cutoff of greater than 16 points: known duration of hypertension, sex, antihypertensive medication dosage, BMI, target organ damage, and size of largest nodule at imaging. Based on the original cohort, the scoring system had 79.2% accuracy of prediction, 84.4% specificity, and 71.3% sensitivity with an AUC of 0.839.[72] The Utsumi nomogram, however, was developed based on 132 Japanese patients with PA managed surgically. Duration of hypertension, preoperative number of antihypertensive drug classes, age, and sex were incorporated into the nomogram with an AUC of 0.83.[74] In a study comparing the predictive validities of the Utsumi nomogram, with that of the ARS and Wachtel et al. systems on 200 patients (91 American, 109 French) who underwent an adrenalectomy for PA, the Utsumi model demonstrated the highest predictive validity with an overall AUC of 0.78.[80]

Medical management of hypertension with MRAs usually takes as long as 4 and 8 weeks for improvement but requires a lifelong dependence on the therapy. The correction of hypokalemia, if coexistent, occurs promptly. The efficacy of MRAs depends on whether sufficient blockade is achieved. Persistent suppression of renin with insufficient doses of MRAs has been correlated with a twofold higher risk for developing myocardial infarction, heart failure requiring hospitalization, stroke, nearly threefold excess risk for cardiovascular events and atrial fibrillation, and a 63% higher risk for death compared with age-matched patients with essential hypertension and similar BP control. By contrast, a substantial rise in renin, brought about in patients with a higher dose of MRAs, produces a risk profile comparable to patients with essential hypertension.[27] Wu et al. have shown that a PRA level <0.6 ng/mL/h or PAC >27 ng/dL at 1 year after starting medical therapy with MRAs could be related to higher risks of long-term incident major adverse cardiovascular events or mortality.[67] The incomplete aldosterone blockade, together with renal insufficiency and underlying medical comorbidities, has been associated with persistent cardiac organ damage.

Studies examining the direct comparisons between a surgical adrenalectomy and MRAs have been limited due to the bias in terms of the varied demographics and clinical presentation of unilateral versus bilateral disease. Comparative longitudinal or interventional studies between the use of MRAs and surgery are lacking, along with standardized recommendations for the titration of MRAs. Patients with unilateral disease often present younger in age and with more severe hypertension. In contrast, patients with bilateral disease often present older in age, with more chronic exposure to elevated aldosterone levels, and are generally more non-White. The few studies performed have suggested improved long-term cardiovascular, renal, and cerebrovascular outcomes, in addition to reduced mortality with an adrenalectomy compared with an MRA regimen.[27,67,68,81,82] Chang et al. showed that patients with PA treated with MRAs had a higher risk of stroke (hazard ratio = 1.83, $p < .001$), while patients who underwent an adrenalectomy had a lower risk of incident stroke (hazard ratio = 0.75) compared to patients with essential hypertension.[82] Patients who underwent an adrenalectomy have more improvement on the left ventricle mass index than those on MRAs, largely due to the reversal of the collagen content in the myocardium and more pronounced and permanent attenuation of the aldosterone effect.[67] The reversal of poor LV diastolic function has been demonstrated after an adrenalectomy for PA with a reduction in the concentric geometry and burden of LV hypertrophy. Rossi et al. had shown that patients treated with MRAs had the highest incidence of atrial fibrillation, compared with patients who underwent an adrenalectomy and those with essential hypertension (pooled OR: 2.83, 95% CI: 1.76-4.57 in the random-effects model; pooled OR: 1.91, 95% CI: 1.11-3.28).[51] Patients with suppressed renin levels from inadequate MR blockade is an indicator of continued aldosterone exposure and consequent cardiometabolic effects.

Functional and anatomical changes in the kidneys occur with hyperaldosteronism due to expansion of extracellular volume, progressive hypertension, increased renal perfusion pressure, with the suppression of renin. Glomerular hypertension, due to the contraction of the efferent arterioles rather than afferent arterioles attributable to aldosterone, is thought to lead to structural damage of the glomerulus. In addition, aldosterone has also been shown to increase the levels of cytokines that include fibronectin and transforming growth factor, β, that lead to renal fibrosis. The increase in global glomerular pressure leads to glomerular hyperfiltration and, in some situations, glomerular hypertrophy. With the removal of the source of hyperaldosteronism, the kidney impairment can be unmasked. The underlying chronic kidney disease can be seen in both surgical and medical therapy of PA but is largely reversible after an adrenalectomy.[83] Independent risk factors that lead to postoperative deterioration of renal function include older age, high preoperative PAC and estimated glomerular filtration rate, and low preoperative serum potassium.

Adrenalectomy has also been reported to significantly lower the utilization of antihypertensive medications, produce higher rates of BP normalization, and improve several indices of quality of life.[84,85] Although distinct from clinical cure, an ARR should be obtained 1 to 2 days after the procedure to confirm a biochemical cure. Similarly, since insufficient MR blockade is coupled with the continued suppression of renin, titration of adequate MRA to target a rise in renin may be the most effective indicator of adequate antagonism. However, the goal of achieving a substantial rise in renin with more aggressive MRA dosing may not always be possible largely due to the antiandrogenic effects of spironolactone (including gynecomastia, erectile dysfunction, and menstrual irregularities), and the risk for hyperkalemia, especially in patients with chronic renal insufficiency.

Eplerenone, associated with fewer adverse side effects but seemingly less effective, is also more expensive and not available in many countries.

WHEN TO REFER/WHEN TO ADMIT

The overall management of patients suspected of having an underlying diagnosis of PA should comprise of a team-based approach that is patient-centered and with systems support for a clinical decision-making algorithm, collaboration, adherence to prescribed regimen, BP monitoring, and timely follow-up care. The team-based care includes the patient, the primary care provider, cardiologist, nephrologist, endocrinologists, nurses, pharmacists, physician assistants, dietitians, social workers, community health workers, and surgeons. Ultimately, all patients with hypertension, both newly diagnosed and chronic, should be screened for workup of PA. The workup should be done in the outpatient setting unless the patient presents with an episode of hypertensive emergency. The referral to a surgical team or specialized centers for further workup should be made if the individual patient has an elevated ARR, if the BP is uncontrolled with maximal medical management, has a positive confirmatory test, workup of an adrenal incidentaloma suggestive of PA, or any appropriate at-risk patients.

A minimally invasive approach to an adrenalectomy for PA has been shown to have a similar overall risk profile to a laparoscopic cholecystectomy.[86] Although the preoperative patient characteristics and indications for operative intervention are distinctly different for an aldosteronoma as opposed to benign biliary disease, the type of procedure has not been shown to influence the rate of complications. Similar to a laparoscopic cholecystectomy, a minimally invasive adrenalectomy is largely an outpatient procedure with postoperative admission occurring in unique circumstances such as in patients with complicated comorbidities, for reimbursement as authorized by insurance companies, or in standard practices by the surgeon.

There should be enhanced communication among and between care providers, both medical and surgical, for better patient outcomes. However, for the algorithm to be successful, there must be a more heightened awareness of PA as a common cause for hypertension and duty to address the major public health issue that results from patients with PA who go untreated.

REFERENCES

1. Kayser SC, Dekkers T, Groenewoud HJ, et al. Study heterogeneity and estimation of prevalence of primary aldosteronism: a systematic review and meta-regression analysis. *J Clin Endocrinol Metab*. 2016;101(7):2826-2835.
2. Funder JW, Carey RM, Mantero F, et al. The management of primary aldosteronism: case detection, diagnosis, and treatment: an endocrine society clinical practice guideline. *J Clin Endocrinol Metab*. 2016;101(5):1889-1916.
3. Conn JW. Presidential address. I. Painting background. II. Primary aldosteronism, a new clinical syndrome. *J Lab Clin Med*. 1955;45(1):3-17.
4. Baudrand R, Guarda FJ, Fardella C, et al. Continuum of renin-independent aldosteronism in normotension. *Hypertension*. 2017;69(5):950-956.
5. Wannachalee T, Lieberman L, Turcu AF. High prevalence of autonomous aldosterone production in hypertension: how to identify and treat it. *Curr Hypertens Rep*. 2022;24(5):123-132.
6. Reincke M, Bancos I, Mulatero P, Scholl UI, Stowasser M, Williams TA. Diagnosis and treatment of primary aldosteronism. *Lancet Diabetes Endocrinol*. 2021;9(12):876-892.
7. Burrello J, Monticone S, Losano I, et al. Prevalence of hypokalemia and primary aldosteronism in 5100 patients referred to a tertiary hypertension unit. *Hypertension*. 2020;75(4):1025-1033.
8. Akasaka H, Yamamoto K, Rakugi H, et al. Sex difference in the association between subtype distribution and age at diagnosis in patients with primary aldosteronism. *Hypertension*. 2019;74(2):368-374.
9. Calhoun DA, Nishizaka MK, Zaman MA, Thakkar RB, Weissmann P. Hyperaldosteronism among black and white subjects with resistant hypertension. *Hypertension*. 2002;40(6):892-896.
10. Nanba K, Omata K, Gomez-Sanchez CE, et al. Genetic characteristics of aldosterone-producing adenomas in blacks. *Hypertension*. 2019;73(4):885-892.
11. Stavropoulos K, Imprialos KP, Patoulias D, Katsimardou A, Doumas M. Impact of primary aldosteronism in resistant hypertension. *Curr Hypertens Rep*. 2022;24(8):285-294.
12. Vaidya A, Mulatero P, Baudrand R, Adler GK. The expanding spectrum of primary aldosteronism: implications for diagnosis, pathogenesis, and treatment. *Endocr Rev*. 2018;39(6):1057-1088.
13. El-Asmar N, Rajpal A, Arafah BM. Primary hyperaldosteronism: approach to diagnosis and management. *Med Clin North Am*. 2021;105(6):1065-1080.
14. Monticone S, Burrello J, Tizzani D, et al. Prevalence and clinical manifestations of primary aldosteronism encountered in primary care practice. *J Am Coll Cardiol*. 2017;69(14):1811-1820.
15. Scholl UI. Genetics of primary aldosteronism. *Hypertension*. 2022;79(5):887-897.
16. Stowasser M. Aldosterone and primary aldosteronism: star performers in hypertension research. *Hypertension*. 2021;78(3):747-750.
17. Meyer LS, Handgriff L, Lim JS, et al. Single-center prospective cohort study on the histopathology, genotype, and postsurgical outcomes of patients with primary aldosteronism. *Hypertension*. 2021;78(3):738-746.
18. Spyroglou A, Piaditis GP, Kaltsas G, Alexandraki KI. Transcriptomics, epigenetics, and metabolomics of primary aldosteronism. *Cancers*. 2021;13(21):5582.
19. Meng Z, Dai Z, Huang K, et al. Long-term mortality for patients of primary aldosteronism compared with essential hypertension: a systematic review and meta-analysis. *Front Endocrinol*. 2020;11:121.
20. Adler GK, Murray GR, Turcu AF, et al. Primary aldosteronism decreases insulin secretion and increases insulin clearance in humans. *Hypertension*. 2020;75(5):1251-1259.
21. Monticone S, D'Ascenzo F, Moretti C, et al. Cardiovascular events and target organ damage in primary aldosteronism compared with essential hypertension: a systematic review and meta-analysis. *Lancet Diabetes Endocrinol*. 2018;6(1):41-50.

22. Murck H, Schlageter L, Schneider A, et al. The potential pathophysiological role of aldosterone and the mineralocorticoid receptor in anxiety and depression: lessons from primary aldosteronism. *J Psychiatr Res.* 2020;130:82-88.
23. Shi S, Lu C, Tian H, Ren Y, Chen T. Primary aldosteronism and bone metabolism: a systematic review and meta-analysis. *Front Endocrinol.* 2020;11:574151.
24. Gomez-Sanchez EP. Third-generation mineralocorticoid receptor antagonists: why do we need a fourth? *J Cardiovasc Pharmacol.* 2016;67(1):26-38.
25. Morimoto S, Ichihara A. Management of primary aldosteronism and mineralocorticoid receptor-associated hypertension. *Hypertens Res.* 2020;43(8):744-753.
26. Chen YL, Xu TY, Xu JZ, Zhu LM, Li Y, Wang JG. A prospective comparative study on cardiac alterations after surgery and drug treatment of primary aldosteronism. *Front Endocrinol.* 2021;12:770711.
27. Hundemer GL, Curhan GC, Yozamp N, Wang M, Vaidya A. Cardiometabolic outcomes and mortality in medically treated primary aldosteronism: a retrospective cohort study. *Lancet Diabetes Endocrinol.* 2018;6(1):51-59.
28. Lin X, Ullah MHE, Wu X, et al. Cerebro-cardiovascular risk, target organ damage, and treatment outcomes in primary aldosteronism. *Front Cardiovasc Med.* 2021;8:798364.
29. Kramers BJ, Kramers C, Lenders JW, Deinum J. Effects of treating primary aldosteronism on renal function. *J Clin Hypertens.* 2017;19(3):290-295.
30. Mancia G, Fagard R, Narkiewicz K, et al. 2013 ESH/ESC guidelines for the management of arterial hypertension: the Task Force for the Management of Arterial Hypertension of the European Society of Hypertension (ESH) and of the European Society of Cardiology (ESC). *Eur Heart J.* 2013;34(28):2159-219.
31. Zeiger MA, Thompson GB, Duh QY, et al. The American Association of Clinical Endocrinologists and American Association of Endocrine Surgeons medical guidelines for the management of adrenal incidentalomas. *Endocr Pract.* 2009;15(Suppl 1):1-20.
32. Leung AA, Nerenberg K, Daskalopoulou SS, et al. Hypertension Canada's 2016 Canadian hypertension education program guidelines for blood pressure measurement, diagnosis, assessment of risk, prevention, and treatment of hypertension. *Can J Cardiol.* 2016;32(5):569-588.
33. Terzolo M, Stigliano A, Chiodini I, et al. AME position statement on adrenal incidentaloma. *Eur J Endocrinol.* 2011;164(6):851-870.
34. Carey RM, Calhoun DA, Bakris GL, et al. Resistant hypertension: detection, evaluation, and management: a scientific statement from the American Heart Association. *Hypertension.* 2018;72(5):e53-e90.
35. Naruse M, Katabami T, Shibata H, et al. Japan Endocrine Society clinical practice guideline for the diagnosis and management of primary aldosteronism 2021. *Endocr J.* 2022;69(4):327-359.
36. Amar L, Baguet JP, Bardet S, et al. SFE/SFHTA/AFCE primary aldosteronism consensus: introduction and handbook. *Ann Endocrinol.* 2016;77(3):179-186.
37. Wu J, Tian W, Zhang L, Zhang J, Zhou B. Assessing the quality of guidelines for primary aldosteronism: which guidelines are worth applying in diverse settings? *J Hypertens.* 2019;37(7):1500-1512.
38. Tanabe A, Naruse M, Takagi S, Tsuchiya K, Imaki T, Takano K. Variability in the renin/aldosterone profile under random and standardized sampling conditions in primary aldosteronism. *J Clin Endocrinol Metab.* 2003;88(6):2489-2494.
39. Mulatero P, Monticone S, Deinum J, et al. Genetics, prevalence, screening and confirmation of primary aldosteronism: a position statement and consensus of the Working Group on Endocrine Hypertension of the European Society of Hypertension. *J Hypertens.* 2020;38(10):1919-1928.
40. Hung A, Ahmed S, Gupta A, et al. Performance of the aldosterone to renin ratio as a screening test for primary aldosteronism. *J Clin Endocrinol Metab.* 2021;106(8):2423-2435.
41. Yamashita T, Shimizu S, Koyama M, et al. Screening of primary aldosteronism by clinical features and daily laboratory tests: combination of urine pH, sex, and serum K. *J Hypertens.* 2018;36(2):326-334.
42. Kietsiriroje N, Wonghirundecha R, Suntornlohanakul O, Murray RD. Construction of a predictive scoring system as a guide to screening and confirmation of the diagnosis of primary aldosteronism. *Clin Endocrinol.* 2020;92(3):196-205.
43. Buffolo F, Burrello J, Burrello A, et al. Clinical score and machine learning-based model to predict diagnosis of primary aldosteronism in arterial hypertension. *Hypertension.* 2021;78(5):1595-1604.
44. Wang K, Hu J, Yang J, et al. Development and validation of criteria for sparing confirmatory tests in diagnosing primary aldosteronism. *J Clin Endocrinol Metab.* 2020;105(7):dgaa282.
45. Park JJ, Park BK, Kim CK. Adrenal imaging for adenoma characterization: imaging features, diagnostic accuracies and differential diagnoses. *Br J Radiol.* 2016;89(1062):20151018.
46. Rossi GP, Rossitto G, Amar L, et al. Clinical outcomes of 1625 patients with primary aldosteronism subtyped with adrenal vein sampling. *Hypertension.* 2019;74(4):800-808.
47. Kempers MJ, Lenders JW, van Outheusden L, et al. Systematic review: diagnostic procedures to differentiate unilateral from bilateral adrenal abnormality in primary aldosteronism. *Ann Intern Med.* 2009;151(5):329-337.
48. Thiesmeyer JW, Ullmann TM, Stamatiou AT, et al. Association of adrenal venous sampling with outcomes in primary aldosteronism for unilateral adenomas. *JAMA Surg.* 2021;156(2):165-171.
49. Rossi GP, Auchus RJ, Brown M, et al. An expert consensus statement on use of adrenal vein sampling for the subtyping of primary aldosteronism. *Hypertension.* 2014;63(1):151-160.
50. Rossi GP, Barisa M, Allolio B, et al. The Adrenal Vein Sampling International Study (AVIS) for identifying the major subtypes of primary aldosteronism. *J Clin Endocrinol Metab.* 2012;97(5):1606-1614.
51. Rossi GP, Maiolino G, Flego A, et al. Adrenalectomy lowers incident atrial fibrillation in primary aldosteronism patients at long term. *Hypertension.* 2018;71(4):585-591.
52. Quencer KB. Adrenal vein sampling: technique and protocol, a systematic review. *CVIR Endovasc.* 2021;4(1):38.
53. Küpers EM, Amar L, Raynaud A, Plouin PF, Steichen O. A clinical prediction score to diagnose unilateral primary aldosteronism. *J Clin Endocrinol Metab.* 2012;97(10):3530-3537.
54. Nanba K, Tsuiki M, Nakao K, et al. A subtype prediction score for primary aldosteronism. *J Hum Hypertens.* 2014;28(12):716-720.
55. Kocjan T, Janez A, Stankovic M, Vidmar G, Jensterle M. A new clinical prediction criterion accurately determines a subset of patients with bilateral primary aldosteronism before adrenal venous sampling. *Endocr Pract.* 2016;22(5):587-594.
56. Kobayashi H, Abe M, Soma M, et al. Development and validation of subtype prediction scores for the workup of primary aldosteronism. *J Hypertens.* 2018;36(11):2269-2276.

57. Nagano H, Kono T, Saiga A, et al. Aldosterone reduction rate after saline infusion test may be a novel prediction in patients with primary aldosteronism. *J Clin Endocrinol Metab.* 2020;105(3):dgz092.
58. Puar TH, Loh WJ, Lim DS, et al. Aldosterone-potassium ratio predicts primary aldosteronism subtype. *J Hypertens.* 2020;38(7):1375-1383.
59. Burrello J, Burrello A, Pieroni J, et al. Development and validation of prediction models for subtype diagnosis of patients with primary aldosteronism. *J Clin Endocrinol Metab.* 2020;105(10):dgaa379.
60. Venos ES, So B, Dias VC, Harvey A, Pasieka JL, Kline GA. A clinical prediction score for diagnosing unilateral primary aldosteronism may not be generalizable. *BMC Endocr Disord.* 2014;14:94.
61. Kocjan T, Vidmar G, Popovic P, Stankovic M. Validation of three novel clinical prediction tools for primary aldosteronism subtyping. *Endocr Connect.* 2022;11(5):e210532.
62. Kitamoto T, Kitamoto KK, Omura M, et al. Precise mapping of intra-adrenal aldosterone activities provides a novel surgical strategy for primary aldosteronism. *Hypertension.* 2020;76(3):976-984.
63. Wu Q, Hong M, Xu J, et al. Diurnal blood pressure pattern and cardiac damage in hypertensive patients with primary aldosteronism. *Endocrine.* 2021;72(3):835-843.
64. Monticone S, Sconfienza E, D'Ascenzo F, et al. Renal damage in primary aldosteronism: a systematic review and meta-analysis. *J Hypertens.* 2020;38(1):3-12.
65. Hundemer GL, Vaidya A. Management of endocrine disease: the role of surgical adrenalectomy in primary aldosteronism. *Eur J Endocrinol.* 2020;183(6):R185-R196.
66. Williams TA, Lenders JWM, Mulatero P, et al. Outcomes after adrenalectomy for unilateral primary aldosteronism: an international consensus on outcome measures and analysis of remission rates in an international cohort. *Lancet Diabetes Endocrinol.* 2017;5(9):689-699.
67. Wu VC, Wang SM, Huang KH, et al. Long-term mortality and cardiovascular events in patients with unilateral primary aldosteronism after targeted treatments. *Eur J Endocrinol.* 2021;186(2):195-205.
68. Aune A, Gerdts E, Kokorina M, et al. Persistent cardiac organ damage in surgically and medically treated primary aldosteronism. *J Hypertens.* 2022;40(6):1204-1211.
69. Mulatero P, Sechi LA, Williams TA, et al. Subtype diagnosis, treatment, complications and outcomes of primary aldosteronism and future direction of research: a position statement and consensus of the Working Group on Endocrine Hypertension of the European Society of Hypertension. *J Hypertens.* 2020;38(10):1929-1936.
70. Jacobsen NE, Campbell JB, Hobart MG. Laparoscopic versus open adrenalectomy for surgical adrenal disease. *Can J Urol.* 2003;10(5):1995-1999.
71. Zarnegar R, Young WF, Jr., Lee J, et al. The aldosteronoma resolution score: predicting complete resolution of hypertension after adrenalectomy for aldosteronoma. *Ann Surg.* 2008;247(3):511-518.
72. Burrello J, Burrello A, Stowasser M, et al. The primary aldosteronism surgical outcome score for the prediction of clinical outcomes after adrenalectomy for unilateral primary aldosteronism. *Ann Surg.* 2020;272(6):1125-1132.
73. Yang Y, Williams TA, Song Y, et al. Nomogram-based preoperative score for predicting clinical outcome in unilateral primary aldosteronism. *J Clin Endocrinol Metab.* 2020;105(12):dgaa634.
74. Utsumi T, Kamiya N, Endo T, et al. Development of a novel nomogram to predict hypertension cure after laparoscopic adrenalectomy in patients with primary aldosteronism. *World J Surg.* 2014;38(10):2640-2644.
75. Wachtel H, Cerullo I, Bartlett EK, et al. Long-term blood pressure control in patients undergoing adrenalectomy for primary hyperaldosteronism. *Surgery.* 2014;156(6):1394-1402; discussion 1402-3.
76. Morisaki M, Kurihara I, Itoh H, et al. Predictors of clinical success after surgery for primary aldosteronism in the Japanese nationwide cohort. *J Endocr Soc.* 2019;3(11):2012-2022.
77. Araujo-Castro M, Paja Fano M, Gonzalez Boillos M, et al. Predictive model of hypertension resolution after adrenalectomy in primary aldosteronism: the SPAIN-ALDO score. *J Hypertens.* 2022;40(12):2486-2493.
78. Kaneko H, Umakoshi H, Ogata M, et al. Machine learning-based models for predicting clinical outcomes after surgery in unilateral primary aldosteronism. *Sci Rep.* 2022;12(1):5781.
79. O'Toole SM, Hornby C, Sze WC, et al. Performance evaluation of scoring systems for predicting post-operative hypertension cure in primary aldosteronism. *Clin Endocrinol (Oxf).* 2021;95(4):576-586.
80. Thiesmeyer JW, Ullmann TM, Greenberg J, et al. Hypertension resolution after adrenalectomy for primary hyperaldosteronism: which is the best predictive model? *Surgery.* 2021;169(1):133-137.
81. Vorselaars W, Nell S, Postma EL, et al. Clinical outcomes after unilateral adrenalectomy for primary aldosteronism. *JAMA Surg.* 2019;154(4):e185842.
82. Chang YH, Chung SD, Wu CH, et al. Surgery decreases the long-term incident stroke risk in patients with primary aldosteronism. *Surgery.* 2020;167(2):367-377.
83. Park KS, Kim JH, Yang YS, et al. Outcomes analysis of surgical and medical treatments for patients with primary aldosteronism. *Endocr J.* 2017;64(6):623-632.
84. Citton M, Viel G, Torresan F, Rossi GP, Iacobone M. Effect of unilateral adrenalectomy on the quality of life of patients with lateralized primary aldosteronism. *BMC Surg.* 2019;18(Suppl 1):105.
85. Katabami T, Fukuda H, Tsukiyama H, et al. Clinical and biochemical outcomes after adrenalectomy and medical treatment in patients with unilateral primary aldosteronism. *J Hypertens.* 2019;37(7):1513-1520.
86. Limberg J, Ullmann TM, Gray KD, et al. Laparoscopic adrenalectomy has the same operative risk as routine laparoscopic cholecystectomy. *J Surg Res.* 2019;241:228-234.

46 Pheochromocytoma & Paraganglioma

Claire E. Graves, MD
Quan-Yang Duh, MD

GENERAL CONSIDERATIONS

Pheochromocytomas and paragangliomas (PPGLs) are chromaffin cell neuroendocrine tumors. In approximately 80% to 85% of cases, these tumors arise from the adrenal medulla and are termed "pheochromocytomas," and in approximately 15% to 20% of cases, the tumors arise from extra-adrenal sites, in which case they are termed "paragangliomas." These extra-adrenal sites include the sympathetic chain ganglia of the thorax, abdomen, or pelvis, as well as the parasympathetic paraganglia of the head and neck. The prevalence of PPGL in patients with hypertension is estimated to be approximately 0.2% to 0.6%, while in patients with an incidental adrenal tumor, it is approximately 3% to 7%. The incidence of PPGLs peaks between the third and fifth decades of life.

PPGLs secrete catecholamines, leading to signs and symptoms of hypertension, anxiety, palpitations, and hyperglycemia. They are best diagnosed by increased levels of catecholamine metabolites (metanephrine and normetanephrine). Some PPGLs are biochemically silent, including approximately 95% of head and neck paragangliomas. They can present as symptomatic tumors, can be diagnosed during screening for familial syndromes, or can be found incidentally on unrelated imaging.

PATHOGENESIS

With over 20 susceptibility genes identified to date, increased recognition of the role of genetic mutations in PPGL has led to a better understanding of its tumorigenesis. Currently identified genes fall into three distinct clusters, each related to different pathways of tumorigenesis: the pseudohypoxic cluster, the kinase signaling cluster, and the Wnt/β-catenin cluster. The pseudohypoxic cluster includes tumors secondary to mutations in the *SDHx, FH, MDH2, SLC25A11, GOT2, DLST*, and *VHL* genes. Mutations of these genes lead to abnormal stabilization of hypoxia-inducible factors (HIFα) and pseudohypoxia state. The activation of the pseudohypoxia pathway stimulates genes responsible for angiogenesis, cell proliferation, epithelial-mesenchymal transition, and cell survival. The kinase signaling cluster includes genetic mutations leading to activation of the mitogen-activated protein kinase (MAPK) and mechanistic target of rapamycin (mTOR) pathways, including mutations of *RET, NF1, TMEM127, MAX, MET, HRAS*, and *MERTK*. The *RET* proto-oncogene, for example, encodes a receptor tyrosine kinase activating the MAPK pathway. Finally, a third cluster demonstrates activation of the tumorigenic Wnt/β-catenin pathway, driven by a fusion gene including mastermind-like transcriptional coactivator 3 (MAML3). Current guidelines recommend discussion regarding genetic screening in all patients with PPGL, as identification of specific gene mutations leads to better understanding of tumorigenesis and tumor behavior, and therefore, directly influences recommended surveillance and follow-up.

EARLY DIAGNOSIS

All patients with incidentally discovered adrenal nodules should undergo biochemical screening for pheochromocytoma (see below, "Laboratory Findings"). Imaging evaluation should also be performed with adrenal protocol CT or MRI to determine the size and characteristics of the tumor, including lipid content (Hounsfield Units on CT or chemical shift on MRI), rapidity of contrast washout, heterogeneity, and tumor margin. Appropriate evaluation of incidentally found adrenal nodules can lead to early diagnosis of pheochromocytomas—often before clinical signs and symptoms are apparent.

Patients with known heritable mutations associated with PPGL should undergo lifelong clinical and biochemical surveillance. The age of recommended initiation of screening varies depending on the specific mutation but can be as early as ages 6 to 8 in children with known *SDHB* mutation.

CLINICAL FINDINGS

Symptoms & Signs

Most clinical manifestations of PPGL are caused by catecholamine secretion from the tumor. Heterogeneity in the type of catecholamine(s) (epinephrine, norepinephrine, or dopamine), as well as the amount and pattern of secretion, leads to wide variability in the signs and symptoms experienced by the patient. Importantly, in up to 10% to 15% of patients, pheochromocytomas are asymptomatic and clinically silent—only identified incidentally on imaging or at autopsy.

The most commonly reported symptoms include palpitations, resulting from the stimulation of β1-adrenergic receptors, paroxysmal headaches from peripheral α-adrenergic receptor-mediated vasoconstriction, and diaphoresis due to α-adrenergic receptor activation on the sweat glands. Additional symptoms include nausea, fever, constipation, and anxiety.

The most common clinical sign associated with PPGL is hypertension, which may be sustained or paroxysmal, with episodes of normal blood pressure. Hypertension is caused by the activation of both α1-adrenergic receptors, which cause vasoconstriction and an increase in peripheral vascular resistance, and β1-adrenergic receptors, which increase myocardial inotropy and chronotropy, and thus, cardiac output. PPGL should be suspected in patients who have unexplained blood pressure variability or unexpected blood pressure responses to drugs, procedures, or anesthesia. Children with hypertension should be evaluated for PPGL, given the high prevalence of PPGL in this patient population. The cardiovascular effects associated with pheochromocytomas, if unrecognized and left untreated, can lead to serious complications including myocardial ischemia, heart failure, arrhythmias, cerebral hemorrhage, and sudden death.

Elevated catecholamines also promote increased insulin resistance and impaired insulin secretion, likely as a result of inhibitory α-adrenergic stimulation in pancreatic β cells, as well as the promotion of increased gluconeogenesis and glycogenolysis through β2-receptor stimulation. Combined, they can have adverse effects on glucose and insulin homeostasis, presenting as glucose intolerance or even frank diabetes mellitus.

In patients being evaluated for possible PPGL, a thorough family history should be obtained. As PPGL is frequently heritable and part of several hereditary syndromes, physicians must additionally seek out other associated features of these syndromes (Table 46–1). Identifying PPGL in one family member may allow for earlier diagnosis and treatment in other family members.

Laboratory Findings

Current Endocrine Society Clinical Practice Guidelines recommend initial biochemical testing for PPGLs with measurements of plasma free metanephrines or urinary fractionated metanephrines due to their high diagnostic accuracy. Plasma free metanephrines, in particular, demonstrate a very high negative predictive value. Thus, when plasma free metanephrines result within the normal range, PPGL can be considered excluded with a very high reliability. Measurement of plasma free metanephrines is preferred over measurement of catecholamines due to the continuous production of these metabolites, as opposed to the episodic secretion of catecholamines. Moreover, free metanephrines are produced within chromaffin cells by catecholamine O-methyltransferase, an enzyme found only in these cells and not in the sympathetic nerves. Because of this, free metanephrines are more specific markers for chromaffin tumors.

Multiple factors can affect the measurement of plasma and urine metanephrines. Liquid chromatography with mass spectrometric or electrochemical assays has shown superior diagnostic performance than other laboratory methods for the diagnosis of PPGL. For plasma metanephrines, stress and upright body position may stimulate the sympathetic nervous system and increase plasma metanephrines. Ideally, blood should be sampled from the supine position after at least 30 minutes of rest to minimize false-positive results. This may be logistically difficult in many centers, and therefore seated-position samples should be carefully interpreted in the setting of an increased likelihood of false-positive results. For urine studies, completeness of urine collection should be ensured by concomitant measurement of urinary creatinine.

Both plasma and urine metanephrines measurements may be affected by multiple drugs, which can interfere with either the analysis of the samples or the pharmacologic results (Table 46–2). Tricyclic antidepressants and sympathomimetic drugs such as ephedrine, cocaine, caffeine, nicotine, or amphetamines are commonly encountered and can significantly elevate plasma and urine normetanephrine (tricyclic antidepressants and sympathomimetics) and/or metanephrines (sympathomimetics), leading to false positive test results.

Importantly, a physiologic increase in sympathetic activity can be seen in many clinical conditions, which can also be a source of falsely elevated plasma metanephrines. This includes patients under considerable physiologic stress, such as in those with heart failure, in alcohol withdrawal, or critically ill patients in intensive care units. In these patients, a reliable biochemical diagnosis is not feasible, and imaging should be considered if there is a high clinical suspicion for PPGL.

Normal plasma or urinary metanephrines can exclude a functioning PPGL with high accuracy. However, positive test results do not necessarily indicate the presence of a tumor. In general, metanephrines that are higher than twice the upper limit of normal are strongly suggestive of PPGL in patients not under physiologic stress or on confounding medications.

Table 46–1. Genes associated with PPGL.

Gene	Syndrome	Protein	Risk of PPGL	Associated Features
SDHx	Hereditary PPGL syndrome			Clear cell RCC, GIST
SDHA		Catalytic subunit A of SDH	10%	+ multiple head/neck paragangliomas, pituitary adenomas
SDHB		Catalytic subunit B of SDH	25%	+ thoracic/abdominal paraganglioma, pituitary adenomas
SDHC		Anchoring subunit C of SDH	Low	+ head/neck paragangliomas
SDHD		Anchoring subunit D of SDH	45%	+ multiple head/neck paragangliomas, pituitary adenomas
SDHAF2		Assembly factor of SDH	Low	head/neck paragangliomas
RET	Multiple Endocrine Neoplasia type 2	Tyrosine kinase receptor	50%	Medullary thyroid carcinoma, primary hyperparathyroidism (MEN2A), mucocutaneous neuromas, skeletal deformities (MEN2B)
VHL	Von Hippel-Lindau syndrome	Von Hippel-Lindau protein	20%	Clear cell RCC, pancreatic NET, CNS hemangioblastomas
NF1	Neurofibromatosis type 1	Neurofibromin 1, regulator of RAS signaling pathway	1-13%	Neurofibromas, CNS gliomas, Lisch nodules, café-au-lait spots, bony abnormalities, GIST
MAX	-	Leucine zipper-type transcription factor	Unknown	-
FH	Hereditary leiomyomatosis and RCC syndrome	Fumarate dehydrogenase	Low	Papillary type RCC, cutaneous leiomyomas, uterine fibroids
EPAS1	-	Hypoxia-inducible factor 2-alpha	Unknown	Polycythemia, somatostatinoma
EGLN1/PHD2	-	Hypoxia-inducible factor prolyl hydroxylase 2	Unknown	Erythrocytosis
TMEM127	-	Transmembrane protein 127	Low	RCC

CNS, central nervous system; GIST, gastrointestinal stromal tumors; RCC, renal cell carcinoma; SDH, succinate dehydrogenase.

Patients with indeterminate results should be assessed for clinical probability of a tumor, as well as drug interference or inappropriate sampling, and re-testing should be considered. The clonidine suppression test, though of historic interest, is rarely used currently.

In patients with normal plasma or urinary metanephrine and normetanephrine, chromogranin A can be an alternative marker of functional activity in patients with a highly suspicious lesion on imaging. PPGL with normal metanephrine/normetanephrine is very rare in the abdomen; this pattern is predominantly seen in head and neck paragangliomas.

Conventional Imaging Studies

When biochemical testing suggests the presence of a PPGL, imaging should be obtained to localize the tumor and

Table 46–2. Drugs or medications that can lead to false elevations in biochemical testing for PPGL.

Drug/Medication
Tricyclic antidepressants
Phenoxybenzamine
Monoamine oxidase inhibitors
Cocaine
Sulphasalazine
Levodopa
Acetaminophen
Labetalol
Antihistamines

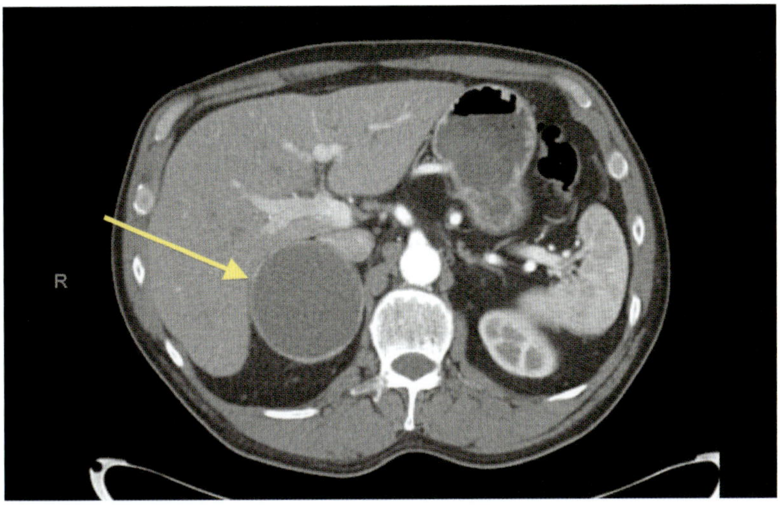

▲ **Figure 46–1.** Contrast-enhanced axial CT demonstrating predominantly cystic right-sided pheochromocytoma (arrow).

determine the optimal approach to surgery. A CT scan of the abdomen and pelvis is recommended as the first-line imaging modality (Figure 46–1). CT has excellent spatial resolution in the abdomen and pelvis, and modern scanners can localize tumors of 5 mm or larger. PPGL on CT may appear homogeneous or heterogeneous, solid, cystic, or necrotic with some calcifications. Most PPGL will have a mean attenuation of more than 10 Hounsfield units on unenhanced images.

In patients with contraindications or relative contraindications for CT, including those with an allergy to iodinated contrast or excessive radiation exposure, children, or pregnant women, an MRI should be obtained. The sensitivity of CT for PPGL decreases in extra-adrenal, recurrent, or metastatic tumors. For this reason, MRI is preferred over CT for detection of extra-adrenal and skull base or neck paragangliomas. High signal intensity on T2-weighted images is characteristic of PPGL and highly sensitive, though lacks specificity.

Functional Imaging Studies

The availability of new radiotracers, along with an increasing understanding of the genetic and molecular basis of PPGL, has led to changes in the use of functional imaging for the diagnosis of PPGL. Radiopharmaceuticals developed to target-specific receptors and metabolic pathways involved in PPGL include ^{131}I/^{123}I-metaiodo-benzylguanidine, 6-^{18}F-fluoro-L-3,4-dihydroxyphenylalanine (^{18}F-DOPA), ^{18}F-FDG, and ^{64}Cu- or ^{68}Ga-DOTA-somatostatin analogs. The North American Neuroendocrine Tumor Society (NANETS) recommends *against* routine use of functional imaging in all patients with primary PPGL. However, if metastatic disease is suspected, ^{64}Cu- or ^{68}Ga-DOTA-somatostatin analogs, most commonly ^{68}Ga-DOTATATE, appear to have the highest per-lesion sensitivity and are currently the first-choice radiotracers for the evaluation of metastatic PPGL and head and neck paragangliomas (Figure 46–2). Somatostatin receptor positron emission tomography (PET)/CT can also be safely used in pediatric patients and patients with known *SDHx* mutations, but in patients with PPGL associated with polycythemia, there is evidence that ^{18}F-DOPA may be preferred. Somatostatin receptor PET/CT can also be used to determine patient suitability for ^{90}Y/^{177}Lu-DOTA-somatostatin analog therapy.

Historically ^{123}I-metaiodobenzylguanidine (MIBG) was the most widely used functional imaging modality, but it has lower sensitivity for detection of metastatic lesions compared to newer PET-based modalities. The role of MIBG imaging is now limited to screening for potential ^{131}I-MIBG therapy (see below, "Prognosis").

DIFFERENTIAL DIAGNOSIS

A clinical presentation that mimics PPGL—including severe paroxysmal episodes of hypertension with no evidence of a trigger, as well as anxiety, sweating, palpitations, and headaches—without any anatomical abnormality and normal or mildly elevated catecholamines or metanephrines has been dubbed "pseudopheochromocytoma" and is an uncommon but recognized phenomenon. Patients with sustained or episodic hypertension should be evaluated for other secondary causes of hypertension, such as renal artery stenosis, renal parenchymal disease, obstructive sleep apnea, hyper- or hypothyroidism, carcinoid syndrome, or anxiety/panic attacks.

Patients with incidentally discovered adrenal masses should undergo a complete biochemical workup to rule out

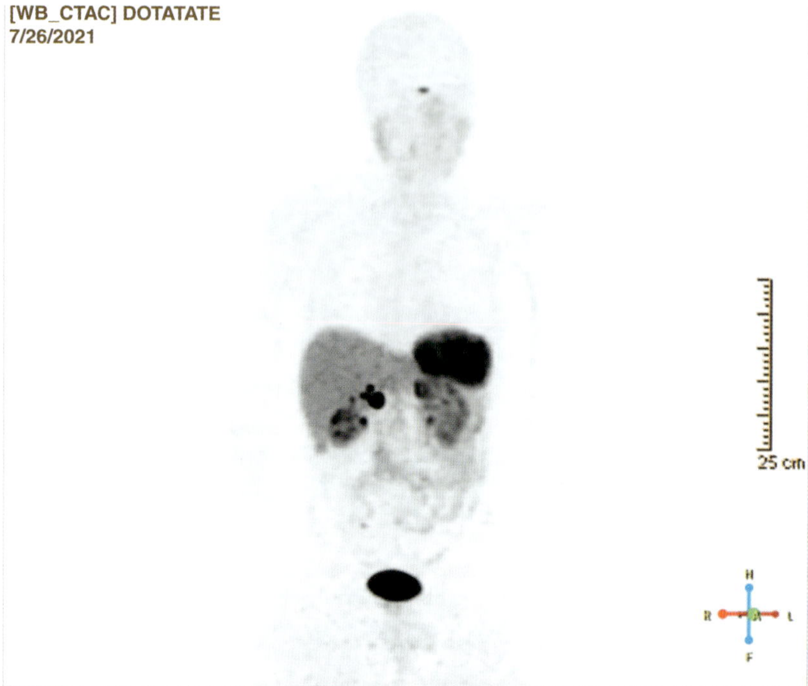

A

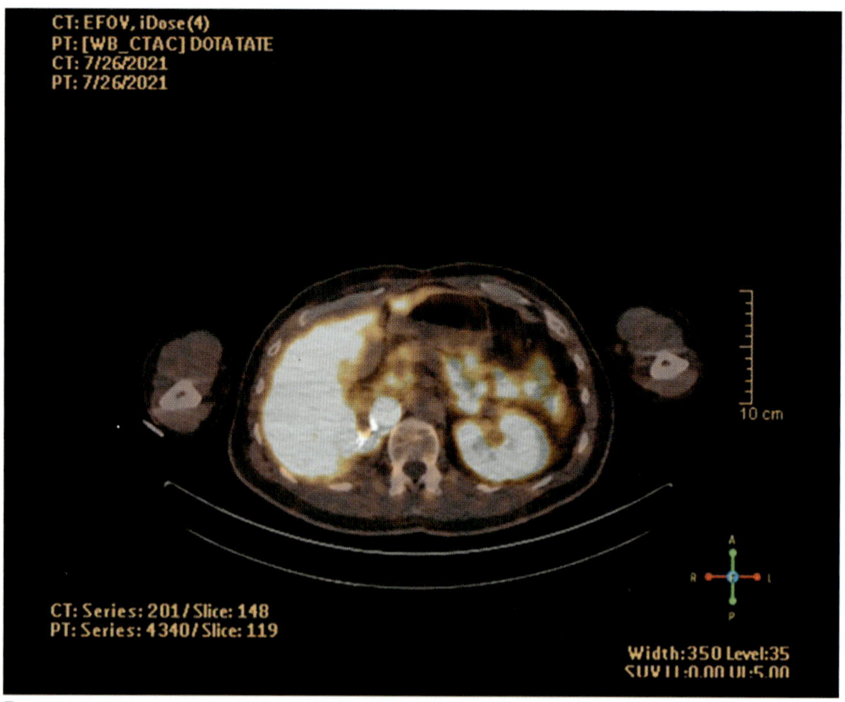

B

▲ **Figure 46–2.** **(A)** Whole-body ^{64}Cu-DOTATE PET image of a 53-year-old man s/p resection of a right-sided pheochromocytoma with recurrent multifocal disease in the right adrenal bed, consistent with pheochromocytomatosis. **(B)** Axial ^{64}Cu-DOTATE PET/CT of the same patient, demonstrating right adrenal bed pheochromocytomatosis.

other functional tumors, such as aldosterone-producing or cortisol-producing adenomas. In patients with large adrenal masses (>4-6 cm), or those with concerning radiographic characteristics, the possibility of adrenocortical carcinoma should be considered. The differential diagnosis of adrenal masses also includes benign cysts, myelolipoma, and metastatic tumors. Depending on the location of a paraganglioma, the differential diagnosis includes metastatic lesions and mesenchymal or nerve sheath tumors.

As mentioned earlier, during biochemical evaluation for PPGL, situational factors such as psychologic or physiologic stress, as well as multiple medications and foods, can lead to false elevations in plasma or urine metanephrines and catecholamines. Repeat testing should be considered, ensuring the absence of these interfering factors.

TREATMENT

Surgery & Preoperative Preparation

Surgical resection is the recommended treatment for PPGL to prevent the clinical sequelae and long-term complications associated with excess catecholamine secretion (Figure 46–3). A minimally invasive approach with laparoscopic (transperitoneal or retroperitoneal) or robotic resection is preferred when feasible, but open resection should be employed for tumors with preoperative evidence of invasion to ensure complete resection, avoid capsular disruption, and prevent local recurrence. For these same reasons, open resection should be considered for large tumors or those at high risk for fracture. Due to the wide variation in location of paragangliomas, the surgical approach should be carefully considered using an individualized plan based on location of the tumor on imaging and patient factors such as size, habitus, and surgical history, as well as availability of surgical expertise.

Partial adrenalectomy (cortex-sparing adrenalectomy) may be an option in some patients with hereditary pheochromocytoma. This approach can obviate the need for steroid replacement in many patients, but there may be an increased risk of recurrent pheochromocytoma from remnant adrenal gland. The risks and benefits of this approach should be carefully weighed by the surgeon and patient.

Because stress, including surgery, can stimulate the sudden, uncontrolled release of catecholamines from the tumor and cause hypertensive crisis, evaluation and preparation by a multidisciplinary team is recommended prior to surgery. A preoperative cardiovascular examination should evaluate the patient for evidence of cardiac injury or dysfunction. Medical preparation with α-adrenergic blockade is recommended for at least 7 to 14 days preoperatively. Alpha blockers counteract the vasoconstrictive effects of catecholamines, leading to decreased peripheral vascular tone and lowered blood pressure. Patients should be encouraged to ingest a high-salt diet and to aggressively hydrate while on alpha blockers to replete their intravascular volume, and

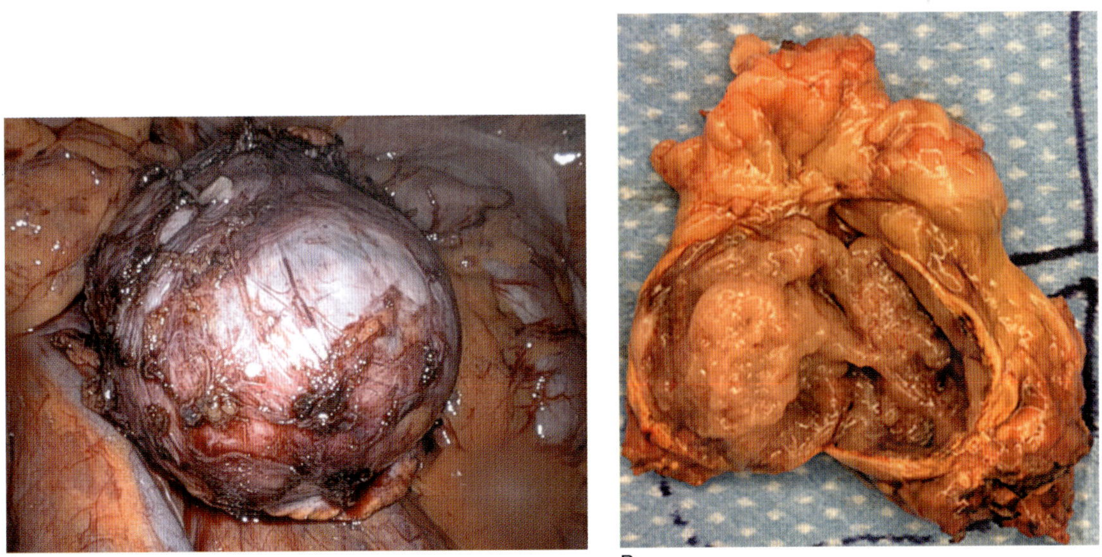

A B

Figure 46–3. **(A)** Resected left-sided pheochromocytoma within the abdomen prior to specimen extraction. Note an area of golden-colored normal adrenal tissue at the inferior border of the tumor. **(B)** Gross appearance of a bisected pheochromocytoma (different specimen from above) with surrounding rim of adrenal cortical tissue.

they should be cautioned regarding symptoms of orthostatic hypotension and advised to monitor their blood pressure at home. The nonselective and noncompetitive α-receptor blocker phenoxybenzamine and the competitive α-1-selective receptor blocker doxazosin are the two most commonly used medications. A recent randomized trial by Buitenwerf et al. between these two medications found no difference in cumulative intraoperative time outside of blood pressure targets. This study did suggest less hemodynamic instability in the phenoxybenzamine group, but notably, the phenoxybenzamine group included more patients on β blockers, and at a higher dose, than the doxazosin group.

β blockers can be effective adjuncts for preoperative preparation in PPGL, decreasing tachycardia and tachyarrhythmias. Importantly, however, β blockers should only be started *after* proper and effective α-blockade is in place. As catecholamines stimulate primarily vasoconstricting α-1 receptors, but also vasodilatory β2 receptors, if β2 receptors are blocked, unopposed α-stimulation can lead to severe and dangerous vasoconstriction and cardiac stress.

Intraoperatively, stimulation of catecholamines, followed by the abrupt cessation of catecholamine secretion following surgical resection, can lead to hemodynamic instability. While preoperative preparation aims to blunt these effects, an experienced anesthesia team, and open communication between the surgical and anesthesia teams, are crucial. Patients are at risk for hypotension postoperatively due to catecholamine withdrawal and should be closely monitored. Liberal fluids and volume resuscitation during and after surgery can counteract the effects of vasodilation and help maintain blood pressure. Importantly, patients with postoperative hypotension may be resistant to drugs typically used for urgent treatment, such as phenylephrine, norepinephrine, or epinephrine, due to chronic catecholamine excess. Vasopressin, a nonadrenergic vasopressor that induces vasoconstriction and increases vascular resistance via V1 receptors in the vascular smooth muscle and increases free water resorption via V2 receptors in the distal convoluted tubule of the kidney, is the optimal drug for catecholamine-resistant hypotension.

In addition, glucose should be monitored postoperatively, as postresection hypoglycemia is a known complication following PPGL resection. Catecholamines inhibit pancreatic insulin secretion, stimulate glycogenolysis and gluconeogenesis, and increase peripheral insulin resistance. With sudden withdrawal of catecholamines, rebound insulin secretion can occur. Moreover, normal responses to hypoglycemia may be dulled due to desensitization from chronically elevated catecholamines. Children are particularly at risk due to decreased muscle mass and lower hepatic glycogen reserve. One positive effect of this phenomenon, however, is that many patients with concurrent diabetes and pheochromocytoma will have a lower insulin requirement following tumor resection, and some even have long-term resolution of their diabetes.

Follow-up

Close monitoring of patients after surgery is critical for their management. Plasma or urine metanephrines should be obtained at 2 to 6 weeks after surgery to assess for complete removal of the tumor. Persistent elevation of metanephrines is concerning for incomplete resection or metastatic disease and should prompt additional imaging.

Germline mutations can be found in up to 40% of cases of PPGL, even if there is no apparent family history. The most common mutations, found in over half of patients with hereditary PPGL, are those of the *SDHx* genes (*SDHA, SDHB, SDHC, SDHD,* and *SDHAF2*). These genes are responsible for encoding the subunits and assembly of succinate dehydrogenase (SDH), a mitochondrial enzyme involved in the Krebs cycle as well as in the transfer of electrons in the mitochondrial respiratory chain. Additionally, PPGL is associated with the autosomal dominant cancer predisposition syndromes neurofibromatosis type 1 (gene: *NF1*), von-Hippel-Lindau (gene: *VHL*), and multiple endocrine neoplasia type 2 (gene: *RET*). Over 20 susceptibility genes have been reported, each of which confers predisposition to clinical phenotypes, such as early forms of the disease (*VHL, RET, SDHD, EPAS1, DLST*), multiple tumors (*SDHD, TMEM127, MAX, DLST, MDH2, GOT2*), or malignancy (*SDHB, FH, SLC25A11*).

All patients with PPGL should be considered for genetic testing—ideally, with the involvement of a genetic counselor to discuss the risks and benefits of testing and the implications for the patient's family. The identification of a germline mutation allows for targeted follow-up and surveillance based on the patient's specific mutation and the known associated genotype-phenotype correlation. In addition, the identification of a mutation allows for early screening of the patient's relatives.

In general, following complete resection, history and physical, blood pressure monitoring, and biochemical surveillance (plasma or urine metanephrines for biochemically active tumors) are recommended after 3 to 12 months, then every 6 to 12 months for the first 3 years after surgery, then annually for at least 10 years. Imaging with abdominal CT or MRI or chest CT should be considered in patients with elevated metanephrines postoperatively or in patients with biochemically inactive tumors (normal metanephrines prior to surgery), or those in whom biochemical testing was not performed prior to surgery. Imaging and biochemical testing should be performed earlier than these recommended times if at any time patients develop symptoms concerning for possible recurrence. In patients with identified genetic mutations, surveillance protocols should be personalized to the known phenotypic patterns of that mutation.

All patients who undergo surgery for PPGL should be followed for at least 10 years to screen for local or metastatic recurrence. Patients with a germline mutation, young age at time of presentation, a large tumor, or a paraganglioma are considered at higher risk for recurrence and should be offered life-long annual follow-up.

PROGNOSIS

Although most PPGL are benign, approximately 15% to 25% of PPGL develop metastatic disease, defined as tumor presence in nonchromaffin-derived tissue. PPGL can have a long latency period, and metastatic disease can be diagnosed as long as 20 years after discovery of the primary tumor. All PPGLs are considered to have some metastatic potential, and the concept of "benign" versus "malignant" PPGL has been replaced by that of gradation of risk for metastasis, with certain features indicating higher or lower risk. Paragangliomas are more likely to metastasize than pheochromocytomas, and PPGLs associated with a familial syndrome tend to be more aggressive and likely to metastasize than sporadic tumors.

Features found to be associated with higher risk of subsequent metastasis include tumors larger than 5 cm, sympathetic paragangliomas, norepinephrine-secreting tumors, tumors with histological evidence of invasion into soft tissue or blood vessels, hypercellularity, large confluent nests, comedo-type necrosis, and high mitotic count or Ki-67 proliferative index. Despite these accepted risk factors, quantification of risk in individual patients remains challenging. The two most commonly used grading systems are the Pheochromocytoma of the Adrenal gland Scaled Score (PASS) and the Grading system for Adrenal Pheochromocytoma and Paraganglioma (GAPP) score. However, these scores have not been rigorously validated, and the PASS score has been shown to demonstrate significant interobserver variability. The addition of germline and somatic tumor markers to clinical and histopathologic data has been suggested to potentially improve scoring systems for individual patient risk. Metastatic disease is rare in patients with MEN2- and VHL-associated PPGL, as well as those with *SDHC*-, *SDHD*-, *SDHAF2*-associated PPGL, but patients with *SDHA* and *SDHB* mutations have a higher risk of metastatic disease.

In patients with locally unresectable or distant metastasis, cross-sectional imaging with CT or MRI is recommended every 3 to 6 months for the first year, and then, if stable, every 6 to 12 months. Somatostatin receptor-based PET should not be used for routine surveillance but can be useful to evaluate for possible therapeutic options. In patients with metastatic, hormonally functional PPGL, plasma metanephrines, as well as symptoms, blood pressure, and heart rate, should be monitored every 3 to 6 months.

Though data are limited, the role for surgery in metastatic PPGL is primarily in cases in which resection will leave no evidence of disease. However, resection of the primary tumor in the setting of metastatic disease is recommended. Moreover, surgical debulking in the setting of known residual foci may help alleviate symptoms in patients with functional tumors and potentially improve the efficacy of additional chemotherapy, targeted therapy, or radionucleotide therapy. Percutaneous image-guided cryo- and radiofrequency ablations have also been described for oligometastatic disease.

Pheochromocytomatosis is a specific type of recurrence caused by tumor rupture during resection leading to adrenal bed and intraperitoneal seeding of tumor cells (Figure 46–4). Re-resection can be difficult and frequently incomplete. This complication is best prevented by meticulous care during initial resection.

Therapeutic options for unresectable metastatic PPGL include chemotherapy, targeted molecular therapy with tyrosine kinase inhibitors, radionuclide therapy, and radiation therapy. Chemotherapy (typically, cyclophosphamide/vincristine/dacarbazine or temozolomide-based) is considered first-line treatment for patients with bulky disease, rapid progression, or symptoms. Tyrosine kinase inhibitors have shown promise in clinical trials of metastatic PPGL but can be associated with cardiovascular toxicity, and patients should be blocked prior to treatment with alpha- and beta-blockers to reduce the risk of catecholamine surges. In patients with MIBG-avid disease, radionuclide therapy with high specific activity ^{131}I-MIBG should be considered. In patients with negative MIBG imaging, but positive somatostatin receptor PET imaging, ^{177}Lu-DOTATATE is a newer therapeutic radionuclide with potential clinical benefit. With both agents, patients should also have hypertension medically managed prior to treatment due to the risk of catecholamine release. Finally, radiation therapy can be effective for local control and pain relief, particularly in metastases to the bone. Additional novel treatments such as immunotherapy are currently being investigated in ongoing clinical trials.

WHEN TO REFER

Patients with PPGL benefit from specialized, multidisciplinary management and are best served by teams with specific expertise. During the course of their diagnosis and treatment, patients are typically evaluated by multiple medical and surgical specialists, including an endocrinologist, endocrine surgeon, anesthesiologist, radiologist, and geneticist/genetic counselor, all of whom should work in concert to provide appropriate evidence-based care. Patients benefit from this team-based care, including discussion at interdisciplinary tumor boards.

As genotype-phenotype correlations in PPGL continue to be elucidated, with distinct biochemical and clinical presentations based on the mutated driver genes present, the management of these rare and diverse tumors will undoubtedly become more and more personalized to the patient's unique genetic signature. Thus, patients will benefit from centers with specific interest and expertise in these tumors, where a variety of diagnostic and therapeutic techniques are available.

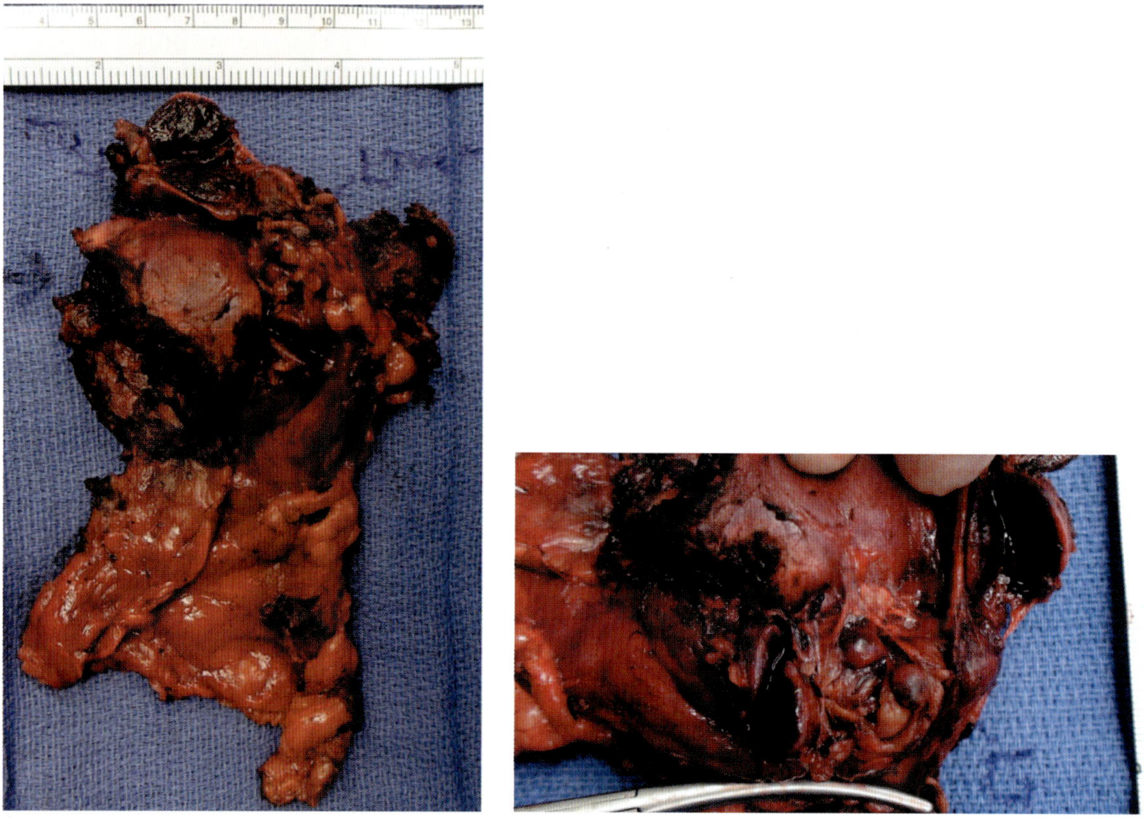

A B

Figure 46–4. **(A)** Specimen from resection of pheochromoctyomatosis in a re-operative right adrenalectomy bed, requiring partial nephrectomy (portion of kidney at mid-left specimen, large arrow). **(B)** This close-up image highlights the multiple small tumor implants, just superior to the clamp and at the top right corner of the specimen.

SUGGESTED READINGS

1. Lenders JWM, Duh Q-Y, Eisenhofer G, et al. Pheochromocytoma and paraganglioma: an endocrine society clinical practice guideline. *J Clin Endocrinol Metab.* 2014;99(6):1915-1942.
2. Shah MH, Goldner WS, Benson AB, et al. Neuroendocrine and adrenal tumors, version 2.2021, NCCN clinical practice guidelines in oncology. *J Natl Compr Canc Netw.* 2021;19(7):839-868.
3. Buffet A, Burnichon N, Favier J, Gimenez-Roqueplo A-P. An overview of 20 years of genetic studies in pheochromocytoma and paraganglioma. *Best Pract Res Clin Endocrinol Metab.* 2020;34(2):101416.
4. Castro-Vega LJ, Letouzé E, Burnichon N, et al. Multi-omics analysis defines core genomic alterations in pheochromocytomas and paragangliomas. *Nat Commun.* 2015;6:6044.
5. Dariane C, Goncalves J, Timsit M-O, Favier J. An update on adult forms of hereditary pheochromocytomas and paragangliomas. *Curr Opin Oncol.* 2021;33(1):23-32.
6. Fishbein L, Leshchiner I, Walter V, et al. Comprehensive molecular characterization of pheochromocytoma and paraganglioma. *Cancer Cell.* 2017;31(2):181-193.
7. Carrasquillo JA, Chen CC, Jha A, et al. Imaging of pheochromocytoma and paraganglioma. *J Nucl Med.* 2021;62(8):1033-1042.
8. Eisenhofer G, Prejbisz A, Peitzsch M, et al. Biochemical diagnosis of chromaffin cell tumors in patients at high and low risk of disease: plasma versus urinary free or deconjugated O-methylated catecholamine metabolites. *Clin Chem.* 2018;64(11):1646-1656.
9. Han S, Suh CH, Woo S, Kim YJ, Lee JJ. Performance of 68Ga-DOTA-conjugated somatostatin receptor-targeting peptide PET in detection of pheochromocytoma and paraganglioma: a systematic review and meta analysis. *J Nucl Med.* 2019;60(3):369-376.
10. Johnbeck CB, Knigge U, Loft A, et al. Head-to-head comparison of 64Cu-DOTATATE and 68Ga-DOTATOC PET/CT: a prospective study of 59 patients with neuroendocrine tumors. *J Nucl Med.* 2017;58(3):451-457.
11. Komada H, Hirota Y, So A, et al. Insulin secretion and insulin sensitivity before and after surgical treatment of pheochromocytoma or paraganglioma. *J Clin Endocrinol Metab.* 2017;102(9):3400-3405.
12. Lenders JWM, Eisenhofer G. Update on modern management of pheochromocytoma and paraganglioma. *Endocrinol Metab.* 2017;32(2):152-161.

13. Neary NM, King KS, Pacak K. Drugs and pheochromocytoma–don't be fooled by every elevated metanephrine. *N Engl J Med.* 2011;364(23):2268-2270.
14. Sbardella E, Grossman AB. Pheochromocytoma: an approach to diagnosis. *Best Pract Res Clin Endocrinol Metab.* 2020;34(2):101346.
15. Mamilla D, Gonzales MK, Esler MD, Pacak K. Pseudopheochromocytoma. *Endocrinol Metab Clin North Am.* 2019;48(4):751-764.
16. Zeiger MA, Thompson GB, Duh Q-Y, et al. American Association of Clinical Endocrinologists and American Association of Endocrine Surgeons Medical Guidelines for the Management of Adrenal Incidentalomas: executive summary of recommendations. *Endocr Pract.* 2009;15(5):450-453.
17. Araujo-Castro M, García Centero R, López-García M-C, et al. Surgical outcomes in the pheochromocytoma surgery. Results from the PHEO-RISK STUDY. *Endocrine.* 2021;74(3):676-684.
18. Beninato T, Kluijfhout WP, Drake FT, et al. Resection of pheochromocytoma improves diabetes mellitus in the majority of patients. *Ann Surg Oncol.* 2017;24(5):1208-1213.
19. Buffet A, Burnichon N, Favier J, Gimenez-Roqueplo A-P. An overview of 20 years of genetic studies in pheochromocytoma and paraganglioma. *Best Pract Res Clin Endocrinol Metab.* 2020;34(2):101416.
20. Buitenwerf E, Osinga TE, Timmers HJLM, et al. Efficacy of α-blockers on hemodynamic control during pheochromocytoma resection: a randomized controlled trial. *J Clin Endocrinol Metab.* 2020;105(7):2381-2391.
21. Chen Y, Hodin RA, Pandolfi C, Ruan DT, McKenzie TJ. Hypoglycemia after resection of pheochromocytoma. *Surgery.* 2014;156(6):1404-1408; discussion 1408-1409.
22. Komada H, Hirota Y, So A, et al. Insulin secretion and insulin sensitivity before and after surgical treatment of pheochromocytoma or paraganglioma. *J Clin Endocrinol Metab.* 2017;102(9):3400-3405.
23. Nölting S, Bechmann N, Taieb D, et al. Personalized management of pheochromocytoma and paraganglioma. *Endocr Rev.* 2022;43(2):199-239.
24. Plouin PF, Amar L, Dekkers OM, et al. European Society of Endocrinology Clinical Practice Guideline for long-term follow-up of patients operated on for a phaeochromocytoma or a paraganglioma. *Eur J Endocrinol.* 2016;174(5):G1e10.
25. Simforoosh N, Soltani MH, Shemshaki H, Bonakdar Hashemi M, Dadpour M, Kashi AH. Symptom resolution and recurrence outcomes after partial versus total laparoscopic adrenalectomy: 13 years of experience with medium-long term follow up. *Urol J.* 2020;18(2):165-170.
26. Wang W, Li P, Wang Y, et al. Effectiveness and safety of laparoscopic adrenalectomy of large pheochromocytoma: a prospective, nonrandomized, controlled study. *Am J Surg.* 2015;210(2):230-235.
27. Fishbein L, Del Rivero J, Else T, et al. The North American Neuroendocrine Tumor Society consensus guidelines for surveillance and management of metastatic and/or unresectable pheochromocytoma and paraganglioma. *Pancreas.* 2021;50(4):469-493.
28. Lam AK-Y. Update on Adrenal Tumours in 2017 World Health Organization (WHO) of Endocrine Tumours. *Endocr Pathol.* 2017;28(3):213-227.
29. Thompson LDR. Pheochromocytoma of the Adrenal gland Scaled Score (PASS) to separate benign from malignant neoplasms: a clinicopathologic and immunophenotypic study of 100 cases. *Am J Surg Pathol.* 2002;26(5):551-566.
30. Turchini J, Cheung VKY, Tischler AS, De Krijger RR, Gill AJ. Pathology and genetics of phaeochromocytoma and paraganglioma. *Histopathology.* 2018;72(1):97-105.
31. Wachtel H, Hutchens T, Baraban E, et al. Predicting metastatic potential in pheochromocytoma and paraganglioma: a comparison of PASS and GAPP scoring systems. *J Clin Endocrinol Metab.* 2020;105(12):e4661-e4670.

47 Adrenocortical Carcinoma, Adrenal Lymphoma, Metastases to the Adrenal Gland

Nicci Owusu-Brackett, MD
Barbra S. Miller, MD

INTRODUCTION

Due to the increasing number of imaging tests performed in the course of evaluation of patients, the identification of adrenal lesions on imaging studies is estimated to be 4% to 10%.[1] The majority of identified incidentalomas are nonfunctioning cortical adenomas. Twenty years ago, patients with primary adrenal malignancies often presented at late stages with signs or symptoms of adrenal hormone excess or sequelae of local compressive effects. Today, more adrenal malignancies are diagnosed incidentally at earlier stages when imaging studies are performed for other reasons.

ADRENOCORTICAL CARCINOMA

General Considerations

Adrenocortical carcinoma (ACC) is rare with an incidence of 0.5 to 2 cases per million in the population.[2-5] ACC represents about 2% of all adrenal incidentalomas. ACC has a bimodal distribution with more cases identified during childhood and between the ages of 40 and 50 years.

Prevention

No screening of the general population is recommended due to the rarity of ACC. However, in patients with personal and family histories suggestive of a possible genetic predisposition, referral to a licensed genetic counselor is encouraged. Lynch, Beckwith-Wiedemann, and Li-Fraumeni syndromes are all associated with the potential for development of ACC.

Clinical Findings

A. Symptoms and Signs

Between 40% and 50% of ACCs produce excess hormones. The hormones most commonly secreted are cortisol and androgens, although increased levels of steroid synthesis intermediaries may also be noted. Aldosterone excess is less common, and estrogen-producing hormones are least common. Some tumors secrete multiple hormones, and these along with cortisol-only producing tumors are associated with worse prognosis. Table 47–1 lists the signs and symptoms associated with each type of hormone excess. Some patients have subclinical disease and exhibit no signs or symptoms. It is important to obtain a comprehensive biochemical panel to determine any degree of autonomous hormone secretion, even when subclinical, as the hormone levels, including steroid intermediaries, can be used as tumor markers during surveillance. Early identification and treatment of excess hormone is critical due to detrimental effects leading to increased morbidity and mortality.[6,7]

In the absence of hormonal excess, patients present with no or only vague tumor-related symptoms such as fatigue, weight gain or loss, abdominal pain, nausea, or lower extremity swelling due to occlusive tumor thrombus in the inferior vena cava. Due to the aggressive nature of the disease, many patients present with advanced local and/or metastatic disease. They may have shortness of breath due to pleural effusions, point tenderness over the spine, or neurologic impairment due to vertebral body fractures or nerve involvement.

ACCs present with a mean tumor size ranging from 7 to 10 cm, are heterogeneous, and are characterized by decreased lipid content and slower contrast washout due to increased neovascularization versus adenomas. Tumors that secrete aldosterone tend to be smaller than the average ACC but larger than benign aldosterone-producing adenomas which normally average 1 to 2 cm. Larger, benign aldosterone-producing adenomas occur but retain imaging and washout characteristics of benign tumors.

B. Laboratory Findings

Evaluation for abnormal production of adrenal hormones should be performed in a consistent and

Table 47–1. Signs and symptoms of hormone excess.

Hormone Overproduction	Signs and Symptoms
Aldosterone	Hypertension, hypokalemia, hypernatremia, edema
Cortisol	Moon facies, facial plethora, buffalo hump, muscular weakness, fatigue, striae, hyperglycemia, weight gain, increased visceral adiposity, hirsutism, easy bruising, hypercoagulability, emotional lability, hypertension, hypokalemia
Androgens and estrogens	Changes in secondary sexual characteristics

comprehensive manner. Nearly 25% of patients with dysregulated adrenal hormone production have subclinical disease, and assessment of patients based on clinical presentation alone can result in missed diagnoses. Table 47–2 lists the typical biochemical evaluation pursued for adrenal tumors. Complete biochemical analysis is imperative, not only to diagnose autonomous hormone secretion, but also to utilize as marker(s) of disease recurrence or progression.

C. Imaging Studies

Characterization of the adrenal tumors by imaging is key not only to determine size and location, but also to differentiate between a benign and indeterminate/possibly malignant lesion. Adrenal protocol CT is the most commonly performed imaging study to evaluate the adrenal glands and is the modality surgeons are usually most comfortable interpreting for preoperative planning. MRI is equally useful in differentiating benign from indeterminate lesions.[8-12] MRI has an added benefit of being able to evaluate heterogeneous lesions, as calculation of washout percentage on CT is not meant for these. MRI has higher specificity regarding vascular invasion and presence of intravenous tumor thrombus than CT. MRI is also more sensitive for identifying liver metastases. Table 47–3 lists characteristics of indeterminate adrenal lesions. Adrenal

Table 47–2. Initial adrenal biochemical evaluation of adrenal lesions.

Metabolic panel, aldosterone, renin
Plasma or 24-hour urine metanephrine and normetanephrine levels
0800 ACTH, 0800 cortisol, DHEA-S, 11-deoxycortisol, and separate 1 mg DST (0800 ACTH, cortisol, quantitative dexamethasone level) and/or late-night salivary cortisol
24-hour urine-free cortisol if overt Cushing syndrome or abnormal DST
Testosterone, estradiol, 17-OH progesterone

Table 47–3. Imaging characteristics concerning for potential malignancy.

Characteristics	Indeterminate
Size (cm)	>4-6 cm with other indeterminate characteristics
Unenhanced CT (Hounsefield units)	>10 with other indeterminate characteristics
Internal attenuation	Heterogeneous
Percentage washout on CT (calculated for homogeneous tumors only)	<60% absolute washout <50% relative washout
Calcification	Present
Necrosis	Present
Borders	Irregular
Invasion of adjacent structures	Present
Intravascular tumor thrombus	Present
Lymphadenopathy	Present

lymphoma often involves both adrenal glands and may be accompanied by "B" symptoms and other findings on imaging. ACC can also involve both adrenal glands, but this is usually later in the disease course. If there is concern for malignancy, at a minimum, a chest CT should be obtained preoperatively to assess for metastatic disease, as evidence of Stage IV disease would most likely change the treatment plan.

In addition to detecting extra-adrenal metastases and nodal involvement, 18-FDG-PET CT can be helpful to further differentiate between benign and malignant adrenal tumors characterized as indeterminate by CT or MRI as the diagnosis may inform selection of operative approach (minimally invasive versus open). The SUV ratio of the adrenal tumor to the liver should be calculated to assist with characterization. Approximately 10% of benign tumors are classified as likely malignant by 18-FDG PET CT but ultimately are found to be benign on final pathology; these are usually oncocytic tumors with a greater number of mitochondria. Renal cell cancer, which is sometimes in the differential, is not associated with increased 18-FDG avidity.[13-16]

Ultimately, if an adrenal mass is unable to be characterized as benign by imaging characteristics, the mass should be treated as an adrenal cancer until final pathology provides a final diagnosis. This has implications for surgical resection, as the technical steps required for adrenalectomy for ACC are different than for a benign adrenal tumor.

D. Fine-Needle Aspiration Evaluation

There are few indications for fine-needle aspiration (FNA) of an adrenal lesion. These are: (1) in the setting of a nonfunctional tumor, the patient is a poor operative candidate and a tissue diagnosis is needed to guide additional medical therapy; (2) nonfunctional borderline or unresectable adrenal cancer that will be treated medically to attempt to improve resectability; (3) other metastatic disease with no other sites amenable to biopsy (lung, liver, etc.); (4) concern for lymphoma confined to the adrenal glands.[17,18] FNA is poor in its ability to reliably differentiate between benign and malignant primary tumors of adrenal origin. In all cases, the surgeon must rule out pheochromocytoma and weigh the risk of hemorrhage or seeding of the needle tract with tumor when considering FNA.[19] While FNA can differentiate between adrenal and nonadrenal tissue, if metastasis to the adrenal gland is in the differential and the adrenal is the only site of metastatic disease, the patient is usually offered surgery given documented survival benefit.

E. Genetics

Given that nearly 10% of ACCs are caused by germline genetic mutations, genetic testing is recommended in any patient diagnosed with ACC. Mutations of the TP53 gene causing Li-Fraumeni syndrome are often the cause of ACC in children. More recently, mutations in the MSH and MLH mismatch repair genes leading to Lynch syndrome have also been described as a cause of ACC; however, screening Lynch patients for ACC is not recommended at this time.[20-22] If no germline mutations are identified, tissue from the tumor can be evaluated for targetable somatic mutations for more personalized systemic therapy, especially if metastatic disease is refractory to first- or second-line therapy.

Staging

The two most commonly used staging systems for ACC are from the American Joint Committee on Cancer (AJCC)[23] and the European Network for the Study of Adrenal Tumors (ENSAT).[24] While different in the past, the two-staging systems are now essentially interchangeable. Addition of certain features to these staging systems has been proposed in the literature, including grade, age, presence of cortisol excess, and mutations noted that are associated with worse outcomes in some studies, but these features have not been included in either the ENSAT or AJCC staging systems. ACC is an aggressive disease with half of patients presenting with Stage IV disease at diagnosis. The two most important prognostic factors in patients who have undergone resection of ACC are disease stage and disease-free margins after resection.

Treatment

When technically feasible, surgery with resection of the primary tumor and any involved lymph nodes and/or adjacent organs is pursued, as this is the only treatment modality alone that can achieve cure. Surgery is usually only pursued in patients in whom complete resection of the primary tumor is anticipated. In rare, highly selected situations, resection of the primary tumor in the setting of metastatic disease may be pursued if all sites of disease can be addressed, whether through medical therapy or surgical intervention. Debulking surgery to control hormone excess is described by some; however, disease often progresses relatively soon thereafter, returning to a state where medical treatment is required. Medication can control high levels of hormone excess relatively well, and higher-risk surgery with often lengthy recovery periods can be avoided when survival is not significantly impacted. Adjuvant therapy is often pursued, depending on patient and tumor characteristics, as well as specifics related to the technical aspects of surgical resection. Systemic therapy alone for treatment of ACC has limited success.

A. Surgical Treatment

1. Preoperative Preparation—Preoperative care focuses on medical control of hormone excess (along with resulting blood pressure, electrolyte, glucose, nutrition, and/or fitness derangements) and determination of optimal surgical approach based on the patient's disease, anatomy, surgical history, and comorbidities.

Numerous medications are available to control adrenal hormone excess (Table 47–4).[25] Metyrapone inhibits

Table 47–4. Medications to control adrenal hormone excess.

Hormone		
Cortisol	**Medication**	**Mechanism of Action**
First-line	Metyrapone	Inhibits 11-beta-hydroxylase
Alternatives	Ketoconazole	Inhibits 11-beta-hydroxylase, 17-hydroxylase, and 17,20-lyase
	Mifepristone	Cortisol receptor blocker
	Etomidate	Inhibits 11-beta-hydroxylase
	Mitotane	Inhibits cholesterol side-chain cleavage enzyme, 11-beta-hydroxylase, 18-hydroxylase, and 3β-hydroxysteroid dehydrogenase
	Osilodrostat	Inhibits 11-β-hydroxylase and aldosterone synthase
Aldosterone	Spironolactone	MR antagonist
	Eplerenone	MR antagonist
	Amiloride	Antikaliuretic-diuretic
Androgens	Spironolactone	Blocks androgen receptor
Estrogens (Males)	Anastrozole	Aromatase inhibitor

11-beta-hydroxylase and is considered first-line therapy for treatment of cortisol excess in patients with ACC (although osilodrostat may eventually be found to have better efficacy). Spironolactone is a mineralocorticoid receptor antagonist and blocks the androgen receptor which can be used to manage aldosterone and androgen excess. Anastrozole can control estrogen excess by inhibiting aromatase.

2. Surgery—Open transabdominal adrenalectomy with multivisceral resection, vascular reconstruction, and/or therapeutic lymphadenectomy when necessary remains the approach of choice for resection of ACC.[24] Much debate has centered on the results achieved with minimally invasive approaches; however, the critical technical steps required for resection of ACC are not easily achieved by minimally invasive approaches. A thoracoabdominal approach is occasionally utilized in patients having had prior surgery in upper quadrants and in patients requiring access to the chest and abdomen, respectively.

3. Operative Approach—

A. Right Adrenalectomy—Although a midline incision can be made, a wide right subcostal incision extending across the midline to the left side is favored. The peritoneal cavity is inspected in a systematic manner. Intraoperative ultrasound of the liver and evaluation of the adrenal vein and vena cava for tumor thrombus may be performed. The attachments to the liver are divided, and the right lobe of the liver is rotated medially. A self-retaining retractor is placed. Through the surface of the posterior peritoneal lining, which should be preserved as the anterior margin over the tumor, the kidney and the adrenal gland are appreciated. If the tumor is found to be invading the posterior aspect of the liver, a rim of normal liver may be resected en-bloc as part of the anterior margin. The dissection, as shown in Figure 47–1, begins inferiorly over the superior half of the kidney, taking the posterior peritoneal lining and any fat over the superior aspect of the kidney to the plane between the adrenal gland and kidney. Removal of the capsule of the kidney, or a partial or complete nephrectomy, may be required if there is invasion of the kidney. As external beam radiation may be pursued postoperatively and the kidney becomes nonfunctional as a result, nephrectomy is of less consequence; however, it should be preserved when not invaded and margins are uninvolved to facilitate optimal renal function, especially considering the frequent need for nephrotoxic

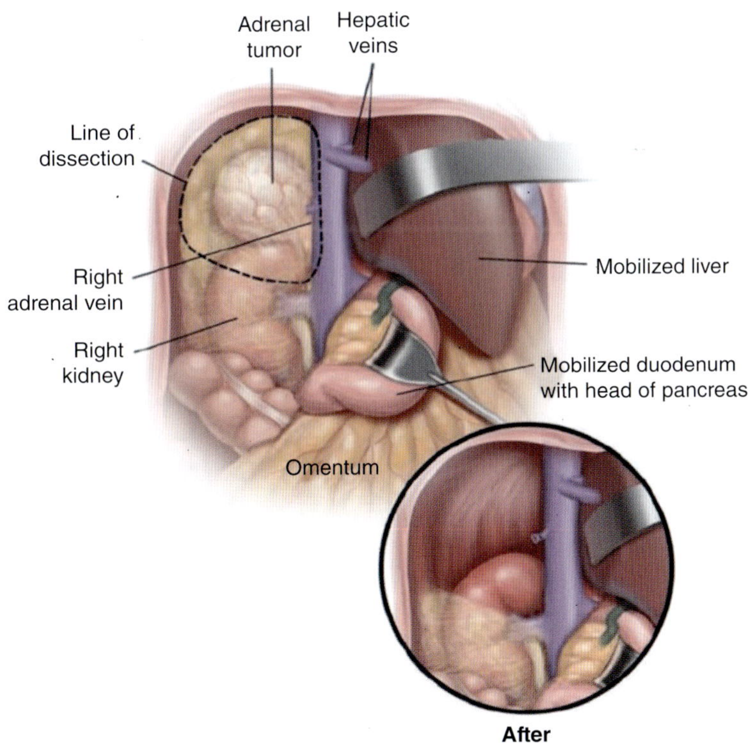

Figure 47–1. Diagram of area of resection when performing right adrenalectomy for known or suspected cancer. Dashed line indicates line of resection to include periadrenal retroperitoneal fat.

systemic therapies (cisplatin) as adjuvant therapy. Dissection proceeds laterally to the sidewall with the removal of all retroperitoneal fat surrounding the tumor as part of the lateral and posterior margins. Dissection continues superiorly to the diaphragm. A portion of the diaphragm may be excised en-bloc if there is evidence of invasion. Any resulting diaphragmatic defect can be closed in standard fashion with a running locking suture or with mesh for a large defect. Medial dissection begins over the anterior aspect of the vena cava. The usually small amount of fat medial to the tumor is then removed as part of the specimen. Fat and abnormal lymph nodes posterior to the renal hilum and vena cava are removed. Working superior to inferior and vice versa, the adrenal vein is identified, ligated, and divided in standard fashion. The junction of the right adrenal vein and retrohepatic vena cava should be examined and palpated to assess for tumor thrombus (ultrasound can be helpful). If invasion of the vena cava is present, resection of vein (partial or circumferential) to obtain negative medial margins or extract tumor thrombus can be achieved. Depending on the amount of vena cava resected, the vena cava may be repaired primarily with a patch (often bovine pericardium), or by replacing the entire segment with ringed polytetrafluoroethylene graft. Venovenous or cardiopulmonary bypass may be needed, and this is determined by the superior extent of the tumor and/or thrombus. The tumor is then removed and marked. Clips are placed at the edges of the resection if radiation therapy will be considered in the future. The abdominal wall is closed in two fascial layers along with suture re-approximation of the deep subcutaneous tissue and closure of the skin with running suture or staples.[26]

B. Left Adrenalectomy—Dissection on the left side proceeds in a similar fashion (Figure 47–2). The main differences are that the stomach, spleen, and pancreas overly the left adrenal gland and must be mobilized. In addition, the peritoneal lining that is preserved over the tumor on the right side does not directly overlie the tumor on the left side, and the surgeon must be careful not to disturb the anterior surface of the tumor. The posterior aspect of the distal pancreas or spleen may be invaded by tumor and should be resected if necessary. The left adrenal vein joins the left renal vein, and both should be examined and palpated (ultrasound is an option) to ensure removal of any tumor thrombus.

An open adrenalectomy via thoracoabdominal approach requires an incision between the ribs that is carried to the midline and inferiorly toward the umbilicus requiring transection of the costal margin and division of the diaphragm. The key technical elements of adrenalectomy remain the same for the thoracoabdominal approach as for the transabdominal approach.

The Operative Standards for Cancer Surgery have standardized the technical aspects of resection for ACC.

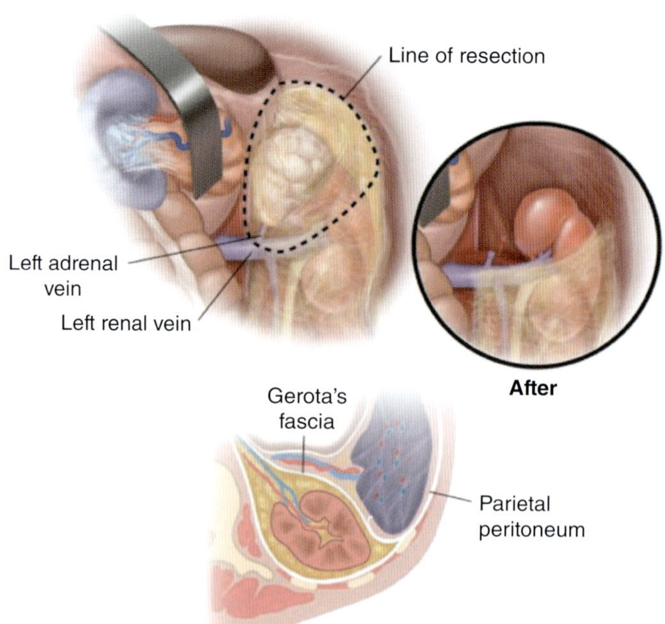

Figure 47–2. Diagram of area of resection when performing left adrenalectomy for known or suspected cancer. Dashed line indicates line of resection to include periadrenal retroperitoneal fat.

Table 47–5. Critical elements of resection of adrenocortical carcinoma.

Element	Description
Exploration	Fully explore the peritoneal cavity unless limited by scar tissue, examine liver surface, consider ultrasound of liver, and vena cava (for right side resection)
Complete R0 resection of the primary tumor	Wide resection, including the periadrenal fat and any peritoneal covering, to microscopically negative margins without disruption of the tumor capsule.
En-bloc resection of involved adjacent organs	Resect adjacent organs (fully or partially) if direct invasion or adherence
En-bloc resection of involved vasculature and/or thrombectomy of tumor thrombus	Dependent on extent, utilize bypass, liver perfusion, and/or circulatory arrest as needed, with or without reconstruction
Therapeutic lymphadenectomy	Abnormal lymph nodes noted on imaging or intraoperatively. Examine peri-adrenal, peri-renal, aortocaval lymph nodes

Table 47–5 lists the critical elements of resection of ACC.[26] R0 resection is of the utmost importance.[27] Fragmentation or morcellation of the tumor is contraindicated as it prevents accurate pathologic examination, and therefore determination of true stage and resection status. Similarly, if the periadrenal fat is not removed with the tumor, assessment for periadrenal invasion and upstaging to Stage 3 is not possible. Patients with locally invasive disease may benefit from at least two cycles of neoadjuvant chemotherapy and mitotane to improve the chance of R0 resection.[27]

Occasionally, metastatic disease may be encountered upon entry into and examination of the peritoneal cavity. The operation is commonly aborted; however, the decision to proceed depends on the volume of disease and resectability of all disease. Debulking can be considered but is associated with poor long-term outcomes. Resection of the primary tumor and all metastatic disease followed by early utilization of mitotane and combination chemotherapy (usually etoposide, doxorubicin, and cisplatin) can be undertaken in carefully selected situations.[28]

4. Postoperative Care—Care after surgery follows routine practices. Monitoring of electrolytes, especially sodium and potassium, along with renal function and hemoglobin is undertaken. Given the position of the adrenal glands and lack of involvement of the gastrointestinal tract, bowel function is usually quick to return, and diets can be resumed early in the postoperative period. Postoperative complications are rare but include bleeding, infection, development of incisional hernias, and renal dysfunction secondary to hypovolemia. If an open adrenalectomy is performed, pain management and respiratory function can be improved with the use of locoregional blocks and/or epidural.

Administration of intravenous hydrocortisone should be assumed necessary postoperatively for those with overt Cushing syndrome. Given the half-life of cortisol, intraoperative administration is not usually necessary. Those undergoing adrenalectomy for mild, "subclinical" excess cortisol secretion may not require glucocorticoid administration, and postoperative testing of the hypothalamic-pituitary-adrenal (HPA) axis should be performed the morning after surgery. The need for and replacement dose of steroid should be determined and managed in conjunction with an experienced endocrinologist.

Patients undergoing bilateral adrenalectomy, or those with adrenal insufficiency awaiting return of HPA axis function are at risk for developing Addisonian crisis if adequate amounts of steroids are not provided. These patients should be monitored closely, educated on actions to take in the event of a health emergency or signs of adrenal insufficiency, and wear a medical alert device.[29]

Operative and pathology reports in those diagnosed with ACC, or where other postoperative questions or concerns arise, should be discussed in a multidisciplinary setting (eg, tumor board).[24]

A. Medical Treatment

Mitotane is an isomer of the insecticide DDT and remains the only drug specifically approved for use in ACC. It inhibits enzymes within the steroid synthesis pathway, and cortisol production in particular. Through an unknown mechanism, it also leads to destruction of the adrenal cortex. Due to these two mechanisms, supplemental steroids should be administered to patients taking mitotane. A serum mitotane level of 14 to 20 mg/L and without signs of toxicity is desirable; however, many patients are unable to reach a therapeutic level due to intolerance of side effects, most commonly gastrointestinal. Mitotane may be used alone as adjuvant treatment in patients at high risk for recurrence. The recent ADIUVO trial revealed no benefit of mitotane in patients with low-risk features for disease recurrence. With disease recurrence or Stage IV disease at presentation, mitotane may be initiated as the sole agent;[30] however, the most common combination regimen is mitotane with etoposide, doxorubicin, and cisplatin (carboplatin if renal insufficiency). Streptozocin and 5-fluorouracil have been used as second-line therapy. Immunotherapy has been found to have benefits in some patients, but less so in those with cortisol-producing tumors.

In those few with borderline resectable disease or small-volume metastatic disease exhibiting regression or stability of disease while being treated with chemotherapy in a neoadjuvant fashion, surgical resection may be of benefit. Conversely, those with progressive disease will likely not see significant benefit from surgical resection.

Lung and liver metastases are most common, followed by bone metastases. Brain metastases are rare and generally occur more than 10 years after diagnosis. The addition of adjuvant radiation to the tumor bed after resection of the primary tumor is considered on an individual basis, but has shown benefit in preventing local recurrence. One study suggests improvement in overall survival.[31]

Reoperative Surgery for ACC

The disease-free interval, quality of the initial resection, location(s) of tumor, tumor grade, anticipated operation required to remove all recurrent disease, and the physiologic status of the patient to tolerate reoperation must be considered when making the complex decision about reoperating for recurrent disease. Even if an operation is technically feasible, the tumor biology may instead dictate avoidance of surgery and pursuit of systemic therapy. Because recurrence after reoperation for an initial recurrence approaches 70% to 90% and the recurrence is often in the same organ,[32] local therapies such as single-beam radiation therapy, radiofrequency ablation, microwave ablation, or cryoablation are increasingly considered for control of small volume metastatic disease to minimize the morbidity of repeated surgical resections. Long-term durability of reoperation to control hormone excess is often poor with a nonsignificant increase in survival (3 to 6 months) when the time for recovery from surgery is considered from a quality-of-life standpoint.[32]

Prognosis

The reported 5-year overall survival in those who have undergone surgical resection with curative intent ranges from 39% to 55%, while 5-year overall survival in patients with stage IV disease is approximately 10%.[24] The most important prognostic factors in patients who have undergone resection of ACC is disease stage and margin-negative resection. High tumor grade and production of excess cortisol are also significant prognostic markers. Regardless of the reported survival data, each patient's case should be reviewed and approached in an individualized fashion. Reported data is difficult to interpret given wide variation in evaluation and management, and often nonstandard, suboptimal care.

When to Refer

The only factors associated with better outcomes for ACC have been guideline-centered care, R0 resection, and treatment at referral centers with a multidisciplinary team having expertise in the management of adrenal malignancies. Adrenalectomy performed by a high-volume adrenal surgeon is associated with shorter length of hospital stay and fewer complications.[33-35] As there is a significant difference in the conduct of adrenalectomy for benign versus malignant adrenocortical tumors, surgeon experience must also be evaluated with this in mind as there are few centers and surgeons truly treating a high volume of patients with ACC.

ADRENAL LYMPHOMA

General Considerations

Lymphoma may metastasize to the adrenal glands, or infrequently, arise from within the adrenal glands. The incidence of secondary adrenal involvement in non-Hodgkin lymphoma (NHL) detectable on computed tomography (CT) scan is ~5%, and 25% to 30% when autopsies are included.[36-38] Primary adrenal lymphoma (PAL) is a rare extranodal form of lymphoma accounting for 1% of NHL cases. PAL most commonly affects older men (median age, 68 years; male-to-female ratio, 2:1) and most often presents with bilateral adrenal masses.[39-41] Unilateral involvement of the adrenal glands is more commonly associated with systemic lymphoma.

Pathogenesis

Adrenal lymphoma is predominantly of large B-cell type. PAL is thought to be of hemopoietic origin in a single adrenal gland which is then attracted to the microenvironment of the contralateral gland. There has been evidence of hematogenous spread from a single focus. Immune dysfunction with past or concurrent malignancy, HIV, EBV autoimmune disease, and mutations in p53 and c-kit genes have all been suggested to be responsible for the development of PAL.[39,42,43]

Clinical Findings

A. Signs & Symptoms

Patients with primary adrenal lymphoma often present with bulky disease. Tumor size ranged from 4 to 17 cm with mean size 8 cm in one series.[39] Patients often present with abdominal or lumbar pain, adrenal insufficiency, or "B" symptoms such as fever, weight loss, and/or night sweats. Less commonly, patients may present with anorexia, nausea/vomiting, diarrhea, neurological symptoms, thrombocytopenia, hemolytic anemia, or hypercalcemia.

B. Laboratory Analysis

Comprehensive evaluation should be pursued as the differential can be wide. A complete blood count, chemistry panel, liver function tests, coagulation studies, LDH, B2 microglobulin, C-reactive protein, ferritin, and adrenal-specific biochemistry should be obtained until the range of diagnoses can be narrowed. Additional tumor markers should be ordered in the setting of a prior malignancy (colon, lung, or other cancers). Elevated LDH is seen in 88% of cases and is associated with bilaterality.[44] LDH levels greater than twice the upper limit of normal are associated with CNS involvement. Patients can be evaluated for adrenal insufficiency by evaluating ACTH and morning cortisol levels or by performing an ACTH stimulation test.

C. Imaging

PALs typically appear as solid, nodular, hypoechoic heterogeneous masses on ultrasound with low density and moderate enhancement on CT scan. MRI demonstrates a T1-hypointense T2-hyperintense pattern, but these are not diagnostic.[45] There are often areas of necrosis and hemorrhage. These tumors are generally 18-FDG avid. Regardless of the differential, if malignancy is suspected to be in the differential of diagnoses, additional full-body imaging should be pursued, most often in the form of PET imaging. FDG-PET imaging identified additional sites of disease in nearly 80% in one study.[46] Other extranodal sites of disease may be involved, including the testicles, pituitary gland, thyroid, and eye. PAL commonly appears to involve the vena cava, renal, and/or splenic vessels.

D. Diagnostic Interventions

Suspected adrenal lymphoma is one of the few circumstances in which patients benefit from biopsy of the adrenal gland. FNA is avoided, and instead core biopsy is pursued to allow for adequate sampling. In cases of systemic lymphoma, other sites may be more amenable to biopsy. If image-guided core biopsy is not technically feasible, minimally invasive approaches to the adrenal gland can be pursued. In cases of PAL, lymph node or bone marrow involvement is rarely identified. Lumbar puncture may be pursued to rule out CNS involvement, especially in the setting of elevated LDH levels.

Differential Diagnosis

ACC can present later in the disease process as bilateral indeterminate masses. Other malignancies may metastasize to the adrenal glands and most commonly include melanoma, lung, renal cell, breast, and some colon cancers. Infectious etiologies such as tuberculosis, histoplasmosis, cryptococcosis, paracoccidiomycosis, and CMV commonly localize within the adrenal gland and should also be considered.

Treatment

First-line therapy for primary adrenal diffuse large B-cell lymphoma is R-CHOP chemotherapy. Achieving complete response with R-CHOP (cyclophosphamide, doxorubicin, vincristine, and prednisone) was a significant predictor of longer overall and progression-free survival while no survival benefit was observed in patients who underwent adrenalectomy prior to chemotherapy.[47] CHOP with rituximab can be considered in cases of CD20+ disease. CNS prophylaxis with intrathecal systemic methotrexate can be offered to patients with concern for CNS involvement as evidenced by LDH level or high international prognostic index score.

Surgery for lymphoma involving the adrenal gland is generally avoided; however, in some cases, adrenalectomy may be pursued when tissue cannot be obtained by image-guided means or there is diagnostic uncertainty after biopsy. Bilateral adrenalectomy can be considered in some younger patients prior to systemic adjuvant chemotherapy, but this is not a common occurrence, and in one French study was of no benefit.[46] Additionally, preservation of some normal adrenal tissue would be advantageous to avoid the need for lifelong steroid replacement when chemotherapy is able to eradicate disease in the adrenal glands. Surgery without adjuvant chemotherapy is associated with poor long-term outcomes. The role of radiation therapy is not well defined but can be considered in some cases.

Prognosis

Prognosis of systemic lymphoma is better than PAL. Overall 5-year survival of systemic regional lymphoma is 64% overall, 73% for regional involvement, and 57% for distant involvement. Prognosis of PAL is poor with 3-, 6-, and 12-month survival rates reported as 67%, 46%, and 20%, respectively.[44]

METASTASIS TO THE ADRENAL GLAND

General Considerations

Patients should undergo comprehensive evaluation, including assessment for malignancy (current diagnosis of active malignancy, signs or symptoms suggestive of a new cancer diagnosis, or prior history of malignancy). Family history of malignancy or other disorders may indicate the potential for germline mutations and a genetic syndrome leading to malignancy. While any malignancy can metastasize to the adrenal gland, the most common are lung (39%), renal cell, breast (35%), melanoma, and lymphoma. Colorectal cancer less commonly metastasizes to the adrenal glands, but the number of reported cases is increasing.[45,48,49] Metastasis to the adrenals is primarily through hematogenous spread and can involve both adrenal glands. It is hypothesized that metastases commonly occur in the adrenals due to the rich sinusoidal blood supply of the glands.[50]

Prevention

Given that any malignancy can theoretically metastasize to the adrenal gland, routine health maintenance exams are of primary importance, including skin, breast, and colon cancer screenings among others. In those with a current or prior malignancy, recommendations for scheduled surveillance should be followed according to accepted guidelines.

Clinical Findings

A. Signs & Symptoms

Most metastatic disease to the adrenal gland is found at the time of initial diagnosis of a malignancy or on surveillance imaging. With growth of adrenal metastases, local symptoms of compression may develop. Adjacent structures may become encased or invaded. Rarely, if both adrenal glands are replaced by metastatic disease, patients may develop signs or symptoms of adrenal insufficiency.

B. Imaging

Imaging is dependent on how metastatic disease to the adrenal gland is first identified. Any adrenal mass should be evaluated in a consistent fashion as previously described. Should the mass be indeterminate by imaging characteristics, additional imaging should be pursued. This often includes CT imaging of the chest. PET imaging is also often indicated. Some malignancies are not FDG avid (eg, renal cell cancer) and this should be kept in mind when interpreting imaging studies.

C. FNA Evaluation

As previously mentioned, FNA has a limited role in the evaluation of an adrenal mass. In the setting of known metastatic disease to the adrenal gland, reasonable data exist to proceed with adrenalectomy if there are no other sites of disease or the other sites will also be treated. FNA can be avoided in these situations. However, if there are multiple sites of metastatic disease, and tissue confirmation is necessary to proceed with selection of systemic therapy, biopsy of an adrenal metastasis is reasonable. Often, other sites of disease are more amenable to biopsy than the adrenal gland.

Treatment

A. Surgical Treatment

Surgical indications in those with metastatic disease to an adrenal gland include: (1) metastatic disease in which the adrenal gland is the only site of disease; and (2) those with concern that the tumor involving the adrenal gland will progress and result in local invasion of adjacent structures and sequelae when other disease is controlled by another treatment modality.[51] Isolated adrenal metastases are rare.[52] Patients with multiple sites of metastatic disease are better served with other treatment modalities such as radiation or chemotherapy. Radiation to adrenal metastases is often performed for patients with metastatic cancer prior to consultation with an adrenal surgeon. Radiation does make subsequent adrenalectomy more difficult, and should the tumor not respond, consideration for adrenalectomy as an alternative treatment should be discussed in a multidisciplinary format prior to selection of definitive treatment. Surgery for metastatic disease to the adrenal glands should ensure a complete, margin-negative resection. Given differences in tumor biology, some cancers metastatic to the adrenal glands can be removed by minimally invasive means.

B. Medical Treatment

Immune checkpoint inhibitors (ICI) are being used with increasing frequency in the management of many types of cancers known to metastasize to the adrenal glands. Interestingly, despite the success of ICIs in the management of the primary cancers, similar responses have not been seen in some metastatic sites.[53] It is believed that the endogenous glucocorticoids within the adrenals impair the efficacy of ICIs, especially given that endogenous glucocorticoids within the tumor microenvironment have been shown to promote CD8+ tumor-infiltrating lymphocyte dysfunction which reduces ICI efficacy.[54]

Prognosis

Overall, patients with metastatic disease have a poor prognosis, but adrenalectomy for singular metastatic disease to an adrenal gland can be associated with improved long-term survival and avoid complications related to invasion of adjacent vital structures.[55,56]

REFERENCES

1. Song JH, Chaudhry FS, Mayo-Smith WW. The incidental adrenal mass on CT: prevalence of adrenal disease in 1,049 consecutive adrenal masses in patients with no known malignancy. *Am J Roentgenol.* 2008;190:5:1163-1168.
2. Kebebew E, Reiff E, Duh QY, Clark OH, McMillan A. Extent of disease at presentation and outcome for adrenocortical carcinoma: have we made progress? *World J Surg.* 2006;30(5):872-878.
3. Kerkhofs TM, Verhoeven RH, Bonjer HJ, et al. Surgery for adrenocortical carcinoma in The Netherlands: analysis of the national cancer registry data. *Eur J Endocrinol.* 2013;169(1):83-89.
4. Almeida MQ, Bezerra-Neto JE, Mendonca BB, Latronico AC, Fragoso M. Primary malignant tumors of the adrenal glands. *Clinics.* 2018;73(Suppl 1):e756s.
5. Fassnacht M, Libe R, Kroiss M, Allolio B. Adrenocortical carcinoma: a clinician's update. *Nat Rev Endocrinol.* 2011;7(6):323-335.
6. Debono M, Bradburn M, Bull M, Harrison B, Ross RJ, Newell-Price J. Cortisol as a marker for increased mortality in patients with incidental adrenocortical adenomas. *J Clin Endocrinol Metab.* 2014;99(12):4462-4470.
7. Bancos I, Alahdab F, Crowley RK, et al. Therapy of endocrine disease: improvement of cardiovascular risk factors after adrenalectomy in patients with adrenal tumors and subclinical Cushing's syndrome: a systematic review and meta-analysis. *Eur J Endocrinol.* 2016;175(6):R283-R295.

8. Petr EJ, Else T. Adrenocortical carcinoma (ACC): when and why should we consider germline testing? *Presse Med.* 2018;47(7-8 Pt 2):e119-e125.
9. Caoili EM, Korobkin M, Francis IR, et al. Adrenal masses: characterization with combined unenhanced and delayed enhanced CT. *Radiology*. 2002; 222(3):629-633.
10. Caoili EM, Korobkin M, Francis IR, Cohan RH, Dunnick NR. Delayed enhanced CT of lipid-poor adrenal adenomas. *AJR Am J Roentgenol.* 2000;175(5):1411-1415.
11. Corwin MT, Navarro SM, Malik DJ, et al. Differences in growth rate on CT of adrenal adenomas and malignant adrenal nodules. *Am J Roentgenol* 2019 213(3):632-636.
12. Haider MA, Ghai S, Jhaveri K, Lockwood G. Chemical shift MR imaging of hyperattenuating (>10 HU) adrenal masses: does it still have a role? *Radiology.* 2004;231:711-716.
13. Elsayes KM, Mukundan G, Narra VR, et al. Adrenal masses: MR imaging features with pathologic correlation. *Radiographics.* 2004;24(Suppl. 1):S73-S86.
14. Caoili EM, Korobkin M, Brown RK, Mackie G, Shulkin BL. Differentiating adrenal adenomas from nonadenomas using (18)F-FDG PET/CT: quantitative and qualitative evaluation. *Acad Radiol.* 2007;14(4):468-475.
15. Groussin L, Bonardel G, Silvéra S, et al. 18F-Fluorodeoxyglucose positron emission tomography for the diagnosis of adrenocortical tumors: a prospective study in 77 operated patients. *J Clin Endocrinol Metab.* 2009;94:1713-1722.
16. Leboulleux S, Dromain C, Bonniaud G, et al. Diagnostic and prognostic value of 18-fluorodeoxyglucose positron emission tomography in adrenocortical carcinoma: a prospective comparison with computed tomography. *J. Clin Endocrinol Metab.* 2006;91:920-925.
17. Khan TS, Sundin A, Juhlin C, Långström B, Bergström M, Eriksson B. 11C-metomidate PET imaging of adrenocortical cancer. *Eur J Nucl Med Mol Imaging.* 2003;30:403-410.
18. Fassnacht M, Arlt W, Bancos I, et al. Management of adrenal incidentalomas: European Society of Endocrinology Clinical Practice Guideline in collaboration with the European Network for the Study of Adrenal Tumors. *Eur J Endocrinol.* 2016;175(2):G1-G34.
19. Bancos I, Tamhane S, Shah M, et al. Diagnosis of endocrine disease: the diagnostic performance of adrenal biopsy: a systematic review and meta-analysis. *Eur J Endocrinol.* 2016; 175(2):R65-R80.
20. Berruti A, Baudin E, Gelderblom H, et al. Adrenal cancer: ESMO Clinical Practice Guidelines for diagnosis, treatment and follow-up. *Ann Oncol.* 2012;23(Suppl 7):vii131-138.
21. Petr EJ, Else T. Genetic predisposition to endocrine tumors: diagnosis, surveillance and challenges in care. *Semin Oncol.* 2016;43(5):582-590.
22. Else T, Kim AC, Sabolch A, et al. Adrenocortical carcinoma. *Endocr Rev.* 2014;35(2):282-326.
23. Amin MB, Greene FL, Edge SB, et al. The eighth edition AJCC cancer staging manual: continuing to build a bridge from a population-based to a more "personalized" approach to cancer staging. *CA Cancer J Clin.* 2017;67(2):93-99.
24. Fassnacht M, Dekkers OM, Else T, et al. European Society of Endocrinology Clinical Practice Guidelines on the management of adrenocortical carcinoma in adults, in collaboration with the European Network for the Study of Adrenal Tumors. *Eur J Endocrinol.* 2018;179(4):G1-G46.
25. Miller BS, Else T, AACE Adrenal Scientific Committee. Personalized care of patients with adrenocortical carcinoma: a comprehensive approach. *Endocr Pract.* 2017;23(6):705-715.
26. Miller BS. Chapter 3: Adrenalectomy including multivisceral resection. In: *Operative Standards for Cancer Surgery*. Vol Volume III, Hepatobiliary, Peritoneal Malignancies, Neuroendocrine, Sarcoma, Adrenal, Bladder. Philadelphia: Lippincott Williams & Wilkins; 2021.
27. Bednarski BK, Habra MA, Phan A, et al. Borderline resectable adrenal cortical carcinoma: a potential role for preoperative chemotherapy. *World J Surg.* 2014;38(6):1318-1327.
28. Hughes MS, Lo WM, Beresnev T, et al. A phase II trial of cytoreduction and hyperthermic intraperitoneal chemotherapy for recurrent adrenocortical carcinoma. *J Surg Res.* 2018;232: 383-388.
29. Miller BS. Management of adrenal cortical tumors. *Cameron.* 2020;12(141):5-13.
30. Gaujoux S, Mihai R, joint working group of ESES and ENSAT. European Society of Endocrine Surgeons (ESES) and European Network for the Study of Adrenal Tumours (ENSAT) recommendations for the surgical management of adrenocortical carcinoma. *Br J Surg.* 2017;104(4):358-376.
31. Gharzai LA, Green MD, Griffith KA, et al. Adjuvant radiation improves recurrence-free survival and overall survival in adrenocortical carcinoma. *J Clin Endocrinol Metab.* 2019; 104:3743-3750.
32. Glenn JA, Else T, Hughes DT, et al. Longitudinal patterns of recurrence in patients with adrenocortical carcinoma. *Surgery.* 2019;165(1):186-195.
33. Palazzo F, Dickinson A, Phillips B, et al. Adrenal surgery in England: better outcomes in high-volume practices. *Clin Endocrinol.* 2016;85(1):17-20.
34. Park HS, Roman SA, Sosa JA. Outcomes from 3144 adrenalectomies in the United States: which matters more, surgeon volume or specialty? *Arch Surg.* 2009;144(11):1060-1067.
35. Lindeman B, Hashimoto DA, Bababekov YJ, et al. Fifteen years of adrenalectomies: impact of specialty training and operative volume. *Surgery.* 2018;163(1):150-156.
36. Paling MR, Williamson BR. Adrenal involvement in non-Hodgkin lymphoma. *AJR Am J Roentgenol.* 1983;141:303-305.
37. Rosenberg SA, Diamond HD, Jaslowitz B, Craver LF. Lymphosarcoma: a review of 1269 cases. *Med.* 1961;40:31-84.
38. Straus DJ, Filippa DA, Lieberman PH, Koziner B, Thaler HT, Clarkson BD. The non-Hodgkin's lymphomas. I. A retrospective clinical and pathologic analysis of 499 cases diagnosed between 1958 and 1969. *Cancer.* 1983;51:101-109.
39. Wang J, Sun NC, Renslo R, et al. Clinically silent primary adrenal lymphoma: a case report and review of the literature. *Am J Hematol.* 1998;58:130-136.
40. Wu HC, Shih LY, Chen TC, Chu SH, Tsai CC. A patient with bilateral primary adrenal lymphoma, presenting with fever of unknown origin and achieving long-term disease-free survival after resection and chemotherapy. *Ann Hematol.* 1999;78: 289-292.
41. Kumar R, Xiu Y, Mavi A, El-Haddad G, Zhuang H, Alavi A. FDG-PET imaging in primary bilateral adrenal lymphoma: a case report and review of the literature. *Clin Nucl Med.* 2005; 30:222-230.
42. Ohsawa M, Tomita Y, Hashimoto M, Yasunaga Y, Kanno H, Aozasa K. Malignant lymphoma of the adrenal gland: its possible correlation with Epstein–Barr virus. *Mod Pathol.* 1996; 9:534-543.
43. Nakatsuka S, Hongyo T, Syaifudin M, Nomura T, Shingu N, Aozasa K. Mutations of p53, c-kit, K-ras, and beta-catenin gene in non-Hodgkin's lymphoma of adrenal gland. *Jpn J Cancer Res.* 2002;93:267-274.

44. Tsujimoto A, Ueda T, Kuge H, et al. Long-term survival after adrenal metastasectomy from colorectal cancer: a report of two cases. *Surg Case Rep*. 2019;5:61.
45. Cunningham JJ. Ultrasonic findings in "primary" lymphoma of the adrenal area. *J Ultrasound Med*. 1983;2:467-469.
46. Laurent C, Casasnovas O, Martin L, et al. Adrenal lymphoma: presentation, management and prognosis. *QJM*. 2017;110(2): 103-109.
47. Coiffier B, Lepage E, Briere J, et al. CHOP chemotherapy plus rituximab compared with CHOP alone in elderly patients with diffuse large-B-cell lymphoma. *N Engl J Med*. 2002;346: 235-242.
48. Klikovits T, Lohinai Z, Fábián K, et al. New insights into the impact of primary lung adenocarcinoma location on metastatic sites and sequence: a multicenter cohort study. *Lung Cancer*. 2018;126:139-148.
49. Blažeković I, Jukić T, Granić R, Punda M, Franceschi M. An unusual case of papillary thyroid carcinoma iodine-131 avid metastasis to the adrenal gland. *Acta Clin Croat*. 2018;57(2): 372-376.
50. Kung AW, Pun KK, Lam K, Wang C, Leung CY. Addisonian crisis as presenting feature in malignancies. *Cancer*. 1990;65:177-179.
51. Romero Arenas MA, Sui D, Grubbs EG, Lee JE, Perrier ND. Adrenal metastectomy is safe in selected patients. *World J Surg*. 2014;38(6):1336-1342.
52. Bradley CT, Strong VE. Surgical management of adrenal metastases. *J Surg Oncol*. 2014;109:31-35.
53. Borgers JSW, Tobin RP, Torphy RJ, et al. Melanoma metastases to the adrenal gland are highly resistant to immune checkpoint inhibitors. *J Natl Compr Canc Netw*. 2021:jnccn20283.
54. Acharya N, Madi A, Zhang H, et al. Endogenous glucocorticoid signaling regulates CD8+ T cell differentiation and development of dysfunction in the tumor microenvironment. *Immunity*. 2020;53:658-671.e6.
55. Krumeich LN, Roses RE, Kuo LE, et al. Survival after adrenalectomy for metastatic lung cancer. *Ann Surg Oncol*. 2022;29(4): 2571-2579.
56. Illuminati G, Pasqua R, D'Ermo G, et al. Results of adrenalectomy for isolated, metachronous metastasis of breast cancer: a retrospective cohort study. *Front Surg*. 2021;8:671424.

Adrenalectomy: Open Approach

48

Bernice Huang, MD
Paul H. Graham, MD

INTRODUCTION

The adrenal glands are two small endocrine glands located in the retroperitoneum immediately superior and medial to the kidneys. They are composed of two distinct layers, the outer cortex and inner medulla, and are responsible for the production of mineralocorticoids, glucocorticoids, secondary sex hormones, and catecholamines. Abnormalities may result from glandular hyperplasia, adenomatous growth, other benign aberrations, or malignant conversion of the gland. The majority of adrenal tumors are benign and commonly come to attention as an incidental finding on unrelated imaging, a true incidentaloma. Alternatively, the clinical manifestations of excess hormone production or local invasion may prompt evaluation. Surgical resection is the primary treatment of various adrenal neoplasia and their associated hormone abnormalities.

PATIENT SELECTION

Preoperative Workup

A. Biochemical Evaluation

Neoplasms of the adrenal gland are assessed for functionality, or excess hormone production. Both benign and malignant neoplasms have the capability of producing excessive levels of adrenal hormone and may present with the characteristic clinical manifestations attributed to the particular hormone irregularity. Biochemical testing for hormone excess confirms the specific functional tumor type and aids in determining the need for further diagnostic tests or localization studies necessary in surgical planning. Additionally, the hormonal evaluation may provide information regarding the clinical behavior of an adrenal neoplasm. For instance, identification of a large adrenal mass with associated hypercortisolism increases the suspicion of malignancy, given over half of adrenocortical carcinomas (ACCs) are associated with excess production of one or more adrenal hormones. Furthermore, adrenocortical carcinomas associated with excess cortisol production have been found to be associated with worse prognosis.[1] Early identification of excess hormone production also allows for medical optimization against the hormonal effects to provide appropriate perioperative stabilization.

B. Imaging

Cross-sectional imaging by computed tomography (CT) or magnetic resonance imaging (MRI) provides essential characterization of features distinctive to benign or malignant adrenal neoplasia, such as size, heterogeneity, and attenuation on unenhanced and enhanced imaging (Table 48–1).[2]

Additionally, for tumors with characteristics concerning for malignancy, cross-sectional imaging provides initial staging of the adrenal neoplasm to help direct the extent of surgical resection and operative approach. Functional imaging with modalities such as fluorodeoxyglucose-positron emission tomography (FDG-PET) can also aid in the detection, characterization, and staging of disease.

CT of the abdomen and pelvis with dedicated adrenal protocol is a frequently used modality in the evaluation of an adrenal mass, in part due to its accessibility and high spatial resolution. MRI can also be performed in place of or complementary to a CT scan, particularly with the use of chemical shift imaging (CSI), which helps detect lipid-rich adenomas, and dynamic contrast-enhanced imaging (DCI), which can be useful when CSI cannot adequately classify an adenoma. On MRI, adrenocortical carcinomas show low signal intensity on T1-weighted images and high signal intensity on T2-weighted images, with strong heterogenous contrast enhancement and slow washout. Adenomas, on the other hand, are more homogenous with low signal intensity on T2-weighted images and demonstrate loss of signal intensity on out-of-phase images with CSI.

Table 48–1. CT imaging characteristics of malignant adrenal neoplasms.

• Large size (>6 cm)
• Heterogeneity
• Calcifications
• Tumor necrosis
• Irregular borders
• Local/vascular invasion
• Lymphadenopathy
• Metastases
• Increased density (>30 HU on unenhanced CT)
• Poor washout on delayed contrast-enhanced CT (<50% at 10 minutes)

HU, Hounsfield units.

Pheochromocytomas can present as solid, cystic, or mixed tumors, with increased heterogeneity as they enlarge in size. On CT, they demonstrate increased attenuation on precontrast images (HU >20), with intense enhancement in the portal venous phase and delayed washout. MRI is particularly helpful in identifying pheochromocytomas, as they can appear slightly hypointense on T1-weighted imaging and have high signal intensity on T2-weighted images. Radionuclide modalities, including metaiodobenzylguanidine (MIBG) scintigraphy, FDG-PET, and PET-DOTATATE, can also be useful in detecting pheochromocytomas when there is diagnostic uncertainty on CT or MRI, or in cases where the risk of extra-adrenal tumors or metastasis is present.

C. Biopsy

Biopsy of adrenal lesions is generally not indicated, except to confirm a metastasis to the adrenal gland if there is no indication for surgical excision or when a nonfunctional retroperitoneal neoplasm, such as lymphoma or sarcoma, is difficult to distinguish from primary adrenal pathology. Importantly, it is imperative to rule out pheochromocytoma prior to performing a biopsy of an adrenal mass to prevent inadvertent catecholamine crisis.

Surgical Indications & Considerations

Resection of an adrenal neoplasm is indicated when the tumor is functional or when there is concern for a primary adrenocortical malignancy. Pheochromocytomas and paragangliomas maintain an inherent potential for local invasion and metastasis as well; therefore, resection is indicated. At times, resection may be indicated for secondary metastases to the adrenal gland or for the diagnosis of indeterminate adrenal masses. The surgical approach to resection is dictated by the etiology and size of the pathology.

Contemporary surgical management of adrenal neoplasia has progressed to a predominant use of minimally invasive approaches to resection. This may be a result of increased identification of incidental small, benign tumors on cross-sectional imaging, surgeon familiarity with minimally invasive approaches, and the enhanced patient recovery and low complication rates associated with these approaches.[3] Open surgical approaches are primarily utilized for adrenal neoplasia of larger size, which may be challenging to remove via a minimally invasive approach, or for neoplasia concerning for malignancy in which local invasion, concomitant organ resection, or the need to prevent tumor rupture necessitates the exposure and tissue handling of an open approach. Though some guidelines allow for a minimally invasive surgical approach to small ACCs in the hands of experienced adrenal surgeons,[4] the risk of earlier disease recurrence by MIS approach in many surgical series lends caution to this approach.[5,6]

When operating for ACC, complete R0 resection with negative margins is of utmost importance in dictating patient outcomes.[7] Capsule disruption and tumor spillage may lead to recurrence. Therefore, invasion of local structures necessitates *en bloc* resection, and concomitant nephrectomy, distal pancreatectomy, splenectomy, or partial liver resection may be necessary. Additionally, tumor thrombus may also extend into the lumen of the renal vein, IVC, or right atrium and should be extracted, which may require venotomy and vascular reconstruction, and even cardiopulmonary bypass on rare occasions. These complex cases may require consultation and coordination with multiple surgical specialties. In certain instances of metastatic or recurrent ACC in which complete resection is not possible, tumor debulking may be helpful to control extreme hormone excess, though the overall prognosis remains poor. There is no clear consensus on the role of regional lymphadenectomy in the treatment of ACC and the extent of lymphadenectomy performed is variable, though could include renal hilum, celiac, para-aortic, and para-caval lymph nodes. There is evidence to suggest, however, that locoregional lymph node dissection may improve tumor staging and oncologic outcomes.[8,9] An open approach facilitates the necessary exposure should *en bloc* resection or lymphadenectomy be utilized.

As with ACC, it is best to avoid capsule rupture during resection of pheochromocytoma as it may predispose patients to recurrence. Most pheochromocytomas can preferably be resected using a minimally invasive approach. However, an open approach should be considered in larger tumors and is the standard of care for those with concern for potential local invasion. Resection of metastatic pheochromocytomas may be considered when feasible and can help improve symptoms of hormone excess, improve the efficacy of subsequent therapies, or prevent or treat complications due to tumor location. In patients with bilateral pheochromocytomas, cortical-sparing adrenalectomy may be considered in an attempt to avoid permanent steroid dependency and may be approached by either open or minimally invasive techniques.[10]

A. Genetic Factors

Advances in genomics over the past decades have allowed us a better understanding of adrenal tumors, their pathophysiology, and their prognosis. While there is still much more to learn, our knowledge to date does have significant implications for the surgical treatment of adrenal tumors.

Although most adrenal tumors are sporadic, certain hereditary cancer syndromes have been associated with ACC. These include Li-Fraumeni syndrome (inactivating p53 mutations), Beckwith-Wiedemann syndrome (abnormalities on chromosome 11 [11p15]), multiple endocrine neoplasia type 1 (inactivating MEN1 mutations), and Lynch syndrome (inactivating mutations on mismatch repair genes). When considering an operation for patients with an adrenal tumor who are known or suspected to have one of these genetic syndromes associated with ACC, it may be prudent to assume malignancy and opt for an open approach to adrenalectomy rather than a minimally invasive approach depending on the size of the lesion and the skill of the surgeon.

Genetic testing is recommended for all patients with a pheochromocytoma. In general, tumors can be classified by their mutations into three primary subtypes, with the most common being the pseudohypoxia subtype, which involves mutations in the tricarboxylic acid cycle. Several hereditary syndromes are associated with pheochromocytomas, including Von Hippel-Lindau (VHL) disease (VHL mutations), multiple endocrine neoplasia (MEN) 2A and 2B (RET mutations), neurofibromatosis (NF mutations), and familial paraganglioma or pheochromocytoma syndromes (SDHB, SDHC, and SDHD mutations). In particular, SDHB mutations have been associated with a greater risk of extra-adrenal disease and aggressive behavior.[11,12] On the other hand, pheochromocytomas associated with MEN2 and VHL disease have low rates of malignancy, though extra-adrenal tumors can be seen in VHL disease. Patients with MEN2, VHL disease, and SDHB/SDHD mutations also have an increased risk for the development of bilateral pheochromocytomas, which can be synchronous or metachronous. Therefore, the preoperative identification of hereditary syndromes in patients with pheochromocytomas can be useful in surgical planning,[13] as an open approach may be preferred in patients with higher risk of malignancy, and cortical sparing techniques may be considered in patients with bilateral tumors.

TECHNIQUE FOR OPEN ADRENALECTOMY

Operative Approach

Given the location of the adrenal glands in the retroperitoneum, various approaches to an open adrenalectomy are feasible, including anterior, flank, or posterior approaches. Patient positioning will vary accordingly and may include supine, lateral decubitus, or prone positioning. In the supine position, exposure may be facilitated by elevating the ipsilateral flank with a bump. Flexing the table at the level of the iliac crest can also improve exposure in lateral decubitus positions. It is important to provide adequate padding and support to prevent nerve injury and postoperative discomfort.

For an anterior approach, the peritoneum can be entered through a midline incision, subcostal incision (unilateral and bilateral/chevron), or modified variations, such as a modified Makuuchi incision, or a thoracoabdominal approach (Figure 48–1). A modified Makuuchi approach facilitates exposure for potential concomitant organ resection. A thoracoabdominal approach, which extends from the abdomen up into the ninth intercostal space, may be utilized in cases with malignant involvement of the diaphragm in which both the abdominal and thoracic cavities are affected. Posterior approaches to open adrenalectomy, although a viable option, are less commonly utilized in the minimally invasive era where indications for open approaches, such as tumor size or invasiveness, often suggest an anterior or lateral approach.

Key Operative Steps

On entry of the abdomen, initial inspection for obvious disseminated metastases along the peritoneal and liver surfaces should be performed in cases of known or suspected malignancy. Due to differences in anatomy and the vascular supply of the left and right adrenal glands, the operative techniques for each side are varied as described in the following section.

A. Left Adrenalectomy

For left-sided adrenal tumors (Figure 48–2), the descending colon is mobilized from its lateral attachments and the splenic flexure to expose the retroperitoneum. The lesser sac may be opened broadly to expose the pancreas. Full medial mobilization of the spleen and distal pancreas from the splenorenal ligament, lateral attachments, and short gastric veins may be necessary for adequate exposure of larger adrenal masses. Once exposure is obtained, the left adrenal gland and left kidney may be visible, but often the organs are obscured by the surrounding Gerota's fat. The fascia over the fat is opened to expose the underlying adrenal gland and kidney, the latter of which may be palpable. The order of the dissection may vary according to the etiology of disease and severity of local invasion but entails full circumferential dissection of the adrenal gland, ideally including a margin of surrounding soft tissue, and control of the venous drainage of the left adrenal vein into the left renal vein. Dissection along the medial aspect of the retroperitoneum is performed to identify the left renal vein, and dissection is carried along the anterior surface toward the renal hilum. The left adrenal vein is encountered entering from superiorly and is isolated for

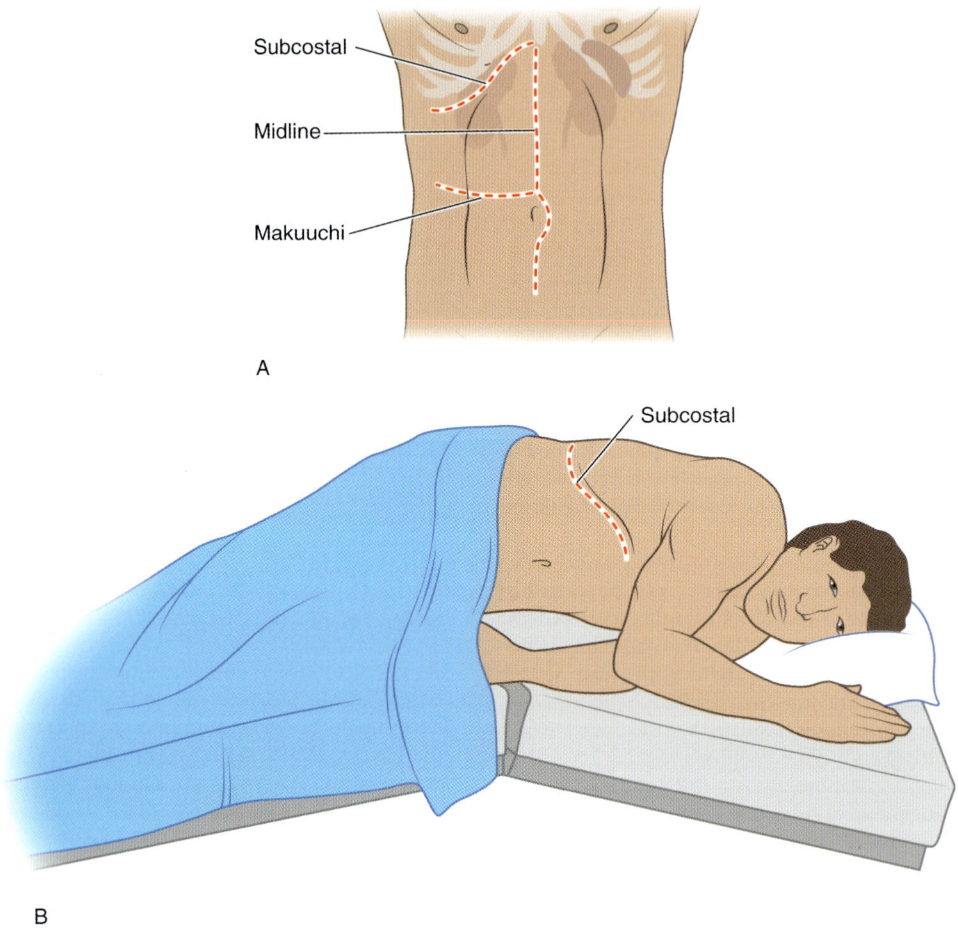

▲ **Figure 48–1.** Surgical approach and common incisions. **(A)** Supine approach with subcostal, midline, and modified Makuuchi incisions. **(B)** Lateral decubitus approach with subcostal incision. (Medical illustrations by David Aten MA, CMI. Copyright © The Board of Regents of the University of Texas System.)

future division. Early division of the adrenal vein may lead to increased tumor congestion and bleeding, and therefore, it may be delayed until the end of the dissection. The medial aspect of the left adrenal gland is dissected superiorly from the left renal vein along the aorta toward the inferior aspect of the pancreas. Small feeding vessels directly from the aorta and retroperitoneal lymphatics are controlled with energy devices, clips, or suture ligation. The superior aspect of the gland is dissected inferiorly away from the pancreas and spleen if no invasion is of concern. The splenorenal ligament is divided if not already done so to allow continued inferior dissection along the lateral aspect of the adrenal gland. The adrenal mass is rotated medially out of the retroperitoneum in the process. Posterior attachments are ligated or controlled with an energy device for hemostasis and sealing of lymphatics. Gerota's fascia and perinephric fat is dissected off the superior aspect of the kidney to complete near-circumferential dissection. At this time, the left adrenal vein may be ligated if not already performed, and dissection distally along the superior aspect of the left renal vein facilitates full mobilization of the left kidney away from the adrenal mass. Any remaining posterior retroperitoneal attachments are divided to complete the circumferential resection.

B. Right Adrenalectomy

Much of the dissection is similar for right-sided masses (Figure 48–3). The right colon and hepatic flexure are mobilized medially to expose the retroperitoneum. The falciform and right triangular ligaments may be divided to facilitate superior and medial retraction of the right lobe of the liver. The duodenum and pancreatic head are kocherized to

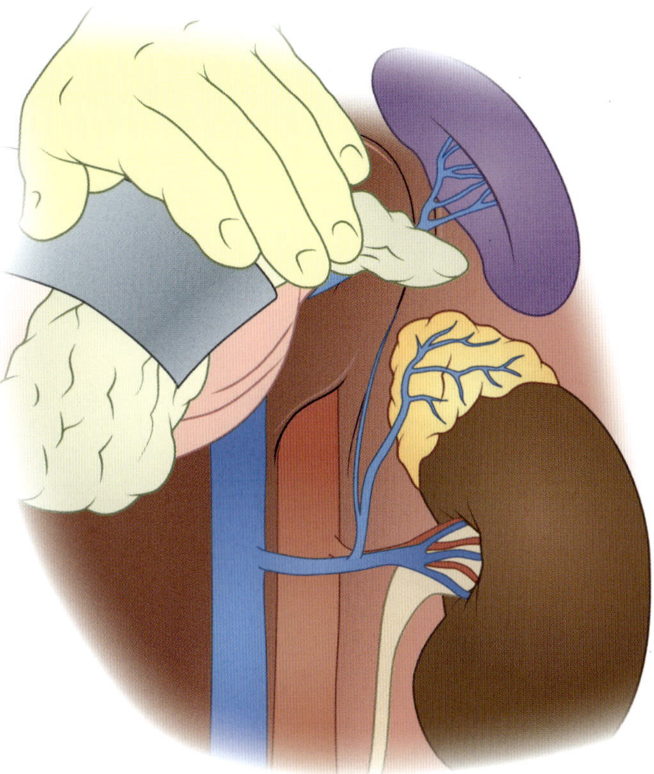

▲ **Figure 48–2.** Mobilization of the left adrenal gland. The left adrenal gland is bordered by the pancreas, spleen, left kidney, renal vessels, and the aorta. (Medical illustration by David Aten MA, CMI. Copyright © The Board of Regents of the University of Texas System.)

facilitate exposure of the inferior vena cava (IVC) and right renal vein. Small veins from the caudate lobe of the liver may be ligated to facilitate further elevation of the liver and exposure of the IVC. The right adrenal gland is separated from the right kidney in similar fashion to the left but without concern of a dominant adrenal vein draining into the right renal vein. The superior aspect of the right gland is dissected away from the inferior liver capsule. Medial dissection of the gland typically occurs from inferior to superior along the IVC. The right adrenal vein is identified as draining directly into the IVC at the superomedial aspect of the gland and is ligated and divided according to length of the vein and surgeon preference. Posterior dissection to complete circumferential mobilization of the gland is carried out in a similar fashion to the left.

COMPLICATIONS

Open adrenal surgery is typically performed with low morbidity and complications according to surgeon experience, with increased experience leading to improved outcomes.[14] Nevertheless, the location of the gland, tumor functionality, or invasiveness of malignancy may lead to advanced resections and associated complications.

Injury to Surrounding Organs

During a left adrenalectomy, care must be taken to avoid injury to the spleen from excessive traction during mobilization. Damage to the pancreatic tail can lead to postoperative pancreatic leak. The transverse and descending colon are also at risk of direct injury or devascularization during mobilization of the splenic flexure. On the right side, the hepatic flexure of the colon and the duodenum may be injured. The liver may also be injured directly or from excessive traction during a right adrenalectomy. In both left and right adrenalectomies, injury to the upper pole of the kidney may occur. Depending on the approach and sometimes due to direct invasion of the tumor, repair of the diaphragm may also be required intraoperatively. An occult diaphragm injury or disrupted repair can present as a pleural effusion or respiratory compromise postoperatively.

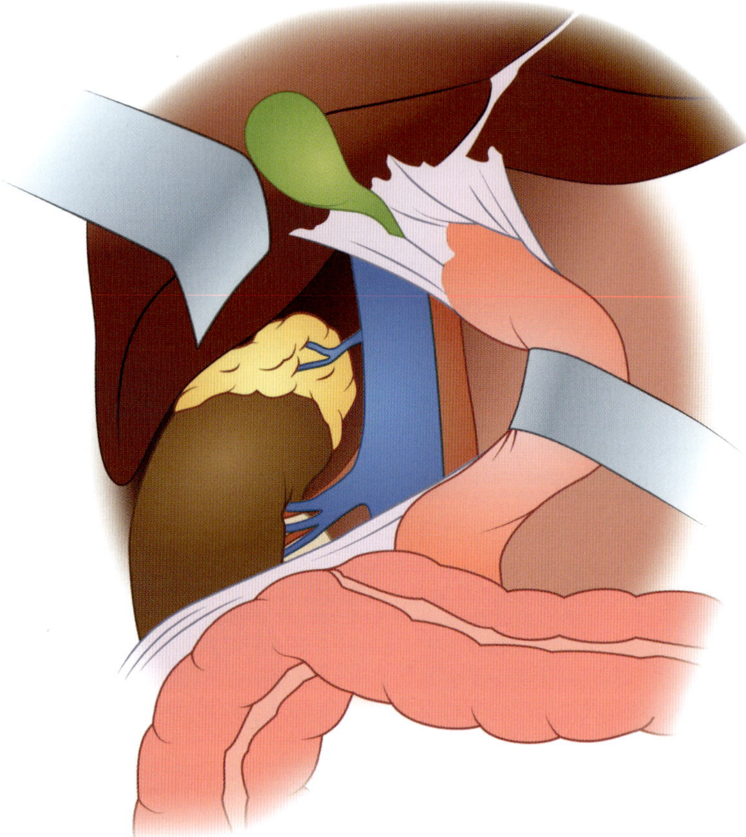

▲ **Figure 48–3.** Mobilization of the right adrenal gland. The right adrenal gland is bordered by the liver, IVC, right kidney, and renal vessels. (Medical illustration by David Aten MA, CMI. Copyright © The Board of Regents of the University of Texas System.)

Vascular Injury

Multiple vascular structures reside in the field of dissection during open adrenalectomies and can result in significant bleeding. In some patients, superior pole renal arteries may be encountered. Larger tumors may approach and even involve the renal hilum and main renal vasculature, putting them at risk during dissection and potentially requiring *en bloc* nephrectomy. Additionally, the hepatic veins are at risk during mobilization of the liver. Excessive traction on the right adrenal vein should also be avoided as it can result in avulsion from the IVC.

Lymphatic Injury

Damage to lymphatic vessels is a potential complication of retroperitoneal surgery and can result in a chyle leak. In general, most postoperative chyle leaks can be managed conservatively with drainage and a low fat with high-protein diet or total parenteral nutrition.[15] On rare occasions, lymphangiography or surgical intervention may be required.[16]

Hemodynamic Variability

Despite adequate preoperative pharmacological blockade, patients undergoing open surgery for pheochromocytoma may still experience some lability in hemodynamics during the intraoperative and immediate postoperative period. Effective communication between the surgical and anesthesia teams is crucial to allow for anticipation of hemodynamic changes during key steps of the operation.

Adrenal Insufficiency

Patients with hyperfunctioning tumors, particularly those with Cushing syndrome, are at higher risk of adrenal insufficiency and hypotension as a result of contralateral gland suppression and the abrupt decrease in corticosteroids after adrenalectomy.[17] At-risk patients typically necessitate supplemental corticosteroids perioperatively, with a gradual taper performed after surgery.

Recurrence

Rates of recurrence after adrenalectomy depend on primary tumor type. Recurrence of ACC after resection is relatively common.[18] Most recurrences after adrenalectomy for ACC occur early within the first few years after surgery, though they can also occur long after treatment.[18,19] The prognosis of patients with recurrent disease is generally poor. Given that chemotherapy and radiation typically have limited efficacy in treating ACC, surgical resection, if feasible and in appropriately selected patients, is the only potentially curative option.[20]

Recurrence after curative resection of pheochromocytoma is possible, even in cases of benign disease. For patients with sporadic pheochromocytoma, a recent study found the rate of recurrence to be around 3%, with a weighted mean time to recurrence of 49 months.[21] Not surprisingly, rates of recurrence or the development of new tumors is increased in patients with hereditary pheochromocytoma.[22] Another recent study noted that predictors of recurrence of pheochromocytomas and paragangliomas included young age, family history of chromaffin tissue neoplasms, mutations in susceptibility genes, larger tumors, and higher risk behavior as measured using the Pheochromocytoma of the Adrenal Gland Scaled Score (PASS).[23] Lifelong follow-up is generally recommended for patients with pheochromocytomas due to the persistent risk of recurrence.

Recurrence of other benign functional tumors, such as aldosteronomas, is rare following either minimally invasive or open adrenalectomy, especially in the absence of intraoperative tumor rupture.

REFERENCES

1. Vanbrabant T, Fassnacht M, Assie G, Dekkers OM. Influence of hormonal functional status on survival in adrenocortical carcinoma: systematic review and meta-analysis. *Eur J Endocrinol.* 2018;179(6):429-436.
2. Albano DA-O, Agnello F, Midiri F, et al. Imaging features of adrenal masses. *Insights Imaging.* 2019;10(1):1.
3. Chen Y, Scholten A, Chomsky-Higgins K, et al. Risk factors associated with perioperative complications and prolonged length of stay after laparoscopic adrenalectomy. *JAMA Surg.* 2018;153(11):1036-1041.
4. Fassnacht M, Dekkers OM, Else T, et al. European Society of Endocrinology Clinical Practice Guidelines on the management of adrenocortical carcinoma in adults, in collaboration with the European Network for the Study of Adrenal Tumors. *Eur J Endocrinol.* 2018;179(4):G1-G46.
5. Delozier OM, Stiles ZE, Deschner BW, et al. Implications of conversion during attempted minimally invasive adrenalectomy for adrenocortical carcinoma. *Annals Surg Oncol.* 2021;28(1):492-501.
6. Huynh KT, Lee DY, Lau BJ, Flaherty DC, Lee J, Goldfarb M. Impact of laparoscopic adrenalectomy on overall survival in patients with nonmetastatic adrenocortical carcinoma. *J Am Coll Surg.* 2016;223(3):485-492.
7. Margonis GA, Kim Y, Prescott JD, et al. Adrenocortical carcinoma: impact of surgical margin status on long-term outcomes. *Annals Surg Oncol.* 2016;23(1):134-141.
8. Deschner BW, Stiles ZE, DeLozier OM, et al. Critical analysis of lymph node examination in patients undergoing curative-intent resection for adrenocortical carcinoma. *J Surg Oncol.* 2020;122(6):1152-1162.
9. Gerry JM, Tran TB, Postlewait LM, et al. Lymphadenectomy for adrenocortical carcinoma: is there a therapeutic benefit? *Annals of Surg Oncol.* 2016;23(Suppl 5):708-713.
10. Neumann HPH, Tsoy U, Bancos I, et al. Comparison of pheochromocytoma-specific morbidity and mortality among adults with bilateral pheochromocytomas undergoing total adrenalectomy vs cortical-sparing adrenalectomy. *JAMA Netw Open.* 2019;2(8):e198898.
11. Jochmanova I, Wolf KI, King KS, et al. SDHB-related pheochromocytoma and paraganglioma penetrance and genotype-phenotype correlations. *J Cancer Res Clin Oncol.* 2017;143(8):1421-1435.
12. Crona J, Lamarca A, Ghosal S, Welin S, Skogseid B, Pacak K. Genotype-phenotype correlations in pheochromocytoma and paraganglioma: a systematic review and individual patient meta-analysis. *Endocr Relat Cancer.* 2019;26(5):539-550.
13. Rossitti HM, Söderkvist P, Gimm OA-OX. Extent of surgery for phaeochromocytomas in the genomic era. *Br J Surg.* 2018;105(2):e84-e98.
14. Leong DA-O, Nyantoro M, Shedzad H, et al. Management of adrenocortical carcinoma in Western Australia: a perspective over 14 years. *ANZ J Surg.* 2021;91(1-2):62-67.
15. Lv S, Wang Q, Zhao W, et al. A review of the postoperative lymphatic leakage. *Oncotarget.* 2017;8(40):69062-69075.
16. Gao J, Jin Y, Chen W. Treatment of lymphatic leakage after retroperitoneal tumor resection by lymphangiography and embolization: a case report. *Oncol Lett.* 2020;20(4):55.
17. Prete A, Paragliola RM, Bottiglieri F, et al. Factors predicting the duration of adrenal insufficiency in patients successfully treated for Cushing disease and nonmalignant primary adrenal Cushing syndrome. *Endocrine.* 2017;55(3):969-980.
18. Amini N, Margonis GA, Kim Y, et al. Curative resection of adrenocortical carcinoma: rates and patterns of postoperative recurrence. *Annals Surg Oncol.* 2016;23(1):126-133.
19. Glenn JA, Else T, Hughes DT, et al. Longitudinal patterns of recurrence in patients with adrenocortical carcinoma. *Surgery.* 2019;165(1):186-195.
20. Tran TB, Maithel SK, Pawlik TM, et al. Clinical score predicting long-term survival after repeat resection for recurrent adrenocortical carcinoma. *J Am Coll Surg.* 2016;223(6):794-803.
21. Holscher I, van den Berg TJ, Dreijerink KMA, Engelsman AF, Nieveen van Dijkum EJM. Recurrence rate of sporadic pheochromocytomas after curative adrenalectomy: a systematic review and meta-analysis. *J Clin Endocrinol Metab.* 2021;106(2):588-597.
22. Amar L, Lussey-Lepoutre C, Lenders JW, Djadi-Prat J, Plouin PF, Steichen O. Management of Endocrine Disease: recurrence or new tumors after complete resection of pheochromocytomas and paragangliomas: a systematic review and meta-analysis. *Eur J Endocrinol.* 2016;175(4):R135-R145.
23. Parasiliti-Caprino M, Lucatello B, Lopez C, et al. Predictors of recurrence of pheochromocytoma and paraganglioma: a multicenter study in Piedmont, Italy. *Hypertens Res.* 2020;43(6):500-510.

SUGGESTED READINGS

Dickson PV, Kim L, Yen TWF, et al. Evaluation, staging, and surgical management for adrenocortical carcinoma: an update from the SSO endocrine and head and neck disease site working group. *Ann Surg Oncol*. 2018;25(12):3460-3468.

Mihai R. Open adrenalectomy. *Gland Surg*. 2019;8(Suppl 1):S28-S35.

Patel D. Surgical approach to patients with pheochromocytoma. *Gland Surg*. 2020;9(1):32-42.

Patel D, Phay JE, Yen TWF, et al. Update on pheochromocytoma and paraganglioma from the SSO endocrine and head and neck disease site working group, Part 2 of 2: perioperative management and outcomes of pheochromocytoma and paraganglioma. *Ann Surg Oncol*. 2020;27(5):1338-1347.

Ruffolo LI, Nessen MF, Probst CP, et al. Open adrenalectomy through a makuuchi incision: a single institution's experience. *Surgery*. 2018;164(6):1372-1376.

Taffurelli G, Ricci C, Casadei R, Selva S, Minni F. Open adrenalectomy in the era of laparoscopic surgery: a review. *Updates Surg*. 2017;69(2):135-143.

Zeiger MA, Thompson GB, Duh QY, et al. American Association of Clinical Endocrinologists and American Association of Endocrine Surgeons Medical Guidelines for the management of adrenal incidentalomas: executive summary of recommendations. *Endocr Pract*. 2009;15(5):450-453.

Adrenalectomy: Transabdominal Laparoscopic Approach

49

Thomas Szabo Yamashita, MD
Vivian E. Strong, MD
Travis J. McKenzie, MD

INTRODUCTION

The adrenal glands are one of the end organs in the hypothalamic-pituitary-adrenal axis (HPAA), and as such are responsible for the production of multiple hormones. The adrenal glands produce various steroid and amine hormones. The cortex of the adrenal produces cortisol, aldosterone, and sex hormones (as well as multiple precursors derived from cholesterol). The adrenal medulla produces catecholamines from the precursor, tyrosine. The adrenal glands are a key component for endocrine homeostasis with intricate biochemical feedback systems.[1]

Widespread use of modern imaging technology has resulted in the common discovery of incidental adrenal masses. In case of hormonally active disease, patients may present with a myriad of symptoms or signs depending on which hormone is being hyper-secreted with persistent hypertension, metabolic derangements, hypercortisol symptoms, and virilization being often seen from excess cortisol, aldosterone, catecholamines, and/or sex hormones, respectively.[1,2]

The transperitoneal laparoscopic adrenalectomy, frequently referred to as laparoscopic transabdominal adrenalectomy (TA), has been used as curative surgical treatment for many adrenal pathologies since its initial description by Gagner and colleagues.[3] It is performed for both diagnostic purposes in cases of indeterminate adrenal masses and therapeutic purposes for hormonally active and inactive neoplastic and hyperplastic processes. Most adrenal masses are of benign pathology, with adrenocortical carcinoma and adrenal metastasis melanoma, renal cell carcinoma, etc. being less common. Bilateral laparoscopic adrenalectomy is performed in selected cases of ACTH-dependent Cushing syndrome from a pituitary source (Cushing disease) or for ectopic production of ACTH from a nonpituitary neoplastic process.[4-6]

The minimally invasive approaches to adrenalectomy are associated with less morbidity, more rapid recovery, and shorter hospital stays. Many centers perform outpatient adrenalectomy in selected patients.[2,7]

Two minimally invasive techniques are currently widely utilized, including laparoscopic transabdominal and retroperitoneoscopic. Either approach may be performed with either conventional laparoscopic equipment or may be performed with robotic assistance with near equivalent results.[6,7] This chapter focuses on the technical aspects of laparoscopic transabdominal adrenalectomy, right and left.

LAPAROSCOPIC TRANSABDOMINAL ADRENALECTOMY—LEFT

General anesthesia is utilized. A urinary catheter and arterial line are placed selectively, depending on pathology and patient characteristics. A decompressive nasogastric tube may be placed as the fundus of the stomach lies in close proximity to the superior and medial aspects of the left adrenal gland. The patient is positioned in lateral decubitus with left side up. It is important that the chest is in approximately 90-degree decubitus position to allow gravity to pull the spleen medially once mobilized. The operating room table is flexed with the interspace of the iliac crest and costal margin being positioned at the point of flexion, thereby allowing this working space to be maximized. The patient is secured to the table at the feet, legs, and chest, with arms extended. A 12-mm optical trocar or Veress needle is utilized to enter the abdominal cavity without pre-insufflation in the left periumbilical space. Once atraumatic entrance into abdominal cavity is assured, a 12 mm sub-xyphoid trocar is placed for the surgeon's left hand. Another 12 mm or 5 mm trocar is placed at left subcostal region near the anterior axillary line for the surgeon's right hand. An assistant 5 mm trocar may be placed near the midaxillary line as needed based on tumor and patient characteristics.

The descending colon is mobilized along the White Line of Toldt and the left mesocolon is released from Gerota's

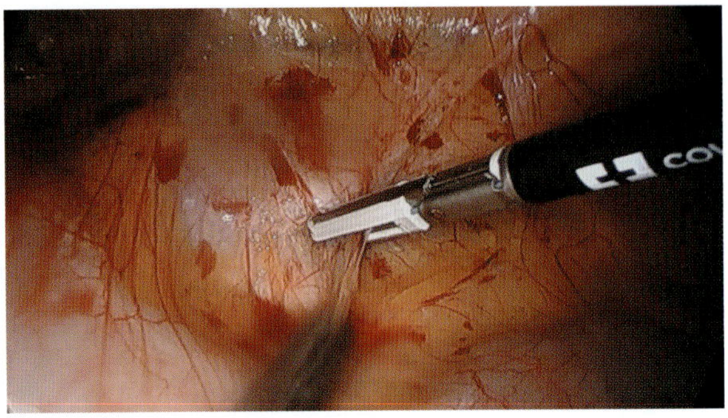

▲ **Figure 49–1.** Mobilization of left colon: left hand is retracting the mesocolon, so the LigaSure can be used to open the White Line of Toldt and mobilize the left colon medial and caudally.

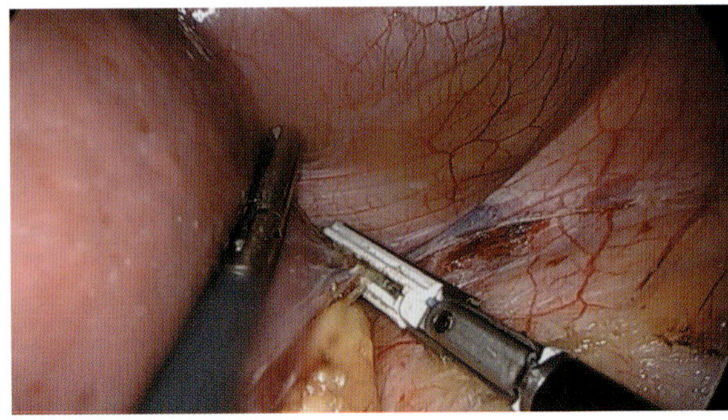

▲ **Figure 49–3.** Mobilization of spleen: left hand gently retracting the spleen medially, allowing the right hand to use the LigaSure to take the splenic attachments. Decubitus positioning allows gravity to assist with rotation of spleen.

fascia. It is a common mistake for trainees to begin mobilization too high, which puts the plane of dissection behind the left kidney, as seen in Figures 49–1 and 49–2. Mobilization of the mesocolon from Gerota's fascia can be performed by gently pulling the mesocolon medially with an atraumatic left-hand grasper and the right hand bluntly dissecting in the avascular plane between the mesocolon and left kidney. This dissection should begin near the inferior pole of the left kidney and proceed proximally along the mesocolon. Routine mobilization of the splenic flexure is not necessary, and usually necessary only for large adrenal masses.

This dissection plane is continued superiorly toward the inferior pole of the spleen, which should be easily visualized. Except for very large or low-lying adrenal masses, it is usually unnecessary to mobilize the transverse colon. Once the descending colon and splenic flexure are released, the surgeon retracts the spleen with a left-handed grasper, such as a bowel grasper or suction. The spleen and perisplenic adhesions are not grasped as the capsule of the spleen can easily be torn with focal traction. The lateral aspect of a closed grasper serves as an atraumatic retractor. The spleen is fully released from its attachments. Near the superior pole of the spleen, care is taken not to thermally injure the fundus of the stomach (Figure 49–3).

As this plane is developed, the kidney and adrenal within Gerota's fascia will be generally identifiable. The posterior aspect of the pancreatic tail will be visible as it is released and rotated medially. Care is taken to identify and avoid injury to the splenic artery and vein in this location (Figure 49–4).

The cleft created by this dissection is deepened and can be likened to the opening of a book. The left page of the book is the colon, mesocolon, spleen, and pancreas tail. The right page of the book is the adrenal and kidney within Gerota's. There are no major vessels crossing from one page to the other. Dissection should proceed in an avascular plane. It can be helpful to identify the inferior phrenic vessels on the

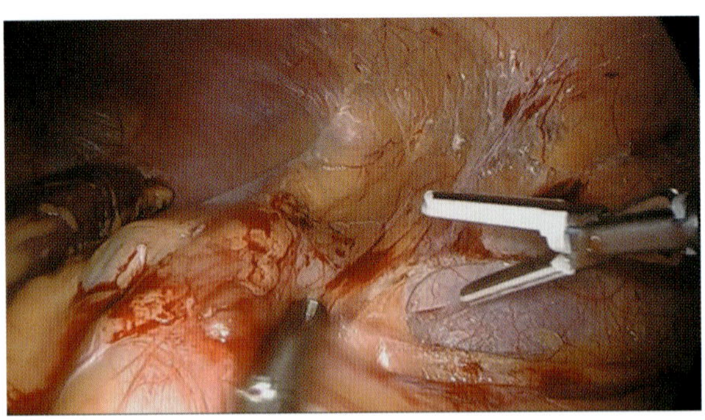

▲ **Figure 49–2.** Exposure of Gerota's fascia: the right-hand grasper is retracting the mesocolon on top of Gerota's fascia, exposing it to be divided with the LigaSure.

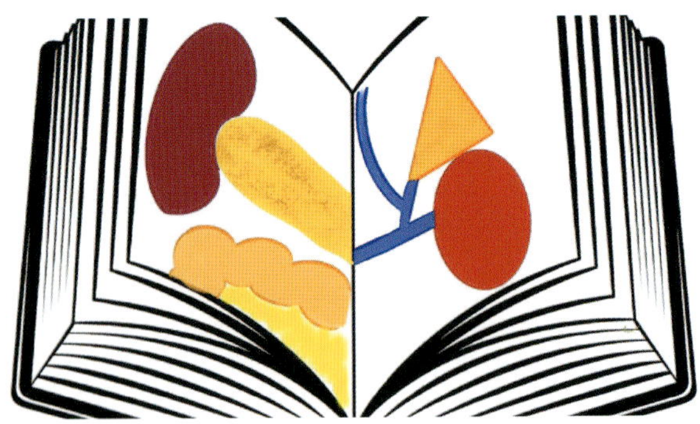

▲ **Figure 49–4.** "Open book" anatomy, with spleen, pancreas and splenic flexure mobilized medially, exposing the left adrenal and kidney.

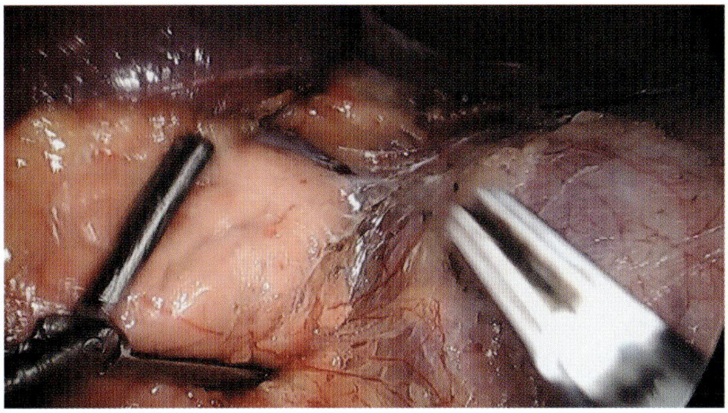

▲ **Figure 49–5.** Mobilization of pancreas: left hand rotating pancreas medially while right hand carries down the dissection.

diaphragm as the phrenic vein will most commonly drain along the cleft created while opening the cleft between pancreas and adrenal prior to confluencing with the adrenal vein (Figure 49–5). They will help guide dissection when working to identify the adrenal vein. Once at this stage, Gerota's Fascia is opened with L-hook cautery and the adrenal gland and left renal vein are visually identified. The adrenal gland can be mobilized away from the superior pole of kidney and off the psoas muscle posteriorly and diaphragm superiorly. This mobilization of the adrenal proceeds along a mostly avascular plane and will facilitate manipulation of the adrenal for division of the adrenal artery branches and adrenal vein (Figure 49–6).

Once Gerota's fascia is fully opened and the left adrenal has been mobilized off the kidney and psoas muscle, the adrenal venous anatomy is delineated. This can be accomplished by dissecting the superior margin of the left renal vein. The adrenal vein will be found confluencing with the superior margin of the left renal vein at the inferior-medial margin of the left adrenal. The left adrenal vein is generally 1 to 3 cm in length and frequently confluences with the inferior phrenic vein prior to confluencing with the left renal vein. Once the adrenal vein is fully viewed, it can be circumferentially dissected with a Maryland or right-angle dissector. The left adrenal vein, once exposed, is clipped with one or two 5 mm titanium clips proximal to the confluence with the phrenic vein. The phrenic vein can be maintained or sacrificed depending on length of the adrenal vein prior to confluence with the phrenic vein. Once clips are in place and secure, the adrenal vein is divided with a clip or the LigaSure device on the adrenal side, leaving the clips in situ. Arterial branches are divided with LigaSure. Arterial branches come from three inflow sources; aorta, inferior phrenic artery, and renal artery. However, the actual arterial branches supplying the adrenal at the capsular border are numerous and generally quite small and not easily visible in many cases. They may be enlarged with large, more complex pathology. The adrenal can be retracted with an open grasper to help expose the arterial branches. However, it is never grasped as the capsule and cortex are fragile and can bleed profusely with injury. As the specimen is further dissected, the retroperitoneal muscles become visible. On inferior dissection of the adrenal it is important to not go lower than the clipped adrenal vein, to protect the renal vein. Intraoperatively ultrasound may be utilized to aid in identification of key structures. Ideally, the left renal vein will be kept in view during this portion of dissection. When dividing medial arterial branches off the aorta and phrenic artery, it is important to be aware that the aorta and the origin of the celiac and SMA are frequently only a few millimeters away from the plane of dissection, which should proceed on the right medial edge of the adrenal. There are no vessels going from the retroperitoneum to the adrenal, so it can be safely taken in combined blunt and with thermal instrument from its posterior margin. The adrenal parenchyma has a different hue of orange/yellow than the retroperitoneal fat. Haptic feedback also helps to delineate the adrenal gland from fat, as it feels denser compared to fat when manipulated with laparoscopic instruments. The specimen can then be removed in a retrieval bag and removed through the most lateral 12 mm trocar. The trocar site may need to be dilated with a dilator in case of larger specimens, in which case its site should be closed with a suture-passer utilizing absorbable suture. If the fascia and abdominal wall muscle are incised to facilitate removal, the fascia is closed in layers with absorbable suture. The adrenal bed is checked for hemostasis, the abdomen is desufflated and skin can be closed. Topical hemostatic agents may be utilized selectively.

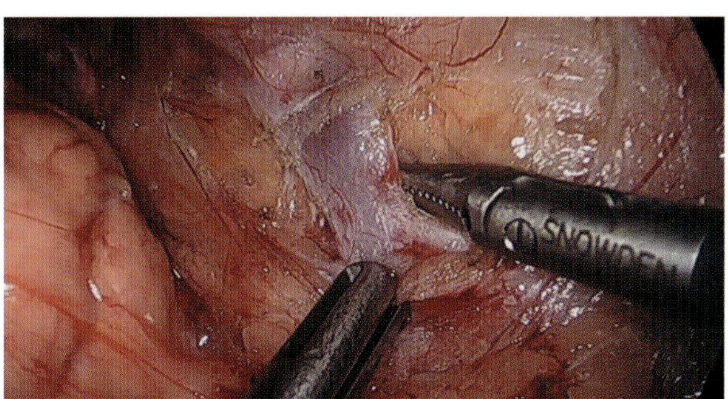

▲ **Figure 49–6.** Dissection of left adrenal vein.

ANTERIOR TRANSPERITONEAL LAPAROSCOPIC ADRENALECTOMY—RIGHT

The patient is positioned in right lateral decubitus with arms out and bed positioned as described above. In the midclavicular line approximately 10 cm below the right costal margin, a 12 mm optical trocar or a Veress needle is placed

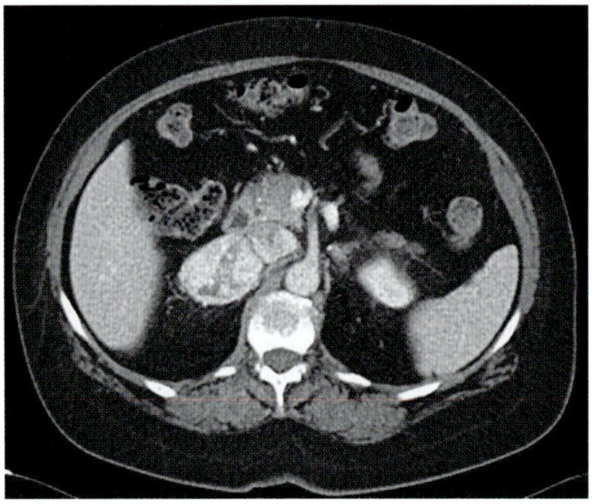

▲ **Figure 49–7.** Axial CT scan with right pheochromocytoma.

without pre-insufflation. A 12 mm trocar is placed in the sub-xiphoid region to the right of the falciform ligament, through which the liver retractor will be used. It is important to place this trocar no further cephalad than the caudal-most portion of segment 4 of the liver. A 5 mm port is placed most laterally in the subcostal region for the surgeon's left hand near the retroperitoneal reflection of the right colon. Finally, a trocar is placed in the right subcostal region near the anterior axillary line.

Through the sub-xiphoid 12 mm trocar, a liver retractor is placed, and the liver is retracted cephalad by exposing the retroperitoneal reflection of the right lobe of the liver and the right triangular ligament. The surgeon can visually identify the hepatic flexure of the colon, duodenum, right kidney, and the subhepatic inferior vena cava (Figures 49–7 and 49–8).

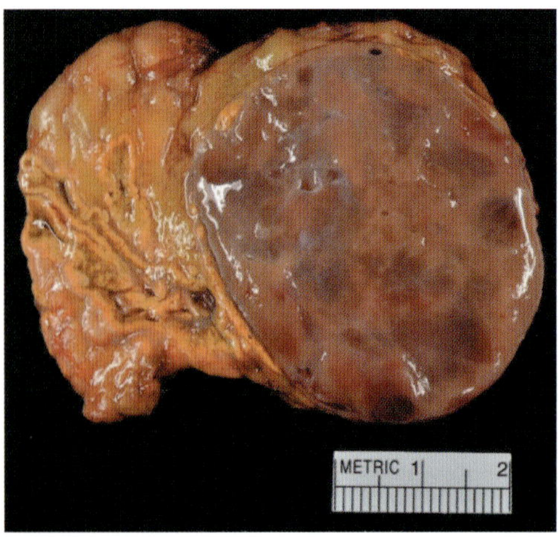

▲ **Figure 49–8.** Specimen of right adrenalectomy for pheochromocytoma.

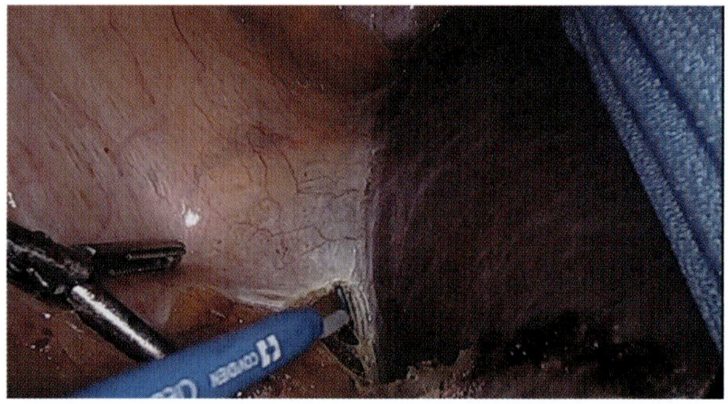

▲ **Figure 49–9.** Mobilization of right liver.

The retroperitoneal attachments to right lobe of liver are divided with electrocautery, protecting the bare area of liver and Glisson's capsule (Figure 49–9). It is important to avoid hepatic parenchyma injury when mobilizing the liver as troublesome bleeding may occur that can obscure visualization during the rest of the procedure. The dissection is carried laterally to the right triangular ligament of the liver, which is divided. The right lobe of the liver should be mobilized to slightly beyond the point where the entire cephalad border of the adrenal can be identified. At this point, the adrenal arterial branches arising off the phrenic artery can be divided with LigaSure or electrocautery.

The IVC should be visually identified and exposed medial to the adrenal gland. When the anterior aspect of the IVC is exposed, it can be readily identified and is an excellent landmark to guide dissection (Figure 49–10). Rather than attempting to mobilize the adrenal away from the IVC and divide the right adrenal vein, the adrenal should be mobilized off the kidney and psoas muscle and diaphragm initially.

This will provide mobility to the adrenal and facilitate later dissection away from the IVC (Figure 49–11). To accomplish this, the right kidney can be retracted caudally,

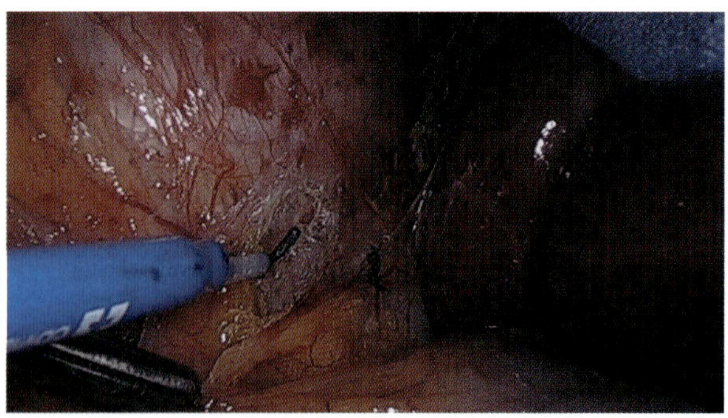

▲ **Figure 49–10.** IVC exposure.

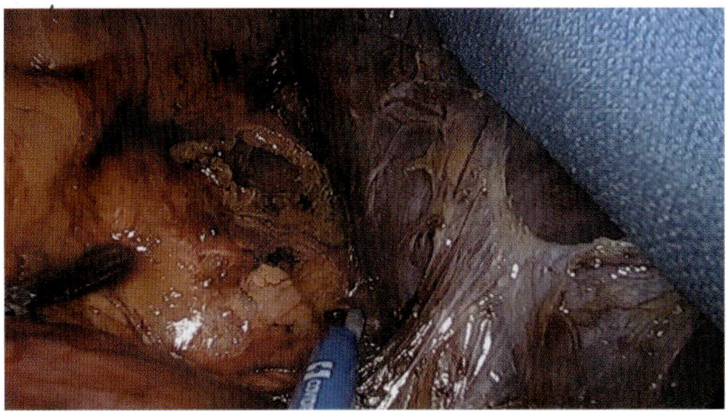

Figure 49–11. Mobilization of adrenal off IVC.

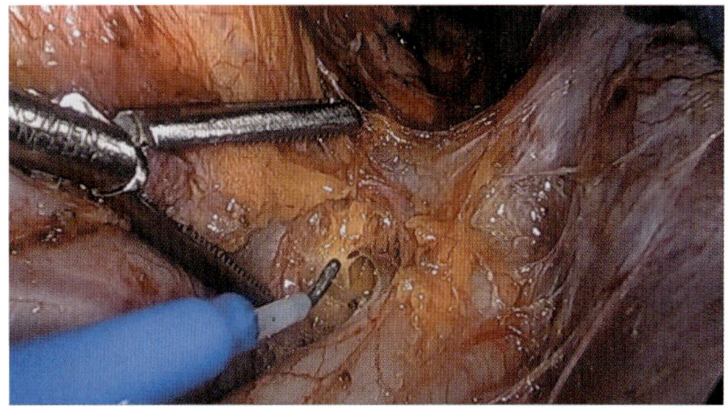

Figure 49–13. Identification and dissection of cephalad portion of adrenal gland.

and a plane is developed between the inferior aspect of the right adrenal and the superior pole of the kidney. This plane of dissection is carried laterally around the adrenal until the plane meets with where the superior aspect of the adrenal was previously mobilized.

Once initial superior, inferior, lateral, and posterior mobilization is complete, the adrenal can easily be pushed away from the IVC facilitating dissection between the adrenal and IVC. As this plane is deepened, arterial branches from the aorta running posterior to the IVC will be encountered and are divided, initially starting low on the medial border of the adrenal (Figure 49–12).

As the surgeon progresses up the medial border, the short adrenal vein will most frequently be identified confluencing with the posterolateral aspect of the IVC near the cephalad portion of the adrenal gland (Figure 49–13).

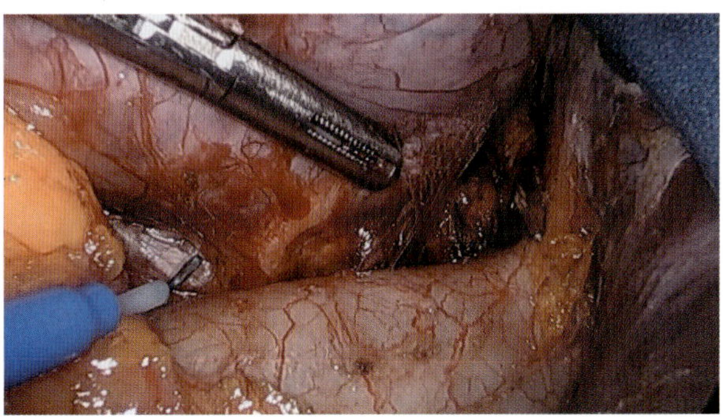

Figure 49–12. Dissection of adrenal arterial branches arising from the aorta.

The adrenal is retracted laterally and slightly inferiorly providing slight tension to the adrenal vein, which is then dissected circumferentially. A single or double 5 mm clip is placed across the right adrenal vein at the confluence with the IVC and the vein is then divided with LigaSure on the specimen side. Finally, any remaining retroperitoneal attachments are divided to fully free the adrenal. The adrenal is placed in a specimen retrieval bag and removed through the lateral-most 12 mm trocar. If dilated or if the fascia is incised to assist with removal, the fascia is closed in layers with absorbable suture.

REFERENCES

1. Nieman LK. Recent updates on the diagnosis and management of Cushing's syndrome. *Endocrinol Metab*. 2018;33(2):139-146.
2. Porterfield JR, Thompson GB, Young WF Jr, et al. Surgery for Cushing's syndrome: an historical review and recent ten-year experience. *World J Surg*. 2008;32(5):659-677.
3. Gagner M, Lacroix A, Bolte E. Laparoscopic adrenalectomy in Cushing's syndrome and pheochromocytoma. *N Engl J Med*. 1992;327(14):1033.
4. Szabo Yamashita T, Sada A, et al. Bilateral adrenalectomy: differences between cushing disease and ectopic ACTH-producing tumors. *Ann Surg Oncol*. 2020;27(10):3851-3857.
5. Szabo Yamashita T, Sada A, et al. Differences in outcomes of bilateral adrenalectomy in patients with ectopic ACTH producing tumor of known and unknown origin. *Am J Surg*. 2021;221(2):460-464.
6. Balla A, Ortenzi M, Palmieri L, et al. Laparoscopic bilateral anterior transperitoneal adrenalectomy: 24 years experience. *Surg Endosc*. 2019;33(11):3718-3724.
7. Di Dalmazi G, Reincke M. Adrenal surgery for Cushing's syndrome: an update. *Endocrinol Metab Clin North Am*. 2018;47(2):385-394.

50 Adrenalectomy: Posterior Retroperitoneoscopic Approach

Martin K. Walz, MD, PhD

INTRODUCTION

The posterior retroperitoneoscopic approach for adrenalectomy (PRA) combines the advantages of the historic posterior open approach with minimally invasive techniques.[1] As the abdominal cavity remains closed, PRA offers reduced postoperative morbidity compared to transabdominal approaches.[2,3] Due to the unusual access and exposure, PRA requires special knowledge of surgical anatomy and surgical techniques. The following chapter is based on the experience of more than 2800 posterior retroperitoneoscopic adrenalectomies.

SURGICAL ANATOMY

The adrenal glands are small retroperitoneal organs (<15 g) positioned on the upper pole of the kidney. They are behind the inferior vena cava (IVC) on the right side, meaning that the gland and/or its tumor are in front of the IVC in PRA. The main landmarks are medially the spine, laterally the peritoneum behind the right liver, and caudally the kidney. The right adrenal gland is always positioned in that triangle but might be covered by variable amounts of retroperitoneal fatty tissue (Figure 50–1). The amount of fatty tissue primarily differentiates between easy and difficult adrenalectomies, as more fatty tissue means a more challenging case. The surgical solution is the concept of *en-bloc* resection of the gland and fatty tissue, removing the whole anatomic triangle. Alternatively, limited liposuction or lipoextraction may be helpful for the identification of essential landmarks.

In addition to the posterior aspect of the IVC, other vascular structures have to be respected, principally the right renal vein that joins the IVC at an oblique angle and the right renal artery that crosses behind the IVC medially. The aorta is always covered by the parts of the crus and, therefore, is not visible in PRA. The same is true for the ureters—they always run caudally from the renal vessels and, therefore, are not in the surgical field. This is even true in large adrenal tumors, which always respect the level of the renal vessels by pushing the kidney toward the pelvis (Figure 50–2).

The perfusion of the adrenal glands is complex as small arteries feed the organs from three directions: medially, caudally, and cranially. They are typically accompanied by paired veins (Figure 50–3), except the right "main adrenal vein" that runs directly into the upper IVC. This vein shows variations in about 10% of cases—typically as a branch of a posterior hepatic vein or rarely as a double vein.[4] The complex perfusion of the adrenal gland means that function-preserving (partial) adrenalectomy is successful if at least one group of vessels can be spared. The pattern of adrenal perfusion makes the traditional pheochromocytoma tactic to cut the main vein first more questionable, as multiple veins exist. In our experience, the dissection of the adrenal arteries is essential in these cases.

On the **left side,** the gland is more anterior to the kidney. Therefore, sufficient exposure of the adrenal needs an extended mobilization of the upper pole of the left kidney. The main landmarks on the left side are medially the spine, laterally the peritoneum behind the spleen, and caudally the kidney. The left adrenal gland is always in that triangle, and—as on the right side—the amount of fatty tissue determines the difficulty of the adrenalectomy. Notably, the fatty tissue on the left usually exceeds the fat volume on the right side (Figure 50–1).

Nevertheless, ideal surgery tries an *en-bloc* removal of the embryologic layers, including the gland in the center. The left adrenal arteries show the same pattern as on the contralateral side. They rise from the renal artery and aorta. As in the view from the right side, the aorta is not visible during left adrenalectomy because of coverage by the muscle layer of the left crus. The main left adrenal vein usually enters the left renal vein opposite to the gonadal veins. Around 2 to 3 cm above the renal and adrenal veins junction, a very predictable diaphragmatic vein joins the adrenal vein, which may be

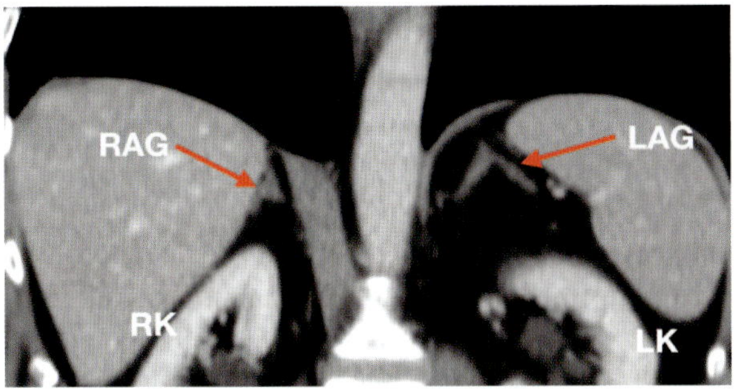

▲ **Figure 50–1.** Computed tomography of the upper abdomen. The amount of periadrenal fatty tissue defines the difficulty of adrenalectomy. LAG: left adrenal gland; LK: left kidney; RAG: right adrenal gland; RK: right kidney.

preserved in surgery if indicated. In the case of a retroaortic position of the left renal vein, the adrenal vein will not run into the renal vein but into some spinal branches.

Further important landmarks for posterior left adrenalectomy include the renal vessels, which are always caudal to adrenal tissue, adrenal tumors, and splenic vessels. Though the latter are usually covered by the anterior Gerota's fascia, they might be very close to the adrenal surface. Especially in cases of anterior adhesions, for example, in adrenal metastases, the dissection of the posterior aspect of both the splenic artery and vein might be necessary.

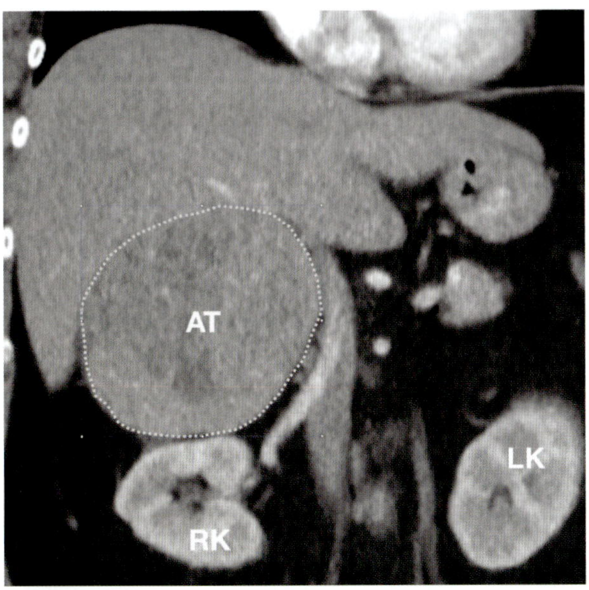

▲ **Figure 50–2.** Computed tomography of the upper abdomen. The right-sided adrenal tumor (AT: dotted line) respects the renal vessels. LK: left kidney; RK: right kidney.

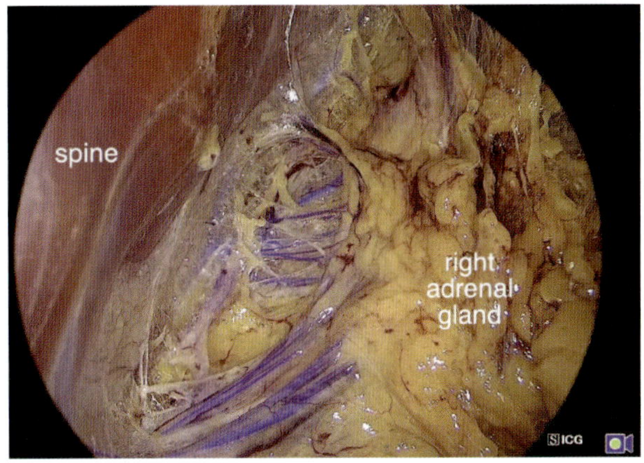

▲ **Figure 50–3.** Posterior retroperitoneoscopic adrenalectomy. View on the retrocaval adrenal vessels visualized with indocyanine green intravenously. Note the multiple pairs of arterial and venous branches (both highlighted).

SURGICAL TECHNIQUES

After introducing general anesthesia, proper prone positioning of the patient is an essential step. The spine has to be horizontal without lordosis. Therefore, hip joints and knees must be flexed (around 120 degrees) to create a sufficient distance between the last rib and the iliac crest. The patient's lateral aspect and the surgical table should be in one vertical line. Pelvic and chest pillows are necessary to allow a hanging of the abdomen. Both arms are positioned laterally-cranially to allow easy access to the peripheral lines (Figure 50–4). After prepping and draping the patient, the first skin incision (2 cm) is performed half-distance between the spine and the lateral aspect of the patient. It is usually found at the tip of the 12th rib. A channel into the retroperitoneal space is created by sharp and partly blunt vertical dissection. The lower edge of the rib should be touched and dissected free directly to the periosteum. This is essential for two reasons: firstly, the balloon port (inserted a bit later) will have a stable fixation even in patients with excess soft tissue (eg, Cushing syndrome or disease); secondly, an injury of the subcostal nerve can be avoided due to its distance to the lateral bone of around 1 to 2 cm. The wound is widened bluntly digitally by the finger that enters the retroperitoneum, trying to feel the tip of the 12th and 11th rib from inside. This finger should not create any space to preserve the anatomy. The second skin incision is placed about 8 cm lateral to the first under finger guidance. A 5-mm port is inserted in the direction of the tip of the finger, usually in the area of the most lateral part of the 11th rib. Again, a close positioning to the port on the periosteum is recommended to avoid injury to the Th11 nerve. After the finger is removed from the first incision, a 10-mm port with an inflatable balloon is inserted. The CO_2 insufflation

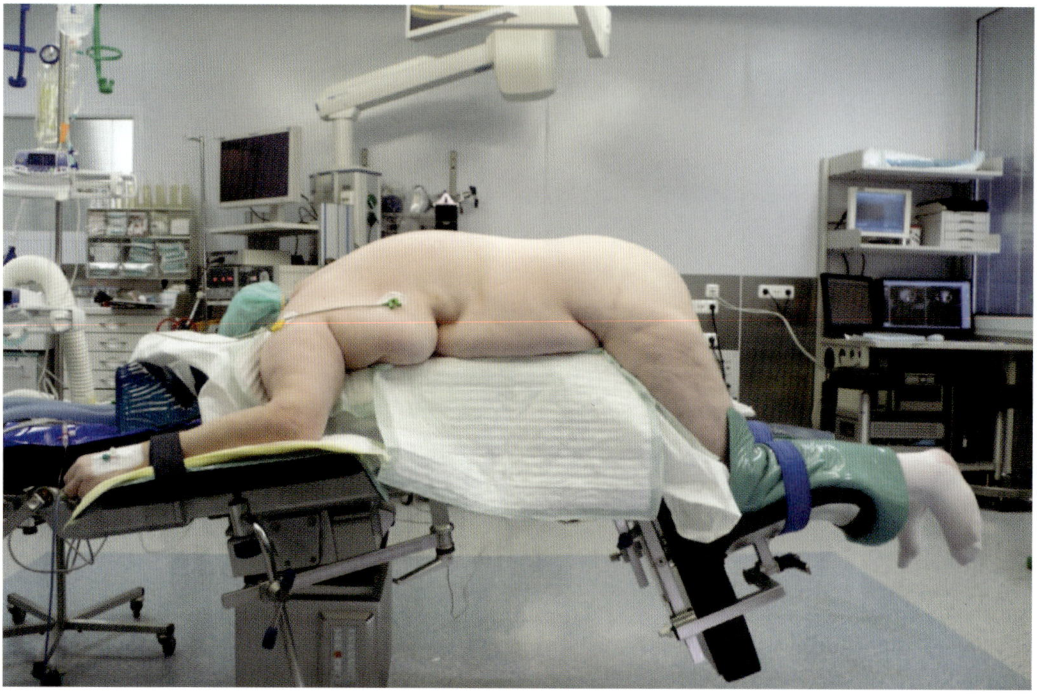

▲ **Figure 50–4.** Posterior retroperitoneoscopic adrenalectomy. Positioning of the patient. Note: The spine is horizontal, and the hip joint and knees are bent.

pressure is routinely fixed at 20 mmHg (Figure 50–5). Variations are used in children (around 15 mmHg) or obese patients (25-30 mmHg). The camera is inserted into the inflatable port and a grasper is placed in the lateral one. The first anatomic structure that comes into view is Gerota's fascia. This has to be opened with the lateral instrument by grasping and rupturing (Figure 50–6). Due to the avascularity of this layer, bleeding will not occur. A space is created by gas insufflation and pushing the fatty tissue down from the posterior abdominal wall (Figure 50–7).

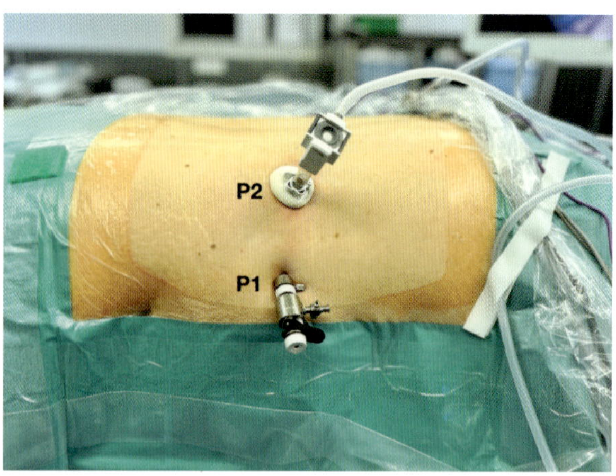

▲ **Figure 50–5.** Right-sided PRA. The initial two ports: P1 inserted under finger guidance at the tip of the 11th rib through the incision for P2.

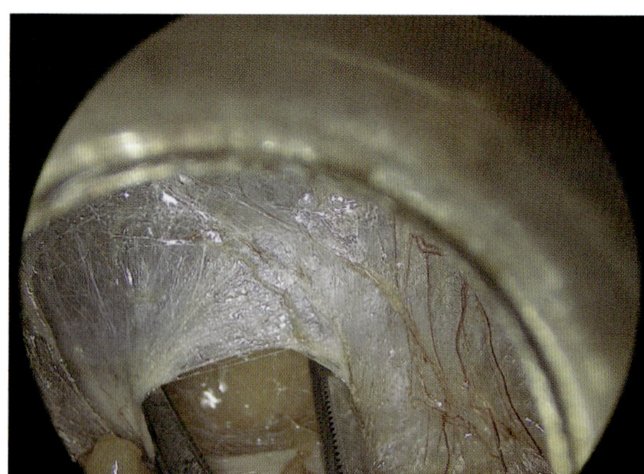

▲ **Figure 50–6.** Right-sided PRA. Opening of Gerota's fascia.

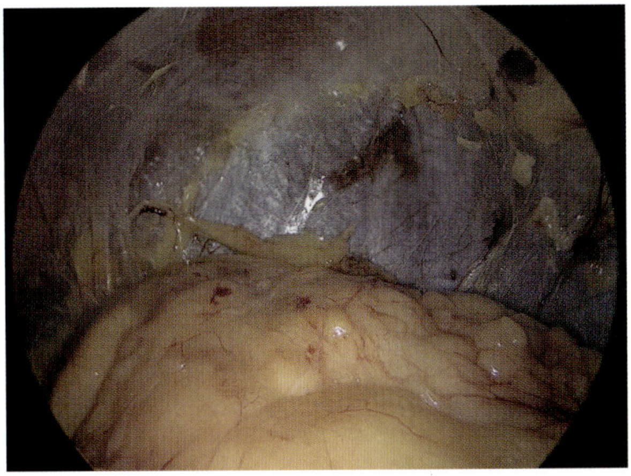

▲ **Figure 50–7.** Right-sided PRA. Creating the retroperitoneal space. All fatty tissue is pushed down (anteriorly).

On the **right** side, this space is surrounded by the spine medially, the peritoneum behind the right lobe of the liver laterally, and the upper pole of the kidney caudally. A third port is inserted under optical control 4 to 5 cm medial to the initial incision at a flat angle (30-45 degrees) and parallel to the spine. As this will be used as the optical port, its dimension depends on the optical system (5 mm or 10 mm) (Figure 50–8). Dissection starts with the mobilization of the right kidney. The upper half should be mobilized, preserving the renal capsule. This means a medial visualization of the renal vessels. Extensive mobilization is essential for a complete view of and approach to the adrenal gland.

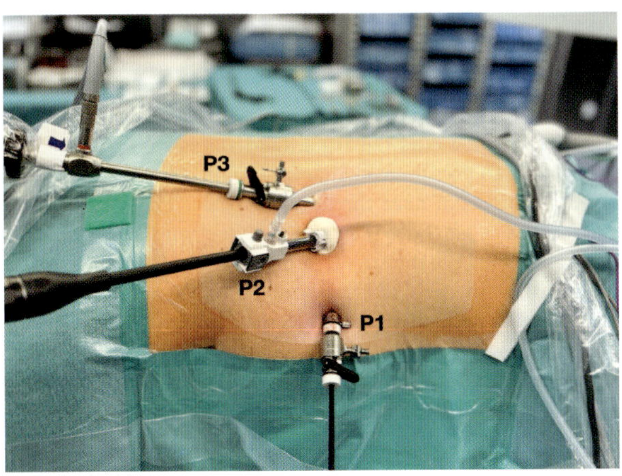

▲ **Figure 50–8.** Right-sided PRA. Three ports: P1 and P2 for surgical instruments. P3 for the camera. The latter is inserted under visual control after creating the retroperitoneal space. Note the asymmetric distance between the ports.

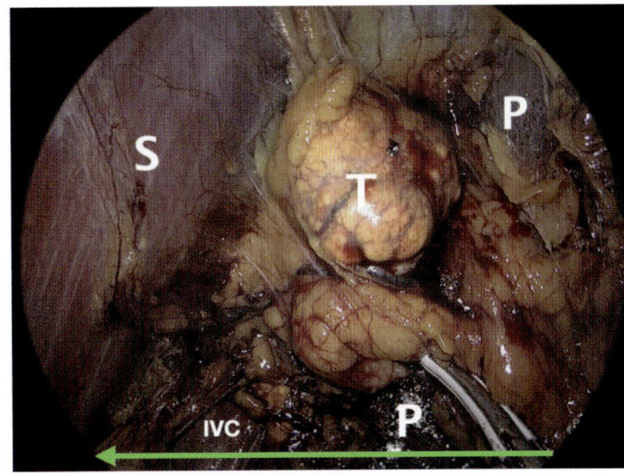

▲ **Figure 50–9.** Right-sided PRA. Horizontal dissection (⟶) between kidney (not visible) and adrenal tumor (T) from 3 to 9". Inferior vena cava (IVC), spine (S), anterior peritoneum (P).

The fatty tissue between the kidney and gland is dissected horizontally ("from 3 to 9 o'clock"), ideally on the anterior Gerota's fascia (Figure 50–9). Medially, the IVC comes into view with the insertion of the right renal vein. By performing this horizontal dissection, all vessels between the renal vessels and the adrenal gland are cut. The next step is the medial vertical transection of the vessels behind the IVC, mainly small arteries running from the aorta (Figure 50–10). As noted previously, the aorta is not visible as the diaphragm covers it. The posterior cava is completely freed. Posterior venous branches are very unusual until the short

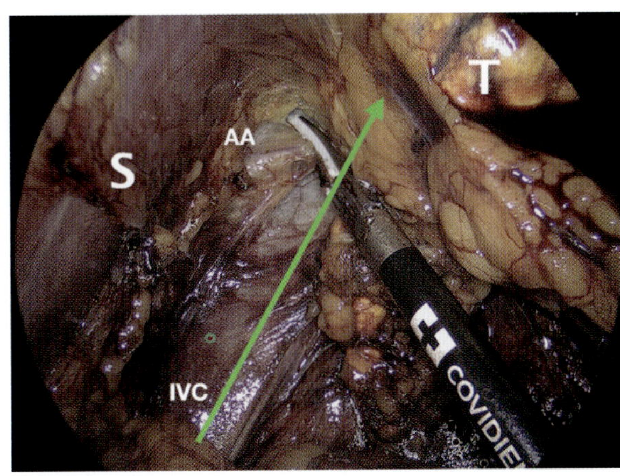

▲ **Figure 50–10.** Right-sided PRA. Vertical dissection (⟶) between the spine (S) and adrenal tumor (T). The posterior aspect of the inferior vena cava (IVC) is freed. AA: adrenal artery.

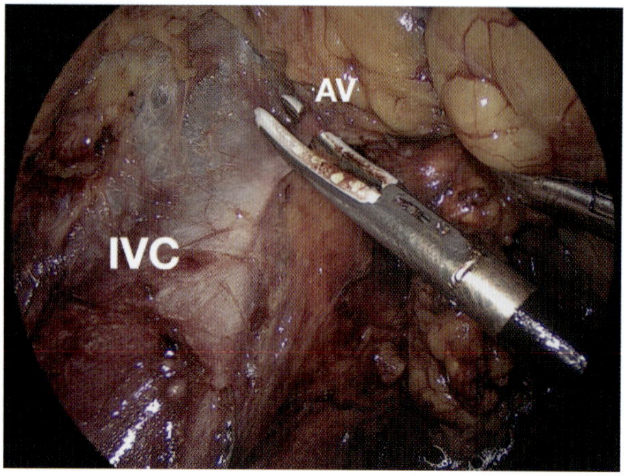

▲ **Figure 50–11.** Right-sided PRA. Dissection of the main adrenal vein (AV). IVC: inferior vena cava (posterior aspect).

main right adrenal vein comes into view. It is always running posteriorly-laterally and cranially. It is circumferentially freed and dissected (Figure 50–11) by using modern bipolar devices or ultrasound-driven devices or by using clips. I avoid clips for occluding the main adrenal veins and use bipolar instruments instead for more than the last 2000 cases. An exception is the presence of a wide adrenal vein, for example, in large pheochromocytomas. In those cases, the use of absorbable clips is safest. Following the dissection of the main adrenal vein, the adrenal gland is mobilized *en-bloc* with the surrounding fatty tissue ventrally and cranially. Finally, small cranial vessels are cut. The completely mobilized specimen is retrieved in a bag (Figure 50–12) through the initial incision. I never widen the skin incision to remove

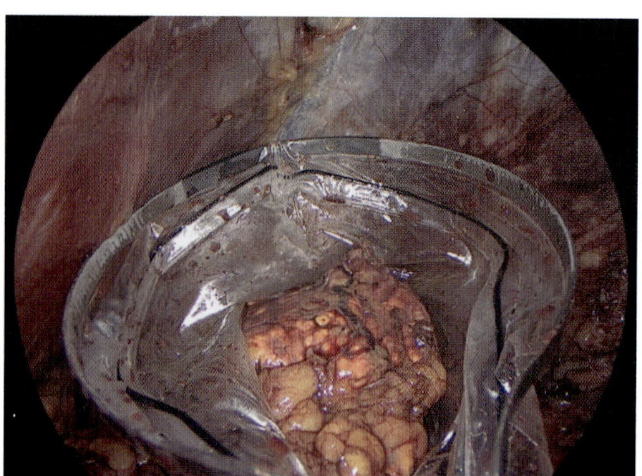

▲ **Figure 50–12.** Right-sided PRA. Adrenal tumor in a retrieval bag.

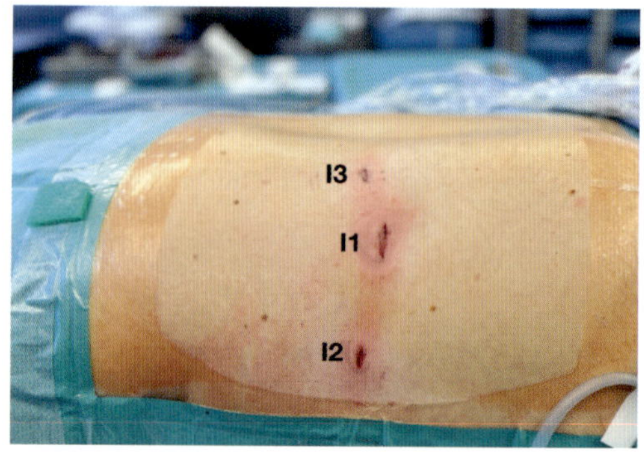

▲ **Figure 50–13.** Right-sided PRA. The final aspect is after the closure of the skin. Distance incision 1 (I1)-I2 about 8 cm, distance I1-I3 about 4 cm.

the adrenal tissue as I fragment the specimen to permit extraction through the initial port site incision. Irrigation of the retroperitoneal space with water solution is followed by the closure of the skin incisions by absorbable and intracutaneous stitches, respectively (Figure 50–13).

On the **left** side, the surgical retroperitoneal space is surrounded by the spine medially, the peritoneum behind the spleen laterally, cranially by Gerota's fascia behind the stomach and the pancreas, and caudally by the kidney. As on the right side, dissection starts on the upper pole of the kidney following the insertion of the third medial camera port (Figure 50–14). As the left adrenal gland is more ventral to the kidney, the mobilization of the upper half of the kidney must be meticulous. Opposite to the right side, the dissection of the fatty tissue starts lateral and continues to medial ("from 9 to 3 o'clock") (Figure 50–15). Medially, the renal vessels might be visualized before the main adrenal vein is identified. A diaphragmatic branch is typically found joining the adrenal vein about 2 to 3 cm from entering the renal vein (Figure 50–16). The next step is the vertical dissection along the spine, which cuts the small medial vessels that enter the gland. I try to preserve the diaphragmatic venous branch and cut the main vein near the adrenal tissue. The stump of the vein serves as a handle for further dissection in the avascular ventral plane. Finally, the cranial adhesions are dissected, and the specimen is retrieved into a bag. The further steps correspond to those on the right side. Finally, the bed of the adrenal tumor is irrigated and controlled for any bleeding before the closure of the incisions (Figure 50–17).

Surgical **modifications** concern the number of approaches (conventional vs single access), the extent of resection (total or partial), the tactic in bilateral cases (sequential or concurrent), and the extent of dissection of neighboring tissue and structures (kidney capsule, peritoneum, Gerota's fascia, renal vein, IVC). A single-access retroperitoneoscopic adrenalectomy **(SARA)** may be used in selected cases with small adrenal tumors and a small amount of periadrenal fatty tissue.[5,6]

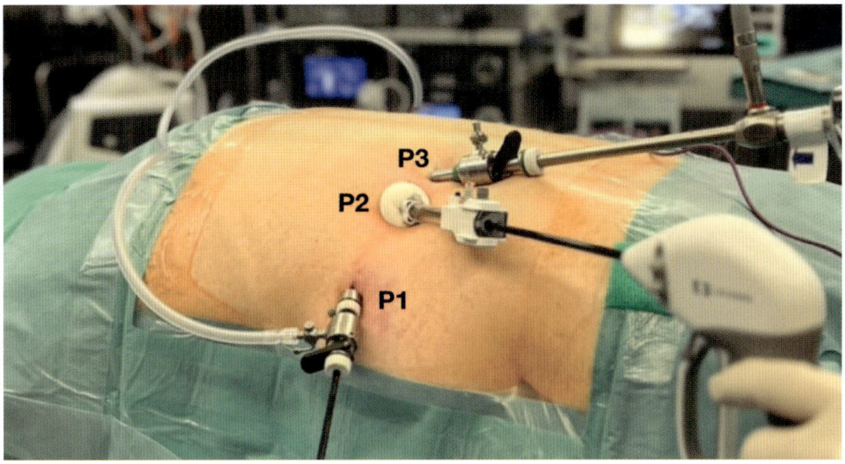

▲ **Figure 50–14.** Left-sided PRA. Three ports: P1 and P2 for surgical instruments. P3 for the camera. Mirrored to Figure 50-14. Note the asymmetric distance between the ports.

The idea is a one-hand dissection through a 5-mm port and another 5-mm port for the camera. Both ports are inserted through a 2.5-cm skin incision located at the same point as the first incision in conventional retroperitoneoscopic adrenalectomy (Figure 50–18). Our results show that one-hand adrenalectomy takes about 15 minutes longer than the conventional two-port method. **Partial adrenalectomy** is technically simple, as the adrenal parenchyma can be dissected in all directions.[7-9] Bleeding from the cutting edge can easily controlled by diathermy and is even less in cases where the main (central) vein can be preserved, as this avoids venous congestion of the remnant. Additionally, the increased CO_2 pressure in PRA is helpful. In bilateral adrenal pathologies, concurrent PRA is our method of choice (CoBRA: *Co*ncurrent *B*ilateral *R*etroperitoneoscopic *A*drenalectomy). Therefore, operating time is shortened to a minimum. Two teams and two towers for minimally invasive surgery are needed (Figure 50–19). Synchronous bilateral insufflation does not show any side effects.

In cases of adrenal tumors (especially in metastases) with potential or real **infiltration of neighboring layers** as the peritoneum (right side), Gerota's fascia (left side), or renal capsule (both sides), these structures should be transected and left on the tumor as a safety margin. On the right side, this may mean the opening of the abdominal cavity, resulting

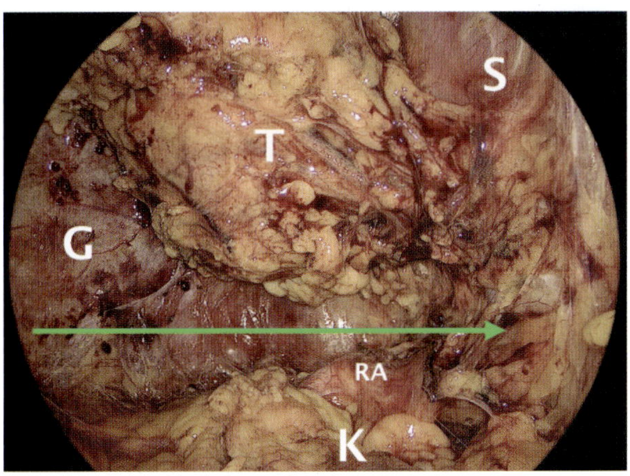

▲ **Figure 50–15.** Left-sided PRA. Horizontal dissection between kidney (K) and adrenal tumor (T). Anterior Gerota's fascia (G), spine (S), renal artery (RA).

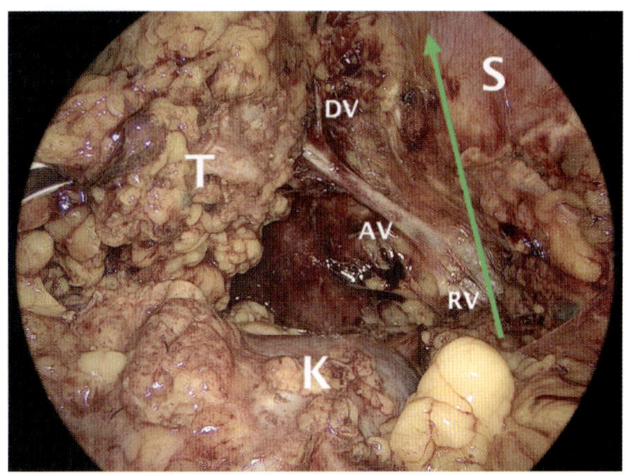

▲ **Figure 50–16.** Left-sided PRA. Vertical dissection between spine (S) and adrenal tumor (T). Main adrenal vein (AV), diaphragmatic branch (DV), kidney (K), renal vein (RV).

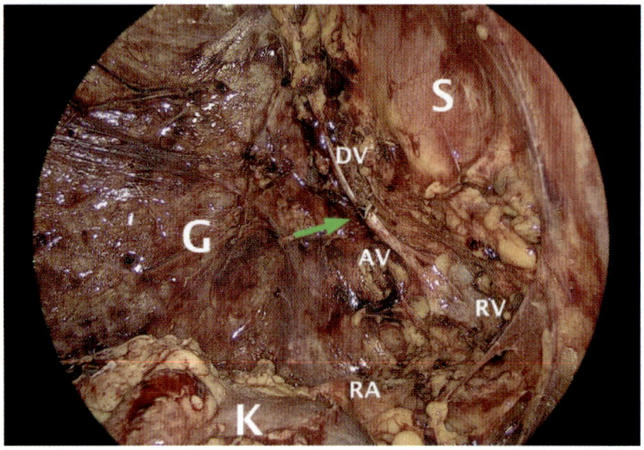

▲ **Figure 50–17.** Left-sided PRA. Bed of the adrenal tumor after adrenalectomy. Kidney (K), renal artery (RA), renal vein (RV), adrenal vein (AV) cut (⟶), diaphragmatic branch (DV), spine (S), anterior Gerota's fascia (G) covering pancreas (not visible).

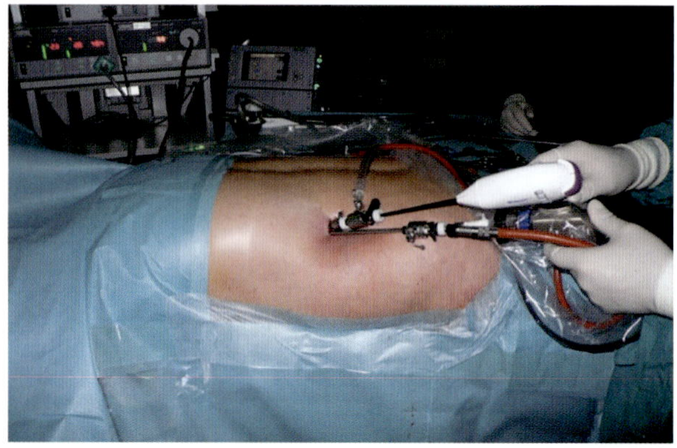

▲ **Figure 50–18.** Right-sided single access retroperitoneoscopic adrenalectomy (SARA).

in reduced operative space. Nevertheless, PRA can be continued, and I never needed to convert because of this reason. On the left side, tumors may be fixed to the anterior Gerota's fascia between the pancreas and retroperitoneum. Transection of this fascia will result in a direct view of the posterior aspect of the pancreas and the splenic vein and artery. Therefore, a meticulous dissection is required. If the adrenal tumor is fixed to the surface of the upper pole of the kidney, a partial renal decapsulation is recommended. Tiny bleeding from the renal parenchyma will stop by itself or can easily be controlled by diathermy. In principle, there is no need for

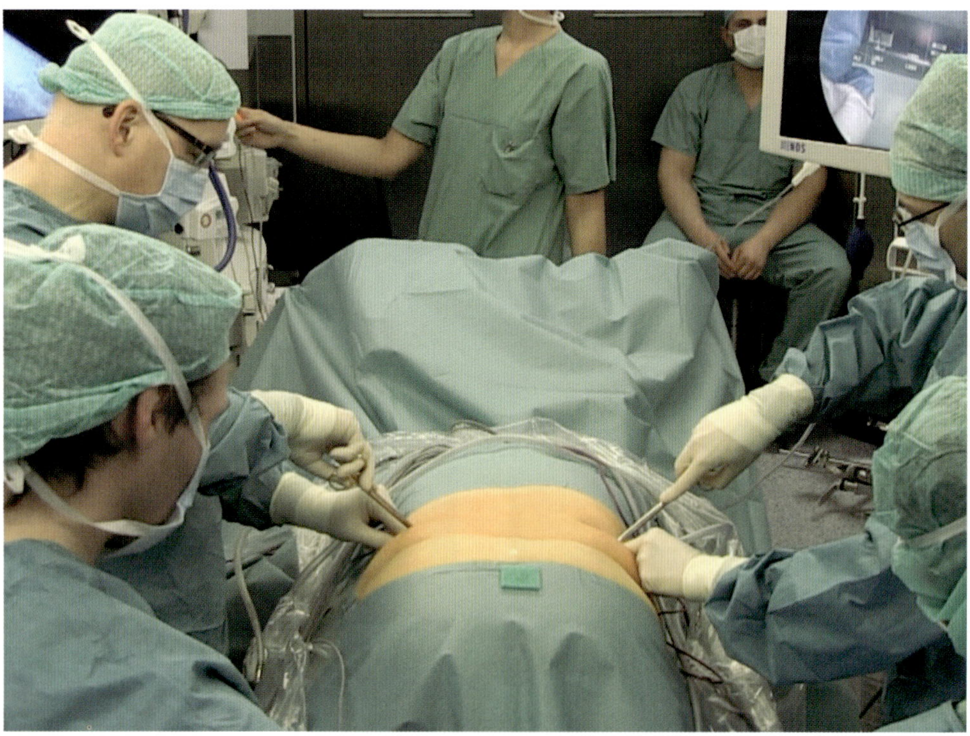

▲ **Figure 50–19.** Concurrent posterior retroperitoneoscopic adrenalectomy (CoBRA). Two teams, two towers.

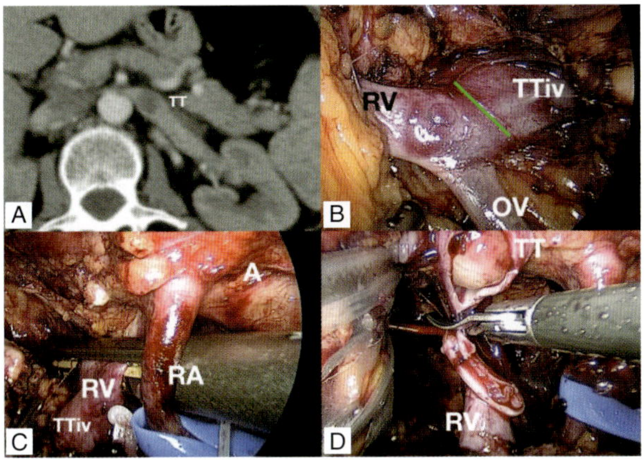

▲ **Figure 50–20.** Left adrenal metastasis with tumor thrombus in the renal vein.
(A) CT scan.
(B) Dissection of renal vein and ovarian vein. Green line: planned lateral transsection of the renal vein.
(C) Medial transsection of the renal vein by stapling anterior-lateral to the aorta.
(D) Lateral transection of renal vein. Tumor thrombus is visible.

A: abdominal aorta; OV: ovarian vein; RA: renal artery; RV: renal vein; TT: tumor thrombus; TTiv: tumor thrombus intravenously.

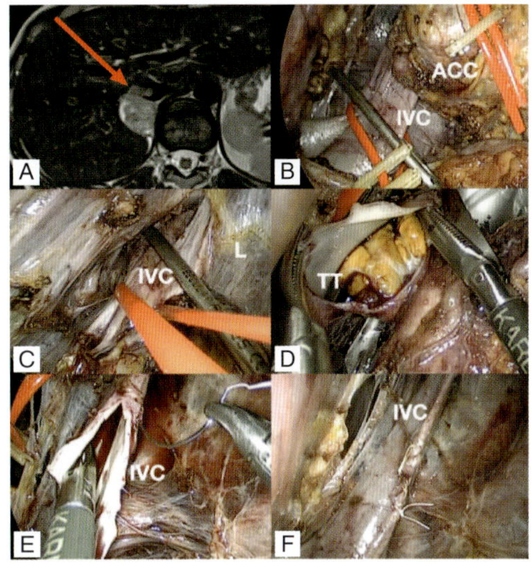

▲ **Figure 50–21** Right adrenocortical carcinoma (ACC) with tumor thrombus in inferior vena cava (IVC).
(A) Magnet resonance imaging. → tumor thrombus.
(B) Clamping of IVC inferiorly to the adrenal vein.
(C) Clamping of IVC superiorly the adrenal vein. L: liver.
(D) IVC opened. Tumor thrombus (TT) visible.
(E) IVC defect after excision of the collar-like adrenal vein with the ACC.
(F) The IVC defect is closed with a running suture.

nephrectomy in adrenal cases as all types of adrenal tumors respect the renal vessels, with one exception on the left side, a **tumor thrombus** growing through the adrenal vein into the renal vein. Even in these rare situations, the oncologic resection can be performed by PRA as long as the thrombus does not reach the IVC. As renal perfusion (and function) can be preserved by a patent left gonadal vein, a tumor thrombus in the renal vein can be removed *en bloc* with a central segment of the vein. Oblique clipping of the lateral renal vein and stapling on the centrally (near the conjunction with the IVC) controls potential bleeding (Figure 50–20A-D). On the right side, an adrenal tumor, especially an adrenocortical cancer, may develop a tumor thrombus into the IVC via the main adrenal vein. PRA is an option if this thrombus is limited to 2 to 3 cm in length and the adrenal tumor is 4 to 5 cm in diameter.[10] The oncologic *en-bloc* resection of the primary tumor and thrombus needs excision of the right main adrenal vein out of the IVC. Therefore, the IVC segment between the renal vein conjunctions and the inferior liver veins has to be isolated and clamped caudally and cranially. This allows an incision of the IVC inferior to the adrenal vein. The thrombus becomes visible, and the excision of the collar-like adrenal vein around the neoplasia allows for resection without tumor cell spillage. After removal of the tumor in a bag, the venous incision will be closed by a running suture before the clamps can be removed (Figure 50–21A-F).

Indications for PRA are all types of adrenal tumors with surgical indications. This includes all functioning neoplasias and nonfunctioning tumors larger than 4 cm except asymptomatic myelolipomas, adrenal cysts, and adrenal metastases. **Limits** are the size of more than 6 to 8 cm in diameter in adrenocortical tumors and pheochromocytomas. In larger tumors, the risk of a capsule lesion increases due to the need for a circumferential dissection in a limited space. Adrenal metastases tend to cause a desmoplastic reaction in the periadrenal fatty tissue. Therefore, *en-bloc* resection is more difficult, and a 5- to 6-cm size limit is recommended.

REFERENCES

1. Walz MK, Peitgen K, Hoermann R, et al. Posterior retroperitoneoscopy as a new minimally invasive approach for adrenalectomy: results of 30 adrenalectomies in 27 patients. *World J Surg.* 1996;20:769-774.
2. Barczynski M, Konturek A, Nowak W. Randomized clinical trial of posterior retroperitoneoscopic adrenalectomy versus lateral transperitoneal laparoscopic adrenalectomy with a 5-year follow-up. *Ann Surg.* 2014;260(5):740-747; discussion 747-8.
3. Cabalag MS, Mann GB, Gorelik A, et al. Comparison of outcomes after laparoscopic versus posterior retroperitoneoscopic

adrenalectomy: a pilot study. *Surg Laparosc Endosc Percutan Tech.* 2014;24:62-66.
4. Walz MK, Peitgen K, Walz MV, et al. Posterior retroperitoneoscopic adrenalectomy: lessons learned within five years. *World J Surg.* 2001;25:728-734.
5. Walz MK, Alesina PF. Single access retroperitoneoscopic adrenalectomy (SARA)—one step beyond in endocrine surgery. *Langenbecks Arch Surg.* 2009;394:447-450.
6. Walz MK, Groeben H, Alesina PF. Single-access retroperitoneoscopic adrenalectomy (SARA) versus conventional retroperitoneoscopic adrenalectomy (CORA): a case-control study. *World J Surg.* 2010; 34(6):1386-1390.
7. Walz MK, Peitgen K, Saller B, et al. Subtotal adrenalectomy by the posterior retroperitoneoscopic approach. *World J Surg.* 1998;22:621-626.
8. Walz MK, Peitgen K, Diesing D, et al. Partial versus total adrenalectomy by the posterior retroperitoneoscopic approach: early and long-term results of 325 consecutive procedures in primary adrenal neoplasias. *World J Surg.* 2004;28:1323-1329.
9. Alesina PF, Hinrichs J, Meier B, et al. Minimally invasive cortical-sparing surgery for bilateral pheochromocytomas. *Langenbecks Arch Surg.* 2012;397:233-238.
10. Walz MK, Jongekkasit I, Alesina P. Retroperitoneoscopic adrenalectomy in adrenocortical carcinoma with tumor thrombus in inferior vena cava: one step further in minimally invasive endocrine surgery. *Video Endocrinol.* 2021;8.

Adrenalectomy: Robotic Approach

51

Aljehani Ashwaq, MD
Alahmed Feras, MD
Brunaud Laurent, MD

INTRODUCTION

The adrenal glands are located in the perirenal compartment of the retroperitoneum.[1] Adrenal tumors involve a broad spectrum of pathological entities; they can vary from a benign adrenocortical adenoma without hormonal secretion to a secretory adrenocortical malignancy.[2] The incidence of adrenal tumors ranges approximately from 1.5% to 9% among the general population. Less than 5% of adrenal tumors are malignant, and about 10% of them are functional.[3]

The adrenal gland can be approached either open or endoscopically, with or without the use of the robotic system.[1] Laparoscopic adrenalectomy was first described in 1992. The laparoscopic approach routinely replaced open operations as the standard treatment for adrenal tumors because of several advantages such as shorter hospital stay, minimally invasive incisions, and less hemorrhage.[3] There has been an accumulation of evidence over the last three decades that showed the safety and efficacy of laparoscopic adrenalectomy, which led to shifting from open to laparoscopic adrenalectomy.[4]

The Food and Drug Administration (FDA) approved the da Vinci robot (Intuitive Surgical, INC., Sunnyvale, CA, USA) over a decade ago, and it has undergone various redesigns by the company. The first robotic-assisted adrenalectomy was reported in 2001 by Horgan et al., and since then, the approach has been increasingly utilized.[5] Robotic adrenalectomy has been increasingly used and has replaced the laparoscopic approach in some medical centers.[3]

Robotic technology offers several advantages such as better ergonomics for surgeons, better camera control, magnified three-dimensional view, and reduced surgeon fatigability, which make it theoretically a better alternative to laparoscopic technology.[6] However, the robotic approach has some disadvantages, such as accessibility and higher cost, which has limited its widespread global adoption.[6]

Indications for Adrenalectomy

Most adrenal masses are diagnosed incidentally due to the use of ultrasound and other radiological imaging.[7] Adrenalectomy is indicated in the case of functional adrenal tumors, tumors suspicious for malignancy, or malignant tumors, including adrenocortical cancer and metastatic tumors.[7] Regardless of the size of hormone-producing tumors, adrenalectomy is indicated for the treatment of such tumors. Adrenalectomy is also indicated for adrenocortical cancer, although malignant tumors are rarely encountered. The adrenal gland is also a common site for metastasis of breast and lung tumors, renal cell cancer, lymphoma, and melanoma. Adrenalectomy is indicated in the treatment of some patients with metastases, but only after discussion with a multidisciplinary team. Regarding nonfunctional adrenal tumors, the main indication for surgery is the risk of malignancy, which is related to the size and imaging characteristics of the tumor, including uptake intensity on PET-FDG. The risk of malignancy is approximately 2% for a lesion smaller than 4 cm, whereas it increases to 6% for lesion size between 4 and 6 cm and it increases to 25% for lesions of 6 cm and larger.[7] In sum, the indications for laparoscopic adrenalectomy with or without the robotic system generally include benign nonfunctional tumors with a size of ≥4 to 5 cm, all functional adrenal tumors, and metastases in selected patients with soft-tissue or solid-organ primary tumors, usually in the setting of mono or oligometastatic disease.[8]

Robotic-Assisted Transperitoneal Adrenalectomy

As with any other surgical procedure, the selection of patients is an important factor for robotic adrenal surgery. Lateral transperitoneal robotic adrenalectomy is the main approach used when the robotic platform is available. The indications for lateral robotic adrenalectomy include pheochromocytomas, hormonal secreting tumors, symptomatic myelolipomas, hormone inactive lesions larger than 3 to 4 cm which show growth overtime and/or FDG uptake, tumors of a diameter larger than 5 cm, and adrenal metastatic tumors.[9] Transabdominal lateral adrenalectomy is usually performed in patients with a tumor larger than 6 cm in diameter, whereas the posterior retroperitoneal approach can be used in patients with tumor diameter of less than 6 cm.[9] Contraindications for lateral robotic adrenalectomy include very large tumors (>10-12 cm) and infiltrative adrenal masses with large vascular structure involvement.[9]

TECHNICAL ASPECTS

The da Vinci Robotic surgical system consists of a robotic manipulator with three or four arms based on the robot version; the camera is held by the central arm, the surgical instruments are held by the other two or three arms and there is a remote console where the first operator is seated during the procedure. Trocars are placed and right and left robot arms are connected once the pneumoperitoneum is created. The robot is controlled by the operating surgeon at the console, whereas the laparoscopic instruments are inserted through one or two accessory trocars by the first assistant. A zero-angle scope is used; however, a 30 degrees is also possible.[10]

The surgical procedure is performed under general anesthesia. The preparation and positioning of the patient is the same as that for laparoscopic adrenalectomy. The patient is positioned in the right or left lateral decubitus side according to the tumor location; right-side adrenal tumors require left decubitus position, whereas for left-side tumors the patient is placed in the right decubitus position. In left adrenalectomy, four trocars are used, whereas right adrenalectomy requires an additional trocar for aiding in liver retraction.[11]

Right-sided Robotic Adrenalectomy

The first port involves an 8- or 12-mm camera port (according to robotic platform version) which is placed between the right costal margin and the umbilicus. The other two ports are two robotic instrument ports; both 8 mm and are placed along a line two fingerbreadths from the costal margin. The liver retraction port is the third port which is a 5- or 10-mm port and it is placed in the midline in the epigastrium. The 10-mm accessory port, which is the fifth port, is placed in the right abdomen through which the assistant can use an endobag.[12]

The dissection of the adrenal space involves the use of a robotic hook and bipolar forceps. The triangular ligament is divided using a robotic monopolar hook, whereas liver retraction is performed by a laparoscopic retractor to provide exposure of the inferior vena cava. The incision of Gerota's fascia is performed at the level of the upper pole of the kidney.[11]

The adrenal gland is identified on the superomedial aspect of the kidney. Direct manipulation of the adrenal gland should be reduced. The periadrenal tissues are removed or grasped with a blunt grasper to facilitate circumferential dissection. It is important to identify the adrenal vein early during the course of dissection to facilitate mobilization.[12]

After precise dissection of vena cava, the identification of the right adrenal vein and the major components such as the psoas muscle in the superior and posterior pole of the right kidney in the anterior takes place (Figure 51–1 A-C). Then, clips are applied on the adrenal vein and the vein is divided. The adrenal dissection with hemostasis is performed, and the gland is then removed using a specimen retrieval bag.[11]

Left-sided Robotic Adrenalectomy

The patient, in this case, is placed in a right lateral decubitus position (Figure 51–2). The exposure of the gland requires mobilizing the splenic flexure of colon, lateral attachments of spleen, and the tail of the pancreas, which are mobilized medially with caution; the mobilization is performed until the gland is identified. Dissection of the periadrenal fat is required for the lateral identification of the superior pole of the kidney, inferior identification of the left renal vein, psoas muscle, and diaphragm at the posterior aspect, and the tail of the pancreas and splenic vessels medially.[11]

Dissection steps of the left adrenal are similar to that of the right adrenal gland. The junction of the left adrenal vein with the left renal vein is generally identified. The inferior phrenic vein, which connects the left adrenal vein medially, also requires dissection clipping and division.[10]

The dissection of the left main adrenal vein is performed with the hook and the vein is controlled using a clip (Figure 51–3 A-D). The adrenal dissection with hemostasis is performed, and the gland is then removed using a specimen retrieval bag.[11] After completing the adrenalectomy, the robot is undocked.[11]

Outcome, Safety & Effectiveness of the Robotic Technique

A study involving 111 patients who underwent transperitoneal adrenalectomy showed that robotic approach was safe and effective with low morbidity and no mortality.[13]

Recently, Materazzi and Rossi (2021) reported that the robotic technique offers advantages to overcome some laparoscopic shortcomings such as loss of 3D vision, rigid instruments, or unstable camera. Thus, the feasibility and the safety of robot-assisted adrenalectomy was investigated in high-volume centers with outcomes comparable to laparoscopic adrenalectomy.[14]

Several case series have evaluated and presented the outcomes of robotic-assisted transabdominal lateral and retroperitoneal posterior adrenalectomy (Table 51–1). There were only three available studies that included more than 50 patients.[15-17] Niglio et al.[18] conducted a large clinical series that reported on 64 patients who underwent a laparoscopic approach and 40 patients who underwent a robotic-assisted

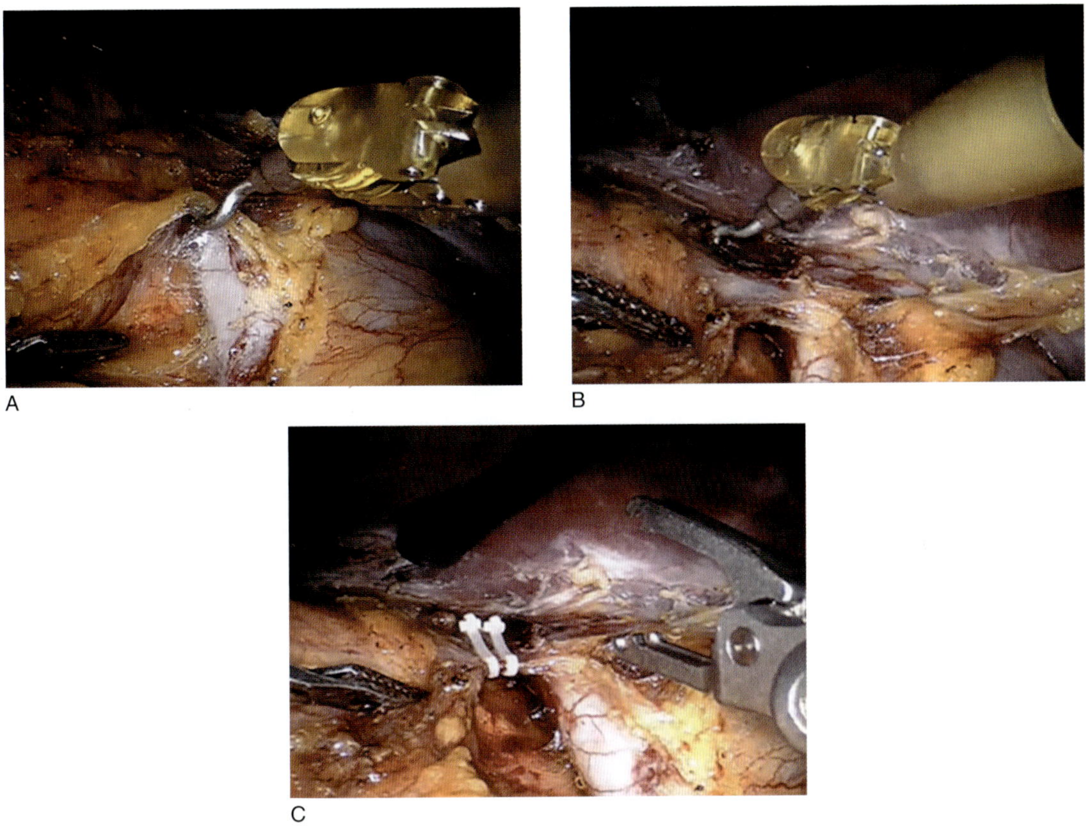

▲ **Figure 51–1.** **(A-C)** Right adrenalectomy in a patient with a 4.2 cm adrenal incidentaloma. **(A)** Dissection along the inferior vena cava. **(B)** The right main adrenal vein. **(C)** Clip on the right adrenal vein.

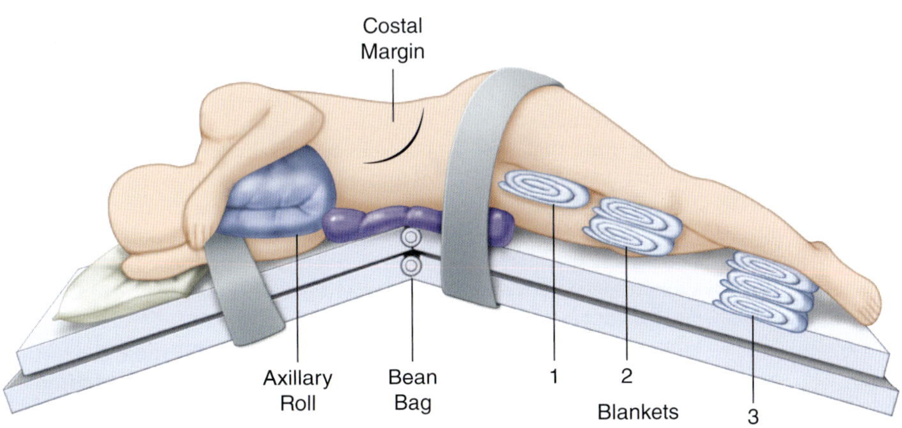

▲ **Figure 51–2.** Lateral decubitus position for transabdominal adrenalectomy. (Reproduced with permission from Madani A, Lee JA. Surgical approaches to the adrenal gland. *Surgical Clin North Am.* 2019;99(4):773-791.)

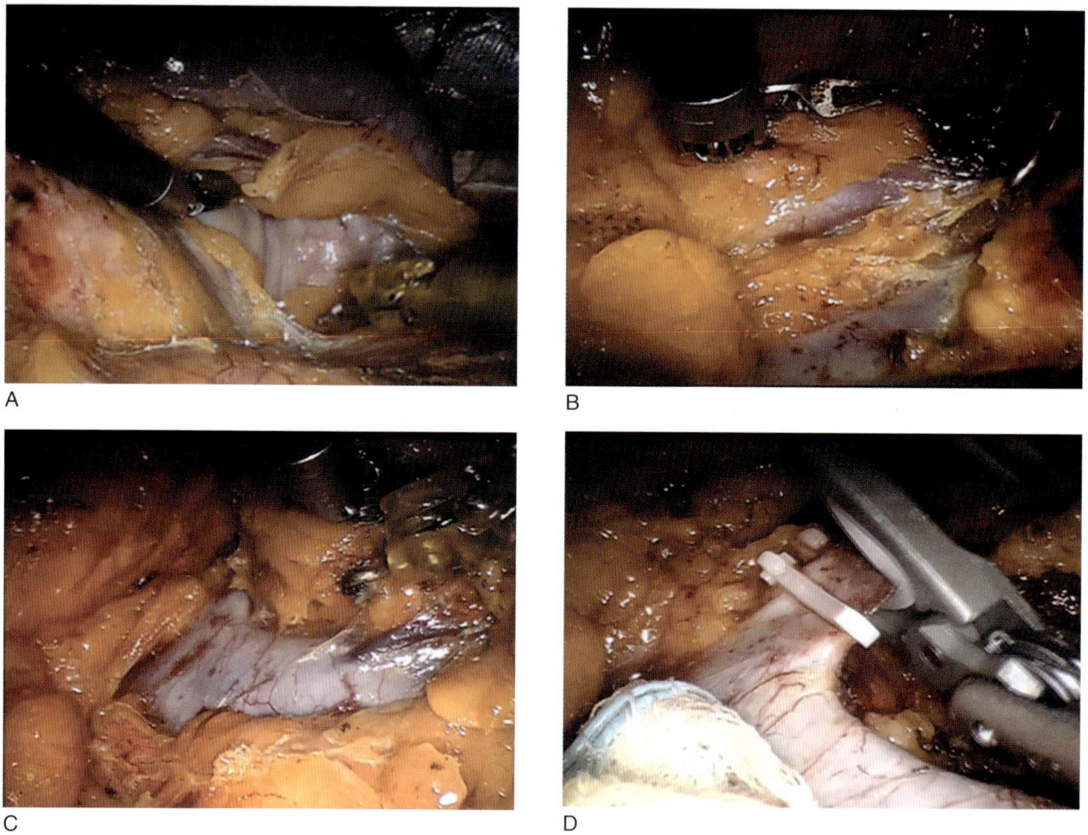

Figure 51–3. **(A-D)** Left adrenalectomy in a patient with 5 cm adrenal cortical tumor. **(A)** Posterior pancreatic dissection and spleen mobilization allowing to expose the posterior aspect of the stomach (anatomical landmark). **(B)** Splenic artery and vein are anatomical landmarks during the dissection behind the pancreatic tail. **(C)** The left renal and the main adrenal veins. **(D)** Clip on the left adrenal vein.

transperitoneal lateral adrenalectomy. The mean operative time for the robotic approach was 102.2 minutes, which was lower compared to previous reported studies.[19-21] Brunaud et al.[17] reported a mean operative time that was 95 minutes. Also, Niglio et al.[18] reported that no conversion occurred in patients that underwent a robotic approach, and this was similar to Brandao,[19] Giulianotti,[22] Winter,[23] and Hanly.[24] The conversion rate ranged from 0%[18,19,22-24] to 8%.[25] The morbidity rate also varied and ranged between 2%[26] and 20%.[19] Other studies that assess the outcome, safety, and effectiveness of robotic adrenalectomy are mentioned in Table 51–1.[27-29]

Robotic Partial Adrenalectomy

Partial adrenalectomy allows the opportunity to avoid the need for steroid replacement and therefore may be desired for bilateral and hereditary adrenal tumors. It can be performed safely when patients are selected carefully. The tumor size should not exceed 3 cm because our experience and that of others has shown that a robotic partial adrenalectomy becomes technically less feasible. Intraoperative assessment of tumor localization within the adrenal gland is also another determinant for the feasibility of robotic partial adrenalectomy. Tumors located anteriorly and on the margin of the adrenal gland can be removed easily compared to posterior tumors and tumors located close to the adrenal vein.[30]

Comparison of Robotic Adrenalectomy & Laparoscopic Adrenalectomy

The large majority of previous studies agree that robotic adrenalectomy is a feasible, effective, and safe surgical approach for benign adrenal tumors, and its results are similar to that of standard laparoscopic surgery, regardless of the patient habitus or robotic system used (Xi or Si).[31,32]

Table 51–1. Studies evaluating robotic-assisted adrenalectomy (with more than 30 patients).

Study	Year	Patients	Type	Operative Time (min)	Conversion Rate (%)	Morbidity (%)
Niglio[18]	2020	40	Trans	102.2	0	—
Kin[15]	2019	61	Retro	138	—	—
Kahramangil[27]	2017	188	Trans & retro	154/136	2.5	4.8
Brandao[19]	2014	30	Trans	120	0	20
Pineda[20]	2013	30	Trans	190	—	—
Aksoy[28]	2013	42	Trans & retro	186	0	4.8
D'annibale[21]	2012	30	Trans	223	3.3	10
Agcaoglu[29]	2012	31	Retro	163	0	—
Karabulut[26]	2012	50	Trans & retro	159	0	2
Nordenstrom[16]	2011	100	Trans	113	7	13
Giulianotti[22]	2011	41	Trans	118	0	4.8
Brunaud[17]	2008	100	Trans	95	5	8
Brunaud[25]	2008	50	Trans	104	8	10
Winter[23]	2006	30	Trans	185	0	7
Hanly[24]	2004	30	Trans	—	0	—

The complications associated with the robotic adrenalectomy also are similar to those in laparoscopic adrenalectomy and they include hemorrhage, hematoma, wound infection, urinary tract infection, and injuries of adjacent organs.[11]

A series that included 300 consecutive patients to assess the risk factors for perioperative complications in robotic-assisted unilateral adrenalectomy showed that conversion to open laparotomy and capsular rupture were each 3%. Postoperative complications occurred in 9.2% of patients. BMI was not a significant risk factor for conversion or postoperative complications, whereas a tumor size of more than 5 cm was a significant factor for conversion to laparotomy. On the other hand, age of the patient and conversion to laparotomy were predictive factors for postoperative complications.[33]

In a systematic review that included 26 series and 1710 patients, it was found that robotic adrenalectomy reduced bleeding compared to laparoscopic and open adrenalectomy. Also, robotic access was significantly associated with a considerably lower duration of hospital stay, whereas the operative duration for open adrenalectomy was lower.[34]

In a meta-analysis of 27 studies, it was found that there was no significant variation between robotic adrenalectomy and laparoscopic adrenalectomy regarding intraoperative and postoperative complications, conversion to laparotomy, blood loss, and mortality. However, shorter hospitalization and significantly longer operating time were noted among patients who underwent robotic adrenalectomy.[35]

The conversion rate was reported to be affected by the tumor size among 200 cases who underwent minimally invasive adrenalectomy (laparoscopic adrenalectomy and robotic adrenalectomy).[36] There has been no specific prospective study conducted on the robotic approach in patients with large tumors (>5 cm), including adrenocortical carcinoma.[37]

In a meta-analysis and systematic review that included 13 studies with 798 patients (379 underwent robotic adrenalectomy and 419 underwent laparoscopic adrenalectomy), it was found that there was significantly less blood loss and shorter hospital stay in the robotic patients compared to patients who underwent laparoscopic adrenalectomy.[38] Also, an analysis of the effectiveness of robotic adrenalectomy and conventional laparoscopic surgery showed similar postoperative outcomes in the management of obese patients.[39]

In one study conducted to compare the outcomes of transperitoneal laparoscopic adrenalectomy (TLA), retroperitoneal laparoscopic adrenalectomy (RLA), and robot-assisted transperitoneal laparoscopic adrenalectomy (RATLA), it was found that the operative time was similar in the first two groups, whereas blood loss was significantly lower for RATLA group compared to TLA group. Also, the length of stay for the RATLA group was significantly shorter compared to the other two groups. The transfusion rate and complication rate were similar between the three groups.[3] Feng et al.[40] compared the outcomes between laparoscopic and robotic-assisted adrenalectomy. The study showed that the robotic group had anesthesia and procedure time similar to the laparoscopic group. The mean duration of hospital stay for robotic laparoscopic was 1.7 days, whereas that of laparoscopic adrenalectomy was 1.9 days, with no significant difference.

A study conducted to investigate the short-term outcomes between robotic adrenalectomy and laparoscopic adrenalectomy using the national inpatient sample database reported that there was no difference in the conversion and complication rates between the two approaches. The only significance found was regarding the shorter hospital stay noted for patients who underwent robotic adrenalectomy.[41] Another study by Fang et al. included 156 adrenalectomy cases; both robotic and conventional laparoscopic approaches resulted in similar rates of complications, blood loss, and length of hospital stay.[42] Also, Perivoliotis et al. in their meta-analysis and trial sequential analysis that included 21 studies and 2997 patients found that laparoscopic adrenalectomy and robotic adrenalectomy were similar in terms of operative duration, positive margin, mortality rate, and complications.[43]

Cost-Effectiveness of Robotic System

The use of robotic system is associated with additional costs (about 2.3 times more expensive), so the laparoscopic adrenalectomy is still widely favored and utilized.[44] Feng et al. reported that an experienced surgical team that limits the number of energy devices and the number of robotic instruments used in the robotic approach could keep the cost of robotic adrenalectomy similar to that of laparoscopic adrenalectomy.[40] The excess cost of robotic adrenalectomy could be balanced by a shorter length of hospital stay, improved postoperative outcomes, and increasing patients referral.[45]

CONCLUSION

The robotic approach is effective and safe for adrenalectomy and its results are similar to that of standard laparoscopic surgery. The robotic approach is associated with a significantly lower duration of hospital stay and lower blood loss. However, shortcomings of robotic adrenalectomy include a longer operative time and higher costs that limit its use as compared to standard laparoscopic surgery.

REFERENCES

1. Madani A, Lee JA. Surgical approaches to the adrenal gland. *Surg Clin North Am*. 2019;99(4):773-791.
2. Nomine-Criqui C, Germain A, Ayav A, Bresler L, Brunaud L. Robot-assisted adrenalectomy: indications and drawbacks. *Updates Surg*. 2017;69(2):127-133.
3. Ji C, Lu Q, Chen W, et al. Retrospective comparison of three minimally invasive approaches for adrenal tumors: perioperative outcomes of transperitoneal laparoscopic, retroperitoneal laparoscopic and robot-assisted laparoscopic adrenalectomy. *BMC Urol*. 2020;20(1):1-6.
4. Grogan RH. Current status of robotic adrenalectomy in the United States. *Gland Surg*. 2020;9(3):840.
5. Feng Z, Feng MP, Feng DP, Solórzano CC. Robotic-assisted adrenalectomy using da Vinci Xi vs. Si: are there differences? *J Robotic Surg*. 2020;14(2):349-355.
6. Ragavan N, Selvaraj N, Raghavan D, et al. Robot assisted laparoscopic adrenalectomy: does size matter? *Cureus*. 2020;12(8).
7. Uludağ M, Aygün N, İşgör A. Surgical indications and techniques for adrenalectomy. *Sisli Etfal Hastan Tip Bull*. 2020;54(1):8.
8. Okoh AK, Berber E. Laparoscopic and robotic adrenal surgery: transperitoneal approach. *Gland Surg*. 2015;4(5):435.
9. Alahmed F, Nomine-Criqui C, Poirier A, et al. Robotic adrenalectomy: updates on lateral transperitoneal approach. *Current Surg Rep*. 2020;8(12):1-6.
10. Brunaud L, Germain A, Zarnegar R, et al. Robot-assisted adrenalectomy. *Surg Laparosc Endosc Percutan Tech*. 2011;21(4): 248-254.
11. Makay O, Erol V, Ozdemir M. Robotic adrenalectomy. *Gland Surg*. 2019;8(Suppl 1):S10.
12. Yiannakopoulou E. Robotic assisted adrenalectomy: surgical techniques, feasibility, indications, oncological outcome and safety. *Int J Surg*. 2016;28:169-172.
13. Ozdemir M, Dural AC, Sahbaz NA, et al. Robotic transperitoneal adrenalectomy from inception to ingenuity: the perspective on two high volume endocrine surgery centers. *Gland Surg*. 2020;9(3):815.
14. Materazzi G, Rossi L. Robot-assisted adrenalectomy: state of the art. *Updates Surg*. 2021;73(3):1131-1146.
15. Kim WW, Lee YM, Chung KW, et al. Comparison of robotic posterior retroperitoneal adrenalectomy over laparoscopic posterior retroperitoneal adrenalectomy: a single tertiary center experience. *Int J Endocrinol*. 2019;2019:9012910.
16. Nordenström E, Westerdahl J, Hallgrimsson P, et al. A prospective study of 100 robotically assisted laparoscopic adrenalectomies. *J Robotic Surg*. 2011;1:1-5.
17. Brunaud L, Ayav A, Zarnegar R, et al. Prospective evaluation of 100 robotic-assisted unilateral adrenalectomies. *Surgery*. 2008;144:995-1001.
18. Niglio A, Grasso M, Costigliola L, et al. Laparoscopic and robot-assisted transperitoneal lateral adrenalectomy: a large clinical series from a single center. *Updates Surg*. 2020;72(1):193-198.
19. Brandao LF, Autorino R, Laydner H, et al. Robotic versus laparoscopic adrenalectomy: a systematic review and metaanalysis. *Eur Urol*. 2014;65:1154-1161.
20. Pineda-Solis K, Medina-Franco H, Heslin M. Robotic versus laparoscopic adrenalectomy: a comparative study in a high-volume center. *Surg Endosc*. 2013;27:599-602.
21. D'annibale A, Lucandri G, Monsellato I, et al. Robotic adrenalectomy: technical aspects, early results and learning curve. *Int J Med Robotics Comput Assist Surg*. 2012.
22. Giulianotti PC, Buchs NC, Addeo P, et al. Robot-assisted adrenalectomy: a technical option for the surgeon? *Int J Med Robotics Comput Assist Surg*. 2011;7:27-32.
23. Winter JM, Talamini MA, Stanfield CL, et al. Thirty robotic adrenalectomies: a single institution's experience. *Surg Endosc*. 2006;20:119-124.
24. Hanly EJ, Talamini MA. Robotic abdominal surgery. *Am J Surg*. 2004;188:19S-26S.
25. Brunaud L, Bresler L, Ayav A, et al. Robotic-assisted adrenalectomy: what advantages compared to lateral transperitoneal laparoscopic adrenalectomy? *Am J Surg*. 2008;195:433-438.
26. Karabulut K, Agcaoglu O, Aliyev S, et al. Comparison of intraoperative time use and perioperative outcomes for robotic versus laparoscopic adrenalectomy. *Surg*. 2012;151:537-542.

27. Kahramangil B, Berber E. Comparison of posterior retroperitoneal and transabdominal lateral approaches in robotic adrenalectomy: an analysis of 200 cases. *Surg Endosc.* 2018;32(4):1984-1989.
28. Aksoy E, Taskin H, Aliyev S, et al. Robotic versus laparoscopic adrenalectomy in obese patients. *Surg Endosc.* 2013;27:1233-1236.
29. Agcaoglu O, Aliyev S, Karabulut K, et al. Robotic vs laparoscopic posterior retroperitoneal adrenalectomy. *Arch Surg.* 2012;147:272-275.
30. Calì B, Nomine-Criqui C, Bihain F, Brunaud L. Robotic approach for partial adrenalectomy. *Updates Surg.* 2021;7:1-8.
31. Agcaoglu O, Karahan SN, Tufekci T, Tezelman S. Single-incision robotic adrenalectomy (SIRA): the future of adrenal surgery? *Gland Surg.* 2020;9(3):853.
32. Fiori C, Checcucci E, Amparore D, et al. Adrenal tumours: open surgery versus minimally invasive surgery. *Current Opin Oncol.* 2020;32(1):27-34.
33. Greilsamer T, Nomine-Criqui C, Thy M, et al. Robotic-assisted unilateral adrenalectomy: risk factors for perioperative complications in 303 consecutive patients. *Surg Endosc.* 2019; 33:802-810.
34. Heger P, Probst P, Hüttner FJ, et al. Evaluation of open and minimally invasive adrenalectomy: a systematic review and network meta-analysis. *World J Surg.* 2017;41:2746-2757.
35. Economopoulos KP, Mylonas KS, Stamou AA, et al. Laparoscopic versus robotic adrenalectomy: a comprehensive meta-analysis. *Int J Surg.* 2017;38:95-104.
36. Calcatera NA, Hsiung-Wang C, Suss NR, et al. Minimally invasive adrenalectomy for adrenocortical carcinoma: five-year trends and predictors of conversion. *World J Surg.* 2018;42:473-481.
37. Ho CH, Liao PW, Lin VC, et al. Laparoendoscopic single-site (LESS) retroperitoneal partial adrenalectomy using a custom-made single-access platform and standard laparoscopic instruments: technical considerations and surgical outcomes. *Asian J Surg.* 2015;38:6-12.
38. Agrusa A, Romano G, Navarra G, et al. Innovation in endocrine surgery: robotic versus laparoscopic adrenalectomy. Meta-analysis and systematic literature review. *Oncotarget.* 2017;8:102392-400.
39. Coste T, Caiazzo R, Torres F, et al. Laparoscopic adrenalectomy by transabdominal lateral approach: 20 years of experience. *SurgEndosc.* 2017;31:2743-51.
40. Feng Z, Feng MP, Feng DP, Rice MJ, Solórzano CC. A cost-conscious approach to robotic adrenalectomy. *J Robot Surg.* 2018;12(4):607-611.
41. Samreen S, Fluck M, Hunsinger M, et al. Laparoscopic versus robotic adrenalectomy: a review of the national inpatient sample. *J Robot Surg.* 2019;13:69-75.
42. Fang AM, Rosen J, Saidian A, et al. Perioperative outcomes of laparoscopic, robotic, and open approaches to pheochromocytoma. *J Robotic Surg.* 2020;14(6):849-854.
43. Perivoliotis K, Baloyiannis I, Sarakatsianou C, Tzovaras G. Comparing the efficacy and safety of laparoscopic and robotic adrenalectomy: a meta-analysis and trial sequential analysis. *Langenbecks Arch Surg.* 2020;405(2):125-135.
44. Al-Qurayshi Z, Robins R, Buell J, et al. Surgeon volume impact on outcomes and costs of adrenal surgeries. *Eur J Surg Oncol.* 2016;42:1483-1490.
45. Mihai R, Donatini G, Vidal O, Brunaud L. Volume-outcome correlation in adrenal surgery—an ESES consensus statement. *Langenbecks Arch Surg.* 2019;404(7):795-806.

52 Adrenal Venous Sampling

Nimesh Shah, FRCR
William Drake, FRCP, DM
Matthew Matson, MRCP, FRCR

INTRODUCTION

Adrenal venous sampling (AVS) is an endovascular technique that allows selective catheterization of the right and left adrenal veins. The most common indication for AVS is primary aldosteronism (PA), sometimes also known as primary hyperaldosteronism (PHA), or (less frequently) Conn syndrome. Hypertension affects over 30% of adults worldwide and significantly impacts morbidity and mortality.[1,2] PA is the commonest surgically curable cause of secondary hypertension,[3] affecting approximately 6% of all patients with hypertension and 20% of those with resistant hypertension, defined as uncontrolled hypertension on three agents or controlled on four or more agents. In addition to the morbidity solely associated with hypertension, PA has effects independent of this. Proinflammatory and profibrotic effects have been noted in the vascular system, the heart and kidneys.[4] The relative risk for stroke, renal damage, myocardial infarction, and atrial fibrillation is higher in PA even after correcting for blood pressure.

Other rare indications for AVS have been for patients with biochemically proven pheochromocytoma where a source was not seen on cross-sectional imaging, but it is vanishingly rare to do this now.[5] It may also be performed, rarely, in cases of ACTH-independent Cushing syndrome with bilateral adrenal masses to ascertain which adrenal gland is the sole or dominant source of cortisol excess.[6] This chapter will focus on PA as the main indication for AVS.

Case Detection & Confirmation

Case detection in PA is a two-stage process. In the first (case finding) stage, patients with hypertension at risk of PA are screened with an aldosterone/renin ratio (ARR); a raised aldosterone level in the presence of a suppressed renin hormone level is suggestive of the diagnosis. The Endocrine Society Guidelines suggest that an ARR should be obtained in patients with sustained blood pressure (BP) above 150/100 mmHg on each of three measurements obtained on different days; hypertension (BP >140/90 mmHg) resistant to three conventional antihypertensive drugs (including a diuretic), or controlled BP (<140/90 mmHg) on four or more antihypertensive drugs; hypertension and spontaneous or diuretic-induced hypokalemia; hypertension and adrenal incidentaloma; hypertension and sleep apnoea; hypertension and a family history of early onset hypertension or cerebrovascular accident at a young age (<40 years); and all hypertensive first-degree relatives of patients with PA.

This is followed by confirmatory testing in most patients. Confirmatory testing usually involves one of four testing procedures: oral sodium loading, saline infusion, fludrocortisone suppression, and captopril challenge. The evidence for confirmatory testing is limited and a gold standard confirmatory test has not been determined. The choice of the confirmatory test offered is determined by local experience and availability.[7]

The second stage is to determine the subtype of PA (adrenal adenoma, unilateral or bilateral adrenal hyperplasia [BAH], adrenal carcinoma or inherited conditions of familial hyperaldosteronism). All patients are recommended to undergo contrast-enhanced CT imaging in the first instance. Imaging findings can include normal appearing adrenal glands, unilateral limb thickening/nodularity, unilateral micronodule (≤1 cm) or macronodule (>1 cm) (Figures 52–1 through 52–4). The poor concordance between adrenal lesions seen on CT imaging and hormone production on AVS has been well described.[8-10] Several factors contribute to the observed discordance. Most aldosterone-producing adenomas (APAs) are found to be less than 1 cm, where detection on CT is challenging. Furthermore, pathological unilateral hyperplasia has been found to comprise up to 45% of unilateral production,[11] where CT has also been found to be insensitive. CT imaging is therefore evaluated with a few considerations: firstly, to assess the presence of a large (>2.5 cm) unilateral adrenal mass, secondly to assess

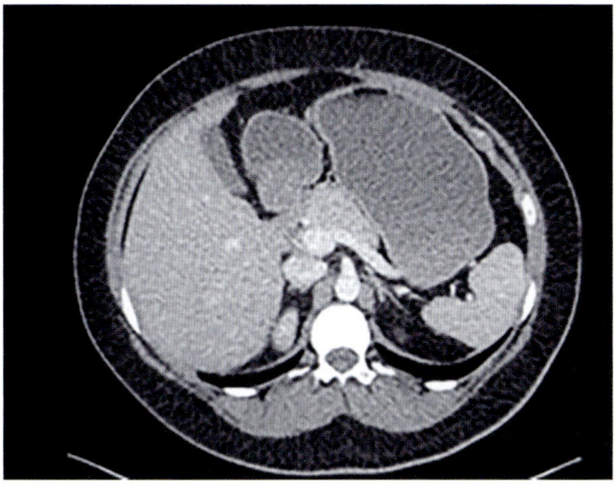

▲ **Figure 52–1.** Normal left adrenal gland.

the anatomy of the right adrenal vein, and finally to provide anatomical guidance to the surgeon in the event of an adrenalectomy (Figure 52–5).

There are a few circumstances in which primary surgical removal can be considered without the need for lateralising the aldosterone production to either adrenal gland with AVS. One such instance is the presence of a large unilateral adrenal mass which may represent an adrenocortical carcinoma. Another such instance is a young patient under 35 with new-onset unequivocal PA evidenced by hypertension, spontaneous hypokalaemia, and clear evidence of a unilateral macronodule on CT imaging with features suggestive of a benign lipid-rich adenoma.[12]

Prior to invasive testing with AVS, patients should be assessed with regard to their potential suitability for an adrenalectomy. If there is no intention to offer surgical

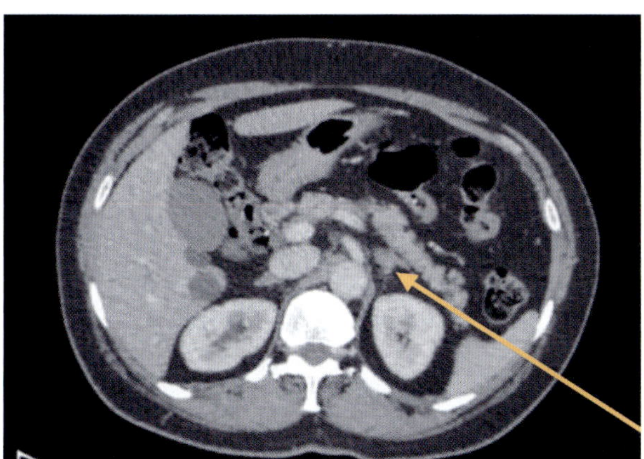

▲ **Figure 52–2.** CT showing a nodular left adrenal gland.

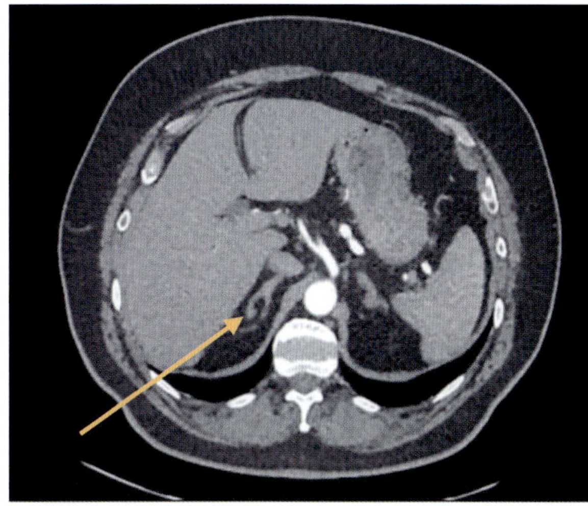

▲ **Figure 52–3.** CT showing right unilateral adrenal microadenoma (<1 cm).

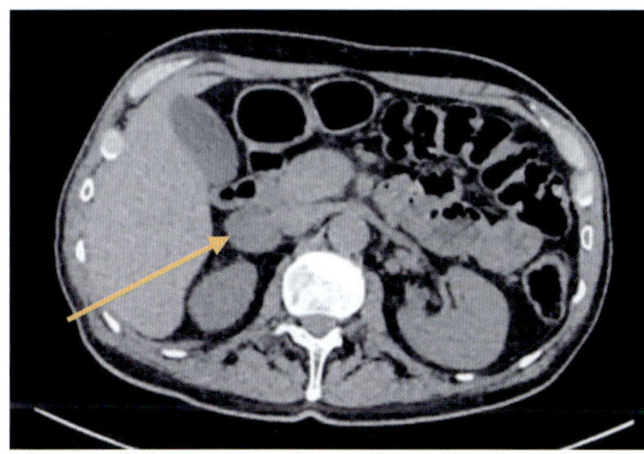

▲ **Figure 52–4.** CT showing right adrenal lesion.

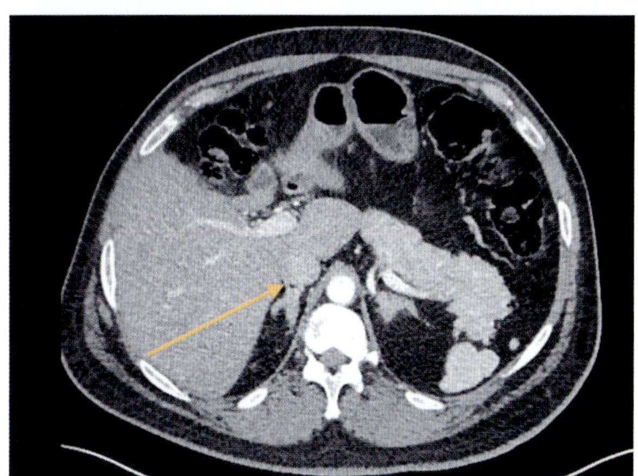

▲ **Figure 52–5.** Right adrenal vein.

intervention following lateralization, then medical treatment with mineralocorticoid receptor antagonists should be used. Patients with unilateral production of aldosterone are suitable for unilateral laparoscopic adrenalectomy, which has a biochemical cure rate of 80% to 100%.

The use of molecular imaging has been advocated for as a noninvasive option for lateralization. Most experience exists with ^{11}C-labeled metomidate as a tracer, with preparatory dexamethasone ensuring that the ligand binds almost exclusively to CYP11B2, the enzyme responsible for the final step of aldosterone synthesis. The results of the MATCH trial, directly comparing AVS with ^{11}C metomidate PET CT, are awaited.[13] Unfortunately, the disadvantage of using ^{11}C metomidate as a tracer is the 20-minutes half-life which necessitates the availability of an onsite radiopharmacy and cyclotron. Promising research with use of 68Ga-Pentixafor as a tracer has been published[14] and a fluorine-labeled compound (18F CETO) very similar to metomidate is also in clinical trials.[15]

ANATOMY

The anatomy of the adrenal veins is notable for its constancy. There is a single central draining vein for both the right and left adrenal veins.[16]

Right Adrenal Vein

The right adrenal vein drains directly into the IVC at the posterolateral aspect (entering the IVC in the 6 o'clock and 9 o'clock position on CT). Cadaver studies have shown the vein averages 3.5 to 5 mm in diameter and ranges from 1 to 15 mm in length, whereas on angiography the vein appears usually around 2 to 3 mm in diameter. The topic of multiple adrenal veins remains controversial and there is evidence to suggest that in a small number of cases (2.4%) they may be present.[17] In addition, the presence of a common origin with an accessory hepatic vein is also disputed. Daunt[18] supports the cadaveric findings[19] in that common origins are not observed but does note some authors have reported adrenal veins entering hepatic venous structures.[20] Our institutional experience supports that common origins are not observed.

Left Adrenal Vein

The left adrenal vein (LAV) joins the more medial inferior phrenic vein to form a common trunk which travels caudally to join the left renal vein.[19] Rarely, less than 1%, the LAV and left inferior phrenic vein enter the left renal vein separately.

Caval and left renal vein variation, which will have been identified on the preprocedure CT, will influence the approach taken within the procedure. A retroaortic left renal vein is the most common variant; this can manifest as a lower positioned left renal vein usually 4 cm lower than a normally sited vein at L3. Other variants include a circumaortic renal vein and bilateral IVCs.[21]

PROCEDURE

AVS can be performed as a day-case procedure. Patients are initially admitted to an endocrine or radiology day-case facility where preprocedure checks are undertaken. If synthetic ACTH is being administered then this can be administered. The procedure is performed in a fluoroscopy suite and they are recovered on the endocrine/day-case ward as per institutional guidance on venous puncture. Local guidelines on cessation of anticoagulation/antiplatelet therapies and clotting should be adhered to.

PATIENT PREPARATION

Medications

Before the patient undergoes AVS, there are several regular medications that should be modified. Particularly, the validity of the results can be affected by hypokalaemia and medications that lead to de-suppression of renin.

Medications which influence potassium and renin should therefore be considered prior to adrenal vein sampling.

Hypokalaemia restrains aldosterone secretion and generous oral supplementation is often required to maintain normo- or near normokalaemia. Derepression of renin has the potential to increase aldosterone production in the contralateral adrenal gland to an APA and therefore obscure lateralization. Positive lateralization can be considered valid, but a negative lateralization may be less reliable and should be approached with caution in the context of hypokalaemia or increased renin.

Historically mineralocorticoid receptors should be withheld for 6 weeks prior to procedure, although with the introduction of eplerenone, a shorter duration of withdrawal may be recommended. Antihypertensive medication adjustments should be made with careful attention to their effect on serum potassium and renin. Therefore, peripheral α1 blockers such as doxazosin and long-acting dihydropyridine or nondihydropyridine calcium-channel blockers such as verapamil are suggested due to their negligible effect on renin.

Patients with drug-resistant hypertension may be on multiple antihypertensive agents including ACE inhibitors, A2RBs, diuretics, and β blockers. Ideally, all these medications should be discontinued prior to AVS, although some consider the use of ACEi, ARBs, and diuretics permissible, so long as renin remains suppressed.[22-24]

Pharmacological Stimulation

There is a diurnal variation in natural ACTH production which has a variable effect on APAs compared with the contralateral adrenal gland. To avoid false negatives, AVS without pharmacological stimulation should occur in the morning when the levels of ACTH are highest.[25] In addition, aldosterone production is pulsatile necessitating bilateral catheterization and simultaneous sampling.

Pharmacological stimulation can be achieved with a synthetic ACTH (synacthen/cosyntropin), which may be given as a bolus or an infusion. This has a number of potential benefits: increased cortisol production from the adrenal glands and increased selectivity index, increased aldosterone produced by the APA, and reduction in stress variations.[24,26] It has also been postulated that synthetic ACTH increases adrenal blood flow, causing venous engorgement, thereby making the cannulation easier.[27]

At our institution synthetic ACTH is given; via a peripheral cannula, 250 μg in 500 mL normal saline is run at 50 μg/h and is given starting 1 hour prior to the sampling.

Analgesia & Anaesthesia

Every effort should be made to make the procedure as least stressful as possible. Activation of the hypothalamic-pituitary-adrenal axis, and subsequently cortisol and aldosterone release from the adrenal glands, is particularly sensitive to emotion and pain-related stress. This causes a reduction in the lateralization index but an increased selectivity index.[28] Local anaesthesia prior to venous puncture is always given. Additional conscious sedation with benzodiazepines (midazolam) and opioids (fentanyl) can also be considered, but patient cooperation and compliance is mandatory for the success of the procedure due to the need for relaxed breathing (to ensure the catheter doesn't disengage) and breath holds.

Equipment

- 6 French vascular sheath
- Vascular contrast media
- Hydrophilic wire
- Right adrenal vein catheters:
    - Renal Double Curve
    - Simmons 1 (SIM1)
    - Cobra C2
    - Multipurpose A2
    - Mikaelsson
- Left adrenal vein catheters:
    - Simmons 2 (SIM2)
    - Simmons 3 (SIM3)
    - Multipurpose A
- Offer catheter alternatives for each side.
    - 2 mL sampling syringes
    - 10 mL sampling syringes

TECHNIQUE

Puncture

Via a right common femoral vein puncture, a 6Fr sheath is introduced using a standard Seldinger technique. If utilising a sequential sampling technique with pharmacological stimulation, then one sheath is sufficient. If simultaneous sampling is required, then a second common femoral vein sheath is inserted ipsilaterally or contralaterally.

Cannulation

A. Right Adrenal Vein

Typically, cannulation of the right adrenal vein (RAV) is the most challenging part of AVS and recognition of the vein is critical. The RAV is therefore usually sampled first if using a sequential technique; since cannulation on the right is more time-consuming than on the left, this minimizes the time between samples.

A number of catheters can be used to cannulate the RAV. The key aim is that the adrenal vein is cannulated superficially to avoid sampling from too deep within the gland and therefore potentially beyond the draining branch vein of an APA. Standard technique suggests forward-facing catheters such as a Renal Double Curve to cannulate the RAV. Reverse curve catheters, such as a SIM1, are adept at cannulating the vein but are more at risk than forward-facing catheters with regard to deep cannulation, so should be used with caution to superficially engage the adrenal vein.[8,29]

Once the suspected vein has been cannulated, care must be taken when injecting contrast not to inject too quickly or forcefully, as there is a risk of discomfort and adrenal hemorrhage (see Figure 52–10 later). The aim is simply to demonstrate the successful cannulation of the adrenal vein. There is a large degree of variation in the appearance of an adrenal venogram, with the most common appearance being a gland-like appearance with a main central stem and spidery branches (Figure 52–6).

A common pitfall is the misrecognition of the inferior accessory hepatic vein (IAHV) as the RAV (Figure 52–7). Careful interrogation of the venogram should be made to assess for any sinusoidal staining or draining veins toward the main hepatic veins/IVC which indicates cannulation of the hepatic vein. If the IAHV is cannulated, it should be used as a marker for the position of the RAV. The RAV origin is reliably found within 5 mm in 70% of patients and not more than 20 mm away. The literature suggests that when the IAHV is found the RAV is successfully cannulated in 92% of cases.[30] The adrenal vein has several communications with emissary veins extending to the perirenal fat. On the right, the emissary veins can course laterally, medially, inferiorly and can communicate with the right renal vein (see Figure 52–11 later), intercostal veins, and phrenic veins.

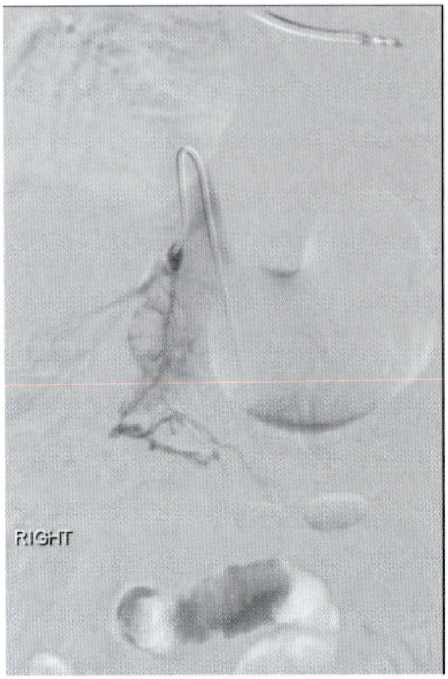

▲ **Figure 52–6.** Right adrenal venogram.

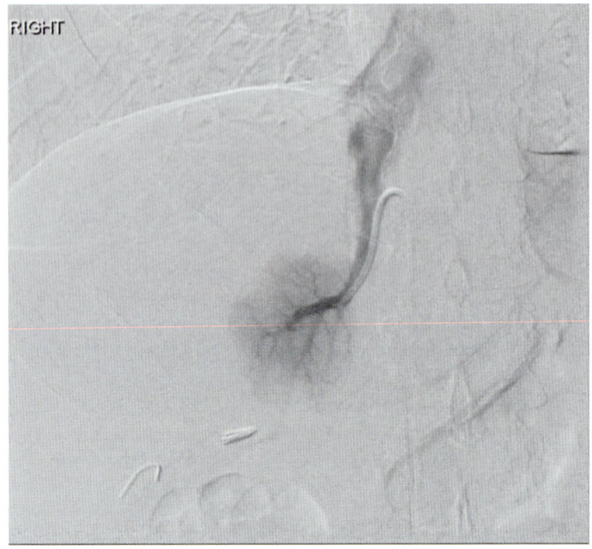

▲ **Figure 52–8.** Inferior accessory hepatic vein.

The appearance of an emissary vein is a reliable sign with a sensitivity of 86% (Figure 52–8).[31]

If there is doubt regarding whether the adrenal vein has been cannulated, a sample should be taken. A confirmatory venogram on completion of the sampling should be taken to ensure that the catheter has not moved and that an adequate sample has been obtained.

B. Left Adrenal Vein

The cannulation of the left adrenal vein (LAV) is typically more straightforward. The consistency with which the vein drains into the superior aspects of the renal vein means that following cannulation of the renal vein, cannulation of the adrenal vein is uncomplicated.

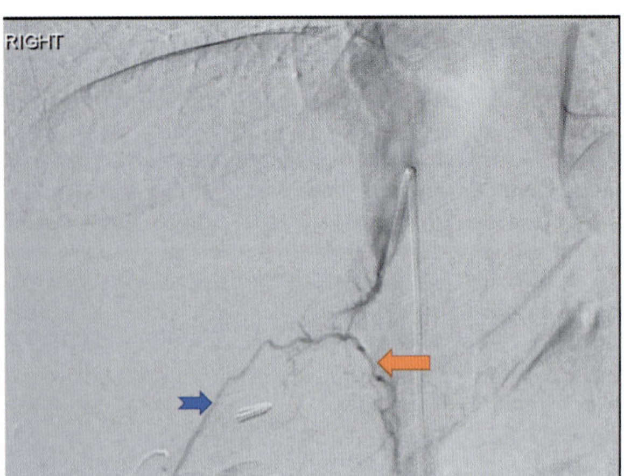

▲ **Figure 52–7.** Lateral (blue arrow) and inferior (orange).

A reverse-curve catheter, for example, SIM2 or SIM3 is most commonly used to cannulate the LAV. After cannulation of the RAV, the catheter can be brought down to the IVC bifurcation and a wire passed into the contralateral iliac vein. A SIM2 catheter can be formed over the IVC bifurcation, obviating the need to form the SIM2 in the right atrium and the subsequent risks of intracardiac catheter manipulation.

The SIM2 catheter is used to cannulate the renal vein and on slow withdrawal, the catheter will usually jump forward into the adrenal vein and the sample can be taken (Figure 52–9). This is generally around the level of the left paraspinal line. If the catheter does not engage, a SIM3 may fit better. Alternatively, the catheter can be withdrawn to close to the origin of the left renal vein and a 0.035″ hydrophilic angled wire advanced into the adrenal vein to guide the catheter. If none of these techniques work, the reverse catheter can be exchanged over a wire in the renal vein for a forward-facing catheter such as a multipurpose with side-holes (MPA2).

Care must be taken not to advance the catheter too far which may inadvertently select the more medial inferior phrenic vein or, as with the RAV, bypass a branch vein from an aldosterone-producing adenoma.

Sampling

The sampling protocol involves taking multiple venous samples from the right and left adrenal veins which are

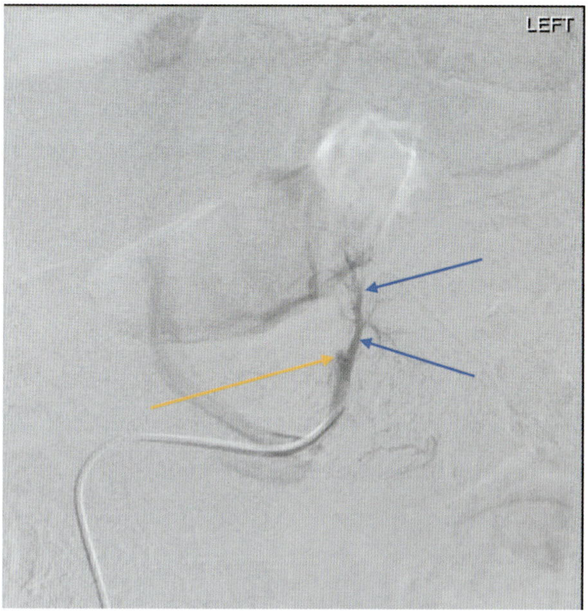

▲ **Figure 52–9.** Left common trunk cannulation. Left adrenal vein and gland seen on venography (blue arrows). Orange arrow highlights the insertion of the phrenic vein.

compared with peripheral samples taken from the vascular sheath. A sampling protocol should be established with the local endocrine team and laboratory.

Some centres have intraprocedural PCC (plasma cortisol concentration) available, which allows confirmation of cannulation of the adrenal vein in real time.[32,33] Mostly, the success of the procedure is assessed when the results are available. Comparison of the hormone levels between the adrenal vein samples and the peripheral circulation are evaluated.

SAFETY & COMPLICATIONS

Procedural complications include adrenal vein rupture, thrombosis, and adrenal hemorrhage. The most severe complication is that of adrenal hemorrhage which was reported up to 10% in early studies,[34] but more recent literature suggests that the rate is approximately 0.6%.[35] This improvement has been attributed to a reduction in the volume of contrast injected and not performing routine diagnostic adrenal venography. Interestingly, it is noted that the rate of complications is inversely proportional to the number of cases a particular operator and centre has performed. Patients with PA or Cushing disease are thought to have a greater degree of vein fragility increasing their susceptibility to adrenal hemorrhage.[20] Adrenal hemorrhage is recognized

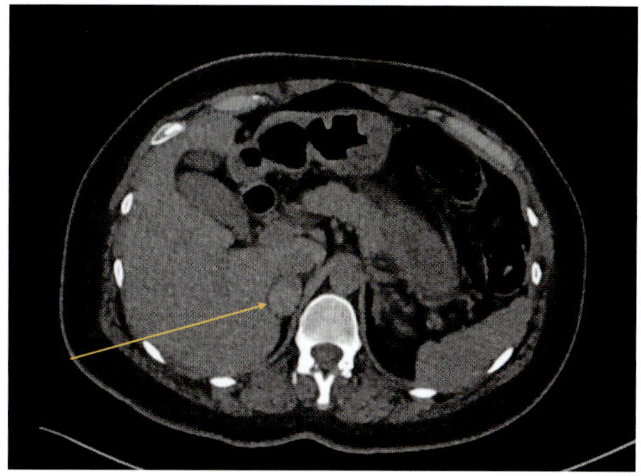

▲ **Figure 52–10.** Noncontrast CT shows right adrenal hemorrhage.

by persistent flank pain after the cessation of contrast injection, often increasing to a peak within 30 to 60 minutes. If suspected, it should be investigated and confirmed with noncontrast CT imaging (Figure 52–10). The pain can be associated with a fever that can last up to 48 hours and is treated with supportive measures. Adrenal hemorrhage

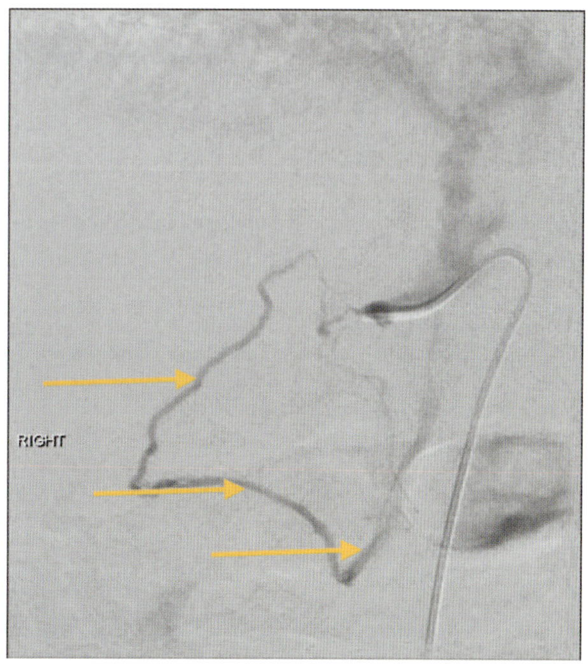

▲ **Figure 52–11.** Right adrenal venogram shows communication with a lateral emissary vein draining into the right renal vein.

Table 52–1. Variations in adrenal vein sampling protocol.

Study	Cosyntropin Use	Sequential vs Simultaneous	Selectivity Index	Lateralization Index
SPARTICUS[36]	Cont. infusion	Sequential	≥3	≥4.0 w/ CSI ≤1
Deipolyi[37]	Cont. infusion	sequential	>3	>4
Kocjan[38]	Cont. infusion	sequential	>5	>4
Pasternak[39]	Cont. infusion	sequential	NR	≥4
Ota[40]	Bolus 250 μg, sample 15 min later	Simultaneous	≥5	NR
Miotti[11,41]	No stim	Simultaneous	≥1.1	≥2.0
Conn[42]	No stim	Sequential	≥2	≥3
Wolley[43]	No stim	Sequential	≥3	≥2* with CSI ≤1
Lee[44] Bellavance[45]	Pre and post 250 μg bolus	Simultaneous	≥3 Pre ≥5 Post	>2 Precosyntropin >4 Postcosyntropin
Teng[46]	Pre and post (bolus + infusion)	Sequential	>2 Precosyntropin >3 Postcosyntropin	>3 Precosyntropin >4 Postcosyntropin
Webb[47]	Pre and post (bolus + infusion)	Simultaneous	>5	>4
Japanese Endocrine[48]	250 μg cosyntropin bolus	Simultaneous	≥5 and ≥200 μg/dL cortisol	≥2.6 or unilateral aldosterone ≥14,000 pg/mL
Funder[7]	No conclusive rec	No conclusive rec	>5 with cosyntropin >2 without cosyntropin	>4 with cosyntropin >2 without cosyntropin
Expert Consensus[24]	No conclusive rec	No conclusive rec	≥3 with cosyntropin ≥2 without cosyntropin	≥4 with cosyntropin ≥2 without cosyntropin

NR = not reported.
*Wolley et al. used a modified lateralization index of (Dominant Adrenal Aldosterone/Cortisol)/(IVC Aldosterone/Cortisol) ≥2 and a CSI ≤1.

can further complicate the situation as there is a suggestion that leads to retroperitoneal adhesions which makes laparoscopic adrenalectomy a more complicated procedure.[24]

RESULTS INTERPRETATION

There is a great degree of heterogeneity between sampling technique and cutoff values used in interpreting sensitivity index (SI) and lateralization index (LI). These are summarized in a systematic review published by Quencer et al. (Table 52–1).[22] This highlights the variation that exists in performing AVS and its interpretation. The values used below are therefore a pragmatic guideline.

Selectivity Index (SI) = "adrenal vein" cortisol/ peripheral vein cortisol

SI is used to determine sample adequacy and the success in cannulating the adrenal veins by assessing the cortisol gradient between the adrenal venous samples and the peripheral venous samples. SIs of more than 2 and more than 5 for unstimulated and stimulated procedures, respectively, are most commonly used to indicate successful cannulation. The cutoffs must be met bilaterally before the laterality index is applied.

Lateralization Index (LI) = dominant adrenal vein aldosterone ÷ cortisol/nondominant adrenal vein aldosterone ÷ cortisol).

The LI is used to determine whether the production of aldosterone is unilateral or bilateral. LIs of more than 2 and more than 4 for unstimulated and stimulated patients are suggestive of unilateral production. The literature supports that the greater the laterality index, the higher the chance of biochemical cure in patients who undergo adrenalectomy.

CONCLUSION

AVS is a critical tool in subtyping PA and allows the patient to be commenced on their most appropriate treatment pathway. It is a procedure that can, in experienced hands, be performed safely and quickly with minimal risk.

REFERENCES

1. Mills KT, Stefanescu A, He J. The global epidemiology of hypertension. *Nat Rev Nephrol.* 2020;16(4):223-237.
2. Oparil S, Zaman MA, Calhoun DA. Pathogenesis of hypertension. *Ann Int Med.* 2003;139(9):761-776.
3. Byrd JB, Turcu AF, Auchus RJ. Primary aldosteronism: practical approach to diagnosis and management. *Circulation.* 2018;138(8):823-835.
4. Brown NJ. Contribution of aldosterone to cardiovascular and renal inflammation and fibrosis. *Nat Rev Nephrol.* 2013;9(8):459-469.
5. Freel EM, Stanson AW, Thompson GB, et al. Adrenal venous sampling for catecholamines: a normal value study. *J Clin Endocrinol Metabol.* 2010;95(3):1328-1332.
6. Kaltsas G, Mukherjee JJ, Kola B, et al. Is ovarian and adrenal venous catheterization and sampling helpful in the investigation of hyperandrogenic women? *Clin Endocrinol.* 2003; 59(1):34-43.
7. Funder JW, Carey RM, Mantero F, et al. The management of primary aldosteronism: case detection, diagnosis, and treatment: an endocrine society clinical practice guideline. *J Clin Endocrinol Metabol.* 2016;101(5):1889-1916.
8. Young Jr WF, Stanson AW, Thompson GB, Grant CS, Farley DR, van Heerden JA. Role for adrenal venous sampling in primary aldosteronism. *Surgery.* 2004;136(6):1227-1235.
9. Nwariaku FE, Miller BS, Auchus R, et al. Primary hyperaldosteronism: effect of adrenal vein sampling on surgical outcome. *Arch Surg.* 2006;141(5):497-503.
10. Kempers MJ, Lenders JWM, van Outheusden L, et al. Systematic review: diagnostic procedures to differentiate unilateral from bilateral adrenal abnormality in primary aldosteronism. *Ann Int Med.* 2009;151(5):329-337.
11. Citton M, Viel G, Rossi GP, Mantero F, Nitti D, Iacobone M. Outcome of surgical treatment of primary aldosteronism. *Langenbeck's Arch Surg.* 2015;400(3):325-331.
12. Küpers EM, Amar L, Raynaud A, Plouin PF, Steichen O. A clinical prediction score to diagnose unilateral primary aldosteronism. *J Clin Endocrinol Metabol.* 2012;97(10):3530-3537.
13. Brown M. *Is Metomidate PET-CT Superior to Adrenal Venous Sampling in Predicting Outcome From Adrenalectomy in Patients With Primary Hyperaldosteronism.* 2021.
14. Ding J, Tong A, Zhang Y, et al. Functional characterization of adrenocortical masses in nononcologic patients using 68Ga-Pentixafor. *J Nucl Med.* 2022;63(3):368-375.
15. Thomas M. *CETO First in Human Trial.* 2020.
16. Gagnon R. The venous drainage of the human adrenal gland. *Rev Can Biol.* 1956;14(4):350-359.
17. Scholten A, Cisco RM, Vriens MR, Shen WT, Duh QY. Variant adrenal venous anatomy in 546 laparoscopic adrenalectomies. *JAMA Surg.* 2013;148(4):378-383.
18. Daunt N. Adrenal vein sampling: how to make it quick, easy, and successful. *Radiographics.* 2005;25(suppl_1):S143-S158.
19. Monkhouse W, Khalique A. The adrenal and renal veins of man and their connections with azygos and lumbar veins. *J Anat.* 1986;146:105.
20. Bookstein J. The roles of angiography in adrenal disease. *Abram's Angiography.* 1983:1395-1424.
21. Trigaux JP, Vandroogenbroek S, De Wispelaere JF, Lacrosse M, Jamart J. Congenital anomalies of the inferior vena cava and left renal vein: evaluation with spiral CT. *J Vasc Interv Radiol.* 1998;9(2):339-345.
22. Quencer KB. Adrenal vein sampling: technique and protocol, a systematic review. *CVIR Endovasc.* 2021;4(1):1-11.
23. Rossi GP. A comprehensive review of the clinical aspects of primary aldosteronism. *Nat Rev Endocrinol.* 2011;7(8):485-495.
24. Rossi GP, Auchus RJ, Brown M, et al. An expert consensus statement on use of adrenal vein sampling for the subtyping of primary aldosteronism. *Hypertension.* 2014;63(1):151-160.
25. Rossi GP, Pitter G, Bernante P, Motta R, Feltrin G, Miotto D. Adrenal vein sampling for primary aldosteronism: the assessment of selectivity and lateralization of aldosterone excess baseline and after adrenocorticotropic hormone (ACTH) stimulation. *J Hypertension.* 2008;26(5):989-997.
26. Rossitto G, Amar L, Azizi M, et al. Subtyping of primary aldosteronism in the AVIS-2 study: assessment of selectivity and lateralization. *J Clin Endocrinol Metabol.* 2020;105(6):2042-2052.
27. Violari EG, Arici M, Singh CK, et al. Adrenal vein sampling with and without cosyntropin stimulation for detection of surgically remediable aldosteronism. *Endocrinol, Diabetes Metabol.* 2019;2(2):e00066.
28. Seccia TM, Miotto D, Battistel M, et al. A stress reaction affects assessment of selectivity of adrenal venous sampling and of lateralization of aldosterone excess in primary aldosteronism. *Eur J Endocrinol.* 2012;166(5):869.
29. Tan SYT, Ng KS, Tan C, Chuah M, Zhang M, Puar TH. Bilateral aldosterone suppression in patients with right unilateral primary aldosteronism and review of the literature. *J Endocr Soc.* 2020;4(4):bvaa033.
30. Trerotola SO, Smoger DL, Cohen DL, Fraker DL. The inferior accessory hepatic vein: an anatomic landmark in adrenal vein sampling. *J Vasc Interv Radiol.* 2011;22(9):1306-1311.
31. Kohi MP, Agarwal VK, Naeger DM, et al. The inferior emissary vein: a reliable landmark for right adrenal vein sampling. *Acta Radiologica.* 2015;56(4):454-457.
32. Mengozzi G. Rossato D, Bertello C, et al. Rapid cortisol assay during adrenal vein sampling in patients with primary aldosteronism. *Clin Chem.* 2007;53(11):1968-1971.
33. Rossi E, Regolisti G, Perazzoli F, et al. Intraprocedural cortisol measurement increases adrenal vein sampling success rate in primary aldosteronism. *Am J Hypertension.* 2011;24(12):1280-1285.
34. Walters N, Thomson K. *Urogenital venography.* Practical Interventional Uroradiology. Edward Arnold: Edinburgh, Scotland; 1993.
35. Rossi GP, Barisa M, Allolio B, et al. The Adrenal Vein Sampling International Study (AVIS) for identifying the major subtypes of primary aldosteronism. *J Clin Endocrinol.* 2012;97(5):1606-1614.
36. Dekkers T, Prejbisz A, Kool LJS, et al. Adrenal vein sampling versus CT scan to determine treatment in primary aldosteronism: an outcome-based randomised diagnostic trial. *Lancet Diabetes Endocrinol.* 2016;4(9):739-746.
37. Deipolyi AR, Bailin A, Wicky S, Alansari S, Oklu R. Adrenal vein sampling for Conn's syndrome: diagnosis and clinical outcomes. *Diagnostics.* 2015;5(2): 254-271.
38. Kocjan T, Jensterle M, Vidmar G, Vrckovnik R, Berden P, Stankovic M. Adrenal vein sampling for primary aldosteronism: a 15-year national referral center experience. *Radiol Oncol.* 2020;54(4):409-418.
39. Pasternak JD, Epelboym I, Seiser N, et al. Diagnostic utility of data from adrenal venous sampling for primary aldosteronism despite failed cannulation of the right adrenal vein. *Surgery.* 2016;159(1):267-274.

40. Ota H, Seiji K, Kawabata M, et al. Dynamic multidetector CT and non-contrast-enhanced MR for right adrenal vein imaging: comparison with catheter venography in adrenal venous sampling. *Eur Radiol.* 2016;26(3):622-630.
41. Miotto D, Toni RD, Pitter G, et al. Impact of accessory hepatic veins on adrenal vein sampling for identification of surgically curable primary aldosteronism. *Hypertension.* 2009;54(4):885-889.
42. Vonend O, Ockenfels N, Gao N, et al. Adrenal venous sampling: evaluation of the German Conn's registry. *Hypertension.* 2011;57(5):990-995.
43. Wolley MJ, Gordon RD, Ahmed AH, Stowasser M. Does contralateral suppression at adrenal venous sampling predict outcome following unilateral adrenalectomy for primary aldosteronism? A retrospective study. *J Clin Endocrinol Metabol.* 2015;100(4):1477-1484.
44. Lee J, et al. Clinical outcomes of primary aldosteronism based on lateralization index and contralateral suppression index after adrenal venous sampling in real-world practice: a retrospective cohort study. *BMC Endocr Disord.* 2020;20(1):114. Published 2020 Jul 29.
45. Bouchard-Bellavance R, Perrault F, Soulez G, et al. Adrenal vein sampling: external validation of multinomial regression modelling and left adrenal vein-to-peripheral vein ratio to predict lateralization index without right adrenal vein sampling. *Clin Endocrinol.* 2020;93(6):661-671.
46. Teng J, Hutchinson ME, Doery DCG, et al. Role of adrenal vein sampling in primary aldosteronism: the Monash Health experience. *Int Med J.* 2015;45(11):1141-1146.
47. Webb R, Mathur A, Chang R, et al. What is the best criterion for the interpretation of adrenal vein sample results in patients with primary hyperaldosteronism? *Ann Surg Oncol.* 2012;19(6):1881-1886.
48. Nishikawa T. The Task Force Committee on Primary Aldosteronism, the Japan Endocrine Society. Guidelines for the diagnosis and treatment of primary aldosteronism—the Japan Endocrine Society 2009. *Endocr J.* 2011;58:711-721.

Pancreatic Anatomy & Physiology

53

Angela E. Thelen, MD, MHPE
Christopher R. McHenry, MD

GENERAL CONSIDERATIONS

The pancreas is an endocrine and exocrine organ that plays an important role in both glucose homeostasis and digestion. While the endocrine and exocrine pancreas are often thought of as separate portions of the gland, they have a sophisticated regulatory feedback system for digestive enzyme and hormone secretion. In this chapter, we describe the embryology, anatomy, and physiology of the pancreas, focusing on important aspects that relate to endocrine surgery. A thorough understanding of the anatomy of the pancreas and its relationship to adjacent viscera and blood vessels is important for the surgeon who treats endocrine pancreatic neoplasms and performs adrenalectomy. Important aspects of pancreatic imaging and pancreatic surgical procedures for neuroendocrine tumors of the pancreas are reviewed in general terms only, as the evaluation and management of specific neuroendocrine tumors of the pancreas are discussed elsewhere in the textbook.

EMBRYOLOGY

The embryology of the pancreas is important to help understand normal pancreatic anatomy and the relationship of the pancreas to other adjacent structures as well as common anatomic variations, particularly in pancreatic ductal anatomy. The pancreas derives from the foregut. Pancreatic development begins during the fifth week of gestation from two endodermal outpouchings, a dorsal pancreatic bud from the duodenum and a smaller ventral pancreatic bud from the hepatic diverticulum (Figure 53–1). Pancreatic acinar and islet cells differentiate from the endodermal cells of these embryonic buds. The first glucagon-producing cells, or alpha (A) cells appear in the third week of gestation. The first organized islets appear in the tenth week of gestation. There is subsequently a significant increase in endocrine cell numbers, particularly beta (B) or insulin-producing cells. Postnatally, there is a surge of B-cell proliferation in the first two years of life, with minimal B-cell proliferation thereafter.[1]

The ventral bud develops into the inferior portion of the head and uncinate process of the pancreas. The duct from the ventral bud connects directly to the common bile duct, ultimately forming part of the main pancreatic duct, known as the *duct of Wirsung* (Figure 53–1). The larger dorsal pancreatic bud develops into the neck, body, tail, and the remainder of the head of the pancreas. The duct from the dorsal pancreatic bud drains directly into the duodenum, part of which becomes the accessory pancreatic duct, known as the *duct of Santorini* (Figure 53–1). During the eighth week of gestation with gut rotation, the ventral pancreatic bud rotates clockwise, posteriorly around the duodenum to fuse with the dorsal pancreatic bud. The ductal system of each bud fuses together in the pancreatic head, such that the majority of the pancreas drains via the duct of Wirsung, which joins common bile duct to form a common channel before emptying into the duodenum (Figure 53–1).[2]

Failure of the duct of Wirsung and duct of Santorini to fuse results in *pancreas divisum*, a congenital anatomic variation, which occurs in approximately 4% to 10% of patients.[3] In this anatomic variant, the majority of the pancreas drains through the duct of Santorini and the minor papilla while the inferior portion of the pancreatic head and uncinate process drain via the duct of Wirsung and major papilla. While this most commonly occurs as an asymptomatic anatomic variant, a minority of patients can develop pancreatitis from a relative outflow obstruction if the minor papilla is inadequate to handle the flow of pancreatic juices from the majority of the gland.[2] Pancreas divisum leading to pancreatitis can sometimes require treatment with sphincteroplasty of the minor papilla.[3,4]

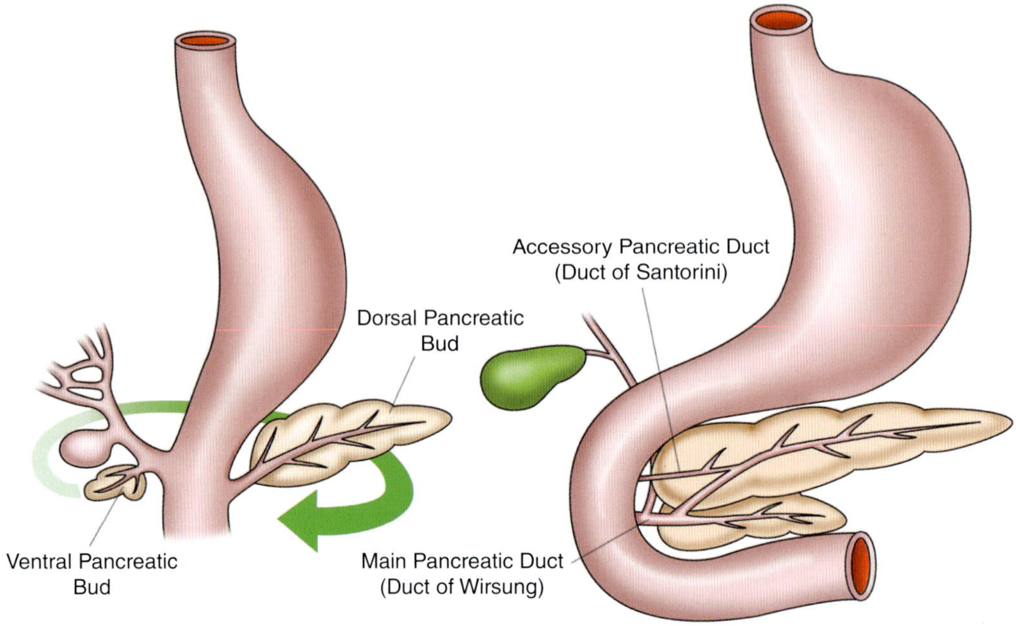

▲ **Figure 53–1.** Embryologic development of the pancreas from a dorsal and a ventral pancreatic bud. **(A)** The ventral pancreatic bud rotates clockwise, posteriorly around the duodenum (indicated by the arrow). **(B)** Anatomic relationship of the pancreatic primordia and the ductal system following posterior migration of the ventral pancreatic bud, fusion of the dorsal and ventral pancreatic buds, and coalescence of the ducts.

SURGICAL ANATOMY

Gross Anatomy

The pancreas is a retroperitoneal organ. Inflammatory or neoplastic conditions of the pancreas may present with epigastric, left upper quadrant, or back pain, but because of the retroperitoneal location of the pancreas, pain originating from pancreatic pathology is typically poorly localized and often ill-defined in nature. The pancreas is 15 to 20 cm in length, 3 cm in width, and 1.5 cm in thickness and weighs 75 to 100 g in an adult.

The pancreas lies in a transverse oblique position anterior to the second lumbar vertebrae, extending upward from the C-loop of the duodenum on the right where it is fixed, to the splenic hilum on the left where it is mobile (Figure 53–2). The root of the transverse mesocolon lies along the anterior margin of the gland. The stomach is anterior to the pancreas. The inferior vena cava, aorta, portal vein, mesenteric vessels, and left adrenal gland are posterior to the pancreas. The pancreas is separated into five main divisions: the head, uncinate process, neck, body, and tail.

A. Divisions of the Pancreas (Figure 53–2)

1. Head—The head of the pancreas is the part of the gland that is nestled in the C-loop of the duodenum, posterior to the transverse mesocolon. The pancreatic head lies to the right of the superior mesenteric artery (SMA). Posterior to the head of the pancreas are the inferior vena cava (IVC), the right renal artery, and both renal veins. The common bile duct runs in a deep groove on the posterior aspect of the pancreatic head until it passes through the parenchyma of the pancreas to join the main pancreatic duct at the ampulla of Vater.[5]

2. Uncinate Process—The uncinate process is a posterolateral projection of the inferior portion of the head of the pancreas. With the pancreatic head, the uncinate process wraps around the right side of the portal vein to end posteriorly near the space between the SMA and superior mesenteric vein (SMV), passing behind the retropancreatic vessels and remaining anterior to the IVC and aorta. The venous branches draining the head and uncinate process enter along the right lateral and posterior sides of the portal vein.

3. Neck—The neck of the pancreas is defined as the short segment overlying the superior mesenteric vessels, which divides the pancreas into approximately two equal parts. The confluence of the superior mesenteric and splenic veins forming the portal vein is present at the inferior border of the neck of the pancreas. Typically, there are no anterior venous tributaries to the portal vein and a plane can be developed

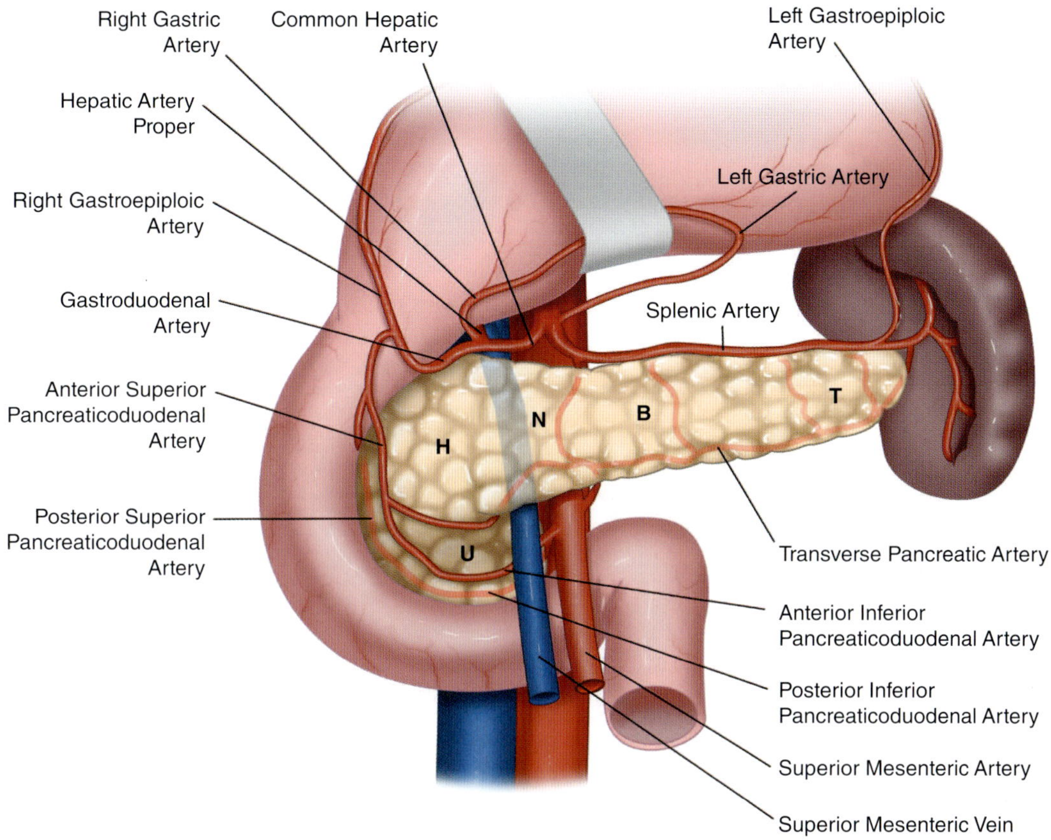

▲ **Figure 53–2.** Anatomy of the pancreas demonstrating its relationship to surrounding structures and its arterial blood supply. B, body; H, head; N, neck; T, tail; U, uncinate process.

between the neck of the pancreas and the portal vein and SMV during pancreatic resection, unless a tumor is invading the vein anteriorly.

4. Body—The body of the pancreas lies just anterior to the splenic vessels and to the left of the superior mesenteric vessels. Division of the gastrocolic omentum exposes the body and tail of the pancreas in the lesser sac, posterior to the stomach. The base of the transverse mesocolon attaches to the inferior margin of the body and tail of the pancreas. The anterior surface of the body is covered by peritoneum.

Pancreatic pseudocysts that occur in the body of the pancreas can be drained into the posterior wall of the stomach. The splenic artery traverses along the posterior superior edge of the body and tail of the pancreas. The splenic vein runs in a groove on the posterior surface of the pancreas and runs parallel and inferior to the artery. The splenic vein is fed by multiple fragile venous branches from the pancreatic parenchyma that must be divided when performing a spleen-preserving distal pancreatectomy.

5. Tail—The tail of the pancreas is the segment of the gland continuous with the body of the pancreas and intimately related to the hilum of the spleen. The tail of the pancreas is anterior to the splenic vessels, the left adrenal gland, and the left kidney. It is important to be aware of the pancreatic tail's relationship to surrounding viscera, as its position nestled in the hilum of the spleen makes it easy to injure during splenic mobilization during a left adrenalectomy or mobilization of the splenic flexure of the colon. The pancreas may also be confused for the left adrenal gland during laparoscopic left adrenalectomy.

Ductal Anatomy (Figure 53–3)

A. Pancreatic Duct of Wirsung

The pancreatic duct of Wirsung, or the main pancreatic duct, forms from the coalescence of the ducts from the dorsal and ventral pancreatic buds (Figure 53–1). It is usually approximately 2 to 3 mm in diameter. It is present midway between

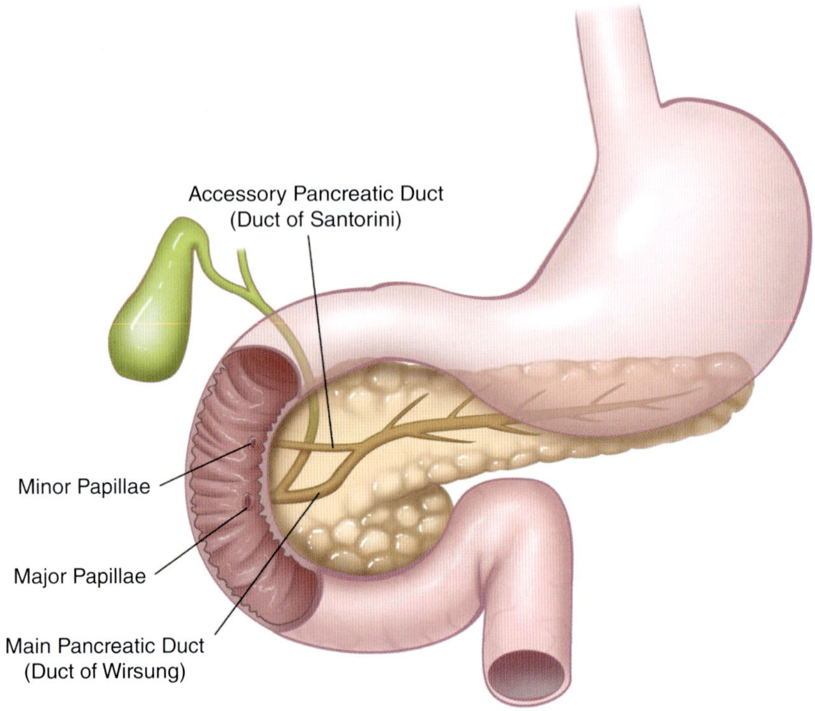

Figure 53–3. Pancreatic ductal anatomy and the major and minor papillae.

the superior and inferior borders of the pancreas. It begins in the tail of the pancreas and travels through the parenchyma to the head where it merges with the common bile duct to form a common channel. The pancreatic duct of Wirsung drains the majority of the pancreas.[5]

The pressure in the main pancreatic duct is about twice that of the common bile duct, which is thought to prevent reflux of bile into the pancreatic duct. The duct usually runs closer to the posterior surface of the gland than the anterior surface. Together with the common bile duct, the pancreatic duct of Wirsung empties into the duodenum at the hepatopancreatic ampulla, commonly known as the ampulla of Vater, located on the major duodenal papilla. The major papilla is on the medial aspect of the second portion of the duodenum. The muscle fibers around the ampulla form the sphincter of Oddi, which controls the flow of pancreatic and biliary secretions into the duodenum.

B. Accessory Duct of Santorini

The accessory duct of Santorini, or the lesser pancreatic duct, forms from the embryological dorsal pancreatic bud. The accessory duct of Santorini drains the uncinate process and the inferior portion of the head of the pancreas. In most patients, the accessory duct drains directly into the duodenum through the minor papilla, which is located approximately 2 cm proximal to the ampulla of Vater. The minor papilla is most often posterior to the gastroduodenal artery (GDA) and is at risk of injury during surgery for peptic ulcer disease. However, anatomic variation in the course and drainage pattern of the lesser pancreatic duct is common.

C. Common Channel

The common channel is formed when the pancreatic duct of Wirsung merges with the common bile duct. The length of this channel can be variable, with some patients having a true common channel present for several millimeters while in others the two ducts empty directly into the major papilla. The common channel empties into the duodenum via the ampulla of Vater.[5]

Neurovascular Supply

A. Arterial Supply (Figure 53–2)

The arterial supply of the pancreas derives from multiple branches of the celiac artery and the SMA. From the celiac trunk, the common hepatic artery gives rise to the GDA before continuing toward the porta hepatis as the proper hepatic artery. The right gastric artery branches off the GDA just superior to the duodenum, and the GDA travels inferiorly, anterior to the pancreas and posterior to the duodenal bulb. At the inferior border of the duodenum, the GDA divides into the right gastroepiploic artery and the superior pancreaticoduodenal artery, which further branches into the anterior and posterior superior pancreaticoduodenal arteries. As the SMA passes behind the pancreas, it gives off the inferior pancreaticoduodenal artery at the inferior margin of the neck of the pancreas. This divides into the anterior and posterior inferior pancreaticoduodenal arteries. The head of the pancreas is supplied by an arcade of vessels from the superior and inferior pancreaticoduodenal arteries.[6]

The body and tail of the pancreas are supplied by the splenic artery. The splenic artery arises from the celiac trunk and courses along the superior border of the body and tail of the pancreas, giving off multiple branches to the gland along its path toward the spleen. The first branch coming off the splenic artery, and usually the most prominent branch, is the dorsal pancreatic artery. The next two branches are the greater pancreatic artery and the caudal pancreatic artery. These vessels run perpendicular to the splenic artery and connect with the inferior pancreatic artery, also known as the transverse pancreatic artery, along the inferior border of the pancreas. The inferior pancreatic artery typically arises from the SMA and runs parallel to the splenic artery, also supplying the body and tail of the pancreas. The arcades formed by this network of vasculature within the body and tail of the pancreas help account for the rich blood supply of the gland.[6]

Variations in the arterial anatomy around the pancreas are common. In up to 15% of patients, the right hepatic artery will arise from the SMA and travel upward toward the liver along the posterior aspect of the head of the pancreas, known as a *replaced right hepatic artery*. Similarly, the common hepatic artery and GDA can also arise from the SMA.[7] Finally, the origin of the dorsal pancreatic artery can be variable. While most commonly originating from the splenic artery, variations have been described where it originates from the common hepatic artery, the celiac trunk, or, less frequently, the SMA. It is important to recognize these anatomic variants on preoperative imaging and in the operating room to avoid iatrogenic injury.[8]

B. Venous Drainage

The venous drainage of the pancreas parallels the arterial supply. However, there can be significant variability in the number, location, and pattern of drainage for the veins of the pancreas.[6] It is important to recognize that the veins are typically thin-walled and fragile and can be easily injured.

The head and uncinate process of the pancreas are drained by an anterior and posterior venous arcade, with the anterior superior and both inferior pancreaticoduodenal veins draining into the SMV and the posterior superior pancreaticoduodenal vein draining into the portal vein just above the neck of the pancreas. The veins terminate in the lateral and posterior aspects of the portal vein and SMV. There are numerous other additional venous branches coming from the pancreatic parenchyma that drain directly into the lateral and posterior aspect of the portal vein, which may be injured during retraction of the head of the pancreas.

The anterior inferior pancreaticoduodenal vein joins the right gastroepiploic vein and middle colic vein to form a common venous trunk, which enters the SMV. Traction on the transverse mesocolon can tear these veins, which then retract into the parenchyma of the pancreas, making bleeding difficult to control.

Multiple venous tributaries from the neck, body, and tail of the pancreas drain superiorly into the splenic vein and inferiorly into the transverse pancreatic vein. The transverse pancreatic vein joins the inferior mesenteric vein before it joins with the splenic vein to become the SMV. Ligation of the splenic vein during distal pancreatectomy or en bloc resection of an adrenal cortical carcinoma or as a result of an injury during left adrenalectomy requires a splenectomy. Comparatively, ligation of the splenic artery does not necessarily require splenectomy, since the spleen still has blood supply from the short gastric arteries.

C. Lymphatic Drainage

The lymphatic drainage of the pancreas follows the course of the blood vessels. The head and uncinate process of the pancreas are drained by pancreaticoduodenal and pyloric lymph nodes and the lymph nodes along the common bile duct and hepatic artery proper. The neck, body, and tail of the pancreas are drained by superior and inferior pancreaticosplenic lymph nodes. They are present along the inferior border of the pancreatic body and along the splenic artery and vein. Anterior and superior peripancreatic lymph nodes drain to the celiac lymph node basin and the posterior and inferior peripancreatic lymph nodes drain to the superior mesenteric and periaortic nodal basins. Both drainage pathways ultimately drain into the cisterna chyli at the lower end of the thoracic duct. Peripancreatic lymphatics also communicate with the lymph nodes of the transverse mesocolon and mesentery of the proximal jejunum.[9]

D. Nerve Innervation

The pancreas has both sympathetic and parasympathetic nerve innervation via the abdominopelvic splanchnic nerves and the celiac branch of the vagus nerve, respectively. Sympathetic and parasympathetic nerves carry visceral afferent (sensory) and visceral efferent (motor) fibers to the pancreas, which are involved with regulation of blood flow, cell secretion, and pain sensation. The parasympathetic nervous system stimulates endocrine and exocrine secretion, and the sympathetic system inhibits secretion, although endocrine and exocrine pancreatic secretion is primarily under hormonal control. Nerves pass from the celiac and superior mesenteric plexus and follow the pancreatic blood vessels to give rise to intrapancreatic periacinar nerve plexuses.[10] The pancreas also has a rich supply of visceral afferent or sensory nerve fibers that are responsible for the intense pain associated with pancreatitis. The somatic fibers travel superiorly to the celiac ganglia, and interruption of these somatic fibers by chemical splanchnicectomy, that can be accomplished using image-guidance or at operation to help reduce the transmission of pain.

MICROSCOPIC ANATOMY & PHYSIOLOGY

The pancreatic gland is predominantly made up of hormone-secreting endocrine cells and digestive enzyme-secreting acinar cells, with accompanying vasculature and lymphatics. The exocrine pancreas acts as an accessory digestive organ through the secretion of digestive enzymes. Meanwhile, the primary physiologic role of the endocrine pancreas is regulation of glucose homeostasis.

Exocrine Secretion

The exocrine pancreas makes up approximately 85% of pancreatic gland mass and produces pancreatic juice that enters the duodenum through the pancreatic duct. The pancreas secretes 500 to 800 cc of pancreatic juice per day. Pancreatic juice is a colorless, odorless, alkaline, isosmotic fluid that is a combination of acinar cell and ductal cell secretions. The major constituents of pancreatic juice include amylase, proteases, and lipases, which are the enzymes responsible for the digestion of carbohydrates, proteins, and fats, respectively. An overview of these enzymes and their function is provided in Table 53–1.

A. Histomorphology (Figure 53–4)

The exocrine pancreas is made up of acinar cells and ductal cells. Acinar cells secrete the pancreatic enzymes that facilitate digestion. Each individual acinar cell synthesizes all the types of pancreatic digestive enzymes in the endoplasmic reticulum. The specific ratio of enzymes released by the acinar cells is adjusted based on the composition of food ingested.

Approximately 40 acinar cells are arranged in a spherical unit called an *acinus*. Acinar cells are pyramid-shaped with their apices facing the lumen of the acinus. Near the apex of each cell, enzyme-containing zymogen granules fuse with the apical cell membrane to release pancreatic enzymes into the lumen of the acinus via exocytosis. Proteins combine with water and bicarbonate secretions from centroacinar cells, and the pancreatic juice then travels into small intercalated ducts, several of which combine to form interlobular ducts.

Ductal cells in the interlobular ducts contribute fluid and electrolytes to the pancreatic fluid. The interlobular ducts then join to form secondary ducts, which empty into the main pancreatic duct. The destruction of this branching ductal tree from inflammation or scarring can contribute to damage of the exocrine pancreas and exocrine pancreatic insufficiency.[11]

B. Carbohydrate Digestion

Pancreatic amylase, the enzyme responsible for the digestion of carbohydrates, is secreted in its active form. The digestion of starch and glycogen is initiated by salivary amylase and is completed by pancreatic amylase. The two amylase enzymes have the same activity, both hydrolyzing starch and glycogen to glucose, maltose, maltotriose, and dextrins. The simple sugars can then be transported across the brush border of intestinal epithelial cells via active transport.

C. Protein Digestion

Proteolytic enzymes, responsible for the digestion of proteins, are produced as proenzymes that require activation.

Table 53–1. Function of exocrine pancreatic enzymes.

Pancreatic Enzymes			
Enzyme	**Activated By**	**Active Form**	**Function**
Carbohydrate			
Amylase	NA	NA	Breaks down starch and glycogen into simple sugars
Protein			
Trypsinogen	Enterokinase	Trypsin	Cleave bonds between amino acids
Chymotrypsinogen	Enterokinase, Trypsin	Chymotrypsin	Cleave bonds between amino acids
Proelastase	Enterokinase, Trypsin	Elastase	Cleave bonds between amino acids
Procarboxypeptidase A&B	Enterokinase	Carboxypeptidase A&B	Cleave amino acids from end of peptide chains
Lipid			
Pancreatic lipase	NA	NA	Hydrolyzes triglycerides to 2-monoglycerides and two fatty acids
Phospholipase A2	Trypsin	Phospholipase A2	Hydrolyzes phospholipids
Cholesterol esterase	NA	NA	Hydrolyzes neutral lipids

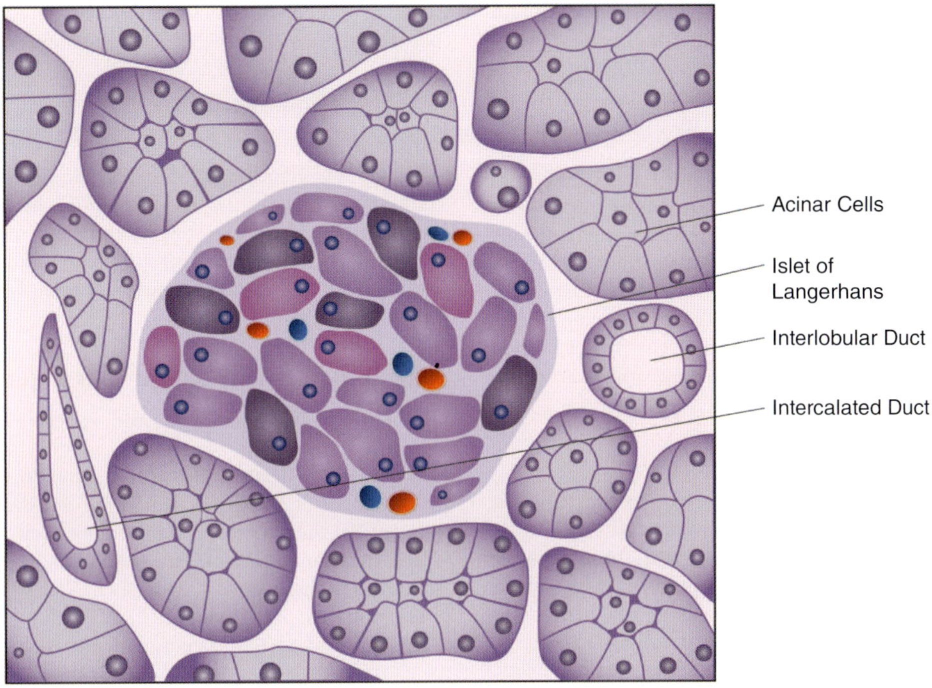

Figure 53–4. Histomorphology of the pancreas.

These proenzymes are packaged into secretory vesicles and secreted into the duodenum within the pancreatic juice. Once in the duodenum, they are converted into their active form.

Enterokinase, a brush-border glycoprotein produced by duodenal mucosal cells, first activates trypsinogen to its active form, trypsin, through the hydrolysis of the N-terminal fragment of the molecule. Trypsin then catalyzes the activation of the rest of the proteolytic enzymes. The inhibition of trypsinogen activation within the pancreas ensures that other proteolytic enzymes remain in their precursor state before they enter the intestine. Trypsinogen is kept in its inactive form within the pancreas by pancreatic secretory trypsin inhibitor, also known as *serine protease inhibitor Kazal type 1* (SPINK1), which is secreted by acinar cells.[12] Failure to express a normal trypsinogen inhibitor or a mutation in the *PRSS1* gene encoding for cationic trypsinogen are common causes of hereditary pancreatitis[12,13]

Additional proteolytic enzymes produced by the pancreas include chymotrypsin, elastase, carboxypeptidase A and B, and phospholipase. Together, these enzymes break down proteins into single amino acids and small peptides. Specifically, trypsin, chymotrypsin, and elastase cleave amino acid bonds within target peptide chains. Carboxypeptidase A and B cleave amino acids at the end of peptide chains. Individual amino acids and small dipeptides are transported into intestinal epithelial cells through active transport mechanisms.

D. Lipid Digestion

Fat digestion is primarily completed by pancreatic lipase, which is secreted in an active form. Triglycerides cannot be directly absorbed through the intestinal mucosa. Pancreatic lipase hydrolyzes triglycerides to 2-monoglyceride and two fatty acids. The activity of pancreatic lipase is facilitated by colipase, which is also secreted by the pancreas. The digestion of fats requires the presence of bile salts in the lumen of the intestine, which aid in the emulsification of triglycerides.

Additional pancreatic enzymes involved in lipid digestion include phospholipase A2, carboxylic ester hydrolase, and cholesterol esterase. Phospholipase A2 is secreted by the pancreas as a proenzyme that is activated by trypsin in the duodenum. Its primary function is to hydrolyze phospholipids. Carboxylic ester hydrolase and cholesterol esterase hydrolyze neutral lipid substrates including cholesterol esters, fat-soluble vitamins, and triglycerides. Hydrolyzed fat is packaged into micelles for transport into the intestinal epithelial cells, where fatty acids are reassembled and packaged inside chylomicrons for transport through the lymphatic system and into the bloodstream.

E. Additional Fluid and Electrolytes

Centroacinar and intercalated duct cells secrete the water and electrolytes present in pancreatic juice. Centroacinar cells are located near the center of the acinus. They contain the enzyme carbonic anhydrase, which is required for bicarbonate secretion. A higher concentration of bicarbonate is secreted as the pancreatic secretory rate increases, whereas chloride secretion has an inverse relationship with bicarbonate secretion. Sodium and potassium concentrations are kept constant regardless of secretory rates. Secretin, released from cells in the duodenal mucosa in response to acidic chyme passing through the pylorus, is a major stimulant for bicarbonate secretion. This buffers the acidic fluid entering the duodenum from the stomach. Cholecystokinin (CCK) potentiates secretin-stimulated bicarbonate secretion. Gastrin and acetylcholine stimulate gastric acid secretion, which is also a weak stimulus of pancreatic bicarbonate secretion.[14]

F. Regulation

A complex system regulates exocrine pancreatic function including type of digestion, rate, processing, and distribution of absorbed nutrients. The endocrine pancreas, through physical approximation of islets with the exocrine pancreas, presence of specific islet hormone receptors on plasma membranes of pancreatic acinar cells, and existence of an islet-acinar portal blood system, influences the adjacent exocrine pancreatic secretions. Insulin stimulates exocrine secretion, amino acid transport, and protein and enzyme synthesis. On the other hand, glucagon inhibits those activities. Somatostatin and pancreatic polypeptide (PP) also inhibit exocrine secretion.

Endocrine Secretion

Whereas the exocrine pancreas makes up approximately 85% of pancreatic gland mass, the endocrine pancreas makes up only approximately 2% of pancreatic gland mass, 10% is made up of extracellular matrix, and 3% is made up of blood vessels. Endocrine cell secretion enters directly into the bloodstream to complete its primary role of glucose homeostasis and regulation.

A. Histomorphology of Islet Cells (Figure 53–4)

There are approximately 1 million islets of Langerhans in the normal adult pancreas varying in size from 40 to 900 μm. Most islets contain around 3000 to 4000 cells of the five major islet cell types, which are not evenly distributed throughout the pancreas. The five major cell types, with their major hormone products, are outlined in Table 53–2. These cell types include alpha (A), beta (B), delta (D), epsilon (E), and pancreatic polypeptide (PP) or F cells.

In contrast to acinar cells, which secrete the full breadth of exocrine enzymes, each islet cell type secretes predominantly one hormone. A cells make up approximately 10% of islet cell mass and secrete glucagon. They are located at the

Table 53–2. Pancreatic islet cell types and function.

Islet Cell	Location Within Pancreas	Major Hormones Secreted	Function
Alpha (A) cell	Evenly distributed	Glucagon	• Promote gluconeogenesis, glycogenolysis, fatty acid breakdown, ketogenesis • Inhibit glucose uptake, glycogenesis, protein synthesis
Beta (B) cell	Body/tail	Insulin	• Promote glucose uptake, glycogenesis, protein synthesis • Inhibit gluconeogenesis, glycogenolysis, fatty acid breakdown, ketogenesis
		Amylin (IAPP)	• Promote satiety and delay gastric emptying • Inhibit glucagon secretion
		Pancreastatin	• Promote glucagon secretion • Inhibit insulin and somatostatin secretion
Delta (D) cell	Evenly distributed	Somatostatin Vasoactive Inhibitory Polypeptide (VIP)	• Inhibit secretion of other hormones in the gastrointestinal tract • Stimulate insulin release • Stimulate water secretion into pancreatic juice • Inhibit gastric acid secretion • Induce smooth muscle relaxation
Epsilon (E) cell	Evenly distributed	Ghrelin	• Stimulate appetite • Inhibit insulin secretion
PP cell (F cell)	Head and uncinate process	Pancreatic polypeptide	• Stimulate gastric acid secretion • Inhibit pancreatic exocrine secretion • Facilitate hepatic effect of insulin

periphery of the islet and are evenly distributed throughout the pancreas. B cells make up about 70% of total islet cell mass and secrete insulin. They are generally located in the central portion of each islet and are concentrated in the body and tail of the pancreas. D cells make up 5% of islet cell mass and secrete somatostatin. They are evenly distributed throughout the islet and are concentrated in the body and tail of the pancreas. E cells make up less than 1% of islet cell mass and secrete ghrelin. PP cells, also known as F cells, make up approximately 15% of total islet mass and secrete pancreatic polypeptide. They are located peripherally within the islet and are heavily concentrated within the uncinate process of the pancreas.

The composition of the islets varies based on their location within the pancreas. As aforementioned, A and D cells are both evenly distributed throughout the pancreas. Islets in the head and uncinate process have a greater proportion of PP cells and fewer A cells, whereas islets in the body and tail of the pancreas contain more A cells and fewer PP cells. This diversity in distribution becomes clinically relevant, as a pancreatoduoudenectomy removes a significant share of the PP cells within the pancreas. This may, in part, account for the increased incidence of glucose intolerance after this operation compared to a distal pancreatectomy with equivalent amounts of tissue resected. Similarly, the predominance of A cells in the body and tail of the pancreas explains the typical location of glucagonomas.

Islet cell hormones are secreted directly into the bloodstream. Larger islets are located closer to major arterioles and smaller islets are embedded more deeply in the parenchyma of the pancreas. The portal microcirculation of pancreatic islets allows for hormonal regulation through endocrine-to-endocrine cell signaling. Afferent arterioles enter the islet in the periphery. The islet is then perfused from the B cell core outward, so the B cells are perfused first, followed by the A and lastly the D cells. The order of intraislet vascular perfusion allows B cells to inhibit A cell secretion and A cells to stimulate D cell secretion.[15]

B. Insulin

Insulin is a 56-amino-acid polypeptide that was first discovered in 1920 by an orthopedic surgeon, Frederick Banting, and a medical student, Charles Best, who shared a Nobel Prize in Physiology and Medicine for their work.[16] Insulin is synthesized and secreted by B cells in response to glucose. It has two chains, an alpha and a beta chain, which are joined by two disulfide bridges. The location of these disulfide bridges is highly conserved between species.

Insulin is first synthesized as a precursor peptide called proinsulin. Proinsulin is made in the endoplasmic reticulum of the beta cell and transported to the Golgi complex. The alpha and beta chains, in addition to being joined by the disulfide bridges, are connected by a C-peptide which is cleaved in the Golgi complex. After cleavage of the C-peptide, insulin is moved via microtubules and packaged into secretory granules. It is subsequently released directly into the bloodstream via exocytosis. Insulin and C-peptide are secreted into the bloodstream in equimolar amounts. This is important since patients with an insulinoma have elevated insulin, proinsulin, and C-peptide levels, whereas patients with surreptitious insulin injection have elevated insulin levels, but with proinsulin and C-peptide levels that are not elevated.

The primary function of insulin is the regulation of glucose. Insulin promotes the storage of energy by facilitating the transport of glucose into cells, inhibiting glycogenolysis and fatty acid breakdown, and stimulating protein synthesis, thereby decreasing plasma glucose levels. There are two phases of insulin secretion in response to glucose. The first is an immediate response with a short burst of stored insulin lasting about 4 to 6 minutes. Second is a longer, sustained release that requires the active production of new insulin in the beta cell.

Insulin binds a specific glycoprotein cell surface receptor. Insulin receptors have been well characterized, and consist of dimeric, tyrosine kinase transmembrane proteins. The stimulation of insulin receptors is dependent on the concentration of insulin. After stimulation of the insulin receptor, glucose is actively transported across the cell membrane by membrane-bound transporters. Several classes of glucose transporters exist throughout the body with varying affinities for glucose. Insulin is primarily metabolized by the liver and has a half-life of approximately 4 to 6 minutes.

Insulin synthesis and secretion are highly regulated, with the most significant factor being changes to glucose concentration. Insulin release is maximally stimulated at blood glucose concentrations of 400 to 500 mg/dL. The administration of oral glucose has a greater effect on insulin secretion than an equivalent amount of intravenous glucose, even if blood levels are similar, as oral glucose also stimulates the release of enteric hormones that augment the release of insulin. These insulinotropic factors are termed *incretins.*

Incretins act on beta cells to stimulate the release of insulin and include glucagon, gastric inhibitory polypeptide (GIP), glucagon-like peptide-1 (GLP-1), cholecystokinin (CCK), amino acids (arginine, lysine, and leucine), and free fatty acids. Humoral inhibitors of insulin secretion include somatostatin, amylin, leptin, and pancreastatin.[14,17] Vagal (cholinergic) neural signals and beta sympathetic fibers additionally stimulate insulin release.[18] Conversely, alpha sympathetic fibers strongly inhibit the release of insulin.

There is a significant functional reserve in the secretory capacity of insulin. If the remnant gland is healthy, up to 80% to 85% of the pancreas can be resected without a patient developing diabetes. However, in patients with chronic pancreatitis or other pancreatic diseases, a larger remnant may be present after pancreatic resection and can still lead to the development of diabetes.

Diabetes can be the result of insulin deficiency, as seen in type 1 diabetes mellitus or the result of insulin resistance, as seen in type 2 diabetes. Insulin resistance can be secondary to a decreased number of insulin receptors or a decreased affinity of receptors for insulin. Insulin resistance or type 2 diabetes is associated with a downregulation of insulin receptors and a relative hyperinsulinemia. Conversely, insulin deficiency results in the upregulation of insulin receptors, leading to an enhanced sensitivity to insulin which can increase the risk of insulin-induced hypoglycemia. Additional types of diabetes are associated with select impairments of hepatic or peripheral insulin receptors (ie, pancreatogenic diabetes or maturity-onset diabetes of the young [MODY]).[12]

C. Glucagon

Glucagon is secreted by A cells and is the major counterregulatory hormone to insulin. It is a 29-amino-acid straight chain polypeptide. The primary function of glucagon is to elevate blood glucose levels, which it facilitates through the promotion of hepatic glycogenolysis, gluconeogenesis, and lipolysis. Like insulin, the synthesis and release of glucagon is primarily regulated by serum glucose levels but in an inverse fashion. An increase in blood glucose has a strong suppressive effect on glucagon secretion. A low blood glucose and the amino acids arginine and alanine stimulate the release of glucagon. Insulin, somatostatin, GLP-1, and GIP inhibit glucagon secretion via a paracrine effect within the islet.[19]

Neural fibers regulate the secretion of glucagon in a similar fashion to insulin, with cholinergic and beta sympathetic fibers stimulating glucagon release and alpha sympathetic fibers inhibiting glucagon release. The loss of pancreatic innervation in the setting of pancreatic or islet cell transplantation can lead to changes in the pattern and quality of insulin and glucagon secretion. Excessive levels of glucagon, as seen in glucagonomas, can lead to hyperglycemia. On the other hand, insufficient glucagon can lead to profound hypoglycemia, and the loss of glucagon responsiveness to a fall in blood glucose levels in pancreatogenic diabetes (type 3c) increases the risk for hypoglycemia.[20]

D. Somatostatin

Somatostatin is secreted by D cells and is a 14-amino-acid polypeptide. It was originally isolated from the hypothalamus and has a wide anatomic distribution. Somatostatin plays a fundamental role in the regulation of processes throughout the body. There is one gene that encodes a common precursor of somatostatin, which is then differentially processed to create two tissue-specific bioactive products, somatostatin-14 and somatostatin-28. The primary pancreatic role of these peptides is the inhibition of endocrine and exocrine secretion. They also affect neurotransmission, gastrointestinal and biliary motility, intestinal absorption, vascular tone, and cell proliferation.

Five different somatostatin receptors (SSTRs) have been characterized, all of which are G-protein-coupled receptors with seven highly conserved transmembrane domains and unique amino and carboxy termini. Somatostatin-28 is selective for SSTR5, while octapeptide analogues of somatostatin such as octreotide bind to SSTR2, SSTR3, and SSTR5. Synthetic analogues have a longer serum half-life than endogenous somatostatin, and their inhibitory effect is often utilized to treat endocrine and exocrine pancreatic disorders including secretory diarrhea, enteric and pancreatic fistulas, and endocrine hypersecretory syndromes. Early research examining the efficacy of octreotide in the reduction of pancreatic and enteric fistulae output and improved time to healing was promising. However, current studies have failed to find strong evidence for its use.[21-23] In addition, multiple randomized controlled trials have failed to demonstrate a decrease in the incidence of postoperative pancreatic fistulae with the use of prophylactic octreotide.[24-26]

E. Pancreatic Polypeptide

Pancreatic polypeptide (PP) is a 36-amino-acid straight chain polypeptide, which is secreted by F cells. It was discovered in 1968 during the process of insulin purification. PP is a part of the peptide YY/neuropeptide Y family of polypeptides. PP functions in the modulation of food intake and energy homeostasis, with its greatest role appearing to be in glucose regulation through the regulation of hepatic insulin receptor gene expression. It has also been shown to inhibit bile secretion, gallbladder contraction, and pancreatic exocrine secretion.

Infusion of PP in humans leads to loss of appetite, and decreased levels of PP have been noted in obesity. Cholinergic stimulation secondary to hypoglycemia is a strong stimulant for PP secretion and is the predominant regulator of PP. Similarly, protein and fatty acids in the duodenum also stimulate PP release. Vagotomy effectively ablates the increased PP typically seen after a meal.[27]

F. Ghrelin

Ghrelin is a 28-amino acid peptide hormone produced by endocrine cells in the gastrointestinal tract. While primarily synthesized in the gastric mucosa, ghrelin-producing cells, also termed E cells, have been found in low numbers within the pancreatic islet. Ghrelin functions in metabolic regulation and energy balance. It inhibits the release of insulin from the pancreas and blocks the effects of insulin on the liver, thereby increasing hepatic glucose production.

Ghrelin is an orexigenic or appetite-stimulating peptide, and increased plasma levels have been noted in obesity. In diet-induced obesity, ghrelin exacerbates hyperglycemia and leads to impaired glucose tolerance. In starvation or severe calorie restriction, ghrelin increases blood glucose concentrations to maintain glucose homeostasis. Ghrelin also stimulates growth hormone secretion via growth hormone-releasing hormone secretion from the pituitary gland.[15]

Other Peptide Products of Islet Cells

A. Amylin

Amylin, also known as islet amyloid polypeptide (IAPP), is a 37-amino acid polypeptide predominantly secreted by B cells. It is a regulatory peptide that functions to inhibit the secretion of both insulin and glucagon within the islet as well as their function at distant binding sites. It was first discovered due to its ability to aggregate in islets as amyloid deposits, which have been noted in patients with type 2 diabetes. The cytotoxic effects of IAPP deposits are thought to contribute to the loss of B cells in type 2 diabetes.

B. Pancreastatin

Pancreastatin is a 49-amino acid regulatory polypeptide derived from the processing of chromogranin A. The primary role of pancreastatin is the modulation of energy metabolism via a counterregulatory effect to insulin. It induces hepatic glycogenolysis and lipolysis in adipocytes. Increased levels of pancreastatin have been found in insulin-resistance conditions including gestational diabetes and hypertension, and the peptide may play an important role in the pathophysiology of these diseases.

C. Neuropeptides

There are a number of neuropeptide products of islet cells including vasoactive intestinal peptide (VIP), galanin, and serotonin. VIP is a 28-amino acid polypeptide that stimulates insulin release and inhibits gastric secretion. It is found throughout the gastrointestinal and respiratory tract where it causes vasodilation and bronchodilation.[28] Galanin is a 29-amino acid peptide that acts as a sympathetic neurotransmitter of the islets. Its effects therefore correlate with the effect of sympathetic stimulation, inhibiting insulin release and stimulating glucagon secretion.

DIAGNOSTIC IMAGING FOR PANCREATIC NEUROENDOCRINE TUMORS

In recent years, there has been a significant increase in diagnosis of pancreatic neuroendocrine tumors (PNETs) as a result of incidental identification on imaging studies done for other reasons. Most PNETs are found in asymptomatic patients.[29] Regardless of presentation, these patients require a clinical assessment for pain and signs and symptoms of excess hormone secretion, hormone measurement based on clinical suspicion, and further cross-sectional or more advanced imaging to localize the PNET. Typically, the first step in localization is cross-sectional imaging with computed tomography (CT) or magnetic resonance imaging (MRI).

Computed Tomography (CT) (Figure 53–5)

CT is most often the first-line imaging modality for diagnosis and characterization of a PNET. In addition to being a fast and widely available method, CT provides excellent anatomic characterization of the pancreas. A complete CT sequence includes multiphase imaging with precontrast views and arterial, pancreatic, and venous phases after the administration of intravenous contrast.[30] Due to the rich vascular supply of PNETs, these tumors appear as a hyperenhancing mass.

The sensitivity of CT for the localization of a PNET depends on the size of the tumor, and therefore thinner collimation techniques are critical to better identify the tumors. The sensitivity of CT for identifying PNETs is approximately 82%, with a lower sensitivity for tumors less than 1.5 cm.[31] The sensitivity of CT for the localization of insulinomas and duodenal gastrinomas is also lower, as these tumors are

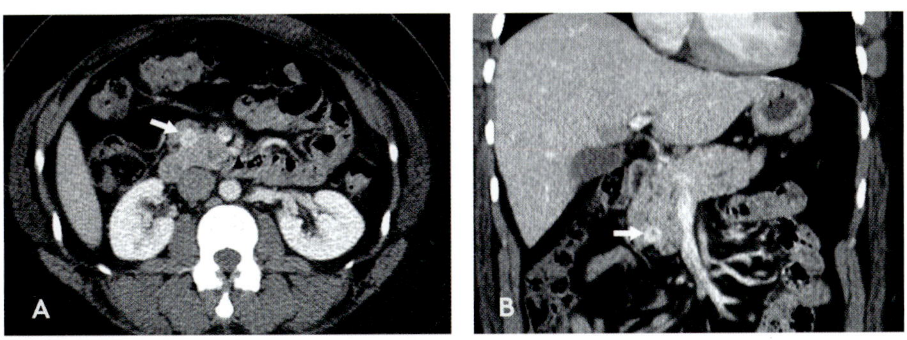

Figure 53–5. Axial **(A)** and coronal **(B)** computed tomograms with IV contrast demonstrating a PNET (arrow) that is characteristically hyperenhancing compared to the remainder of the pancreas. This hyperenhancement is best seen during the arterial phase of contrast.

typically smaller at presentation. CT is also used for the identification of liver metastases from PNETs.[32,33]

Magnetic Resonance Imaging (MRI) (Figure 53–6)

MRI is also commonly used for the localization of PNETs, especially in patients for which radiation exposure is a concern. Complete MRI includes T1- and T2-weighted sequences, dynamic three-dimensional imaging with venous, arterial, and delayed sequences before and after gadolinium contrast administration, and diffusion-weighted sequences.[30] On T1-weighted imaging, PNETs are typically hypointense compared to the rest of the pancreas. On T2-weighted images, PNETs demonstrate relative hyperintensity. However, less frequently they can be T2 hypointense.

PNETs characteristically demonstrate arterial enhancement on dynamic gadolinium-enhanced images. Similar to CT, the sensitivity of MRI for the detection of PNETs is dependent on tumor size. While the overall sensitivity of MRI for the detection of PNETs is approximately 79%, it is less for smaller tumors. MRI with diffusion-weighted sequences is superior to CT in the characterization of hepatic metastases.[32-34]

Endoscopic Ultrasound (EUS)

EUS is a commonly used imaging modality for PNETs that cannot be localized on CT scan or MRI. EUS has a sensitivity of approximately 90% for tumors of all sizes and allows for better visualization of the morphological features and spatial relationships of the tumor.

Typically, PNETs appear as a sonolucent mass of uniform consistency on EUS. Like MRI, there is no exposure to radiation with EUS. Fine-needle aspiration biopsy may also be performed under EUS guidance to obtain a pathologic diagnosis.[32] EUS has a lower sensitivity for the detection of lesions in the pancreatic tail, a limited ability to examine the liver for metastases, and it is invasive and operator dependent.[30]

Somatostatin Receptor Scintigraphy (SRS)

Somatostatin receptors are expressed by 80% to 100% of well-differentiated PNETs, with the exception of insulinomas, which carry a lower rate of expression. SRS uses radiolabeled somatostatin analogues targeting somatostatin receptors (SSTR2 > SSTR3 and SSTR5), which are overexpressed by PNETs. It is a useful adjunct for the localization of tumors not evident of CT or MRI.

SRS has a sensitivity of approximately 80% for PNETs; however, sensitivity is affected by tumor size. Poorly differentiated PNETs typically do not express somatostatin receptors and are rarely identified by SRS.[32] SRS is limited in defining the exact localization of PNETs. Rather, it provides information on the general vicinity of the tumor, most often within a few centimeters. It does not offer the same anatomic precision seen with CT, MRI, or EUS, thereby limiting its usefulness for surgical planning. Physiologic somatostatin uptake and uptake as a result of benign conditions may also occur. In many institutions, 68-Ga DOTATATE positron emission tomography (PET)/CT has replaced somatostatin scintigraphy as the preferred functional imaging study for evaluation of PNETs.[33,35]

68-Ga DOTATATE Positron Emission Tomography (PET)/CT (Figure 53-7)

68-Ga DOTATATE PET/CT uses DOTATATE labeled with the radioisotope gallium-68. Similar to SRS, DOTATATE binds to somatostatin receptors overexpressed by PNETs. 68-Ga DOTATATE PET/CT is the functional imaging modality of choice for the localization of PNETs, as it has many advantages over SRS and other imaging techniques. First, DOTATATE scans have a higher sensitivity than other imaging modalities, with a sensitivity of approximately 93%. In addition, the tracer has a higher affinity for SSTRs, increasing the diagnostic accuracy and detection of PNETs. The PET scan provides whole-body imaging at one time,

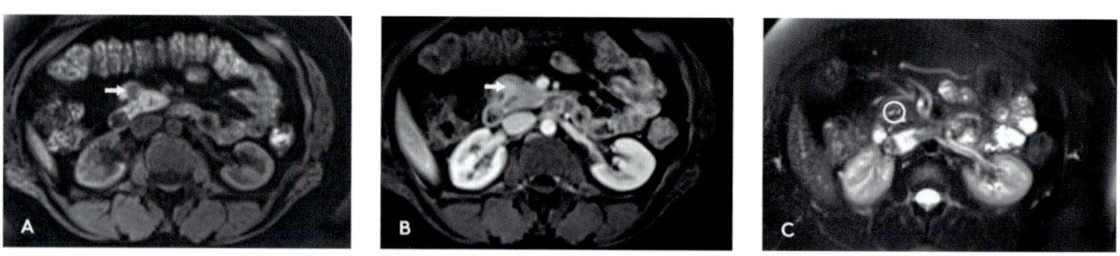

▲ **Figure 53–6.** Pre- **(A)** and postcontrast **(B)** T1 with fat saturation and T2 with fat saturation **(C)** magnetic resonance images demonstrating the characteristic appearance of a PNET. **(A)** A PNET (arrow) is hypointense compared to the remainder of the normal pancreas which is bright on a precontrast T1 image related to pancreatic exocrine function. **(B)** A PNET (arrow) is relatively hyperintense on a T1 image after contrast administration due to hypervascularity. **(C)** PNETs may also have internal cystic degeneration, which manifest as areas of focal increased T2 signal on this T2 image with fat saturation.

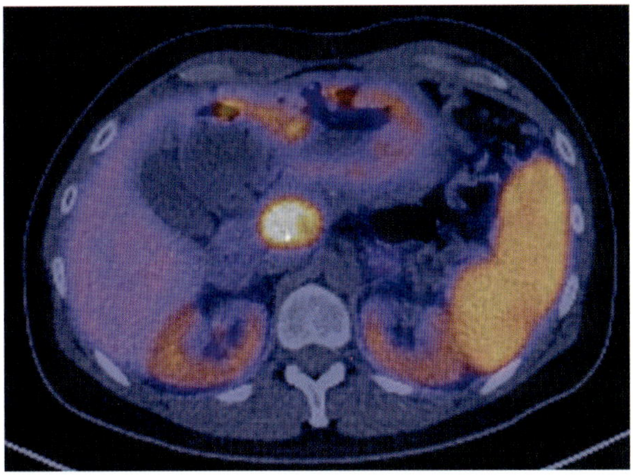

▲ **Figure 53–7.** 68-Ga DOTATATE positron emission tomographic image demonstrating uptake in a PNET in the head of the pancreas.

allowing for the detection of distant metastases. Ga DOTATATE PET/CT also requires a lower dose of radiation and 68-Ga DOTATATE has a shorter half-life than other radiolabeled tracers, allowing for faster scanning. Finally, the resolution of the scan is higher, providing more precise anatomic localization. However, a contrast-enhanced CT or MRI is still necessary for surgical planning.[32,33,36]

Fluorodeoxyglucose (FDG) PET

FDG-PET scans are rarely used for the imaging of PNETs, because PNETs do not have avid glucose uptake secondary to their slow growth. Therefore, the somatostatin receptor functional imaging modalities are significantly more useful for the detection and localization of PNETs. However, FDG-PET scanning can be useful for the imaging of poorly differentiated PNETs. As aforementioned, poorly differentiated PNETs are less likely to express somatostatin receptors and therefore do not always show up well on SRS or 68-Ga DOTATATE PET/CT. In addition, they can be faster-growing tumors with a higher avidity for glucose uptake, making FDG-PET a better imaging technique for poorly differentiated PNETs.[32,36]

OPERATIONS FOR NEUROENDOCRINE TUMORS

The primary treatment of PNETs is surgical resection. The surgical approach and extent of pancreatic resection is determined by the type of tumor, tumor location, extent of disease, whether the tumor is sporadic or a manifestation of Multiple Endocrine Neoplasia type I (MEN I), as well as patient factors. The goal in most patients is to remove the primary tumor and regional lymph nodes while preserving normal pancreatic parenchyma.[37] Surgical options for resection include simple enucleation, distal pancreatectomy with or without splenectomy, pancreatoduodenectomy (Whipple procedure), and, rarely, total pancreatectomy.[38] For patients with gastrinoma and MEN I, duodenotomy and resection of duodenal gastrinomas, distal pancreatectomy, enucleation of tumors in the head, and uncinate process of the pancreas and lymphadenectomy are performed. PNETs are often small and noninvasive, making them amenable to minimally invasive laparoscopic or robotic approaches.[39]

Exposure of the Pancreas

Exposure of the pancreas in patients with a PNET can be obtained through an open approach using an upper midline or bilateral subcostal incision. Alternatively, a minimally invasive approach with or without robotic assistance can be used. For a minimally invasive approach, the patient can be placed in the supine, lithotomy, or left semilateral decubitus position for lesions in the head or uncinate process of the pancreas or supine, lithotomy, or right lateral decubitus position for lesions in the pancreatic tail.

Operation for a PNET is begun by exploring the abdomen for extrapancreatic disease, with special attention to the liver and peritoneal surfaces looking for metastases. The entire pancreas is examined. PNETs may be small (<2 cm) and multiple. Intraoperative ultrasound is a useful adjunct for detecting small PNETs and defining the relationship of a PNET to the pancreatic duct and adjacent vascular structures.[40] It is also useful for evaluation of the liver for metastatic disease. The duodenum and peripancreatic lymph nodes are also examined for extrapancreatic neuroendocrine tumors.

Ninety percent of gastrinomas are found in the gastrinoma triangle (Figure 53–8). The boundaries of the gastrinoma triangle are the junction of the cystic duct and common bile duct superiorly, the second and third portions of the duodenum inferiorly, and the junction of the neck and body of the pancreas medially. Nonfunctional PNETs and insulinomas are evenly distributed throughout the pancreas. Glucagonomas most commonly occur in the tail of the pancreas.

The neck, body, and tail of the pancreas are exposed by dividing the gastrocolic ligament while the stomach is retracted upward and the transverse colon is retracted downward. The peritoneum along the inferior border of the pancreas is incised, separating the base of the transverse mesocolon from the inferior margin of the body and tail of the pancreas medially to the middle colic vein and laterally to the splenic flexure of the colon. The splenocolic ligament is divided and the splenic flexure of the colon is mobilized. This allows access to the posterior surface of the pancreas and the splenic artery and splenic vein.

Exposure of the head of the pancreas is obtained by performing a complete Kocher maneuver, which allows for bi-digital palpation of the head and uncinate process of

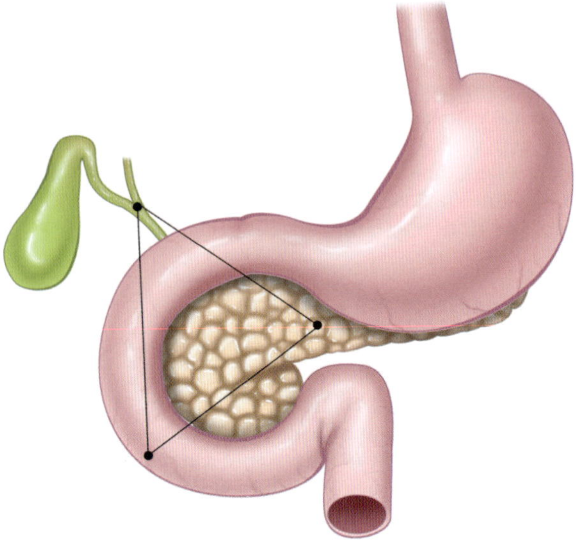

▲ **Figure 53–8.** Anatomic boundaries of the gastrinoma triangle where 90% of gastrinomas are found.

the pancreas during an open procedure or evaluation with the laparoscopic ultrasound during a minimally invasive approach. The lateral peritoneal attachments of the second portion of the duodenum are divided. The hepatic flexure of the colon can be mobilized to facilitate duodenal mobilization. Proximal and superior duodenal mobilization is completed by division of the avascular portion of the hepatoduodenal ligament. Distal and inferior duodenal mobilization allows for exposure of the IVC and the aorta.

Enucleation (Figure 53–9)

One of the major advantages of performing an enucleation procedure is the preservation of normal pancreatic parenchyma. Insulinomas, 90% of which are benign, and other small PNETs that can be excised without injury to the main pancreatic duct or larger superficial lesions are the most common indications for enucleation. The rate of postoperative pancreatic fistula is higher for enucleation compared to other resection options.[40,41]

Pancreatic enucleation can be performed through an open or minimally invasive approach. Intraoperative ultrasound is of value to help locate the PNET within the pancreas and define its relationship to the pancreatic duct. It is also used to rule out any additional lesions. A spatula, which is used to perform carotid endarterectomy, is used in combination with electrocautery or an energy device to perform enucleation. Part of the omentum is freed from the transverse colon and can be used to pack the defect in the pancreas created by enucleation of the PNET. A closed suction drain is placed.

Distal Pancreatectomy, Pancreaticoduodenectomy, & Total Pancreatectomy

Distal pancreatectomy and pancreaticoduodenectomy are performed for PNETs that are large, that involve or are in close proximity to the main pancreatic duct, or are deep in the pancreatic parenchyma and not amenable to enucleation. A distal pancreatectomy with or without a splenectomy is indicated for PNETs in the neck, body, or tail of the pancreas. Pancreaticoduodenectomy, or a Whipple procedure, is indicated for PNETs in the head and uncinate process of the pancreas that are not amenable to enucleation.[39]

Total pancreatectomy is rarely the index operation for patients with PNETs because of the high morbidity associated with endocrine and exocrine insufficiency. However, it is an option for patients with MEN I, who characteristically have multifocal disease, but it is most often reserved for patients with recurrent disease. However, even with recurrent disease, pancreas-preserving procedures including re-resection of the pancreatic neck or enucleations are preferred options. Distal pancreatectomy with enucleation of tumors in the head and uncinate process of the pancreas, duodenotomy for removal of duodenal gastrinomas and peripancreatic lymph node dissection is another option for patients with MEN I who have multifocal disease (Figure 53–9).[39]

The importance of performing a distal pancreatectomy with splenic preservation remains controversial, as spleen-preserving techniques have lower lymph node yields. Although lymph node dissection allows for a better determination of prognosis, its therapeutic value has not been proven.[42] Splenic preservation is reasonable in most cases if the tumor is remote from the splenic hilum and suspicion of lymph node metastases is low.[39]

Distal pancreatectomy with or without splenectomy can be performed through an open or minimally invasive approach with split leg positioning. The gastrocolic ligament is divided widely to open the lesser sac and expose the pancreas. If performing a splenectomy, gentle traction is applied to the spleen medially to divide the splenocolic and splenorenal ligaments. The short gastric arteries are ligated, and the stomach is retracted superomedially. Both the spleen and pancreas are mobilized from their retroperitoneal attachments and the inferior mesenteric vein is divided. The spleen and pancreas are dissected free medially to the confluence of the SMV and the splenic vein. The splenic vessels are ligated, and the pancreas can then be transected at the neck with a stapler.

If performing a spleen-sparing distal pancreatectomy, the inferior margin of the pancreas is mobilized by developing the plane between the root of the transverse colon and the anterior fascia of the pancreas. The pancreas is carefully elevated from the retroperitoneum, and the splenic vessels

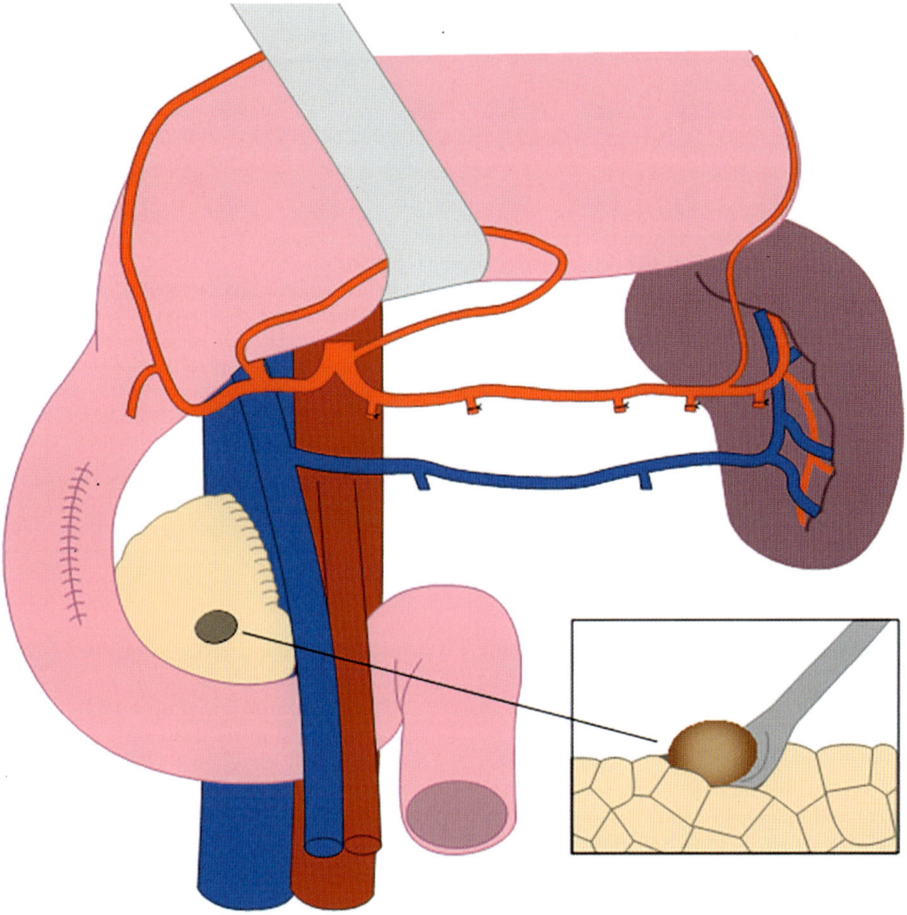

▲ **Figure 53–9.** Completed operation for MEN I gastrinoma included: a distal pancreatectomy with splenic preservation, enucleation of PNETs in the head and uncinate process of the pancreas, duodenotomy, and excision of duodenal gastrinomas from the second portion of the duodenum, and regional lymphadenectomy.

are identified and isolated. A plane is created between the pancreas and the splenic vessels, and the pancreas is transected with a stapler device. The resected pancreas is then dissected from the retroperitoneum, taking care to divide the multiple small tributaries between the splenic vessels and the pancreas. The pancreatic staple line or main pancreatic duct is reinforced, and a closed suction drain is placed adjacent to the staple line.

Pancreaticoduodenectomy is associated with a higher risk of perioperative morbidity. Furthermore, when pancreaticoduodenectomy is performed for a PNET, the pancreatic duct is small and the surrounding pancreatic parenchyma is soft. As a result, pancreaticoduodenectomy may be associated with a higher risk for pancreatic leak and fistula formation. Although technically more challenging, laparoscopic and robotic approaches are gaining popularity.[43,44]

COMPLICATIONS OF SURGERY ON THE PANCREAS

Surgery of the pancreas is associated with a high morbidity rate. While rates of morbidity vary based on the specific procedure, any surgical intervention on the pancreas requires a thorough understanding of the anatomy, specialized training, and technical expertise. The most significant consequences of removing part of or the entire pancreas include pancreatic fistula, exocrine insufficiency, and endocrine insufficiency.

Pancreatic Fistula

In 2005, the International Study Group of Pancreatic Surgery (ISGPS) established a standard definition for pancreatic fistula. A postoperative pancreatic fistula is defined as any measurable volume of fluid output in an operatively

Table 53–3. International Study Group of Pancreatic Surgery Grading System for Postoperative Pancreatic Fistula.[45]

ISGPS Grade	Definition	Impact
Biochemical Leak (formerly Grade A)	Amylase >3× upper limit of normal serum value without any clinical impact on the patient	• No deviation in normal postoperative care • Does not affect postoperative length of stay • May require operative drain to remain in place after discharge up to 3 weeks
Grade B	Properly defined fistula with increased amylase activity from any drain in association with a clinically relevant condition	• Extended period of operative drain requirement >3 weeks • Interventional percutaneous or endoscopic procedure required to manage undrained fluid collection • Postoperative transfusion or angiography to control postoperative fistula-related hemorrhage or pseudoaneurysm • Infection requiring antibiotic management without signs of organ failure • May require the patient to be kept NPO or supported with enteral or parenteral nutrition • May require therapeutic treatment with somatostatin analogues
Grade C	Grade B postoperative pancreatic fistula leading to reoperation, organ failure, or death	• Need for reoperation • Signs of organ failure and/or clinical instability • Death • Often requires excessively prolonged hospital stay

placed drain with amylase activity greater than 3 times the upper limit of normal serum value. ISGPS updated their consensus grading system in 2016, which is outlined in Table 53–3.[45]

The most important risk factors for the occurrence of a postoperative pancreatic fistula include the presence of a soft pancreas and a small main pancreatic duct. In most PNETs, the surrounding normal pancreas has a soft texture and the diameter of the pancreatic duct is normal, increasing the risk of pancreatic fistula after partial pancreatectomy.[46,47] Tumor enucleation is also considered a risk factor for the development of pancreatic fistula; however, the overall complication rate is comparable to standard partial pancreatectomy.[48] As tumor enucleation is a parenchyma-sparing procedure, the rates of endocrine and exocrine insufficiency are low for this procedure.

Exocrine & Endocrine Insufficiency

Exocrine insufficiency is defined as the persistent need for pancreatic enzyme supplementation for at least 6 months after surgery. It typically presents as steatorrhea and bloating due to the decreased ability of the gastrointestinal tract to absorb fats and nutrients. Endocrine insufficiency is defined as the development of diabetes mellitus postoperatively. More specifically, it can be classified as the need for a new pharmacological intervention postoperatively with either oral hypoglycemic medications or insulin. If a patient undergoing pancreatic surgery already has signs of exocrine or endocrine insufficiency preoperatively, these conditions may worsen after surgery and require escalation in management. Patients with postoperative exocrine and endocrine insufficiency report reduced quality of life compared to the general population.[49]

Parenchymal-preserving resections, including enucleation, were first introduced with the aim of reducing physiologic insufficiency postoperatively. Whipple procedures have been shown to be higher risk for the development of both exocrine and endocrine insufficiency postoperatively compared to tumor enucleation or distal pancreatectomy. At least 20% of normal pancreas is required to prevent postoperative physiologic insufficiency. However, in many patients undergoing surgical resection the remnant pancreas is not normal, and exocrine and endocrine insufficiency can develop with smaller portions of the gland removed. Patients with a higher body mass index, a family history of diabetes mellitus, or a preexisting diagnosis of diabetes mellitus are at a significantly higher risk of developing postoperative endocrine insufficiency.[50]

REFERENCES

1. Gregg BE, Moore PC, Demozay D, et al. Formation of a human β-cell population within pancreatic islets is set early in life. *J Clin Endocrino Metab*. 2012;97(9):3197-3206.
2. Dimitriou I, Katsourakis A, Nikolaidou E, Noussios G. The main anatomical variations of the pancreatic duct system: review of the literature and its importance in surgical practice. *J Clin Med Res*. 2018;10(5):370-375.
3. Gutta A, Fogel E, Sherman S. Identification and management of pancreas divisum. *Expert Rev Gastroenterol Hepatol*. 2019;13(11):1089-1105.
4. Ferri V, Vicente E, Quijano Y, et al. Diagnosis and treatment of pancreas divisum: a literature review. *Hepatobiliary Pancreat Dis Int*. 2019;18(4):332-336.

5. Sherifi F, Bexheti S, Gashi Z, Bajraktari I, Shatri J, Lahu A. Anatomic variations of pancreaticobiliary union. *Open Access Maced J Med Sci*. 2018;6(6):988-991.
6. Henry BM, Skinningsrud B, Saganiak K, Pękala PA, Walocha JA, Tomaszewski KA. Development of the human pancreas and its vasculature: an integrated review covering anatomical, embryological, histological, and molecular aspects. *Ann Anat*. 2019;221:115-124.
7. Farghadani M, Momeni M, Hekmatnia A, Momeni F, Baradaran Mahdavi MM. Anatomical variation of celiac axis, superior mesenteric artery, and hepatic artery: evaluation with multidetector computed tomography angiography. *J Res Med Sci*. 2016;21:129.
8. Baranski AG, Lam H-D, Braat AE, Schaapherder AF. The dorsal pancreatic artery in pancreas procurement and transplantation: anatomical considerations and potential implications. *Clin Transplant*. 2016;30(10):1360-1364.
9. Cesmebasi A, Malefant J, Patel SD, et al. The surgical anatomy of the lymphatic system of the pancreas. *Clin Anat*. 2015;28(4): 527-537.
10. Lin EE, Scott-Solomon E, Kuruvilla R. Peripheral innervation in the regulation of glucose homeostasis. *Trends Neurosci*. 2021; 44(3):189-202.
11. Singh VK, Yadav D, Garg PK. Diagnosis and management of chronic pancreatitis: a review. *JAMA*. 2019;322(24):2422-2434.
12. Wynne K, Devereaux B, Dornhorst A. Diabetes of the exocrine pancreas. *J Gastroenterol Hepatol*. 2019;34(2):346-354.
13. Girodon E, Rebours V, Chen JM, et al. Clinical interpretation of PRSS1 variants in patients with pancreatitis. *Clin Res Hepatol Gastroenterol*. 2021;45(1):101497.
14. Williams JA. Cholecystokinin (CCK) regulation of pancreatic acinar cells: physiological actions and signal transduction mechanisms. *Compr Physiol*. 2019;9(2):535-564.
15. Barreto SG, Carati CJ, Toouli J, Saccone GTP. The islet-acinar axis of the pancreas: more than just insulin. *Am J Physiol-Gastrointest*. 2010;299(1):G10-G22.
16. Hegele RA, Maltman GM. Insulin's centenary: the birth of an idea. *Lancet Diabetes Endocrinol*. 2020;8(12):971-977.
17. Haeusler RA, McGraw TE, Accili D. Biochemical and cellular properties of insulin receptor signalling. *Nat Rev Mol Cell Biol*. 2018;19(1):31-44.
18. Makhmutova M, Weitz J, Tamayo A, et al. Pancreatic β-cells communicate with vagal sensory neurons. *Gastroenterol*. 2021; 160(3):875-888.e11.
19. Müller TD, Finan B, Clemmensen C, DiMarchi RD, Tschöp MH. The new biology and pharmacology of glucagon. *Physiol Rev*. 2017;97(2):721-766.
20. Janah, Kjeldsen, Galsgaard, et al. Glucagon receptor signaling and glucagon resistance. *IJMS*. 2019;20(13):3314.
21. Boike GM, Sightler SE, Averette HE. Treatment of small intestinal fistulas with octreotide, a somatostatin analog. *J Surg Oncol*. 1992;49(1):63-65.
22. Gans SL, van Westreenen HL, Kiewiet JJS, Rauws EA, Gouma DJ, Boermeester MA. Systematic review and meta-analysis of somatostatin analogues for the treatment of pancreatic fistula. *Br J Surg*. 2012;99(6):754-760.
23. Paran H, Neufeld D, Kaplan O, Klausner J, Freund U. Octreotide for treatment of postoperative alimentary tract fistulas. *World J Surg*. 1995;19(3):430-433; discussion 433-434.
24. El Nakeeb A, ElGawalby A, A Ali M, et al. Efficacy of octreotide in the prevention of complications after pancreaticoduodenectomy in patients with soft pancreas and non-dilated pancreatic duct: a prospective randomized trial. *Hepatobiliary Pancreat Dis Int*. 2018;17(1):59-63.
25. Garg PK, Sharma J, Jakhetiya A, Chishi N. The role of prophylactic octreotide following pancreaticoduodenectomy to prevent postoperative pancreatic fistula: a meta-analysis of the randomized controlled trials. *Surg J (N Y)*. 2018;4(4):e182-e187.
26. Kurumboor P, Palaniswami KN, Pramil K, et al. Octreotide does not prevent pancreatic fistula following pancreatoduodenectomy in patients with soft pancreas and non-dilated duct: a prospective randomized controlled trial. *J Gastrointest Surg*. 2015;19(11):2038-2044.
27. Khandekar N, Berning BA, Sainsbury A, Lin S. The role of pancreatic polypeptide in the regulation of energy homeostasis. *Mol Cell Endocrinol*. 2015;418 Pt 1:33-41.
28. Iwasaki M, Akiba Y, Kaunitz JD. Recent advances in vasoactive intestinal peptide physiology and pathophysiology: focus on the gastrointestinal system. *F1000Res*. 2019;8:F1000 Faculty Rev-1629.
29. Dasari A, Shen C, Halperin D, et al. Trends in the incidence, prevalence, and survival outcomes in patients with neuroendocrine tumors in the United States. *JAMA Oncol*. 2017;3(10):1335-1342.
30. Dromain C, Déandréis D, Scoazec J-Y, et al. Imaging of neuroendocrine tumors of the pancreas. *Diagn Interv Imaging*. 2016;97(12):1241-1257.
31. Scott AT, Howe JR. Evaluation and management of neuroendocrine tumors of the pancreas. *Surg Clin North Am*. 2019;99(4):793-814.
32. Lee L, Ito T, Jensen RT. Imaging of pancreatic neuroendocrine tumors: recent advances, current status, and controversies. *Expert Rev Anticancer Ther*. 2018;18(9):837-860.
33. Sundin A, Arnold R, Baudin E, et al. ENETS Consensus Guidelines for the Standards of Care in Neuroendocrine Tumors: Radiological, Nuclear Medicine & Hybrid Imaging. *Neuroendocrinology*. 2017;105(3):212-244.
34. Lo GC, Kambadakone A. MR imaging of pancreatic neuroendocrine tumors. *Magn Reson Imaging Clin N Am*. 2018;26(3):391-403.
35. Hope TA, Bergsland EK, Bozkurt MF, et al. Appropriate use criteria for somatostatin receptor PET imaging in neuroendocrine tumors. *J Nucl Med*. 2018;59(1):66-74.
36. Ito T, Jensen RT. Molecular imaging in neuroendocrine tumors: recent advances, controversies, unresolved issues, and roles in management. *Curr Opin Endocrinol Diabetes Obes*. 2017;24(1):15-24.
37. Liu JB, Baker MS. Surgical management of pancreatic neuroendocrine tumors. *Surg Clin North Am*. 2016;96(6):1447-1468.
38. Ma Z-Y, Gong Y-F, Zhuang H-K, et al. Pancreatic neuroendocrine tumors: a review of serum biomarkers, staging, and management. *World J Gastroenterol*. 2020;26(19):2305-2322.
39. Howe JR, Merchant NB, Conrad C, et al. The North American Neuroendocrine Tumor Society Consensus Paper on the Surgical Management of Pancreatic Neuroendocrine Tumors. *Pancreas*. 2020;49(1):1-33.
40. Bartolini I, Bencini L, Risaliti M, Ringressi MN, Moraldi L, Taddei A. Current management of pancreatic neuroendocrine tumors: from demolitive surgery to observation. *Gastroenterol Res Pract*. 2018;2018:9647247.
41. Zhou Y, Zhao M, Wu L, Ye F, Si X. Short- and long-term outcomes after enucleation of pancreatic tumors: an evidence-based assessment. *Pancreatology*. 2016;16(6):1092-1098.
42. Lopez-Aguiar AG, Zaidi MY, Beal EW, et al. Defining the role of lymphadenectomy for pancreatic neuroendocrine tumors: An Eight-Institution Study of 695 Patients from the US Neuroendocrine Tumor Study Group. *Ann Surg Oncol*. 2019;26(8):2517-2524.

43. Nassour I, Winters SB, Hoehn R, et al. Long-term oncologic outcomes of robotic and open pancreatectomy in a national cohort of pancreatic adenocarcinoma. *J Surg Oncol.* 2020;122(2):234-242.
44. Kornaropoulos M, Moris D, Beal EW, et al. Total robotic pancreaticoduodenectomy: a systematic review of the literature. *Surg Endosc.* 2017;31(11):4382-4392.
45. Bassi C, Marchegiani G, Dervenis C, et al. The 2016 update of the International Study Group (ISGPS) definition and grading of postoperative pancreatic fistula: 11 years After. *Surgery.* 2017;161(3):584-591.
46. Ecker BL, McMillan MT, Allegrini V, et al. Risk factors and mitigation strategies for pancreatic fistula after distal pancreatectomy: analysis of 2026 resections from the International, Multi-institutional Distal Pancreatectomy Study Group. *Ann Surg.* 2019;269(1):143-149.
47. Kawaida H, Kono H, Hosomura N, et al. Surgical techniques and postoperative management to prevent postoperative pancreatic fistula after pancreatic surgery. *World J Gastroenterol.* 2019;25(28):3722-3737.
48. Jilesen APJ, van Eijck CHJ, Busch ORC, van Gulik TM, Gouma DJ, van Dijkum EJMN. Postoperative outcomes of enucleation and standard resections in patients with a pancreatic neuroendocrine tumor. *World J Surg.* 2016;40(3):715-728.
49. Stoop TF, Ateeb Z, Ghorbani P, et al. Impact of endocrine and exocrine insufficiency on quality of life after total pancreatectomy. *Ann Surg Oncol.* 2020;27(2):587-596.
50. Kusakabe J, Anderson B, Liu J, et al. Long-term endocrine and exocrine insufficiency after pancreatectomy. *J Gastrointest Surg.* 2019;23(8):1604-1613.

Diagnosis & Management of Nonfunctional Pancreatic Neuroendocrine Tumors

54

Alexander Manzella, MD, MPH
Amanda M. Laird, MD, FACS
Steven K. Libutti, MD, FACS

GENERAL CONSIDERATIONS

PANCREATIC NEUROENDOCRINE TUMORS: FUNCTIONAL & NONFUNCTIONAL

Pancreatic neuroendocrine tumors (pNETs) are a group of tumors derived from neuroendocrine cells in the pancreas. They are a subset of neuroendocrine neoplasms in the gastroenteropancreatic tract and as such they may secrete hormones, which led to their discovery and classification based on systemic effects of hormone secretion.[1] They may be classified as functional when excess hormone secretion causes systemic symptoms or nonfunctional in the absence of symptoms. Nonfunctional pancreatic neuroendocrine tumors (NF-pNETs) are not associated with hypersecretion syndromes like functional pNETs. Their lack of function may come from an absence of detectable hormone secretion or secretion of inactive hormones such as Chromogranin A.[1,2] Like functional pNETs, they are a rare neoplasm, but their lack of symptoms from excessive hormone secretion allows them to remain undetected for longer, leading to delayed diagnosis.

Epidemiology of NF-pNETs

pNETs are rare, only accounting for 2% of all pancreatic neoplasms and 7% of all neuroendocrine tumors with an age-adjusted incidence of 0.5 to 1 case per 100,000 individuals.[2,3] This incidence has increased over the past 50 years, attributed to the increased use of imaging allowing for identification of previously silent tumors (Figure 54–1). Of the total population of pNETs, NF-pNETs are the most common type, comprising anywhere from 50% to 90% of all cases.[1,2] NF-pNETs are slightly more common in women than men, and while they can occur at any age, they predominantly appear in patients between the ages of 40 and 65. Most NF-pNETs are sporadic, with 10% being attributed to genetic syndromes.[4]

Staging & Grading of NF-pNETs

NF-pNETs are graded and staged using site-specific systems developed by the European Neuroendocrine Tumor Society (ENETS) and endorsed by the World Health Organization (WHO) and American Joint Commission on Cancer (AJCC). Using the ENETS tumor-grading system, pNETs are graded as low (G1), intermediate (G2), or high (G3) grade, determined histologically by cellular features and measuring mitotic index and Ki-67 activity (Table 54–1).[5-8] Ki-67 expression is associated with proliferation, and the degree of Ki-67 activity helps to determine tumor grade as well as being a possible marker to predict tumor response to therapy.[5,8] G1 and G2 tumors are then classified as well-differentiated while G3 tumors comprise a heterogeneous group of tumors with poor prognosis.[9] G3 tumors may be poorly differentiated and classified as neuroendocrine carcinomas (NECs), or they may be well differentiated but with a high proliferative rate and Ki-67 expression.[8] Analysis of these two groups of G3 tumors has shown different responses to chemotherapeutic agents between poorly and well differentiated tumors as well as inferring different levels of prognosis.[9] This information is combined with the Tumor-Node-Metastasis (TNM) staging system where T is determined by tumor size and local invasion, N correlates to nodal disease status, and M is based on the presence of distant metastatic disease, to improve prognostication and guide clinical management (Table 54–2).

Association With Genetic Syndromes

pNETs, and by extension NF-pNETs, are associated with multiple genetic syndromes including multiple endocrine neoplasia Type 1 (MEN1), Von-Hippel-Lindau syndrome (VHL), neurofibromatosis 1 (NF1), and tuberous sclerosis (TS).[1,10] MEN1 is caused by a mutation in the tumor-suppressing *Menin* gene on chromosome 11q13 and is associated with hyperparathyroidism, pancreatic neoplasms, and anterior pituitary tumors. MEN1 is the most common

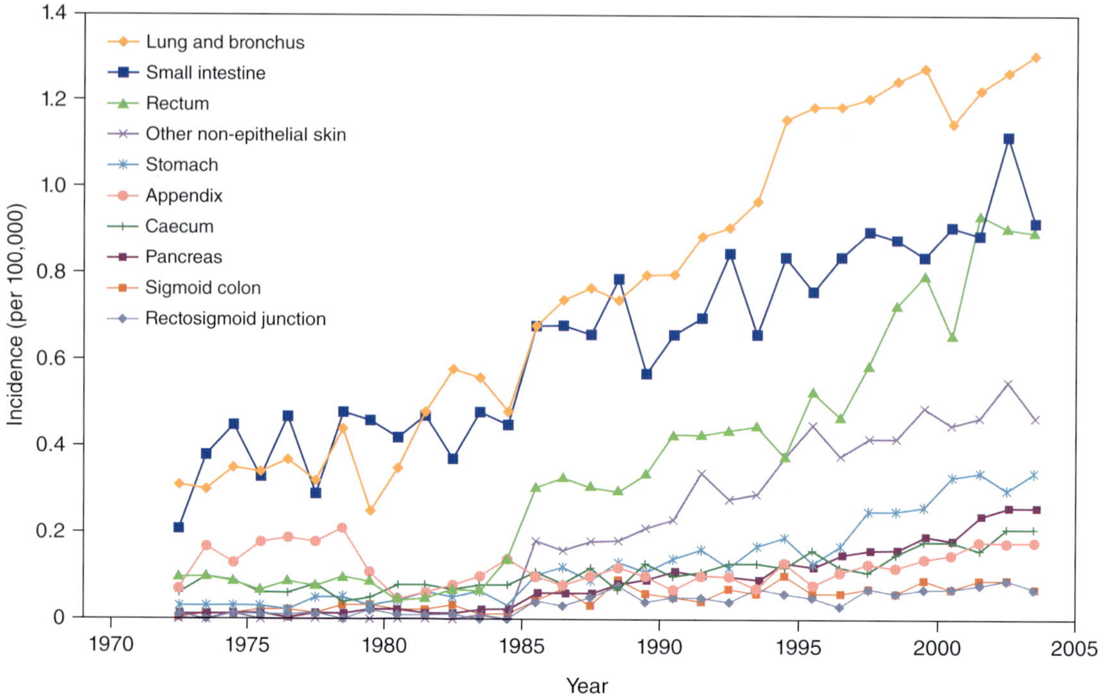

▲ **Figure 54–1.** Increased incidence of carcinoid tumors, US population 1973-2005. Reproduced with permission from Modlin IM, Oberg K, Chung DC, et al. Gastroenteropancreatic neuroendocrine tumors. *Lancet Oncol*. 2007;9(1):61-72.

genetic syndrome associated with pNETs, accounting for 10% of all cases.[11] pNETs are the second most common manifestation of MEN1, with an estimated incidence of 90% of all MEN1 patients by the age of 75, and represent a significant risk for morbidity and mortality.[12] Large NF-pNETs have been found in MEN1 patients as young as 10 years old, leading to screening recommendations that will be discussed later in this chapter.[11] While NF-pNETs in MEN1 patients tend to occur at younger ages and are more likely to occur as multiple tumors than in sporadic patients, they are more likely to show an indolent growth pattern.[10,12] pNETs and NF-pNETs are also found in 10% of patients with VHL and less frequently can be associated with NF1 and TS. These associations are not as clear as those between MEN1 and pNETs, and as a result, do not carry special management or screening recommendations.

Screening

There are no screening recommendations for NF-pNETs for the general population. Because of the high incidence of NF-pNETs with significant risks for morbidity and mortality, all patients with a diagnosis of MEN1 should undergo screening for NF-pNETs using CT, MRI, or endoscopic ultrasound (EUS).[4,10,12] Given that patients as young as 10 have been diagnosed with clinically relevant NF-pNETs requiring surgical intervention, the age at which screening can be initiated may begin as early as before the age of 10 for first imaging, but most recent studies recommend beginning screening in the second decade of life.[12,13] The intervals between imaging screening in asymptomatic patients are currently under debate, with some groups recommending yearly screening, but the final decision is left to the discretion of each MEN1 center. The decision for initiating and maintaining screening must be individualized to the patient and consider the psychological burden, cumulative radiation exposure, and invasive nature of screening tests. While some centers perform biochemical screening for NF-pNETs by checking chromogranin A, neuron-specific enolase, progastrin-releasing peptide, glucagon, or pancreatic polypeptide levels, there is insufficient evidence to recommend for biochemical screening.[8]

Clinical Findings

A. Signs & Symptoms

The majority of NF-pNETs are diagnosed incidentally in patients undergoing cross-sectional imaging for other pathologies. When patients do present with symptoms from an NF-pNET, it is generally related to local mass effects from

Table 54–1. WHO 2017 grading criteria for pancreatic neuroendocrine neoplasms.

Classification	Mitotic Rate*	Ki-67 Proliferation Index (%)**	Distribution of Cases (%)
Well-Differentiated p-NENs:			
NET G1	<2	<3	31%
NET G2	2-20	3-20	33%
NET G3	>20	>20	13%
Poorly Differentiated p-NENs:			
NEC G3	>20	>20	23%

*The mitotic rate is based on the evaluation of mitoses in 50 high-power fields in areas of higher density and is expressed as mitoses per 10 high-power fields.

**The Ki-67 proliferation index is based on the evaluation of >500 cells in areas of high nuclear labeling.

G, grading; NEC, neuroendocrine carcinoma; NET, neuroendocrine tumor; p-NENs, pancreatic neuroendocrine neoplasms; WHO, World Health Organization.

Source: Adapted from Yang M, Zeng L, Ke NW, et al. World Health Organization grading classification for pancreatic neuroendocrine neoplasms: a comprehensive analysis from a large Chinese institution. *BMC Cancer.* 2020;20(1):906.

an advanced tumor.[14] This can present as abdominal or back pain, early satiety, anorexia, nausea, weight loss, pancreatitis, biliary obstruction, or bowel obstruction depending on what organ is compressed by the mass (Table 54–3).[14-16] Patients found to be symptomatic from NF-pNETs are more likely to have advanced disease given the indirect nature of symptoms from tumor mass effect.

Table 54–2. Definitions of American Joint Committee on Cancer and European Neuroendocrine Tumor Society staging for pancreatic neuroendocrine tumors.

	AJCC 8th and ENETS Staging Classification
T1	Tumor limited to the pancreas, ≤2 cm
T2	Tumor limited to the pancreas, 2-4 cm
T3	Tumor limited to the pancreas, >4 cm, or invading the duodenum or common bile duct
T4	Tumor invades adjacent structures
N0	No regional lymph node metastasis
N1	Regional lymph node metastasis
M0	No distant metastasis
M1	Distant metastasis
M1a	Metastasis confined to liver
M1b	Metastasis in at least one extrahepatic site
M1c	Both hepatic and extrahepatic metastases

Table 54–3. Signs and symptoms of nonfunctional pancreatic neuroendocrine tumors.

Sign or Symptom	Percent of Patients
Abdominal pain	37%-78%
Weight loss	20%-35%
Anorexia and nausea	45%
Intra-abdominal hemorrhage	4%-20%
Jaundice	17%-50%
Palpable mass	7%-40%

Source: Adapted from Falconi M, Plockinger U, Kwekkeboom DJ, et al. Well-differentiated pancreatic nonfunctioning tumors/carcinoma. *Neuroendocrinology.* 2006;84(3):196-211.

Laboratory Findings

General laboratory findings in patients presenting with NF-pNETs are most likely associated with their symptomatology. While rare, patients may present with liver function abnormalities, pancreatic enzymes may be elevated in patients with pancreatitis, and asymptomatic patients may have no laboratory abnormalities at all.[16] Potential specialized laboratory tests for chromogranin A, glucagon, and pancreatic polypeptide are being investigated as potential biochemical aids in diagnosis, but there is insufficient evidence at this time for strong recommendations for their use.[5,16,17] The most well studied of these tests is chromogranin A which has less than 50% sensitivity and specificity for NF-pNETs, but when found to be elevated in patients with NF-pNETs can be used to monitor response to therapy.[16,17]

Imaging Studies

A. CT

As many NF-pNETs are discovered incidentally on cross-sectional imaging, the most common first scan is a CT given their ubiquitous use for diagnosing intra-abdominal pathologies.[18,19] CT scan sensitivity decreases drastically for tumors smaller than 2 cm and is less specific for differentiating NF-pNETs versus pancreatic adenocarcinoma than imaging options described in the following section (Table 54–4).[18-20] Optimal CT protocol for pancreatic mass evaluation involves four stages of contrast exposure: unenhanced, pancreatic arterial phase, venous phase, and late phase. CT is the best modality for evaluating for metastatic lesions of the lung, which is a rare manifestation of NF-pNETs.[3,20,21]

B. MRI

MRI is a more sensitive modality than CT for the evaluation of smaller pancreatic masses as well as providing better

Table 54–4. Differential for solid pancreatic masses.

Differential for Solid Pancreatic Masses
Neoplasm
Pancreatic adenocarcinoma
Pancreatic neuroendocrine tumor, nonfunctional or functional
Pseudopapillary tumor
Acinar cell carcinoma
Periampullary tumor (ampullary adenocarcinoma/adenoma, duodenal adenocarcinoma, GISTS, distal cholangiocarcinoma)
Metastatic disease (renal cell carcinoma, non-small-cell lung cancer, breast cancer, sarcoma, melanoma, colon cancer)
Inflammatory Diseases
Sequelae of chronic pancreatitis
Autoimmune pancreatitis

Source: Adapted from Yamashita Y, Kitano M. Endoscopic ultrasonography for pancreatic solid lesions. *J Med Ultrason (2001)*. 2020;47(3): 377-387.

imaging of hepatic lesions, a common site of metastases for NF-pNETs.[5,16,18,19] The diagnostic value of MRI is similar to that of EUS for direct evaluation of pancreatic lesions and the adjacent region as described below but is significantly less invasive.[19] Evaluation of T1-weighted, T2-weighted, and diffusion-weighted imaging (DWI) MRI with and without Gadolinium contrast are the imaging modalities of choice when evaluating for metastatic liver lesions, the most common site of NF-pNET metastasis.[8,22] Frequently MRI is used in conjunction with EUS to evaluate tumors less than 2 cm.[19,23]

C. FDG PET

Fluorodeoxyglucose (FDG)-positron emission topography (PET) CT has long been a standard imaging modality for the staging of numerous neoplasms for its ability to identify metabolically active loci throughout the body.[18] FDG-PET CT has limited use in the diagnosis and staging of NF-pNETs as it has poor sensitivity for well-differentiated tumors and only moderate sensitivity for the most aggressive poorly differentiated tumors. The ability to detect a poorly differentiated NF-pNET via FDG-PET CT may be indicative of an extremely aggressive tumor.[18,24]

D. Radiolabeled Somatostatin Analog PET CT

Somatostatin analogs such as octreotide, octreotate, and lanreotide have been combined with the chelator tetraazacyclododecane tetraacetic acid (DOTA) to produce somatostatin analogs that can be radiolabeled for functional imaging of somatostatin expressing neuroendocrine tumors. DOTA-octreotate (DOTATATE) has replaced DOTA-octreotide and DOTA-lanreotide to be the most utilized somatostatin analog.[3,19,24-26] DOTATATE is frequently labeled with Gallium 68 similar to FDG labeling in PET CT. NF-pNETs frequently express type 2 somatostatin receptors as neuroendocrine tumors at a higher concentration than normal tissues.[6] This allows 68Ga-DOTATATE to selectively bind in larger amounts to NF-pNETs, leading to a higher sensitivity for detecting G1, G2, and G3 tumors compared to traditional FDG-PET scans which have poor sensitivity to well-differentiated tumors.[5,19,25] Therefore, 68Ga-DOTATATE scans are integral for evaluating disease burden and recurrences.[27,28] Additionally, DOTATATE can be used therapeutically in combination with peptide receptor radionuclide therapy (PRRT) to treat select NF-pNETs.[6]

E. EUS

Endoscopic ultrasound (EUS) performed as part of an esophagogastroduodenoscopy (EGD) is the most sensitive modality for evaluating pancreatic masses and performing regional assessments during the workup of NF-pNETs.[20,23,29-31] Fine-needle aspiration (FNA) may be performed under imaging guidance during EUS to provide tissue samples for diagnosis. As EUS with EGD requires sedation and procedural intervention, it is the most invasive of the imaging modalities described here, and as such requires a careful consideration of patient factors prior to utilization. EUS can be used to identify the location and imaging characteristics of a pancreatic mass as well as utilizing contrast, elastography, and FNA to differentiate between pNETs and adenocarcinoma (Table 54–4).[20,30] EUS can also identify vascular or lymph node involvement. A limitation to EUS is that the ability to detect lesions decreases when moving from the head of the pancreas toward the tail, unlike other imaging modalities such as MRI which provide equal imaging throughout the body.[31] For this reason, MRI and EUS-FNA are often both performed when working up pancreatic masses less than 2 cm.[5]

Specialized Tests

A. NETest

NETest is a "liquid biopsy," a type of genetic molecular test where blood samples are searched for tumor transcriptome patterns based on circulating tumor mRNAs.[32] This test has shown to be highly specific and sensitive for detecting and differentiating pNETs from other forms of pancreatic neoplasm or disease (Table 54–4).[8,32] There has been shown to be a small profile overlap between pNETs and intraductal papillary mucinous neoplasms of the pancreas.[32] This test has high specificity and sensitivity for diagnosing disease, predicting the success of treatments such as PRRT, and monitoring responses to therapy.[33]

Management

A. Observation

Surgical intervention for resectable NF-pNETs <2 cm is not associated with prolonged survival compared to observation and may be more harmful given complication rates of 14% to 45% of pNET surgeries.[13,17,28,34-37] Therefore, ENETS Consensus Guidelines recommend performing active surveillance for asymptomatic low-grade (G1, G2) NF-pNETs that are less than 2 cm in size.[5,7,16] Surveillance may be continued every 6 to 12 months using the imaging methods discussed previously to monitor for tumor growth.[19,28] The Response Evaluation Criteria in Solid Tumors (RECIST) version 1.1 can be used to monitor NF-pNET response to therapy. RECIST 1.1 defines progressive disease as a 20% increase of at least 5 mm in the sum of diameters of the target lesion.[22,38] If tumors are noted to grow more than 0.5 cm in an interval period, show evidence of progressive disease by RECIST 1.1 criteria, or have a total size larger than 2 cm, then surgery should be considered.[22,38] Observation of high-grade (G3) NF-pNETs of any size is not recommended given their high risk for locoregional spread and metastases.[36]

B. Surgery

Patients with asymptomatic NF-pNETs of any grade that are greater than 2 cm have a survival benefit from surgery compared to observation or adjuvant therapy and should be evaluated for surgical intervention.[5,6,8,17,36,37]

Patients with low grade, solitary tumors that are distant from vasculature and pancreatic ducts are candidates for enucleation.[5,6,17,36] This is because there is little evidence of lymphatic spread of disease.[39] Enucleation has a higher risk for pancreatic fistula formation (but a less morbid grade of fistula) but equal survival in small, low-grade tumors.[1,34,35,40] Enucleation can be performed open or laparoscopically with ultrasound to confirm tumor position relative to pancreatic ducts and vasculature.[36]

Central pancreatectomy is an option for resection of a central NF-pNET of any grade when a tumor is too high grade or associated with other pancreatic structures to undergo enucleation.[28,36] This is a difficult and morbid procedure with high risk of pancreatic fistula formation but has lower risk of causing exocrine and endocrine dysfunction than larger resections.[34,35,40]

Distal pancreatectomy is an option for resection for NF-pNETs located in the distal body or tail of the pancreas.[6,8,28] Since there is low evidence that lymphatic dissection improves survival, the distal pancreatectomy may be performed without splenectomy when there is no direct involvement of the splenic vessels or hilum, and no signs of lymphadenopathy.[36] In the setting of NF-pNET involvement of the spleen or local lymphadenopathy, then a splenectomy should be performed as part of the distal pancreatectomy to obtain pathologic information regarding nodal metastases to all for the most accurate staging.[36]

Pancreaticoduodenectomy, also known as the Whipple procedure, is an option for resection of NF-pNETs located in the head of the pancreas or involving the Ampulla of Vater.[5,6,17] The execution of a Whipple procedure for NF-pNET is more challenging than performing one for pancreatic adenocarcinoma as the pathology of NF-pNET is less likely to cause tissue changes to the pancreas and cause ductal obstruction.[34,35] As a result, the pancreatic parenchyma is often soft and the ducts are of normal caliber, both features make the procedure more technically challenging and increase the risk for complications.[34,35]

Laparoscopic surgery has been studied and shown to be equivalent to an open approach in trained laparoscopic hepatobiliary surgeons; therefore, all the above procedures may be performed laparoscopically or open on a case-by-case basis.[5,34,35] Robotic surgery has yet to be studied at the same volume as laparoscopic surgery, but early reports indicate that it is also a feasible alternative to laparoscopic surgery with experienced surgeons.

C. Locally Advanced and Metastatic Disease

NF-pNETs present with locally advanced or metastatic disease in 50% to 60% of cases.[7,21] The most common site of metastases is the liver and the most common cause of death in patients with metastatic disease is liver failure.[21] Surgical intervention in these cases must be tailored to the individual patient, the potential for achieving an R0 resection, and adjuvant treatment options.[17,36,39] Patients with isolated metastatic disease that is resectable are recommended to undergo synchronous surgical intervention as resection of isolated metastases and primary tumor is associated with increased survival. Patients with more diffuse metastatic disease to the liver may benefit from debulking procedures such as wedge resection and ablation. Patients with an average of 20% of liver parenchyma replaced by a tumor that can undergo at least a 70% reduction in metastatic hepatic tumor burden have an improved progression-free and overall survival compared to those not undergoing surgical intervention.[41]

The role of surgical intervention in patients with diffuse metastatic disease is limited. Outside select cases of localized hepatic disease, there is no survival benefit for diffuse metastatic disease, but palliative intervention for the alleviation of gastric outlet obstruction or biliary obstruction may be considered on a case-by-case basis.[36,41]

Medical Management

A. Somatostatin Analogues

Somatostatin analogues such as octreotide, pasireotide, and lanreotide are utilized in symptom management for functional pNETs and have been shown to slow tumor growth in low and intermediate-grade pNETs.[8,15,42] The CLARINET trial demonstrated prolonged progression-free survival in patients with grade 1 or 2 metastatic pNETs using lanreotide, leading to the recommendation of somatostatin analogs for the treatment of high-burden, well-differentiated NF-pNETs in patients who either are not candidates for surgical intervention or have unresectable disease.[43] The most common side effects of this class of medications are nausea, bloating, diarrhea, cholestasis, and/or steatorrhea but these symptoms may improve over time.[17] Patients that are expected to be treated with somatostatin analogues after surgical intervention may benefit from prophylactic cholecystectomy during surgery to avoid gallbladder-associated morbidity from cholestasis.[17]

B. Targeted Therapies and Chemotherapeutic Agents

Multiple chemotherapeutic agents are under investigation for treatment of pNETs including mTOR inhibitors, tyrosine kinase inhibitors, VEGF inhibitors, cytotoxic chemotherapeutic agents, alkylating chemotherapeutic agents, and combinations of agents from different categories.[1,6,8,44] There is a paucity of research specifically studying the effects of many of these agents solely on NF-pNETs, instead the majority of testing and recommendations are for the whole class of pNETs.[6,44] Most agents are second-line treatments following the use of somatostatin analogues and tend to be more effective against well-differentiated tumors than poorly differentiated ones.[27,33]

C. mTOR Inhibitors

One of the most common agents in use for management of locally advanced or metastatic pNETs is everolimus, an mTOR inhibitor shown to increase survival in low- and intermediate-grade disease.[5,6,42] Side effects include hyperglycemia, stomatitis, pneumonitis, dyslipidemia, hypertension, and headache.[6]

D. Tyrosine Kinase Inhibitors

Sunitinib has been shown to prolong survival in patients with well-differentiated metastatic pNETs.[6,8,44] Side effects include hypertension, thyroid and renal dysfunction, thromboembolism, liver toxicity, and impaired wound healing.[6]

E. VEGF Inhibitors

There is limited data supporting the use of VEGF inhibitors for pNETs.[6] Pazopanib, a kinase inhibitor that targets VEGF receptors, and surufatinib, a VEGF receptor inhibitor, are two VEGF inhibitors under investigation as potential agents.[6] Bevacizumab, a VEGF inhibitor, has been studied in combination with temisirolimus, an mTOR inhibitor, and has shown to cause radiologic response to treatment, but has not been shown to prolong survival.[15]

F. Cytotoxic and Alkylating Chemotherapeutic Agents

Streptozocin, an alkylating agent, was used in combination with 5-FU and increased overall survival and progression-free survival in patients with advanced and high-grade pNETs but was limited by streptozocin's cumulative renal toxicity.[6] Streptozocin has now predominantly been replaced by temozolomide as the chemotherapeutic agent of choice for pNETs. It may be used as a monotherapy but frequently is used in combination with bevacizumab and capecitabine.[1,27] The combination of capecitabine and temozolomide (CAPTEM) currently shows a tumor response rate of 70% with increases in overall survival.[28,42] Side effects of CAPTEM are neutropenia, thrombocytopenia, and lymphopenia.

G. Peptide Receptor-Targeted Radiotherapy (PRRT) and Radiotherapy

PRRT involves tagging a radionuclide, such as 177-Lutetium or 90-Yttrium, to a chelator and a receptor-binding analog to deliver localized radiation therapy.[6] PRRT is therefore a treatment option for patients with NF-pNETs that have high somatostatin receptor expression which can be identified by functional scans such as 68Ga-DOTATATE. Following the NETTER-1 trial that demonstrated improved progression-free survival in patients with metastatic midgut neuroendocrine tumors, 177-Lu-DOTATATE has been approved for the treatment of metastatic pNETs.[5,6,8] Somatostatin receptor expression has been shown to be elevated in most low- and intermediate-grade pNETs, and new research suggests it may be elevated in larger amounts of poorly differentiated pNETs than previously believed.[45] Patients with metastatic low- or intermediate-grade pNETs have been shown to have a survival benefit from PRRT and research is currently ongoing on the efficacy of PRRT in poorly differentiated pNETs.[45,46] At this time, patients with NF-pNETs of any grade can be considered for PRRT given functional imaging that confirms high somatostatin receptor expression.[46] The side effect profile for PRRT is typically milder than that of targeted or chemotherapeutic agents but does present the potential for myelodysplastic disorders, acute kidney injury, and hepatotoxicity.[46] PRRT is a new technology that potentially boasts better survival outcomes, safer side effect profile, and increased ability to treat poorly differentiated cancers when compared to current chemotherapeutic agents, and it is possible it will become a more common second-line treatment for metastatic NF-pNETs as a result.[45,46]

There is limited data on the use of external beam radiotherapy for NF-pNETs and its use is not recommended at this time.[6]

Interventional Treatment of Metastatic Lesions

In addition to the previously mentioned surgical approaches to treating locally advanced and isolated metastatic NF-pNET disease, several therapeutic options are available for the treatment of liver metastases. Treatments such as tumor ablation, hepatic artery embolization, chemoembolization, and radioembolization have been utilized in patients with functional pNETs with metastatic liver disease for symptom control in the setting of hormonal secretion.[5-8,17] It is unclear if these therapies offer a survival benefit and therefore may have limited utility in the treatment of NF-pNETs.[21,47] Patients with NF-pNETs who may benefit from interventional treatment of metastatic hepatic disease should be evaluated on a case-by-case basis.

Prognosis

Prognosis for patients with NF-pNETs is primarily determined by tumor grade and stage.[7,9] Compared to other sites in the body, pNETs have poor prognosis, and NF-pNETs tend to have worse prognosis than their functional counterparts.[7] This may be explained by the symptomatic nature of functional pNETs causing symptoms and prompting a workup at an earlier stage of disease compared to the asymptomatic nature of NF-pNETs until local invasion, metastatic disease, or tumor size results in symptoms.[3,17]

Tumor grade is associated with 5-year survival rates of 80%, 67%, and 13% for G1, G2, and G3 tumors, respectively.[7] In the absence of metastatic disease, 5-year survival is 78% regardless of tumor grade.[39] Patients with distant metastatic disease have poor prognosis with a 5-year survival rate of 27%.[39]

Surgical intervention increases survival in all patients, but the survival benefit in patients with T1 disease is smaller than that in patients with more advanced disease, leading to discussions about the benefit of active surveillance in patients with T1 disease mentioned previously.[6,36,37] The increase in overall survival from surgical intervention is greater than the survival benefits of PRRT, chemotherapy, somatostatin analog therapy, and targeted therapy but there is likely selection bias for surgical patients.[33,36,48]

When to Refer

Patients found to have a pancreatic mass that may be a NF-pNET should be referred immediately to a center with surgical oncology, endocrine surgery, interventional gastroenterology, and medical oncology to facilitate the appropriate oncologic workup described earlier.

When to Admit

Patients with a known history of NF-pNET should be admitted when the development of symptoms can potentially be attributed to disease progression. These patients should undergo prompt imaging and multidisciplinary evaluation if imaging findings show unexpected progression of disease. In addition, patients may be admitted in the setting of intractable symptoms to facilitate palliation and hospice care when appropriate.

REFERENCES

1. Perri G, Prakash LR, Katz MHG. Pancreatic neuroendocrine tumors. *Curr Opin Gastroenterol.* 2019;35(5):468-477.
2. Wu J, Sun C, Li E, et al. Non-functional pancreatic neuroendocrine tumours: emerging trends in incidence and mortality. *BMC Cancer*. 2019;19:334.
3. Dasari A, Shen C, Halperin D, et al. Trends in the incidence, prevalence, and survival outcomes in patients with neuroendocrine tumors in the United States. *JAMA Oncol.* 2017;3(10):1335-1342.
4. Klein Haneveld MJ, van Treijen MJC, Pieterman CRC, et al. Initiating pancreatic neuroendocrine tumour (pNET) screening in young MEN1 patients: results from the DutchMEN Study Group. *J Clin Endocrinol Metab.* 2021;106(12):3515-3525.
5. Falconi M, Eriksson B, Kaltsas G, et al. ENETS Consensus Guidelines Update for the Management of Patients with Functional Pancreatic Neuroendocrine Tumors and Non-Functional Pancreatic Neuroendocrine Tumors. *Neuroendocrinology*. 2016; 103(2):153-171.
6. Akirov A, Larouche V, Alshehri S, Asa SL, Ezzat S. Treatment options for pancreatic neuroendocrine tumors. *Cancers (Basel).* 2019;11(6):828.
7. Cavalcanti MS, Gönen M, Klimstra DS. The ENETS/WHO grading system for neuroendocrine neoplasms of the gastroenteropancreatic system: a review of the current state, limitations and proposals for modifications. *Int J Endocr Oncol.* 2016;3(3):203-219.
8. Ma ZY, Gong YF, Zhuang HK, et al. Pancreatic neuroendocrine tumors: a review of serum biomarkers, staging, and management. *World J Gastroenterol.* 2020;26(19):2305-2322.
9. Yang M, Zeng L, Ke NW, et al. World Health Organization grading classification for pancreatic neuroendocrine neoplasms: a comprehensive analysis from a large Chinese institution. *BMC Cancer.* 2020;20(1):906.
10. van Treijen MJC, van Beek DJ, van Leeuwaarde RS, Vriens MR, Valk GD. Diagnosing nonfunctional pancreatic NETs in MEN1: the evidence base. *J Endocr Soc.* 2018;2(9):1067-1088.
11. Niederle B, Selberherr A, Bartsch DK, et al. Multiple endocrine neoplasia Type 1 and the pancreas: diagnosis and treatment of functioning and non-functioning pancreatic and duodenal neuroendocrine neoplasia within the MEN1 syndrome—An International Consensus Statement. *Neuroendocrinology.* 2021;111(7):609-630.
12. Kamilaris CDC, Stratakis CA. Multiple endocrine neoplasia Type 1 (MEN1): an update and the significance of early genetic and clinical diagnosis. *Front Endocrinol (Lausanne).* 2019;10:339.
13. Pieterman CRC, de Laat JM, Twisk JWR, et al. Long-term natural course of small nonfunctional pancreatic neuroendocrine tumors in MEN1-results from the Dutch MEN1 study group. *J Clin Endocrinol Metab.* 2017;102(10):3795-3805.
14. Vinik AI, Woltering EA, Warner RR, et al. NANETS consensus guidelines for the diagnosis of neuroendocrine tumor. *Pancreas*, 2010;39(6):713-734.
15. Ramírez-Rentería C, Ferreira-Hermosillo A, Marrero-Rodríguez D, Taniguchi-Ponciano K, Melgar-Manzanilla V, Mercado M. An update on gastroenteropancreatic neuroendocrine neoplasms: from mysteries to paradigm shifts. *Arch Med Res.* 2020;51(8):765-776.

16. Garcia-Carbonero R, Sorbye H, Baudin E, et al. ENETS Consensus Guidelines for High-Grade Gastroenteropancreatic Neuroendocrine Tumors and Neuroendocrine Carcinomas. *Neuroendocrinology*. 2016;103(2):186-194.
17. Falconi M, Plockinger U, Kwekkeboom DJ, et al. Well-differentiated pancreatic nonfunctioning tumors/carcinoma. *Neuroendocrinology*. 2006;84(3):196-211.
18. Guarneri G, Gasparini G, Crippa S, Andreasi V, Falconi M. Diagnostic strategy with a solid pancreatic mass. *Presse Med*. 2019;48(3 Pt 2):e125-e145.
19. Yu R, Wachsman A. Imaging of neuroendocrine tumors: indications, interpretations, limits, and pitfalls. *Endocrinol Metab Clin North Am*. 2017;46(3):795-814.
20. Dietrich CF, Sahai AV, D'Onofrio M, et al. Differential diagnosis of small solid pancreatic lesions. *Gastrointest Endosc*. 2016;84(6):933-940.
21. Maxwell JE, Sherman SK, O'Dorisio TM, Bellizzi AM, Howe JR. Liver-directed surgery of neuroendocrine metastases: what is the optimal strategy? *Surgery*. 2016;159(1):320-335.
22. Eisenhauer EA, Therasse P, Bogaerts J, et al. New response evaluation criteria in solid tumours: revised RECIST guideline (version 1.1). *Eur J Cancer*. 2009;45(2):228-247.
23. Fujimori N, Osoegawa T, Lee L, et al. Efficacy of endoscopic ultrasonography and endoscopic ultrasonography-guided fine-needle aspiration for the diagnosis and grading of pancreatic neuroendocrine tumors. *Scand J Gastroenterol*. 2016;51(2):245-252.
24. Panagiotidis E, Alshammari A, Michopoulou S, et al. Comparison of the impact of 68Ga-DOTATATE and 18F-FDG PET/CT on clinical management in patients with neuroendocrine tumors. *J Nucl Med*. 2017;58(1):91-96.
25. Moradi F, Jamali M, Barkhodari A, et al. Spectrum of 68Ga-DOTA TATE uptake in patients with neuroendocrine tumors. *Clin Nucl Med*. 2016;41(6):e281-e287.
26. Watanabe H, Ide R, Yamazaki Y, et al. Quantitative digital image analysis of somatostatin receptor 2 immunohistochemistry in pancreatic neuroendocrine tumors. *Med Mol Morphol*. 2021;54(4):324-336.
27. Shah MH, Goldner WS, Halfdanarson TR, et al. NCCN Guidelines Insights: Neuroendocrine and Adrenal Tumors, Version 2.2018. *J Natl Compr Canc Netw*. 2018;16(6):693-702.
28. Scott AT, Howe JR. Evaluation and management of neuroendocrine tumors of the pancreas. *Surg Clin North Am*. 2019;99(4):793-814.
29. Glasbey J, et al. Effect of COVID-19 pandemic lockdowns on planned cancer surgery for 15 tumour types in 61 countries: an international, prospective, cohort study. *Lancet Oncol*. 2021;22(11):1507-1517.
30. Yamashita Y, Kitano M. Endoscopic ultrasonography for pancreatic solid lesions. *J Med Ultrason (2001)*. 2020;47(3):377-387.
31. Zilli A, Arcidiacono PG, Conte D, et al. Clinical impact of endoscopic ultrasonography on the management of neuroendocrine tumors: lights and shadows. *Dig Liver Dis*. 2018;50(1):6-14.
32. Modlin IM, Kidd M, Malczewska A, et al. The NETest: The clinical utility of multigene blood analysis in the diagnosis and management of neuroendocrine tumors. *Endocrinol Metab Clin North Am*. 2018;47(3):485-504.
33. Lee L, Ito T, Jensen RT. Prognostic and predictive factors on overall survival and surgical outcomes in pancreatic neuroendocrine tumors: recent advances and controversies. *Expert Rev Anticancer Ther*. 2019;19(12):1029-1050.
34. Jilesen AP, van Eijck CH, Busch OR, et al. Postoperative outcomes of enucleation and standard resections in patients with a pancreatic neuroendocrine tumor. *World J Surg*. 2016;40(3):715-728.
35. Jilesen AP, van Eijck CH, in't Hof KH, et al. Postoperative complications, in-hospital mortality and 5-year survival after surgical resection for patients with a pancreatic neuroendocrine tumor: a systematic review. *World J Surg*. 2016;40(3):729-748.
36. Liu JB, Baker MS. Surgical management of pancreatic neuroendocrine tumors. *Surg Clin North Am*. 2016;96(6):1447-1468.
37. Rosenberg AM, Friedmann P, Del Rivero J, et al. Resection versus expectant management of small incidentally discovered nonfunctional pancreatic neuroendocrine tumors. *Surgery*. 2016;159(1):302-309.
38. Schwartz LH, Litière S, de Vries E, et al. RECIST 1.1-Update and clarification: from the RECIST committee. *Eur J Cancer*. 2016;62:132-137.
39. Genc CG, Klumpen HJ, van Oijen MGH, et al. A nationwide population-based study on the survival of patients with pancreatic neuroendocrine tumors in the Netherlands. *World J Surg*. 2018;42(2):490-497.
40. Nell S, Borel Rinkes IHM, Verkooijen HM, et al. Early and late complications after surgery for MEN1-related nonfunctioning pancreatic neuroendocrine tumors. *Ann Surg*. 2018;267(2):352-356.
41. Morgan RE, Pommier SJ, Pommier RF. Expanded criteria for debulking of liver metastasis also apply to pancreatic neuroendocrine tumors. *Surgery*. 2018;163(1):218-225.
42. Cives M, Ghayouri M, Morse B, et al. Analysis of potential response predictors to capecitabine/temozolomide in metastatic pancreatic neuroendocrine tumors. *Endocr Relat Cancer*. 2016;23(9):759-767.
43. Caplin ME, Pavel M, Ćwikła JB, et al. Lanreotide in metastatic enteropancreatic neuroendocrine tumors. *N Engl J Med*. 2014;371(3):224-233.
44. Faivre S, Niccoli P, Castellano D, et al. Sunitinib in pancreatic neuroendocrine tumors: updated progression-free survival and final overall survival from a phase III randomized study. *Ann Oncol*. 2017;28(2):339-343.
45. Sorbye H, Kong G, Grozinsky-Glasberg S. PRRT in high-grade gastroenteropancreatic neuroendocrine neoplasms (WHO G3). *Endocr Relat Cancer*. 2020;27(3):R67-R77.
46. Strosberg J, El-Haddad G, Wolin E, et al. Phase 3 trial of ^{177}Lu-Dotatate for midgut neuroendocrine tumors. *N Engl J Med*. 2017;376(2):125-135.
47. Haugvik SP, Janson ET, Osterlund P, et al. Surgical treatment as a principle for patients with high-grade pancreatic neuroendocrine carcinoma: a nordic multicenter comparative study. *Ann Surg Oncol*. 2016;23(5):1721-1728.
48. Li X, Gou S, Liu Z, Ye Z, Wang C. Assessment of the American Joint Commission on cancer 8th edition staging system for patients with pancreatic neuroendocrine tumors: a surveillance, epidemiology, and end results analysis. *Cancer Medicine*. 2018;7(3):626-634.

Functional Pancreatic Neuroendocrine Tumors (pNETs): Insulinoma

55

John D. Allendorf, MD
Christine E. Kolwitz, DO
Despoina Daskalaki, MD
Matthew A. Krell, MD

GENERAL CONSIDERATIONS

Insulinoma is the most common functional neuroendocrine pancreatic tumor (pNET), with an incidence of 0.4%.[1] Insulinomas are functioning tumors that arise from the insulin-producing beta cells of the pancreas. The median age at diagnosis is approximately 50 years. They are most commonly solitary, benign, well-differentiated lesions and are often diagnosed when they are small (5 mm-2 cm), due to symptoms caused by the excessive endogenous insulin secretion.[2] Although the vast majority are solid tumors, cystic variants have been reported. Insulinomas are mostly sporadic tumors, but they are also associated with Type 1 multiple endocrine neoplasia syndrome (MEN1).[2,3] MEN1-associated lesions occur in younger patients, tend to be multifocal, and may recur.[3,4] Malignant insulinomas are rare entities that represent less than 6% of all insulinomas and have a worse prognosis.[5-7]

Clinical Findings

A. Symptoms and Signs

Patients with insulinoma typically present with fasting hypoglycemia. Overall, the signs and symptoms of hypoglycemia are not specific. They are both neuroglycopenic and autonomic. Some patients initially are misdiagnosed with a neurologic or psychiatric disorder before confirming the insulinoma-induced hypoglycemia.[8] Common neuroglycopenic symptoms comprise confusion, personality changes, dizziness, weakness, blurred vision, diplopia, headache, and dysarthria. They can be as severe as paresis, convulsions, and even coma. Weight gain occurs due to the relief of symptoms after a meal. The most common autonomic symptoms are diaphoresis, palpitations, and tremors. Typically, the symptoms disappear after ingestion of carbohydrates or intravenous administration of glucose, but up to 17% of patients can have symptoms not related to meals.[9,10]

	Symptoms
Neuroglycopenia	Mild • Confusion • Personality change • Dizziness • Weakness • Blurred vision • Diplopia • Headache • Dysarthria Severe • Paresis • Convulsions (Seizures??) • Coma
Autonomic	• Trembling • Palpitations • Sweating • Anxiety • Hunger • Nausea • Tingling

B. Laboratory Findings

Endogenous insulin does not get suppressed in insulinoma-induced hypoglycemia. This results in elevated levels of insulin, in combination with low blood glucose levels. Suggestive laboratory findings are blood glucose <55 mg/dL in patients having symptoms and <40 mg/dL without symptoms. Hyperinsulinemia, with insulin level >6 mcU/mL and serum insulin to plasma glucose ratio >0.3, suggests an insulin-mediated cause. Proinsulin is secreted by the pancreatic cells and is the precursor of insulin. It is formed by an alpha and a beta chain that are connected by the C-peptide. The modification of proinsulin to insulin occurs only in the beta cells of the pancreas. Pharmaceutical insulin only consists of the beta chain, hence if normal proinsulin and C-peptide levels are found, excess administration of exogenous insulin (factitious hypoglycemia) should be suspected. Proinsulin levels ≥5 pmol/L and C-peptide level ≥0.6 ng/mL are suggestive of insulinoma. Historically, the gold standard for diagnosis is the 72-hour observed fasting test. Individuals who are asymptomatic at the time of evaluation require hospital admission. More than 95% of patients with an insulinoma will develop symptoms within 48 hours. Blood glucose levels are monitored through finger sticks, and insulin, proinsulin, and c-peptide levels are measured every 6 hours, in the presence of hypoglycemia and in the presence of symptoms. A C-peptide suppression test is indicated if the patient remains asymptomatic after 72 hours of fasting and the plasma glucose level after an overnight fast is higher than 50 mg/dL. Patients with insulinoma fail to suppress their C-peptide levels to normal (<1.2 ng/mL) during insulin infusion (0.1 U/kg/h).[11,12]

Lab	Normal	Diagnostic of Insulinoma
Glucose	<100 mg/dL	<55 mg/dL
Insulin	<3 microU/dL	≥3 microU/mL
Proinsulin	<5 pmol/L	≥5 pmol/L
C-peptide	<0.2 nmol/mL	≥0.2 nmol/L

C. Imaging Studies

After confirmatory diagnostic laboratory tests, an insulinoma must be accurately localized with imaging. Preoperative localization is imperative for operative planning, and helps the surgeon know where to assess the tumor as many of these tumors are not palpable because of their size or because of their depth within the pancreas.

Noninvasive Imaging Modalities

A. Transabdominal Ultrasound

Sensitivity for transabdominal ultrasound for insulinoma localization is only 9% to 64%. This imaging modality therefore is not commonly recommended.

B. Computed Tomography (CT)

One noninvasive localization strategy is CT scan, which is an excellent way to localize an insulinoma because there are characteristic features with which this type of tumor is associated when CT imaging is utilized. CT is 80% sensitive for localization of pNETs in general[13] and 33% to 64% sensitive when used to localize insulinoma[11] and the diagnostic sensitivity is known to be as high as 94.4%.[13] The advantage of CT is that it delineates the relationship of the insulinoma to surrounding structures, such as the portal vein and superior mesenteric artery. It also allows for one to detect the presence of metastases.[11]

Typical CT appearance of insulinoma is hypervascular and hyperenhancing (compared to surrounding pancreatic parenchyma) during the arterial phase (Figures 55-1 and 55-2). Atypical appearance consistent with insulinoma includes a hypovascular and hypoenhancing lesion (compared to surrounding pancreatic parenchyma) in the

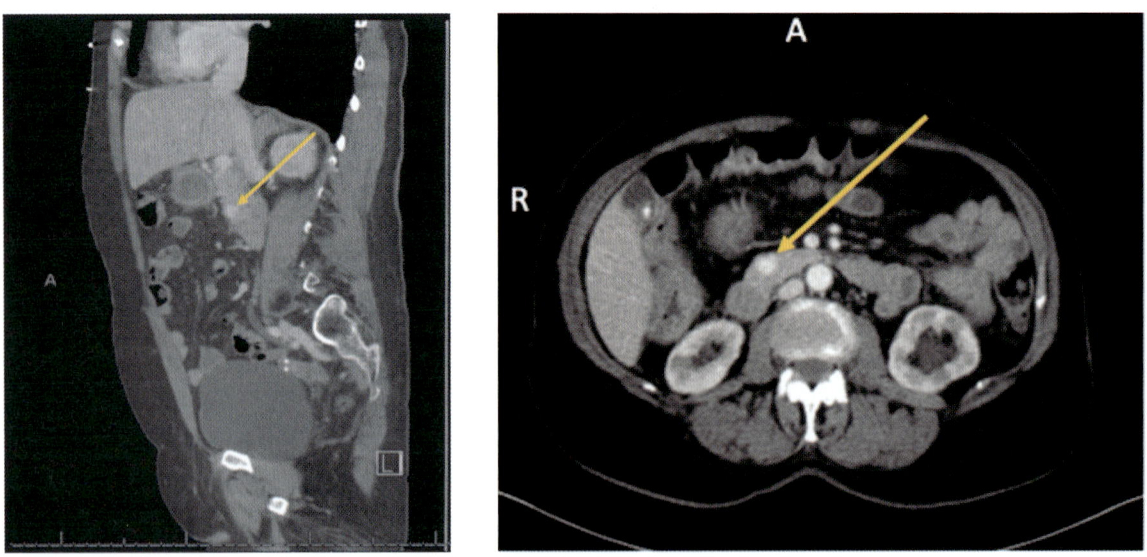

▲ **Figure 55–1.** IV contrast-enhanced CT showing a 1.5 cm hyperattenuating lesion within the head of the pancreas, consistent with a pancreatic neuroendocrine tumor, in an 83-year-old female.

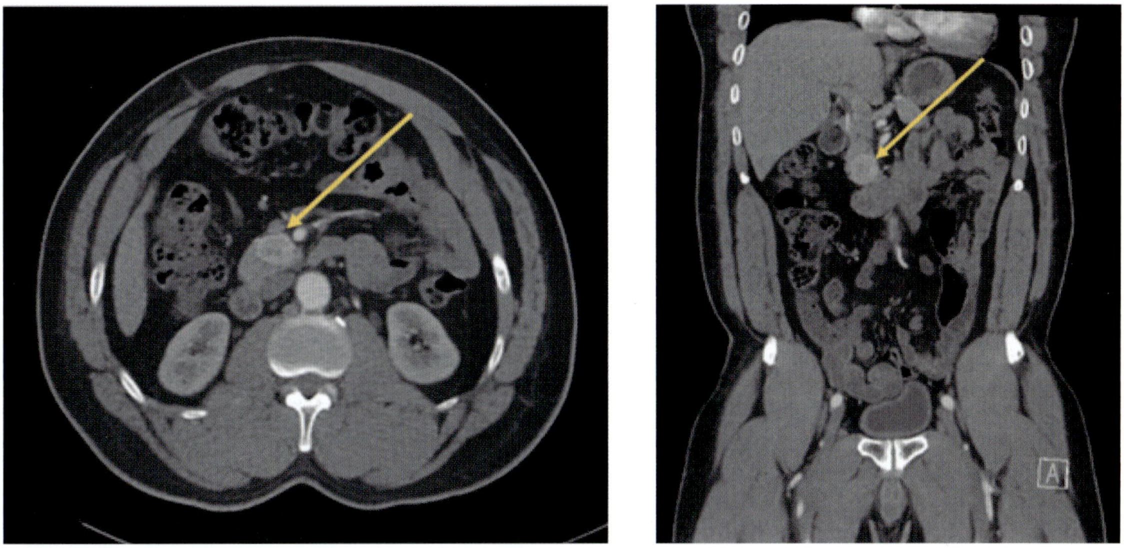

▲ **Figure 55–2.** IV contrast-enhanced CT of a 64-year-old male patient showing 2.5 cm arterially enhancing mass in the region of the uncinate process of the pancreas, consistent with neuroendocrine tumor.

washout phase.[11] These lesions can also rarely appear as hyperdense before contrast, as cystic masses, or as calcified masses. Calcification is more commonly seen when the insulinoma is malignant rather than in benign lesions.[11]

CT is also excellent at identifying liver metastases of pNETs including insulinoma, with a sensitivity of 75% to 100% and very successful at differentiating them from metastases that originate from GI adenocarcinoma based on imaging characteristics.[14]

C. Magnetic Resonance Imaging (MRI)

MRI is another imaging modality that is safe, effective, and noninvasive. MRI like CT can identify liver metastases and has characteristic imaging findings associated with insulinoma. Insulinomas are most often found to be high intensity when using T1-weighted imaging and low intensity when using T2-weighted imaging. Sensitivity can be increased by using gadolinium contrast-enhanced imaging techniques.[11] The main benefit of MRI over CT is that the patient is able to avoid ionizing radiation with the former. MRI sensitivity for detecting insulinoma is 10% to 85% and 67% to 100% for detection of associated liver metastases.[14]

D. DOTATATE PET/CT

Dodecane tetraacetic acid (DOTA) octreotate (TATE), or DOTATATE for short, is a peptide that is bonded with Gallium-68 creating a radioactive molecule that is injected intravenously into a patient with suspected insulinoma. This molecule has a high affinity for somatostatin receptor 2 which is highly concentrated in pNETs, although only in about 80% of insulinoma. On positron emission tomography (PET)/CT scan the insulinoma should be highly active and hyperenhancing.[15]

The benefit of this modality is that the overall radiation exposure is less than other localizing nuclear medicine tests that are available, as well as having a higher sensitivity for pNET localization, about 90%.[16] It also allows for the identification of metastatic disease and the ability to rule out synchronous neuroendocrine lesions, specifically in those patients with MEN1 syndrome.[15]

The sensitivity in localization of insulinoma is much less than other pNETs, cited at about 25% likely because about 20% of insulinomas have low levels of somatostatin subtype receptors 2 expression.[15]

The best use of DOTATATE scan is when other imaging modalities such as CT or MRI are unable to localize insulinoma in a patient who has been diagnosed based on other clinical findings. This imaging modality is especially helpful in identifying small tumors that are not seen on CT/MRI, but does not offer much diagnostic information when used in addition to CT/MRI.[15]

E. Somatostatin Receptor Scintigraphy

Somatostatin receptor scintigraphy was previously the test of choice for localizing pNETs. This imaging modality uses octreotide radiolabels with Indium 111 as the radiotracer and is a type of SPECT/CT imaging. Because of its higher radiation exposure to patients and lower sensitivity, it has been mostly replaced by DOTATATE scans.[11]

Invasive Imaging Modalities

A. Endoscopic Ultrasound

Endoscopic ultrasound (EUS) has become the invasive test of choice. In the hands of an experienced endoscopist, an EUS allows localization of very small tumors that may not have been easily localized on CT/MRI due to their small size.[11] The overall sensitivity for detection of insulinoma by EUS is 89.5%. The sensitivity of EUS is, however, somewhat dependent on the location of the tumor within the pancreas, with much higher sensitivity in the head of the pancreas (92.6%) when compared to the body and tail, at 78.9% and 40.0%, respectively.[17]

The appearance of insulinoma on EUS is easily recognizable with a round shape, hypoechogenicity, and well-defined circumferential margins. Occasionally this type of lesion can be missed on endoscopic ultrasound because it can appear isoechoic to the surrounding pancreas. This is more common in women, young patients, and those who have little excess adipose tissue.[11] The quality of the exam is mostly dependent on the operator's abilities and experience.[11]

B. Selective Arterial Calcium Stimulation

This is a test that is performed by a specialized interventional radiologist, and much like EUS, the outcomes and interpretation of the test are heavily operator dependent. Different arterial branches that supply distinct portions of the pancreas are targeted individually angiographically by the operator. Calcium is then injected into a single branch at a time, and at 10 and 180 seconds following injections, a sample is taken from the hepatic vein. It is expected that if the portion of the pancreas in which the insulinoma resides is stimulated a recognizable increase in insulin will be seen in the sample from the hepatic vein.

The accuracy of this test is >90%. This is a test that should be reserved for only those patients in whom noninvasive localization strategies have failed.[18] This can be especially helpful in those patients whose tumors reside outside of the head of the pancreas, as sensitivity of EUS drops substantially when the tumor is located in the body or tail of the pancreas as stated previously.[18]

Differential Diagnosis

A few other conditions need to be taken into consideration when evaluating a patient presenting with hypoglycemia and hyperinsulinemia.

Nesidioblastosis and noninsulinoma pancreatogenous hypoglycemic syndrome (NIPHS) are similar rare disorders characterized by diffuse hypertrophy and hyperfunction of the islet cells, with dysregulation of the beta cells. It can be diffuse or localized in one part of the pancreas. Biochemically the findings are comparable to those of insulinomas. Selective imaging techniques need to be used to exclude the presence of an insulinoma. Clinically, it is characterized by postprandial hypoglycemia, with symptoms occurring approximately 2 to 4 hours after meals. The treatment is surgical resection and the final diagnosis is made on histopathology.[14,19]

Nesidioblastosis after Roux-en-Y gastric bypass. There have been cases described in the literature of patients developing pancreatic islet abnormalities after bariatric surgery. It is still a matter of debate whether the diffuse proliferation of the beta cells results from the obesity and antecedes the procedure, or it develops as a consequence.[20,21]

Factitious hypoglycemia is a condition characterized by hypoglycemia due to excessive exogenous administration of insulin or oral hypoglycemic medications in individuals with or without diabetes mellitus. It is more common in adolescent females. Even though it might be challenging to diagnose initially, laboratory findings are typical. Contrary to insulinomas that are characterized by low blood glucose levels associated with elevation in insulin, proinsulin, and C-peptide levels, in the case of factitious hypoglycemia there is hyperinsulinemia with low proinsulin and C-peptide concentrations.[22,23]

Sulfonylurea-induced hypoglycemia. Sulfonylureas are common oral hypoglycemic agents that inhibit potassium channels on the membrane of the pancreatic beta cells and cause exocytosis of insulin granules. The insulin secretion is independent of the blood glucose level and hypoglycemia is a common complication that is unrelated to meals or fasting. Plasma or urine sulfonylurea testing should be requested when there is a suspicion of sulfonylurea-induced hypoglycemia.[23]

Insulin autoimmune syndrome is a rare condition, more commonly found in Asian populations. It is characterized by hyperinsulinemic hypoglycemia, high insulin or insulin-receptor antibody titers, normal pancreatic islet cells, and no history of prior exposure to exogenous insulin. This syndrome may develop spontaneously or be related to certain drug or virus exposure. The hypoglycemia can develop both during fasting and after meals. The symptoms are usually mild and self-limiting. Laboratory testing for insulin and insulin receptor antibodies should be ordered to differentiate it from other forms of hyperinsulinemic hypoglycemia.[24]

Treatment

A. Surgical Treatment

Surgery is the treatment of choice for insulinoma. Surgery is indicated to relieve symptoms, avoid malignant transformation, and in the rare cases of malignant insulinoma, improve survival. Preoperative imaging should be used as a guide to surgical planning.[1,10,25,26]

The extent of the resection may vary depending on the size of the mass, the proximity to the main pancreatic duct, the number of lesions, cellular differentiation, mitotic rate, Ki-67 index, and association familial syndromes.

Intraoperative imaging with ultrasound should be used to confirm the location of the tumor, evaluate its relationship to the main pancreatic duct, examine the liver to rule out potential metastatic lesions, and assess the peri-pancreatic region for possible enlarged lymph nodes. The detection rate of insulinomas using intraoperative ultrasound is as high as 97%. We also find it useful to evaluate the pancreas with the ultrasound after resecting the tumor, for example in case of an enucleation, to confirm the integrity of the pancreatic duct and bile duct.

Pancreas-sparing resections, such as *enucleation*, are ideal for single, small insulinomas (<2 cm) that are not in close proximity to the main pancreatic duct (>2 mm). The two most important considerations for the surgeon during this operation are avoiding damage to the pancreatic duct, and preservation of the tumor capsule to achieve an adequate margin. This procedure is safe and feasible using minimally invasive techniques, such as a laparoscopic or robotic approach, with comparable postoperative and pathologic outcomes to open surgery.[1,26-29] Postoperative pancreatic fistula (POPF) is the main concern after such a procedure. It has been reported that the rate of POPF is correlated with the distance between mass and pancreatic duct, as well as with operative time. It is our preference to leave a drain in proximity of the resection plane to monitor and control a POPF. If the main pancreatic duct is damaged during the procedure, a pancreaticojejunostomy can be performed at the site of excision to avoid a high-output POPF, or the procedure can be converted to a formal pancreatic resection.

Formal pancreatic resections are necessary in certain cases. These include large tumors, tumors involving or abutting the duct of Wirsung, locally advanced disease, and in patients with MEN1 syndrome, due to a higher chance of recurrence. Pancreaticoduodenectomy is preferred for tumors of the head of the pancreas and uncinate process. Distal pancreatectomy is favored for lesions of the body and tail of the pancreas. Spleen preservation is feasible and acceptable in most cases, given the benign nature of most insulinomas. Central pancreatectomy is performed less frequently, but it could be ideal for small tumors of the neck and proximal body of the pancreas, in an attempt to preserve more parenchyma. Total or subtotal pancreatectomy might be necessary for multifocal disease or, rarely, for large malignant tumors. Debulking surgery can be performed in patients with widespread disease to improve the symptoms and the efficacy of loco-regional or systemic treatment.[1,2,4,10,26-31]

Routine formal pancreatic resection with regional lymphadenectomy is not necessary in every case of insulinoma. While lymph node involvement is associated with worse prognosis, the value of routine regional lymphadenectomy remains a matter of debate. Formal oncologic resection with lymphadenectomy should be considered in case of malignant insulinoma and in patients with MEN1 syndrome.[4,5,25,31]

Minimally invasive pancreatic surgery has gained favor over the past 20 years. Several articles have been published in the literature confirming the safety and feasibility of both the laparoscopic and robotic approaches. Even complex pancreatic resections, such as pancreaticoduodenectomies, are often performed using minimally invasive methods. Postoperative and oncologic outcomes are comparable to the open approach. In addition, minimally invasive techniques have been shown to have some improved outcomes, such as lower blood loss, less postoperative pain, and shorter hospital stay.[1,26,28]

When metastatic disease is present, surgery should be considered in cases of a resectable primary tumor and isolated, resectable secondary lesions (eg, isolated liver metastases).[5,7,11] The procedures can be staged, or synchronous. Noncurative debulking surgery might be considered in selected cases, but is not usually a consideration in cases of insulinoma.[32]

B. Medical Treatment

Nonsurgical treatment is another option for the management of insulinomas. It should be considered in patients that are not medically fit for surgery, patients who refuse surgery, in cases of a missed insulinoma after an initial operation, in cases of symptomatic recurrent disease, or in cases of unresectable, or disseminated metastatic disease.[2,3,6,34]

Diazoxide inhibits insulin release from pancreatic beta cells by opening potassium channels. It is considered the first line of treatment and it can be used in association with somatostatin analogues. Approximately half the patients develop side effects, most commonly, fluid retention, weight gain, hirsutism, and gastrointestinal symptoms.[12,39]

Somatostatin analogues, such as octreotide and lantreotide, are considered second-line agents, but can be used as first-line medical treatment in malignant insulinomas. They are more effective in tumors that have high expression of somatostatin receptor expression. Side effects include gastrointestinal symptoms and gallstone formation.[12,33,34]

Oral corticosteroids decrease insulin synthesis and glucose uptake, increase insulin resistance and gluconeogenesis. They should be considered if the first two lines of treatment are ineffective. A low starting dose is usually effective.[12]

Everolimus is an mTOR inhibitor that causes peripheral insulin resistance and reduces proinsulin secretion. It can be used to improve severe hypoglycemia in patients with unresectable or metastatic insulinoma, without producing antitumor effects. It may result in severe toxicity (eg, opportunistic infections, neutropenia) and is reserved only for selected cases.[35]

Verapamil, a calcium channel blocker, and phenytoin, an anticonvulsant medication, both decrease insulin secretion and have been used in an attempt to control and treat hypoglycemia, but their efficacy is questionable.

Peptide receptor radionuclide therapy (PRRT) acts with a similar mechanism to somatostatin analogues and may be an option for patients with inoperable or metastatic disease. The somatostatin analogue is labeled with a radioactive isotope, which allows for targeted systemic radiation therapy. Somatostatin analogue administration needs to be discontinued prior to PRRT.[12] ^{177}Lu-DOTA-TATE, currently the most commonly used radionuclide, is then administered. The optimal treatment is three cycles with a 10- to 12-week interval between cycles. Side effects include nausea, vomiting, anemia, and renal toxicity. Disease control rates have been reported as high as 80% in patients with inoperable, malignant insulinoma.[36,37]

Chemotherapy, with agents such as doxorubicin, streptozocin, and a combination of streptozocin and 5-fluorouracil, can be attempted in cases of undifferentiated tumors or rapidly progressive, inoperable tumors with uncontrolled symptoms.[38] Approximately one-third of the patients can achieve a radiologic response of 30% reduction of the initial tumor load.

Transcatheter arterial embolization with or without selective hepatic artery infusion chemotherapy is an option for patients who present with liver metastases and unresectable disease, or symptomatic patients who are not candidates for surgical resection.[40,41] The goal is necrosis of the tumor, which has blood supply from the hepatic artery, and preservation of the normal hepatic parenchyma, which derives blood from the portal vein.

There are three common types of transcatheter arterial embolization used in the treatment of neuroendocrine liver metastases, bland transarterial embolization (TAE), transarterial chemoembolization (TACE), and transarterial radioembolization (TARE).[41] These therapies utilize the hypervascular composition of these neuroendocrine liver metastases to achieve effectiveness. TAE relies on ischemia to induce damage to the tumor. TACE and TARE utilize a combination of local administration of chemotherapy or radiation therapy with ischemia directed specifically toward the tumor. There is still debate about which is the appropriate choice for specific patient types. A recent meta-analysis from studies over the last 10 years has shown no high-quality evidence to support one over the other. TACE has a slight overall survival benefit and has been more frequently utilized, but TARE has the added ability to treat a complete liver lobe or diffuse liver disease with less toxicity.[41] While surgical therapy has traditionally been the preferred method of treatment of neuroendocrine liver metastases, there is growing interest in some of these less invasive procedures for a population with a limited 5-year survival in hopes of increasing quality of life. There has been proven efficacy for symptomatic and unresectable neuroendocrine liver metastases. TARE has some support for its advantage over TACE, but available literature has mixed findings.[41,42] These therapies will likely become more expansive in their applications as the oncology community grows more familiar with them.

Radiofrequency ablation (RFA), percutaneous or laparoscopic, can be used to treat liver metastases of smaller size.[42] There have also been reports in the literature of primary insulinomas and other pancreatic neuroendocrine tumors being treated with RFA, as an alternative to surgical resection.[14,39-42]

Endoscopic ultrasound-guided radiofrequency ablation (EUS-RFA) induces tumor mass thermal necrosis and is a potentially curative treatment with low periprocedural risks.[26,42] A recent systematic review found the overall effectiveness of EUS-RFA to be about 96% without a difference between functional and nonfunctional pNETs. The authors also noted that a greater tumor dimension was predictive of treatment failure. Another study found that for pNETs sized 1-1.5 cm compared to 1.5-2 cm showed a success of EUS-RFA rate of 88.9% versus 78% respectively without a statistically significant difference.[11,26] This approach can be considered for insulinomas that are a safe distance from the main pancreatic duct. Larger scale studies are needed to confirm the true efficacy of this procedure, and the long-term outcomes.[11,26,42]

Surveillance

The National Comprehensive Cancer Network (NCCN) guidelines version 1.2015 recommends a history and physical examination 3 to 12 months after resection, as well as biochemical markers, if clinically indicated and imaging with CT or MRI. Subsequently, from 1 to 10 years postresection, the same evaluation is recommended every 6 to 12 months. If asymptomatic loco-regional or metastatic disease develops, with low tumor burden and stable disease, the patient can be monitored every 3 to 12 months with markers and imaging. Alternatively, treatment with somatostatin analogues can be initiated.

Prognosis

Patients with benign insulinoma who undergo surgical resection are cured. Their overall survival is comparable to the general population. Recurrence after resection occurs in up to 5% of patients with sporadic disease at 10 years, and up to 20% of patients with MEN1 syndrome.

Malignant insulinomas have a survival rate of approximately 60% at 5 years. A recent multicenter study found that prognostic factors associated with better overall survival are surgery and Ki-67 ≤10%, whereas an insulin level >60 μU/mL is a negative prognostic factor.[7]

When to Refer/When to Admit

Patients who are suspected of having an insulinoma should be referred to an endocrinologist. If MEN syndrome is suspected, the patient should also visit a geneticist. After the proper biochemical workup and imaging has been completed, the patient should be advised to see a surgeon who specializes in pancreatic pathology. Admission, other than at the time of surgery, could be required if there is a need for 72-hour fasting test or a C-peptide suppression test. In patients affected by malignant insulinoma, consultation with an oncologist and radiation specialist should be obtained.

REFERENCES

1. Belfiori G, Wiese D, Partelli S, et al. Minimally invasive versus open treatment for benign sporadic insulinoma comparison of short-term and long-term outcomes. *World J Surg.* 2018;42(10):3223-3230.
2. Brown E, Watkin D, Evans J, Yip V, Cuthbertson DJ. Multidisciplinary management of refractory insulinomas. *Clin Endocrinol (Oxf).* 2018; 88(5):615-624.
3. Giannis D, Moris D, Karachaliou GS, et al. Insulinomas: from diagnosis to treatment. A review of the literature. *J BUON.* 2020;25(3):1302-1314.
4. Ratnayake CBB, Pt Loveday B, Windsor JA, Lawrence B, Pandanaboyana S. Patient characteristics and clinical outcomes following initial surgical intervention for MEN1 associated pancreatic neuroendocrine tumours: a systematic review and exploratory meta-analysis of the literature. *Pancreatology.* 2019;19(3):462-471.
5. Sada A, Glasgow AE, Vella A, Thompson GB, McKenzie TJ, Habermann EB. Malignant insulinoma: a rare form of neuroendocrine tumor. *World J Surg.* 2020;44(7):2288-2294.
6. Spiro AJ, Shakir MKM, Hoang TD. Successful long-term medical management of unresectable insulinomas. *Case Rep Oncol.* 2020;13(2):948-954.
7. Veltroni A, E Cosaro, F Spada, et al. Clinico-pathological features, treatments and survival of malignant insulinomas: a multicenter study. *Eur J Endocrinol.* 2020;182(4):439-446.
8. Censi S, Mian C, Betterle C. Insulin autoimmune syndrome: from diagnosis to clinical management. *Ann Transl Med.* 2018;6(17):335.
9. Dizon AM, Kowalyk S, Hoogwerf BJ. Neuroglycopenic and other symptoms in patients with insulinomas. *Am J Med.* 1999;106(3):307-310.
10. Fahmy JN, Varsanik MA, Hub D, Eguia E, Abood G, Knab LM. Pancreatic neuroendocrine tumors: surgical outcomes and survival analysis. *Am J Surg.* 2021;221(3):529-533.
11. Lopes AA, Miranda AC, Maior MS, de Mello RV, Bandeira FA. Nesidioblastosis associated with pancreatic heterotopia as a differential diagnosis of hypoglycemia: a literature review and case report. *Am J Case Rep.* 2020;21:e922778.
12. Bansal N, Weinstock RS. Non-diabetic hypoglycemia. In: Feingold KR, et al, eds. *Endotext.* South Dartmouth (MA); 2000.
13. Lee CH, Won JGS, Tseng HS. Pancreatogenous hypoglycemic syndrome—insulinoma or non-insulinoma origin (NIPHS). InTech. 2011.
14. Klein-Schwartz W, Stassinos GL, Isbister GK. Treatment of sulfonylurea and insulin overdose. *Br J Clin Pharmacol.* 2016;81(3):496-504.
15. De Herder WW, Zandee WT, Hofland J. Insulinoma. In: Feingold KR, et al, eds. *Endotext.* South Dartmouth (MA); 2000.
16. Okabayashi T, Shima Y, Sumiyoshi T, et al. Diagnosis and management of insulinoma. *World J Gastroenterol.* 2013;19(6):829-837.
17. Malik S, Mitchell JE, Steffen K, et al. Recognition and management of hyperinsulinemic hypoglycemia after bariatric surgery. *Obes Res Clin Pract.* 2016;10(1):1-14.
18. Mulla CM, Storino A, Yee EU, et al. Insulinoma after bariatric surgery: diagnostic dilemma and therapeutic approaches. *Obes Surg.* 2016;26(4):874-881.
19. Cappellani D, Macchia E, Falorni A, Marchetti P. Insulin autoimmune syndrome (Hirata disease): a comprehensive review fifty years after its first description. *Diabetes Metab Syndr Obes.* 2020;13:963-978.
20. Landoni L, Marchegiani G, Pollini T, et al. The evolution of surgical strategies for pancreatic neuroendocrine tumors (Pan-NENs): time-trend and outcome analysis from 587 consecutive resections at a high-volume institution. *Ann Surg.* 2019;269(4):725-732.
21. Schwarz JL, Hogg ME. Current state of minimally invasive pancreatic surgery. *J Surg Oncol.* 2021;123(6):1370-1386.
22. Ore AS, Barrows CE, Solis-Velasco M, Shaker J, Moser AJ. Robotic enucleation of benign pancreatic tumors. *J Vis Surg.* 2017;3:151.
23. Liu R, Wakabayashi G, Palanivelu C, et al. International consensus statement on robotic pancreatic surgery. *Hepatobiliary Surg Nutr.* 2019;8(4):345-360.
24. Jin JB, Qin K, Li H, et al. Robotic enucleation for benign or borderline tumours of the pancreas: a retrospective analysis and comparison from a high-volume centre in Asia. *World J Surg.* 2016;40(12):3009-3020.
25. Mehrabi A, Fischer L, Hafezi M, et al. A systematic review of localization, surgical treatment options, and outcome of insulinoma. *Pancreas.* 2014;43(5):675-686.
26. Tanaka M, Heckler M, Mihaljevic AL, et al. Systematic review and metaanalysis of lymph node metastases of resected pancreatic neuroendocrine tumors. *Ann Surg Oncol.* 2021; 28(3):1614-1624.
27. Memeh KO, Vaghaiwalla T, Keutgen XM. Surgical treatment of non-functioning pancreatic neuroendocrine tumors: current controversies and challenges. *Journal of Pancreatology.* 2020;3(2):51-58.
28. Kaltsas G, Caplin M, Davies P, et al. ENETS Consensus Guidelines for the Standards of Care in Neuroendocrine Tumors: pre- and perioperative therapy in patients with neuroendocrine tumors. *Neuroendocrinology.* 2017;105(3):245-254.
29. Dimitriadis GK, Weickert MO, Randeva HS, Kaltsas G, Grossman A. Medical management of secretory syndromes related to gastroenteropancreatic neuroendocrine tumours. *Endocr Relat Cancer.* 2016;23(9):R423-R436.
30. Bernard V, Lombard-Bohas C, Taquet MC, et al. Efficacy of everolimus in patients with metastatic insulinoma and refractory hypoglycemia. *Eur J Endocrinol.* 2013;168(5): 665-674.
31. Bodei L, Schöder H, Baum RP, et al. Molecular profiling of neuroendocrine tumours to predict response and toxicity to peptide receptor radionuclide therapy. *Lancet Oncol.* 2020; 21(9):e431-e443.
32. Bushnell DL, Bodeker KL. Overview and current status of peptide receptor radionuclide therapy. *Surg Oncol Clin N Am.* 2020;29(2):317-326.
33. Ito T, Jensen RT. Perspectives on the current pharmacotherapeutic strategies for management of functional neuroendocrine tumor syndromes. *Expert Opin Pharmacother.* 2021;22(6):685-693.
34. Herrera-Martinez AD, Hofland J, Hofland LJ, et al. Targeted systemic treatment of neuroendocrine tumors: current options and future perspectives. *Drugs.* 2019;79(1):21-42.
35. Gupta S. Intra-arterial liver-directed therapies for neuroendocrine hepatic metastases. *Semin Intervent Radiol.* 2013;30(1):28-38.

36. Dermine S, Palmieri LJ, Lavolé J, et al. Non-pharmacological therapeutic options for liver metastases in advanced neuroendocrine tumors. *J Clin Med.* 2019;8(11).
37. Gillams A, Cassoni A, Conway G, Lees W. Radiofrequency ablation of neuroendocrine liver metastases: the Middlesex experience. *Abdom Imaging.* 2005;30(4):435-441.
38. Yao C, Wang X, Zhang Y, et al. Treatment of insulinomas by laparoscopic radiofrequency ablation: case reports and literature review. *Open Med (Wars).* 2020;15:84-91.
39. Imperatore N, de Nucci G, Mandelli ED, et al. Endoscopic ultrasound-guided radiofrequency ablation of pancreatic neuroendocrine tumors: a systematic review of the literature. *Endosc Int Open.* 2020;8(12):E1759-E1764.
40. Oleinikov K, Dancour A, Epshtein J, et al. Endoscopic ultrasound-guided radiofrequency ablation: a new therapeutic approach for pancreatic neuroendocrine tumors. *J Clin Endocrinol Metab.* 2019;104(7):2637-2647.
41. Ngo L, Elnahla A, Attia AS, et al. Chemoembolization versus radioembolization for neuroendocrine liver metastases: a meta-analysis comparing clinical outcomes. *Ann Surg Oncol.* 2021;28(4):1950-1958.
42. Chandan S, Dhaliwal AJ, Mohan BP, et al. Sa1475 Does tumor size or location affect outcomes of endoscopic ultrasound guided radiofrequency ablation (EUS-RFA) in pancreatic neuroendocrine tumors: a systematic review; meta-analysis. *Gastrointestinal Endoscopy.* 2020;91(6) Supplement: AB207. https://www.sciencedirect.com/science/article/pii/S001651072031511X.

56 Functional Pancreatic Neuroendocrine Tumors (PNETs): Gastrinoma & Zollinger-Ellison Syndrome

Rosyli F. Reveron-Thornton, MD, MS
Deshka S. Foster, MD, PhD
Jeffrey A. Norton, MD

INTRODUCTION

Definition

Gastrinoma is a type of gastrointestinal neuroendocrine tumor (GI-NET) that secretes excessive gastrin. More specifically, gastrinomas belong to a subset of GI-NETs known as functional NETs (F-NETs) that synthesize biologically active peptides/hormones leading to a functional clinical syndrome (F-NETs). The clinical syndrome is called Zollinger-Ellison syndrome (ZES).

Gastrin

Gastric antrum G cells synthesize and release gastrin, which is a hormone that induces enterochromaffin-like cells (ECL cells) to produce and release histamine. Histamine subsequently binds to histamine-2 receptors (H2R) on the parietal cells stimulating acid secretion. Chronically elevated gastrin levels produce both stimulatory and trophic effects on the parietal cells, gastric enterochromaffin-like cells (ECL), and other gastric mucosal cells that result in an elevation in basal acid output (BAO) and an increased maximal ability to secrete acid (MAO).[1]

Gastrin-associated acid hypersecretion in the setting of a gastrinoma leads to the development of refractory peptic ulcer disease (PUD). ZES was first described in 1955 by Drs. Robert Zollinger and Edwin Ellison and was originally thought to be due to gastric acid hypersecretion and PUD in the setting of a nonbeta islet cell tumor of the pancreas. As we discuss later in the chapter, gastrinomas are located in either the pancreas or duodenum. ZES-associated ulcers most commonly arise in the proximal duodenum but can also be found in other areas of the gastrointestinal (GI) tract including the stomach, distal duodenum, and jejunum. Gastrinoma gastric acid hypersecretion can also cause severe gastroesophageal reflux disease (GERD), secretory diarrhea, and weight loss. When acid secretion is controlled with proton pump inhibitors (PPI), all the symptoms of ZES resolve.

Classes of ZES

Two main classes of ZES exist and are classified based on the presence of genetic mutations (sporadic ZES) and multiple endocrine neoplasia (MEN1/ZES).

A. Sporadic ZES (75%-80%)

Sporadic ZES tumors are usually small, located in the duodenum and pancreas, and are less than 1 cm in diameter. Typically, the duodenal tumors are more common and very small (3-4 mm).

B. MEN1/ZES (20%-25%)

MEN1 is inherited as an autosomal dominant disorder in which patients develop tumors in various endocrine glands, in addition to those commonly occupied by gastrinomas (duodenum and pancreas). Most commonly, MEN1 patients develop multiple parathyroid adenomas (98%-100%), GI-NETs (80%-100%), and pituitary adenomas (50%-60%). To a lesser extent, these patients also develop tumors in the adrenal glands (adenomas/carcinomas [27%-36%]), carcinoid tumors (bronchial/lung [0%-8%]), nonendocrine tumors of the skin (angiofibromas [60%-90%], gastric carcinoids [7%-35%], thymic carcinoids [0%-8%]), central nervous system (CNS) (meningiomas, schwannomas, [0%-8%]), and smooth muscle tumors (leiomyomas/leiomyosarcomas [1%-7%]).

Incidence

Global incidence of gastrinomas is estimated to be 0.5 to 3 cases/million/year. Gastrinomas are the second most common functional pancreatic neuroendocrine tumor (F-pNETs). ZES is relatively rare, accounting for 0.1% to 1%

of PUD and 2% of refractory PUD cases. Sporadic gastrinomas are frequently diagnosed between the ages of 20 and 50 and are more common in men. MEN1-associated gastrinomas present at an earlier age, between 10 and 30 years.

Behavior

Although gastrinomas are slow-growing tumors, 60% to 90% are malignant. In 25% of cases, these tumors may pursue an aggressive course. Thirty-five percent of pancreatic gastrinomas metastasize to the liver, while only a small percentage of duodenal gastrinomas exhibit this propensity for the liver. Although, duodenal gastrinomas do tend to have a higher incidence of lymph node metastasis than pancreatic gastrinomas.[2]

Tumor Distribution

Approximately 80% of gastrinomas occur within the "gastrinoma triangle," an area bordered by the junction of cystic and common bile ducts (superiorly), the second and third parts of the duodenum (inferiorly), and the neck and body of the pancreas (medially) (Figure 56–1). Although gastrinomas are the second most common functional pancreatic neuroendocrine tumor (panNET), recent studies estimate that duodenal gastrinomas are three- to ninefold more frequent than pancreatic gastrinomas. Approximately two-thirds of sporadic gastrinomas are found in the duodenum and are usually less than 1 cm in size, while ~20-25% arise in the head of the pancreas (pancreatic neuroendocrine tumor [pan-NET]), and the remaining 5% are found in other ectopic locations (eg, heart, liver, ovary) (Figure 56–2).[3] In one series,[4] 10% of sporadic/MEN1 patients had a primary lymph node gastrinoma. Similar to sporadic gastrinomas, 85% to 100% of MEN1/ZES-associated gastrinomas occur in the duodenum with a smaller proportion (0%-15%) reported in the pancreas.[5] While it is not uncommon to have another coinciding pancreatic NET in MEN1/ZES patients with a duodenal primary, many of these tumors are nonfunctional (NF-panNETs). In terms of pancreatic primaries in MEN1 patients, 80% to 100% of MEN1/ZES patients develop microscopic NF-panNETs (0%-13% being symptomatic) and 54% cause ZES (range 20%-61%).

Metastasis

While both duodenal and pancreatic gastrinomas can develop lymph node metastases (30%-70%), pancreatic gastrinomas metastasize to the liver at a much higher rate, negatively affecting long-term survival. On average, 34% (range 13%-53%) of sporadic gastrinomas have already metastasized to the liver at the time of diagnosis. Most gastrinoma hepatic metastases are distributed diffusely, spanning both hepatic

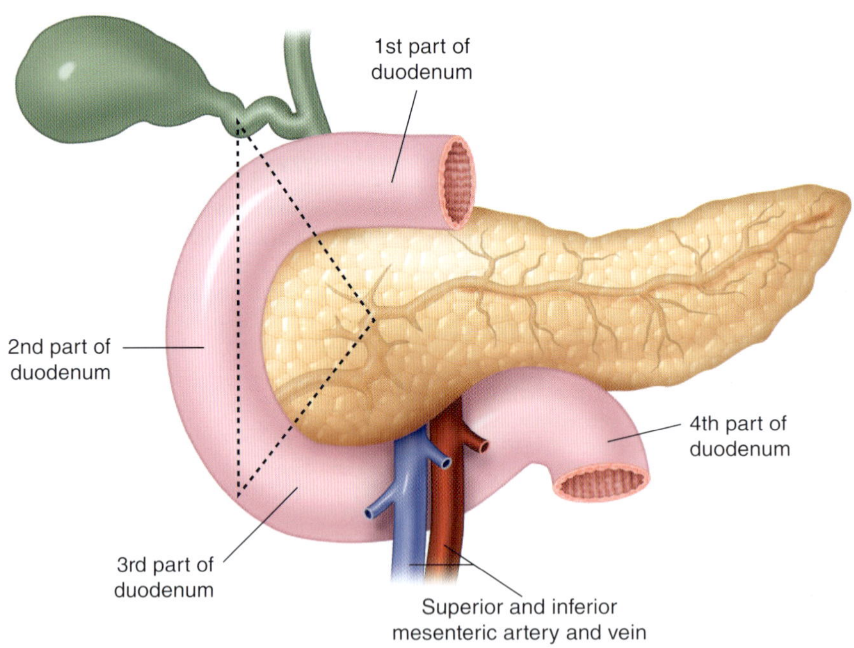

Figure 56–1. Diagram of the gastrinoma triangle. Gastrinoma triangle is centered on the head of the pancreas. It is bordered by the junction of cystic and common bile ducts (superiorly), the second and third parts of the duodenum (inferiorly), and the neck and body of the pancreas (medially).

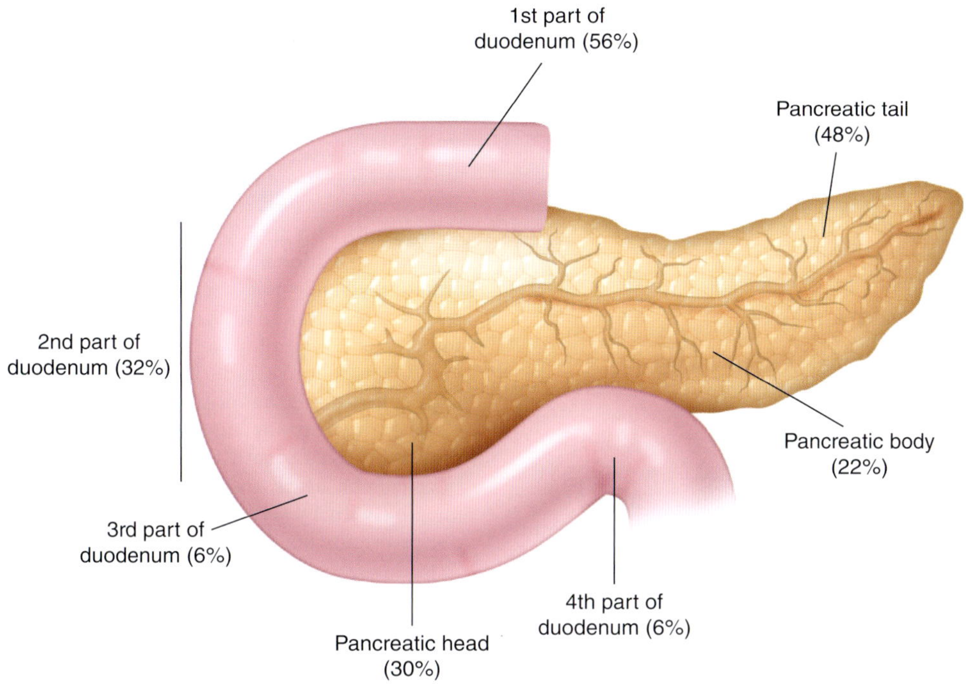

Figure 56–2. Location of surgically identified gastrinomas in the duodenum and pancreas. Gastrinomas are most commonly found throughout the duodenum in decreasing density from proximal to distal. They are also found in the pancreas uniformly distributed throughout the entire pancreas.

lobes, 5% to 15% of patients with metastatic pancreatic gastrinomas have localized hepatic disease.

SYMPTOMS

Sporadic ZES

The presenting clinical symptoms of ZES are entirely due to the gastric acid hypersecretion. The most common symptoms are abdominal pain (73%-98%), diarrhea (60%-75%), heartburn (52%-56%), weight loss (7%-53%), and dysphagia. If untreated, the stigmata of gastric acid hypersecretion can result in potentially life-threatening complications (such as bleeding, strictures, perforation). Up to 10% of ZES patients initially present with a perforated ulcer.

MEN1/ZES

MEN1/ZES patients most commonly present with hypercalcemia secondary to primary hyperparathyroidism or symptoms related to other p-NETs (like hypoglycemia from insulinomas). There are certain cardinal signs that when present should warrant a workup for ZES. These include distal duodenum or jejunal ulcers, multiple or recurrent ulcers, and ulcers associated with diarrhea. High suspicion should be given to any patient with PUD or family history of PUD, hyperparathyroidism, nephrolithiasis, or family history of MEN1.

DIAGNOSIS

A diagnosis of ZES is commonly made several years (often >5 years) after the initial symptom presentation, often in the setting of inadequate medical therapy. This is due to the rare nature of ZES, nonspecific presenting symptoms, and achlorhydric causes of elevated gastrin. ZES is diagnosed by demonstrating an elevated basal fasting serum gastrin concentration in the setting of elevated gastric acid (either by measuring a gastric pH ≤2 or elevated gastric acid output).

Serum Gastrin

A fasting serum gastrin (FSG) level more than normal (100 pg/mL) and often even 10 times the upper limit of normal with a gastric pH less than 2 is diagnostic of ZES. A BAO can also be used in place of gastric pH; elevation is defined as >15 mEq/h or >5 mEq/h if in setting of prior acid-reducing surgery. Of note, patients on PPIs or H2 blockers should discontinue these medications 3 to 7 days before gastrin and acid level testing.

Table 56–1. Causes of hypergastrinemia that mimic ZES.

Atrophic gastritis
PPI or H2RA
Pernicious anemia
Renal insufficiency
Gastric outlet obstruction
G-cell hyperplasia
Retained gastric antrum

Secretin Stimulation Test

Secretin stimulation tests (SSTs) are useful in equivocal cases that cannot distinguish gastrinomas from other causes of hypergastrinemia (Table 56–1). ZES patients have a paradoxical increase in serum gastrin levels in response to secretin while normal gastric G cells are inhibited by secretin. SST is performed by measuring serum gastrin before and after (2-, 5-, 10-, and 15-minute timepoints) a 0.4 μg/kg rapid IV infusion of secretin is given (give over 1 minute). Gastrin levels usually peak 10 to 20 minutes after infusion. The diagnosis of ZES is made with a >200 pg/mL increase in serum gastrin level over the basal level. Unfortunately, STT can be affected by PPI-induced hypo/achlorhydria, and therefore, cannot be reliably performed in patients on PPI or with hypo- or achlorhydria. PPIs should be discontinued as mentioned previously.

LOCALIZATION STUDIES

Tumor localization studies provide pertinent information for surgical planning and staging including tumor location and the presence of metastatic disease. Localization typically begins with an upper endoscopic ultrasound followed by a cross-sectional imaging modality (helical, contrast-enhanced, triple-phase computed tomography [CT] or magnetic resonance imaging [MRI]). This is followed by somatostatin receptor scintigraphy (SRS) or integrated PET/CT (Gallium Ga-68 DOTATATE). SRS and CT scan with contrast are the most utilized studies to identify primary and metastatic disease in ZES patients given their sensitivity. Recall that ZES can also arise outside of the GI tract (in the heart, ovaries, etc.); therefore, full-body CT imaging with DOTATATE is required and is the study of choice (Figure 56–3).

Conventional Studies

Computed tomography (CT), magnetic resonance imaging (MRI), endoscopic ultrasound (EUS), and Gallium Ga-68

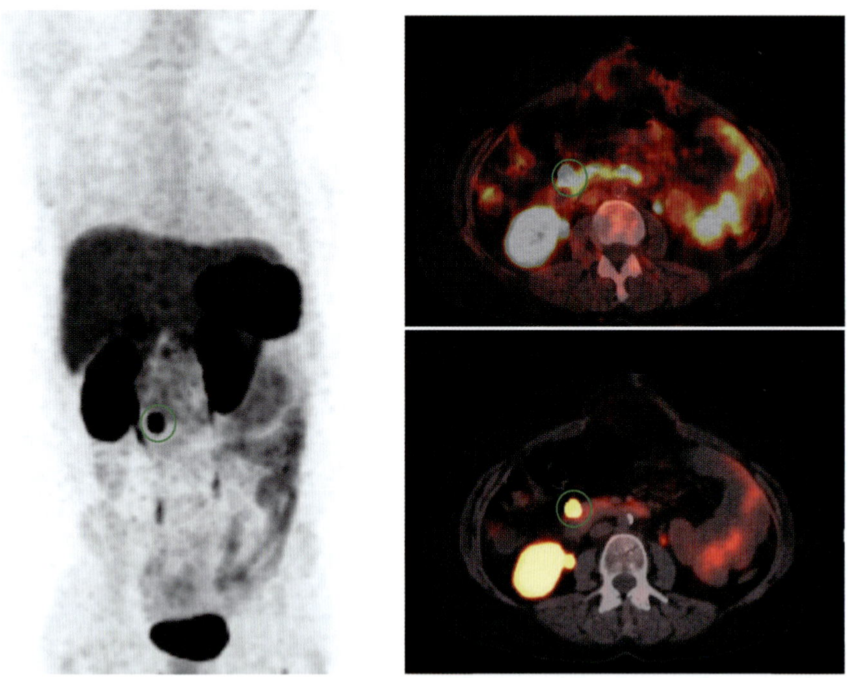

Figure 56–3. Gallium Ga-68 DOTATATE of lymph nodes within the gastrinoma triangle in a patient with ZES. Gallium Ga-68 DOTATATE PET scan that shows a bright image in the head of the pancreas region which is a gastrinoma metastasis to a lymph node. This represents localized nodal metastasis. Duodenal transillumination failed to identify a duodenal tumor, but duodenotomy identified a small duodenal gastrinoma that was excised.

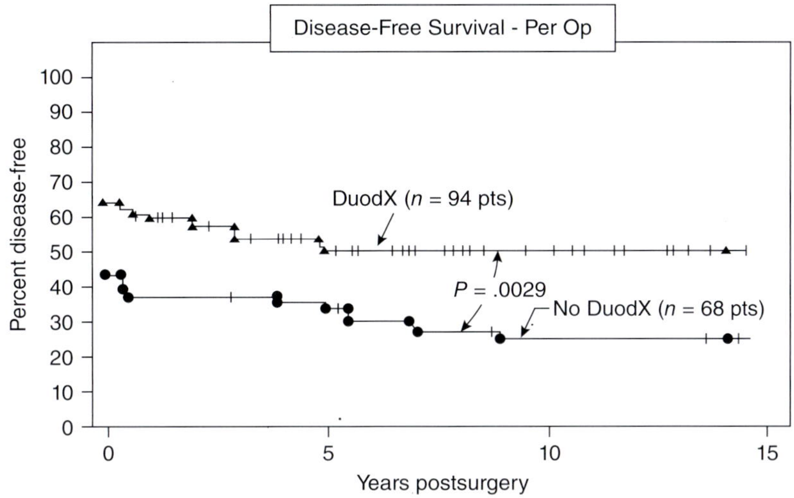

Figure 56–4. Duodenotomy increases the cure rate of sporadic ZES patients. (Reproduced with permission from Norton JA, et al. Does the use of routine duodenotomy (DUODX) affect rate of cure, development of liver metastases or survival in patients with Zollinger-Ellison Syndrome (ZES)? *Ann Surg.* 2004;239(5):617-625.)

DOTATATE PET scan are the fundamental modalities for tumor localization in ZES patients.

A. Localized Disease

Despite the increasing sensitivities of the aforementioned modalities, the small size (<1.0 cm) of the most common primary gastrinoma (duodenal primary) makes them a challenge to image preoperatively. Prospective studies demonstrate an average of 10% to 40% sensitivity of primary gastrinomas for conventional imaging studies, MRI with gadolinium being the most sensitive of the traditional imaging modalities. While EUS is particularly sensitive for intrapancreatic lesions, it has a low sensitivity for detection of duodenal gastrinoma. Given the fact that it is the most common location for a primary gastrinoma studies during surgery have been used to identify these tumors. Duodenotomy is the single best method to identify duodenal tumors and it has increased the disease-free survival rate after surgical excision (Figure 56–4).

B. Metastatic Disease

Two prospective studies demonstrated that 14% to 54% of patients with metastatic gastrinomas to the liver were successfully identified on CT and ultrasound. In patient with liver metastasis, MRI is also very sensitive, identifying 60% to 75% of metastatic disease in gastrinomas patients (Figure 56–5).

Somatostatin Receptor Scintigraphy (SRS) & Gallium Ga-68 DOTATATE PET

Somatostatin receptor scintigraphy (SRS) has the highest sensitivity and therefore is the localization study of choice for primary and metastatic ZES plus combining it with PET makes it even more sensitive. SRS is based on the principle that gastrinomas overexpress somatostatin receptors (SSTR) primarily SSTR subtype 2 (sst2). Once injected systemically, radiolabeled stomatostatin analogue 111-In pentetreotide binds to the sst2 revealing the location of the tumor. SRS has an average sensitivity of 69% to 72% for primary gastrinomas, equal to all conventional imaging studies combined, and has changed the management in 47% of cases. SRS (like conventional studies) correlates closely with tumor size. In a study of 35 ZES patients undergoing SRS followed by exploratory laparotomy, SRS detected 30% of gastrinomas ≤1.1 cm, 64% of those 1.1 to 2 cm, and 96% of those >2 cm and missed primarily small duodenal tumors (Figure 56–5). SRS also identifies patients with metastatic disease who may be eligible for peptide receptor radiation therapy (PRRT).

Intraoperative Localization Studies

The utility of intraoperative studies for detecting gastrinomas is dependent on whether or not the tumor is located in the pancreas or duodenum. Gastrinomas in the pancreas are best identified by intraoperative ultrasound (IOUS) directly on the pancreas with a high-resolution short focal distant ultrasound probe. Tumors appear sonolucent compared to the more echo-dense pancreas. Gastrinomas within the duodenum are important in that these tumors have the highest probability of being missed. They are most commonly located in the first portion of the duodenum (Figure 56–2). These tumors may be identified by endoscopic transillumination and/or duodenotomy. Opening the duodenum is the single best modality because tumors on the medial wall

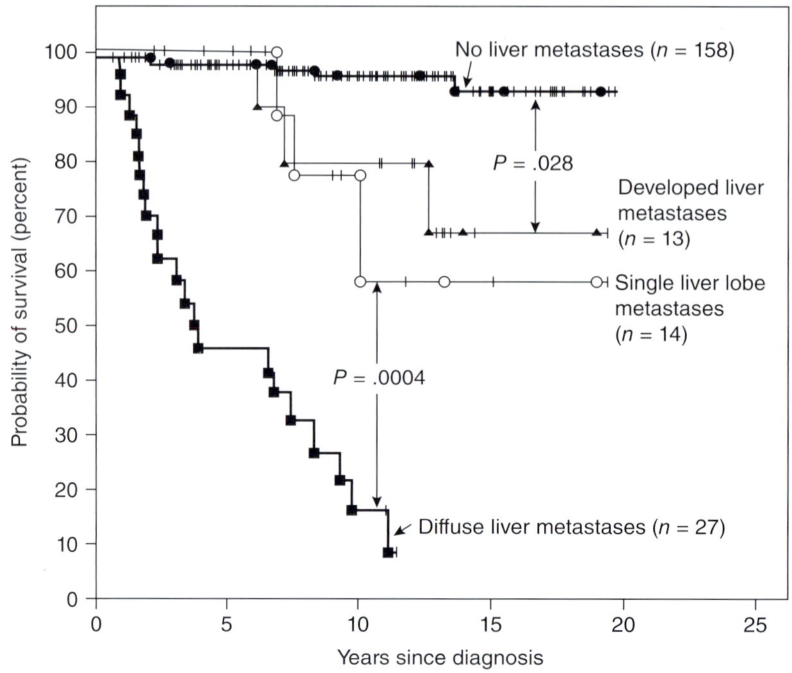

Figure 56–5. Liver metastases decrease survival of gastrinoma patients. Impact of liver metastases on survival of gastrinoma patients. No liver metastases had the best survival, localized liver metastases had intermediate survival and diffuse metastases had the worse survival. (Reproduced with permission from Yu F, et al. Prospective study of the clinical course, prognostic factors, causes of death, and survival in patients with long-standing Zollinger-Ellison syndrome. *J Clin Oncol.* 1999;17(2):615-30.)

cannot be transilluminated. Duodenal gastrinomas commonly metastasize to lymph nodes so that part of the operation periduodenal lymph nodes should be sampled. They less often metastasize to pancreas. Duodenotomy increases the surgical cure rate.

TREATMENT

Like treatments of other F-NETs, treatment of gastrinoma must address two problems: first, control of the indirect effects of the tumor (gastrin-mediated acid hypersecretion) and second, treatment of the possibly malignant tumor.

Gastric Acid Hypersecretion Control—Medical Management of Sporadic ZES & MEN1/ZES

Although initially ZES gastric acid hypersecretion management centered around surgery (total gastrectomy), the development of medical therapies (particularly high-dose PPIs) with improved short- and long-term gastric acid suppression led to their establishment as the primary treatment of choice for ZES patients. Benefits of PPIs are applicable to all medications in the class—omeprazole, esomeprazole, lansoprazole, pantoprazole, rabeprazole. These include daily or twice daily dosing because of its long duration of action. There is less tachyphylaxis compared to histamine receptor antagonists. As a result, we are able to achieve adequate acid hypersecretion in ZES without requiring dose titration in every patient. The usual dose is twice the normal dose of PPI twice daily. For example, if uses omeprazole, the dose is 40 mg twice daily. PPIs are safe and effective for long-term treatment of the symptoms of ZES.

Of note, there are other medical issues when treating acid hypersecretion in patients with MEN1/ZES. Because MEN1/ZES patients most commonly present initially with symptoms related to primary hyperparathyroidism it has been established that elevated serum calcium levels and parathyroid hormone levels worsen the ability to control the acid hypersecretion. These patients require subtotal parathyroidectomy first before surgery focused on the gastrinoma. In fact, in some MEN1/ZES patients, parathyroidectomy completely ameliorates all the signs and symptoms of ZES. Further, MEN-1/ZES patients who have been on a PPI for > 10 years may develop type 2 gastric carcinoid tumors that are malignant and may require gastrectomy to resect these tumors and lymph nodes.

Tumor Directed Therapy—Tumor Surgery for Sporadic ZES

Although presently the approach to gastric acid hypersecretion has shifted from surgical to medical therapy, the approach to the tumor itself has become increasingly surgical. Current guidelines (European Neuroendocrine Tumor Society [ENET), North American Neuroendocrine Tumor Society [NANET], European Society for Medical Oncology, and the National Comprehensive Cancer Network [NCCN]) recommend surgical resection in sporadic ZES if complete tumor removal is possible and there are no accompanying medical conditions limiting life expectancy or increasing surgical risks to unacceptable levels. This recommendation also extends to metastatic disease; if most or all imageable tumor is resectable, surgery is recommended if there are no additional medical conditions precluding surgery. If possible, the preferred surgical approach according to the different guidelines includes enucleation, local resection for pancreatic head lesions, or distal pancreatectomy. Surgery may include mesenteric resection and reconstruction if the tumor invades the mesenteric and/or portal veins. Lymph nodes within the gastrinoma triangle should also be removed when primary gastrinomas are within the triangle.

Several reasons have been offered to explain the favorable shift in management toward surgical resection. First, advancements in imaging modalities have improved tumor localization and staging capabilities, preventing unnecessary surgery. Second, more recent studies report increased disease-free rates in patient undergoing surgery even if preoperative imaging was negative.[3] Third, importantly, studies show that surgical resection in Sporadic ZES patients lead to a decrease in the rate of liver metastasis, an important long-term survival determinant. Fourth, gastrinomas within the duodenum are found in a larger percentage of patients. Fifth, another study demonstrated that even in sporadic ZES patients with negative preoperative imaging, an experienced surgeon was able to successfully locate a gastrinoma in 98% of patients, rendering 50% of these patients' disease free. Sixth, although the presence of lymph node primary gastrinomas are controversial, routine lymphadenectomy in sporadic ZES is now routinely recommended after multiple studies have demonstrated increased long-term (up to 20 years) disease-free survival following resection of only a single lymph node. In addition, two studies demonstrated a lower recurrence rate in patient's achieving disease-free status after primary lymph node gastrinomas resections compared to those with resections of duodenal or pancreatic primary gastrinomas. Therefore, routine lymphadenectomy can increase the disease-free survival rate, with lymph node positivity or lymph node ratio holding prognostic significance in panNETs including gastrinomas.

Controversial surgical approaches to gastrinomas include Whipple resections and laparoscopic approaches. Aggressive surgical procedures like a Whipple pancreaticoduodenectomy have been traditionally reserved for large pancreatic head or duodenal lesions that are not amendable to enucleation. However, more extensive surgeries were thought to increase the chances of rendering patients' disease-free given an estimated 20% to 70% of cases containing lymph node metastasis. Although studies have reported an increased disease-free rate after Whipple resections in sporadic ZES, the long-term complications along with the excellent prognosis of patients with smaller operations support our lack of recommendation for these aggressive procedures. While a laparoscopic approach is more frequently utilized for the surgical management of panNETs (especially localized tumors, NF-NETs, and MEN1), only a small number of sporadic gastrinomas are treated laparoscopically. This is largely due to the need for an extensive exploration of the gastrinoma triangle, liver, and duodenum.

Tumor-Directed Therapy—Nonsurgical—MEN1/ZES and Sporadic ZES

MEN1/ZES and Sporadic ZES patients with unresectable, distant metastatic disease have decreased survival. Therefore, a multimodal approach similar to that utilized in other advanced NETs is taken. This includes utilization of medical therapy (everolimus or tyrosine kinase inhibitors), peptide receptor radionuclide therapy (PRRT) with luteium-177–labeled somatostatin, chemotherapy, and/or liver-directed therapies (chemo-embolization).

FOLLOW-UP

Medical Management Follow-up—Sporadic ZES and MEN-1

Although various surgical societies such as ENET NANET and the Endocrine Society, currently recommend conservative treatment for small panNETs (< 1.5–2.0 cm) in patients with NF-panNETS or MEN1 as discussed earlier, there is no consensus as to how best accomplish this. For intrapancreatic NETs, studies have shown EUS to be the most sensitive modality to assess changes over repeated examinations in MEN1 patients. Furthermore, panNETs <2 cm have been shown to relatively stable and uncommonly increase in size. However, sporadic and MEN1 patients who still have elevated gastrin levels postsurgery will need to stay on the same dose of PPI.

Given the limited sensitivity of EUS in nonintrapancreatic NETs, these patients are typically followed with cross-sectional imaging studies. Cross-sectional imaging can have a sensitivity below 50% for lesions <1.5 cm; while SRI has a higher sensitivity, it has not been established as a reliable measure of serial changes in tumor sizes of MEN1 patients. 68Ga-DOTATATE-PET/CT has even greater sensitivity than cross-sectional imaging but its role in the follow-up period is controversial in MEN1 patients.

OUTCOMES

Outcomes—Overall

In sporadic panNETs, the World Health Organization's tumor grading by pathology has been shown to be one of the few systems to have important prognostic value. One of the primary determinants of long-term survival in gastrinoma is the presence of metastatic disease particularly to the liver. As such, pancreatic gastrinomas confer a worse prognosis compared to duodenal sites of disease given their propensity for spread to the liver. Patients with liver metastases have a 15% 10-year survival after surgery. Furthermore, patients without liver metastases have a 95% 20-year survival. Although lymph node metastases are seen at an increased frequency with duodenal gastrinomas, patients without liver metastases did not demonstrate a decrease in survival. SRS imaging has not been found to increase the disease-free rate even though it has the highest sensitivity of all the localizing modalities combined (Figure 56–3). The use of a duodenotomy during surgery had a significant positive effect on disease-free status in sporadic ZES patients.[6] Reoperations for recurrent or persistent disease occurred in 23% of patients and an average of 6 years after the initial operation. Patients who undergo reoperation typically experience extended survival, and a quarter of them may achieve a cure through additional surgery. This underscores the importance of routine imaging for all patients with Zollinger-Ellison syndrome following resection. If a tumor recurs, it is advisable to consider repeat surgery.[7]

Outcomes—MEN1/ZES

As described earlier, there are several challenges to medically and surgically treating MEN1/ZES patients. First, the often-concurrent hyperparathyroidism affects the activity of hormone states (gastrin/acid hypersecretion) and should be dealt with first. Second, microscopic NF-panNETs are often present in addition to primary gastrinomas or FpanNETs. Third, MEN/ZES duodenal gastrinomas are often, small, multiple, and associated with lymph node metastases. Fourth, the natural history of these patients is still largely unknown. Finally, other malignant tumors like thymic carcinoids are now increasingly described in MEN1 patients. Preliminary studies in MEN1 patients suggest that histological grade of tumors has predictive value; however, most (>80%) are G1, yet some will go on to pursue an aggressive course. A more recent predictor of value is Fludeoxyglucose F-18 (18F-FDG) PET/CT; studies demonstrate that 18F-FDG PET/CT is negative in most well-differentiated (G1, G2) NETs and positive in those with more aggressive behaviors (G3) (sensitivity of 86% and specificity of 95%). Lastly, while there are a few known genotype-phenotype correlations with prognostic value in MEN1 patients (JunD, CHES1, CDNK1B B109 G polymorphism, truncation mutations in the N or C-terminal of *MEN1* gene, and missense mutations in *MEN1* gene), they have not been well studied prospectively and are not widely used presently. The mean age at death of MEN1 patients is shortened at 55 to 60 years old in several studies. While MEN1 patients are rarely dying of acid hypersecretion as noted in earlier studies, other aggressive tumors such as thymic carcinoids have been increasingly described and attributed to an increasing percentage of deaths.

REFERENCES

1. Fraker DL, Norton JA, Saeed ZA, Maton PN, Gardner JD, Jensen RT. A prospective study of perioperative and postoperative control of acid hypersecretion in patients with Zollinger-Ellison syndrome undergoing gastrinoma resection. *Surgery*. 1988;104(6):1054-1063.
2. Norton JA, Fraker DL, Alexander HR, et al. Surgery to cure the Zollinger–Ellison syndrome. *New England Journal of Medicine*. 1999;341(9):635-644.
3. Norton JA, Fraker DL, Alexander HR, Jensen RT. Value of surgery in patients with negative imaging and sporadic Zollinger-Ellison syndrome. *Ann Surg*. 2012;256(3):509-517.
4. Norton JA, Alexander HR, Fraker DL, Venzon DJ, Gibril F, Jensen RT. Possible primary lymph node gastrinoma: occurrence, natural history, and predictive factors: a prospective study. *Ann Surg*. 2003;237(5):650-657; discussion 657-659.
5. Norton JA, Alexander HR, Fraker DL, Venzon DJ, Gibril F, Jensen RT. Comparison of surgical results in patients with advanced and limited disease with multiple endocrine neoplasia type 1 and Zollinger-Ellison syndrome. *Ann Surg*. 2001;234(4):495-505; discussion 505-496.
6. Norton JA, Alexander HR, Fraker DL, Venzon DJ, Gibril F, Jensen RT. Does the use of routine duodenotomy (DUODX) affect rate of cure, development of liver metastases, or survival in patients with Zollinger-Ellison syndrome? *Ann Surg*. 2004;239(5):617-625; discussion 626.
7. Norton JA, Krampitz GW, Poultsides GA, et al. Prospective evaluation of results of reoperation in Zollinger-Ellison syndrome. *Ann Surg*. 2018;267(4):782-788.

Functional Pancreatic Neuroendocrine Tumors (PNETs): Somatostatinoma, VIPoma, PPoma, & Other PNETs

57

Alison P. Woods, MD
Jennifer F. Tseng, MD, MPH
Douglas B. Evans, MD

GENERAL CONSIDERATIONS

Epidemiology

Pancreatic neuroendocrine tumors (PNETs) remain rare but are increasing in incidence largely due to the widespread use of abdominal imaging. Recent work employing the Surveillance, Epidemiology, and End Results (SEER) Program database by Dasari et al. and Sonbol et al. has estimated an annual incidence of approximately 1 per 100,000 people.[1,2] About 10% to 25% of PNETs are functional, and the majority of these functional tumors represent insulinomas or gastrinomas.[3,4] This chapter will focus on somatostatinoma, VIPoma, PPoma, and other rare tumors that comprise the remainder of these functional PNETs.

General Diagnostic Framework

Though each subtype of functional PNET has distinct diagnostic criteria, a common framework connects each tumor type. To be designated as "functional," a PNET must cause a related clinical syndrome, regardless of serum or histopathologic markers. However, biochemical testing (for subtype-specific markers) and localization studies can and should be used to aid in diagnosis. In addition to careful clinical history-taking to elucidate the patient's symptoms, gathering information on family history is essential. In cases where an inherited genetic syndrome is suspected based on this family history (multiple endocrine neoplasia type 1 [MEN1], von Hippel Lindau [VHL] disease, neurofibromatosis type 1 [NF1]), definitive diagnosis is important, as management strategies for PNETs associated with a genetic syndrome are distinct from those of sporadic tumors.

Typical initial localization studies include triple-phase or pancreas-protocol computed tomography (CT) or magnetic resonance imaging (MRI). Historically, endoscopic ultrasound (EUS) with fine-needle aspiration or core biopsy was the preferred approach and offered the additional benefit of simultaneously addressing any tumor-related biliary obstruction if present.[5,6] More recently, gallium-68 DOTATATE positron emission tomography (PET)/CT has been used to diagnose of PNETs, most of which express the somatostatin receptor. DOTATATE imaging is particularly helpful with small PNETs (2 cm in size or smaller), which are uniformly well differentiated and have a low Ki67 index. In such cases, a biopsy is unnecessary; a positive DOTATATE scan secures the diagnosis of a PNET. DOTATATE imaging has also greatly improved radiographic staging as it often discloses small liver, bone, and lymph node metastases not clearly seen with conventional cross-sectional imaging. As gallium-68 DOTATATE imaging increases in availability, guidelines like those from the North American Neuroendocrine Tumor Society (NANETS) have shifted away from octreotide scans using single-photon emission CT (SPECT) technology.[6] CT, MRI, and DOTATATE have become so accurate in diagnosing and staging functional PNETs that angiographic techniques using selective venous sampling with calcium stimulation are rarely performed. Most importantly, the surgeon should never be in the operating room searching for a PNET without accurate preoperative localization. Finally, because functional PNETs are often resected regardless of size, it is important to separate the diagnostic evaluation from the localization process to prevent overinterpretation of incidental findings—a fundamental principle of endocrine surgery.

Table 57–1. The 2022 World Health Organization Epithelial Neuroendocrine Neoplasms Classification.

Neuroendocrine Neoplasm	Classification	Diagnostic Criteria
Gastrointestinal and Pancreatobiliary Tract		
Well-differentiated neuroendocrine tumor (NET)	NET, grade 1	<2 mitoses/2 mm^2 and/or Ki67 <3%
	NET, grade 2	2-20 mitoses/2 mm^2 and/or Ki67 3-20%
	NET, grade 3	>20 mitoses/2 mm^2 and/or Ki67 >20%
Poorly differentiated neuroendocrine carcinoma (NEC)	Smal-cell-NEC	>20 mitoses/2 mm^2 and/or Ki67 >20% (often >70%), and small cell cytomorphology
	Large-cell-NEC	>20 mitoses/2 mm^2 and/or Ki67 >20% (often >70%), and large cell cytomorphology

Source: Reproduced with permission from Rindi G, Mete O, Uccella S, et al. Overview of the 2022 WHO Classification of Neuroendocrine Neoplasms. *Endocr Pathol*. 2022;33(1):115-154.

Tumor Staging & Grading Systems

PNETs are classified by both grade and tumor, node, metastasis (TNM) stage. Currently, the 2022 World Health Organization (WHO) schema is the most widely used grade classification system based on tumor mitotic rate and Ki67 index determined by immunohistochemical methods (Table 57–1).[7] Notably, the WHO classification system separates well-differentiated PNETs, even if high grade, from poorly differentiated tumors, which since the 2017 WHO grading system have now been referred to as poorly differentiated pancreatic neuroendocrine carcinomas (pNECs). The American Joint Committee on Cancer (AJCC) 8th edition staging system, released in 2017, provides a revised clinical and pathologic staging system (Table 57–2).[8] This update emphasized the importance of distinguishing PNETs from exocrine pancreatic cancer and aligned the AJCC system with the European Neuroendocrine Tumor Society classification.[9] Both WHO grade—particularly, its Ki67 component[10–12]—and TNM stage[13,14] have been correlated with survival and other prognostic indicators across various of studies.

A Surgical Disease

Functional PNETs are generally best managed by surgery whenever possible. By definition, a functional tumor is causing a clinical syndrome, and resection enables restoration of normal physiology. In addition, most noninsulinoma PNETs are either malignant or have a high potential to become malignant. Surgery, therefore, also offers an opportunity for cure, optimal local disease control, and prolonged survival. Regional lymphadenectomy has not been formally studied in the rarer classes of functional PNETs but has been found beneficial in nonfunctional PNETs and gastrinoma and is typically performed.[15] Patients with sporadic insulinoma appear to not benefit from removing regional lymph nodes; patients with all other PNETs ≥2 cm in size may benefit from regional lymphadenectomy. When possible, upfront surgery is the most common treatment sequence, but neoadjuvant treatments may be considered for borderline resectable and locally advanced tumors where a reduction in tumor size may make the operation easier and safer. Finally, the use of gallium-68 DOTATATE scans has recently allowed clinicians to detect smaller and smaller tumors, and there is increasing evidence that nonfunctional PNETs <2 cm in size may be managed with an active surveillance protocol, including imaging every 6 to 12 months. Though active surveillance has not yet been studied in rare functional PNETs, it may play a greater role in PNET management in the future,

Table 57–2. The American Joint Committee on Cancer 8th Edition TNM Staging Classification for PNETs.

Stage	Definition		
I	T1	N0	M0
II	T2 or T3	N0	M0
III	T4	N0	M0
III	Any T	N1	M0
IV	Any T	Any N	M1

Category	Criteria
T Classification	
T1	Tumor limited to the pancreas, <2 cm
T2	Tumor limited to the pancreas, 2-4 cm
T3	Tumor limited to the pancreas, >4 cm or tumor invading the duodenum or common bile duct
T4	Tumor invading adjacent organs (stomach, spleen, colon, adrenal gland) or the wall of large vessels (celiac axis or superior mesenteric artery)
N Classification	
N0	No regional lymph node metastasis
N1	Regional lymph node metastasis
M Classification	
M0	No distant metastasis
M1	Distant metastasis
M1a	Hepatic metastasis only
M1b	Extrahepatic metastasis only
M1c	Hepatic and extrahepatic metastasis

particularly in patients with limited symptoms (eg, those with a PPoma) and those of advanced age or with significant medical comorbidities. The specifics of operative management are discussed in greater detail in the section on Surgical Treatment.

PATHOGENESIS

PNETs are primarily believed to originate in the pancreatic islets within endocrine cells. Frequently mutated genes include *MEN1*, *ATRX*, and *DAXX*, all of which play a role in chromatin remodeling and collectively are mutated in most PNETs in some series.[16,17] Additional mutations have been described in genes related to deoxyribonucleic acid (DNA) damage repair, mammalian target of rapamycin (mTOR) signaling pathways, and telomere maintenance.[18] Most PNETs occur sporadically but can also be associated with MEN1, VHL, NF1, and tuberous sclerosis.

PREVENTION

Relatively little is known about risk factors for developing PNETs in the absence of a germline mutation resulting in an inherited endocrinopathy. A case-control study by Halfdanarson et al. found that patients with PNETs were more likely to report diabetes mellitus, less likely to report alcohol use, and similarly likely to report tobacco use compared to controls.[19] However, a case series of several patients diagnosed simultaneously with PPoma and diabetes mellitus found that all had improvement in diabetes after resection, raising the question of elevated pancreatic polypeptide bringing about associated diabetes rather than diabetes contributing to PNET risk.[20] Finally, a family history of PNET that does not fall within an inherited syndrome has still been found to confer excess risk of developing a PNET, as did a family history of sarcoma or gallbladder, gastric, or ovarian cancer.[19]

TYPES OF RARE FUNCTIONAL PNETs

Somatostatinoma

Somatostatinomas may be located in either the pancreas (most commonly the head) or the duodenum (periampullary) and are most often malignant. Patients may present with steatorrhea, diabetes, and cholelithiasis. Because of the initially insidious onset of these relatively nonspecific symptoms, these tumors, when in the pancreas, are frequently diagnosed at a more advanced stage. Accordingly, patients may often have developed abdominal pain or obstructive jaundice, owing either to local tumor effects or as a complication of associated cholelithiasis. Fasting plasma somatostatin will typically be elevated, and electrolyte abnormalities, including hypochloremia, may be present. A recent case series by Luna et al. of 23 pancreatic and duodenal tumors with immunoreactivity primarily or exclusively to somatostatin and clinically associated with aspects of the somatostatinoma syndrome illustrated the heterogeneity of this tumor and its close relationship with nonfunctional PNETs.[21] Though all patients with metastatic disease had elevated plasma somatostatin, this was not the case among those with nonmetastatic tumors. In addition, few patients exhibited all or nearly all of the clinical findings classically associated with somatostatinoma. Treatment algorithms are typically the same as for nonfunctional PNETs or PPomas. Somatostatinomas have long been known to be associated with NF1. When associated with NF1, somatostatinomas are more commonly duodenal or periampullary in location. Within the last decade, these tumors have also been found to comprise part of a syndrome including somatostatinomas, paragangliomas/pheochromocytomas, and polycythemia related to mutations in the hypoxia-inducible factor 2 alpha (*HIF2A*) gene.[22] Table 57–3 provides an overview of somatostatinoma and the other functional PNETs discussed in this chapter.

VIPoma

Functional PNETs secreting vasoactive intestinal peptide (VIP), commonly known as VIPomas, originate in D2 cells of the pancreatic islets and are primarily found in the body and tail of the pancreas; the majority are malignant. VIPomas cause a characteristic clinical phenotype known as Verner-Morrison syndrome or WDHA syndrome (so named for "watery diarrhea, hypokalemia, and achlorhydria"). The associated iso-osmotic, secretory diarrhea causes the underlying VIPoma-related electrolyte disturbances. Stool volumes can be profoundly elevated and exceed 3 L or 20 bowel movements per day. Weight loss, dehydration, and crampy abdominal pain are also often reported due to hyperperistalsis and rapid gastrointestinal transit. Laboratory findings include markedly elevated fasting VIP (a recent systematic review and meta-analysis reported a median of >600 pg/mL[23]), hypokalemia, hypochloremia, and metabolic acidosis owing to stool bicarbonate losses. Initial treatment of patients with VIPomas requires careful management of diarrhea and electrolyte disturbances. Tumors are typically responsive to somatostatin analogs and the tyrosine kinase inhibitor sunitinib. Though the vast majority of patients will initially respond well to somatostatin analogs and have a marked decrease in stool output, progressive dose increases, including the use of long-acting depot formulations, are usually required. At these high doses, patients must be monitored for somatostatin analog-induced hypertension and pancreatic exocrine insufficiency, which is treated with pancreatic enzyme replacement. Finally, though VIP-secreting tumors have also been reported in pediatric patients, in this population, they are typically found in extrapancreatic, retroperitoneal locations in the adrenal glands or along the sympathetic chain.[24]

Table 57–3. Overview of the rare functional PNETs.

Tumor Type	Predominant Location	Key Clinical Symptoms or Signs	Key Laboratory Findings
Somatostatinoma	Head, duodenum (periampullary)	Steatorrhea, diabetes mellitus, cholelithiasis	Elevating fasting somatostatin, hypochloremia
VIPoma	Body, tail	High-volume secretory diarrhea	Elevated fasting VIP, hypokalemia, achlorhydria
PPoma	Head	Related to tumor burden (abdominal pain, obstructive jaundice)	Elevated pancreatic polypeptide
Glucagonoma	Body, tail	NME, diabetes mellitus, dermatitis, DVT, depression	Elevated fasting glucagon, hyperglycemia
ACTH-secreting tumor	Tail, head	Cushing syndrome	Elevated ACTH, elevated cortisol, hyperglycemia

ACTH, adrenocorticotropic hormone; DVT, deep vein thrombosis; NME, necrolytic migratory erythema; PP, pancreatic polypeptide; VIP, vasoactive intestinal peptide.

PPoma

Tumors secreting pancreatic polypeptide (PP) are known as PPomas. They are exceedingly rare in incidence, and the body of knowledge about patients with PPomas is based largely on case reports. Because excess pancreatic polypeptide does not cause a specific clinical syndrome, PPomas are often classified as nonfunctional PNETs and treated as such. Clinical symptoms due to PPomas are typically related to tumor burden and mass effect, with pain, obstructive jaundice, and bulky metastasis-related hepatomegaly being commonly reported. Watery diarrhea has also been described. In addition, recent reports have raised the possibility of an association between MEN1 and PPoma.[25,26] Because of their lack of a specific clinical syndrome, many PPomas are diagnosed after metastasis has occurred; therefore, overall survival is inferior to truly functional PNETs which are typically diagnosed when the primary tumor is small and often localized to the pancreas. Laboratory findings include a high circulating pancreatic polypeptide level, which is typically >3 times the upper limit of the normal range.

Glucagonoma

Glucagonomas originate in pancreatic alpha cells and most commonly are located in the body or tail of the pancreas. Glucagonomas are typically malignant and occur with a slight female predominance. These tumors classically cause the "4 D's" of diabetes mellitus, dermatitis, deep vein thrombosis (DVT), and depression. Weight loss, diarrhea, glossitis, and angular stomatitis are also frequently reported. The characteristic skin finding of necrolytic migratory erythema (NME) is a specific and often early sign of glucagonoma (Figure 57–1); in a recent large meta-analysis by Song et al., 80% of patients exhibited NME.[27] The underlying etiology of this skin lesion is felt to be related to overproduction of glucagon, which in turn causes depletion of amino acids and vitamin/mineral deficiencies, particularly zinc deficiency.[28] Laboratory studies should include fasting glucagon levels (typically >1000 pg/mL) and careful monitoring of serum glucose and hemoglobin A1c. Glucagon secretion can be reduced with somatostatin analogs such as octreotide and lanreotide.[29] In addition, treatment of diabetes with oral antihyperglycemic agents or insulin plays an important role in management before resection or in cases of metastatic or refractory disease. Finally, given the association between glucagonoma and DVT, careful attention to thrombotic prophylaxis is required in patients with this type of PNET.

ACTH-Secreting Tumors

Adrenocorticotropic hormone (ACTH)-secreting PNETs, also known as ACTHomas, present clinically with Cushing syndrome. Patients may exhibit a combination of the classic Cushing-related signs and symptoms, including obesity, dorsocervical fat pad, facial plethora, easy bruising, abdominal striae, hirsutism, menstrual irregularities, depression, and proximal muscular weakness. Laboratory findings will reveal substantially elevated ACTH and frequently also show hyperglycemia. Cushing syndrome can be more formally evaluated via 24-hour urine-free cortisol, late-night salivary cortisol, or overnight 1 mg dexamethasone suppression testing; however, the clinical symptoms are usually those of profound cortisol excess. Initial management often requires expeditious control of hypercortisolism with steroidogenesis-inhibiting agents, including metyrapone, ketoconazole, or mitotane. Bilateral adrenalectomy is sometimes required for control of hypercortisolism in cases of refractory or unresectable ACTH-secreting PNETs and is supported by

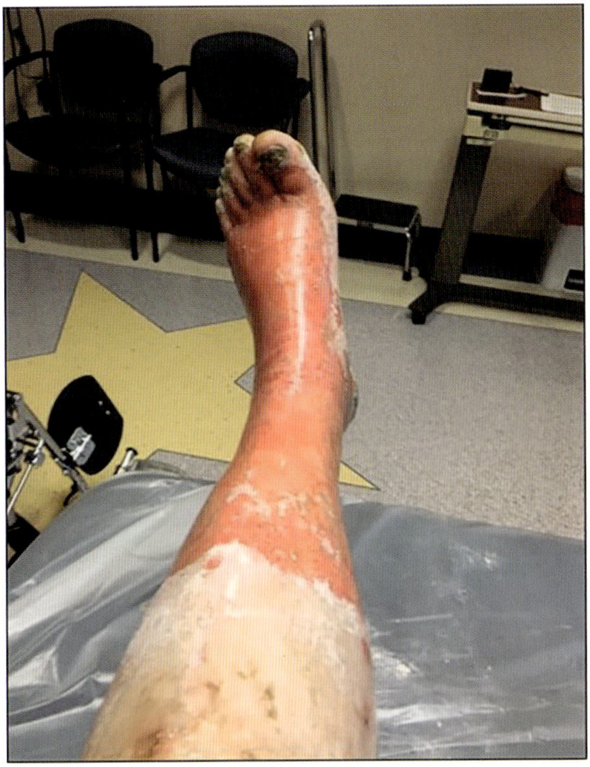

▲ **Figure 57–1.** Necrolytic migratory erythema associated with glucagonoma. Clinical image of necrolytic migratory erythema exhibiting a large area of eroded skin surface. Earlier clinical presentations include erythematous or scaly lesions. NME most commonly affects the lower extremities and intertriginous areas. (Photograph obtained by Dr. Callisia Clarke, Medical College of Wisconsin and reprinted with permission from Fischer JE, et al, eds. *Fischer's Master of Surgery*. 7th ed. Philadelphia, PA: Wolters Kluwer; 2019.)

NANETS guidelines.[29] In fact, a delay in bilateral adrenalectomy is much more common than the over-application of this operation. A minimally invasive bilateral adrenalectomy can sometimes be a life-saving procedure for patients with ectopic ACTH produced by a neuroendocrine tumor. Multiple recent series and retrospective reports have confirmed the aggressive nature of ACTH-secreting PNETs.[30-32]

DIFFERENTIAL DIAGNOSIS

Differential diagnoses for functional PNETs can be split into two categories: other types of pancreatic or duodenal masses that can appear similar on imaging and other causes of the clinical syndromes that are associated with functional PNETs.

Distinguishing Imaging Characteristics of PNETs

As the most commonly encountered pancreatic tumor, pancreatic ductal adenocarcinoma (PDAC) must be differentiated from PNET to ensure the correct course of therapy. Clinically, because PDAC arises from ductal epithelium itself and PNETs arise from the endocrine cells of the pancreas, PDAC is more likely to cause obstructive jaundice. On imaging with CT or MRI, most PNETs are hypervascular and show enhancement on arterial and venous contrast images, while PDAC classically appears hypovascular. Larger PNETs may exhibit cystic or necrotic changes. Serous cystic neoplasms (SCNs) tend to be more completely cystic than PNETs, with lower density on non-contrast CT and high intensity on T2-weighted MRI.[33,34] Similarly, necrotic solid-pseudopapillary neoplasms tend to have a larger area of internal necrosis, seen as heterogeneous densities on cross-sectional imaging. Other cystic neoplasms (including intraductal papillary mucinous neoplasms and mucinous cystic neoplasms) and pancreatic pseudocysts are typically thin-walled without enhancement, while PNETs feature thicker tumor walls with potential enhancement.[33] PNETs have a typical radiographic appearance on CT imaging and are usually positive on gallium-68 DOTATATE PET. They can occasionally be cystic, yet even when cystic, they usually appear positive on DOTATATE. Renal cell carcinoma (RCC) metastatic to the pancreas and the occasional accessory spleen (splenule) can mimic a PNET; a tagged red blood cell scan (Technetium 99m-labeled red cells) will differentiate a splenule and if both kidneys are in place, one can typically exclude metastatic RCC.

The location of a pancreatic mass may also impact differential diagnostic considerations. Very rarely, a duodenal gastrointestinal stromal tumor may be confused with a PNET in the pancreatic head as they both possess a hypervascular pattern on CT and MRI. Arterial phase attenuation value may offer a differentiating factor between these two entities, as does the visualization of a fat plane between the pancreas and tumor, if present.[35] In the pancreatic tail, both intrapancreatic accessory spleens and PNETs appear hypervascular as mentioned above.[36]

Alternative Etiologies for Functional PNET Clinical Syndromes

Functional PNETs cause a constellation of clinical symptoms with a broad array of potential underlying etiologies. Diarrhea, as seen prominently in VIPoma as well as somatostatinoma, may also be related to infectious or noninfectious causes. A myriad of noninfectious causes exist, from medication side effects to primary gastrointestinal conditions such as inflammatory bowel disease, celiac disease, microscopic colitis, and irritable bowel syndrome. Notably, VIPoma will produce secretory diarrhea, while somatostatinoma leads to steatorrhea by reducing pancreatic exocrine activity.

Most cases of diabetes mellitus, as can be seen in glucagonoma, somatostatinoma, and ACTH-secreting tumors, are related to progressive insulin resistance and dysfunction of pancreatic beta cells. When present, the characteristic skin findings of necrolytic migratory erythema are highly suggestive of an underlying glucagonoma. Finally, the elements of Cushing syndrome—among them obesity, dorsocervical fat pad, menstrual irregularities, easy bruising, abdominal striae—may also be related to Cushing disease (pituitary adenoma), primary adrenal cortical adenoma or bilateral adrenal hyperplasia, or ectopic ACTH secretion, most commonly from a primary lung cancer or bronchial neuroendocrine tumor (NET). Despite the broad initial differential for many symptoms seen in functional PNETs, elevation in the relevant serum polypeptide in combination with imaging showing a pancreatic mass can often easily distinguish alternative diagnoses from a functional PNET.

INHERITED CONDITIONS

Though most PNETs are sporadic, at least 10% are associated with a defined genetic syndrome.[37] In some cases, this can affect management strategies, particularly regarding thresholds for surgical resection.

Multiple Endocrine Neoplasia Type 1

Multiple endocrine neoplasia type 1 (MEN1) is the inherited syndrome most frequently associated with PNETs. Recent work by Ito et al. investigating a Japanese population found that 4.9% of patients with functional PNETs had MEN1.[38] Gastrinoma and insulinoma remain the functional PNETs most commonly associated with MEN1, but other functional PNETs such as those described in this chapter are also possible. MEN1 is an autosomal dominant condition involving a mutation of the tumor suppressor gene *MEN1* found on chromosome 11. This gene encodes the protein menin, which regulates transcription, genome stability, cellular division, and proliferation.[37] The classic clinical syndrome includes hyperparathyroidism, pituitary adenoma, and pancreatic tumors. Because MEN1 predisposes to multifocal PNETs, whether synchronous or metachronous, the surgical management of PNETs in patients with MEN1 strives to minimize both the risk of metastatic disease and insulin-dependent diabetes mellitus. Functional PNETs in patients with MEN1 should, in general, be surgically removed; however, we occasionally observe asymptomatic patients with low-level gastrin elevations in the absence of a pancreatic mass. Among nonfunctional PNETs, recent NANETS guidelines have recommended resection for tumors >2 cm and observation for tumors <1 cm, with the management of intermediate, 1 to 2 cm tumors, dependent on physician and patient preference.[6] Almost all PNETs in patients with MEN1 have the biological ability to metastasize to extrapancreatic sites (most notably the liver), where they are then, in general, incurable. Therefore, total pancreatectomy or pancreaticoduodenectomy (the "Whipple" procedure) is a very reasonable consideration in some patients based on tumor burden, especially in those with functional tumors (Figure 57–2). In fact, removal of the distal stomach and duodenum may reduce trophic hormones and lessen the risk of subsequent metastatic disease. No safe size criteria for observation have been proposed for the functional, extremely rare, and frequently malignant tumors discussed in this chapter. Unfortunately, in the case of multifocal tumors in patients with MEN1, it may also be impossible to define which lesion is the source of hormonal function preoperatively. Testing for MEN1 germline mutations is typically recommended for all patients with multifocal PNETs, a PNET and another MEN1-associated tumor, or a gastrinoma.[29,39] Current guidelines do not specify a consensus surveillance protocol once a patient has been diagnosed with MEN1. We begin imaging in teenagers and continue at 18- to 24-month intervals for the pancreas and at 3-year intervals for the chest to evaluate for bronchial carcinoid tumors.[6] Finally, patients with MEN1 of childbearing age should be counseled to consider in-vitro fertilization and preimplantation genetic testing to prevent MEN1 in subsequent generations.

Von Hippel Lindau Syndrome

Von Hippel Lindau (VHL) syndrome predisposes to PNETs along with a wide variety of other tumors, including retinal and central nervous system hemangioblastoma, pheochromocytoma, benign cystic neoplasms of the pancreas, and RCC. VHL exhibits autosomal dominant inheritance caused by the *VHL* gene on chromosome 3, a tumor suppressor gene that regulates angiogenesis. VHL-associated PNETs have a better prognosis than sporadically occurring PNETs[40] and are nearly always nonfunctional.[6] Thus, risk stratification and management algorithms based on tumor diameter, genotyping, location, and/or growth rate have been proposed by Tirosh et al. and Keutgen et al. to guide decisions for surgical intervention and frequency of surveillance imaging in these nonfunctional tumors.[41,42] Importantly, all patients with VHL should be screened for pheochromocytoma before any intervention. In those with a history of treatment for RCC, a hypervascular pancreatic mass could be a metastasis from RCC or a PNET; DOTATATE imaging could be positive in both cases, and an EUS-guided FNA may be indicated in this situation.

Tuberous Sclerosis

Tuberous sclerosis is an autosomal dominant condition related to mutations in the *TSC1* or *TSC2* tumor suppressor genes located on chromosomes 9 and 16, respectively. The encoded proteins, hamartin and tuberin, form a complex that plays a role in mTOR pathway regulation. Patients primarily develop

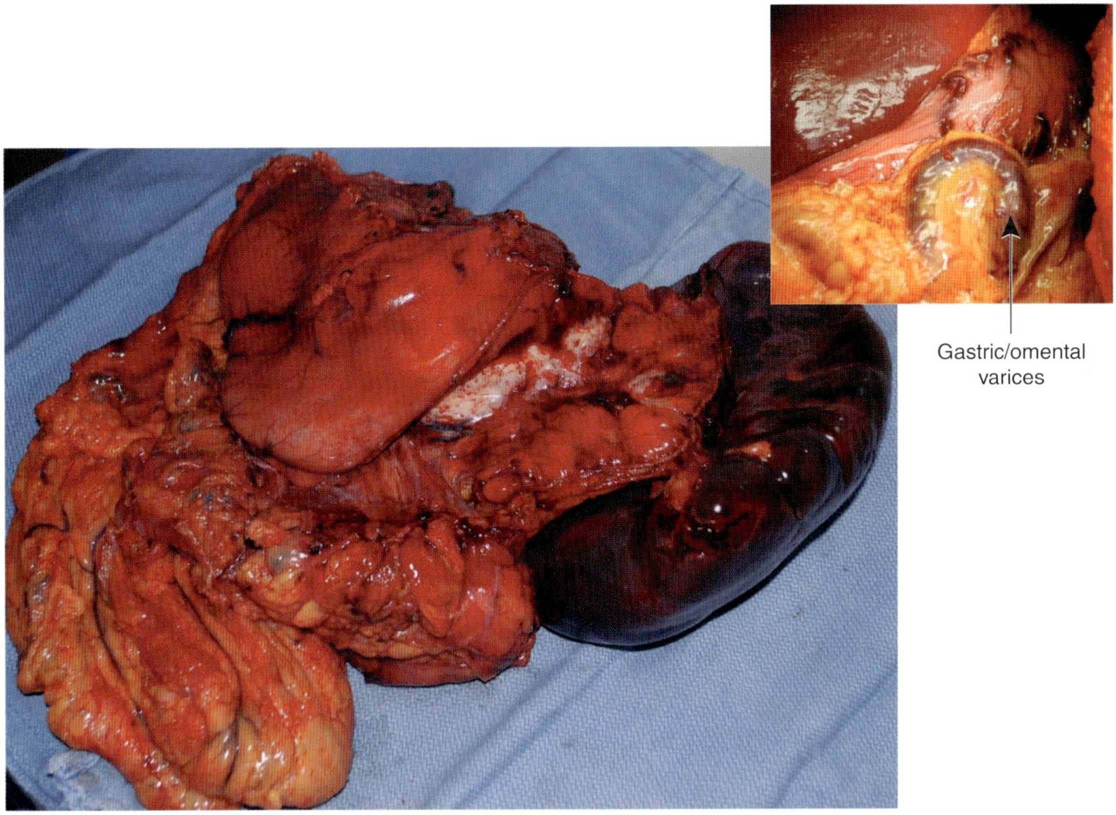

▲ **Figure 57–2.** Total pancreatectomy performed for T3N0 PNET. This patient with a T3N0 tumor (Ki67 2%) underwent total pancreatectomy with temporary mesocaval bypass and replacement of the superior mesenteric vein-portal vein confluence using the left internal jugular vein. At >10 years follow-up, the patient continues to have no evidence of disease. (Images courtesy of Dr. Douglas Evans, Department of Surgical Oncology, Medical College of Wisconsin.)

benign hamartomas within diverse organ systems, neurological disorders, and characteristic skin findings, and rarely, can also develop PNETs. Most tuberous sclerosis-associated PNETs are small, benign, functional, and located in the body or tail of the pancreas, with insulinoma being a relatively frequent subtype.[6] Given the relative infrequency of TSC-associated PNETs, no disease-specific PNET surveillance and management guidelines exist. However, many patients with TSC undergo routine cross-sectional imaging surveillance for other disease-associated tumors, and PNETs are often found incidentally in this manner.[43,44]

Neurofibromatosis Type 1

Neurofibromatosis type 1 (NF1) is an autosomal dominant condition caused by mutations of the *NF1* gene on chromosome 17. Neurofibromin, the encoded protein, helps regulate the tuberous sclerosis complex as described earlier. Patients with this condition develop neurofibromas (benign tumors that occur primarily along the peripheral nerves) and cutaneous findings such as café-au-lait spots. Patients with NF1 can develop periampullary duodenal somatostatinomas as well as PNETs. Because of the risk of biliary obstruction with periampullary tumors and the fact that a substantial proportion of these are malignant, resection (via pancreaticoduodenectomy or more localized resection) is typically recommended whether or not an associated tumor is clinically functional.[6] Patients with NF1 can also develop pheochromocytoma which should be screened for before any intervention.

SURGICAL TREATMENT

After diagnosis, preoperative optimization often presents the next challenge, as patients with functional tumors frequently have derangements in fluid, electrolyte, and/or glycemic status. In many cases, the associated clinical syndrome can be controlled with somatostatin analogs. In general, whenever possible, functional tumors should be surgically excised. Individualized patient factors such as medical comorbidities, age, and functional status are important to consider, particularly in nonfunctional tumors and PNETs of smaller size.

Surgery for Early-Stage Tumors

Surgical options for early-stage PNETs hinge on tumor size and location within the pancreas. Notably, National Comprehensive Cancer Network (NCCN) guidelines allow for consideration of enucleation or local excision with or without regional lymphadenectomy, or even observation alone, in tumors <2 cm in size that are nonfunctional, as well as PPomas, ACTHomas, or somatostatinomas.[45] For larger tumors located in the pancreatic head, pancreaticoduodenectomy is usually required, and those in the body and tail are treated with distal pancreatectomy. Regional lymphadenectomy is an important part of the operation as lymph node metastases are frequently found and if not removed, can grow substantially in the future (Figure 57–3). Whether the spleen should be preserved in patients undergoing distal pancreatectomy who do not have involvement of the spleen or its vessels is uncertain. We favor spleen-preserving distal or total pancreatectomy in young patients; this most often involves patients with MEN1. "Young" is obviously hard to define and somewhat of a moving target. Blood loss is usually slightly greater with spleen preservation due to the need to separate the pancreas from the splenic vessels. We would advise against spleen-preserving distal pancreatectomy with ligation of both the splenic artery and vein. However, the spleen will usually survive on the short gastric (left gastric arterial inflow with or without the right gastroepiploic artery) as long as the splenic vein is intact. The splenic vein outflow is much more important than the arterial inflow for splenic preservation. Recent NANETS guidelines suggest consideration of splenic preservation whenever favorable tumor features are present. These features include smaller size (<3 cm), lower risk of nodal metastases (potentially missed if resection is limited by splenic preservation), and lack of chronic pancreatitis or postneoadjuvant therapy inflammation.[6] The goal of surgical resection should be to obtain negative margins, and a complete gross resection of the tumor is important whenever possible. There is no universally accepted appropriate number of lymph nodes to be sampled in the regional lymphadenectomy. However, the above-referenced recent NANETS guidelines propose harvesting 11-15, and European Neuroendocrine Tumor Society (ENETS) guidelines recommend at least 12 lymph nodes,[46] similar to PDAC. The number of lymph nodes in the pathology report is a function of both the extent of surgery and the rigor of the pathologic assessment of the surgical specimen.

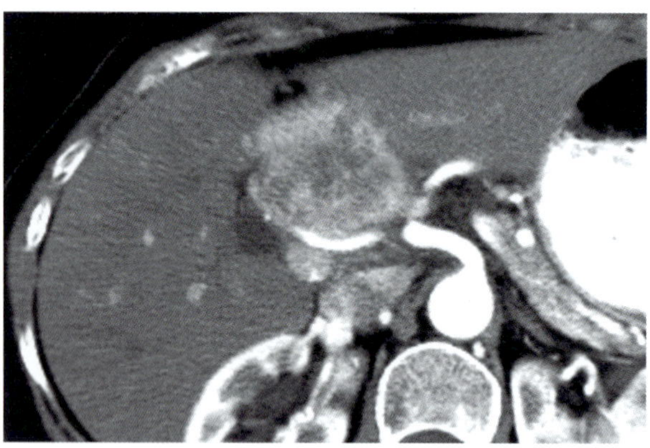

Figure 57–3. The importance of lymphadenectomy and long-term follow-up. This patient underwent a pancreaticoduodenectomy for low-grade PNET. Surveillance imaging >10 years later revealed recurrence in a lymph node along the common hepatic artery, as shown above. Common hepatic artery lymph nodes can and should be removed at the time of index pancreaticoduodenectomy for the treatment of PNETs. (Image courtesy of Dr. Douglas Evans, Department of Surgical Oncology, Medical College of Wisconsin and Dr. James Yao, Department of Gastrointestinal Medical Oncology, M.D. Anderson Cancer Center.)

Minimally invasive surgical techniques, whether laparoscopic or robotic, have been safely used for distal pancreatectomy for PNETs and other pancreatic tumors with similar oncologic results in limited PNET-specific data, and similar or sometimes improved postoperative morbidity.[47-52] For pancreaticoduodenectomy, multicenter data from Zureikat et al. suggests that robotic resection may offer similar or even improved morbidity at highly experienced centers.[53] However, the safety of laparoscopic pancreaticoduodenectomy has recently been called into question by the LEOPARD-2 randomized controlled trial.[54] Though several prospective studies have now examined drain placement in pancreatic resections, only a small minority of patients had PNETs in these experiences. With a more extensive lymphadenectomy, one may want to consider routine drain placement due to the risk for postoperative ascites, which will resolve in 1 to 3 weeks. Given rates of cholelithiasis and related complications in some functional PNETs—particularly somatostatinomas—and the need for long-term somatostatin analog use in almost all patients with advanced disease, incorporating a cholecystectomy should always be considered whenever the abdomen is opened. Reported rates of postoperative pancreatic fistula are substantial among patients who require pancreatectomy for PNET given their relatively normal surrounding pancreatic parenchyma. Finally, though it is becoming rare to have unexpected intraoperative findings in the era of gallium-68 DOTATATE imaging, small liver metastases may still be found at the time of operation directed at the primary tumor. The patient should always be made aware of this possibility, and the surgical team should always be prepared to remove or ablate liver metastases when technically possible. As mentioned earlier, remove the gallbladder and be prepared to deal with small liver metastases in all patients.

Surgery for Advanced or Metastatic Tumors

PNETs are frequently borderline resectable, locally advanced, or metastatic at diagnosis. However, even though most patients will not experience a long-term cure, surgery as part of a multimodality treatment program for these more advanced and even metastatic tumors plays an important role for two reasons: control of symptoms and improvement in survival duration. PNETs are unusual in that the surgical reduction of the overall tumor burden benefits survival duration. It remains very important that the timing of surgical intervention is optimal and that surgery is accompanied by low morbidity and close to zero mortality. Borderline resectability is typically defined for patients with PNETs as it is for patients with PDAC, incorporating vascular abutment and encasement status. Interestingly, we and others have observed that vessel abutment does not always require vascular resection and reconstruction; the portal venous anatomy and the visceral arteries can often (but not always) be separated from the primary tumor.[55] For these borderline resectable or locally advanced tumors, neoadjuvant medical therapy may in some cases allow for a safer operation if overall tumor size can be reduced. Various treatment options have been described, including favorable responses to temozolomide and capecitabine (Figure 57–4)[56] and the regimen of 5-fluorouracil, doxorubicin, and streptozocin.[57] Neoadjuvant peptide receptor radionuclide therapy (PRRT) has largely been delivered after incomplete surgical resection, and the optimal treatment sequencing of such emerging therapies remains under active investigation.

Because progression of liver metastases is the leading cause of death in patients with PNETs, efforts should be made to address hepatic metastases with medical or surgical therapy. Management of hepatic metastases in patients with well-differentiated PNETs without widely metastatic extra-abdominal disease is complex (Figure 57–5). Often, these tumors metastasize not as a solitary focus but as multiple lesions in a bilobar distribution, and care must be taken to ensure that an adequate liver remnant remains. However, when possible, resection of hepatic metastases has been associated with improved survival, as demonstrated in a recent meta-analysis by Yuan et al.[58] Historically, metastasectomy has been performed in cases of 90% or greater anticipated cytoreduction, but more recently, a threshold of 70% or greater cytoreduction has also been associated with significantly improved survival.[59-61] Again, it is critically important that such operations be performed safely and that the patient recovers to allow for consideration of adjuvant systemic therapy, liver-directed therapy, and potentially PRRT. When and in what order to apply liver resection/ablation, liver-directed therapy, systemic therapy, and PRRT remains unresolved, and each patient poses an often unique set of treatment challenges. If the primary tumor and liver metastases are resectable, we favor initially resecting the primary tumor. We then consider hepatic metastasectomy during the same operation if the patient is doing well and the primary tumor resection was uncomplicated. As mentioned, given the long survival duration of patients with even metastatic PNETs, ensuring no undue operative morbidity and mortality is

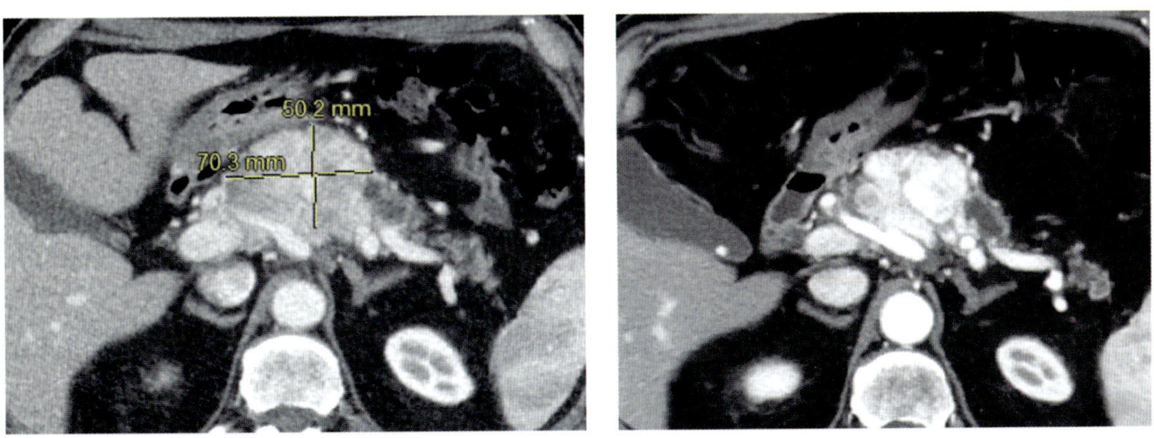

Figure 57–4. Tumor response to neoadjuvant capecitabine-temozolomide and lanreotide. Computed tomography images of a PNET in a patient in his 70s who required 3 months of cardiology workup and treatment before surgery, before *(left)*, and after *(right)* 4 months of neoadjuvant therapy. (Images courtesy of Dr. Douglas Evans, Department of Surgical Oncology, Medical College of Wisconsin.)

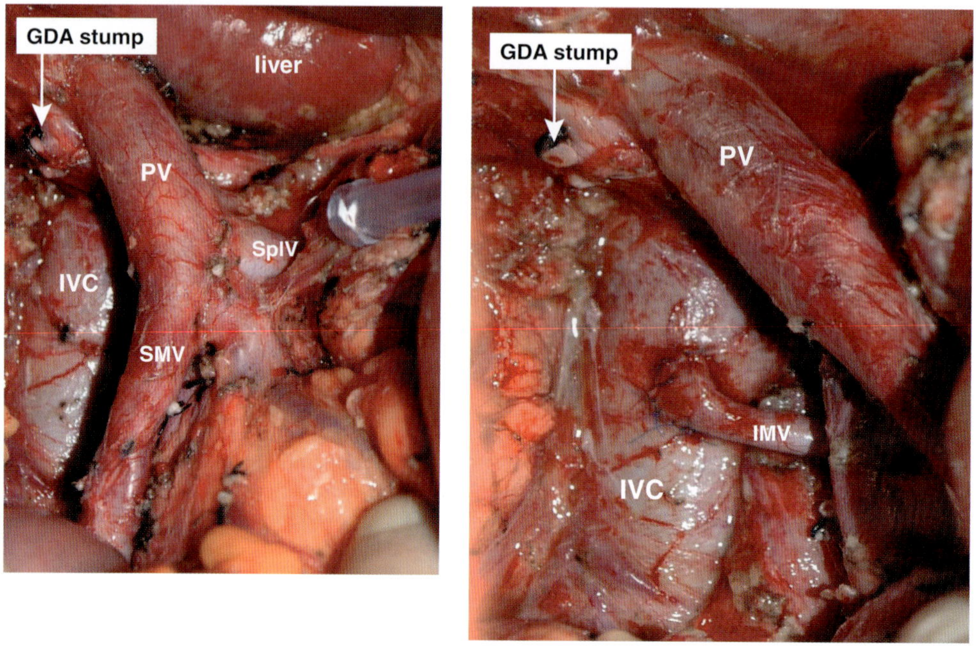

▲ **Figure 57–5.** Mesocaval shunt performed during pancreaticoduodenectomy after multimodal treatment of hepatic metastases. This patient presented with metastatic liver dominant disease and was initially treated with neoadjuvant systemic therapy and an extended right hepatectomy. At the time of her pancreaticoduodenectomy, she produced significant ascites (due to prior liver resection and hepatotoxicity of extensive systemic therapy on her liver remnant), which was addressed by placing a low-volume central shunt using the IMV to decompress the PV. GDA, gastroduodenal artery; IMV, inferior mesenteric vein; IVC, inferior vena cava; PV, portal vein; SMV, superior mesenteric vein; SplV, splenic vein. (Images courtesy of Dr. Douglas Evans, Department of Surgical Oncology, Medical College of Wisconsin.)

the most important guiding principle. For this reason, we encourage surgeons to consider a simultaneous pancreas and liver resection very carefully. In cases where unresectable metastatic disease coexists with a resectable primary tumor, selected patients may still benefit from resection of solely the primary tumor to decrease functional symptoms, avoid the risks of local pancreatic tumor progression, and possibly improve response to PRRT.[62] There is little definitive data on the value of resection of the primary tumor or hepatic metastases in the setting of peritoneal carcinomatosis or extensive bone metastases. There is also little data to guide specifics of the timing of cytoreductive surgery if performed.

Finally, liver transplant has also been performed for patients with metastatic PNETs, albeit rarely. This remains controversial, as similar survival with less morbidity may be achievable with modern optimal multimodal management. In addition, given the shortage of donor organs, liver transplant candidates for other indications are often perceived to have better survival compared to those with even relatively indolent metastatic malignancy. However, a recent analysis by Mazzaferro et al. of patients with gastroentero-pancreatic neuroendocrine tumors (about one-third of which were PNETs) using propensity score-matched patients selected according to Milan-NET criteria showed dramatically improved survival at 5 and 10 years.[63]

ADVANCES IN NONSURGICAL THERAPIES

Various nonsurgical treatment options exist for functional PNETs. These include systemic medical therapies, nuclear medicine treatments, and liver-directed procedures such as ablation and embolization. There is little data to specifically guide treatment sequencing besides physician experience, although somatostatin analogs are often used initially given their relatively favorable side effect profile. This is particularly true for functional syndromes, where patients may see symptomatic benefit in their tumor-related clinical manifestations.

Systemic Medical Therapies

A. Somatostatin Analogs

Somatostatin analogs, such as octreotide and more recently lanreotide and pasireotide, have long played an important role in reducing functional polypeptide section in patients with functional PNETs. These compounds have now been shown to benefit disease progression as well. The placebo-controlled randomized PROMID trial, which was conducted in patients with metastatic mid-gut NETs, found that long-acting octreotide lengthened the time to tumor progression.[64] Although long-term overall survival results were similar, most patients in the placebo group had eventually crossed over to treatment with octreotide.[65] The CLARINET trial, in which over 40% of patients had PNETs, also showed significant benefits in progression-free survival (PFS), with a median of 18 months in the placebo group[66] compared to an ultimate PFS of over 38 months in the treatment group-only analysis of the open-label extension trial.[67]

B. Targeted Therapies

Targeted medical therapies for PNETs include mTOR and tyrosine kinase inhibitors. The RADIANT series of trials investigated the mTOR inhibitor everolimus. In the placebo-controlled phase III RADIANT-3 trial, which examined over 400 patients with progressive PNETs, Yao et al. reported that median PFS was significantly longer at 11 months in the everolimus group compared to 4.6 months in the placebo group.[68] Similar PFS results and equivalent quality of life across everolimus and placebo groups were subsequently confirmed in the additional phase III RADIANT-4 trial.[69,70] Sunitinib, a tyrosine kinase inhibitor that acts on the vascular endothelial growth factor (VEGF) receptor and other downstream receptors, has also been examined in treating PNETs. A phase III randomized controlled trial of 171 patients with advanced and/or metastatic well-differentiated PNETs by Raymond et al. was discontinued early in favor of the sunitinib arm, which exhibited a PFS of 11.4 months compared to 5.5 months in the placebo group.[71]

C. Cytotoxic Chemotherapy

Cytotoxic chemotherapy has historically not produced impressive results in patients with PNETs, perhaps owing to the well-differentiated nature of the majority of these tumors. Until relatively recently, streptozocin-based regimens were often considered the standard.[29] However, temozolomide and temozolomide plus capecitabine-based regimens have demonstrated promise in retrospective analyses, with 30% to 70% objective response rates.[72-74] The Eastern Cooperative Oncology Group (ECOG) E2211 randomized study of temozolomide versus temozolomide and capecitabine in patients with advanced PNETs is ongoing, with early results showing significant improvements in interim PFS (22.7 months in the combined group vs 14.4 months in the temozolomide monotherapy group) and overall survival.[75]

Peptide Receptor Radionuclide Therapy

PRRT is a nuclear medicine therapy that employs radiolabeled (often lutetium-177) somatostatin analogs such as octreotide or octreotate. The phase III NETTER-1 trial showed significant benefits in patients with metastatic mid-gut NETs in terms of PFS, overall survival, and time to deterioration in quality of life, including response rates of 18% in the ^{177}Lu-DOTATATE arm and 3% in the control arm.[76,77] Though no randomized trials have evaluated PRRT in PNETs, observational studies have reported favorable results.[78,79] Zandee et al. recently analyzed 34 patients at a single center with metastatic functional PNETs (65% of whom had progressive disease at baseline) treated with PRRT, reporting an overall response rate of nearly 60%; most patients also experienced a reduction in symptoms.[80] Monitoring for complications of PRRT remains important, as a substantial minority of patients develop bone marrow, renal, or other toxicities. Long-term therapeutic risks include the development of PRRT-induced myeloid neoplasms.

Liver-Directed Therapy

A. Hepatic Artery Embolization

Hepatic artery embolization takes advantage of the fact that metastases are supplied primarily by the hepatic artery while normal liver parenchyma has a dual blood supply that includes the portal system. Hepatic artery embolization thus selectively devascularizes the tumor as distinct from the normal liver. Transarterial chemoembolization (the liver-directed injection of cytotoxic agents before embolization, known as TACE) may also comprise part of the embolization procedure, and functional NETs appear to be particularly sensitive to TACE.[81] Radioembolization using the injection of yttrium-90 microspheres has also been described and may have an advantage in patients with a biliary-enteric anastomosis, where embolization can frequently lead to hepatic abscess formation.[82] The preference for TACE or radioembolization is often institution specific and based on physician experience;[83,84] current guidelines do not recommend a preferred embolization method.[29,85] Regardless of the specific technique chosen, embolization is best performed at a highly experienced center by physicians who perform these therapies frequently. Hepatic artery embolization is typically carried out on one hepatic lobe (or less) at a time to minimize the risk of severe adverse events such as hepatic insufficiency.

B. Hepatic Ablation

Hepatic ablation is either performed as a standalone procedure via a percutaneous approach or combined with surgical metastasectomy. Either radiofrequency or microwave ablative techniques may be used. Although limited data is available, recent studies have generally found comparable disease control rates across different ablative techniques and similar survival following hepatic resection with or without ablation.[86,87] Importantly, as mentioned, patients with a prior biliary-enteric anastomosis (eg, as part of a pancreaticoduodenectomy) are generally not good candidates for ablation or embolization procedures. Because biliary-enteric anastomoses allow for colonization of bile with gut flora, ablation and embolization place patients at high risk for hepatic abscess in the devascularized portion of the liver. We therefore strongly recommend determining an overall treatment strategy upfront in patients presenting with a PNET in the pancreatic head in the setting of unresectable hepatic metastases.

PROGNOSIS

The prognosis for patients with PNETs has long been known to be more favorable than that for patients with PDAC. With recent changes in the nomenclature of these neoplasms, however, there has been a growing recognition that essentially all pancreatic neuroendocrine neoplasms have the potential to display malignant behavior. Despite this, prognosis can vary widely, as tumors range from indolent to highly aggressive. Patients with grade 1 or 2 PNETs have a substantially better prognosis than those with grade 3 PNETs. In turn, poorly differentiated neuroendocrine carcinomas are now felt to be of an entirely distinct cellular lineage from grade 3 (or other) PNETs, and such patients have a poor prognosis, similar to or worse than that for PDAC.[88,89] As with most cancers, the components of the TNM stage—tumor size, nodal spread, and distant metastasis—also aid in prognostication, with smaller and localized tumors signaling a relatively better prognosis. Recent work by Dasari et al. using the SEER database included patients with PNETs of all grades and found an overall survival of 3.6 years.[1] However, in the same study, even among grade 1 or 2 PNETs with distant spread, median survival was 5 years. Another recent SEER-based study by Keutgen et al. specifically focused on malignant functional PNETs by subtype;[90] nearly half of the included patients had distant disease at diagnosis, 59% underwent surgery, and 81% had grade 1 or 2 tumors. Median survival was 7.7 years among 52 patients with glucagonoma and 7.9 years among 24 patients with VIPoma; too few patients had somatostatinomas to report survival results. A recent single-institution series by Fahmy et al. examining 87 primarily nonfunctional PNETs reported concordant results. They again emphasized the importance of grade in determining prognosis, with median survival for patients with grade 1 tumors of 7.9 years, compared to 4.5 years for grade 2 tumors and 1.9 years for grade 3 tumors.[91] Finally, a meta-analysis of 36 patients with pancreatic somatostatinoma found a median survival of nearly 48 months.[92] Encouragingly, recent results suggest survival has improved in the modern era.[1] This may be related to earlier detection of tumors but probably also reflects improvements in therapy.

WHEN TO REFER & WHEN TO ADMIT

When to Refer

Given the extremely low prevalence of somatostatinoma, VIPoma, PPoma, and other rare functional PNETs, we favor routine referral to tertiary centers for patients suspected or proven to have these diagnoses. Although research on rare functional PNETs is lacking, a large body of work demonstrates improved outcomes associated with higher-volume centers and surgeons in resecting PDAC and other hepatopancreatobiliary and complex upper gastrointestinal surgeries.[93-98] These results would also apply to operations for functional PNETs. In addition, multidisciplinary tumor boards and advanced gastroenterology capabilities are invaluable in the diagnosis and nonsurgical aspects of treatment. Most importantly, the patient's story with a PNET, even if metastatic, is told over years—often many years—and survival will be optimized if the many available treatments are applied in the best possible sequence. Management of such patients is very complicated, and new therapies are made available every year.

When to Admit

Patients with rare functional PNETs may require hospital admission for any of several reasons; first, clinical symptoms requiring admission may be associated with their primary tumor, including uncontrolled hyperglycemia related to diabetes, severe dehydration or electrolyte abnormalities secondary to large-volume diarrhea, obstructive jaundice caused by tumor mass effect or choledocholithiasis (as in somatostatinoma), and abdominal pain related to a bulky primary tumor or metastatic disease. Second, patients may require admission due to toxicity related to disease treatment. The complexity of the operative management of pancreatic or duodenal disease or of hepatic metastases often mandates an inpatient stay to ensure that an operation has been completed safely without hemorrhage, anastomotic breakdown, or other early postoperative problems. In addition, pain control, monitored progression of diet, education related to any new insulin dependence caused by pancreatic resection, and oftentimes physical or occupational therapy for postoperative deconditioning are often best initiated in an inpatient setting.

REFERENCES

1. Dasari A, Shen C, Halperin D, et al. Trends in the incidence, prevalence, and survival outcomes in patients with neuroendocrine tumors in the United States. *JAMA Oncol.* 2017;3(10):1335-1342.
2. Sonbol MB, Mazza GL, Starr JS, Hobday TJ, Halfdanarson TR. Incidence and survival patterns of pancreatic neuroendocrine tumors over the last two decades: a SEER database analysis. *J Clin Oncol.* 2020;38(4_suppl):629-629.

3. Zerbi A, Falconi M, Rindi G, et al. Clinicopathological features of pancreatic endocrine tumors: a prospective multicenter study in Italy of 297 sporadic cases. *Am J Gastroenterol.* 2010; 105(6):1421-1429.
4. Halfdanarson TR, Rabe KG, Rubin J, Petersen GM. Pancreatic neuroendocrine tumors (PNETs): incidence, prognosis and recent trend toward improved survival. *Ann Oncol Off J Eur Soc Med Oncol.* 2008;19(10):1727-1733.
5. James PD, Tsolakis AV, Zhang M, et al. Incremental benefit of preoperative EUS for the detection of pancreatic neuroendocrine tumors: a meta-analysis. *Gastrointest Endosc.* 2015;81(4):848-856.e1.
6. Howe JR, Merchant NB, Conrad C, et al. The North American Neuroendocrine Tumor Society consensus paper on the surgical management of pancreatic neuroendocrine tumors: *Pancreas.* 2020;49(1):1-33.
7. Rindi G, Mete O, Uccella S, et al. Overview of the 2022 WHO classification of neuroendocrine neoplasms. *Endocr Pathol.* 2022;33(1):115-154.
8. Amin MB, Edge S, Greene F, et al., eds. *AJCC Cancer Staging Manual.* 8th ed. Springer International Publishing; 2017. Accessed September 8, 2021. https://www.springer.com/gp/book/9783319406176
9. Klöppel G, Rindi G, Perren A, Komminoth P, Klimstra DS. The ENETS and AJCC/UICC TNM classifications of the neuroendocrine tumors of the gastrointestinal tract and the pancreas: a statement. *Virchows Arch Int J Pathol.* 2010;456(6):595-597.
10. Kankava K, Maisonneuve P, Mangogna A, et al. Prognostic features of gastro-entero-pancreatic neuroendocrine neoplasms in primary and metastatic sites: grade, mesenteric tumour deposits and emerging novelties. *J Neuroendocrinol.* 2021;33(8):e13000.
11. Fujimori N, Miki M, Lee L, et al. Natural history and clinical outcomes of pancreatic neuroendocrine neoplasms based on the WHO 2017 classification: a single-center experience of 30 years. *Pancreatology.* 2020;20(4):709-715.
12. Asano D, Kudo A, Akahoshi K, et al. Curative surgery and Ki-67 value rather than tumor differentiation predict the survival of patients with high-grade neuroendocrine neoplasms. *Ann Surg.* 2022;276(2):e108-e113.
13. Schmocker RK, Wright MJ, Ding D, et al. Duodenal, ampullary, and pancreatic neuroendocrine tumors: oncologic outcomes are driven by tumor biology and tissue of origin. *J Surg Oncol.* 2021;123(2):416-424.
14. You Y, Jang JY, Kim SC, et al. Validation of the 8th AJCC cancer staging system for pancreas neuroendocrine tumors using Korean nationwide surgery database. *Cancer Res Treat.* 2019;51(4):1639-1652.
15. Shah MH, Goldner WS, Benson AB, et al. Neuroendocrine and Adrenal Tumors, Version 2.2021, NCCN Clinical Practice Guidelines in Oncology. *J Natl Compr Cancer Netw JNCCN.* 2021;19(7):839-868.
16. Jiao Y, Shi C, Edil BH, et al. DAXX/ATRX, MEN1 and mTOR pathway genes are frequently altered in pancreatic neuroendocrine tumors. *Science.* 2011;331(6021):1199-1203.
17. Chan CS, Laddha SV, Lewis PW, et al. ATRX, DAXX or MEN1 mutant pancreatic neuroendocrine tumors are a distinct alpha-cell signature subgroup. *Nat Commun.* 2018;9:4158.
18. Scarpa A, Chang DK, Nones K, et al. Whole-genome landscape of pancreatic neuroendocrine tumours. *Nature.* 2017; 543(7643):65-71.
19. Halfdanarson TR, Bamlet WR, McWilliams RR, et al. Risk factors for pancreatic neuroendocrine tumors: a clinic-based case-control study. *Pancreas.* 2014;43(8):1219-1222.
20. Maxwell JE, O'Dorisio TM, Bellizzi AM, Howe JR. Elevated pancreatic polypeptide levels in pancreatic neuroendocrine tumors and diabetes mellitus: causation or association? *Pancreas.* 2014;43(4):651-656.
21. Luna IE, Monrad N, Binderup T, et al. Somatostatin-immunoreactive pancreaticoduodenal neuroendocrine neoplasms: twenty-three cases evaluated according to the WHO 2010 classification. *Neuroendocrinology.* 2016;103(5):567-577.
22. Därr R, Nambuba J, Del Rivero J, et al. Novel insights into the polycythemia-paraganglioma-somatostatinoma syndrome. *Endocr Relat Cancer.* 2016;23(12):899-908.
23. Schizas D, Mastoraki A, Bagias G, et al. Clinicopathological data and treatment modalities for pancreatic VIPomas: a systematic review. *J BUON Off J Balk Union Oncol.* 2019; 24(2):415-423.
24. Yeh PJ, Chen SH, Lai JY, et al. Rare cases of pediatric vasoactive intestinal peptide secreting tumor with literature review: a challenging etiology of chronic diarrhea. *Front Pediatr.* 2020; 8:430.
25. Ilić I, Katić V, Randjelović P, Stojanović N, Antovic A, Ilić R. Pancreatic polypeptide-secreting tumour of the proximal pancreas (PPoma)-ultra rare pancreatic tumour: clinically malign, histologically benign. *Med Kaunas Lith.* 2019;55(9):E523.
26. Mosenia A, Ward C, Yee A, Qorbani A, Corvera C. Multifocal pancreatic PPoma in the setting of MEN1: case report and review of literature. *Int J Surg Case Rep.* 2021;83:106008.
27. Song X, Zheng S, Yang G, et al. Glucagonoma and the glucagonoma syndrome. *Oncol Lett.* 2018;15(3):2749-2755.
28. John AM, Schwartz RA. Glucagonoma syndrome: a review and update on treatment. *J Eur Acad Dermatol Venereol JEADV.* 2016;30(12):2016-2022.
29. Halfdanarson TR, Strosberg JR, Tang L, et al. The North American Neuroendocrine Tumor Society consensus guidelines for surveillance and medical management of pancreatic neuroendocrine tumors. *Pancreas.* 2020;49(7):863-881.
30. Zhang C, Jin J, Xie J, et al. The clinical features and molecular mechanisms of ACTH-secreting pancreatic neuroendocrine tumors. *J Clin Endocrinol Metab.* 2020;105(11):dgaa507.
31. Davi' MV, Cosaro E, Piacentini S, et al. Prognostic factors in ectopic Cushing's syndrome due to neuroendocrine tumors: a multicenter study. *Eur J Endocrinol.* 2017;176(4):453-461.
32. Wu Y, Xiong G, Zhang H, Wang M, Zhu F, Qin R. Adrenocorticotropic hormone-producing pancreatic neuroendocrine neoplasms: a systematic review. *Endocr Pract Off J Am Coll Endocrinol Am Assoc Clin Endocrinol.* 2021;27(2):152-157.
33. Lee NJ, Hruban RH, Fishman EK. Pancreatic neuroendocrine tumor: review of heterogeneous spectrum of CT appearance. *Abdom Radiol.* 2018;43(11):3025-3034.
34. Park HS, Kim SY, Hong SM, et al. Hypervascular solid-appearing serous cystic neoplasms of the pancreas: differential diagnosis with neuroendocrine tumours. *Eur Radiol.* 2016;26(5):1348-1358.
35. Ren S, Chen X, Wang J, et al. Differentiation of duodenal gastrointestinal stromal tumors from hypervascular pancreatic neuroendocrine tumors in the pancreatic head using contrast-enhanced computed tomography. *Abdom Radiol.* 2019;44(3):867-876.
36. Lo GC, Kambadakone A. MR imaging of pancreatic neuroendocrine tumors. *Magn Reson Imaging Clin N Am.* 2018;26(3): 391-403.

37. Geurts JL. Inherited syndromes involving pancreatic neuroendocrine tumors. *J Gastrointest Oncol.* 2020;11(3).
38. Ito T, Igarashi H, Nakamura K, et al. Epidemiological trends of pancreatic and gastrointestinal neuroendocrine tumors in Japan: a nationwide survey analysis. *J Gastroenterol.* 2015;50(1):58-64.
39. Hampel H, Bennett RL, Buchanan A, Pearlman R, Wiesner GL, Guideline Development Group, American College of Medical Genetics and Genomics Professional Practice and Guidelines Committee and National Society of Genetic Counselors Practice Guidelines Committee. A practice guideline from the American College of Medical Genetics and Genomics and the National Society of Genetic Counselors: referral indications for cancer predisposition assessment. *Genet Med Off J Am Coll Med Genet.* 2015;17(1):70-87.
40. de Mestier L, Gaujoux S, Cros J, et al. Long-term prognosis of resected pancreatic neuroendocrine tumors in von hippel-lindau disease is favorable and not influenced by small tumors left in place. *Ann Surg.* 2015;262(2):384-388.
41. Tirosh A, Sadowski SM, Linehan WM, et al. Association of VHL genotype with pancreatic neuroendocrine tumor phenotype in patients with von Hippel–Lindau disease. *JAMA Oncol.* 2018;4(1):124-126.
42. Keutgen XM, Hammel P, Choyke PL, Libutti SK, Jonasch E, Kebebew E. Evaluation and management of pancreatic lesions in patients with von Hippel–Lindau disease. *Nat Rev Clin Oncol.* 2016;13(9):537-549.
43. Mortaji P, Morris KT, Samedi V, Eberhardt S, Ryan S. Pancreatic neuroendocrine tumor in a patient with a TSC1 variant: case report and review of the literature. *Fam Cancer.* 2018;17(2):275-280.
44. Mowrey K, Northrup H, Rougeau P, et al. Frequency, progression, and current management: report of 16 new cases of nonfunctional pancreatic neuroendocrine tumors in tuberous sclerosis complex and comparison with previous reports. *Front Neurol.* 2021;12:627672.
45. Shah MH, Golder WS, Benson AB. NCCN Clinical Practice Guidelines in Oncology: Neuroendocrine and Adrenal Tumors, Version 3.2021. NCCN. Accessed October 3, 2021. https://www.nccn.org/guidelines/guidelines-detail
46. Partelli S, Bartsch DK, Capdevila J, et al. ENETS consensus guidelines for the standards of care in neuroendocrine tumours: surgery for small intestinal and pancreatic neuroendocrine tumours. *Neuroendocrinology.* 2017;105(3):255-265.
47. Najafi N, Mintziras I, Wiese D, Albers MB, Maurer E, Bartsch DK. A retrospective comparison of robotic versus laparoscopic distal resection and enucleation for potentially benign pancreatic neoplasms. *Surg Today.* 2020;50(8):872-880.
48. Guerrini GP, Lauretta A, Belluco C, et al. Robotic versus laparoscopic distal pancreatectomy: an up-to-date meta-analysis. *BMC Surg.* 2017;17(1):105.
49. Björnsson B, Larsson AL, Hjalmarsson C, Gasslander T, Sandström P. Comparison of the duration of hospital stay after laparoscopic or open distal pancreatectomy: randomized controlled trial. *Br J Surg.* 2020;107(10):1281-1288.
50. de Rooij T, van Hilst J, van Santvoort H, et al. Minimally invasive versus open distal pancreatectomy (leopard): a multicenter patient-blinded randomized controlled trial. *Ann Surg.* 2019;269(1):2-9.
51. Drymousis P, Raptis DA, Spalding D, et al. Laparoscopic versus open pancreas resection for pancreatic neuroendocrine tumours: a systematic review and meta-analysis. *HPB.* 2014;16(5):397-406.
52. Xourafas D, Tavakkoli A, Clancy TE, Ashley SW. Distal pancreatic resection for neuroendocrine tumors: is laparoscopic really better than open? *J Gastrointest Surg.* 2015; 19(5):831-840.
53. Zureikat AH, Postlewait LM, Liu Y, et al. A multi-institutional comparison of perioperative outcomes of robotic and open pancreaticoduodenectomy. *Ann Surg.* 2016;264(4):640-649.
54. van Hilst J, de Rooij T, Bosscha K, et al. Laparoscopic versus open pancreatoduodenectomy for pancreatic or periampullary tumours (LEOPARD-2): a multicentre, patient-blinded, randomised controlled phase 2/3 trial. *Lancet Gastroenterol Hepatol.* 2019;4(3):199-207.
55. Norton JA, Harris EJ, Chen Y, et al. Pancreatic endocrine tumors with major vascular abutment, involvement, or encasement and indication for resection. *Arch Surg Chic Ill 1960.* 2011;146(6):724-732.
56. Ambe CM, Nguyen P, Centeno BA, et al. Multimodality management of "borderline resectable" pancreatic neuroendocrine tumors: report of a single-institution experience. *Cancer Control J Moffitt Cancer Cent.* 2017;24(5):1073274817729076.
57. Prakash L, Bhosale P, Cloyd J, et al. Role of fluorouracil, doxorubicin, and streptozocin therapy in the preoperative treatment of localized pancreatic neuroendocrine tumors. *J Gastrointest Surg Off J Soc Surg Aliment Tract.* 2017;21(1):155-163.
58. Yuan CH, Wang J, Xiu DR, et al. Meta-analysis of liver resection versus nonsurgical treatments for pancreatic neuroendocrine tumors with liver metastases. *Ann Surg Oncol.* 2016;23(1):244-249.
59. Maxwell JE, Sherman SK, O'Dorisio TM, Bellizzi AM, Howe JR. Liver-directed surgery of neuroendocrine metastases: what is the optimal strategy? *Surgery.* 2016;159(1):320-333.
60. Morgan RE, Pommier SJ, Pommier RF. Expanded criteria for debulking of liver metastasis also apply to pancreatic neuroendocrine tumors. *Surgery.* 2018;163(1):218-225.
61. Scott AT, Breheny PJ, Keck KJ, et al. Effective cytoreduction can be achieved in patients with numerous neuroendocrine tumor liver metastases (NETLMs). *Surgery.* 2019;165(1):166-175.
62. Bertani E, Fazio N, Radice D, et al. Resection of the primary tumor followed by peptide receptor radionuclide therapy as upfront strategy for the treatment of G1-G2 pancreatic neuroendocrine tumors with unresectable liver metastases. *Ann Surg Oncol.* 2016;23(Suppl 5):981-989.
63. Mazzaferro V, Sposito C, Coppa J, et al. The long-term benefit of liver transplantation for hepatic metastases from neuroendocrine tumors. *Am J Transplant Off J Am Soc Transplant Am Soc Transpl Surg.* 2016;16(10):2892-2902.
64. Rinke A, Müller HH, Schade-Brittinger C, et al. Placebo-controlled, double-blind, prospective, randomized study on the effect of octreotide LAR in the control of tumor growth in patients with metastatic neuroendocrine midgut tumors: a report from the PROMID study group. *J Clin Oncol Off J Am Soc Clin Oncol.* 2009;27(28):4656-4663.
65. Rinke A, Wittenberg M, Schade-Brittinger C, et al. Placebo-controlled, double-blind, prospective, randomized study on the effect of octreotide LAR in the control of tumor growth in patients with metastatic neuroendocrine midgut tumors (PROMID): results of long-term survival. *Neuroendocrinology.* 2017;104(1):26-32.
66. Caplin ME, Pavel M, Ćwikła JB, et al. Lanreotide in metastatic enteropancreatic neuroendocrine tumors. *N Engl J Med.* 2014;371(3):224-233.

67. Caplin ME, Pavel M, Phan AT, et al. Lanreotide autogel/depot in advanced enteropancreatic neuroendocrine tumours: final results of the CLARINET open-label extension study. *Endocrine*. 2021;71(2):502-513.
68. Yao JC, Shah MH, Ito T, et al. Everolimus for advanced pancreatic neuroendocrine tumors. *N Engl J Med*. 2011;364(6):514-523.
69. Yao JC, Fazio N, Singh S, et al. Everolimus for the treatment of advanced, non-functional neuroendocrine tumours of the lung or gastrointestinal tract (RADIANT-4): a randomised, placebo-controlled, phase 3 study. *Lancet Lond Engl*. 2016;387(10022):968-977.
70. Pavel ME, Singh S, Strosberg JR, et al. Health-related quality of life for everolimus versus placebo in patients with advanced, non-functional, well-differentiated gastrointestinal or lung neuroendocrine tumours (RADIANT-4): a multicentre, randomised, double-blind, placebo-controlled, phase 3 trial. *Lancet Oncol*. 2017;18(10):1411-1422.
71. Raymond E, Dahan L, Raoul JL, et al. Sunitinib malate for the treatment of pancreatic neuroendocrine tumors. *N Engl J Med*. 2011;364(6):501-513.
72. de Mestier L, Walter T, Evrard C, et al. Temozolomide alone or combined with capecitabine for the treatment of advanced pancreatic neuroendocrine tumor. *Neuroendocrinology*. 2020;110(1-2):83-91.
73. Strosberg JR, Fine RL, Choi J, et al. First-line chemotherapy with capecitabine and temozolomide in patients with metastatic pancreatic endocrine carcinomas. *Cancer*. 2011;117(2):268-275.
74. Cives M, Ghayouri M, Morse B, et al. Analysis of potential response predictors to capecitabine/temozolomide in metastatic pancreatic neuroendocrine tumors. *Endocr Relat Cancer*. 2016;23(9):759-767.
75. Kunz PL, Catalano PJ, Nimeiri H, et al. A randomized study of temozolomide or temozolomide and capecitabine in patients with advanced pancreatic neuroendocrine tumors: A trial of the ECOG-ACRIN Cancer Research Group (E2211). *J Clin Oncol*. 2018;36(15_suppl):4004-4004.
76. Strosberg J, El-Haddad G, Wolin E, et al. Phase 3 trial of 177Lu-dotatate for midgut neuroendocrine tumors. *N Engl J Med*. 2017;376(2):125-135.
77. Strosberg J, Wolin E, Chasen B, et al. Health-related quality of life in patients with progressive midgut neuroendocrine tumors treated with 177Lu-dotatate in the phase III NETTER-1 trial. *J Clin Oncol Off J Am Soc Clin Oncol*. 2018;36(25):2578-2584.
78. Ramage J, Naraev BG, Halfdanarson TR. Peptide receptor radionuclide therapy for patients with advanced pancreatic neuroendocrine tumors. *Semin Oncol*. 2018;45(4):236-248.
79. Fröss-Baron K, Garske-Roman U, Welin S, et al. 177Lu-dotatate therapy of advanced pancreatic neuroendocrine tumors heavily pretreated with chemotherapy: analysis of outcome, safety, and their determinants. *Neuroendocrinology*. 2021;111(4):330-343.
80. Zandee WT, Brabander T, Blažević A, et al. Symptomatic and radiological response to 177Lu-dotatate for the treatment of functioning pancreatic neuroendocrine tumors. *J Clin Endocrinol Metab*. 2019;104(4):1336-1344.
81. Marrache F, Vullierme MP, Roy C, et al. Arterial phase enhancement and body mass index are predictors of response to chemoembolisation for liver metastases of endocrine tumours. *Br J Cancer*. 2007;96(1):49-55.
82. Elf AK, Andersson M, Henrikson O, et al. Radioembolization versus bland embolization for hepatic metastases from small intestinal neuroendocrine tumors: short-term results of a randomized clinical trial. *World J Surg*. 2018;42(2):506-513.
83. Do Minh D, Chapiro J, Gorodetski B, et al. Intra-arterial therapy of neuroendocrine tumour liver metastases: comparing conventional TACE, drug-eluting beads TACE and yttrium-90 radioembolisation as treatment options using a propensity score analysis model. *Eur Radiol*. 2017;27(12):4995-5005.
84. Chen JX, Rose S, White SB, et al. Embolotherapy for neuroendocrine tumor liver metastases: prognostic factors for hepatic progression-free survival and overall survival. *Cardiovasc Intervent Radiol*. 2017;40(1):69-80.
85. Kennedy A, Bester L, Salem R, Sharma RA, Parks RW, Ruszniewski P. Role of hepatic intra-arterial therapies in metastatic neuroendocrine tumours (NET): guidelines from the NET-liver-metastases consensus conference. *HPB*. 2015;17(1):29-37.
86. Takahashi H, Kahramangil B, Berber E. Local recurrence after microwave thermosphere ablation of malignant liver tumors: results of a surgical series. *Surgery*. 2018;163(4):709-713.
87. Perrodin SF, Renzulli MM, Maurer MH, et al. Can microwave ablation be an alternative to resection for the treatment of neuroendocrine liver metastases? *Endocr Pract Off J Am Coll Endocrinol Am Assoc Clin Endocrinol*. 2020;26(4):378-387.
88. Taskin OC, Clarke CN, Erkan M, Tsai S, Evans DB, Adsay V. Pancreatic neuroendocrine neoplasms: current state and ongoing controversies on terminology, classification and prognostication. *J Gastrointest Oncol*. 2020;11(3):548-558.
89. Basturk O, Yang Z, Tang LH, et al. The high-grade (WHO G3) pancreatic neuroendocrine tumor category is morphologically and biologically heterogenous and includes both well differentiated and poorly differentiated neoplasms. *Am J Surg Pathol*. 2015;39(5):683-690.
90. Keutgen XM, Nilubol N, Kebebew E. Malignant-functioning neuroendocrine tumors of the pancreas: a survival analysis. *Surgery*. 2016;159(5):1382-1389.
91. Fahmy JN, Varsanik MA, Hubbs D, Eguia E, Abood G, Knab LM. Pancreatic neuroendocrine tumors: surgical outcomes and survival analysis. *Am J Surg*. 2021;221(3):529-533.
92. Mastoraki A, Schizas D, Papoutsi E, et al. Clinicopathological data and treatment modalities for pancreatic somatostatinomas. *In Vivo*. 2020;34(6):3573-3582.
93. de Geus SW, Woods AP, Papageorge MV, et al. Combined hepatopancreaticobiliary volume and hepatectomy outcomes in hepatocellular carcinoma patients at low-volume liver centers. *J Am Coll Surg*. 2021;232(6):864-871.
94. Hata T, Motoi F, Ishida M, et al. Effect of hospital volume on surgical outcomes after pancreaticoduodenectomy: a systematic review and meta-analysis. *Ann Surg*. 2016;263(4):664-672.
95. Macedo FIB, Jayanthi P, Mowzoon M, Yakoub D, Dudeja V, Merchant N. The impact of surgeon volume on outcomes after pancreaticoduodenectomy: a meta-analysis. *J Gastrointest Surg Off J Soc Surg Aliment Tract*. 2017;21(10):1723-1731.
96. Toomey PG, Teta AF, Patel KD, Ross SB, Rosemurgy AS. High-volume surgeons vs high-volume hospitals: are best outcomes more due to who or where? *Am J Surg*. 2016;211(1):59-63.
97. Sheetz KH, Nuliyalu U, Nathan H, Sonnenday CJ. Association of surgeon case numbers of pancreaticoduodenectomies vs related procedures with patient outcomes to inform volume-based credentialing. *JAMA Netw Open*. 2020;3(4):e203850.
98. de Geus SWL, Hachey KJ, Nudel JD, et al. Volume of pancreas-adjacent operations favorably influences pancreaticoduodenectomy outcomes at lower volume pancreas centers. *Ann Surg*. 2022;276(2):e102-e107.

58 Pancreatic Surgery: Pancreaticoduodenectomy (Whipple Procedure)

Gopal Menon, MBBS, MD
John A. Chabot, MD

INTRODUCTION

Pancreaticoduodenectomy (PD) remains the cornerstone of managing periampullary tumors. Since its description in the early 1900s, the technique, operative, and postoperative management have evolved, and overall survival has improved.[1] In addition, with the advent of newer chemotherapy and radiation regimens, lesions previously deemed unresectable have increasingly come under the purview of surgery. This chapter describes the relevant anatomy, primary indications, surgical technique, and complications of pancreaticoduodenectomy. Pancreatic neuroendocrine tumors (PNETs) make up a relatively small proportion of neoplasms requiring pancreaticoduodenectomy. However, the unique aspects of PNETs will be emphasized.

Relevant Anatomy

The pancreas is a retroperitoneal organ closely related to the duodenum, stomach, and transverse colon. The head and uncinate process are typically resected in a PD, with the neck of the pancreas forming the transection zone. The pancreas and duodenum share a common, extensively linked blood supply, which necessitates removing the two in continuity. The pylorus and distal antrum are more proximally resected in a classical PD while spared in a pylorus-preserving PD. The common bile duct passes posterior to the duodenum before entering the pancreatic parenchyma and joining the main pancreatic duct to form a common channel of variable length, which opens into the duodenum through the major duodenal papilla (ampulla of Vater). The majority of tumors arise in this region (Figure 58–1).

The relationship between the pancreas and the abdominal vasculature is vital to both the technical aspects of PD and in determining resectability. The splenic vein and superior mesenteric vein (SMV) join posterior to the pancreatic neck to form the portal vein (PV), which runs cranially in the posterior aspect of the hepatoduodenal ligament. In particular, the pancreatic head and uncinate process are directly apposed to the vein, with a variable number of small venous tributaries draining the pancreatic parenchyma. Thus, the degree of involvement of both the SMV and PV are crucial to determining resectability. More recently, portal and/or SMV resection and reconstruction have been accepted as tolerable risk operations, but this needs to be planned and performed by a highly experienced surgeon.

The arterial supply to the pancreas arises from both the celiac axis and the superior mesenteric artery (SMA). The common hepatic artery is closely related to the superior border of the pancreas. Further to the right, the gastroduodenal artery (GDA) branches off at 90 degrees to run directly inferiorly, entering the pancreatic parenchyma as the superior pancreaticoduodenal artery, forming an extensive collateral network with the inferior pancreaticoduodenal artery, a branch of the SMA. The splenic artery (SA) runs posterosuperior along the length of the pancreas, providing various branches along its course. In general, the larger vessels run longitudinally within the pancreatic parenchyma. In addition, it is crucial to maintain an awareness of common variations in vascular anatomy during pancreatic resection.[2,3]

Indications

Periampullary tumors, including ductal adenocarcinoma, distal cholangiocarcinoma, ampullary adenocarcinoma, and duodenal adenocarcinoma, constitute the primary indications for PD for malignancy. Other indications include neuroendocrine tumors and various less common tumors. In addition, intraductal mucinous papillary neoplasms (IPMN), chronic pancreatitis, and pancreatic trauma are some of the benign etiologies that sometimes require a PD.

Primary surgical resection is the standard of care for clearly resectable tumors that are operative candidates, although this notion is being challenged by recent trials.[4,5] Tumors encroaching on the PV, SMV, or branches of the celiac axis may be deemed "borderline resectable," a situation

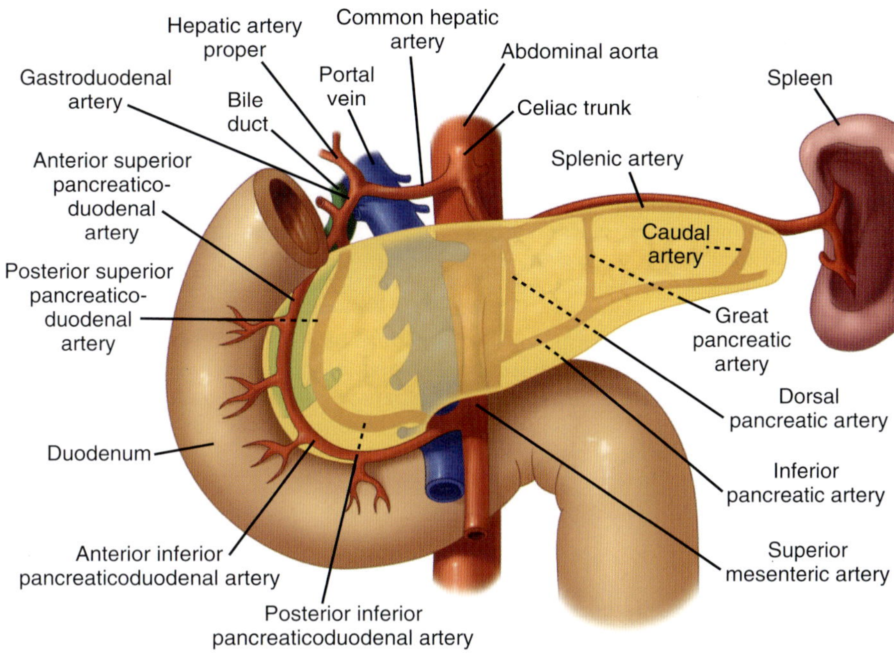

Figure 58–1. Gross anatomy of the pancreas with its relationship to surrounding structures. Note the proximity of the duodenal loop to the pancreatic head and the important vascular structures in the vicinity. (Reproduced with permission from Brunicardi FC, Andersen DK, Billiar TR, et al, eds. *Schwartz's Principles of Surgery*. 11th ed. New York: McGraw Hill; 2019.)

where neoadjuvant therapy (chemotherapy or chemoradiation) is increasingly advocated. PD is contraindicated in nonresectable cases or in cases where metastatic spread is noted.[6] Neoadjuvant therapy is rarely helpful for neuroendocrine tumors.[7] Therefore, venous resection and reconstruction are employed as needed (Table 58–1).

SURGICAL TECHNIQUES

The surgical technique for pancreatic resection varies between surgeons but follows similar basic principles. The operation can be divided into three phases: abdominal exploration, extirpation, and reconstruction. The importance of careful preoperative imaging review to ascertain resectability, identify possible metastases and vascular anomalies cannot be overstated. The following steps describe a typical approach to PD in our institution.

Positioning

The patient is positioned supine, and preoperative antibiotics and chemoprophylaxis for deep vein thrombosis are routinely administered. An ultrasound probe is always available, especially for smaller tumors. In addition, we routinely prep

Table 58–1. Criteria for resectability for pancreatic tumors based on international consensus.

Vessel	Resectable	Borderline Resectable	Unresectable
PV/SMV	No contact, <180°, no vein contour irregularity	>180°, <180° with contour irregularity or thrombosis allowing safe reconstruction	Unreconstructable obstruction
CHA	No tumor contact	Contact without extension to CA or HA bifurcation	Extension to CA or HA bifurcation
CA	No tumor contact	No contact (head), contact <180° body and tail	Contact >180°, any contact with aorta
SMA	No tumor contact	Contact <180°	Contact >180°, any contact with aorta

CA, celiac axis; CHA, common hepatic artery; HA, hepatic artery; PV, portal vein; SMA, superior mesenteric artery; SMV, superior mesenteric vein.

the left neck for a potential internal jugular vein harvest if a PV reconstruction is a possibility.

Diagnostic Laparoscopy

Diagnostic laparoscopy is routinely performed for adenocarcinoma. Abdominal insufflation is achieved with a Verres needle at Palmer's point. Two five-millimeter ports are placed at the planned upper midline incision poles, typically above the umbilicus and in the sub-xiphoid region. A 5-mm camera and a blunt-tip grasper are used to carefully inspect the peritoneal surfaces, with close attention to the liver, omentum, and abdominal wall surfaces. Any suspicious lesions are biopsied with immediate frozen section analysis. Confirmation of a metastatic lesion terminates the operation, saving the patient from an extensive resection with no mortality benefit. Bulky PNETs will often benefit from resection of the primary in the setting of low-volume liver metastases, so this step is omitted.

Open Exploration

An upper midline incision is made, typically terminating above the umbilicus. In the preperitoneal space, the falciform ligament is detached from the abdominal wall and the umbilicus to fashion a flap that is used to cover the GDA stump after ligation. Once the peritoneal cavity is opened, the peritoneal surfaces and tumor are palpated again to confirm resectability. We typically use a Bookwalter retractor for exposure.

Duodenal Dissection

The hepatic flexure is separated from Gerota's fascia and the incision is extended to the lateral border of the duodenum. The duodenum is then Kocherized, typically till the inferior vena cava (IVC) is completely exposed. At this stage, the pancreas should be palpable between the thumb and fore-fingers, with the fingers passing behind the pancreatic head. In addition, a replaced right hepatic artery, if present, will be palpable posterior to the pancreas.

Creation of Retropancreatic Tunnel

The lesser sac is then entered by opening the gastrocolic ligament while maintaining the gastroepiploic arcade. Once the anterior surface of the pancreas is exposed, the mesocolic attachment is mobilized. The SMV is then identified by passing beneath the pancreatic neck and its identification can be aided by following the middle colic vein to its insertion into the SMV. The anterior surface of the SMV is then separated from the pancreatic neck, creating a tunnel beneath the pancreas. Sharp dissection with a gentle snip and spread motion with anterosuperior retraction of the pancreas greatly aids this process. Care must be taken to handle the vein gently and to ligate draining branches (Figure 58–2).

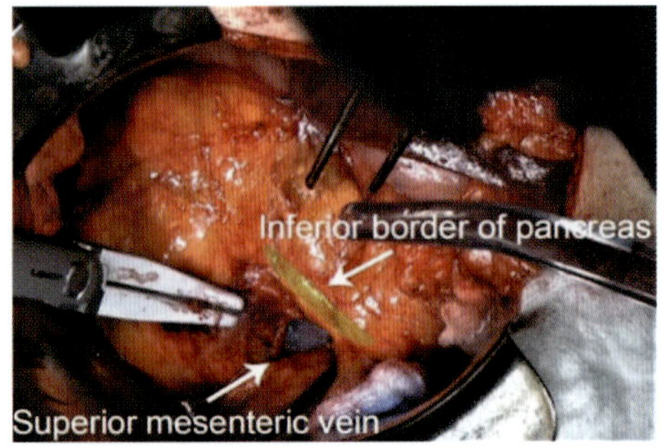

Figure 58–2. Relationship of the pancreatic neck to the superior mesenteric vein running directly posteriorly. The pancreas is elevated off the SMV during the creation of the retro-pancreatic tunnel. (Image used with permission from the Department of Surgery, Columbia University Irving Medical Center.)

Cholecystectomy

Once the inferior portion of the tunnel is complete, we typically proceed to cholecystectomy top-down, identifying and ligating the cystic duct and artery. The cystic duct leads to the common bile duct, aiding in its identification.

Dissecting the Hepatoduodenal Ligament

We then turn our attention to dissecting the hepatoduodenal ligament. First, the common hepatic artery is identified by dividing the thin lymphatic tissue overlying it. Next, we ensure that the lymphatic tissue is dissected off the artery and included in the final specimen. The origin of the GDA is then identified and encircled. We then occlude the GDA and palpate the hepatic artery distal to the take-off of the GDA. This ensures that the hepatic artery is not relying on the GDA for flow (via pancreaticoduodenal collaterals with SMA). Once hepatic artery flow is confirmed, the GDA is double-ligated with 0-Silk ties and divided, leaving a small stump.

Once the GDA is divided, the anterior surface of the PV is visible. Dissection is continued along the anterior surface of the PV toward the superior margin of the pancreas. Staying on the anterior surface of the PV, the pancreas is separated from the vein to meet the inferior portion of the tunnel over the SMV. The CBD is then encircled and divided proximal to the cystic duct insertion. Care is taken to avoid skeletonizing the CBD, thereby preserving its blood supply (Figure 58–3).

Jejunal Mobilization

We then turn our attention to dissecting the fourth portion of the duodenum. The transverse mesocolon is elevated to identify the ligament of Treitz. A suitable point roughly 8 cm

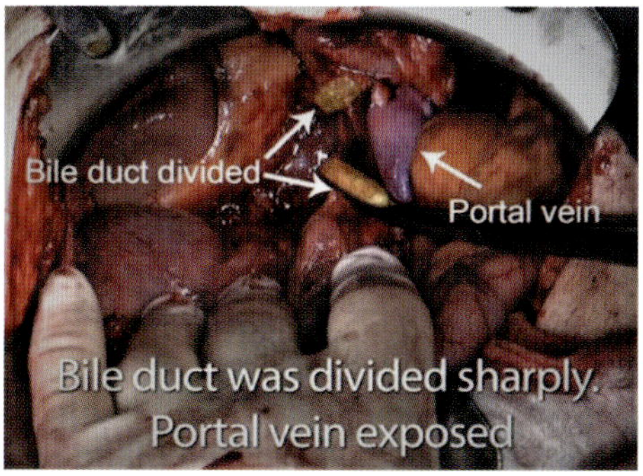

Figure 58–3. Portal vein lying posteriorly after the division of the common bile duct. The cranial portion of the retro-pancreatic tunnel is created by separating the pancreatic neck from the portal vein-SMV confluence. (Image used with permission from the Department of Surgery, Columbia University Irving Medical Center.)

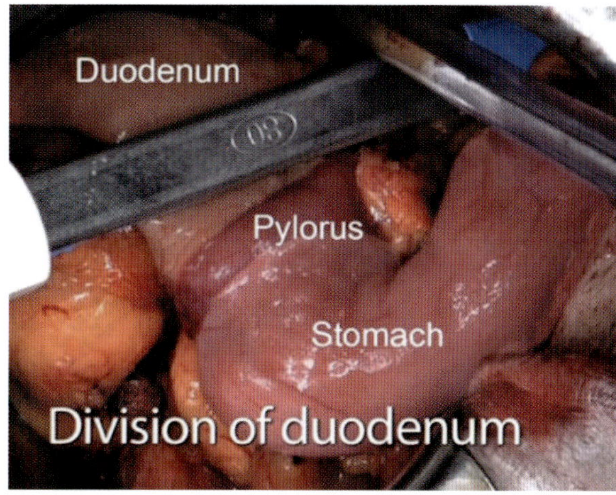

Figure 58–4. Division of the proximal duodenum with a linear stapler in a pylorus-preserving PD. In a classical PD, the stomach is divided just proximal to the pylorus. (Image used with permission from the Department of Surgery, Columbia University Irving Medical Center.)

distal to the ligament is selected and the proximal jejunum is transected with a 3.5-mm stapler. Following this, the small bowel mesentery is divided, taking care to stay close to the specimen. We typically use a Ligasure device to seal vessels. Once the duodenum is freed from its vasculature at the ligament of Treitz, the specimen can typically be pushed through this window to the supramesocolic compartment. We typically close the mesocolic defect with a few interrupted sutures.

Dividing the Pancreas

The proximal resection margin is either just proximal or distal to the pylorus, depending on whether a pylorus-preserving PD is performed or not. Next, the stomach is divided with a stapling device and retracted superiorly.

In preparation for dividing the pancreas, "figure of 8" sutures are placed at the superior and inferior margin of the pancreas, on either side of the proposed line of division with 2-0 Silk (Figure 58–4). The pancreas is then divided sharply, taking care not to injure the underlying SMV/PV. Brisk bleeding from the pancreatic cut surface is usually controlled with 4-0 silk sutures.

Uncinate Dissection

The uncinate dissection is commenced by gently dissecting the pancreatic parenchyma off the SMV/PV. Smaller bleeders are controlled using a Ligasure, while larger vessels are suture ligated. Extreme caution must be taken to avoid injury to the SMA and the PV, especially before activating the Ligasure. At the end of the dissection, the lateral margin of the SMA should be free of pancreatic tissue.

Pancreaticojejunostomy

Reconstruction typically begins with a pancreaticojejunostomy. The stapled end of the jejunal loop is brought through the base of the transverse mesocolon, usually to the right of the middle colic artery and oriented in a candy-cane fashion, with the cut surface of the pancreas opposing the jejunal sidewall. We typically perform a single-layer continuous duct to mucosa anastomosis except in cases where the PD is extremely small, in which case the cut surface is dunked into the jejunum. For the more common duct-to-mucosa anastomosis, a small jejunotomy is created. Two 5-0 Maxon/PDS sutures are placed posteriorly between the duct and jejunostomy with knots on the inside. In a running fashion, the pancreatojejunostomy continues until the anastomosis is completed anteriorly. Once complete, two sutures are placed at the superior and inferior portion of the anastomosis to fold the jejunum over the pancreas, to buttress the anastomosis.

Choledochojejunostomy

Further along the jejunal limb, roughly 10-cm distal to the P-J, an end-to-side choledochojejunostomy is performed similarly to the PJ, that is, single layer, continuous duct-to-mucosa anastomosis (Figure 58–5). In cases where the duct is small, we use interrupted Vicryl sutures instead.

Gastrojejunostomy

The gastrojejunostomy is performed in an antecolic fashion. A loop of jejunum is brought up above the transverse colon.

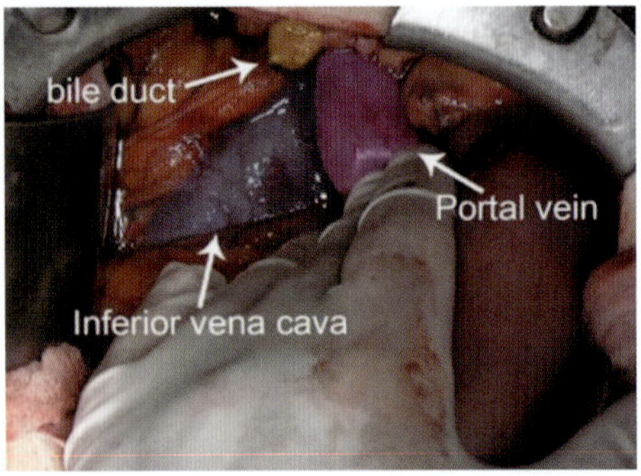

Figure 58–5. Exposure of the portal vein and inferior vena cava after specimen removal. (Image used with permission from the Department of Surgery, Columbia University Irving Medical Center.)

The gastric staple line is excised, and a longitudinal jejunostomy is created. A single-layer suture anastomosis using 3-0 Monocryl is typically performed.

Once the anastomoses are finished and hemostasis achieved, two Blake drains are placed anterior and posterior to the PJ. The falciform flap that was created is interposed between the GDA and PJ. The abdomen is irrigated and closed.

Postoperative Care

We typically follow an ERAS protocol for patients undergoing PD. The nasogastric tube is removed on postoperative day 1 (POD 1). Drain fluid is sent for amylase levels on POD 2 and 4 and removed if less than three times the upper limit of normal. Patients are placed on a multimodal pain regimen, and DVT prophylaxis is continued (Figure 58–6).

POSTOPERATIVE COMPLICATIONS

Postoperative Pancreatic Fistula

Postoperative pancreatic fistula (POPF) is a result of an anastomotic leak at the PJ. The reported incidence ranges from 10% to 30%. The main risk factors for POPF include a small pancreatic duct and a soft pancreas. It is more common to encounter a small duct and soft pancreas, hence operating for PNET than adenocarcinoma. The severity of POPF has been graded by the International Study Group on Pancreatic Fistula (ISGPF).[8-10] Grade A is a biochemical leak (diagnosed by drain amylase levels more than three times the upper limit of normal) with minimal clinical symptoms and requires no intervention. Grade B is symptomatic POPF, which may require long-term nutritional support and/or external/internal drainage. Grade C POPF refers to uncontrolled leakage of pancreatic fluid, causing organ failure and/or requiring reoperation. In general, the vast majority of POPF is treated with prolonged drainage and appropriate nutritional support.

Delayed Gastric Emptying

Delayed gastric emptying (DGE) is defined as the inability to tolerate oral intake 1 week after surgery. The incidence of delayed gastric emptying varies from 12% to 45%, depending on the series published.[11] It is a clinical diagnosis, with patients presenting with nausea, vomiting, and increased abdominal distension. A CT scan is often performed to rule out a mechanical cause and/or peripancreatic collection. Management typically includes nasogastric decompression and the use of prokinetic agents such as metoclopramide or azithromycin. Severe or prolonged DGE may necessitate long-term enteric decompression and institution of total parenteral nutrition.

Bleeding & Visceral Artery Pseudoaneurysm

Bleeding is a relatively common complication of PD. The majority of bleeding can be managed by withholding prophylactic anticoagulation and transfusion as needed. If a reoperation is required, an active source of bleeding is seldom found.[12] A unique complication of PD that requires extreme vigilance and prompt diagnosis and treatment to prevent mortality is a pseudoaneurysm of the GDA. The pseudoaneurysm is typically formed in the setting of a pancreatic leak where the ligated stump of the GDA is exposed to the digestive action of pancreatic enzymes. Patients may present with a herald or sentinel bleed; however, a significant portion of patients will present with hemorrhagic shock. Management of a ruptured pseudoaneurysm involves urgent, visceral angiography with embolization. A preexisting agreement with interventional radiology to treat this condition as an absolute emergency avoids additional diagnostic procedures and potentially lethal delays in these situations. In rare cases where an operation is required, the mortality rate is exceedingly high.

Conclusion

Pancreaticoduodenectomy, despite its morbidity, continues to be the gold standard in the management of pancreatic neoplasms. Refinements in surgical technique, patient selection, postoperative and anesthesia care, and management of complications have greatly improved operative outcomes. In addition, advances in systemic therapy have shifted the paradigm of care, and further research in these areas is likely to yield even more significant benefits in the coming years.

ColumbiaDoctors
Department of Surgery

The Pancreas Center

Whipple Procedure Enhanced Recoverhy Pathway

	Day Before Surgery	Day of Surgery in the OR	Recovery Room/POD-0
Diet	Regular diet as tolerated plus *Impact advanced recovery* × 3	NPO	NG tube to low wall suction
Labs		Confirm active T&S	CBC, BMP
Actions	(Outpatient team: click ERAS in case request order)	Order blood on hold Review imaging and operative plan with attending	Drain(s) to gravity
Medications/Orders			
Neuro/Pain	Gabapentin 300 mg at noon and 8 pm	Methadone 0.2 mg/kg IV up to a max of 20 mg Toradol 30 mg IV post-op Toradol 15 mg IV post-op if age >75 or GFR <50	Dilaudid PCA Standing rectal Tylenol 650 mg q6h Continue standing Toradol 30 mg IV q6h, or 15 mg q8h if age >75 or GFR <50
Cardiac	Stop ACE-inhibitors* Stop ARBs**		Home medications or equivalents as needed
Heme	If on Lovenox: take AM dose day before surgery, hold PM dose day before surgery, hold AM dose day of surgery	Pre-op SQ Heparin 5000u	
GI		Dexamethasone 6 mg IV	IV PPI PRN Zofran
ID		Pre-op Zosyn 4.5 mg IV within 1 h of incision Pre-op Levaquin 500 mg IV/Flagyl 500 mg IV if TRUE PCN allergy	Zosyn 4.5 g IV q8h × 3 doses Flagyl 500 mg IV q8 × 3 if TRUE PCN allergy

	POD-1	POD-2	POD-3	POD-4	POD-5 Discharge Criteria	Post-Discharge
Diet	Clear liquid diet	Continue clears	*Modified fiber/GI diet (in Epic)* unless nauseated or distended	Continue *Modified fiber/GI diet*	Eating 40% normal volume	E-mail communication between floor PA and outpatient PA/NP Phone call from outpatient PA/NP next business day Post-op visit following week VNS if drain still in place
Labs	CBC, BMP, Mg, LFTs Don't order Phos or Coags	• CBC; LFTs if venous recon. • Drain amylase unless fluid bilious or turbid	Labs only if specific concern	• Labs only if specific concern • Repeat drain amylase if drain still present	CBC	
Actions	• If NG <250cc, pull; if 250-500cc, pull and start Reglan 10 mg IV q8h, or Azithromycin 500 mg IV q24h if age >75; if NG output >500cc, discuss with attending • Remove Foley	• PT consult • Social work for dispo planning • Drain removal if: clear or serosanguineous & <200cc & drain amylase <411 U/L • Start home medications	• Check with insurance company for coverage of NOACs for DVT prophylaxis • Resume pancreatic enzymes if taking pre-operatively	• If considering discharge POD5 • Discuss drain removal		
Counseling	Encourage out of bed Encourage ambulation	Ambulation × 4	Continue ambulation Stair practice	Lovenox teaching if not cleared for oral DVT prophylaxis	Ambulating comfortably Flatus +/– BM, no major distension No wound issues	
Medications/Orders						
Neuro/Pain	• Start Gabapentin 300 mg q8h • Switch to PO Tylenol 650 mg q6h • Continue Toradol	• Stop PCA • Continue Gabapentin, Tylenol, Toradol • Add Tramadol 50 mg PO q6h PRN breakthrough pain	Continue standing Gabapentin, Tylenol, Toradol Continue PRN Tramadol	• Continue standing Gabapentin, Tylenol, PRN Tramadol • STOP Toradol • Start Naproxen 500 mg q12h, unless age >75 or GFR <50	Continue standing Gabapentin, Tylenol, Naproxen (unless age >75, GFR <50) Continue PRN Tramadol	**Discharge Medications:** Tylenol 650 mg q6h × 7d Naproxen 500 mg q12h × 7d unless age >75, GFR <50 Tramadol 50 mg q6h PRN × 4d – call for refill if needed PO PPI × 30d PRN Zofran Reglan if started in hospital For a total of 28 days if cancer: Pradaxa 220 mg qD OR Eliquis 2.5 mg BID OR Lovenox 40 mg SQ qD Unless GFR < 30, then discuss prophylaxis with attending
Heme	Start Lovenox 40 mg q24h Start Heparin 5000u SQ q8h if age > 75, GFR <30	Continue Lovenox or Heparin	Continue lovenox or Heparin	Continue Lovenox or Heparin	Continue Lovenox or Heparin	
GI	Switch to PO PPI Continue PRN Zofran	Continue PO PPI Continue PRN IV Zofran Continue Reglan or Azithromycin if started	Continue PO PPI Switch to PO Zofran PRN Swith to PO Reglan or PO Azithromycin if started	Continue PO PPI Continue PRN Zofran Continue Reglan or Azithromycin if started	Continue PO PPI Continue PRN Zofran Continue Reglan or Azithromycin if started	

▲ **Figure 58–6.** Enhanced recovery pathway used at our institution. (Reproduced with permission from the Department of Surgery, Columbia University Irving Medical Center.)

REFERENCES

1. Are C, Dhir M, Ravipati L. History of pancreaticoduodenectomy: early misconceptions, initial milestones and the pioneers. *HPB*. 2011;13(6):377-384.
2. Rebelo A, Michalski CW, Ukkat J, Kleeff J. Pancreatic cancer surgery with vascular resection: current concepts and perspectives. *J Pancreatol*. 2019;2(1):1-5.
3. Zhang Q, Wu J, Tian Y, et al. Arterial resection and reconstruction in pancreatectomy: surgical technique and outcomes. *BMC Surg*. 2019;19(1):141.
4. Cloyd JM, Heh V, Pawlik TM, et al. Neoadjuvant therapy for resectable and borderline resectable pancreatic cancer: a meta-analysis of randomized controlled trials. *J Clin Med*. 2020;9(4):1129.
5. Versteijne E, Vogel JA, Besselink MG, et al. Meta-analysis comparing upfront surgery with neoadjuvant treatment in patients with resectable or borderline resectable pancreatic cancer. *Br J Surg*. 2018;105(8):946-958.
6. Mavros MN, Moris D, Karanicolas PJ, Katz MHG, O'Reilly EM, Pawlik TM. Clinical trials of systemic chemotherapy for resectable pancreatic cancer: a review. *JAMA Surg*. 2021; 156(7):663-672.
7. Pavel M, Öberg K, Falconi M, et al. Gastroenteropancreatic neuroendocrine neoplasms: ESMO Clinical Practice Guidelines for diagnosis, treatment and follow-up. *Ann Oncol*. 2020; 31(7):844-860.
8. Isaji S, Mizuno S, Windsor JA, et al. International consensus on definition and criteria of borderline resectable pancreatic ductal adenocarcinoma 2017. *Pancreatology*. 2018;18(1):2-11.
9. Bassi C, Marchegiani G, Dervenis C, et al. The 2016 update of the International Study Group (ISGPS) definition and grading of postoperative pancreatic fistula: 11 years after. *Surgery*. 2017;161(3):584-591.
10. Wente MN, Bassi C, Dervenis C, et al. Delayed gastric emptying (DGE) after pancreatic surgery: a suggested definition by the International Study Group of Pancreatic Surgery (ISGPS). *Surgery*. 2007;142(5):761-768.
11. Wente MN, Veit JA, Bassi C, et al. Postpancreatectomy hemorrhage (PPH): an International Study Group of Pancreatic Surgery (ISGPS) definition. *Surgery*. 2007;142(1):20-25.
12. Brodie B, Kocher HM. Systematic review of the incidence, presentation and management of gastroduodenal artery pseudoaneurysm after pancreatic resection. *BJS Open*. 2019; 3(6):735-742.

Neuroendocrine Tumors of the Thymus

59

Polina V. Zmijewski, MD, MA
Peter J. Mazzaglia, MD, FACS

GENERAL CONSIDERATIONS

First described in 1972 by Rosai and Higa,[1,2] primary neuroendocrine tumors of the thymus (NETTs) are an extremely rare as well as aggressive tumor type with an incidence in the United States of 0.18/1,000,000 persons. NETTs are biologically aggressive, demonstrating an approximately 80% rate of malignancy.[3] They are a tumor of thymic origin most commonly arising in the anterior mediastinal space.[4] The tumors are most commonly found in male patients with the highest incidence between 40 and 60 years of age.[2,5]

Surgical management remains the gold standard for treatment of these complex tumors, with chemoradiotherapy utilized in cases of incomplete resection or invasive, high-grade disease. Even when completely resected, NETTs have a poor prognosis, due to the highly aggressive nature of the disease. Outcomes can be optimized with appropriate staging, meticulous surgical resection, and management of concomitant associated endocrinopathies.[2]

PREVENTION

NETTs are generally sporadic, and no modifiable risk factors have been identified in the literature. Approximately 5% to 10% of patients with diagnosed NETT will also have multiple endocrine neoplasia type I syndrome (MEN1). Interestingly, male patients with NETTs are significantly more likely to have MEN1 than female patients (10:1).[6] NETTs are a major cause of death in MEN1 patients, so much so that some authors recommend a concomitant thymectomy in MEN1 patients undergoing parathyroidectomy as a preventative measure.[2,7-10]

CLINICAL FINDINGS

Symptoms & Signs

Approximately 30% of patients are asymptomatic on presentation and are diagnosed through a chest imaging performed for other reasons. The remaining patients are diagnosed while investigating the source of symptoms related to mass effect, distant metastatic disease, or aberrant hormonal secretion.[2,10]

Chest compressive symptoms associated with NETTs can include cough, pain, dyspnea, or, in severe cases, superior vena cava syndrome.[10] Hoarseness due to involvement of the recurrent laryngeal nerve or elevation of the hemidiaphragm due to phrenic nerve invasion are uncommon presenting signs.[2]

Approximately half of NETTs are functional and secrete active hormones resulting in symptomatic endocrinopathies.[10] These most commonly include Cushing syndrome, acromegaly, and hypertrophic osteoarthropathy. Classic carcinoid syndrome, with characteristic flushing, diarrhea, valvular heart disease, and wheezing, though very uncommon, can be experienced by patients with thymic carcinoids.[6]

Laboratory Findings

Chromogranin A is the most sensitive laboratory marker for the detection of neuroendocrine tumors (NETs), with elevation in 60% to 100% of patients with both functional and nonfunctional NETs.[6,11-14] Urinary 5-hydroxyindoleacetic acid, though useful in diagnosing NETs of the GI tract, is rarely elevated in thoracic NETs. Other tumor markers that can be found immunohistochemically include synaptophysin, CD56, and neuron-specific amylase.[6,15]

Imaging Studies

Diagnostic imaging workup generally includes a chest X-ray (CXR) and a chest CT scan. The characteristic appearance of a NETT on anteroposterior and lateral CXR can be seen in Figure 59–1. On a chest CT, NETTs often appear as an anterior mediastinal mass with associated hemorrhage or necrosis. A NETT on chest CT scan is shown in Figure 59–2.

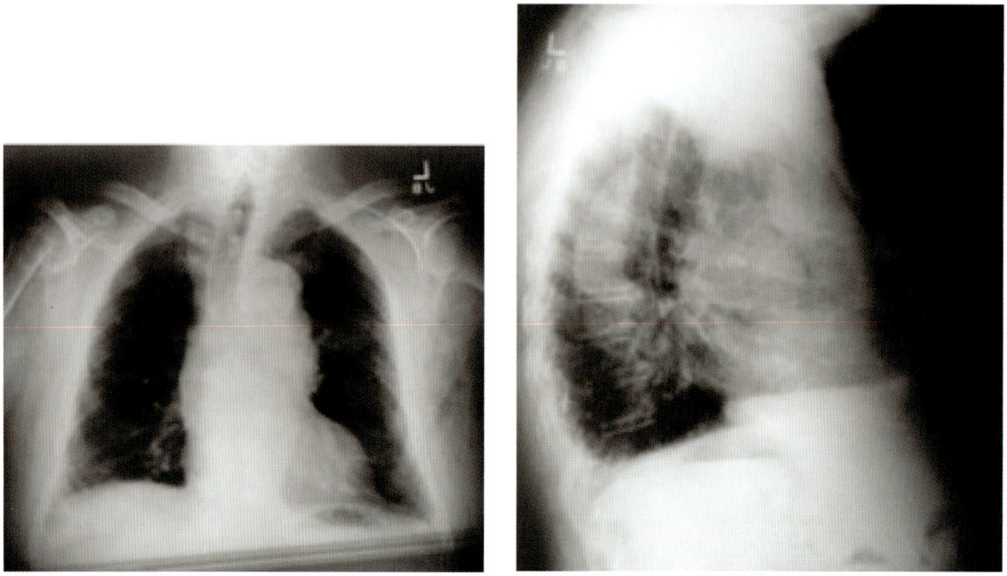

A B

▲ **Figure 59–1.** Patient with large primary NETT on chest radiograph with mass effect on trachea. **(A)** Anteroposterior view. **(B)** Lateral view. (Reproduced with permission from Chaer R, Massad MG, Evans A, et al. Primary neuroendocrine tumors of the thymus. *Ann Thorac Surg*. 2002;74(5):1733-1740.[10])

111- Indium-diethylenetriamine pentacetic acid-D-phenylalanine-octreotide (Octreoscan) scintigraphy can be helpful, as the tumors can express somatostatin receptors. FDG-PET can be a useful adjunct, especially in highly proliferative tumors. MRI is used to rule in or rule out invasion into neighboring structures and for operative planning.[2]

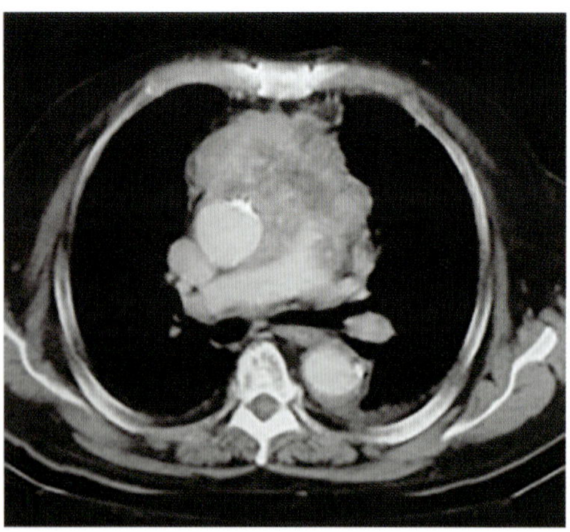

▲ **Figure 59–2.** CT scan of chest demonstrating a large anterior mediastinal NETT with para-aortic lymphadenopathy. (Reproduced with permission from Chaer R, Massad MG, Evans A, et al. Primary neuroendocrine tumors of the thymus. *Ann Thorac Surg*. 2002;74(5):1733-1740.[10])

DIFFERENTIAL DIAGNOSIS

Table 59–1 provides a list of thymic masses that can be mistaken for NETTs. These masses include a broad spectrum of benign and malignant disease. Because these masses can be

Table 59–1. The differential diagnosis of thymic neuroendocrine tumors.

Congenital or acquired thymic cyst
True thymic hyperplasia
Thymic (follicular) lymphoid hyperplasia
Thymolipoma
Thymic Hodgkin disease (granulomatous thymoma)
Thymic non-Hodgkin lymphoma
Thymic carcinoma
Thymic neuroendocrine carcinoma (cylindromatous thymoma)
Seminomatous thymoma
Nonseminomatous germ cell tumor
Teratoma

Source: Reproduced with permission from Chaer R, Massad MG, Evans A, et al. Primary neuroendocrine tumors of the thymus. *Ann Thorac Surg*. 2002;74(5):1733-40.[10]

very hard to differentiate based on radiographic characteristics, tissue confirmation is required.

If the diagnosis of NETT is suspected based on imaging, histologic confirmation is recommended prior to resection via a core needle biopsy or a parasternal mediastinotomy.[2]

OPERATIVE MANAGEMENT

Surgical resection remains the treatment of choice for patients with a confirmed diagnosis of NETT. Approximately 28% to 100% (mean 86%) of diagnosed tumors are deemed resectable on diagnosis with invasion into the heart, great vessels, aorta, phrenic nerves, or trachea prohibiting complete resection. There is no role for surgical debulking of this tumor.[1]

A median sternotomy is the most common surgical approach, though thoracotomy is also often utilized. Mediastinal lymphadenectomy is always performed to allow for staging of the disease, so there is no role for tumor removal via a cervical thymectomy.[6] A complete thymectomy with resection of all fatty tissue to the level of the phrenic nerves is typical.[16] A gross pathologic specimen postresection can be seen in Figure 59–3. All resection attempts should be performed at an experienced center with access to multidisciplinary care, and with the help of a trained thoracic surgeon.

ADJUVANT THERAPIES

Very limited data exist in the literature studying the effectiveness of adjuvant therapies in the treatment of this rare malignancy. As previously stated, complete surgical resection remains the mainstay of treatment,[6,17,18] and surgical resection alone can be sufficient for tumors of the less aggressive, well-differentiated type.[6]

Chemotherapy and radiation are administered based on stage and grade of NETT. A treatment algorithm is included in Figure 59–4. Both the staging and the grading of NETTs are controversial, with no consensus definition.

Staging is most commonly performed via the Masaoka-Koga system[6,19-21] (Table 59–2) though other classification systems have been proposed,[22] including a TNM classification system (Table 59–3).[23]

The most widely used grading system was developed in 2015 by the World Health Organization (WHO) (Table 59–4). The WHO classification categorized NETTs as a type of thymic carcinoma with well-differentiated/low-grade (typical and atypical carcinoids) and poorly differentiated/high-grade (small and large cell) phenotypes. Grade is determined by presence of necrosis and mitoses per high power field.[2,6,24,25] A recent study by Dinter et al. used whole genome sequencing and immunohistochemical studies to create a three-tiered morpho molecular grading classification system for improved prognostication.[26]

Various chemotherapeutic agents, used as single agents or in combination with others have been attempted but have not shown significant improvement in survival. Likewise, radiation therapy has not been shown to improve survival in NETT patients.[5,21,27,28]

Despite lack of proven survival benefit, for NETTs that are high stage, or of the "poorly differentiated" or "high-grade" subtype, platinum-based chemotherapy agents can be used to attempt to optimize outcome, especially in patients with metastatic or unresectable disease. Other agents described in the literature include streptozocin, carmustine, VP-16, 5-flurouracil, and everolimus.[10,17,18,29-35] Chemotherapy can be given in an adjuvant fashion or as an induction therapy to allow for surgical resection. In addition, it can be useful as a form of palliation, though the effectiveness of chemotherapy in all settings is poorly studied.[35] Lastly, polypeptide receptor radionuclide therapy has been used in the systemic treatment of metastatic disease in patients who are not operative candidates or have unresectable tumors.[2]

NETTs can very rarely present with carcinoid syndrome. Somatostatin analogs can be useful inhibitors of secreted bioactive compounds. Acromegaly is a rare endocrinopathy that can result from growth-hormone secreting NETTs, and can also be managed medically with somatostatin.[6] NETTs can present with Cushing syndrome, due to cortisol secretion from the tumor. The symptoms of Cushing syndrome in the context of NETT are most often treated medically, with ketoconazole, aminoglutethimide, etomidate, mitotane, mifepristone, or metyrapone. Lastly, interferon α 2a and 2b can also be administered to degrade secreted hormones.[6]

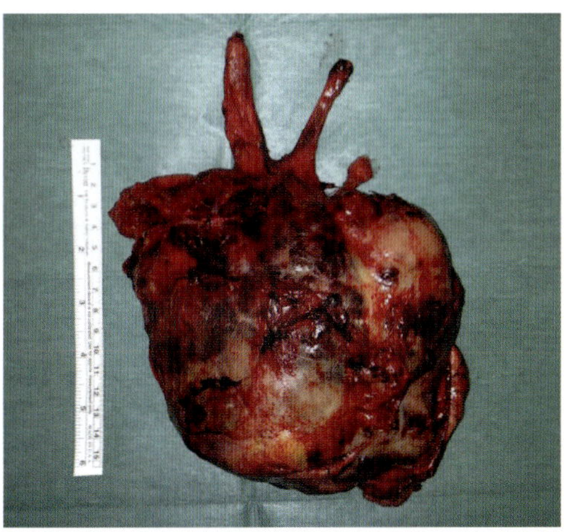

▲ **Figure 59–3.** 15 cm NETT. (Reproduced with permission from Filosso PL, Ruffini E, Solidoro P, et al. Neuroendocrine tumors of the thymus. *J Thorac Dis.* 2017;9(Suppl 15): S1484-S1490.[2])

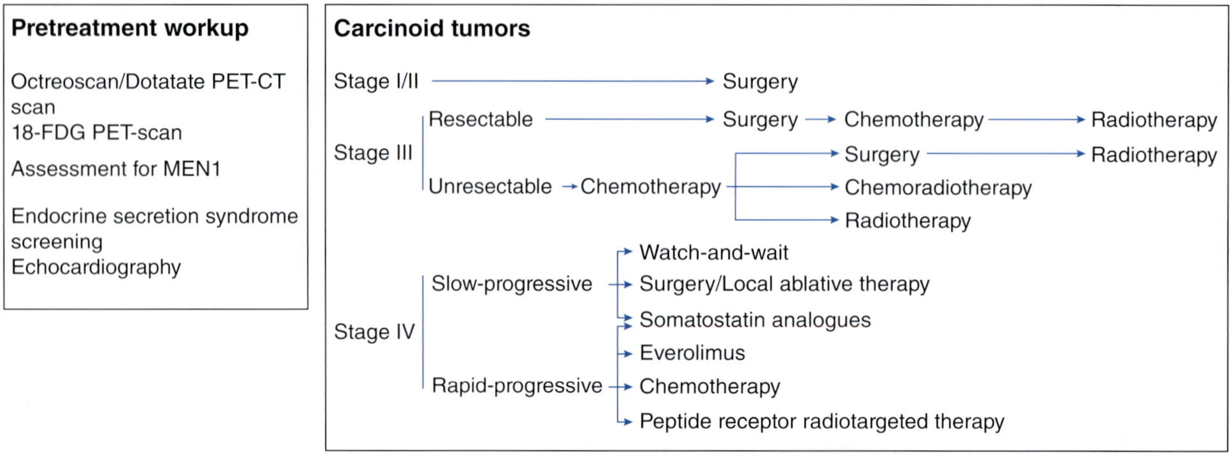

Figure 59–4. Diagnostic workup and treatment by stage of NETT. (Reproduced with permission from Girard N. Neuroendocrine tumors of the thymus: the oncologist point of view. *J Thorac Dis.* 2017;9(15):S1491-S1500.[35])

MANAGEMENT OF ADVANCED DISEASE

Metastatic spread is present in approximately 20% of neuroendocrine thymic carcinoids and up to 80% of small-cell NETTs. For highly aggressive, poorly differentiated NETTs (small-cell and large-cell types), treatment regimens with cisplatin, anthracycline, and etoposide are often administered. Carboplatin and paclitaxel have also been proposed as a regimen, but both regimens are poorly studied and have unclear effects on patient outcome. For metastatic carcinoid NETTs, varied treatment approaches are utilized, ranging from "watch-and-wait," surgery, local ablative approaches, and somatostatin analogues. Everolimus is used in cases of failure of treatment in typical and atypical carcinoids and has shown some success in studies including gastrointestinal and pancreatic NETs. Antiangiogenics, such as sunitinib have also been described as an option in patients with advanced disease.[35]

Table 59–2. The combined Masaoka[19]-Koga[20] classification system.

Stage	Definition
I	Grossly and microscopically completely encapsulated tumor
IIa	Microscopic transcapsular invasion
IIb	Macroscopic invasion into thymic or surrounding fatty tissue or grossly adherent to but not breaking through mediastinal pleura or pericardium
III	Macroscopic invasion into neighboring organ (ie, pericardium, great vessel, or lung)
IVa	Pleural or pericardial metastasis
IVb	Lymphogenous or hematogenous metastasis

Source: Reproduced with permission from Huang J, Detterbeck FC, Wang Z, et al. [Standard outcome measures for thymic malignancies]. *Zhongguo Fei Ai Za Zhi.* 2014;17(2):122-129.[39]

Table 59–3. TNM classification of thymic neuroendocrine tumors.

Classification	Description
Tumor Extension	
T1	Completely encapsulated, no microscopic invasion
T2	Extracapsular invasion into surrounding fatty tissue or mediastinal pleura
T3	Invasion into neighboring organs such as pericardium, great vessels, lung
T4	Pleural or pericardial dissemination
Nodal Involvement	
N0	No lymph node metastasis
N1	Metastasis to anterior mediastinal lymph nodes
N2	Metastasis to intrathoracic lymph nodes outside the anterior mediastinum
N3	Metastasis to extrathoracic lymph nodes
Distant Metastasis	
M0	No hematogenous metastasis
M1	Hematogenous spread to other organs

Source: Reproduced with permission from Yamakawa Y, Masaoka A, Hashimoto T, et al. A tentative tumor-node-metastasis classification of thymoma. *Cancer.* 1991;68(9):1984-1987.[23]

Table 59–4. The World Health Organization 2015 classification of NETTs.

Differentiation	Nomenclature	Grade	Histopathology
Well differentiated (Carcinoid)	Typical carcinoid	Low	No necrosis, <2 mitosis per 2 mm^2 (10 HPF)
	Atypical carcinoid	Intermediate	Necrosis present and/or 2-10 mitoses per 2 mm^2 (10 HPF)
Poorly differentiated (Neuroendocrine carcinoma)	Large cell	High	Nonsmall cell neuroendocrine carcinoma with >10 mitoses per 2 mm^2 (10 HPF)
	Small cell	High	Small-cell cytology

Source: Adapted from Marx A, Chan JK, Coindre JM, et al. The 2015 World Health Organization classification of tumors of the thymus: continuity and changes. *J Thorac Oncol.* 2015;10(10):1383-1395[24] and Corsini EM, Mitchell KG, Sceusi EL, et al. Multidisciplinary treatment of thymic neuroendocrine tumors: surgery remains a key component. *J Thorac Dis.* 2019;11(8):3391-3398.[40]

PROGNOSIS

Though related to NETs of the gastrointestinal tract and lung, NETTs have significantly more aggressive biologic behavior. Neoplasms of this nature found in the mediastinum are malignant in more than 80% of patients.[2,3]

Lymph node metastasis is present in approximately 28% of thymic carcinoid patients and positive lymph nodes are associated with poor patient outcomes.[16,36] Lymph node dissection, though helpful in establishing prognosis of patients and assisting in multidisciplinary treatment planning, has not been shown to improve survival.[34]

In a surveillance, epidemiology, and end results (SEER) database study in 2017 performed by Sullivan et al., 254 patients with diagnosed NETTs were identified and outcomes were retrospectively analyzed. They found a median overall survival time of 73 months and a 5-year survival rate of 56%. In their analysis, Masaoka-Koga stage, surgical resection, and size of tumor were the most significant predictors of survival. Surgery was a significant predictor of survival, with patients who underwent resection having 109 months of survival versus 38 months in the nonoperative group ($p = 0.003$).[21]

In an earlier, smaller, 2010 study of 160 patients by Gaur and colleagues, also querying the SEER database, they found that tumors >5 cm portended a higher rate of regional and distant spread.[5] Masaoka-Koga stage was predictive of a poor prognosis, which has been supported in multiple other studies.[21,28,37,38]

The significance of grade in prognosis is controversial, with studies by Sullivan et al.[21] as well as Filosso and colleagues[28] stating high grade is not associated with poor prognostic outcome, while the Gaur[5] study does identify a correlation.

The most recent study using the SEER database, published in 2020 by Tang et al., looked at 254 patients carrying a NETT diagnosis and attempted to design a prognostic nomogram. In their analysis, low-grade (well differentiated) histologic subtype, early stage, and tumors treated with surgery alone (nonchemotherapy) were associated with improved survival.[25]

WHEN TO REFER/ADMIT

Patients with suspected NETT should be referred routinely to a multidisciplinary setting at an experienced center due to the multimodal treatment often required to treat these complex and highly aggressive malignancies.[2,35]

REFERENCES

1. Rosai J, Higa E. Mediastinal endocrine neoplasm, of probable thymic origin, related to carcinoid tumor. Clinicopathologic study of 8 cases. *Cancer.* 1972;29(4):1061-1074.
2. Filosso PL, Ruffini E, Solidoro P, et al. Neuroendocrine tumors of the thymus. *J Thorac Dis.* 2017;9(Suppl 15):S1484-S1490.
3. Klemm KM, Moran CA. Primary neuroendocrine carcinomas of the thymus. *Semin Diagn Pathol.* 1999;16(1):32-41.
4. Dusmet ME, McKneally MF. Pulmonary and thymic carcinoid tumors. *World J Surg.* 1996;20(2):189-195.
5. Gaur P, Leary C, Yao JC. Thymic neuroendocrine tumors: a SEER database analysis of 160 patients. *Ann Surg.* 2010;251(6): 1117-1121.
6. Phan AT, Oberg K, Choi J, et al. NANETS consensus guideline for the diagnosis and management of neuroendocrine tumors: well-differentiated neuroendocrine tumors of the thorax (includes lung and thymus). *Pancreas.* 2010;39(6):784-798.
7. Teh BT. Thymic carcinoids in multiple endocrine neoplasia type 1. *J Intern Med.* 1998; 243(6):501-504.
8. Trump D, Farren B, Wooding C, et al. Clinical studies of multiple endocrine neoplasia type 1 (MEN1). *Qjm.* 1996;89(9):653-669.
9. Teh BT, Zedenius J, Kytölä S, et al. Thymic carcinoids in multiple endocrine neoplasia type 1. *Ann Surg.* 1998;228(1):99-105.
10. Chaer R, Massad MG, Evans A, et al. Primary neuroendocrine tumors of the thymus. *Ann Thorac Surg.* 2002;74(5):1733-1740.
11. Bajetta E, Ferrari L, Martinetti A, et al. Chromogranin A, neuron specific enolase, carcinoembryonic antigen, and hydroxyindole acetic acid evaluation in patients with neuroendocrine tumors. *Cancer.* 1999;86(5):858-865.
12. Goebel SU, Serrano J, Yu F, et al. Prospective study of the value of serum chromogranin A or serum gastrin levels in the assessment of the presence, extent, or growth of gastrinomas. *Cancer.* 1999;85(7):1470-1483.

13. Bernini GP, Moretti A, Ferdeghini M, et al. A new human chromogranin 'A' immunoradiometric assay for the diagnosis of neuroendocrine tumours. *Br J Cancer*. 2001;84(5):636-642.
14. Nehar D, Lombard-Bohas C, Olivieri S, et al. Interest of chromogranin A for diagnosis and follow-up of endocrine tumours. *Clin Endocrinol (Oxf)*. 2004;60(5):644-652.
15. Ruffini E, Oliaro A, Novero D, et al. Neuroendocrine tumors of the thymus. *Thorac Surg Clin*. 2011;21(1):13-23, v.
16. Cheufou DH, Valdivia D, Puhlvers S, et al. Lymph node involvement and the surgical treatment of thymic epithelial and neuroendocrine carcinoma. *Ann Thorac Surg*. 2019; 107(6): 1632-1638.
17. Fukai I, Masaoka A, Fujii Y, et al. Thymic neuroendocrine tumor (thymic carcinoid): a clinicopathologic study in 15 patients. *Ann Thorac Surg*. 1999;67(1):208-211.
18. de Montpréville VT, Macchiarini P, Dulmet E. Thymic neuroendocrine carcinoma (carcinoid): a clinicopathologic study of fourteen cases. *J Thorac Cardiovasc Surg*. 1996; 111(1):134-141.
19. Masaoka A, Monden Y, Nakahara K, et al. Follow-up study of thymomas with special reference to their clinical stages. *Cancer*. 1981;48(11):2485-2492.
20. Koga K, Matsuno Y, Noguchi M, et al. A review of 79 thymomas: modification of staging system and reappraisal of conventional division into invasive and non-invasive thymoma. *Pathol Int*. 1994;44(5):359-367.
21. Sullivan JL, Weksler B. Neuroendocrine tumors of the thymus: analysis of factors affecting survival in 254 patients. *Ann Thorac Surg*. 2017;103(3):935-939.
22. Gamondès JP, Balawi A, Greenland T, et al. Seventeen years of surgical treatment of thymoma: factors influencing survival. *Eur J Cardiothorac Surg*. 1991;5(3):124-131.
23. Yamakawa Y, Masaoka A, Hashimoto T, et al. A tentative tumor-node-metastasis classification of thymoma. *Cancer*. 1991;68(9):1984-1987.
24. Marx A, Chan JK, Coindre JM, et al. The 2015 World Health Organization classification of tumors of the thymus: continuity and changes. *J Thorac Oncol*. 2015;10(10):1383-1395.
25. Tang JY, Gao HJ, Shi GD, et al. Development and validation of a nomogram prognostic model for patients with neuroendocrine tumors of the thymus. *Thorac Cancer*. 2020;11(9): 2457-2464.
26. Dinter H, Bohnenberger H, Beck J, et al. Molecular classification of neuroendocrine tumors of the thymus. *J Thorac Oncol*. 2019;14(8):1472-1483.
27. Cardillo G, Rea F, Lucchi M, et al. Primary neuroendocrine tumors of the thymus: a multicenter experience of 35 patients. *Ann Thorac Surg*. 2012;94(1):241-245; discussion 245-6.
28. Filosso PL, Yao X, Ruffini E, et al. Comparison of outcomes between neuroendocrine thymic tumours and other subtypes of thymic carcinomas: a joint analysis of the European Society of Thoracic Surgeons and the International Thymic Malignancy Interest Group. *Eur J Cardiothorac Surg*. 2016;50(4): 766-771.
29. Moran CA, Suster S. Neuroendocrine carcinomas (carcinoid tumor) of the thymus. A clinicopathologic analysis of 80 cases. *Am J Clin Pathol*. 2000;114(1):100-110.
30. Wick MR, Carney JA, Bernatz PE, et al. Primary mediastinal carcinoid tumors. *Am J Surg Pathol*. 1982;6(3):195-205.
31. Gal AA, Kornstein MJ, Cohen C, et al. Neuroendocrine tumors of the thymus: a clinicopathological and prognostic study. *Ann Thorac Surg*. 2001;72(4):1179-1182.
32. Valli M, Fabris GA, Dewar A, et al. Atypical carcinoid tumour of the thymus: a study of eight cases. *Histopathology*. 1994;24(4):371-375.
33. Economopoulos GC, Lewis JW, Jr., Lee MW, et al. Carcinoid tumors of the thymus. *Ann Thorac Surg*. 1990;50(1):58-61.
34. Wang DY, Chang DB, Kuo SH, et al. Carcinoid tumours of the thymus. *Thorax*. 1994; 49(4):357-360.
35. Girard N. Neuroendocrine tumors of the thymus: the oncologist point of view. *J Thorac Dis*. 2017;9(Suppl 15):S1491-S1500.
36. Viti A, Bertolaccini L, Terzi A. What is the role of lymph nodal metastases and lymphadenectomy in the surgical treatment and prognosis of thymic carcinomas and carcinoids? *Interact Cardiovasc Thorac Surg*. 2014;19(6):1054-1058.
37. Cardillo G, Carleo F, Giunti R, et al. Predictors of survival in patients with locally advanced thymoma and thymic carcinoma (Masaoka stages III and IVa). *Eur J Cardiothorac Surg*. 2010;37(4):819-823.
38. Ahmad U, Yao X, Detterbeck F, et al. Thymic carcinoma outcomes and prognosis: results of an international analysis. *J Thorac Cardiovasc Surg*. 2015;149(1):95-100, 101.e1-2.
39. Huang J, Detterbeck FC, Wang Z, et al. [Standard outcome measures for thymic malignancies]. *Zhongguo Fei Ai Za Zhi*. 2014;17(2):122-129.
40. Corsini EM, Mitchell KG, Sceusi EL, et al. Multidisciplinary treatment of thymic neuroendocrine tumors: surgery remains a key component. *J Thorac Dis*. 2019; 11(8):3391-3398.

60 Neuroendocrine Tumors of the Stomach

Stephanie Davis, MD
Robert McIntyre, Jr., MD

INTRODUCTION

Gastric neuroendocrine tumors (NETs) are neoplasms that arise from enterochromaffin-like cells in the gastric mucosa. They are categorized into three subtypes (types I, II, and III) based on pathophysiology and behavior. They are most often sporadic but also may occur as part of multiple endocrine neoplasia Type I syndrome (MEN I). Diagnosis consists primarily of endoscopy with biopsies, as well as measurement of fasting serum gastrin and gastric pH levels. Treatment depends on the tumor subtype. Generally, endoscopic resection can manage small lesions, and larger lesions or those with high-risk features require surgical resection.

The overall prognosis is good for type I and II lesions, whereas type III lesions, given the high rate of metastatic disease at presentation, have a similar prognosis to gastric adenocarcinoma.

EPIDEMIOLOGY

Gastric NETs are rare lesions that comprise around 1.8% of all gastric neoplasms and around 8% of all gastrointestinal NETs. The incidence of gastric NETs has increased more than 10-fold over the last 30 years. This is likely attributable to the more widespread use of cross-sectional imaging and endoscopy.

A study from 2015 using data from worldwide cancer registries estimated the prevalence to be per 10,000 in the United States, 0.32 per 10,000 in Europe, and 0.05 per 10,000 in Japan. Gastric NETs are more common in women.

CLINICAL PATHOPHYSIOLOGY

Gastric NETs are neoplasms that arise from enterochromaffin-like cells in the gastric mucosa. They are categorized into three subtypes (types I, II, and III) based on pathophysiology and behavior.

Type I

Type I gastric NETs are the most common type (Table 60–1). They comprise 70% to 80% of all gastric NETs. They tend to be small (<1 cm) and multiple, located in the gastric fundus or body. They are associated with hypergastrinemia secondary to autoimmune chronic atrophic gastritis. The destruction of parietal cells seen in chronic atrophic gastritis leads to achlorhydria, which in turn causes hypergastrinemia (a physiologic hypergastrinemia). The high gastrin stimulation of the gastric mucosa generates hypertrophy and hyperplasia of the enterochromaffin-like cells. Histologic analysis commonly shows atrophic underlying mucosa. Gastric pH levels will be elevated secondary to the achlorhydria. Proton pump inhibitor (PPI) use is also characterized by hypergastrinemia secondary to achlorhydria and may increase the incidence of gastric NETs, but the data are inconclusive. These tumors are often associated with pernicious anemia due to the presence of anti-parietal cells or anti-intrinsic factor antibodies, which leads to decreased vitamin B12 absorption, resulting in megaloblastic anemia. Type I tumors are typically indolent in nature.

Type II

Type II tumors are the least common and comprise 5% to 10% of all gastric NETs (Table 60–1). They tend to be small (<1 cm) and multiple, located primarily in the gastric fundus or body. Like type I tumors, they are associated with hypergastrinemia, but the hypergastrinemia occurs in the setting of a gastrinoma or other nonphysiologic means of elevated gastrin secretion. Gastric NETs occur more commonly in patients with MEN I and Zollinger-Ellison syndrome (ZES) than in patients with sporadic gastrinomas. The high gastrin stimulation of the gastric mucosa generates hypertrophy and hyperplasia of the enterochromaffin-like cells. These NETs are characteristically associated with hyperchlorhydria and, thus, low gastric pH. Histologic analysis commonly shows hypertrophic underlying mucosa. Type II tumors are typically indolent in nature but more aggressive than type I tumors, with a higher incidence of lymph node metastases (up to 30%).

Type III

Type III tumors comprise 10% to 15% of all gastric NETs (Table 60–1). They are typically sporadic and not associated with underlying gastric conditions or hypergastrinemia. They tend to be characterized by larger (>2 cm) solitary lesions located most commonly in the gastric fundus or body. They are associated with normal gastric pH levels. Histologic analysis shows normal surrounding mucosa. Type III tumors are the most aggressive subtype and behave similarly to gastric adenocarcinoma. They are associated with metastatic disease in over 50% of cases. The liver is the most common site of metastatic disease.

CLINICAL PRESENTATION

Gastric NETs are commonly asymptomatic and diagnosed incidentally. Patients may present with symptoms such as abdominal pain, upper gastrointestinal tract bleeding, or anemia, which might prompt further workup and diagnosis of a gastric NET.

Patients with type II tumors may present with peptic ulcer disease in addition to abdominal pain and diarrhea (ZES). Furthermore, they may present with other sequelae of MEN I syndrome, such as pituitary tumors or primary hyperparathyroidism.

Patients with type III tumors may present with carcinoid syndrome if there is metastatic disease to the liver. The carcinoid syndrome is characterized by intermittent flushing, diarrhea, wheezing (from bronchoconstriction), and rarely right-sided heart failure (from valvular fibrosis of right-sided heart valves). This occurs due to the secretion of vasoactive substances (such as serotonin, histamine, and kallikrein) into the systemic circulation.

DIAGNOSIS, LABORATORY, & IMAGING STUDIES

Diagnosis is made with upper endoscopy and biopsies. Biopsies should be taken of the lesion(s), the surrounding mucosa, and the antrum.

Gastric NETs typically appear as submucosal lesions on endoscopy (Figures 60–1A, 60–1B). Endoscopic ultrasound (EUS) is recommended for larger lesions (>1 cm) and for all type III lesions to identify depth of tumor invasion and possible lymph node involvement (Figure 60–2). Fasting gastrin levels should always be measured (PPIs should be discontinued for >1 week if the patient can tolerate it, as PPIs can elevate gastrin levels), and the gastric pH level should also be measured. These tests aid in identifying the subtype of gastric NET (types I, II, or III).

Table 60–1. Gastric neuroendocrine tumor subtypes.

	Type I	Type II	Type III
Prevalence (%)	70-80	5-10	15-20
Association	Chronic atrophic gastritis	Gastrinoma (MEN I syndrome)	Normal mucosa
Size	Small (1-2 cm)	Small (1-2 cm)	Large (>2 cm)
Number	Multiple	Multiple	Single
Mucosa	Atrophic	Hypertrophic	Normal
Histopathology	ECL hyperplasia	ECL hyperplasia	Mucosa normal
Serum gastrin levels	Elevated	Elevated	Poor
Gastric pH	High	Low	
Prognosis	Excellent	Very good	

For patients with type I tumors, vitamin B12 levels should be checked, given the association with pernicious anemia. Cross-sectional imaging is not commonly recommended. Patients with type II tumors should have cross-sectional imaging (abdominal multiphasic CT or MRI) (Figure 60–3), somatostatin receptor scintigraphy (SRS), and/or ^{68}Ga-DOTATATE PET/CT or PET/MR imaging to localize the gastrinoma and detect lymph node metastasis. They should also be worked up for MEN I syndrome, if not already done. They should be screened for primary hyperparathyroidism (serum calcium and parathyroid hormone), pituitary tumors (prolactin, insulin-like growth factor-1), and other enteropancreatic NETs (glucose, insulin, proinsulin, glucagon, chromogranin A, pancreatic polypeptide). Genetic testing should be considered to evaluate for germline mutations in the MEN I gene. Patients with type III tumors should have EUS, multiphasic abdominal imaging, and ^{68}Ga-DOTATATE PET/CT or PET/MR imaging.

NETs are classified by stage and grade. The American Joint Committee on Cancer uses tumor, node, and metastasis (TNM) staging to classify the anatomic extent of disease to help guide management and predict prognosis. The World Health Organization (WHO) classification system of gastroenteropancreatic NETs was originally developed in 2010 and revised in 2017 (Table 60–2). This classification system categorizes tumors based on grade (mitotic rate and Ki-67 index) and differentiation status. The grade is a better predictor of outcomes.

MANAGEMENT

Management depends on the tumor subtype, size and/or depth of invasion, and presence of any metastatic disease (lymph nodes and/or distant sites). Guidelines from the

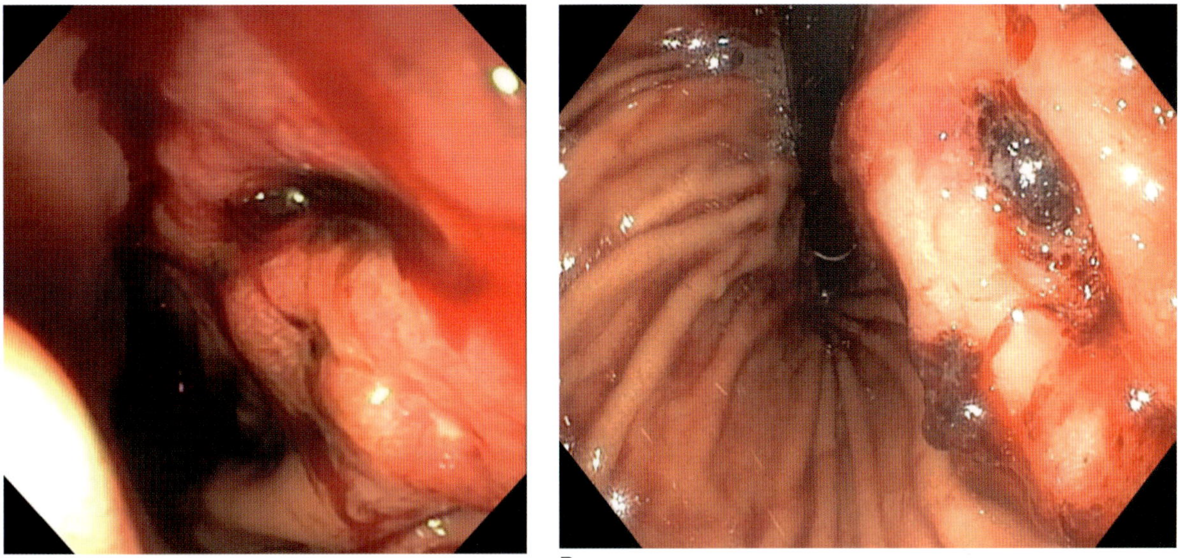

▲ **Figure 60–1.** **(A)** A 43-year-old female with MEN 1 presented with upper gastrointestinal tract bleeding: Upper endoscopy showing a submucosal gastric NET. **(B)** A 43-year-old female with MEN 1 presented with upper gastrointestinal tract bleeding: Upper endoscopy (retroflexed view) showing a submucosal gastric NET.

National Comprehensive Cancer Network (NCCN), the North American Neuroendocrine Tumor Society (NANETS), and the European Neuroendocrine Tumor Society (ENETS) vary slightly and utilize tumor type and grade in the management recommendations.

Type I

Type I gastric NETs should undergo endoscopic mucosal resection (EMR) of lesions that are >1 cm. Lesions smaller than this can undergo observation with endoscopic surveillance every 1 to 3 years. Recurrence of type I lesions is common because hypergastrinemia and the underlying enterochromaffin-like cell changes persist.

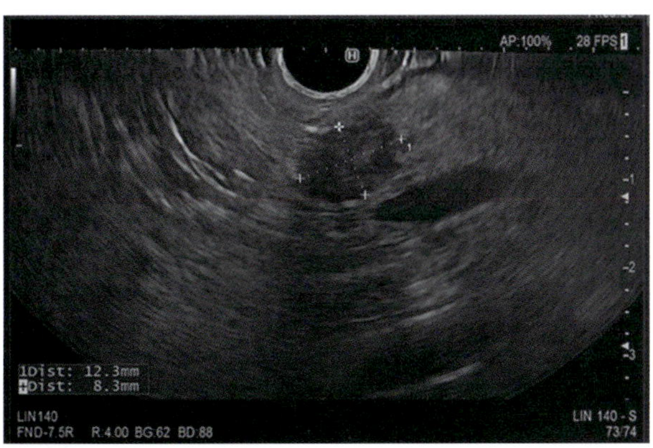

▲ **Figure 60–2.** Endoscopic ultrasound (EUS) showing a hypoechoic lesion in the gastric submucosa.

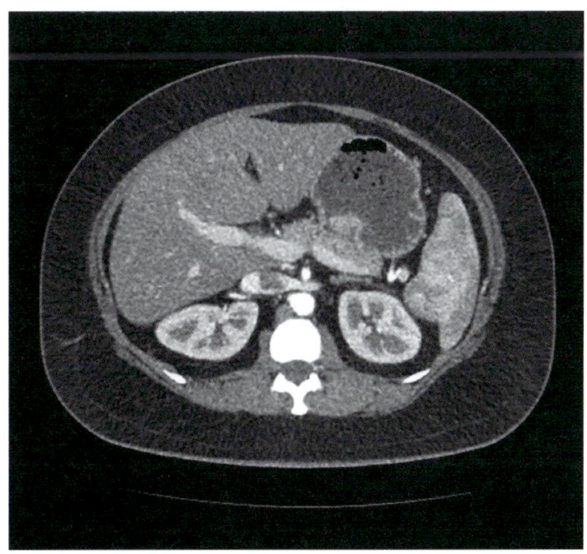

▲ **Figure 60–3.** CT axial imaging showing a mass arising in the gastric wall. Additionally, a pancreatic NET was seen in the pancreatic body.

Table 60–2. 2017 WHO classification of gastroenteropancreatic neuroendocrine tumors.

Type	Grade	Mitotic Rate	Ki-67 Index (%)	Differentiation
NET				
G1	Low	<2	<3	Well differentiated
G2	Intermediate	2-20	3-20	Well differentiated
G3	High	>20	>20	Well differentiated
NEC				
SCNEC	High	>20	>20	Poorly differentiated
LCNEC	High	>20	>20	Poorly differentiated
MiNEN	Variable	Variable	Variable	Well or poorly differentiated

LCNEC, large-cell neuroendocrine carcinoma; MiNEN, mixed neuroendocrine non-neuroendocrine neoplasm; NEC, neuroendocrine carcinoma; NET, neuroendocrine tumor; SCNEC, small-cell neuroendocrine carcinoma.

Type I lesions that are large (>2 cm), numerous (>6 polyps), or invade beyond the submucosa as seen on EUS should be considered for surgical resection. Gastric resection should include antrectomy to reduce the source of the hypergastrinemia (antral G cells) and prevent ongoing enterochromaffin-like cell hyperplasia and hypertrophy.

Somatostatin analogs (SSA) have an antiproliferative action, but their routine use is controversial. The gastrin/cholecystokinin-2 receptor antagonist, netazepide, has been shown to reduce the number and size of gastric NETs in patients with type I gastric NETs. However, tumors recur once it is discontinued.

Type II

The primary gastrinoma associated with type II lesions should be localized. Resection of the gastrinoma will often lead to resolution of the gastric NET. If the gastrinoma is not resectable, the management of type II lesions is similar to the management of type I lesions.

Type III

Type III lesions are treated similarly to gastric adenocarcinoma. This involves oncologic resection, which can include total or subtotal gastrectomy with lymphadenectomy. The lymphadenectomy should include perigastric nodes and those along the celiac trunk, common hepatic artery, and splenic artery (D2 lymphadenectomy) (Figures 60–4A and 60–4B). Small lesions (<1 cm) with low-risk pathologic features (well differentiated, no lymphovascular invasion, no lymph node metastases) can be managed with endoscopic resection or surgical wedge resection.

TREATMENT OF METASTATIC DISEASE

Treatment of metastatic disease depends on symptoms and overall tumor burden. If complete resection is possible, resection of the primary and all metastatic lesion(s) is recommended. If the patient is asymptomatic with a low tumor burden, observation with surveillance imaging or treatment with SSAs (octreotide or lanreotide) is recommended. Resection of an asymptomatic primary lesion in the setting of unresectable metastatic disease is not indicated.

Liver metastasis can be treated with surgical resection, locoregional therapies, or systemic therapy. Liver resection may involve anatomic resection or techniques that spare liver volume, such as wedge resection, enucleation, or ablation. Guidelines recommend resection of grade I and grade II NETs, whereas grade III NETs are less favorable and should only be resected if the lesion is isolated and resectable with very low morbidity. Locoregional therapies include radiofrequency ablation (RFA) and transarterial embolization or chemoembolization. RFA can be done alone or in combination with resection. Transarterial embolization or chemoembolization is most often done in patients who are not good surgical candidates.

If there is a clinically significant or unresectable tumor burden, it is recommended to treat with SSAs and/or alternative therapies. If a patient exhibits disease progression while being treated with SSA or has clinically significant or unresectable tumor burden, alternative therapies consist of the mTOR inhibitor everolimus, peptide receptor radionuclide therapy (PRRT) with ^{177}Lu-DOTATATE (if the tumor displays somatostatin receptors on imaging), radiation therapy for symptomatic bone metastases, or cytotoxic chemotherapy (primarily for patients with high-grade tumors or if no other options are feasible). Cytotoxic chemotherapy consists of a combination of cisplatin with etoposide or 5-fluorouracil or capecitabine with oxaliplatin or irinotecan.

PROGNOSIS

The prognosis of patients with gastric NETs depends on the tumor subtype, tumor grade, and stage. Type I lesions have excellent survival (90%-95% survival at 5 years). Type II lesions have a slightly worse prognosis than type I due to the higher risk of lymph node metastases, but generally still have a very good overall survival (70%-90% at 5 years).

Type III lesions have a poor prognosis (similar to that of gastric adenocarcinoma). More than 50% of patients have metastatic disease at diagnosis. Five-year survival is typically <35%.

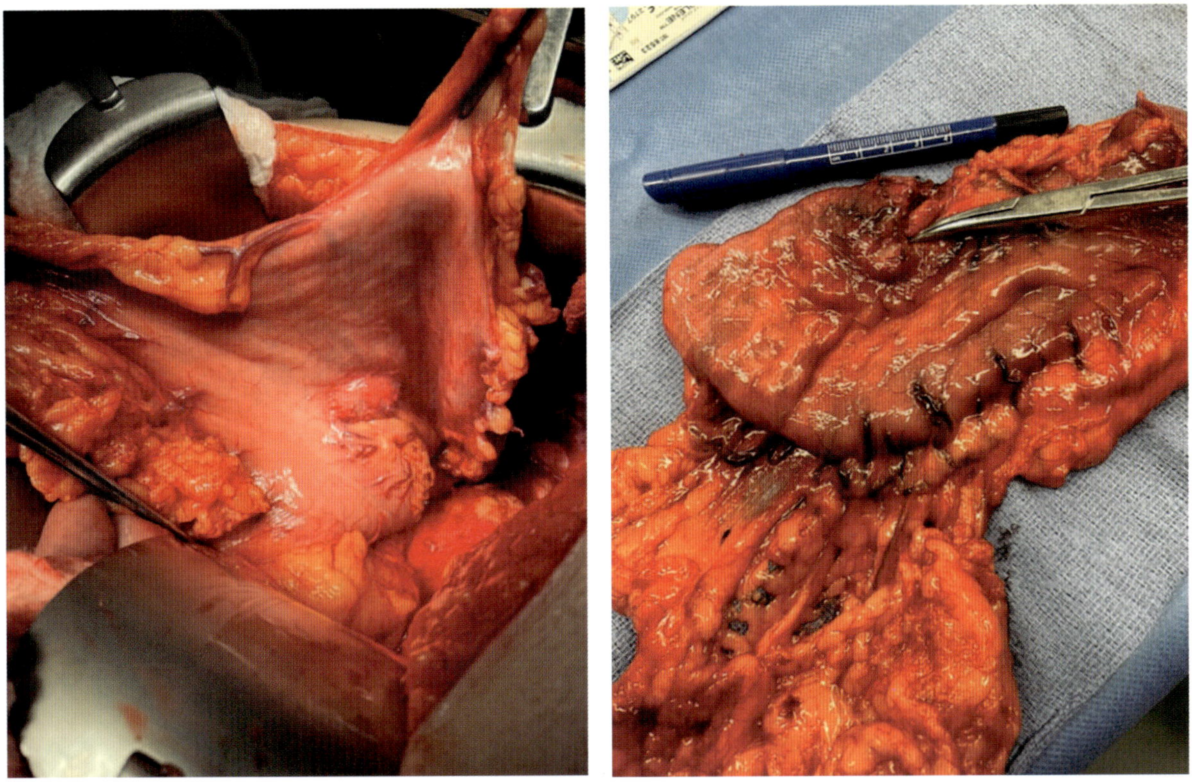

A B

▲ **Figure 60–4.** **(A)** The gastric neuroendocrine tumor is visualized on the posterior border of the lesser curvature. **(B)** Subtotal gastrectomy was done in combination with lymphadenectomy and distal pancreatectomy. The instrument points to the gastric NET.

SUGGESTED READING

Ahmed M. Gastrointestinal neuroendocrine tumors in 2020. *World J Gastrointest Oncol*. 2020;12(8):791-807.

Boyce M, Moore AR, Sagatun L, et al. Netazepide, a gastrin/cholecystokinin-2 receptor antagonist, can eradicate gastric neuroendocrine tumours in patients with autoimmine chronic atrophic gastritis. *Br J Clin Pharmacol*. 2017;83(3):466-475.

Boyce M, Thomsen L. Gastric neuroendocrine tumors: prevalence in Europe, USA, and Japan, and rationale for treatment with a gastrin/CCK2 receptor antagonist. *Scand J Gastroenterol*. 2015;50(5):550-559.

Caplin ME, Pavel M, Ćwikła JB, et al. Lanreotide in metastatic enteropancreatic neuroendocrine tumors. *N Engl J Med*. 2014;371(3):224-233.

Cives M, Strosberg J. Gastroenteropancreatic neuroendocrine tumors. *CA Cancer J Clin*. 2018;68(6):471-487.

Crosby DA, Donohoe CL, Fitzgerald L, et al. Gastric neuroendocrine tumors. *Dig Surg*. 2012;29:331-348.

Dasari A, Shen C, Halperin D, et al. Trends in the incidence, prevalence, and survival outcomes in patients with neuroendocrine tumors in the United States. *JAMA Oncol*. 2017;3(10):1335-1342.

Delle Fave G, OToole D, Sundin A, et al. ENETS consensus guidelines update for gastroduodenal neuroendocrine neoplasms. *Neuroendocrinology*. 2016;103:119-124.

Felder S, Jann H, Denecke T, et al. Gastric neuroendocrine neoplasias: manifestations and comparative outcomes. *Endocr Relat Cancer*. 2019;26(9):751-763.

Grozinsky-Glasberg S, Alexandraki K, Angelousi A, et al. Gastric carcinoids. *Endocrinol Metab Clin North Am*. 2018;47(3):645-660.

Karakas Y, Lacin S, Esin E, et al. Prognostic value of the 2017 World Health Organization Classification System for gastric neuroendocrine tumors: a single-center experience. *Turk J Gastroenterol*. 2020;31(2):91-98.

Kim BS, Park YS, Yook JH, Kim B-S. Comparison of the prognostic values of the 2010 WHO classification, AJCC 7th edition, and ENETS classification of gastric neuroendocrine tumors. *Medicine* (Baltimore). 2016;95(30):e3977.

Kunz PL, Reidy-Lagunes D, Anthony LB, et al. Consensus guidelines for the management and treatment of neuroendocrine tumors. *Pancreas*. 2013;42(4):557-577.

Li T, Qiu F, Qian ZR, Wan J, Qi X-K, Wu B-Y. Classification, clinicopathologic features and treatment of gastric neuroendocrine tumors. *World J Gastroenterol*. 2014;20(1):118-125.

Liu D, Fu X, Liu W, et al. Clinicopathological, treatment, and prognosis study of 43 gastric neuroendocrine carcinomas. *World J Gastroenterol.* 2017;23(3):516-524.

Rinke A, Wittenberg M, Brittinger CS, et al. Placebo-controlled, double-blind, prospective, randomized study on the effect of octreotide LAR in the control of tumor growth in patients with metastatic neuroendocrine midgut tumors (PROMID): results of long-term survival. *Neuroendocrinology.* 2017;104(1): 26-32.

Roberto GA, Rodrigues C, Peixoto RA, Younes RN. Gastric neuroendocrine tumor: a practical literature review. *World J Gastrointest Oncol.* 2020;12(8):850-856.

Sato Y, Hashimoto S, Mizuno KI, Takeuchi KI, Terai S. Management of gastric and duodenal neuroendocrine tumors. *World J Gastroenterol.* 2016 Aug;22(30):6817-6828.

Schmidt B, Yoon SS. D1 versus D2 lymphadenectomy for gastric cancer. *J Surg Oncol.* 2013;107(3):259-264.

Schreckenbach T, Hubert H, Koch C, et al. Surgical resection of neuroendocrine tumor liver metastases as part of multimodal treatment strategies: a propensity score matching analysis. *Eur J Surg Oncol.* 2019;45(5):808-815.

Shah MH, Goldner WS, Halfdanarson TR, et al. NCCN Guidelines insights: neuroendocrine and adrenal tumors, version 2.2018. *J Natl Compr Canc Netw.* 2018;16(6):693-702.

Shen C, Chen H, Chen H, et al. Surgical treatment and prognosis of gastric neuroendocrine neoplasms: a single- center experience. *BMC Gastroenterol.* 2016;16(1):111.

Yang Z, Wang W, Lu JF, et al. Gastric neuroendocrine tumors (G-NETS): Incidence, prognosis and recent trend toward improved survival. *Cell Physiol Biochem.* 2018;45(1):389-396.

Yao JC, Fazio N, Singh S, et al. Everolimus for the treatment of advanced, non-functional neuroendocrine tumours of the lung or gastrointestinal tract (RADIANT-4): a randomised, placebo-controlled, phase 3 study. *Lancet.* 2016;387(10022):968-977.

Neuroendocrine Tumors of the Small Intestine

61

Jessica E. Maxwell, MD, MBA
James R. Howe, MD

INTRODUCTION

Neuroendocrine tumors (NETs) derive from enterochromaffin cells of the diffuse endocrine system and can thus arise in a variety of locations throughout the body. The location of the primary tumor, disease stage, and grade dictate management. The most common sites are the rectum, small intestine, pancreas, and lungs.[1] In recent years, NETs located within the jejunum and ileum (SBNETs) have surpassed adenocarcinoma as the most common malignancy of the midgut, representing approximately 39% to 45% of all cases.[2]

Historically named "carcinoid tumors" for their histologically benign appearance,[3] at high-volume centers in the United States more than 60% of patients may present with advanced disease.[4,5] Patients with SBNETs who present with localized or locoregional disease are treated surgically for curative intent. In advanced disease, surgical resection of the primary tumor with or without metastasectomy may be considered, as it is associated with enhanced survival, symptom control, and prevention of future morbidity in carefully selected populations. There are few systemic therapies approved for this tumor type, which emphasizes the need for experienced, multidisciplinary care to ensure proper ordering of therapies, of which there is no consensus. This chapter discusses current diagnostic and management strategies for patients with SBNETs, with an emphasis on surgical management.

GENERAL CONSIDERATIONS

Epidemiology

NETs are rare but increasing in incidence across all primary tumor sites, stage, and grade. The incidence of SBNETs is estimated to be 1.2 per 100,000, which is a doubling of the incidence of SBNETs in the 1990s. Examined by stage, the increase in incidence is most significant in those with localized disease,[1] which may be in part explained by the increased use and sensitivity of cross-sectional imaging.

Studies correlating behavioral risk factors with SBNET development are mixed. Early reports failed to find an association between common risk factors such as smoking and obesity to tumorigenesis.[9] More recently, a systematic literature review reported that a family history of any cancer, family history of colorectal cancer, any alcohol use, or any smoking history correlated with SBNET development, although the authors acknowledged a great degree of study heterogeneity.[10] More studies with well-defined cohorts will be required to investigate this further. SBNETs are not associated with a known familial syndrome, although families with multiple affected members have been described.[11]

Classification & Nomenclature

The nomenclature for neuroendocrine neoplasms (NENs) has evolved and modern terminology incorporates a tumor's histopathologic appearance and grade, which by extension communicates a patient's prognosis and underlying tumor biology (Figure 61–1). The larger group of neuroendocrine lesions is termed "neuroendocrine neoplasms," which is agnostic of malignant potential, cellular differentiation or grade. NENs are then divided into groups based on cellular differentiation. Well-differentiated NENs are referred to as NETs and this category encompasses the majority of NENs. Poorly differentiated NENs are more commonly known as neuroendocrine carcinomas (NECs). Differentiating a NET from a NEC is extremely important, as prognosis and management strategies are vastly different. NETs are further categorized by their grade. This is typically determined using an IHC method that reports the percentage of neoplastic cells that stain for the proliferation antigen Ki-67, and/or the mitotic rate. The three grades (G1, G2, and G3) correlate with prognosis. Poorly differentiated NECs are uniformly G3.[12]

Disease stage is assigned based on the location of the primary tumor using the American Joint Committee on Cancer

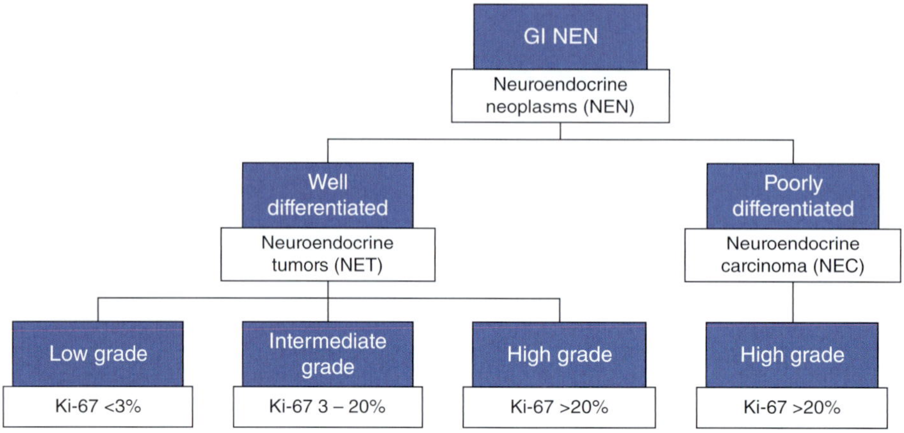

Figure 61–1. Nomenclature classification for neuroendocrine tumors.

(AJCC) tumor node metastasis (TNM) system (Table 61–1). Well-differentiated SBNETs are classified within the standard jejunal/ileal neuroendocrine classification, whereas poorly differentiated small-bowel NECs are classified by the small-bowel adenocarcinoma system.

CLINICAL FINDINGS

Symptoms & Signs

Patients with localized SBNETs are typically asymptomatic. Some patients may relate episodes of vague abdominal cramping or alterations of bowel habits that may be difficult to correlate with imaging. Symptomatology may be more striking once the disease involves mesenteric lymph nodes or distant metastatic sites such as the liver or peritoneum. Large intraluminal primary tumors may cause gastrointestinal (GI) bleeding or intestinal obstruction. Patients with a heavy burden of mesenteric lymph nodes that encase the vasculature may suffer from chronic mesenteric ischemia. Carcinoid syndrome, the most common NET hormonal syndrome, is found in approximately 20% of patients with advanced disease and is associated with diarrhea, cutaneous flushing, and wheezing. In severe cases, patients may present with carcinoid heart disease, which features a cardiac murmur or right-sided heart failure.

Biomarkers

Biomarkers can be used to monitor response to therapy, disease progression, or recurrence. None confer the specificity or sensitivity necessary to be used for diagnosis, especially if the pretest probability is low. For ileal and jejunal NETs, the North American Neuroendocrine Tumor Society (NANETS) has historically suggested measurement of Chromogranin A (CgA) and urine 5-HIAA (u5-HIAA),[13] although more recent literature suggests that the biomarkers pancreastatin (PST) and neurokinin A (NKA) may be of greater utility and possess superior prognostic ability.

Chromogranin A is a secretory protein that is found in endocrine, neuroendocrine, and immune cells. Serum levels correlate with tumor burden, and thus it can be used as a marker to assess the completeness of surgical cytoreduction, and suggest recurrence or progression.[14] Despite its widespread use, it has a number of limitations. In patients with disease confirmed by imaging, its sensitivity and specificity are only 71% and 50%, respectively.[15] Its levels can be altered by numerous pathologic conditions (eg, hypertension, renal failure, cardiac failure, sepsis, or inflammatory bowel disease) as well as by common medications such as proton pump inhibitors.[16]

Urine 5-HIAA is a metabolite of serotonin with high sensitivity (>95%) for gastrointestinal NETs, but with low specificity. It is commonly used to confirm the diagnosis of carcinoid syndrome, but its levels do not correlate with tumor burden or symptom severity and thus it is not useful for disease surveillance.[17] Further complicating its interpretation, the levels can be artificially elevated by medications such as acetaminophen or 5-fluorouracil, caffeine, wine, or tryptophan-rich foods such as tomato and pineapple.[18]

Neurokinin A and PST are two nontraditional biomarkers that are being increasingly incorporated into the care of NET patients and may be especially useful to the NET surgeon. Neurokinin A is a tachykinin that influences gastrointestinal motility, vasodilation, and flushing. Elevated plasma levels are found in 46% of patients with SBNET, and multivariate analyses have demonstrated this marker to be an independent predictor of prognosis. In patients treated with somatostatin analogues (SSA), those in whom NKA stabilized or fell had superior survival compared to those in whom NKA continued to rise despite treatment.[19]

Table 61–1. American Joint Committee on Cancer (AJCC) TNM staging system (8th ed, 2017) or G1/G2 (and rare G3) well-differentiated small bowel neuroendocrine tumors.

	Jejunum/Ileum			
TX	Tumor cannot be evaluated			
T0	No evidence of tumor			
T1	≤1 cm and extends into lamina propria or submucosa			
T2	>1 cm or extends into the muscularis propria			
T3	Invades into but not through subserosa			
T4	Tumor extends beyond serosa, or invades nearby organs			
NX	Regional lymph nodes cannot be assessed			
N0	No regional lymph node metastasis			
N1	Regional lymph node metastases <12 lymph nodes			
N2	Large mesenteric masses (>2 cm) and/or ≥12 nodal deposits, especially those that encase the superior mesenteric vessels			
MX	Distant metastases cannot be assessed			
M0	No distant metastases			
M1a	Metastases confined to the liver			
M1b	Metastases in at least one extrahepatic site			
M1c	Both hepatic and extrahepatic metastases			
	Stage I	**Stage II**	**Stage III**	**Stage IV**
Jejunum/Ileum	T1 N0 M0	T2-3 N0 M0	Any T N1-2 M0 T4 N0 M0	Any T Any N M1

For any T, add (m) for multiple tumors. For multiple tumors with different Ts, use the highest. Per WHO/AJCC guidelines, poorly differentiated neuroendocrine carcinomas (Ki-67 >20%) are staged using the staging classifications for adenocarcinomas at the individual primary tumor sites, not as well-differentiated NETs.

Pancreastatin, a subunit of CgA, holds potentially the greatest value to the NET surgeon. Its levels are less susceptible to those factors affecting CgA and the assay is standardized.[20] Elevated PST levels correlate with poor progression-free survival (PFS) and overall survival (OS) in patients with small bowel or pancreatic NETs.[21] In surgically managed patients, the trajectory of postoperative PST value was prognostic and was superior to CgA in discriminating patient outcome. In those who began with elevated PST values and experienced a biochemical response after surgical resection and/or cytoreduction, a significantly longer 5-year OS (94%) was seen compared to those who did not (58%, $P < .01$).[14]

The NETest is a blood-based test that uses transcriptomal profiling to predict site of origin, estimate tumor burden, monitor therapeutic efficacy, and predict prognosis.[22] In a study of 179 GI and PNETs, the test accurately identified 93% of SBNETs.[23] The test can be used to estimate the completeness of surgical cytoreduction as scores correlate with tumor burden. A small study that included 15 GI NET patients undergoing an operation for curative intent demonstrated a 100% decrease in NETest scores postoperatively. The test was repeated 1 month postoperatively and 4 patients had elevated scores despite a normal CgA level. By 6 months after surgery, these 4 patients had locoregional disease recurrence detected on somatostatin receptor imaging.[24]

Imaging

High-quality imaging studies are required for the workup, staging, and surveillance of SBNETs. Endoscopy can be used for localization and biopsy of SBNETs but it is not a therapeutic modality as complete excision and simultaneous lymphadenectomy cannot be performed. Colonoscopy may find tumors in the terminal ileum, but is rarely useful for more proximal lesions. Balloon enteroscopy or video capsule endoscopy can be employed in cases where an SBNET is suspected, but has escaped localization by other modalities. In this context, the diagnostic yield of balloon enteroscopy is 33%.[25] The value of video capsule endoscopy is less clear.

Some studies estimate a localization rate in SBNET patients as high as 45%, but this rate is unsubstantiated as not all patients included in the study had the lesion confirmed pathologically or even with alternative imaging modalities.[26] Studies including all small-bowel histologies estimate the diagnostic yield of video capsule endoscopy to be between 2% and 9%,[27] and for larger lesions there is risk of obstruction from the capsule itself.

The most common diagnostic and surveillance imaging modality for SBNETs is CT. Often, the diagnosis is suggested by the presence of a cicatrizing, calcified mesenteric mass that is located within the lymphatic drainage basin of the intraluminal primary tumor (Figure 61–2). Strategically, obtaining a triple phase (arterial, portal venous, and delayed phases) "liver protocol" CT of the abdomen and pelvis with intravenous contrast is likely to be the highest yield preoperative imaging study, as it provides excellent visualization of hypervascular NET hepatic metastases and of the mesenteric vasculature. The addition of oral contrast may identify an intraluminal tumor, but the sensitivity of the modality for this indication is rather low. This can be improved using neutral oral contrast agents (like water) as in CT enterography. Even if it cannot be identified radiographically, the location of the primary tumor is suggested by the distribution of the mesenteric lymphadenopathy.

MRI provides superior detail of NET hepatic metastases compared to CT or somatostatin imaging,[28] and is helpful as an adjunctive imaging modality when hepatic resection or cytoreduction is planned. Optimal imaging requires use of IV gadolinium contrast, as most NET metastases are hyperintense on arterial phases. This modality can also be used for surveillance of the abdomen and pelvis in patients who have renal failure or an allergy to iodinated contrast.

Somatostatin receptor imaging is unique to NET. Somatostatin is an endogenous hormone secreted by the delta cells of the gastric antrum, duodenum, and pancreas that binds to somatostatin receptors (SSTR) expressed in the central nervous system, pancreas, endocrine tissues, and gastrointestinal tract. Approximately 80% of well-differentiated NETs express SSTR, which serves as the basis for somatostatin-targeted

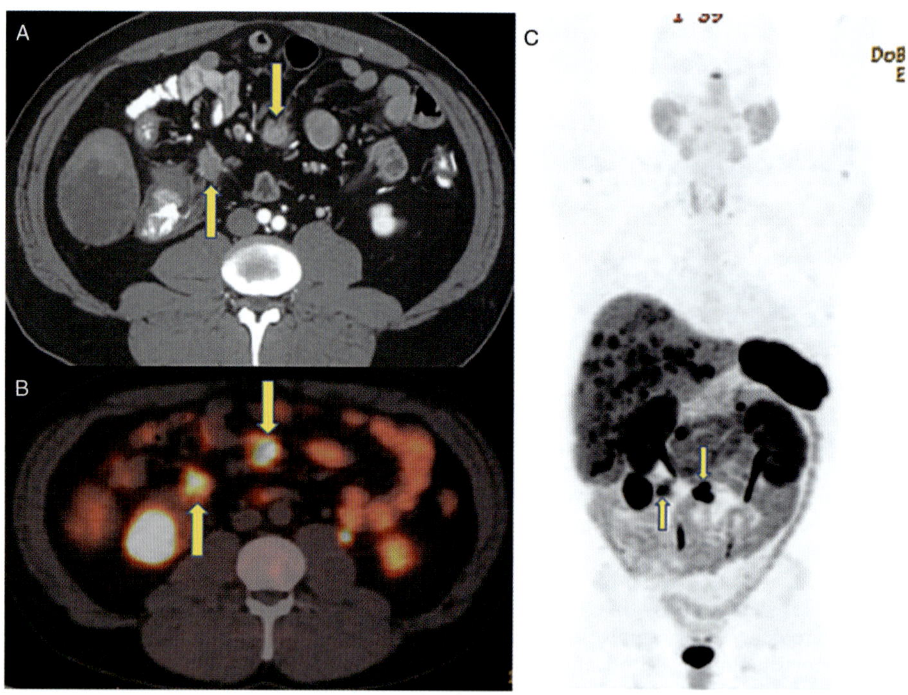

▲ **Figure 61–2.** A 51-year-old patient with a metastatic SBNET. **(A)** Arterially enhanced CT scan demonstrating two mesenteric masses (arrows) and an intraluminal tumor in the cecum/terminal ileum. The mass nearest the primary tumor is causing tethering of the bowel, which contributed to the patient's obstructive symptoms. There is a large tumor in segment 6 of the liver. **(B)** ^{68}Ga-DOTATATE colocalized with a noncontrast CT scan. The mesenteric masses (arrows) and cecal tumor enhance. There is physiologic uptake in the left ureter. **(C)** Planar ^{68}Ga-DOTATATE demonstrating innumerable hepatic metastases, two mesenteric masses (arrows), and the primary tumor. There is a metastasis in the pancreatic head and a retroperitoneal lymph node metastasis. Physiologic uptake is seen in the pituitary, salivary glands, axillary lymph nodes, thyroid, kidneys, ureters, and bladder.

imaging and therapy. An early iteration of this modality, the Octreoscan, used ^{111}In-labeled diethylenetriamine penta-acetic acid octreotide (DTPA-D-Phe^{1}-octreotide) to visualize tumors with a sensitivity and specificity in GI NETs of 85% and 95%, respectively.[29] The Octreoscan has been largely replaced by a type of positron emission tomography (PET) that uses a ^{68}Ga-labelled radioligand conjugated to a somatostatin analogue (^{68}Ga-DOTATOC, ^{68}Ga-DOTANOC, ^{68}Ga-DOTATATE). Anatomic localization is enhanced by fusing this PET with either CT or MRI (Figure 61–2). It has an estimated sensitivity of 97% in gastroenteropancreatic NETs, and can localize intraluminal SBNETs, although the lower limit of detection is approximately 1 cm. It is most appropriately used for initial staging after histological diagnosis of a NET, localization of a primary tumor in patients with metastatic disease but an unknown primary, and to select patients for SSTR-targeted peptide receptor radionuclide therapy (PRRT).[30]

Biopsy

Histopathologic evaluation is required to confirm a diagnosis of SBNET, although biopsy is not required in every case. If clinical history and imaging strongly suggest a diagnosis of NET, and the disease is amenable to surgical cure, histologic confirmation can be obtained from the surgical specimen. In cases of advanced disease that may be amenable to surgical cytoreduction, biopsy of an easily accessed metastasis may aid the multidisciplinary team in determining whether resection or systemic therapy may be the most appropriate. When the location of the primary site is unknown, or the patient is unlikely to be a surgical candidate, a biopsy is recommended. Immunohistochemistry can be used on biopsies of NET metastases to aid in determining the primary tumor site, in cases where it is not localized on imaging (Table 61–2).

Table 61–2. Immunohistochemical markers to identify neuroendocrine tumors.

Marker	Significance
Synaptophysin	Presynaptic vesicle membrane glycoprotein, present on normal and neoplastic neuroendocrine cells
Chromogranin A	Universal marker for neuroendocrine tissue
INSM1 (insulinoma-associated protein 1)	General neuroendocrine marker. Useful for differentiating NET from NEC (positive in NEC)
CDX2 (caudal type homeobox 2)	Transcription factor expressed by epithelial cells of the small bowel. Expression is especially sensitive for jejunoileal or appendiceal NETs
PAX6 (paired box gene 6)	Transcription factor critical for islet development that is useful for identifying pancreatic NET (and to rule out SBNET)
Islet1 (insulin gene enhancer binding protein Isl-1)	Expressed in the mesenchymal cells of the pancreas, in islet cells, chromaffin cells, and in some central nervous system tissue. A marker for pancreatic, rectal, and duodenal NETs
PrAP (prostate (specific) acid phosphatase)	Frequently tested in cases of primary or unknown origin. For well-differentiated NET, is indicative of pancreatic NET and negative predictor for SBNET

IHC testing may be especially helpful in cases where a GI NET is assumed, but the primary site is unknown.[6-8]

DIFFERENTIAL DIAGNOSIS

- Jejunal/ileal neuroendocrine tumor
- Jejunal/ileal adenocarcinoma
- Lymphoma
- Gastrointestinal stromal tumor
- Metastases to the small bowel
- GI conditions associated with chronic diarrhea (eg, irritable bowel syndrome, inflammatory bowel disease, food intolerances, celiac sprue, bacterial overgrowth, parasitic infections)

COMPLICATIONS

Carcinoid Heart Disease

Carcinoid heart disease is the initial manifestation of carcinoid syndrome in 10% to 20% of patients and has been found in up to 50% of patients with carcinoid syndrome in some series.[31] As the cardiac valves normally express high levels of serotonin receptors on their surface, the pathophysiology is ascribed to the elevated levels of circulating serotonin seen in most patients with carcinoid syndrome and the resultant inflammatory response. This results in the development of plaque-like deposits and endocardial thickening on the tricuspid and pulmonary valve leaflets. Over time, this can lead to valvular regurgitation or right heart failure that is manifested by dyspnea on exertion, ascites, peripheral edema, and pleural effusions. All patients with SBNETs should be screened by serum pro-brain natriuretic protein level, and if elevated or there is clinical suspicion of heart disease, a transthoracic echocardiogram (TTE). If valvular disease is present, repeat TTE should be obtained if there is a change in clinical status or every 3 to 6 months, depending on the severity of the underlying heart disease.[32] Surgical valve replacement can improve survival and symptoms. In one early series, the median 2-year survival in patients with severe carcinoid heart disease treated with valve replacement was 40%, compared to only 8% in those who were managed medically.[33] As a greater understanding of which patients are likely to benefit from surgical intervention has grown, outcomes have likewise improved with the 1- and 5-year OS reported at 69% and 35%, respectively.[34] Preoperatively, if valve disease is severe and the patient has minimal GI symptoms, valve replacement should precede resection and/or cytoreductive surgery of the SBNET and metastases.

Carcinoid Crisis

Carcinoid crisis is a controversial hemodynamic phenomenon that is associated with patients diagnosed with carcinoid syndrome. As with carcinoid heart disease, it is thought to be caused by elevated levels of circulating serotonin and other vasoactive substances such as bradykinins and tachykinins.[35] There is no consensus on the definition of carcinoid crisis, and thus the true prevalence is unknown. The incidence in reports in patients undergoing surgical cytoreduction of their NET ranges from 0% to 35%.[36,37] Patients suffering from crisis may display a variety of symptoms that can include cutaneous flushing, diarrhea, prolonged and refractory hypotension, or cardiac arrythmias. It has been reported in patients undergoing a variety of invasive procedures—surgical resection, hepatic artery embolization (HAE), selective internal radiation therapy (SIRT), PRRT, and tumor biopsy. Given its similarity to carcinoid syndrome, treatment or prophylaxis includes administration of octreotide, an intermediate-acting somatostatin analogue, most commonly as an infusion for higher-risk procedures. However, prospective studies have recently called the efficacy of this treatment into question.[35,37] Vasopressin and phenylephrine should be used as needed to improve the hypotension that may occur intraoperatively.

TREATMENT

Localized & Locoregional Disease

Patients with localized or limited locoregional disease may be cured with surgical resection. The standard of care in these patients is an open operation that includes manual palpation of the entire small bowel from the ligament of Treitz to the ileocecal valve. Neither purely robotic-assisted, nor laparoscopic assessment of the small bowel is sufficient because these tumors are often subcentimeter, occult on imaging and gross intraoperative inspection, and multifocal. In two reports from a high-volume NET center, 45% to 56% of explored patients had multifocal disease (Figure 61–3). In the majority of these patients, the presence of multifocal tumors was not detected on preoperative imaging.[38,39] If minimally invasive surgical approaches are used, it is important to manually palpate the entire bowel through the incision used for the extracorporeal anastomosis. Approximately three-quarters of SBNETs are found within the most distal 100 cm of the small intestine (Figure 61–4).[39]

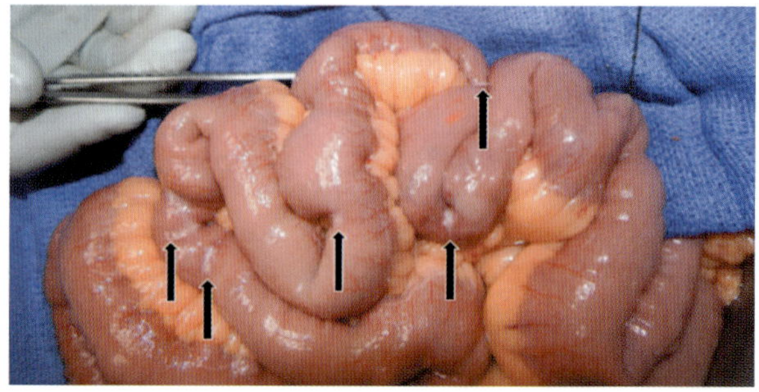

Figure 61–3. Multifocal SBNETs. Intraoperative photo of a segmental bowel resection that includes six primary SBNETs, indicated by arrows. These small tumors may be associated with the white, plaque-like tissue puckering, but can also be invisible externally and only found by manual palpation.

An oncologically complete operation includes a full exploration of the abdomen with inspection and palpation of all peritoneal surfaces, the liver, the entire GI tract from the stomach to the rectum, the ovaries, and the mesentery. The primary SBNET is treated with segmental resection and regional lymphadenectomy (Figure 61–5). Inclusion of a minimum of 12 lymph nodes is required for proper staging,[40] although node count can be misleading in cases of mesenteric masses representing a conglomeration of mesenteric nodes. High ligation of segmental mesenteric vessels should be performed. A common challenge is lymphadenopathy tracking along the mesenteric vessels into the root of the mesentery. These nodes may encase the vasculature and cause venous congestion or bowel ischemia as the disease progresses. The main trunks of the superior mesenteric artery and vein must be preserved,[41] but in many cases the nodes can be dissected off these vessels with great care. If this is not possible, as in the case of matted, intensely fibrotic, or calcified nodes extending proximally along these trunks, sometimes the best course of action is to divide the mass at the origin of the segmental branch. The ileocolic artery can be sacrificed as long as there are a sufficient number of jejunal branches preserved. In contrast to a segmental resection of a jejunal or ileal adenocarcinoma, SBNETs typically produce a vigorous desmoplastic response, which causes tethering of surrounding loops of small bowel and difficulty isolating and ligating a single vascular pedicle associated with the mesenteric mass. Prior to dividing any bowel, the entire length of small intestine should be measured, and the points of transection should be estimated and marked with a stitch to determine the length of bowel remaining once the resection is performed. Most people have 500 to 700 cm of small intestine. Resecting more than 100 cm may be necessary in patients with multifocal disease and large mesenteric masses. Leaving a patient with less than 200 cm of small intestine, especially

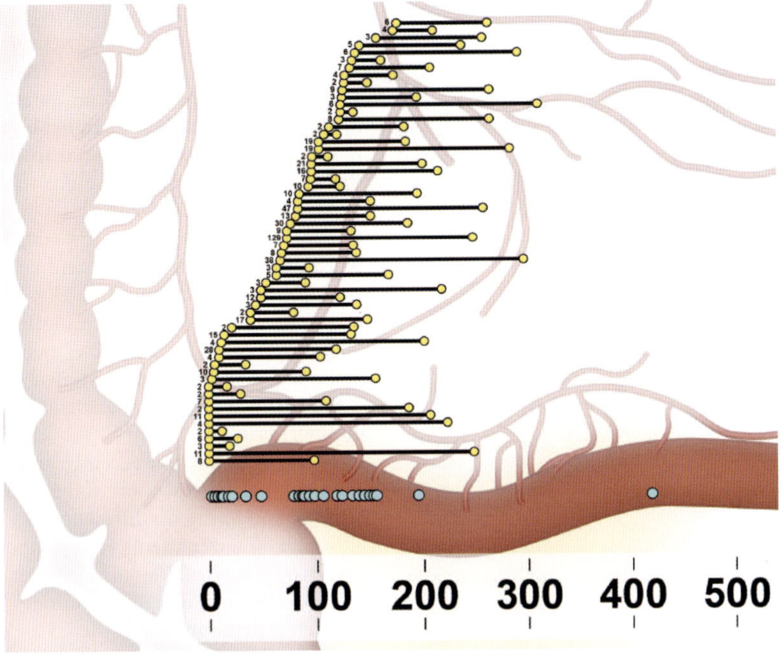

▲ **Figure 61–4.** Tumor location in the small bowel. The bowel length was standardized to 500 cm with the ileocecal valve designated as 0 and the ligament of Treitz designated as 500. The location of unifocal tumors is displayed in blue. The span of multifocal tumors is displayed by black lines with yellow markers at each end with the number of tumors in that span noted to the left. (Reproduced with permission from Keck KJ, Maxwell JE, Utria AF, et al. The distal predilection of small bowel neuroendocrine tumors. *Ann Surg Oncol.* 2018;25:3207-3213.)

when the ileocecal valve is sacrificed, can have a profoundly negative impact on a patient's quality of life. The vasculature involved by the tumor can be dissected out, traced to the SMA or SMV, and then test clamped to ensure that ligation will not leave the remaining bowel compromised. A vascular doppler is helpful to identify surrounding vascular branches and arcades that can be carefully mobilized and preserved.

Metastatic Disease

The goal for treating metastatic SBNET is improvement of quality of life and survival. There are a number of treatment modalities that can be employed—either directed at the liver alone or systemically. No consensus exists on the optimal ordering of these therapies, and thus specialized, multidisciplinary care is required.

Surgical Cytoreduction

Surgical cytoreduction can be useful to palliate symptoms, prevent complications, and possibly improve survival. These operations frequently involve multiple disease sites throughout the abdomen and the risks and benefits must be considered carefully. In advanced disease, an R0 resection is not possible in most cases,[42] and even when achieved, recurrence is near universal. As well, the potential morbidity of a cytoreductive operation must be considered as surgical complications can impact the survival and quality of life in a group of patients who may otherwise survive many years with their disease *in situ*. For these reasons, the operations are best performed at high-volume NET centers where the most complicated cases can be considered by a multidisciplinary team that includes surgeons with experience in these operations and managing these unique patients perioperatively.

Palliative resection of an SBNET primary is reasonable even in the context of unresectable metastatic disease.[43] The most common reasons for an operation in this context are bleeding, obstruction, symptoms of intestinal angina, or when cytoreduction of the primary and associated mesenteric lymph nodes can provide relief of debilitating secretory or mesenteric ischemic symptoms.

In the scenario where the primary tumor is asymptomatic and the distant disease is unresectable, resection may prevent future complications. Prepalliative bowel resection was recently studied in retrospective population-based matched cohort design. Of 1000 patients identified with metastatic SBNET, 785 had resection of their primary only. Compared to those managed nonoperatively, patients undergoing prepalliative resection had lower 3-year risk of hospital

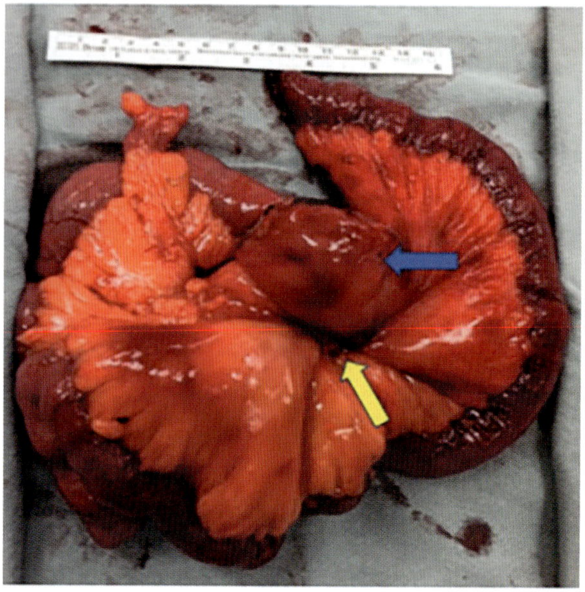

▲ **Figure 61–5.** Intraoperative photo of a segmental bowel resection specimen for an SBNET. The blue arrow indicates the large mesenteric mass, and the yellow arrow demonstrates the desmoplastic puckering that is often seen. This inflammatory response tethered nearby mesenteric vessels, requiring a more extensive bowel resection than otherwise expected from preoperative imaging.

readmission (72.6% vs 86.4%, $p < 0.001$; HR 0.72 [95% CI 0.57-0.91]). Also, upfront resection was associated with a decreased risk of subsequent small-bowel-related surgery (15.4% vs 40.3%, $p < 0.001$; HR 0.44 [95% CI 0.29-0.67]).[44]

The association between primary tumor resection in patients with advanced disease and survival is less clear, and conclusions are limited by the retrospective nature of the studies performed. An interesting analysis by the UKINETS study group evaluated outcomes for a group of 238 SBNET patients with advanced disease who were eligible for surgical resection at presentation. Patients able to undergo the planned operation demonstrated improved survival (median OS 9.92 y, n = 210) compared to those who were taken to the operating room but could only undergo small-bowel bypass (median OS 5.61 y, n = 12), had their procedure aborted (median OS 6.74 y, n = 17), or could not proceed to the operating room due either to oncologic factors or comorbidities (median OS 4.73 y, n = 80).[45] A more recent meta-analysis of six studies examining the issue of survival in patients with unresectable metastases suggested that in patients with metastatic jejunoileal or pancreatic NETs, there was a survival advantage associated with palliative resection of their primary tumor.[46] Propensity-matched studies are less clear. One compared early versus late (>6 months after diagnosis) or no resection of the primary tumor for stage IV SBNET, and found no difference in survival between groups, although 56% of patients who did not undergo an operation within 6 months of diagnosis eventually proceeded to the OR for resection and/or cytoreduction.[47]

Metastatectomy is considered for patients with functional and nonfunctional tumors, and in retrospective analyses of well-selected patients, cytoreduction correlates with improved survival (Table 61–3; Figure 61–6). The most common site of metastases is the liver and the majority of analyses focus on the benefits of hepatic cytoreduction. In this context, recent studies suggest survival benefits and symptomatic relief when at least 70% of tumor bulk can be removed or ablated. One large study included 800 patients with advanced GI NETs who underwent 1001 cytoreductive operations. Sixty-five percent (n = 516) had a primary SBNET. In a subgroup analysis including only those with SBNETs, patients were divided into groups based on the estimated tumor bulk treated intraoperatively—<70%, 70%-89%, 90%-98%, and 99%-100%. The overall survival for those patients included in the groups where more than 70%

Table 61–3. Comparison of survival outcomes of metastatic SBNET patients.

	G1/G2 Stage IV SBNET (SEER)[1]	Woltering et al. 2017[48]	Maxwell et al. 2016[49]	Wonn et al. 2021[53]
Patient population	G1/G2 SBNET n = 14,657	All SBNETs n = 516	G1/G2 SBNETs n = 80	G1/G2 SBNETs with peritoneal carcinomatosis n = 98
Therapeutic intervention	Surgical + Medical	Surgical cytoreduction (any intraabdominal site)	Liver-directed surgery or ablation +/− resection of primary tumor	Peritoneal debulking to Lyon 0 +/− liver-directed surgery +/− resection of primary tumor
Median overall survival (months)	103	161	Not reached	135

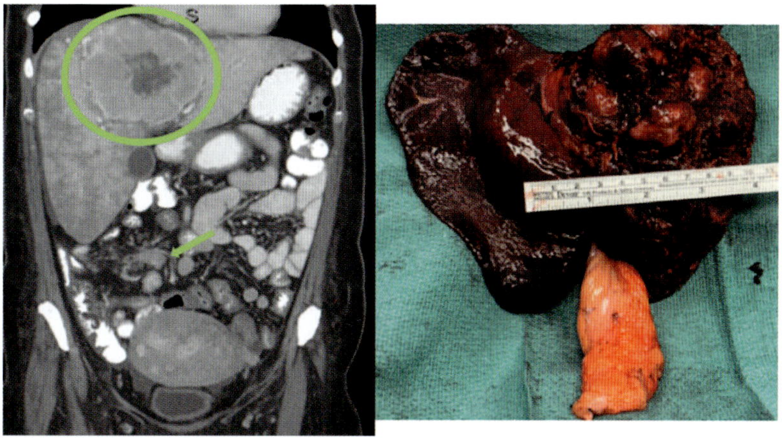

Figure 61–6. A 54-year-old woman with a functional SBNET and large central liver metastasis. Her symptoms included flushing and diarrhea. In addition to carcinoid syndrome, she developed carcinoid heart disease and required replacement of her pulmonic and tricuspid valves. Prior to her cardiac surgery, bland embolization of the dominant hepatic metastasis was performed, and her symptoms decreased in frequency and severity within 1 week. Approximately 3 months after her cardiac surgery, she underwent an extended left hepatectomy to remove the large liver metastasis (circle). The SBNET primary was removed at her third operation after she had recovered from the hepatic resection.

of their tumor could be debulked were similar and exceeded 12.3 years. Patients who were able to have 99%-100% of their tumor debulked had a median survival that was not reached. In comparison, patients who had <70% of their tumor bulk resected had a median survival of only 7.4 years.[48] This 70% minimum threshold has been supported in other recent studies and is used by many high-volume NET surgeons around the country.[49-52]

The benefit of peritoneal cytoreduction has been less well documented but is frequently done as a part of SBNET operations. Of 323 SBNET patients taken to the operating room for metastasectomy, 30% were found to have peritoneal metastases. Cytoreduction of this disease was achieved via omentectomy, peritonectomy, fulguration, or segmental bowel resection. In these well-selected patients, the majority achieved clinically meaningful surgical cytoreduction of their peritoneal disease as scored using the Lyon system, and in those cases, improved survival was noted (Table 61–3).[53]

Orthotopic liver transplantation is another viable, but less widely used surgical approach for treating SBNET patients with liver metastases. The Milan criteria define transplant eligibility (Table 61–4). Mazzaferro et al. reported the long-term results of 42 transplanted patients. A significant survival advantage was seen in the transplanted group compared to the nontransplant group at 5 and 10 years. This advantage persisted when the analysis was adjusted by propensity score.[54] A systematic review of 64 studies that included 1216 patients suggested that enhanced survival may be achieved, although recurrence was reported as 31.3% to 56.8%. Poor prognostic factors included high Ki-67, transplantation when there was >50% tumor involvement, and pancreatic primary tumor location.[57] The scarcity of grafts, high rates of recurrence, and lack of high-level evidence leave this intervention under debate.

Somatostatin Analogues

Somatostatin analogues (SSAs) are often the first-line therapy for symptomatic or metastatic NETs. Available in intermediate- (octreotide) and long-acting (lanreotide)

Table 61–4. Milan criteria for liver transplantation in patients with neuroendocrine liver metastases.[54-56]

Inclusion criteria
• Confirmed histological diagnosis of well-differentiated (G1, G2) NET
• Primary tumor drained by portal system
• Metastatic replacement of liver parenchyma ≤50%
• Good response or stable disease for at least 6 months
• Age ≤60 years
Exclusion criteria
• Small-cell carcinoma or high-grade (poorly differentiated) neuroendocrine carcinoma
• Other medical/surgical conditions contraindicating liver transplantation, including previous tumors
• Primary tumor is a non-GI NET/is not drained by the portal system

formulations, these medications are synthetic versions of the endogenous hormone somatostatin and have demonstrated efficacy mitigating symptoms secondary to hormonal secretion and slowing tumor growth.[58-60] In the landmark, prospective PROMID (octreotide) and CLARINET (lanreotide) trials, these medications were tested in NET patients with advanced disease. The median times to progression were 14.3 months (vs 6.0 months) and not reached (vs 18 months), respectively.[58,59] There are no prospective studies supporting their use in the neoadjuvant setting, although they are occasionally used for this off-label purpose in patients who require symptom stabilization prior to an operation, or in patients who will eventually come to resection, are at risk for progression, but require perioperative optimization and thus have a planned delay.

Peptide Receptor Radionuclide Therapy

Radiolabeled SSAs were approved for use in patients with advanced GI NETs by the FDA in 2018. ^{177}Lutetium is a β- and γ-emitter that is conjugated to the DOTA linker on the SSA ((O)Tyr3) octreotate (DOTATATE), which is administered intravenously to treat widespread disease. The phase III trial (NETTER-1) comparing treatment with ^{177}Lu-DOTATATE versus high-dose long-acting octreotide in patients with low-grade, well-differentiated advanced midgut NETs demonstrated significantly improved PFS (median not reached in PRRT arm vs 8.4 months in octreotide arm). There was a response rate of 18% in the PRRT arm.[61] It is currently the most effective and reliable medical therapy for metastatic SBNETs. There is growing interest in using PRRT as a neoadjuvant therapy, but prospective trials have not been carried out. The majority of retrospective neoadjuvant studies have evaluated patients with pancreatic NET and included few or no patients with metastatic SBNET.

Hepatic Arterial Embolization & Chemoembolization

The rationale behind hepatic embolization of dominant liver metastases is that these tumors receive more than 80% of their blood supply from the hepatic arterial circulation. There are three distinct techniques for hepatic embolotherapy—microparticles alone (bland), chemoembolization (TACE, microparticles mixed with chemotherapy), and drug-eluting bead transarterial chemoembolization (DEB-TACE), although the superiority of one technique over another has not been conclusively demonstrated. There is a randomized trial ongoing to answer this question, but it should be noted that the DEB-TACE arm closed early due to unacceptable toxicity.[62] The most common adverse effect of hepatic embolization is "postembolization syndrome," which is self-limited and is characterized by pain, gastrointestinal distress, fever, leukocytosis, and transaminitis. Major complications such as renal failure, gallbladder perforation, cholangitis and liver abscess, or peptic ulcer hemorrhage are rare.[63] Liver necrosis is likewise rare, but associated with previous bile duct instrumentation or portal vein thrombosis.[64]

Selective Internal Radiation Therapy

Hepatic intra-arterial radioembolization is similar in technique to hepatic embolization, but rather than causing ischemia, delivers smaller particles conjugated to radioactive yttrium-90 (^{90}Y) to unresectable liver metastases. It is minimally embolic due to the size of the infused particle, allowing for more directed therapy and thus repeated treatments, which is advantageous for NET patients who may require multiple treatments over several years.[65] Treatment may result in objective radiographic responses, improved symptoms, decreased tumor marker levels, and also correlates with improved OS (mean 70 months).[66,67] Serious complications are rare, but care must be taken preoperatively to assess hepatic arterial anatomy and the potential for collateral vessels to the lung and stomach to minimize delivery of radioactive particles to nontarget organs. The most common complications are abdominal pain, nausea, vomiting, and fatigue. In one study where follow-up was greater than 1 year, treated patients developed imaging changes suggestive of cirrhosis and portal hypertension (29%). These patients were more likely to have developed transaminitis, but changes in total bilirubin, albumin, platelet count, or leukocyte count were not observed. The clinical relevance of these imaging changes was not defined,[67] but an ongoing controversy is whether patients who receive both radioembolization and PRRT have a higher potential for radiation-induced liver injury.

Everolimus

Everolimus is an inhibitor of the mammalian target of rapamycin (mTOR) pathway and was FDA-approved for use in well-differentiated, nonfunctional, advanced NETs in 2016. Evaluated for efficacy in this group in the prospective, phase III RADIANT-4 trial, everolimus was associated with a 52% decrease in the estimated risk of progression or death ($p < 0.00001$). The improvement of PFS in the everolimus group over placebo was relatively modest (11.0 vs 3.9 months). Severe side effects were present in less than 10% of the treated group, but included stomatitis, diarrhea, infections, anemia, fatigue, and hyperglycemia.[68]

PROGNOSIS

The prognosis of SBNETs is determined by the tumor's histopathologic characteristics and disease stage. When localized, patients with SBNETs have a median OS of approximately 14 years. Patients presenting with advanced SBNET (of all grades) demonstrate a median OS of nearly 6 years. If only well-differentiated G1/G2 advanced SBNETs are considered, the median OS increases to approximately 8.5 years.[1]

The duration of survival for these patients across stages emphasizes the prudent sequencing of therapies and the importance of experienced multidisciplinary teams in creating personalized treatment regimens.

REFERENCES

1. Dasari A, Shen C, Halperin D, et al. Trends in the incidence, prevalence, and survival outcomes in patients with neuroendocrine tumors in the United States. *JAMA Oncol.* 2017;3:1335-1342.
2. Pedersen KS, Raghav K, Overman MJ. Small bowel adenocarcinoma: Etiology, presentation, and molecular alterations. *J Natl Compr Canc Netw*. 2019;17:1135-1141.
3. Oberndorfer S. Karzinoide Tumoren Des Dundarms. *Frankf Z Pathol.* 1907;1:426-432.
4. Norlen O, Stalberg P, Oberg K, et al. Long-term results of surgery for small intestinal neuroendocrine tumors at a tertiary referral center. *World J Surg*. 2012;36:1419-1431.
5. Dahdaleh FS, Calva-Cerqueira D, Carr JC, et al. Comparison of clinicopathologic factors in 122 patients with resected pancreatic and ileal neuroendocrine tumors from a single institution. *Ann Surg Oncol.* 2012;19:966-972.
6. Maxwell JE, Sherman SK, Stashek KM, et al. A practical method to determine the site of unknown primary in metastatic neuroendocrine tumors. *Surgery*. 2014;156:1359-1365; discussion 1365-1356.
7. Bellizzi AM. An algorithmic immunohistochemical approach to define tumor type and assign site of origin. *Adv Anat Pathol.* 2020;27:114-163.
8. Bellizzi AM. Assigning site of origin in metastatic neuroendocrine neoplasms: a clinically significant application of diagnostic immunohistochemistry. *Adv Anat Pathol*. 2013;20:285-314.
9. Hassan MM, Phan A, Li D, et al. Risk factors associated with neuroendocrine tumors: a U.S.-based case-control study. *Int J Cancer*. 2008;123:867-873.
10. Haugvik S-P, Basim Ibrahim I, Hedenström P, et al. Smoking, alcohol and family history of cancer as risk factors for small intestinal neuroendocrine tumors: a systematic review and meta-analysis. *Scand J Gastroenterol*. 2017;52:797-802.
11. Sei Y, Zhao X, Forbes J, et al. A hereditary form of small intestinal carcinoid associated with a germline mutation in inositol polyphosphate multikinase. *Gastroenterology*. 2015;149:67-78.
12. Klimstra DS, Modlin IR, Coppola D, et al. The pathologic classification of neuroendocrine tumors: a review of nomenclature, grading, and staging systems. *Pancreas*. 2010;39:707-712.
13. Vinik AI, Woltering EA, Warner RRP, et al. Nanets consensus guidelines for the diagnosis of neuroendocrine tumor. *Pancreas*. 2010;39:713-734.
14. Tran CG, Sherman SK, Scott AT, et al. It is time to rethink biomarkers for surveillance of small bowel neuroendocrine tumors. *Ann Surg Oncol*. 2021;28:732-741.
15. Vezzosi D, Walter T, Laplanche A, et al. Chromogranin A measurement in metastatic well-differentiated gastroenteropancreatic neuroendocrine carcinoma: screening for false positives and a prospective follow-up study. *Int J Biol Markers*. 2011;26:94-101.
16. Mahata SK, Corti A. Chromogranin A and its fragments in cardiovascular, immunometabolic, and cancer regulation. *Ann N Y Acad Sci*. 2019;1455:34-58.
17. Zandee WT, Kamp K, van Adrichem RC, et al. Effect of hormone secretory syndromes on neuroendocrine tumor prognosis. *Endocr Relat Cancer*. 2017;24:R261-R274.
18. Maxwell JE, O'Dorisio TM, Howe JR. Biochemical diagnosis and preoperative imaging of gastroenteropancreatic neuroendocrine tumors. *Surg Oncol Clin N Am*. 2016;25:171-194.
19. Turner GB, Johnston BT, McCance DR, et al. Circulating markers of prognosis and response to treatment in patients with midgut carcinoid tumours. *Gut*. 2006;55:1586-1591.
20. O'Dorisio TM, Krutzik SR, Woltering EA, et al. Development of a highly sensitive and specific carboxy-terminal human pancreastatin assay to monitor neuroendocrine tumor behavior. *Pancreas*. 2010;39:611-616.
21. Sherman SK, Maxwell JE, O'Dorisio MS, et al. Pancreastatin predicts survival in neuroendocrine tumors. *Ann Surg Oncol.* 2014;21:2971-2980.
22. Modlin IM, Kidd M, Malczewska A, et al. The NETest: the clinical utility of multigene blood analysis in the diagnosis and management of neuroendocrine tumors. *Endocrinol Metabol Clin N Am*. 2018;47:485-504.
23. Modlin IM, Kidd M, Bodei L, et al. The clinical utility of a novel blood-based multi-transcriptome assay for the diagnosis of neuroendocrine tumors of the gastrointestinal tract. *Am J Gastroenterol*. 2015;110:1223-1232.
24. Modlin IM, Frilling A, Salem RR, et al. Blood measurement of neuroendocrine gene transcripts defines the effectiveness of operative resection and ablation strategies. *Surgery*. 2016;159:336-347.
25. Bellutti M, Fry LC, Schmitt J, et al. Detection of neuroendocrine tumors of the small bowel by double balloon enteroscopy. *Dig Dis Sci*. 2009;54:1050-1058.
26. van Tuyl SA, van Noorden JT, Timmer R, et al. Detection of small-bowel neuroendocrine tumors by video capsule endoscopy. *Gastrointest Endosc*. 2006;64:66-72.
27. Yoon JY, Kumta NA, Kim MK. The role of endoscopy in small bowel neuroendocrine tumors. *Clin Endosc*. 2021;54:818-824.
28. Dromain C, de Baere T, Lumbroso J, et al. Detection of liver metastases from endocrine tumors: a prospective comparison of somatostatin receptor scintigraphy, computed tomography, and magnetic resonance imaging. *J Clin Oncol*. 2005;23:70-78.
29. Krenning EP, Kwekkeboom DJ, Bakker WH, et al. Somatostatin receptor scintigraphy with [111in-Dtpa-D-Phe1]- and [123i-Tyr3]-Octreotide: the rotterdam experience with more than 1000 patients. *Eur J Nucl Med*. 1993;20:716-731.
30. Hope TA, Bergsland E, Bozkurt MF, et al. Appropriate use criteria for somatostatin receptor pet imaging in neuroendocrine tumors. *J Nucl Med*. 2018;59:66-74.
31. Hassan SA, Palaskas NL, Agha AM, et al. Carcinoid heart disease: a comprehensive review. *Curr Cardiol Rep*. 2019;21:140.
32. Davar J, Connolly HM, Caplin ME, et al. Diagnosing and managing carcinoid heart disease in patients with neuroendocrine tumors: an expert statement. *J Am Coll Cardiol.* 2017;69:1288-1304.
33. Connolly HM, Nishimura RA, Smith HC, et al. Outcome of cardiac surgery for carcinoid heart disease. *J Am Coll Cardiol.* 1995;25:410-416.
34. Connolly HM, Schaff HV, Abel MD, et al. Early and late outcomes of surgical treatment in carcinoid heart disease. *J Am Coll Cardiol*. 2015;66:2189-2196.
35. Condron ME, Pommier SJ, Pommier RF. Continuous infusion of octreotide combined with perioperative octreotide bolus does not prevent intraoperative carcinoid crisis. *Surgery*. 2016;159:358-365.
36. Fouche M, Bouffard Y, Le Goff MC, et al. Intraoperative carcinoid syndrome during small-bowel neuroendocrine tumour surgery. *Endocr Connect*. 2018;7:1245-1250.

37. Kinney MAO, Nagorney DM, Clark DF, et al. Partial hepatic resections for metastatic neuroendocrine tumors: perioperative outcomes. *J Clin Anesth*. 2018;51:93-96.
38. Choi AB, Maxwell JE, Keck KJ, et al. Is multifocality an indicator of aggressive behavior in small bowel neuroendocrine tumors? *Pancreas*. 2017;46:1115-1120.
39. Keck KJ, Maxwell JE, Utria AF, et al. The distal predilection of small bowel neuroendocrine tumors. *Ann Surg Oncol*. 2018;25:3207-3213.
40. Edge SB, Byrd DR, Compton CC, et al. *AJCC Cancer Staging Manual*. 7th ed. New York, NY: Springer; 2010.
41. Katz MH, Fleming JB, Pisters PW, et al. Anatomy of the superior mesenteric vein with special reference to the surgical management of first-order branch involvement at pancreaticoduodenectomy. *Ann Surg*. 2008;248:1098-1102.
42. Niederhuber JE, Fojo T. Treatment of metastatic disease in patients with neuroendocrine tumors. *Surg Oncol Clin N Am*. 2006;15:511-533, viii.
43. Howe JR, Cardona K, Fraker DL, et al. The surgical management of small bowel neuroendocrine tumors: consensus guidelines of the North American neuroendocrine tumor society. *Pancreas*. 2017;46:715-731.
44. Bennett S, Coburn N, Law C, et al. Upfront small bowel resection for small bowel neuroendocrine tumors with synchronous metastases: a propensity-score matched comparative population-based analysis. *Ann Surg*. 2022;276(5):e450-e458.
45. Ahmed A, Turner G, King B, et al. Midgut neuroendocrine tumours with liver metastases: results of the ukinets study. *Endocr Relat Cancer*. 2009;16:885-894.
46. Almond LM, Hodson J, Ford SJ, et al. Role of palliative resection of the primary tumour in advanced pancreatic and small intestinal neuroendocrine tumours: a systematic review and meta-analysis. *Eur J Surg Oncol*. 2017;43:1808-1815.
47. Daskalakis K, Karakatsanis A, Hessman O, et al. Association of a prophylactic surgical approach to stage IV small intestinal neuroendocrine tumors with survival. *JAMA Oncol*. 2018;4:183.
48. Woltering EA, Voros BA, Beyer DT, et al. Aggressive surgical approach to the management of neuroendocrine tumors: a report of 1,000 surgical cytoreductions by a single institution. *J Am Coll Surg*. 2017;224:434-447.
49. Maxwell JE, Sherman SK, O'Dorisio TM, et al. Liver-directed surgery of neuroendocrine metastases: what is the optimal strategy? *Surgery*. 2016;159:320-333.
50. Scott AT, Breheny PJ, Keck KJ, et al. Effective cytoreduction can be achieved in patients with numerous neuroendocrine tumor liver metastases (Netlms). *Surgery*. 2019;165:166-175.
51. Ejaz A, Reames BN, Maithel S, et al. Cytoreductive debulking surgery among patients with neuroendocrine liver metastasis: a multi-institutional analysis. HPB. 2018;20:277-284.
52. Akyildiz HY, Mitchell J, Milas M, et al. Laparoscopic radiofrequency thermal ablation of neuroendocrine hepatic metastases: long-term follow-up. *Surgery*. 2010;148:1288-1293; discussion 1293.
53. Wonn SM, Limbach KE, Pommier SJ, et al. Outcomes of cytoreductive operations for peritoneal carcinomatosis with or without liver cytoreduction in patients with small bowel neuroendocrine tumors. *Surgery*. 2021;169:168-174.
54. Mazzaferro V, Sposito C, Coppa J, et al. The long-term benefit of liver transplantation for hepatic metastases from neuroendocrine tumors. *Am J Transplant*. 2016;16:2892-2902.
55. Mazzaferro V, Pulvirenti A, Coppa J. Neuroendocrine tumors metastatic to the liver: how to select patients for liver transplantation? *J Hepatol*. 2007;47:460-466.
56. Coppa J, Pulvirenti A, Schiavo M, et al. Resection versus transplantation for liver metastases from neuroendocrine tumors. *Transplant Proc*. 2002;33:1537-1539.
57. Moris D, Tsilimigras DI, Ntanasis-Stathopoulos I, et al. Liver transplantation in patients with liver metastases from neuroendocrine tumors: a systematic review. *Surgery*. 2017;162:525-536.
58. Rinke A, Muller HH, Schade-Brittinger C, et al. Placebo-controlled, double-blind, prospective, randomized study on the effect of octreotide lar in the control of tumor growth in patients with metastatic neuroendocrine midgut tumors: a report from the promid study group. *J Clin Oncol*. 2009;27:4656-4663.
59. Caplin ME, Pavel M, Cwikla JB, et al. Lanreotide in metastatic enteropancreatic neuroendocrine tumors. *N Engl J Med*. 2014;371:224-233.
60. Vinik AI, Chaya C. Clinical presentation and diagnosis of neuroendocrine tumors. *Hematol Oncol Clin N Am*. 2016;30:21-48.
61. Strosberg J, El-Haddad G, Wolin E, et al. Phase 3 Trial of (177) Lu-dotatate for midgut neuroendocrine tumors. *N Engl J Med*. 2017;376:125-135.
62. Chen JX, Wileyto EP, Soulen MC. Randomized embolization trial for neuroendocrine tumor metastases to the liver (Retnet): study protocol for a randomized controlled trial. *Trials*. 2018;19:390.
63. O'Toole D, Ruszniewski P. Chemoembolization and other ablative therapies for liver metastases of gastrointestinal endocrine tumours. *Best Pract Res Clin Gastroenterol*. 2005;19:585-594.
64. Joskin J, de Baere T, Auperin A, et al. Predisposing factors of liver necrosis after transcatheter arterial chemoembolization in liver metastases from neuroendocrine tumor. *Cardiovasc Intervent Radiol*. 2015;38:372-380.
65. Padia SA. Y90 clinical data update: cholangiocarcinoma, neuroendocrine tumor, melanoma, and breast cancer metastatic disease. *Tech Vasc Interv Radiol*. 2019;22:81-86.
66. Kennedy AS, Dezarn WA, McNeillie P, et al. Radioembolization for unresectable neuroendocrine hepatic metastases using resin 90y-microspheres: early results in 148 patients. *Am J Clin Oncol*. 2008;31:271-279.
67. D'Souza D, Golzarian J, Young S. Interventional liver-directed therapy for neuroendocrine metastases: current status and future directions. *Curr Treat Options Oncol*. 2020;21:52.
68. Yao JC, Fazio N, Singh S, et al. Everolimus for the treatment of advanced, non-functional neuroendocrine tumours of the lung or gastrointestinal tract (Radiant-4): a randomised, placebo-controlled, phase 3 study. *Lancet*. 2016;387:968-977.

62 Neuroendocrine Tumors of the Large Intestine: Colon, Rectum, & Appendix

Arthur G. Affleck IV, MD
Rodney F. Pommier, MD, FACS

INTRODUCTION

Neuroendocrine tumors (NETs) are caused by malignant transformation of epithelial cells within the neuroendocrine system that play an integral role in regulating secretions and motility of the gut. NETs can arise in most organs. Many clinical features and characteristics are unique to the site of origin. For many years these neoplasms were referred to as carcinoids, the term first coined as *karzinoid* by Oberndofer in 1907. The North American Neuroendocrine Tumor Society (NANETS) and European Neuroendocrine Tumor Society (ENETS), the two main NET societies, both use "neuroendocrine tumor" or "NET" as the preferable term, followed by the site of origin. NET has a similar incidence to other cancers that affect the central nervous system. In addition, the prevalence of gastroenteropancreatic neuroendocrine tumors (GEP-NETs) is higher than most gastrointestinal cancers, including pancreatic, esophageal, gastric, hepatobiliary, exceeded by colorectal neoplasia. This book chapter will focus on NETs of the large intestine including the colon, rectum, and appendix.

EPIDEMIOLOGY

Colonic & Rectal Nets

NETs of the colon and rectum are known as *hindgut carcinoids* based on their embryologic origins. Colorectal NETs are quite rare, but their incidences are increasing. The surveillance, epidemiology, and end results (SEER) program database was established in 1973 to provide representative cancer incidences and assess survival rates in the United States and Europe.[1] The SEER program covers approximately 15% of the population of the United States and provides data on 5,553,822 cancer cases diagnosed from 1973 to 2007. The SEER database recorded an increase in incidence of colon NETs in the United States from 0.3 new cases per 100,000 per year from 1973 to 1977 to 0.6 new cases per 100,000 per year from 2004 to 2007. It has also seen a 10-fold increase in rectal NETs in the last 35 years. The incidence of rectal NETs increased from 0.09 new cases per 100,000 per year from 1973 to 1977 to 0.97 new cases per 100,000 per year from 2004 to 2007, according to the SEER data.[1]

In the SEER 17 registry (2000-2007), more than half of all NETs were GEP-NETs (61.0%). The rectum and small intestine were the most common primary sites, which account for 17.7% and 17.3%, respectively, of all NETs. The total number of NETs at both of these sites has increased markedly. Colon NETs account for approximately 10.1% of all NETs in the United States of America (USA). Rectal NETs have been shown to have a racial predominance in those of African American (black) and Asian backgrounds. African American patients are 2.3 times more likely to develop rectal NETs than their white counterparts, and Asians are 4.9 times more likely than non-Asians. In Europe and the USA, rectal NETs are between 5% and 27% of all GEP-NETs, while in Japan the incidence of rectal NETs can be as high as 60% of the total.[2]

Appendiceal NETs

The appendix embryologically arises from the midgut, which also encompasses the jejunum, ileum, cecum, ascending, and proximal transverse colon. Appendiceal NETs account for approximately 3.4% of all NETs. The SEER 17 registry (2000-2007) database estimates an incidence of 0.2 new cases per 100,000 annually for appendiceal NETs.[1]

CLINICAL FEATURES

The majority of neuroendocrine tumors of the appendix, colon, and rectum are asymptomatic at time of diagnosis. They are commonly found incidentally on routine endoscopy or at time of surgery. Classic carcinoid syndrome symptoms like flushing and diarrhea are exceedingly rare in colorectal NETs.

Colonic NETs

The average age at diagnosis is 65 years for colon NETs. Most tumors arise in the cecum, followed by ileocecal region, and ascending colon. Symptoms usually only arise with larger tumors (>2 cm) due to the high capacitance of the cecum and ascending colon.[3] When patients with colon NETs have symptoms, they usually include diarrhea, abdominal pain, and/or gastrointestinal (GI) hemorrhage. Obstruction is possible but is exceedingly rare. Patients with colon NETs are typically older with larger tumors that are at an advanced stage at time of diagnosis. Up to 30% to 40% will have distant metastasis at time of diagnosis. Sites of metastasis include the liver, lymph nodes, mesentery, and peritoneum.[3,4]

Rectal NETs

Rectal NETs are less likely to have distant metastasis at time of diagnosis. Sites of metastasis include bone, liver, and lymph nodes. The average age at diagnosis is 56 years. When symptoms are present, bright red blood per rectum is most common. Anorectal symptoms of pain and tenesmus are possible, but rarely seen. More than half of rectal NETs are diagnosed on routine lower endoscopy for surveillance or investigation of unrelated symptoms.[3,4]

Appendiceal NETs

The majority of appendiceal NETs are diagnosed incidentally at the tip of the appendix on pathology after an appendectomy. When located in the proximal or mid appendix, they can cause obstruction leading to appendicitis, though this is uncommon. Functional symptoms secondary to carcinoid syndromes are very rare. Appendiceal NETs are the most common tumor of the appendix, constituting more than 50% of appendiceal neoplasms. They are typically diagnosed in young patients aged 30 to 40.[5,6]

DIAGNOSIS & STAGING

The vast majority of colorectal NETs are diagnosed incidentally on endoscopy evaluation for colorectal cancer or other unrelated symptoms. Colonoscopy remains the gold standard for evaluation of any colorectal lesion. Colonic lesions are often tattooed to help localize lesion if a resection is required based on pathology results. If considering resection for any colorectal or appendiceal NETs a complete colonoscopy should be performed to rule out synchronous lesions or concomitant carcinoma, as this could change surgical management. Most rectal NETs arise in the mid-rectum, 5 to 10 cm above the anal verge. Most of these lesions appear as smooth, beige/yellow-colored, submucosal bulges.[3] Scarring or ulceration could be signs of advanced tumor invasion with a higher rate of lymph node spread.

When a rectal NET is discovered, a full colonoscopy must be performed for proper staging and to rule out concomitant colonic disease and/or synchronous carcinoma. Endoscopic ultrasonography is very useful in evaluating the depth of invasion and local nodal status of rectal NETs. Multiphasic computerized tomography (CT) is the best modality for staging the thorax, abdomen, and pelvis with a sensitivity of 80% to 90%. MRI can help differentiate between uncertain lesions in the liver. Large rectal lesions (>2 cm) should undergo pelvic MRI if considering resection.[3]

Functional imaging studies detecting the somatostatin receptor (SSTR) have revolutionized the detection of NETs. The radio-labeled somatostatin analog Ga-68 tetraazacyclododecanetetraacetic acid-DPhe1-Tyr3-oc-treotate (Ga^{68} DOTATATE) has been shown to have superior affinity to the SSTR compared to Indium-111 (I^{111}) pentetreotide (Octreotide scan), thus providing increased sensitivity and special resolution in the detection of NETs.[7,8] Patients with SSTR-expressing tumors confirmed by Ga^{68} DOTATATE CT/positron emission tomography (PET) can be eligible for alternative medical treatments such as peptide receptor radionucleotide therapy (PRRT). Ga^{68} DOTATATE CT/PET has replaced I^{111} pentetreotide scan as the gold standard for imaging of well-differentiated NETs. Only tumors expressing the SSTR can benefit from this imaging modality and/or PRRT. One study showed they could increase the expression of SSTRs with administration of histone deacetylase (HDAC) inhibitors to pancreatic NETs with little to no SSTR expression initially.[7,8] Determining the utility of this requires further randomized trials; however, it could be promising in the evaluation/treatment of colorectal NETs, as the expression of the SSTR is typically low.

Colorectal NETs have their own TNM classification system. T1 tumors are confined to the submucosa and are <2 cm in size. T1a refers to lesions <1 cm, T1b refers to lesions 1 to 2 cm. T2 tumors either invade the muscularis propria or are >2 cm, or both. T3 and T4 are identical to the T-staging in colorectal adenocarcinoma, with T3 lesions involving the peri-colorectal tissues and T4 lesions penetrating the visceral peritoneum (Table 62-1).

Appendiceal NETs are staged based on size and depth of invasion T1: ≤2 cm; T2: >2 cm and ≤4 cm; T3: >4 cm or there is an invasion into serosa or the mesoappendix regardless of size; and T4: serosal perforation or direct invasion of adjacent organs. Serum serotonin and 5-hydroxyindoleacetic acid (5-HIAA; a byproduct of serotonin) are some common markers associated with many NETs but have little utility in colorectal NETs. These tumors rarely produce serotonin or other bioactive hormones. Chromogranin A/B can be elevated in patients with metastatic disease. Chromogranin A can also be falsely elevated by patients on proton pump inhibitors (PPIs). PPIs should be stopped at least 1 month before drawing levels. Rectal NETs can show elevated carcinoembryonic antigen (CEA) and prostate-specific antigen

Table 62–1. Staging of NETs of the Colon and Rectum based on the American Joint Committee on Cancer (AJCC).

Stage	Primary Tumor (T)		
Tx	Primary tumor cannot be assessed		
T0	No evidence of primary tumor		
T1	Tumor invades mucosa or submucosa and size ≤2 cm		
T1a	Tumor size <1 cm		
T1b	Tumor size 1-2 cm		
T2	Tumor invades muscularis propria or size >2 cm		
T3	Tumor invades muscularis propria into subserosa or pericolic or perirectal tissue		
T4	Tumor invades visceral peritoneum or other organs		
	Regional Lymph Nodes (N)		
Nx	Regional lymph nodes cannot be assessed		
N0	No regional lymph node involvement		
N1	Regional lymph node metastasis present		
	Distant Metastases (M)		
M0	No distant metastasis		
M1	Distant metastasis		
Stage	**T**	**N**	**M**
I	T1	N0	M0
IIA	T2	N0	M0
IIB	T3	N0	M0
IIIA	T4	N0	M0
IIIB	Any T	N1	M0
IV	Any T	Any N	M1

(PSA), but these markers are mostly used as a means for surveillance, not diagnosis (Table 62-2).[5]

PATHOLOGY & PROGNOSIS

Colonic NETs

According to the WHO 2019 classification of gastrointestinal tumors in the colon are subdivided into NET, neuroendocrine carcinomas (NEC), and mixed-neuroendocrine non-neuroendocrine neoplasms (MiNECs). MiNECs are mixed neoplasms that demonstrate morphologic characteristics of both neuroendocrine and non-neuroendocrine components.[9,10] The non-neuroendocrine components usually correspond with adenocarcinoma. The neuroendocrine component can be NET or NEC. NEC and MiNEC are aggressive neoplasms, but are extremely rare. NETs are histologically classified by differentiation and grade (G). The differentiation is a reflection of the cells' appearance under the microscope which provides insight into how the tumor will behave. Grade is a reflection of how fast tumor cells are dividing and growing measured by mitotic index and/or Ki-67 index. Mitotic index is calculated by counting the number of dividing cells (cells in mitosis) within a certain

Table 62–2. Staging of NETs of the appendix based on the AJCC.

Stage	Primary Tumor (T)		
Tx	Primary tumor cannot be assessed		
T0	No evidence of primary tumor		
T1	Size ≤2 cm		
T2	Size >2 cm and ≤4 cm		
T3	Size >4 cm or invades sub-serosa or mesoappendix regardless of size		
T4	Serosal perforation or direct invasion of adjacent organs		
T4a	Tumor invades visceral peritoneum		
T4b	Tumor invades other organs		
	Regional Lymph Nodes (N)		
Nx	Regional lymph nodes cannot be assessed		
N0	No regional lymph node involvement		
N1	Regional lymph node metastasis present		
	Distant Metastases (M)		
M0	No distant metastasis		
M1	Distant metastasis		
Stage	**T**	**N**	**M**
I	T1	N0	M0
II	T2-T3	N0	M0
III	T4	N0	M0
	Any T	N1	M0
IV	Any T	Any N	M1

amount of tissue. Ki-67 index uses the MIB1 monoclonal antibody to stain tumor cell nuclei, then the index is calculated as the percentage of positive tumor cell nuclei in "hot spots" (500-200 cells). G1 tumors have a mitotic count <2 per 10 high-power fields (HPF) and/or Ki-67 <2%. G2 tumors have a mitotic count 2 to 20 per 10 HPF and/or Ki-67 3-20%. G3 tumors have a mitotic count >20 per 10 HPF and/or Ki67 >20%.[10] The biological behavior of well- to moderately differentiated (G1 to G2) NETs are typically indolent, while poorly differentiated NETs (G3) are highly aggressive like NECs and MiNECs. Transformation from low- to high-grade in well-differentiated NETs has been reported, though this is rare and there is not enough evidence to determine their biologic behavior. NECs can be subdivided into small- and large-cell subtypes, large cell being more common in the colon. The colon is the most common site for MiNENs. Histological and immunohistochemical panels are required to differentiate these from poorly differentiated adenocarcinoma.

Colonic NETs have the lowest overall 5-year survival rate of any GEP-NETs at 62%. The 5-year survival rate varies depending on anatomic site and stage at diagnosis; localized disease averages, 76%; regional disease, 71.6%; and tumors with distant metastasis, 30%. The five-year survival rate in tumors located at the cecum is 68%.[9-11]

Rectal NETs

Size is a very important prognostic factor for rectal NETs. The risk of metastasis in tumors <1 cm is 2%. The risk for tumors 1 to 2 cm is 10% to 15%, and tumor size >2 cm markedly increases the metastatic risk to 60% to 80%. The depth of invasion is also an influential factor. Rectal tumors <2 cm showed a risk of metastasis of 2%, with no invasion. The risk of metastasis climbs to 48% with invasion of the muscularis propria present.[11]

Appendiceal NETs

According to the WHO 2019 classification of gastrointestinal tumors in the appendix is also subdivided into NET, NEC, and MiNEC. Appendiceal NETs are also histologically classified by differentiation and grade, where well-differentiated (G1 to G2) account for 80% of cases. Additionally, poorly differentiated (G3) NEC and MiNEC can occur.[6,10]

The prognosis of appendiceal NETs in general is excellent. This is highly influenced by the size and location of the tumor, as well as the presence of lymphovascular and mesoappendix invasion. Appendiceal NETs <1 cm have a 5-year survival rate of 95%. For tumors >2 cm the 5-year survival drops to 70.5%. The majority of appendiceal NETs are located at the tip of the appendix, with only 10% located at the base. Appendiceal NETs are fairly common and do not typically behave aggressively, and most can be cured with appendectomy alone.[6] NEC and MiNEC are aggressive neoplasms; however, these are extremely rare. Prognostic data for these lesions are limited due to the scarcity of the lesions themselves and variable results from the few trials that have investigated them.

ENDOSCOPIC & SURGICAL TREATMENTS

Colonic NETs

Treatment of colorectal NETs is determined by the size of the primary lesion. Colonic lesions <1 cm can be safely excised endoscopically as their risk of lymph node metastasis is low (4%). If lymph node metastasis is present, a segmental colectomy with regional lymphadenectomy is required. Lesions 1 to 2 cm have a 61.5% risk of lymph node metastasis. Patients with high-grade lesions, or if the nodal status is unclear, should undergo surgical resection. Colonic NETs >2 cm are not infrequently discovered. Tumors >2 cm, or if they invade the muscularis propria, should undergo formal segmental colectomy with oncologic lymphadenectomy, similar to what is recommended for adenocarcinoma.[4]

Rectal NETs

Compared to colonic lesions, rectal lesions demonstrate an even lower risk of metastatic spread; therefore, small tumors <1 cm confined only to the mucosa or submucosa can be safely locally excised (endoscopic polypectomy or transanal excision). Tumors <1 cm only require complete excision usually via endoscopic polypectomy. One study demonstrated no recurrences after conventional endoscopic resection in patients with tumors <1 cm that did not invade past the submucosa.[12] There still is a possibility of positive margins after conventional endoscopic resection. However, these lesions do not require negative margins, further resection, workup, or surveillance. Multiple alternative endoscopic techniques have been described such as band ligation, endoscopic submucosal dissection, and aspiration lumpectomy to name a few. Submucosal lesions between 1 and 2 cm should be tattooed after excision in the event a malignant rectal NET is present which may require further intervention. Once the excision site has healed, re-identification of this site can be nearly impossible. For intermittent-sized tumors limited to the submucosa, transanal excision is commonly performed. T2 tumors with invasion in the muscularis propria with endoscopic ultrasound (EUS)-proven lack of nodal involvement are also amenable to transanal excision. Transanal endoscopic microsurgery (TEM) is a minimally invasive technique that provides improved visualization, exposure, and magnification which enables accurate full-thickness resections. TEM can be used to excise lesions up to 20 cm from the anal verge. TEM is often used for 1 to 2 cm lesions that are difficult to excise by conventional means or for excising residual positive margins after polypectomy.[13]

Tumors >2 cm, with invasion of the muscularis propria, or locoregional lymph node involvement should be managed similarly to rectal adenocarcinoma, with TME and low anterior resection or abdominoperineal resection depending on the distance from the anal verge.

Appendiceal NETs

Based on guidelines from NANETS, most appendiceal NETs less than 1 cm can be safely treated with appendectomy. Additionally, tumors less than 2 cm located in the mid to distal appendix with no high-risk features can be safely treated with appendectomy alone. For tumors larger than 2 cm, 1 to 2 cm with mesoappendix invasion, positive regional lymph nodes, high-risk histology (goblet cell carcinoid), or presence of positive margins a right hemicolectomy with regional lymphadenectomy is recommended.[3,5]

POSTOPERATIVE SURVEILLANCE

Recurrence in colorectal NETs can occur many years after resection. Long-term surveillance is often suggested, even though there is a lack of objective data to support this. Many believe that small (<2 cm) T1 tumors limited to the submucosa have a low risk of metastasis, therefore, usually do not require long-term surveillance. T2 or T3 tumors with invasion into or beyond the muscularis propria or positive regional lymph nodes typically undergo long-term endoscopic and radiographic surveillance. The ENETS guidelines recommend tumors 1 to 2 cm or with high-grade features should undergo annual follow-up with endoscopy, EUS, and cross-sectional imaging of the chest, abdomen, and pelvis. High-grade (G3) tumors >2 cm should undergo follow-up with endoscopy, EUS, and cross-sectional imaging in 4 to 6 months in the first year, then annually thereafter. ENETS recommends surveillance for 10 years; NANETS recommends surveillance for 7 years. Chromogranin A/B can be used in surveillance.[3,13]

For appendiceal NETs <2 cm limited to the appendix and treated with appendectomy, no postoperative surveillance is necessary. Tumors with high-risk features such as lymph node positivity that were treated with a hemicolectomy should follow up in 3 to 6 months after resection with CT imaging and chromogranin testing, then 6 to 12 months thereafter, for up to 10 years.[3,13]

TREATMENT OF METASTATIC DISEASE

Surgical Therapies

There are few published randomized trials on management of metastatic colorectal NETs. Recommendations are extrapolated from trials of other GEP-NETs. With the liver being the most common location of distant metastasis, hepatic resection is often considered. Retrospective studies suggest that patients with neuroendocrine tumor liver metastasis (NETLM) who undergo hepatic resection or cytoreduction achieve the best long-term outcomes with improved symptom relief and prolonged survival compared to those not undergoing resection. Five-year survival rate can be as high as 60% to 80% in select patients. One large single-institution review of patients with pancreatic NET with liver metastasis undergoing hepatic resection reported a 5-,10-, and 20-year overall survival (OS) rates of 67%, 51%, and 36%, respectively. Typically the goal of resection is to control disease. Recurrence after resection is common even with a complete resection (R0). One study showed a recurrence of up to 94% in a series of 339 patients who underwent resection for NETLMs.[12,14] The accuracy of cross-sectional imaging and somatostatin receptor for hepatic metastasis <2 cm ranges from 20% to 30%. These data suggest that the high rate of recurrence may be because many patients have unrecognized small metastasis at the time of resection. Mayo and colleagues showed that R0 or R1 (positive microscopic margins) resection was associated with improved overall survival (OS) compared to R2 (gross residual tumor) resection.[15] They also found that margin status was not associated with a significant difference in the rate of recurrence. The NANETS recommends pursuing surgical cytoreduction even when complete resection is not possible. Several studies have demonstrated that debulking 70% or more of gross disease improves symptoms and extends progression-free survival.[15]

For patients with synchronous resectable liver metastasis, resection of the primary tumor either in a staged or combined approach is recommended. Resection of the primary tumor in patients with unresectable metastatic disease depends on the site, functional status, and severity of symptoms caused by the primary. Primary midgut and hindgut NETs potentially can cause obstruction, mesenteric ischemia, and/or GI hemorrhages, and therefore these patients may benefit from a resection even with unresectable metastases. There is no clear evidence showing a benefit of prophylactic resection of a primary NET in the setting of unresectable metastatic disease at this time.

Heated intraperitoneal chemotherapy (HIPEC) is used for cytoreduction of many neoplasms with peritoneal metastasis, but is not currently recommended for treatment of NET peritoneal metastasis. Studies have found a high recurrence rate in patients with NETLM who have undergone liver transplantation; therefore, the role of liver transplant remains controversial.[14]

Medical Therapies

Traditional treatments include somatostatin analogs, interferon alpha (INF-α), and liver-directed therapies to name a few. Somatostatin analogs (SSAs), such as octreotide and lanreotide, work to inhibit symptoms of carcinoid syndrome by inhibiting the secretion of serotonin and other hormones. New evidence also suggests that SSAs can exert an antiproliferative effect and inhibit tumor growth. This was demonstrated in the PROMID trial (placebo-controlled, double-blind, prospective randomized study on the effect of octreotide LAR in the control of tumor growth in patients with metastatic neuroendocrine midgut tumors), a randomized, double-blinded, placebo-controlled clinical trial that showed a significant prolongation in time to tumor progression in patients with metastatic midgut NETs treated with octreotide long-acting repeatable (LAR).[16] Hindgut NETs were not included in these trials. The controlled lanreotide antiproliferative response in neuroendocrine tumors (CLARINET) trial investigated the antiproliferative effects of the long-acting SSA lanreotide in more than 200 patients with nonfunctioning, somatostatin receptor-positive, metastatic enteropancreatic neuroendocrine tumors. This randomized, double-blinded, and multicentered trial showed statistically significant prolonged progression-free survival (PFS) in the group that received lanreotide compared to placebo. Unlike the PROMID trial, the CLARINET trial did include hindgut NETs in their study. Lanreotide is FDA approved for treatment of all GEP-NETs.[17,18]

Everolimus is an oral inhibitor of mammalian target of rapamycin (mTOR) which has been previously shown to have antiproliferative effects on nonpancreatic NETs. The RAD001 in advanced neuroendocrine tumors, fourth trial (RADIANT-4) compared oral everolimus to placebo in advanced, nonfunctioning NET of the lung and gastrointestinal organs (mid- and hindgut). They demonstrated that treatment with everolimus prolonged median PFS by 7.1 months compared to placebo. This study confirms the role of the mTOR pathway in the treatment of lung and gastrointestinal NETs.[19]

PRRT utilizes a radioisotope-labeled somatostatin analog that is a highly effective treatment for many forms of metastatic, well-differentiated, low to intermediate grade of tumors that show a high level of expression of somatostatin receptors 2 and 5. The phase III neuroendocrine tumors therapy (NETTER-1) trial is the only prospective randomized study that evaluated the efficacy of the PRRT ^{177}Lu-DOTATATE plus high-dose SSA compared to high-dose SSA alone in patients with progressive somatostatin-receptor positive midgut NETs.[20] They showed patients treated with ^{177}Lu-DOTATATE plus high-dose SSA had improved PFS compared to high-dose SSAs in metastatic midgut NETs (20 months mean follow-up, progression-free survival was 65.2% for PRRT compared to 10.8%, respectively). Although only midgut NETs were evaluated in this trial, the FDA approved it for use of all progressing GEP-NETs.[20-23] The ENETS currently recommends the use of PRRT in intestinal (midgut) NETs with distant and/or locoregional metastasis as a second- or third-line agent in patients who have progressed on SSAs. The antiproliferative effects of SSA and PRRT are unknown in colorectal NETs. Octreotide LAR and PRRT should be considered for treatment of metastatic colorectal NETs that are proven to have a high level of somatostatin receptor expression. Further randomized clinical trials are needed to determine the true role of these agents in the treatment of colorectal NETs. INF-α agents also have antisecretory and antiproliferative properties; however, these agents often have significant dose-dependent toxicities.

Liver-directed ablation techniques, such as radiofrequency ablation (RFA) and microwave ablation (MWA), are hyperthermic procedures that apply energy to heat tissue to at least 60°C to cause necrosis.[24] Cryotherapy ablation applies energy to cool tissue to −40°C for the same intended effect. RFA and MWA are commonly used to treat primary and metastatic liver lesions. Ablation can be used as an adjunct to resection to improve cytoreduction by targeting smaller (<3 cm) lesions that may not be amendable to resection, while minimizing the loss of normal liver tissue. Compared to RFA, MWA provides a greater zone of necrosis and reduced procedure time due to increased delivery of heat to the target tissue. However, because of this MWA poses a higher risk of complications. Ablation is not recommended for lesions near vital structures or tumors greater than 5 cm in diameter due to increased risk of complications, largely damaging adjacent nontarget organs. RFA and MWA can be performed under ultrasound guidance intraoperatively or via interventional radiology. Based on studies on hepatocellular carcinoma, RFA is the most commonly used ablative technique due to its safety, tolerability, and efficacy.[24]

Liver-directed therapies such as transarterial embolization (TAE) or chemoembolization (TACE) are often considered with the presence of symptomatic hepatic metastasis. The hepatic arteries are thought to be the main source of blood to hepatic tumors. Selective embolization of the hepatic arteries has been shown to improve symptoms and radiographic response. TAE injects small particles intravascularly to obstruct the artery and cause tumor cell ischemia. TACE injects cytotoxic chemotherapy (such as doxorubicin and streptozoin) into the artery before embolization to trigger the same affect, with the idea that ischemia increases chemosensitivity. Hepatic arterial embolization or chemoembolization should be considered in patients with symptomatic or progressive unresectable liver metastasis, particularly when the bulk of metastatic disease is confined to the liver. There is currently no clear data on the superiority of TAE versus TACE.[25,26]

Radioembolization with Yttrium-90 (Y^{90}) glass microspheres is an alternative therapy to TACE, recommended for intermittent stage unresectable liver lesions not amenable to RFA. A systematic review and meta-analysis of 553 patients with unresectable HCC who underwent TACE and Y^{90} radioembolization found similar complete response rates and no significant difference in survival at 4 years between the two groups. Combined treatment with PRRTs like Lu-DOTATATE and Y^{90} radioembolization was commonly used for patients with bulky hepatic disease.[23,27] This regimen was called into question due to concerns for hepatotoxicity. A retrospective study assessed patients treated with PRRT and radioembolization therapy between the years of 2006 and 2016 evaluating efficacy and toxicity defined as radioembolization-induced liver disease (REILD). They found patients with NELM treated with radioembolization after initial PRRT resulted in a disease control rate of 91% at 3 months and the incidence of REILD was 5%. The authors concluded that combined PRRT followed by Y^{90} radioembolization therapy is safe, and that hepatoxicity following this regimen is rare.[23,27-30] Prospective randomized trials are needed to further delineate the role of Y^{90} radioembolization.

REFERENCES

1. Riihimäki M, Hemminki A, Sundquist K, Sundquist J, Hemminki K. The epidemiology of metastases in neuroendocrine tumors. *Int J Cancer*. 2016;139(12):2679-2686.
2. Lawrence B, Gustafsson BI, Chan A, Svejda B, Kidd M, Modlin IM. The epidemiology of gastroenteropancreatic neuroendocrine tumors. *Endocrinol Metab Clin N Am*. 2011;40(1):1-18.
3. Anthony LB, Strosberg JR, Klimstra DS, et al. *The NANETS Consensus Guidelines for the Diagnosis and Management of Gastrointestinal Neuroendocrine Tumors (NETs) Well-Differentiated NETs of the Distal Colon and Rectum*. 2010. www.pancreasjournal.com.
4. Ford MM. Neuroendocrine tumors of the colon and rectum. *Dis Colon Rectum*. 2017;60(10):1018-1021.
5. Bayhan Z, Yildiz YA, Akdeniz Y, et al. Appendix neuroendocrine tumor: retrospective analysis of 4026 appendectomy patients in a single center. *Emerg Med Int*. 2020;2020:1-6.
6. Volante M, Grillo F, Massa F, et al. Neuroendocrine neoplasms of the appendix, colon and rectum. *Pathologica*. 2021;113(1): 19-27.
7. Guenter R, Aweda T, Carmona Matos DM, et al. Overexpression of somatostatin receptor type 2 in neuroendocrine tumors for improved Ga68-DOTATATE imaging and treatment. In: *Surgery (United States)*. Vol 167. Mosby Inc.; 2020:189-196.
8. Crown A, Rocha FG, Raghu P, et al. Impact of initial imaging with gallium-68 dotatate PET/CT on diagnosis and management of patients with neuroendocrine tumors. *J Surg Oncol*. 2020;121(3):480-485.
9. Klimstra DS, Modlin IR, Volkan Adsay N, et al. *Pathology Reporting of Neuroendocrine Tumors: Application of the Delphic Consensus Process to the Development of a Minimum Pathology Data Set*. 2010. http://links.lww.com/PAS/A51.
10. Shah MH, Goldner WS, Benson AB, et al. Neuroendocrine and adrenal tumors, version 2.2021, NCCN Clinical Practice Guidelines in Oncology. *J Natl Compr Cancer Netw*. 2021; 19(7):839-868.
11. You H, Kandathil A, Beg M, de Blanche L, Kazmi S, Subramaniam RM. Ga-68 DOTATATE PET/CT and F-18 FDG PET/CT in the evaluation of low and intermediate versus high-grade neuroendocrine tumors. *Nucl Med Commun*. 2020; 41:1060-1065.
12. Pommier RF. Expert commentary on neuroendocrine tumors of the colon and rectum. *Dis Colon Rectum*. 2017;60(10):1021-1022.
13. Mandair D, Caplin ME. Colonic and rectal NET's. *Best Pract Res Clin Gastroenterol*. 2012;26(6):775-789.
14. Cloyd JM, Wiseman JT, Pawlik TM. Surgical management of pancreatic neuroendocrine liver metastases. *J Gastrointest Oncol*. 2020;11(3):590-600.
15. Mayo SC, de Jong MC, Pulitano C, et al. Surgical management of hepatic neuro-endocrine tumor metastasis: results from an international multi-institutional analysis. *Ann Surg Oncol*. 2010;17(12):3129-3136.
16. Rinke A, Wittenberg M, Schade-Brittinger C, et al. Placebo-controlled, double-blind, prospective, randomized study on the effect of octreotide lar in the control of tumor growth in patients with metastatic neuroendocrine midgut tumors (PROMID): results of long-term survival. *Neuroendocrinology*. 2016;104(1):26-32.
17. Caplin ME, Pavel M, Ćwikła JB, et al. Anti-tumour effects of lanreotide for pancreatic and intestinal neuroendocrine tumours: the CLARINET open-label extension study. *Endocrine-Related Cancer*. 2016;23(3):191-199.
18. Caplin ME, Pavel M, Ćwikła JB, et al. Lanreotide in metastatic enteropancreatic neuroendocrine tumors. *N Engl J Med*. 2014;371(3):224-233.
19. Yao JC, Fazio N, Singh S, et al. Everolimus for the treatment of advanced, non-functional neuroendocrine tumours of the lung or gastrointestinal tract (RADIANT-4): a randomised, placebo-controlled, phase 3 study. *Lancet*. 2016;387(10022):968-977.
20. Strosberg J, Wolin E, Chasen B, et al. Health-related quality of life in patients with progressive midgut neuroendocrine tumors treated with Lu-dotatate in the phase III NETTER-1 trial. *J Clin Oncol*. 2018;36:2578-2584.
21. Strosberg J, El-Haddad G, Wolin E, et al. Phase 3 trial of 177 Lu-dotatate for midgut neuroendocrine tumors. *N Engl J Med*. 2017;376(2):125-135.
22. Lawrence B, Gustafsson BI, Chan A, Svejda B, Kidd M, Modlin IM. The epidemiology of gastroenteropancreatic neuroendocrine tumors. *Endocrinol Metab Clin N Am*. 2011;40(1): 1-18.
23. Guenter R, Aweda T, Carmona Matos DM, et al. Overexpression of somatostatin receptor type 2 in neuroendocrine tumors for improved Ga68-DOTATATE imaging and treatment. In: *Surgery (United States)*. Vol 167. Mosby Inc.; 2020:189-196.
24. Izzo F, Granata V, Grassi R, et al. Radiofrequency ablation and microwave ablation in liver tumors: an update. *Oncologist*. 2019; 24(10):e990-e1005.
25. de Mestier L, Zappa M, Hentic O, Vilgrain V, Ruszniewski P. Liver transarterial embolizations in metastatic neuroendocrine tumors. *Rev Endocr Metab Disord*. 2017;18(4):459-471.
26. Tran CG, Sherman SK, Chandrasekharan C, Howe JR. Surgical management of neuroendocrine tumor liver metastases. *Surg Oncol Clin N Am*. 2021;30(1):39-55.
27. Syed M, Shah J, Montazeri SA, Grajo JR, Geller B, Toskich B. Analysis of dynamic hepatobiliary contrast-enhanced MRI signal intensity after Yttrium-90 radioembolization with glass microspheres for the treatment of hepatocellular carcinoma. *Abdom Radiol*. 2021;46(5):2182-2187.
28. Braat AJAT, Ahmadzadehfar H, Kappadath SC, et al. Radioembolization with 90Y resin microspheres of neuroendocrine liver metastases after initial peptide receptor radionuclide therapy. *Cardiovasc Intervent Radiol*. 2020;43(2):246-253.
29. Saini A, Wallace A, Alzubaidi S, et al. History and evolution of Yttrium-90 radioembolization for hepatocellular carcinoma. *J Clin Med*. 2019;8(1):55.
30. Stueven AK, Kayser A, Wetz C, et al. Somatostatin analogues in the treatment of neuroendocrine tumors: past, present and future. *Int J Mol Sci*. 2019;20(12):3049.

Pituitary Tumors: Prolactinomas, Cushing Disease, Growth Hormone-Producing Tumors, TSH-Secreting Tumors

63

Michael A. Weintraub, MD
Theodore H. Schwartz, MD
Fraser Henderson, Jr., MD
Georgiana A. Dobri, MD

GENERAL CONSIDERATIONS

The prevalence of asymptomatic sellar masses discovered incidentally on imaging studies or on autopsy ranges from 10% to 20%. However, the vast majority of these sellar masses are small, lack hormone-secreting characteristics, and are unlikely to manifest clinically. The prevalence of clinically relevant pituitary adenomas is approximately 1 per 1000 in the general population.[1]

A pituitary adenoma forms through the clonal expansion of a pituitary cell after a somatic mutation or chromosomal abnormality. Adenomas can arise from any type of cell in the anterior pituitary and may hypersecrete a specific hormone or set of hormones. If an adenoma becomes large enough to compress the native pituitary gland, normal pituitary hormone production may become impaired.

A significant portion of pituitary adenomas are clinically nonfunctioning. Historically, tumor classification was based on immunohistochemistry staining. As a more precise cell-lineage-based classification, the 2017 WHO classification system also includes pituitary transcription factors as a more precise cell lineage-based classification. The later approach has reclassified null-cell adenomas to a more precise lineage according to the transcription factors produced.[2,3]

PATHOGENESIS

Pituitary Anatomy & Pathology

The pituitary gland sits at the base of the skull in a cavity of the sphenoid bone named the *sella turcica*, or "turkish saddle" (Figure 63–1). Anterior and inferior to the sella turcica is the sphenoid sinus and posterior is the clinoid process. The gland is surrounded by dura and immediately superior to it is the diaphragma sella, a thin reflection of the dura. The optic chiasm sits superior to the diaphragma sella. The sella is flanked laterally by the cavernous sinuses, which contain the carotid artery and multiple cranial nerves, including cranial nerve VI (abduncens), cranial nerve III (oculomotor), cranial nerve IV (trochlear), the ophthalmic branch of the trigeminal nerve (V1), and the maxillary branch of the trigeminal (V2). The pituitary itself is made up of an anterior, intermediate, and posterior lobe. The pituitary stalk is composed of neuron cell axons that travel from the inferior hypothalamus, pass posterior to the optic chiasm, penetrate the diaphragma sella, and terminate in the posterior pituitary.

Understanding the anatomic relationship of the pituitary gland and its surrounding structures is necessary to appreciate the ability of pituitary adenomas to compress surrounding structures as well as the effects of pituitary surgery. A pituitary adenoma (mostly macroadenomas defined as adenomas 10 mm or greater) can compress the normal pituitary and cause pituitary stalk deviation. Compression of the normal pituitary gland and stalk can cause pituitary insufficiency, discussed in detail later in this chapter. Larger adenomas, typically greater than 15 mm, can exhibit suprasellar extension and compress the optic nerves and chiasm. Compression of the nasal retinal ganglion cells as they cross the optic chiasm to the opposite occipital cortex causes the pathognomonic bitemporal hemianopsia. Other visual field changes are also manifested depending on the tumor location, size, and anatomic relationship of the optic apparatus components and the chiasm. Adenomas can also extend laterally and invade the cavernous sinus and more aggressive tumors can compromise the contained cranial nerves (eg, trigeminal neuralgia).

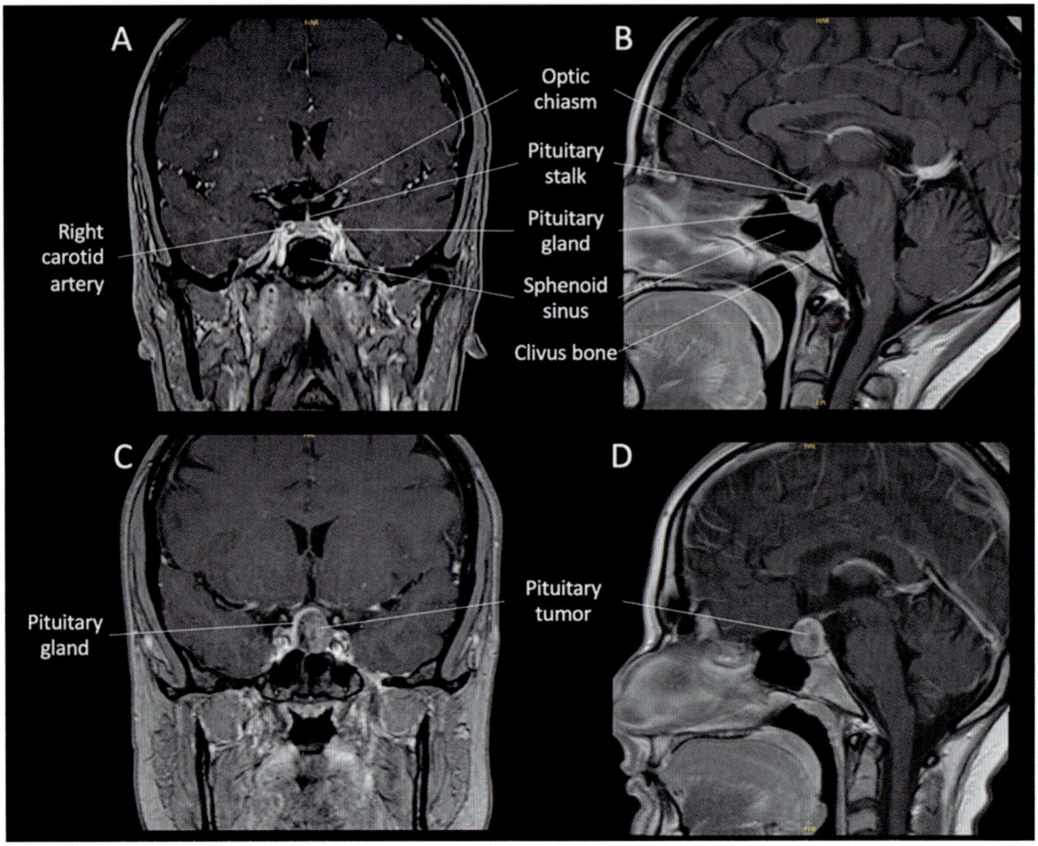

Figure 63–1. Pituitary anatomy. MRI imaging of a patient with normal pituitary is depicted in a coronal **(A)** and sagittal **(B)** view. An MRI of a patient with a 1.6 × 1.4 × 1.2 cm pituitary macroadenoma with signs of compression of the optic chiasm in the coronal **(C)** and sagittal **(D)** view.

Hormone-Secreting Pituitary Adenoma Subtypes

A. Prolactinomas

Also known as lactotroph adenomas, prolactinomas are formed by prolactin-secreting cells. Their prevalence ranges from 40% to 66% of all pituitary adenomas that manifest signs and symptoms and are thus the most common subtype.[4] They occur most frequently as microadenomas in premenopausal women, whereas in men they are more often invasive macroadenomas. They are unique among pituitary adenomas as medical therapy rather than surgery is often attempted first given their excellent response to dopamine agonists.

B. ACTH-secreting Adenomas

These tumors secrete excess adrenocorticotropic hormone (ACTH) which stimulate the adrenal glands to produce excess cortisol. Corticotroph adenomas are rare, comprising 2% to 6% of all pituitary adenomas. Sometimes tumors can be too small to be visualized with imaging but still produce clinical manifestations of Cushing syndrome posing a particular treatment challenge.

C. Growth Hormone-secreting Adenomas

Growth hormone (GH)-secreting adenomas are formed by somatotrophs secreting excess growth hormone, which results in elevated insulin-like growth factor (IGF-1) levels. However, they can cosecrete prolactin and less commonly TSH, given their common origin and transcription factors such as pituitary transcription factor 1 (PIT1). They make up 8% to 16% of all pituitary adenomas.[1,5]

D. TSH-secreting Adenomas

Thyrotroph adenomas, also known as TSH-omas, arise from a clonal expansion of abnormal thyrotrophs autonomously secreting TSH unresponsive to the negative feedback of excess thyroid hormones. Thyrotroph adenomas are extremely rare, accounting for 0.5% to 3% of all pituitary adenomas and for less than 1% of hyperthyroid patients.[6]

CLINICAL FINDINGS

Patients found to have a pituitary adenoma should be evaluated for symptoms and signs of mass effect, impaired pituitary function, and pituitary hypersecretion.

Symptoms & Signs of Mass Effect

A pituitary adenoma's classic visual manifestation is bitemporal hemianopsia. With suprasellar extension of a pituitary tumor, the ipsilateral retinal ganglion cell axons travelling to the occipital cortex are compressed at the level of the optic chiasm and causes blindness of the outer half of each eye's vision. However, depending on the tumor location and portion of optic nerve compression, patients may present only with one eye affected (homonymous hemianopsia) and to variable degrees.

Other vision changes are also caused by pituitary adenomas; thus, an evaluation of the sella should be considered with any vision change. An aggressive pituitary tumor can invade the cavernous sinus and displace the contained third, fourth, and sixth cranial nerve, resulting in diplopia or ptosis. An intrasellar mass can also cause an afferent pupillary defect (Marcus Gunn pupil), where a "swinging flashlight test" will demonstrate a paradoxical pupillary dilation when shining the flashlight at the affected eye. This exam finding is caused by an expanding mass compressing the ipsilateral pupillo-constrictor nerve axons.

Vision changes are due to the tumor compressing the optic chiasm, optic nerves, or tracts. If imaging does not show the tumor abutting the structures of the ophthalmic apparatus, a visual field exam is not necessary.

Headaches are a common presenting symptom due to the stretching and inflammation of the dura mater. They have variable characteristics but can be throbbing and fontal or retro-orbital. The syndrome of sudden onset severe headache, visual impairment, and altered mental status could be from pituitary apoplexy, or a sudden hemorrhage into the pituitary gland. Large adenomas have the potential of halting cerebrospinal fluid flow within the ventricular system causing symptoms and signs of hydrocephalus, including papilledema and proptosis.

Symptoms of Impaired Pituitary Function

Pituitary macroadenomas have an ability to compress normal pituitary tissue and disrupt hormone secretion. Onset of pituitary insufficiency from an adenoma is often gradual as it expands and exerts pressure on normal pituitary cells, but also should be considered in acute settings of adrenal crisis or symptomatic hypothyroidism. Generally, growth hormone and gonadotropin production are lost first, followed by ACTH, TSH, and prolactin production.

Central adrenal insufficiency, the loss of ACTH production and downstream cortisol synthesis by the adrenal glands, produces the most profound clinical manifestations. Symptoms include weakness, anorexia, nausea, and vomiting. Signs of adrenal insufficiency include orthostatic hypotension, fever, and weight loss. Unlike primary adrenal insufficiency, aldosterone-producing zona-glomerulosa of the adrenal gland is still functional as it is regulated by the renin-angiotensin system rather than ACTH. Thus, with a normal functioning renin-angiotensin system, volume depletion and hyperkalemia observed in primary adrenal failure (Addison disease) are usually not seen in central adrenal insufficiency.

Central hypothyroidism, the loss of TSH secretion resulting in loss of thyroid hormone production, can manifest as fatigue, constipation, bradycardia, cold intolerance, dry skin, and brittle hair.

Growth hormone deficiency is the most common hormonal axis deficiency, but symptoms and signs are subtle. Patients exhibit decreased muscle mass, increased fat mass, and decreased quality of life. Loss of gonadotropin production (FSH and LH) causes amenorrhea in women and decreased libido and erectile dysfunction in men. Finally, prolactin deficiency is evident only in postpartum women with the inability to lactate.[7]

An exception to the gradual symptom onset of panhypopituitarism from a pituitary adenoma is pituitary apoplexy. Sudden hemorrhage into the pituitary gland causes a rapid depletion of pituitary hormone production and is life-threatening.

Symptoms & Signs of Hormone-secreting Tumors

A. Prolactinoma

Excess prolactin secretion in premenopausal women results in amenorrhea and galactorrhea. Postmenopausal women, in contrast, rarely exhibit symptoms of prolactin hypersecretion. In men, excess prolactin causes a hypogonadotropic hypogonadism resulting in decreased libido, erectile dysfunction, infertility, and gynecomastia. However, half of the cases of hyperprolactinemia have causes other than a prolactin-secreting adenoma, discussed later in this chapter (see "differential diagnosis of a sellar mass" section).

B. Cushing Syndrome

Hypercortisolism due to a corticotroph adenoma or more commonly from exogenous steroids have a plethora of metabolic, catabolic, reproductive, and psychiatric manifestations. Symptoms range from subclinical to severe depending on the duration and level of hypercortisolism.

Patients have increased abdominal obesity and supraclavicular fat pads along with muscle wasting of the extremities and proximal muscle weakness. Many patients have skin changes such as hirsutism, acne, easy bruising, wide purplish striae, and skin thinning. Skin hyperpigmentation can also occur due to the increased ACTH binding to melanocyte-stimulating hormone receptors. Oligomenorrhea and amenorrhea are common in premenopausal women. Neuropsychiatric symptoms include insomnia, depression, and memory loss.[8]

C. Growth Hormone Tumors

Somatotroph adenomas secrete excess level growth hormone which manifests as gigantism in children and acromegaly in adults. Most common signs and symptoms of elevated growth hormone and insulin-like growth factor-1 (IFG-1) in adults are an insidious enlargement of the hands and feet resulting in increased glove and shoe size, as well as jaw and tongue enlargement. Comorbidities develop as a direct result of excess growth hormone including hypertension, diabetes, hyperlipidemia, cardiomyopathy, sleep apnea, gallstones, kidney stones, and colon polyps, most of which are at least partially reversible with control of growth hormone excess. Due to a delay in diagnosis of an average 8 to 10 years, most patients already exhibit multiple comorbidities on initial presentation.[9] Time to diagnosis is longer in women, who experience worse quality of life with more comorbidities than men.[10,11]

D. TSH-secreting Tumors

The signs and symptoms of hyperthyroidism from a thyrotroph adenoma are the same as other causes of hyperthyroidism, which include palpitations, tremor, heat intolerance, and a diffuse goiter. However, in many cases, patients will be entirely asymptomatic.[12]

E. Gonadotroph Adenomas

Most clinically nonfunctioning pituitary adenomas are gonadotroph adenomas, making them the most common type of pituitary adenoma. These nonfunctioning or "silent" pituitary masses are poorly differentiated and secrete hormone inefficiently. Only rarely do patients present with symptoms of high gonadal function, for example, precocious puberty, irregular menses, or psychiatric manifestations.

Table 63–1. Hormone testing to classify a hormone-producing pituitary tumor.

Tumor	Initial Screening Test	Additional Confirmatory Tests
Prolactinoma	Prolactin	Dilution assay to rule out hook effect if tumor ≥2 cm Macroprolactin (if prolactin elevated but less than 200)
ACTH-secreting adenoma	ACTH 24-hour urine free cortisol Late night salivary cortisol Low-dose dexamethasone suppression test	Dynamic testing to rule out pseudo-Cushing's and explore etiology of ACTH-dependent Cushing's (eg, stimulation test with DDAVP, CRH, or dexamethasone-CRH) Inferior petrosal sinus sampling
GH-secreting adenoma	IGF-1, GH	Oral glucose tolerance test
TSH-secreting adenoma	TSH, free T4, T3	Alpha-subunit to TSH ratio T3 suppression test Thyrotropin-releasing hormone stimulation test

Initial and confirmatory testing to diagnose hormone-secreting pituitary tumors.
ACTH, corticotropin; CHR, corticotropin-releasing hormone; DDAVP, desmopressin; GH, growth hormone; IGF-1, insulin-like growth factor-1; TSH, thyroid-stimulating hormone.

ENDOCRINE EVALUATION & DIFFERENTIAL DIAGNOSIS

Evaluation of a Pituitary "Incidentaloma"

A. Initial Evaluation of Pituitary Hyposecretion

Laboratory evaluation for pituitary hypofunction and hyperfunction begins with the following tests (Table 63–1). A general workup consists of a morning serum cortisol and ACTH level to assess for central adrenal insufficiency. A morning cortisol less than 3 μg/dL at least 24 to 48 hours after any steroid dose is diagnostic of adrenal insufficiency. A low or inappropriately normal ACTH is consistent with central adrenal insufficiency. A cortisol ≥18 μg/dL rules out adrenal insufficiency. When the finding is indeterminate, dynamic stimulation testing may help make a definitive diagnosis. Biochemical evaluation of the hypothalamic-pituitary-adrenal axis also consists of screening for hypercortisolism (eg, late-night salivary cortisol, 24-hour urine-free cortisol).

TSH and free thyroxine (fT4) will assess the hypothalamic-pituitary-thyroid axis. LH and FSH along with the downstream testosterone (men) or estradiol (women) levels and menstrual history will assess for central hypogonadism.[13]

IGF-1 and growth hormone (GH) will assess somatotroph production. GH undergoes pulsatile secretion; thus, a single value may not be useful unless GH is 2.8 μg/L or higher which will rule out GH deficiency. A normal IGF-1 does not rule out GH deficiency and a dynamic stimulation test is indicated in cases where clinical suspicion is high.[14]

A sodium level along with an inquiry about fluid intake and urine output is necessary to evaluate for diabetes insipidus, although posterior pituitary dysfunction is an uncommon presentation of a pituitary adenoma. The presence of hypernatremia in the setting of polyuria and dilute urine should lead to an investigation of alternate etiologies of sellar masses, for example, craniopharyngioma and metastasis.

B. Imaging

MRI is the imaging modality of choice to evaluate pituitary adenomas, superseding CT scans due to its superior resolution and ability to delineate pituitary tumors from normal gland. Gadolinium contrast further aids in differentiating a pituitary tumor, which does not enhance with contrast, compared to normal pituitary tissue which demonstrates enhanced signal intensity. Patients found to have a tumor pressing on the optic apparatus (ie, optic chiasm, optic tract, optic nerve) should be sent for formal visual field testing.[15,16]

Differential Diagnosis of a Sellar Mass

The differential of a sellar mass beyond a functioning and nonfunctioning adenoma is broad (Table 63–2). Considerations include neoplasms such as craniopharyngiomas, meningiomas, germ cell tumors, and metastases. Nonneoplastic cysts can also form in the sella, such as Rathke cleft cysts, epidermoid and dermoid cysts, and arachnoid cysts. Inflammatory syndromes can also affect the sella, such as sarcoidosis, amyloidosis, and IgG4-related disease. The incidence of drug-induced lymphocytic hypophysitis is rising with increased utilization of certain immunotherapies (eg, ipilimumab, nivolumab).[17] Granulomatous hypophysitis can be caused by tuberculosis or fungal infections.

Evaluation of Hormone-secreting Tumors

On discovery of a pituitary incidentaloma, in addition to evaluating for pituitary hypofunction, initial lab work should evaluate for tumor hormone hypersecretion (Table 63–1).

Table 63–3. Causes of hyperprolactinemia.

Physiologic	Pathologic	Medications
Macroprolactin Nipple stimulation Physical stress Pregnancy and lactation Seizures Sexual intercourse	Chest wall lesions (eg, herpes zoster, breast cancer, surgery) Chronic kidney disease Empty sella Inflammatory lesions (eg, hypophysitis, sarcoidosis, tuberculosis) Pituitary stalk compression Polycystic ovary syndrome Primary hypothyroidism Prolactin-secreting adenoma Radiation to the sella Severe liver disease	Antidepressants Antipsychotics Estrogens (eg, oral contraceptives) Methyldopa Opiates Verapamil

A. Prolactinoma

Hyperprolactinemia in the setting of a pituitary adenoma may be due to either a prolactin-secreting adenoma or tumor compression of the pituitary stalk. Prolactin production is constantly inhibited by dopamine transported from the hypothalamus, but compression of the pituitary stalk causes uninhibited prolactin release. It can be challenging but essential to differentiate between the two given first-line treatment of a prolactinoma is a dopamine agonist, and surgery with other tumor types.

Several other physiologic or pathologic conditions can cause hyperprolactinemia, such as pregnancy, primary hypothyroidism, and hepatic or renal failure (Table 63–3). A review of the patient's medication list should also be performed to rule out drug-induced hyperprolactinemia. Generally, a prolactin level greater than 200 μg/L in the absence of other predisposing factors to elevated prolactin levels is suggestive of a prolactinoma.

If large pituitary adenomas (>3 cm) secrete very high levels of prolactin, antibody assays may become saturated by

Table 63–2. Differential diagnosis of a sellar lesion.

Neoplasms	Cystic Masses	Inflammatory	Infectious
Chordoma	Arachnoid cyst	Amyloidosis	Bacterial
Germ cell tumor	Craniopharyngioma	Granulomatosis with polyangiitis	Fungal
Glioma	Dermoid cyst	Langerhans cell histiocytosis	Mycobacterium
Pituitary adenoma	Epidermoid cyst	Lymphocytic hypophysitis	
Meningioma	Rathke cleft cyst	Sarcoidosis	
Metastatic tumor			

the substrate causing an artificially low reported value ("the hook effect"). When clinical suspicion is high for a large prolactinoma, the hook effect can be overcome by rerunning the assay after a 1:100 dilution.

B. Cushing Disease (ACTH-producing Adenoma)

An evaluation for Cushing syndrome begins with an assessment of excess cortisol secretion. Hypercortisolism can be assessed with a 24-hour urine-free cortisol, a dexamethasone suppression test, or a late-night salivary cortisol.[18]

The differential of hypercortisolism is broad (Table 63–4).[19] The most common cause of Cushing syndrome is from exogenous steroids. Pseudo-Cushing's, or non-neoplastic hypercortisolism, can be due to psychiatric disorders, alcohol use disorder, uncontrolled diabetes, or obesity, further complicating the diagnosis. Dynamic testing can be useful to distinguish between ACTH-dependent Cushing's and pseudo-Cushing's, such as with a desmopressin stimulation test.

The next step in evaluating Cushing's is determining whether the source is pituitary, adrenal, or ectopic. An ACTH level can differentiate ACTH-dependent disease (ACTH >15 pmol/L indicating a pituitary or ectopic source) from ACTH-independent disease (ACTH <15 pmol/L indicating an adrenal source).

While conventional MRI can evaluate for a pituitary adenoma in suspected ACTH-dependent Cushing's, these ACTH-producing adenomas are often small with up to 50% of tumors evading detection. Alternative MR sequences (eg, dynamic MRI) and hybrid imaging (eg, PET combined with MRI) have recently been developed to aid tumor localization but are not yet widely adopted.[20] Furthermore, an adenoma found on imaging may not be the cause of the hypercortisolism given the high prevalence of nonfunctioning microadenomas. Inferior petrosal sinus sampling (IPSS) should be performed to confirm a pituitary source in all patients with lesions <6 mm. In this catheter-based endovascular procedure, desmopressin or corticotropin-releasing hormone (CRH) is administered and ACTH levels are measured in the inferior petrosal sinuses and compared to levels in the periphery (ie, the vena cava). A stimulated petrosal sinus to vena cava ratio ≥3:1 is diagnostic of a pituitary source even in the absence tumor visualization on MRI. It is essential that the patient be hypercortisolemic at the time of IPSS to ensure correct interpretation of the results.[21]

Table 63–4. Causes of hypercortisolism.

Cushing Syndrome	Non-neoplastic Hypercortisolism (Pseudo-Cushing's)
Adrenal tumor (adenoma, carcinoma)	Acute illness/hospitalization
Adrenal hyperplasia	Alcoholism
Ectopic ACTH secretion	Anorexia
Exogenous glucocorticoids	Conditions that raise corticosteroid-binding globulin (eg, pregnancy)
Pituitary adenoma (Cushing disease)	Mood disorders (eg, depression, anxiety, obsessive-compulsive disorder)
	Polycystic ovary syndrome
	Uncontrolled diabetes mellitus
	Severe obesity

C. Growth Hormone-producing Tumors

Initial screening for acromegaly begins with an IGF-1 serum measurement. Growth hormone measurement is not as diagnostic given its pulsatile secretion unless low (<0.4 μg/L) when it can rule out the diagnosis. If IGF-1 is less than twofold the upper level of normal, an oral glucose tolerance test should be conducted to confirm diagnosis as a mild elevation in IGF-1 can occur outside of acromegaly (eg, insulin resistance). Acromegaly is consistent with GH levels failing to suppress less than 1 μg/L after an oral glucose load when using older polyclonal hormone assays. A lower cutoff of 0.4 μg/L has been proposed when using a highly sensitive GH assay and this cutoff can be used even in patients with altered glucose metabolism.[22]

Nearly 95% of patients with acromegaly have a growth hormone-producing pituitary tumor, with the remainder of cases due to an ectopic growth hormone-producing neuroendocrine tumor.

D. TSH-secreting Tumors

Thyroid function tests will show an elevated free thyroxine (fT4) and triiodothyronine (T3) in the setting of elevated or inappropriately normal TSH. Etiologies of hyperthyroidism other than a TSH-oma (also known as a thyrotropinoma) can be ruled out with a detectable TSH. However, high fT4 and a normal or high TSH could also be observed in poor adherence to levothyroxine and should be suspected in patients with this history.

It is necessary to differentiate TSH-omas from thyroid hormone resistance due to a mutation in *thyroid hormone receptor beta* (*THRB*). Elevated levels of the serum glycoprotein hormone alpha-subunit (alpha-GSU) are observed in 70% of TSH-omas, particularly macroadenomas. A molar ratio of alpha-GSU to TSH greater than 1 is observed in 80% of TSH-omas. In unclear cases, dynamic testing can be helpful.[23,24]

TREATMENT & PROGNOSIS

Once a pituitary adenoma is discovered, an evaluation for mass effect, pituitary hypofunction, and pituitary hyperfunction is performed to determine the appropriate treatment (Figure 63–2). Except for prolactinomas, transsphenoidal surgery is first-line for hormone-secreting pituitary adenomas.

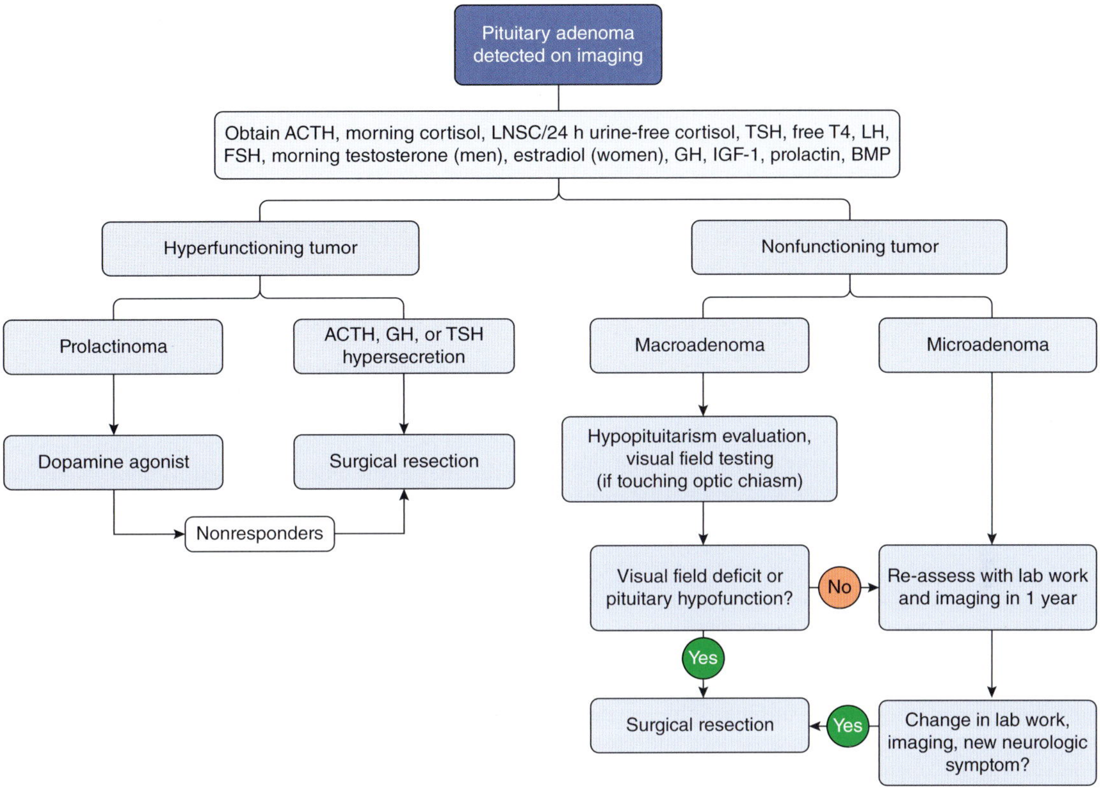

Figure 63–2. Workup of an incidental pituitary adenoma. ACTH, adrenocorticotropic hormone; BMP, basic metabolic panel; FSH, follicle-stimulating hormone; free T4, free thyroxine; GH, growth hormone; IGF-1, insulin-like growth factor-1; LH, luteinizing hormone; LNSC, late-night salivary cortisol; TSH, thyroid-stimulating hormone.

Generally, nonfunctioning microadenomas can be monitored with serial imaging and hormone evaluation. Nonfunctioning macroadenomas, particularly those compressing the optic apparatus or causing pituitary hypofunction, should be removed in good surgical candidates.

Surgical Technique

Surgery for pituitary adenomas has gone through several evolutionary stages. Early surgeons vacillated between a craniotomy and a transsphenoidal approach. Eventually, the transsphenoidal approach became the standard of care, which was performed with the aid of the microscope. The microscope, coopted for this purpose by Jules Hardy, provides stereoscopic vision. However, its use has been gradually supplanted by the two- and three-dimensional endoscope since the reports of Roger Jankowski and Hae-Dong Jho for its panoramic visualization which overcomes the restricted view and long narrow corridor inherent in the transsphenoidal approach.[25] Angled scopes can be employed to further widen the field of view. This improved visualization becomes especially beneficial for adenomas that extend laterally into cavernous sinuses or superiorly into the suprasellar spaces. Given the recent appreciation that adenomas often invade the adjacent dura of the cavernous sinus, surgery in this area becomes mandatory to increase the chance of remission.[26] Comparative series has gradually shown improved rates of gross total resection from an endoscopic versus microscopic approach, and this advantage is more pronounced for tumors extending beyond the sella in which removal of the tuberculum sella and planum sphenoidale may be required.[27]

Preoperative radiographic observations guide the specific surgical approach. A displaced pituitary stalk may signal the location of the adenoma. CT or MRI assessment of nasal sinus anatomy may inform the need for septal repair. Sphenoid sinuses occur in three classic patterns: sellar, presellar, and rarely, conchal (1%-2%). All are amenable to the transsphenoidal approach, but neuronavigation aids especially in the extensive clivus drilling required for the latter. The empty sella sign may also alert the surgeon to increased risk of fistula formation, prompting the harvesting of a nasoseptal flap or possibly a lumbar drain.[28]

Surgery is performed under general anesthesia in the supine position with the head above the patient's heart. Perioperative antibiotics target common nasal flora and may be broadened further for cases in which a high-flow cerebrospinal fluid leak is anticipated. Corticosteroids may be given in stress dose to all patients except those with Cushing disease. Intranasal pledgets soaked in vasoconstrictive agents (topical cocaine or oxymetazoline) reduce intraoperative bleeding along with submucosal injection of epinephrine. Postoperative CSF leak risk may be mitigated by preoperative placement of a lumbar drain.[29]

Surgical techniques vary according to surgeon preference and dictated by specific anatomy. A direct endonasal approach is typically performed by an otorhinolaryngologist who performs a posterior septectomy before removing the anterior sphenoid via enlargement of the natural ostia. This approach permits bimanual surgery and operation through both nares.

The microscopic approach uses either a sublabial incision or an endonasal transseptal approach, and in both of these instances, a nasal speculum is introduced to deviate the septum and out-fracture the turbinates from medial toward lateral. During the endoscopic approach surgeons may elect to remove portions of the middle turbinates to increase instrument maneuverability. The sphenoid face and posterior ethmoid cells are opened and septations are removed to expose a smooth posterior sphenoid wall with complete visualization from cavernous sinus to cavernous sinus, and from tuberculum to clivus.

Once the bony face of the sella is removed, the dura is opened and the tumor may be debulked. The key to successful intrasellar pituitary surgery often relies on the surgeon's ability to identify and maintain the pseudocapsule, which maximizes the chances of a gross total resection and minimizes the occurrence of an intraoperative CSF leak.[30] Extended approaches may be pursued to remove tumor extending into the suprasellar cistern, clivus, and cavernous sinuses. Close attention to hemostasis within the surgical bed helps prevent postoperative hematoma. Craniotomy for pituitary adenoma remains a surgical option for select circumstances.[31]

Risks of transsphenoidal surgery include CSF leak, compressive hemorrhage causing visual deterioration, infection, epistaxis, and dysfunction of the normal pituitary gland. Meticulous hemostasis must be sought, and the tumor cavity may be packed with fat, muscle, or synthetic hemostatic material, taking care to avoid materials that will expand upward and compress the optic apparatus. Fibrin glue sealant may be used to hold packing in place, or to pin a vascularized nasoseptal flap over the skull base defect. A variety of closure techniques have been described to reduce the chance of postoperative CSF leak, chief among these being the use of a vascularized nasoseptal flap and liberal fat grafting. In cases where more extensive bony exposure has been required, a rigid "gasket seal" has been useful. Finally, displaced turbinates and septum are reoriented.

We perform an early MRI during the admission to establish a new baseline for future comparison and to evaluate for presence of an intrasellar hematoma. The next scan is performed 3 months after surgery to definitively assess for residual tumor once surgical products have resolved. Subsequent scans can be obtained annually, then every few years depending on the risk of recurrence, which may be indirectly presumed from the Ki-67.[32]

Immediate Postoperative Management

Different postoperative management approaches are taken in different institutions; in our center, the patients are recovered in the step-down unit for the first 24 hours. Foley catheters and arterial lines remain in place to monitor urine output and blood pressure. Patients are mobilized out of bed the morning after surgery unless there was intraoperative CSF leak, in which case they remain on bedrest for the first 24 hours. Patients are moved to a regular floor bed for the second night and aim to be discharged on postoperative day 2.

Monitoring for Surgical Complications

A. Cavity Hemorrhage & Visual Compromise

Postoperative hemorrhage may manifest by visual deterioration or decline in consciousness after surgery and is a surgical emergency. Therefore, postoperative care requires frequent testing of visual acuity and confrontational fields, and subjective patient reports may be especially useful in detecting the early stages of a decline. Visual compromise is rare: in our series of 1200 consecutive endoscopic endonasal transsphenoidal cases, 8 cases (6 of which were adenomas) of vision deficit referable to postoperative hematoma were identified. All patients experienced improved vision after immediate reoperation to decompress the optic apparatus.[33]

B. Meningitis

Infection is rare during the immediate postoperative period. Prophylactic antibiotics are administered for the first 24 hours. The risk of meningitis increases significantly if there is a postoperative CSF leak, which should be treated as rapidly as possible. Patients in whom a postoperative CSF leak develops are presumed to have meningitis until proven otherwise. Lumbar puncture should be performed prior to initiating antibiotics and attempting a repair.

C. Epistaxis

Minor postoperative epistaxis should be expected. Rarely, additional intranasal hemostatic may be required during recovery, and even more rarely, a patient may be taken back to the operating room for definitive control of a persistent bleed. Delayed epistaxis may rarely occur several weeks after surgery and is often localized to a septal branch of the sphenopalatine artery. In cases of arterial bleeding, packing may be helpful, but definitive management involves cauterization, clipping, or embolization.

D. Cerebrospinal Fluid Fistula

Postoperative CSF leak must be distinguished from expected postoperative nasal drainage. True CSF leak may be identified by beta transferrin assay when available or from obvious dripping of clear fluid when postured forward. CT should be performed to evaluate the presence and degree of pneumocephalus as a baseline. Specific patterns of pneumocephalus may be predictive of CSF leak. In the presence of a nasoseptal flap and absence of pneumocephalus, repair with lumbar drainage may be considered in lieu of return to the operating room. Re-exploration for defect repair and repacking of the tumor bed may be required, particularly in the setting of pneumocephalus or if a nasoseptal flap has not been used in the first closure. Occult leaks may be identified with intrathecal fluorescein injection.[34]

E. Postoperative Sinusitis

The incidence of postoperative sinusitis after the endoscope endonasal approach ranges from 5% to 12%. The use of a week of prophylactic antibiotics has not been shown to impact postoperative nasal quality of life. Patients are seen approximately 1 to 2 weeks after surgery by an otolaryngologist during which time the cavity is inspected and gentle debridement is performed. During later visits, synechiae may be identified and divided to prevent long-term obstruction. Generally, the more extended the approach the more hands-on the postoperative nasal care should be to ensure optimal healing.[35-37]

Postoperative Endocrine Changes

Multidisciplinary care by neurosurgery, endocrinology, and critical care is needed for optimal postoperative management. Close monitoring of vital signs, fluid intake and urine output, and electrolytes is necessary immediately following transsphenoidal surgery to evaluate for diabetes insipidus (DI), syndrome of inappropriate antidiuretic hormone secretion (SIADH), and hypopituitarism.

A. Diabetes Insipidus

Disorders of water metabolism are common after transsphenoidal surgery. Increased urine volume and decreased urine osmolality are suggestive of DI. Hypernatremia is not always present if the patient has an intact thirst mechanism. Onset is typically abrupt and within 24 hours of surgery for most patients. Monitoring for DI consists of measuring fluid intake, urine output, urine specific gravity, and serum sodium every 6 to 8 hours.

Most cases of DI are mild and transient and can be managed by ensuring adequate fluid intake provided patients have an intact thirst mechanism. Desmopressin (DDAVP) is reserved for more severe cases.

B. Hyponatremia

Hyponatremia can occur following transsphenoidal surgery due to an inappropriate release of preformed antidiuretic hormone. Symptoms range from mild nausea and headache to more severe altered mental status and seizures. Usually occurring between postoperative day (POD) 5 and 8, hyponatremia is a common cause of hospital readmission. This may be averted through routine use of 1 L fluid restriction as early as POD 4 with easing of fluid restriction following a normal serum sodium, checked on POD 5 to 8.[38] Mild hyponatremia from SIADH often corrects with fluid restriction and salt tablets. More severe hyponatremia (<125 mEq/L) warrants readmission for close monitoring and cautious sodium correction with furosemide and/or hypertonic saline that is not too rapid to avoid central pontine myelinolysis.

C. Adrenal Insufficiency

Evaluation and treatment of both central adrenal insufficiency and central hypothyroidism are critical immediately following pituitary surgery. Evaluation for central adrenal insufficiency is accomplished by obtaining serum cortisol at approximately 8 AM on postoperative day 1 and 2. The cortisol level should be checked at least 24 hours from the last steroid dose as exogenous steroids corrupt the ability to evaluate the pituitary-adrenal axis. A serum cortisol level below 13 mg/dL is suggestive of adrenal insufficiency and should be treated with glucocorticoid replacement.

Either hydrocortisone dosed two or three times daily (15-25 mg per day orally) or daily prednisone (5 mg per day orally) are typically prescribed. The hypothalamic-pituitary-adrenal axis should be again evaluated 4 to 8 weeks after surgery to test for restored function.[39-41]

D. Central Hypothyroidism

It may take several days for central hypothyroidism to become evident on laboratory analysis. It is advisable to check serum-free thyroxine level on POD 5 or later. Treatment of central hypothyroidism is the same as primary hypothyroidism, although the patient's levothyroxine requirement may be less than if they had complete primary thyroid failure. The levothyroxine dose varies depending on sex, age, and concomitant therapy (eg, estrogens and growth hormone). A typical starting dose is 50 to 75 μg and uptitrated based on symptoms and goal fT4 in the middle to upper end of the reference range.[42]

Of note, treatment of hypothyroidism in patients with panhypopituitarism without properly treating the adrenal insufficiency may precipitate adrenal crisis. Patients with concurrent adrenal insufficiency must therefore be treated with glucocorticoids prior to levothyroxine initiation.

E. Growth Hormone Deficiency & Hypogonadism

Evaluation and treatment of growth hormone deficiency and hypogonadism is not necessary immediately post-op and should be reserved for outpatient follow-up (approximately 4-6 weeks after surgery).[43,44]

Management of Hormone-secreting Tumors

A. Prolactinoma

Dopamine agonists (DAs) decrease prolactin secretion and tumor size and are first-line therapy for prolactin-secreting microadenomas and macroadenomas. Indications include prolactinomas with current or imminent optic chiasm compression, prolactin-induced hypogonadism, irregular menses, or galactorrhea. Microprolactinomas not causing hypogonadism may be only monitored since significant growth of microprolactinomas is uncommon.

Cabergoline has a superior efficacy and safety profile compared to bromocriptine, the first DA to be developed (Table 63–5). The most common side effects of DAs are nausea, postural hypotension, and brain fog. Patients receiving DAs have also experienced impulse control disorders.[45] An association of DAs with cardiac valvulopathies has been reported, but it may not be clinically relevant with the low doses typically required for prolactinomas.[46,47] Carbergoline is initiated at 0.25 to 0.5 mg once or twice weekly and up-titrated at 1 to 2 monthly intervals depending on prolactin levels, symptoms, and tumor size.

Table 63–5. Dopamine agonists for the treatment of prolactin-secreting pituitary adenomas.

Drug Name	Usual Oral Dosages	Adverse Effects
Bromocriptine	1.25 to 10 mg total daily dose, given once or twice daily	Nausea, vomiting, dizziness, headache, nasal congestion, constipation, digital vasospasm, vivid dreams, anxiety, depression, impulsivity
Cabergoline	0.5 to 2.0 mg or more total per week, given several times per week or daily	Similar to bromocriptine (often less severe side effects), cardiac valvulopathy at high doses (>3 mg/day)
Quinagolide*	0.075 to 0.9 mg total daily dose, given once or twice daily	Similar to bromocriptine
Pergolide**	0.05 to 0.1 mg total daily dose, given once per day	Similar to bromocriptine**

*Not currently FDA approved.

**Withdrawn in the United States in 2007 due to cardiac valvulopathy risk.

Transsphenoidal surgery is indicated in patients who experience resistance or intolerance to DAs, pituitary apoplexy, or CSF leakage. Surgery is an option first line in women who desire fertility in the near future and in women with concerning macroadenomas who are planning a pregnancy. Cystic tumors typically do not fully respond to DAs, so surgery may be an initial treatment option.

Given the continued advances in the safety and efficacy of transsphenoidal surgery, it may be on par or even superior to DAs, as reported in a recent meta-analysis surveying literature on disease remission rates and can be considered in individualized cases as first line.[48]

Visual deficit that does not improve within a month of medical therapy, macroadenomas that do not decrease in size, CSF fistula while on medical treatment or drug intolerance are reasons to surgically resect a prolactinoma. It is vital to discriminate correctly between hyperprolactinemia from stalk effect resulting from a nonfunctioning macroadenoma versus hyperprolactinemia from a functioning prolactinoma, as the former is likely a surgical candidate, but the latter may benefit from attempting medical therapy first.

Prolactinomas that have been medically treated tend to become firmer and more fibrous. Normoprolactinemia is reported in 74% of macroprolactinomas and 71% to 100% of micropolactinomas who underwent surgery, with variations correlating to center caseload. Postoperative hypopituitarism after selective adenomectomy occurred in 12/171 patients (7%) and this risk correlated with size of the tumor. Hyperprolactinemia-related low testosterone and menstrual cycle dysfunction usually resolves with normalization of prolactin.[49]

B. ACTH-producing Pituitary Adenoma

Surgery for Cushing disease seeks long-term disease remission through gross total resection which may be achieved reliably in approximately 80% of ACTH-producing adenomas. Those at least 2 mm in size contain a pseudocapsule whose boundaries may be preserved during careful dissection, though larger tumors may require central debulking first. Nevertheless, detection may be difficult. Preoperative imaging may direct the initial exploration, but when imaging fails to localize a suspected Cushing tumor, bilateral petrosal sinus sampling (IPSS) is a technique to confirm the diagnosis and may lateralize the tumor to one wing of the gland. In the absence of radiographic guidance, many surgeons begin dissection on the side correlating with IPSS results. Another systematic method is to make vertical slices sequentially through the gland until the adenoma is encountered. The gland may be divided into quadrants, for example, taking biopsies from each and sending for frozen section analysis. When no adenoma is encountered, removal of half or even the majority of the gland may be considered. Patients suffering from obesity and impaired healing capacity secondary to Cushing disease may be at particular risk of CSF leak, requiring particular attention to strength of closure.

Perioperative thromboembolism is 10 times higher in Cushing patients relative to patients with a nonfunctioning adenoma indicating the need for nonpharmacologic thromboprophylaxis measures (ie, compression stockings, early ambulation).[50] Optimal pharmacologic thromboprophylaxis is not yet clear, but may be considered in high-risk patients with decreased mobility to about 1 month after surgery.[51]

Patients undergo serial morning cortisol and ACTH measurements to determine biochemical remission and to monitor for need for acute steroid supplementation. Take back for further surgery has been advocated for cases in which cortisol levels remain persistently elevated. While earlier reoperation is technically easier than late reoperation, delayed remissions have been reported. Repeat surgery after recurrence achieves postoperative remission in at least 69% of 51 patients in the series by Laws, and as high as 87% in the most recent cohort, reported with an overall variability of 38% to 90%, and hypopituitarism may occur in 19% to 64% of repeat surgeries that are necessarily more aggressive.[52,53] The strength of these results relies on performance of surgery at an experienced center.

Patients with Cushing disease continue to have a higher mortality rate despite successful adenomectomy. Rates of sepsis, stroke, and thromboembolism are significantly higher than the general population even years from remission, underscoring the continued unmet need of these patients. Treatment goals include not only normalizing biochemical markers, but also reversing clinical features, improving quality of life, and preventing long-term recurrence.

Medical therapies are used in persistent or recurrent disease despite surgery, to treat severe hypercortisolism or patients with contraindications for surgery. Drugs with different mechanisms are available including pituitary-directed agents, glucocorticoid receptor blockers, and steroidogenesis inhibitors (Table 63–6). Each have their advantages and side effects and can be used in combination to control hypercortisolism and tumor size. For example, adrenal steroidogenesis inhibitors such as ketoconazole rapidly decrease cortisol production but do not alter tumor size and carry the risk of severe side effects including hepatotoxicity. The somatostatin receptor ligand, pasireotide, produces tumor shrinkage and reduction in

Table 63–6. Medications for the treatment of Cushing disease.

Mechanism	Drug Name	Dose	Adverse Effects
Pituitary-directed agents	Pasireotide (subcutaneous and long-acting release)	0.6 to 1.8 mg total daily dose, given twice daily subcutaneously 10 to 30 mg every 4 weeks, intramuscularly	Nausea, vomiting, diarrhea, hyperglycemia, cholelithiasis
Glucocorticoid receptor blocker	Cabergoline†	0.5 to 7 mg total daily dose, given in divided doses orally	Gastrointestinal side effects, dizziness, headache, nasal congestion, impulsivity, cardiac valvulopathy
	Mifepristone	300 to 1200 mg total daily dose, given once per day orally	Fatigue, headache, nausea, hypokalemia, endometrial thickening, pregnancy termination, abnormal thyroid function tests, hyperlipidemia
Steroidogenesis inhibitors	Osilodrostat	4 to 60 mg total daily dose, given twice daily orally	Nausea, headache, fatigue, hirsutism, hypokalemia, hypertension
	Levoketoconazole	300 to 1200 mg total daily dose, given twice daily orally	Nausea, vomiting, increased liver enzymes, fatigue
	Ketoconazole†	400 to 1600 mg total daily dose, given twice or three times daily orally	Nausea, dyspepsia, rash, increased liver enzymes, hypogonadism, gynecomastia
	Metyrapone†	500 to 6000 mg total daily dose, given three or four times per day orally	Nausea, dizziness, hirsutism, hypertension, edema, hypokalemia
	Mitotane†	500 to 5000 mg total daily dose, given three times per day orally	Nausea, diarrhea, dizziness, ataxia, confusion, increased liver enzymes, rash, gynecomastia
	Etomidate†	0.025 to 0.1 mg/kg/h intravenously	Sedation

†Not currently FDA approved.

hypercortisolism. However, high rates of hyperglycemia, which can be severe, have been observed. Glucocorticoid receptor blockers, for example, mifepristone, can treat hypercortisolism regardless of the cause. Since cortisol concentrations are not affected, they cannot be used to monitor treatment response.[54-56]

For patients unresponsive to surgery and medical therapies, bilateral adrenalectomy and radiosurgery are reasonable options.

C. GH-producing Tumors

Transsphenoidal surgery is first-line for GH-producing tumors, even among the elderly.[57,58] Though most effective for microadenomas, surgery achieves normalization of IGF-1 and GH in a majority of macroadenoma cases as well. Furthermore, surgery provides immediate relief of symptoms resulting from mass effect. Of 81 patients in a contemporary single-institution series, 73% experienced biochemical remission at 1 year after surgery, and 54% experienced long-term remission. Of the initial remissions, 31% recurred during the mean follow-up of 100 months. Reoperation may be required in approximately 26% of cases, achieving long-term remission in 33%.[59]

A random GH on POD 1 less than 1 ng/mL can predict successful resection. However, an IGF-1 level 6 to 12 weeks after surgery is a more accurate measure of remission. A GH nadir after an oral glucose load is also recommended to assess for remission considering the appropriate GH nadir reference range for the type of assay used (frequently <0.4 ng/mL).[60]

After transsphenoidal surgery patients can develop significant polyuria, independent of diabetes insipidus, due to the resolution of GH-related fluid retention.

For patients without biochemical control after surgery, medical therapy is recommended (Table 63–7). Drugs with different mechanisms and routes of administration are utilized including SRLs (eg, injectable and oral octreotide, lanreotide depot, injectable pasireotide), a growth hormone receptor antagonist (pegvisomant), and a dopamine receptor agonist (cabergoline).

First-line medical therapy is typically long-acting octreotide or lanreotide, although other classes can be trialed first as the treatment approaches become more individualized. These SLRs normalize IGF-1 levels in 30% to 55% of cases and reduce tumor size by over 20% in half of cases. An oral delayed-release octreotide formulation, approved in the United States in 2020, is noninferior to the subcutaneous administration at controlling IGF-1 levels and may have improved patient-reported outcomes for fatigue, swelling, satisfaction, and convenience. Pasireotide is more effective than the other SLRs likely due to its higher affinity to somatostatin receptor 5, but with an appreciable rate of hyperglycemia in 70% of patients. Pegvisomant, a second-line treatment in patients without adequate control on SRLs, acts by blocking liver IGF-1 production. Since it does not act directly on the pituitary, tumor size is not reduced and can rarely increase it. Cabergoline is a low-cost oral alternative but lacks FDA approval for the treatment of acromegaly. Combination therapy with an SLR and pegvisomant can have better outcomes and may be more cost-effective than monotherapy at higher dose.[58,61]

Table 63–7. Medications for the treatment of acromegaly.

Mechanism	Drug	Dose	Adverse Effects
Somatostatin receptor ligand	Octreotide acetate	140-1500 µg total daily dose, given three times per day subcutaneously	Gastrointestinal side effects, cholelithiasis, hyperglycemia, hypoglycemia, bradycardia, alopecia
	Octreotide capsule	40-80 mg total daily dose, given twice daily orally	Same as octreotide acetate. Needs to be taken on empty stomach
	Octreotide LAR	10-40 mg every 4 weeks intramuscularly	Similar to octreotide acetate
	Lanreotide depot	60-120 mg every 4 weeks subcutaneously	Similar to octreotide acetate
	Pasireotide LAR	20-60 mg every 4 weeks intramuscularly	Same as octreotide acetate. Higher risk of hyperglycemia (50%)
Growth hormone receptor antagonist	Pegvisomant	5-40 mg total daily dose, given daily subcutaneously	Lipodystrophy, skin rash, hepatotoxicity
Dopamine receptor agonist	Cabergoline*	0.5-7.0 mg total per week, given several times per week or daily orally	Nausea, vomiting, dizziness, headache, nasal congestion, constipation, digital vasospasm, vivid dreams, anxiety, depression, impulsivity; high doses (>3 mg/d) have been associated with cardiac valvulopathy

*Not currently FDA approved.

Radiotherapy is a third-line option after surgery and medical therapy. It controls tumor growth in over 90% and normalizes IGF-1 levels over 60% of cases but at a risk of complications, both endocrine (ie, hypopituitarism) and nonendocrine (eg, secondary tumors, cranial nerve palsy, optic apparatus injury).

Improved medical and surgery therapies have led to a substantial reduction in overall mortality which is on par with the general population.[62] Despite biochemical control, however, over two-thirds of patients still report acromegaly symptoms and decreased quality of life. There is a shift away from solely treating to normalize IGF-1 levels and a focus on targeting comorbidities and quality-of-life measures.[63]

D. TSH-secreting Tumors

Surgery for TSH-secreting adenomas is a first-line treatment that seeks to maintain normal pituitary function, minimize thyroid dysfunction, and alleviate compressive syndromes like visual loss. Presurgical treatment with antithyroid medications and beta blockers can restore normal thyroid function. Additionally, preoperative somatostatin analogs can reduce tumor size in addition to normalizing thyroid function.[64]

Remission rates in surgical series vary from 30% to 96%. A meta-analysis comprising 536 patients reported pooled biochemical remission in the postoperative period of 69.7%. As with most tumors, size and cavernous sinus invasion predict likelihood of gross total resection, which has been achieved in 54% of reported cases.[65]

After surgery, patients with residual tumors may benefit from somatostatin analogs to control thyrotoxicosis as well as tumor growth. Other strategies after unsuccessful transsphenoidal surgery and life-threatening hyperthyroidism are pituitary radiotherapy or thyroidectomy.[66]

REFERENCES

1. Daly AF, Beckers A. The epidemiology of pituitary adenomas. *Endocrinol Metab Clin North Am.* 2020;49(3):347-355.
2. Inoshita N, Nishioka H. The 2017 WHO classification of pituitary adenoma: overview and comments. *Brain Tumor Pathol.* 2018;35(2):51-56.
3. Osamura RY LM, Grossman A, Kontogeorgos G, Trouillas J. *World Health Organization Classification of Tumours of Endocrine Organs.* 4th ed. World Health Organization; 2017.
4. Vroonen L, Daly AF, Beckers A. Epidemiology and management challenges in prolactinomas. *Neuroendocrinology.* 2019;109(1):20-27.
5. Molitch ME. Diagnosis and treatment of pituitary adenomas: a review. *JAMA.* 2017;317(5):516-524.
6. Beck-Peccoz P, Giavoli C, Lania A. A 2019 update on TSH-secreting pituitary adenomas. *J Endocrinol Invest.* 2019;42(12):1401-1406.
7. Higham CE, Johannsson G, Shalet SM. Hypopituitarism. *Lancet.* 2016;388(10058):2403-2415.
8. Nieman LK. Cushing's syndrome: update on signs, symptoms and biochemical screening. *Eur J Endocrinol.* 2015;173(4):M33-M38.
9. Petrossians P, Daly AF, Natchev E, et al. Acromegaly at diagnosis in 3173 patients from the Liège Acromegaly Survey (LAS) Database. *Endocr Relat Cancer.* 2017;24(10):505-518.
10. Lenders NF, McCormack AI, Ho KKY. Management of endocrine disease: does gender matter in the management of acromegaly? *Eur J Endocrinol.* 2020;182(5):R67-R82.
11. Gadelha MR, Kasuki L, Lim DST, Fleseriu M. Systemic complications of acromegaly and the impact of the current treatment landscape: an update. *Endocr Rev.* 2019;40(1):268-332.
12. Beck-Peccoz P, Giavoli C, Lania A. A 2019 update on TSH-secreting pituitary adenomas. *J Endocrinol Invest.* 2019;42(12):1401-1406.
13. Bhasin S, Brito JP, Cunningham GR, et al. Testosterone therapy in men with hypogonadism: an endocrine society clinical practice guideline. *J Clin Endocrinol Metab.* 2018;103(5):1715-1744.
14. Yuen KCJ, Biller BMK, Radovick S, et al. American Association of Clinical Endocrinologists and American College of Endocrinology Guidelines for management of growth hormone deficiency in adults and patients transitioning from pediatric to adult care. *Endocr Pract.* 2019;25(11):1191-1232.
15. Chen CC, Carter BS, Wang R, et al. Congress of neurological surgeons systematic review and evidence-based guideline on preoperative imaging assessment of patients with suspected nonfunctioning pituitary adenomas. *Neurosurgery.* 2016;79(4):E524-E526.
16. Fleseriu M, Bodach ME, Tumialan LM, et al. Congress of neurological surgeons systematic review and evidence-based guideline for pretreatment endocrine evaluation of patients with nonfunctioning pituitary adenomas. *Neurosurgery.* 2016;79(4):E527-E529.
17. Faje A. Immunotherapy and hypophysitis: clinical presentation, treatment, and biologic insights. *Pituitary.* 2016;19(1):82-92.
18. Galm BP, Qiao N, Klibanski A, Biller BMK, Tritos NA. Accuracy of laboratory tests for the diagnosis of Cushing syndrome. *J Clin Endocrinol Metab.* 2020;105(6):dgaa105.
19. Loriaux DL. Diagnosis and differential diagnosis of Cushing's syndrome. *N Engl J Med.* 2017;376(15):1451-1459.
20. Senanayake R, Gillett D, MacFarlane J, et al. New types of localization methods for adrenocorticotropic hormone-dependent Cushing's syndrome. *Best Pract Res Clin Endocrinol Metab.* 2021;35(1):101513.
21. Fleseriu M, Auchus R, Bancos I, et al. Consensus on diagnosis and management of Cushing's disease: a guideline update. *Lancet Diabetes Endocrinol.* 2021;9(12):847-875.
22. Dobri G, Niwattisaiwong S, Bena JF, et al. Is GH nadir during OGTT a reliable test for diagnosis of acromegaly in patients with abnormal glucose metabolism? *Endocrine.* 2019;64(1):139-146.
23. Beck-Peccoz P, Giavoli C, Lania A. A 2019 update on TSH-secreting pituitary adenomas. *J Endocrinol Invest.* 2019;42(12):1401-1406.
24. Soh SB, Aw TC. Laboratory testing in thyroid conditions–pitfalls and clinical utility. *Ann Lab Med.* 2019;39(1):3-14.
25. Cavallo LM, Somma T, Solari D, et al. Endoscopic endonasal transsphenoidal surgery: history and evolution. *World Neurosurg.* 2019;127:686-694.
26. Oldfield EH. Cushing's disease: lessons learned from 1500 cases. *Neurosurgery.* 2017;64(CN_suppl_1):27-36.
27. Singh H, Essayed WI, Cohen-Gadol A, Zada G, Schwartz TH. Resection of pituitary tumors: endoscopic versus microscopic. *J Neurooncol.* 2016;130(2):309-317.

28. Cellina M, Gibelli D, Floridi C, et al. Sphenoid sinuses: pneumatisation and anatomical variants—what the radiologist needs to know and report to avoid intraoperative complications. *Surg Radiol Anat.* 2020;42(9):1013-1024.
29. Cohen S, Jones SH, Dhandapani S, Negm HM, Anand VK, Schwartz TH. Lumbar drains decrease the risk of postoperative cerebrospinal fluid leak following endonasal endoscopic surgery for suprasellar meningiomas in patients with high body mass index. *Oper Neurosurg (Hagerstown).* 2018; 14(1):66-71.
30. Taylor DG, Jane JA, Oldfield EH. Resection of pituitary macroadenomas via the pseudocapsule along the posterior tumor margin: a cohort study and technical note. *J Neurosurg.* 2018;128(2):422-428.
31. Younus I, Gerges MM, Godil SS, et al. Incidence and risk factors associated with reoperation for sellar hematoma following endoscopic transsphenoidal pituitary surgery. *J Neurosurg.* 23 2019:1-7.
32. Gerges MM, Rumalla K, Godil SS, et al. Long-term outcomes after endoscopic endonasal surgery for nonfunctioning pituitary macroadenomas. *J Neurosurg.* 2020;134:535-546.
33. Carnevale JA, Babu CS, Goldberg JL, Fong R, Schwartz TH. Visual deterioration after endonasal endoscopic skull base surgery: causes, treatments, and outcomes. *J Neurosurg.* 2021:1-11.
34. Raza SM, Banu MA, Donaldson A, Patel KS, Anand VK, Schwartz TH. Sensitivity and specificity of intrathecal fluorescein and white light excitation for detecting intraoperative cerebrospinal fluid leak in endoscopic skull base surgery: a prospective study. *J Neurosurg.* 2016;124(3):621-626.
35. Pledger CL, Elzoghby MA, Oldfield EH, Payne SC, Jane JA Jr. Prospective comparison of sinonasal outcomes after microscopic sublabial or endoscopic endonasal transsphenoidal surgery for nonfunctioning pituitary adenomas. *J Neurosurg.* 2016;125(2):323-333.
36. Cho J, Grayson JW, Christensen J, et al. Long-term sinonasal function following transnasal pituitary surgery: a comparison of surgical approach. *Am J Rhinol Allergy.* 2020;34(3): 361-368.
37. Little AS, Kshettry VR, Rosen MR, et al. Postoperative oral antibiotics and sinonasal outcomes following endoscopic transsphenoidal surgery for pituitary tumors study: a multicenter, prospective, randomized, double-blinded, placebo-controlled study. *Neurosurgery.* 2021;89(5):769-776.
38. Winograd D, Staggers KA, Sebastian S, Takashima M, Yoshor D, Samson SL. An effective and practical fluid restriction protocol to decrease the risk of hyponatremia and readmissions after transsphenoidal surgery. *Neurosurgery.* 2020;87(4): 761-769.
39. Polovina TS, Kraljevic I, Solak M, et al. Early basal cortisol level as a predictor of hypothalamic-pituitary-adrenal (HPA) axis function after pituitary tumor surgery. *Exp Clin Endocrinol Diabetes.* 2020;128(11):709-714.
40. Fleseriu M, Hashim IA, Karavitaki N, et al. Hormonal replacement in hypopituitarism in adults: an endocrine society clinical practice guideline. *J Clin Endocrinol Metab.* 2016; 101(11): 3888-3921.
41. Gruber LM, Bancos I. Secondary adrenal insufficiency: recent updates and new directions for diagnosis and management. *Endocr Pract.* 2022;28(1):110-117.
42. Beck-Peccoz P, Rodari G, Giavoli C, Lania A. Central hypothyroidism: a neglected thyroid disorder. *Nat Rev Endocrinol.* 2017;13(10):588-598.
43. van Bunderen CC, Olsson DS. Growth hormone deficiency and replacement therapy in adults: impact on survival. *Rev Endocr Metab Disord.* 2021;22(1):125-133.
44. Melmed S. Pathogenesis and diagnosis of growth hormone deficiency in adults. *N Engl J Med.* 2019;380(26):2551-2562.
45. Dogansen SC, Cikrikcili U, Oruk G, et al. Dopamine agonist-induced impulse control disorders in patients with prolactinoma: a cross-sectional multicenter study. *J Clin Endocrinol Metab.* 2019;104(7):2527-2534.
46. Stiles CE, Tetteh-Wayoe ET, Bestwick J, Steeds RP, Drake WM. A meta-analysis of the prevalence of cardiac valvulopathy in hyperprolactinemic patients treated with Cabergoline. *J Clin Endocrinol Metab.* 2018.
47. Samson SL, Ezzat S. AACE/ACE disease state clinical review: dopamine agonists for hyperprolactinemia and the risk of cardiac valve disease. *Endocr Pract.* 2014;20(6):608-616.
48. Zamanipoor Najafabadi AH, Zandbergen IM, deVries F, et al. Surgery as a viable alternative first-line treatment for prolactinoma patients. A systematic review and meta-analysis. *J Clin Endocrinol Metab.* 2020;105(3):e32-e41.
49. Honegger J, Nasi-Kordhishti I, Aboutaha N, Giese S. Surgery for prolactinomas: a better choice? *Pituitary.* 2020;23(1):45-51.
50. Papakokkinou E, Olsson DS, Chantzichristos D, et al. Excess morbidity persists in patients with Cushing's disease during long-term remission: a swedish nationwide study. *J Clin Endocrinol Metab.* 2020;105(8):dgaa291.
51. Varlamov EV, Langlois F, Vila G, Fleseriu M. Management of endocrine disease: cardiovascular risk assessment, thromboembolism, and infection prevention in Cushing's syndrome: a practical approach. *Eur J Endocrinol.* 2021;184(5):R207-R224.
52. Burke WT, Penn DL, Repetti CS, Iuliano S, Laws ER. Outcomes after repeat transsphenoidal surgery for recurrent Cushing disease: updated. *Neurosurgery.* 2019;85(6):E1030-E1036.
53. Braun LT, Rubinstein G, Zopp S, et al. Recurrence after pituitary surgery in adult Cushing's disease: a systematic review on diagnosis and treatment. *Endocrine.* 2020;70(2):218-231.
54. Fleseriu M, Auchus R, Bancos I, et al. Consensus on diagnosis and management of Cushing's disease: a guideline update. *Lancet Diabetes Endocrinol.* 2021;9(12):847-875.
55. Pivonello R, Ferrigno R, De Martino MC, et al. Medical treatment of Cushing's disease: an overview of the current and recent clinical trials. *Front Endocrinol (Lausanne).* 2020;11:648.
56. Capatina C, Hinojosa-Amaya JM, Poiana C, Fleseriu M. Management of patients with persistent or recurrent Cushing's disease after initial pituitary surgery. *Expert Rev Endocrinol Metab.* 2020;15(5):321-339.
57. Sasagawa Y, Hayashi Y, Tachibana O, et al. Transsphenoidal surgery for elderly patients with acromegaly and its outcomes: comparison with younger patients. *World Neurosurg.* 2018;118:e229-e234.
58. Giustina A, Barkhoudarian G, Beckers A, et al. Multidisciplinary management of acromegaly: a consensus. *Rev Endocr Metab Disord.* 2020; 21(4):667-678.
59. Asha MJ, Takami H, Velasquez C, et al. Long-term outcomes of transsphenoidal surgery for management of growth hormone-secreting adenomas: single-center results. *J Neurosurg.* 2019:1-11.
60. Schilbach K, Gar C, Lechner A, et al. Determinants of the growth hormone nadir during oral glucose tolerance test in adults. *Eur J Endocrinol.* 2019;181(1):55-67.
61. Fleseriu M, Biller BMK, Freda PU, et al. A Pituitary Society update to acromegaly management guidelines. *Pituitary.* 2021; 24(1):1-13.

62. Bolfi F, Neves AF, Boguszewski CL, Nunes-Nogueira VS. Mortality in acromegaly decreased in the last decade: a systematic review and meta-analysis. *Eur J Endocrinol.* 2019;181(5):L5-L16.
63. Fleseriu M, Molitch M, Dreval A, et al. Disease and treatment-related burden in patients with acromegaly who are biochemically controlled on injectable somatostatin receptor ligands. *Front Endocrinol (Lausanne).* 2021;12:627711.
64. Fukuhara N, Horiguchi K, Nishioka H, et al. Short-term preoperative octreotide treatment for TSH-secreting pituitary adenoma. *Endocr J.* 2015;62(1):21-27.
65. Cossu G, Daniel RT, Pierzchala K, et al. Thyrotropin-secreting pituitary adenomas: a systematic review and meta-analysis of postoperative outcomes and management. *Pituitary.* 2019; 22(1):79-88.
66. Mouslech Z, Somali M, Sakali AK, Savopoulo C, Mastorakos G, Hatzitolios AI. TSH-secreting pituitary adenomas treated by gamma knife radiosurgery: our case experience and a review of the literature. *Hormones (Athens).* 2016;15(1):122-128.

Familial Nonmedullary Thyroid Cancer

64

Gustavo Romero-Velez, MD
Allan Siperstein, MD

INTRODUCTION

In recent years, there has been an increase in the incidence of thyroid cancer. Currently, it is the most frequent endocrine-related malignancy, with up to 14.3 cases per 100,000 individuals.[1] A key component while addressing any concept associated with thyroid cancer is the understanding of its distinct embryological origins. During its embryologic development, the thyroid is made up of endoderm which will constitute the epithelial cells. On the other hand, there is controversy regarding the origin of the parafollicular C cells, which traditionally were believed to arise from the neural crest but most recently had been traced to be derived from the endoderm as well.[2] Abnormal proliferation of the C cells can result in the development of medullary thyroid cancer (MTC), which comprises less than 5% of all thyroid malignancies.[3] On the other hand, the malignant transformation of epithelial cells comprises the majority of thyroid malignancies (~95%), sometimes referred to as nonmedullary thyroid cancer (NMTC), and can be further classified as papillary, follicular, Hürthle cell, poorly differentiated, and anaplastic sub-types.

While MTC is less frequent, it has been well studied given its worse prognosis and the fact that up to 25% of the cases have a familial inheritance pattern with a well-described mutation in the *RET* proto-oncogene.[4] The *RET* mutation is inherited in an autosomal dominant fashion and can have either a syndromic (multiple endocrine neoplasia type 2) or nonsyndromic (familial MTC) presentation. Although epithelial-derived tumors constitute most thyroid cancers, the presence of familial susceptibility has only been a matter of discussion over the past 20 years. This entity is commonly referred to as familial nonmedullary thyroid cancer (FNMTC), and it is believed to represent 5% to 15% of follicular cell-derived thyroid cancers.[3,5]

Despite the fact that most of the research on FNMTC has occurred recently, the first evidence of an inherited pattern of NMTC was published in 1954 by Robinson and Orr.[6] In their original report, they describe two identical twins affected with papillary thyroid cancer (PTC) at age 24. A few more reports of kindreds followed, demonstrating the possibility of an inherited pattern; however, it was not until 1999 that Malchoff and Malchoff introduced the term FNMTC.[7,8] Though current knowledge of FNMTC is growing, there are still gaps in understanding and even conflicting evidence, which will be described and addressed in the following sections.

DEFINITION & GENETICS

The linkage of the *RET* proto-oncogene to MEN2 in 1991 has facilitated the identification of individuals with familial forms of MTC.[9] In the case of FNMTC, no individual gene has been identified as the target culprit, making it more difficult to categorize which individuals are affected by a familial form and which ones have sporadic nonmedullary thyroid cancer (SNMTC). Some studies suggest that FNMTC has an autosomal dominant inheritance pattern with variable penetrance, while others consider it to be a polygenic disorder with a high degree of molecular heterogeneity.[3,10]

As in the familial form of MTC, FNMTC can present in a syndromic or nonsyndromic fashion. Syndromic forms are easier to classify as they are part of a well-described entity with diagnostic criteria, and in most of them, there is a specific gene mutation that allows for their identification. The typical syndromes associated with FNMTC are familial adenomatous polyposis (FAP), Cowden syndrome, Carney complex, Werner syndrome, and DICER 1 syndrome.[5,10,11] Although these described syndromes have a well-known association with FNMTC, it is important to note that these constitute less than 3% of the familial cases of NMTC, as shown in Figure 64–1.

FAP has an autosomal dominant inheritance pattern attributed to the *APC* gene on 5q21-22. This condition is

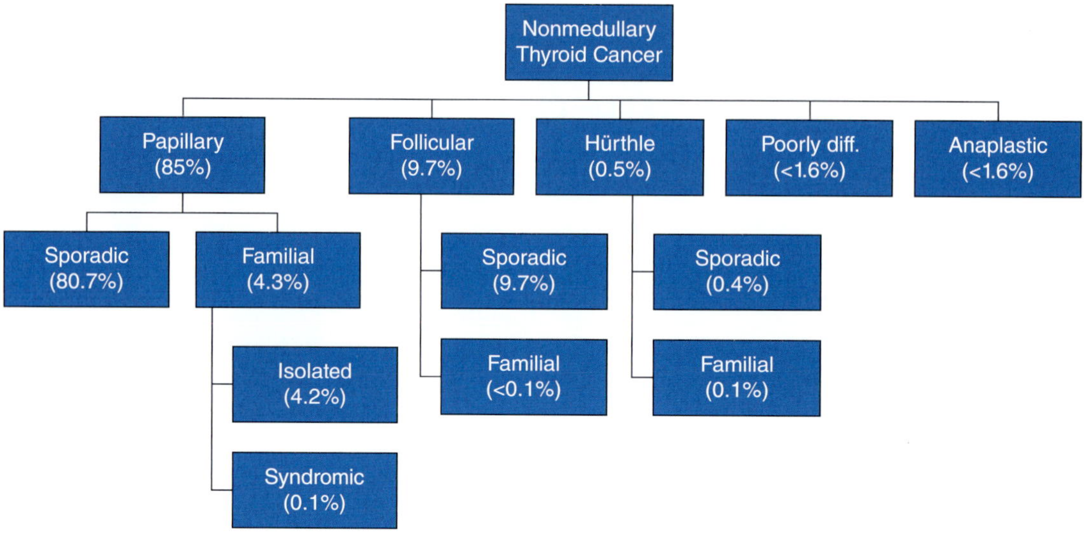

Figure 64–1. Distribution of cases of nonmedullary thyroid cancer. (Adapted from Hińcza K, Kowalik A, Kowalska A. Current knowledge of germline genetic risk factors for the development of nonmedullary thyroid cancer. *Genes*. 2019;10(7):482.)

better known for its risk of colonic and duodenal cancers. Thyroid cancer is the third most common malignancy in patients with FAP, with an incidence between 1% and 7.3%.[12] These patients tend to present before 30 years old with multifocal tumors and typically are found to have PTC with cribriform morula histology.[3,5,13] In our institutional experience, FAP patients screened with neck ultrasound had an incidence of thyroid nodules and thyroid cancer in 38% and 2.6%, respectively.[14] Although it is currently recommended to perform yearly thyroid ultrasound screening for FAP patients beginning in their teenage years, those with nodules are more likely to progress to thyroid cancer compared to those with normal baseline ultrasounds, which might suggest that follow-up can be less frequent in the presence of normal baseline screening.[12]

Cowden syndrome, also referred to as PTEN-hamartoma tumor syndrome, has an autosomal dominant inheritance due to a mutation of *PTEN* on 10q22-23. It is characterized by developmental disorders, gastrointestinal hamartomas, mucocutaneous lesions, and breast, endometrial, and genitourinary cancers. Thyroid cancer can be present in more than 10% of the affected individuals and is usually PTC, but cases of follicular thyroid cancer (FTC) and anaplastic thyroid cancer have also been described.[11] Multinodular goiter is quite prevalent in Cowden syndrome, affecting up to three-quarters of these patients. Current screening guidelines for this population recommend yearly thyroid ultrasounds starting at 18 years old.[15] However, given their high risk of thyroid cancer and the difficulties of performing fine-needle aspiration (FNA) biopsies on those who have concomitant developmental disorders, prophylactic total thyroidectomy has also been suggested as an alternative.[16]

Pleuropulmonary blastoma familial tumor and dysplasia syndrome, more commonly referred to as **DICER 1 syndrome**, is rare and has an autosomal dominant inheritance attributed to mutations of the *DICER1* gene in 14q32. As its name implies, it presents with pleuropulmonary blastoma and other tumors, including Sertoli-Leydig cell, gynandroblastoma, embryonal rhabdomyosarcoma, and presacral malignant teratoma, among others.[17] Thyroid ultrasound screening is recommended starting at age 8 as 13% to 32% of the individuals will have multinodular goiter, and another 16% will have PTC and FTC.[11,18]

Carney complex also has an autosomal dominant inheritance pattern attributed to mutations in the *PRKAR1A* gene at 17q24. Clinically, it is characterized by endocrine manifestations, including nodular adrenocortical disease with manifestations of Cushing syndrome, pituitary growth hormone tumors responsible for acromegaly, and other non-endocrine manifestations such as cutaneous pigmentation, and myxomas of the heart, breast, and skin. Thyroid disease is common, with 75% of patients showing thyroid lesions and 25% having thyroid tumors, of which follicular adenomas are the most common.[19] Nevertheless, PTC and FTC can occur in 2.5% of the patients.[20] There are no current recommendations regarding when to screen for thyroid cancer, but it has been shown that thyroid nodules appear during the first 10 years of life and can be found as early as 2 years.[21]

Werner syndrome shows an autosomal recessive inheritance associated with the gene *WRN* in 8p12. Clinical characteristics include the presence of features of normal aging such as graying of the scalp hair, ocular cataracts, and cancer predisposition to melanoma, meningioma, and soft tissue sarcomas.[22] Thyroid neoplasms are also a common occurrence in this disease. A Japanese study reported that 18% of their patients with Werner syndrome had thyroid cancer, of which 48% was FTC, 35% PTC, and 13% anaplastic.[23] There are no current recommendations regarding when to screen for thyroid cancer, but routine thyroid US screening is recommended.[24]

Hereditary nonpolyposis colorectal cancer (HNPCC) or **Lynch syndrome** is a well-described hereditary cancer syndrome with an autosomal dominant inheritance. Although the Amsterdam criteria had been widely used for its characterization, a responsible germline mutation in the mismatch repair genes (*MLHL, MSH2, MSH6, PMS2,* and *EPCAM*) has facilitated its diagnosis. Microsatellite instability is rare in thyroid cancer and is usually associated with aggressive variants. Until recently, no association with HNPCC had been found, but Aswath et al. were the first to describe a family with Lynch syndrome affected by PTC.[25] Even though an *MSH2* variant was identified in the family, the authors could not link the microsatellite instability as the causative factor accounting for the development of FNMTC.

In the case of nonsyndromic FNMTC, a specific gene mutation has not been identified, as previously mentioned. The clustering of thyroid cancer in kindreds has made it possible to look for a susceptible gene mutation using different techniques, including linkage analysis, genome-wide association studies, and whole-genome sequencing analysis. Some of the candidate identified genes include *HABP2* in 10q25.3, *SRGAP1* in 12q14, *FOXE1* in 9pq22.33, *TITF-1/NKX2*.1 in 14q13, *MAP2K5* in 15q23, *fPTC/PRN1* in 1p13.2, *NMTC1* in 2q21, *MNG1* in 14q32, and *MYO1F* in 19p13.2.[3,10] It is important to note that genetic mutations such as *BRAF, RAS, RET/PTC, TRK,* and *PPAR* γ that are commonplace in SNMTC have not been found in familial forms.[5]

Given the absence of a genetic basis to characterize FNMTC, the currently accepted definition of FNMTC is the occurrence of follicular cell-derived cancer in two or more first-degree relatives of the index patient.[5,10,26] However, an important consideration is that individuals with a family history of any type of cancer are more likely to develop the same type of cancer compared to the rest of the population and this does not necessarily imply a hereditary form.[27] In the case of thyroid cancer, this increased risk can be up to ninefold, which is among the highest for all types of cancers, and one must also consider the interaction of environmental factors with genetic susceptibility.[5,28,29]

A population-based study including patients from five Nordic countries found a cumulative risk of thyroid cancer based on the number of affected relatives. In their study, the risk increased from 2.1% for patients with a single relative affected up to 24.1% for those who had two relatives affected.[29] This idea was also demonstrated in the study by Charkes, who used the Bernoulli trials model applied to the Surveillance Epidemiology and End Results database and found that families with two members with thyroid cancer had a 69% chance of having sporadic cancers. In comparison, families with three affected members and more than three affected members had only a 6% and 4% chance, respectively, of the cancer being sporadic.[30] As a result of this, other authors have suggested that a minimum of three first-degree relatives is needed to make a diagnosis of FNMTC.[31]

The definition of FNMTC based on the number of affected first-degree relatives could be rather simplistic. In 1999, Musholt et al. proposed a more robust definition of FNMTC.[32] Their study consisted of a review and meta-analysis of the literature looking for factors associated with FNMTC. Based on those results, their predictive criteria for FNMTC were applied to 282 patients who underwent treatment for PTC at their institution. They found 12 potential families with FNMTC; some of the family members were further investigated, and 11 individuals in those families were finally diagnosed with PTC. The authors concluded that factors other than a mere familial history of thyroid cancer could aid in identifying kindreds of FNMTC (Table 64–1).

SCREENING

Screening programs are intended to find susceptible individuals at an early stage of their disease. Optimal screening programs need to demonstrate that the early detection of

Table 64–1. Predictive criteria for identification of FNMTC.

Preconditions
• Exclusion of previous radiation exposure
• Exclusion of neoplasia syndromes associated with PTC
• Exclusion of somatic genetic alterations in the tumor DNA
Primary criteria
• PTC in two or more first-degree blood relatives
• Multinodular goiter in at least three first-degree or second-degree relatives of a PTC patient
Secondary criteria
• Diagnosis in patients younger than 33 years
• Multifocal of bilateral PTC
• Organ-exceeding tumor growth (pT4)
• Lymph node metastasis (pN1) or distant metastases (M1)
• Familial accumulation of adolescent-onset thyroid disease
Hereditary predisposition to PTC is considered in the following is present
• Two primary criteria or
• One primary criterion plus three secondary criteria

FNMTC, familial nonmedullary thyroid cancer; PTC, papillary thyroid cancer; DNA, deoxyribonucleic acid.

Source: Reproduced with permission from Musholt TJ, Musholt PB, Petrich T, Oetting G, Knapp WH, Klempnauer J. Familial papillary thyroid carcinoma: genetics, criteria for diagnosis, clinical features, and surgical treatment. *World J Surg*. 2000;24(11):1409-1417.

the disease positively impacts the disease outcome. In 2017, the United States Preventive Services Task Force (USPSTF) recommended against thyroid cancer screening in asymptomatic adults as they found a negative net effect as a result of overdiagnosis and overtreatment.[33] In hereditary cancer syndromes, individuals with certain clinical characteristics are evaluated for the presence of a specific genetic mutation, which allows for the identification of a hereditary component and further evaluation of the rest of their families. The lack of a specific genetic mutation in FNMTC poses great difficulties when evaluating the benefits of screening in this population. In fact, the 2015 American Thyroid Association (ATA) guidelines do not recommend for or against thyroid ultrasound screening of families with suspected FNMTC, as there is no evidence that this would affect the disease outcome.[34] They do suggest that patients with a familial history of thyroid cancer have a careful history and directed neck examination at their routine health assessments.[34]

Syndromic variants of FNMTC have recommendations for using neck ultrasound to screen individuals affected with that particular syndrome, as mentioned in the prior section. On the other hand, performing screening neck ultrasounds on family members of patients with two affected relatives with thyroid cancer is unlikely to be cost-effective. Based on the study by Charkes, this theoretical screening would likely have a high sensitivity to detect FNMTC but will lack specificity as only 31% of the patients with two affected individuals have a familial inheritance pattern.[30]

In a prospective cohort study by the National Institutes of Health (NIH), Klubo-Gwiezdzinska et al. prospectively enrolled kindreds with FNMTC to perform a neck ultrasound. Screening was done on 109 at-risk individuals from 25 families. Thyroid nodules were found in 50.5% of them, and after guideline-based FNA biopsy, thyroid cancer was found in 4.6% of at-risk individuals with two family members affected and in 22.7% of at-risk individuals with three or more family members affected.[35] Based on these results, some authors deem it reasonable to perform US screening starting at age 20 or 10 years before the earliest age at diagnosis in those who have more than three affected family members.[5]

Authors who support screening for FNMTC base their opinion on the fact that these patients have an earlier presentation and more aggressive behavior, but this is still a matter of controversy in the literature.[31] Nonetheless, no study has prospectively demonstrated that screening programs in this population have decreased mortality or improved quality of life.[5] Table 64–2 summarizes some of the available recommendations for screening in FNMTC.

Table 64–2. Screening recommendations.

a) Nonsyndromic FNMTC	
Two affected family members	Careful history and directed neck examination at their routine health assessments.[34]
More three affected family members	Thyroid US screening starting at age 20 or 10 years before the earliest age at diagnosis.[5]
b) Syndromic FNMTC	
Familial adenomatous polyposis	Yearly thyroid US beginning in the teenage years.[12]
Cowden syndrome	Yearly thyroid US starting at 18 years old.[15]
DICER 1 syndrome	Thyroid US screening starting at age 8.[11,18]
Carney complex	No current recommendation but thyroid nodules appear in the first 10 years of life.[21]
Werner syndrome	No current recommendation but routine thyroid US screening is recommended.[24]
Lynch syndrome	No current recommendation.

FNMTC, familial nonmedullary thyroid cancer; US, ultrasound.

PRESENTATION

Syndromic forms of FNMTC share similar clinical characteristics, such as an early age onset, as well as multifocal and bilateral tumors.[14,16,31] Conversely, the lack of genetic testing to accurately diagnose nonsyndromic FNMTC creates much heterogeneity in the results of studies addressing the clinical and pathological aspects of the disease. Conflicting evidence in the literature can be partially explained by the different methods and definitions used in each study. Most of the studies are either case-control or cohort studies derived from institutional databases of thyroidectomy patients, and while most use the accepted definition considering as familial those with more than two family members affected, three others use a less strict definition, including all of those with at least one family member affected.[44-52]

Age at Onset

Most studies have not seen an early age of onset of FNMTC compared to SNMTC. However, Moses et al. studied 30 patients with two or more first-degree relatives affected by thyroid cancer. They compared them to those without a family history and found an earlier age of onset for those with a positive family history (43 years old vs 48 years old, $p < 0.002$).[38] Similarly, Mazeh et al. found an earlier age of onset for those with more than one family member affected (43 years old vs 49 years old, $p = 0.04$).[48] In their sub-analysis, they compared one affected relative versus two or more, and although those with two affected members seemed to be younger (40 years old vs 44 years old), this did not reach statistical significance ($p = 0.4$). Using the same definition of more than one family member affected, Tavarelli et al. also found that FNMTC presents at a younger age, 45 years old, compared to SNMTC at 48 years old ($p < 0.005$).[51]

In contrast, McDonald et al. compared 41 patients with three or more affected family members to 531 patients with no family history and found no difference regarding the age of presentation (43 years old vs 44 years old, $p = 0.14$), and their results are supported by other groups who have also found no age difference.[39-42,44-47,49,50,52] As a result of this discrepancy in the literature, a meta-analysis was conducted, which included 990 patients with FNMTC and compared them to SNMTC, and found that familial cases had a standard mean difference of −0.91 years of age at presentation ($p = 0.01$), which although statistically significant, is not of important clinical significance.[53] As some authors have pointed out, it is impossible to know if the difference observed is due to true biological anticipation or is just the result of increased screening of relatives following a cancer diagnosis.[31]

Sex

Traditionally speaking, NMTC is more frequent in females compared to males, with ratios ranging from 2:1 to 4:1. However, mortality by gender is almost equal, and in fact, newer studies based on autopsies suggest the prevalence between sexes could be the same.[54] In the case of FNMTC, none of the published series found differences in the female-to-male ratio compared to SNMTC.[36-52]

Multifocal Tumors

Multifocal tumors are found in 32% to 39% of NMTC cases and are sometimes used as an independent prognostic factor.[55] Most studies have found that FNMTC has a higher percentage of multifocal tumors than SNMTC. The meta-analysis by Wang et al. showed that FNMTC has a 1.5 times higher risk of harboring multifocal tumors and a 1.29 times higher risk for bilateral tumors.[53] As the National Comprehensive Cancer Network (NCCN) guidelines recommend completion of thyroidectomy in cases with macroscopic multifocal disease, the higher risk for multifocal and bilateral tumors should be discussed during the preoperative counseling of patients with FNMTC.

Primary Tumor Size

Only two studies have suggested that FNMTC patients have larger primary tumors.[41,49] A study by Park et al., comparing the mean size of tumors in SNMTC versus FNMTC, found that FNMTC had smaller tumors (1.2 cm vs 1.4 cm, $p < 0.05$).[49] In contrast, a study by Lei et al. compared groups by tumor size >4 cm and found that FNMTC had a greater percentage of T3 tumors (36.4% vs 12.4%, $p = 0.002$).[41] A full analysis that included 10,417 patients from five different studies found no difference regarding the size ($p = 0.74$).[53]

Extra Thyroidal Extension

Extra thyroidal extension could represent either T3b tumors with invasion to the strap muscles or T4 tumors that have invaded other nearby structures. Although the majority of individual studies have not shown FNMTC to be associated with higher rates of extrathyroidal extension, Wang et al. included 6403 patients from eight studies and found that FNMTC had a 1.2 times higher risk of extrathyroidal extension.[53] Three independent studies also found a higher incidence of extrathyroidal extension in FNMTC.[41,42,48] One study showed that in those with two or more family members affected, local invasion was present in 11% compared to 5.5% when only one member was affected and 0.6% for those with no family history.[48] Meanwhile, the study by Lei showed that in patients with FNMTC, local invasion was present in up to 81% of the cases compared to 23% for SNMTC.[41] Finally, an analysis by Zhang et al. found that capsule invasion was more frequent in familial cases (64% vs 48%, $p = 0.0006$).[42]

Locoregional Spread

In four studies, familial cases presented with locoregional metastatic disease more frequently.[41,42,48,51] Three of those studies had a concomitant higher rate of local tumor invasion in the familial group, putting into question if the higher prevalence of locoregional metastatic disease is a result of the familial form itself or if it is just a consequence of that group exhibiting higher rates of local invasion.[41,42,48] Interestingly, the study by Tavarelli et al. demonstrated N1 disease in 26% of the FNMTC group compared to 17% in the SNMTC group with no other concomitant differences in other prognostic characteristics.[51] Finally, the meta-analysis by Wang et al. showed a 1.18 times higher risk of lymph node metastasis for familial cases.[53]

PROGNOSIS

Before the case-control and cohort studies were published, case series had already reported more aggressive disease in familial cases.[7] Overall, the majority of the studies suggest that FNMTC has a worse prognosis compared to its counterpart, SNMTC. When combining studies, FNMTC patients had higher recurrence rates (OR 1.72 95% CI 1.34-2.20) and lower disease-free survival (HR 2.9 95% CI 1.88-2.79) with moderate heterogeneity among studies.[53] Although differences in their baseline clinical characteristics such as the age of onset, presence of multifocal tumors, size of the primary tumor, extrathyroidal extension, and presence of lymph node metastasis could explain these findings, in some studies, there is not much difference at baseline, and still, FNMTC patients exhibit a worse prognosis (Table 64–3).[36,41,44,45,47-51]

Four studies addressed this concern and performed a matched analysis of patients with more than two affected family members by age, gender, and stage.[36,37,43] Only Alsanea et al. found differences in recurrence (44% vs 17%, $p < 0.001$) and mean disease-free survival (63 months vs 88 months, $p < 0.05$) while comparing 48 familial cases to

144 matched controls.[36] Although, in their study, the treatment also varied between familial cases and matched controls in terms of rate of total thyroidectomy (73% vs 94%, $p < 0.0001$), rate of modified radical neck dissection (46% vs 22%, $p < 0.01$), iodine 131 therapy (60% vs 85%, $p < 0.001$) and mean iodine dose received (88mCi vs 119mCi, $p < 0.01$). Maxwell et al. compared 24 familial cases to 24 matched controls with no difference in the baseline characteristics or surgical treatment and found similar recurrence rates (4.5% vs 5.8%, $p = 0.70$).[37] Cao et al. included 372 FNMTC

Table 64–3. Summary of studies comparing FNMTC vs SNMTC.

Author	Year	Country	Definition	Sample	Age	Sex	Multifocal	Size	Extra Thyroidal	Lymph Node Metastasis	Prognosis
Alsanea et al.[36]	2000	Japan USA	>2	FNMTC = 48 SNMTC = 144	Yes	No*	No*	No*	No*	No*	Yes
Uchino et al.[44]	2002	Japan	>1	FNMTC = 258 SNMTC = 6200	No	No	Yes	No	No	No	Yes
Maxwell et al.[37]	2004	Canada	>2	FNMTC = 24 SNMTC = 519	No*	No*	No*	No*	No*	No*	No
Capezzone et al.[45]	2008	Italy Greece	>1	FNMTC = 34 SNMTC = 235	No	No	Yes	No	No	No	Yes
Ito et al.[46]	2009	Japan	>1	FNMTC = 273 SNMTC = 5742	No	No	Yes	No	No	No	No
Moses et al.[38]	2010	USA	>2	FNMTC = 12 SNMTC = 124	Yes	No	No	No	No	No	No
McDonald et al.[47]	2011	Canada	>1	FMNTC = 91 SNMTC = 521	No	No	No	No	No	No	Yes
Robenshtok et al.[39]	2011	Israel	>2	FNMTC = 67 SNMTC = 375	No	No	No	No	No	No	No
Mazeh et al.[48]	2011	USA	>1	FNMTC = 37 SNMTC = 321	Yes	No	Yes	No	Yes	Yes	Yes
Park et al.[49]	2012	Korea	>1	FNMTC = 318 SNMTC = 2733	No	No	Yes	Yes	No	No	Yes
Lee et al.[50]	2014	Korea	>1	FNMTC = 113 SNMTC = 1149	No	No	Yes	No	No	No	Yes
Pinto et al.[40]	2014	Portugal	>2	FNMTC = 107 SNMTC = 107	No	No	Yes	No	No	No	No
Lei et al.[41]	2015	China	>2	FNMTC = 22 SNMTC = 226	No	No	Yes	Yes	Yes	Yes	Yes
Tavarelli et al.[51]	2015	Italy	>1	FNMTC = 151 SNMTC = 643	Yes	No	Yes	No	No	Yes	Yes
Cao et al.[52]	2016	China	>1	FNMTC = 372 SNMTC = 372	No*	No*	Yes	No*	No*	No*	No
Zhang et al.[42]	2016	China	>2	FNMTC = 78 SNMTC = 3445	No	No	No	No	Yes	Yes	No
Shafiei et al.[43]	2021	Iran	>2	FNMTC = 66 SNMTC = 66	No*	No*	No*	No*	No*	No*	No

Yes, indicates a difference between groups was found.

*Matched controls; FNMTC, familial nonmedullary thyroid cancer; SNMTC, sporadic nonmedullary thyroid cancer.

Source: Adapted from Nixon IJ, Suárez C, Simo R, et al. The impact of family history on non-medullary thyroid cancer. *European Journal of Surgical Oncology (EJSO)*. 2016;42(10):1455-1463.

patients and, using matched controls, found no statistically significant difference in recurrence (7.8% vs 5.38%), but the treatment in the groups differed in terms of the extent of thyroidectomy and use of iodine radiotherapy.[52] Lastly, in the study by Shafiei et al., 66 familial cases who underwent radioiodine therapy were compared to 66 matched controls and no difference was found in terms of response to therapy; however, familial cases took a longer time to respond (26 months vs 15 months, $p = 0.01$).[43]

TREATMENT

The treatment for FNMTC is as controversial as its presentation. Authors who found FNMTC to be more aggressive suggest a concomitant, more aggressive treatment, while those who consider it to be similar to SNMTC recommend treatment based on current guidelines. However, there is no clear evidence to support one approach or the other, and treatment should likely be individualized for each patient.

In the case of familial MTC, the benefit of prophylactic thyroidectomy has been proven, and its use is recommended.[56] On the other hand, for FNMTC, there is no available evidence to support prophylactic thyroidectomy, and it should not be done. Patients determined to be at risk and considered candidates for screening should undergo neck US and receive appropriate treatment based on their findings and current ATA guidelines.[34] As mentioned before, in the case of Cowden syndrome, it has been proposed to perform a prophylactic thyroidectomy, given the high risk of thyroid cancer and the difficulties of performing FNA biopsies on those who have concomitant developmental disorders.[16]

Once the diagnosis of NMTC has been made and a familial case is suspected based on the patient's family history, the treatment should be tailored based on current guidelines, as there is no evidence that patients with FNMTC respond differently to the treatment recommended for a specific disease stage.[5,34] Special preoperative consideration should be given to the extent of the procedure (total thyroidectomy vs lobectomy, central lymph node dissection vs not). Based on the possibility that there is a higher prevalence of multifocal tumors, extrathyroidal extension, lymph node metastasis, and the potential risk of leaving disease behind, some authors favor a total thyroidectomy and consideration for a prophylactic central lymph node dissection.[31]

CONCLUSIONS

FNMTC is an increasingly recognized entity with a still unknown susceptible genetic background, although advances have been made in this field. Up to 15% of the cases of NMTC can be familial, and a diagnosis of FNMTC should be considered when two or more first-degree relatives are diagnosed. Given the lack of available genetic testing, the literature has great variability regarding screening, presentation, and treatment. Evidence suggests that FNMTC could have a more aggressive behavior compared to sporadic disease, but treatment should be individualized to follow current guidelines for each patient. More research is needed to elucidate the best approach to this disease.

REFERENCES

1. Olson E, Wintheiser G, Wolfe KM, Droessler J, Silberstein PT. Epidemiology of thyroid cancer: a review of the national cancer database, 2000-2013. *Cureus*. 2019;11(2):e4127.
2. Policeni BA, Smoker WRK, Reede DL. Anatomy and embryology of the thyroid and parathyroid glands. *Seminars in Ultrasound, CT and MRI*. 2012;33(2):104-114.
3. Hińcza K, Kowalik A, Kowalska A. Current knowledge of germline genetic risk factors for the development of non-medullary thyroid cancer. *Genes*. 2019;10(7):482.
4. Yeganeh MZ, Sheikholeslami S, Hedayati M. RET proto oncogene mutation detection and medullary thyroid carcinoma prevention. *Asian Pac J Cancer Prev*. 2015;16(6):2107-2117.
5. Capezzone M, Robenshtok E, Cantara S, Castagna MG. Familial non-medullary thyroid cancer: a critical review. *J Endocrinol Invest*. 2021;44(5):943-950.
6. Robinson DW. Carcinoma of the thyroid and other diseases of the thyroid in identical twins. *Arch Surg*. 1955;70(6):923.
7. Loh KC. Familial nonmedullary thyroid carcinoma: a meta-review of case series. *Thyroid*. 1997;7(1):107-113.
8. Malchoff CD, Malchoff DM. Familial nonmedullary thyroid carcinoma. *Semin Surg Oncol*. 1999;16(1):16-18.
9. Donis-Keller H, Dou S, Chi D, et al. Mutations in the RET proto-oncogene are associated with MEN 2A and FMTC. *Hum Mol Genet*. 1993;2(7):851-856.
10. Diquigiovanni C, Bonora E. Genetics of familial non-medullary thyroid carcinoma (FNMTC). *Cancers*. 2021;13(9):2178.
11. Cameselle-Teijeiro JM, Mete O, Asa SL, LiVolsi V. Inherited follicular epithelial-derived thyroid carcinomas: from molecular biology to histological correlates. *Endocr Pathol*. 2021;32(1):77-101.
12. Monachese M, Mankaney G, Lopez R, et al. Outcome of thyroid ultrasound screening in FAP patients with a normal baseline exam. *Fam Cancer*. 2019;18(1):75-82.
13. Cetta F, Montalto G, Gori M, Curia MC, Cama A, Olschwang S. Germline mutations of the APC gene in patients with familial adenomatous polyposis-associated thyroid carcinoma: results from a European cooperative study. *J Clin Endocrinol Metab*. 2000;85(1):286-292.
14. Jarrar AM, Milas M, Mitchell J, et al. Screening for thyroid cancer in patients with familial adenomatous polyposis. *Ann Surg*. 2011;253(3):515-521.
15. Tischkowitz M, Colas C, Pouwels S, Hoogerbrugge N, PHTS Guideline Development Group, European Reference Network GENTURIS. Cancer Surveillance Guideline for individuals with PTEN hamartoma tumour syndrome. *Eur J Hum Genet*. 2020;28(10):1387-1393.
16. Milas M, Mester J, Metzger R, et al. Should patients with Cowden syndrome undergo prophylactic thyroidectomy? *Surgery*. 2012;152(6):1201-1210.
17. González IA, Stewart DR, Schultz KAP, Field AP, Hill DA, Dehner LP. DICER1 tumor predisposition syndrome: an evolving story initiated with the pleuropulmonary blastoma. *Mod Pathol*. 2022;35(1):4-22.
18. Mirshahi UL, Kim J, Best AF, et al. A genome-first approach to characterize DICER1 pathogenic variant prevalence, penetrance, and phenotype. *JAMA Netw Open*. 2021;4(2):e210112.

19. Bouys L, Bertherat J. Management of endocrine disease: Carney complex: clinical and genetic update 20 years after the identification of the CNC1 (PRKAR1A) gene. *Eur J Endocrinol.* 2021;184(3):R99-R109.
20. Bertherat J, Horvath A, Groussin L, et al. Mutations in regulatory subunit type 1A of cyclic adenosine 5'-monophosphate-dependent protein kinase (PRKAR1A): phenotype analysis in 353 patients and 80 different genotypes. *J Clin Endocrinol Metab.* 2009;94(6):2085-2091.
21. Stratakis CA, Kirschner LS, Carney JA. Clinical and molecular features of the Carney complex: diagnostic criteria and recommendations for patient evaluation. *J Clin Endocrinol Metab.* 2001;86(9):4041-4046.
22. Oshima J, Martin GM, Hisama FM. Werner syndrome. In: Adam MP, Ardinger HH, Pagon RA, et al., eds. *GeneReviews®*. University of Washington, Seattle; 1993. Accessed October 29, 2021. http://www.ncbi.nlm.nih.gov/books/NBK1514/
23. Ishikawa Y, Sugano H, Matsumoto T, Furuichi Y, Miller RW, Goto M. Unusual features of thyroid carcinomas in Japanese patients with Werner syndrome and possible genotype-phenotype relations to cell type and race. *Cancer.* 1999;85(6): 1345-1352.
24. Son EJ, Nosé V. Familial follicular cell-derived thyroid carcinoma. *Front Endocrinol.* 2012;3:61.
25. Aswath K, Welch J, Gubbi S, et al. Co-occurrence of familial non-medullary thyroid cancer (FNMTC) and hereditary non-polyposis colorectal cancer (HNPCC) associated tumors—a cohort study. *Front Endocrinol.* 2021;12:653401.
26. Malchoff CD, Malchoff DM. Familial nonmedullary thyroid carcinoma. *Cancer Control.* 2006;13(2):106-110.
27. Frank C, Fallah M, Sundquist J, Hemminki A, Hemminki K. Population landscape of familial cancer. *Sci Rep.* 2015;5(1): 12891.
28. Yoon JH. Updates in familial non-medullary thyroid cancer. *Korean J Endocr Surg.* 2015;15(1):6-9.
29. Fallah M, Pukkala E, Tryggvadottir L, et al. Risk of thyroid cancer in first-degree relatives of patients with non-medullary thyroid cancer by histology type and age at diagnosis: a joint study from five Nordic countries. *J Med Genet.* 2013;50(6): 373-382.
30. Charkes ND. On the prevalence of familial nonmedullary thyroid cancer in multiply affected kindreds. *Thyroid.* 2006;16(2):181-186.
31. Nixon IJ, Suárez C, Simo R, et al. The impact of family history on non-medullary thyroid cancer. *Eur J Surg Oncol.* 2016;42(10):1455-1463.
32. Musholt TJ, Musholt PB, Petrich T, Oetting G, Knapp WH, Klempnauer J. Familial papillary thyroid carcinoma: genetics, criteria for diagnosis, clinical features, and surgical treatment. *World J Surg.* 2000;24(11):1409-1417.
33. US Preventive Services Task Force, Bibbins-Domingo K, Grossman DC, et al. Screening for thyroid cancer: US preventive services task force recommendation statement. *JAMA.* 2017; 317(18):1882.
34. Haugen BR, Alexander EK, Bible KC, et al. 2015 American Thyroid Association Management guidelines for adult patients with thyroid nodules and differentiated thyroid cancer: the American Thyroid Association guidelines task force on thyroid nodules and differentiated thyroid cancer. *Thyroid.* 2016;26(1):1-133.
35. Klubo-Gwiezdzinska J, Yang L, Merkel R, et al. Results of screening in familial non-medullary thyroid cancer. *Thyroid.* 2017;27(8):1017-1024.
36. Alsanea O, Wada N, Ain K, et al. Is familial non-medullary thyroid carcinoma more aggressive than sporadic thyroid cancer? A multicenter series. *Surgery.* 2000;128(6):1043-1051.
37. Maxwell EL, Hall FT, Freeman JL. Familial non-medullary thyroid cancer: a matched-case control study. *Laryngoscope.* 2004;114(12):2182-2186.
38. Moses W, Weng J, Kebebew E. Prevalence, clinicopathologic features, and somatic genetic mutation profile in familial versus sporadic nonmedullary thyroid cancer. *Thyroid.* 2011;21(4):367-371.
39. Robenshtok E, Tzvetov G, Grozinsky-Glasberg S, et al. Clinical characteristics and outcome of familial nonmedullary thyroid cancer: a retrospective controlled study. *Thyroid.* 2011;21(1):43-48.
40. Pinto AE, Silva GL, Henrique R, et al. Familial vs sporadic papillary thyroid carcinoma: a matched-case comparative study showing similar clinical/prognostic behaviour. *Eur J Endocrinol.* 2014;170(2):321-327.
41. Lei S, Wang D, Ge J, et al. Single-center study of familial papillary thyroid cancer in China: surgical considerations. *World J Surg Oncol.* 2015;13:115.
42. Zhang Q, Yang S, Meng XY, Chen G, Pang RZ. Clinical analysis of familial nonmedullary thyroid carcinoma. *World J Surg.* 2016;40(3):570-573.
43. Shafiei S, Sadrolodabaei M, Aghaei A, et al. Longer time to reach excellent response to treatment in familial versus sporadic non-medullary thyroid cancer (NMTC): a matched case-control study. *Int J Endocrinol Metab.* 2021;19(2):e108781.
44. Uchino S, Noguchi S, Kawamoto H, et al. Familial nonmedullary thyroid carcinoma characterized by multifocality and a high recurrence rate in a large study population. *World J Surg.* 2002;26(8):897-902.
45. Capezzone M, Marchisotta S, Cantara S, et al. Familial non-medullary thyroid carcinoma displays the features of clinical anticipation suggestive of a distinct biological entity. *Endocr Relat Cancer.* 2008;15(4):1075-1081.
46. Ito Y, Kakudo K, Hirokawa M, et al. Biological behavior and prognosis of familial papillary thyroid carcinoma. *Surgery.* 2009;145(1):100-105.
47. McDonald TJ, Driedger AA, Garcia BM, et al. Familial papillary thyroid carcinoma: a retrospective analysis. *J Oncol.* 2011;2011:948786.
48. Mazeh H, Benavidez J, Poehls JL, Youngwirth L, Chen H, Sippel RS. In patients with thyroid cancer of follicular cell origin, a family history of nonmedullary thyroid cancer in one first-degree relative is associated with more aggressive disease. *Thyroid.* 2012;22(1):3-8.
49. Park YJ, Ahn HY, Choi HS, Kim KW, Park DJ, Cho BY. The long-term outcomes of the second generation of familial nonmedullary thyroid carcinoma are more aggressive than sporadic cases. *Thyroid.* 2012;22(4):356-362.
50. Lee YM, Yoon JH, Yi O, et al. Familial history of non-medullary thyroid cancer is an independent prognostic factor for tumor recurrence in younger patients with conventional papillary thyroid carcinoma. *J Surg Oncol.* 2014;109(2):168-173.
51. Tavarelli M, Russo M, Terranova R, et al. Familial non-medullary thyroid cancer represents an independent risk factor for increased cancer aggressiveness: a retrospective analysis of 74 families. *Front Endocrinol.* 2015;6:117.
52. Cao J, Chen C, Chen C, Wang QL, Ge MH. Clinicopathological features and prognosis of familial papillary thyroid carcinoma—a large-scale, matched, case-control study. *Clin Endocrinol.* 2016;84(4):598-606.

53. Wang X, Cheng W, Li J, et al. Endocrine tumours: familial nonmedullary thyroid carcinoma is a more aggressive disease: a systematic review and meta-analysis. *Eur J Endocrinol.* 2015;172(6):R253-R262.
54. LeClair K, Bell KJL, Furuya-Kanamori L, Doi SA, Francis DO, Davies L. Evaluation of gender inequity in thyroid cancer diagnosis: differences by sex in us thyroid cancer incidence compared with a meta-analysis of subclinical thyroid cancer rates at autopsy. *JAMA Intern Med.* 2021;181(10):1351-1358.
55. Wang F, Yu X, Shen X, et al. The prognostic value of tumor multifocality in clinical outcomes of papillary thyroid cancer. *J Clin Endocrinol Metab.* 2017;102(9):3241-3250.
56. Wang TS, Opoku-Boateng A, Roman SA, Sosa JA. Prophylactic thyroidectomy: who needs it, when, and why. *J Surg Oncol.* 2015;111(1):61-65.

65 Familial Syndromes Associated With Thyroid Cancer

Anderson Lee, BA
Wilson M. Alobuia, MD, MS
Electron Kebebew, MD, FACS

GENERAL CONSIDERATIONS

The prevalence of thyroid cancer has been increasing worldwide, with papillary thyroid cancer (PTC) encompassing nearly 90% of all cases. While the majority of thyroid cancer cases are sporadic, familial thyroid cancer represents approximately 15% of all thyroid cancer cases.[1] The association of thyroid cancer with multiple endocrine neoplasia (MEN) types 2A and 2B has been well documented in patients with medullary thyroid cancer and this type of familial cancer syndrome is addressed in the chapters "Medullary Thyroid Carcinoma" and "Multiple Endocrine Neoplasia Type 2 Syndrome (MEN 2A and MEN 2B)" elsewhere in this book. Familial nonmedullary thyroid cancer (FNMTC) represents a group of cancers that arise from follicular thyroid cells and include papillary (85%), follicular (11%), Hürthle cell (3%), and anaplastic (1%).[1] FNMTC may be syndromic (a component of an inherited familial cancer syndrome) or nonsyndromic (isolated cases of nonmedullary thyroid cancer occurring in kindred with multiple generations affected). Nonsyndromic FNMTC is diagnosed in a patient with follicular cell-derived thyroid cancer who also has a history of thyroid cancer in two or more first-degree relatives in the absence of other predisposing hereditary or environmental causes. It is inherited in an autosomal dominant fashion with incomplete penetrance. Nonsyndromic FNMTC accounts for approximately 90% of all familial thyroid cancer diagnoses and is thought to be more aggressive compared to sporadic nonmedullary thyroid cancer.[1] In syndromic FNMTC, the patient commonly has a history of other diseases due to germline mutations in tumor suppressor genes. Syndromic FNMTCs include familial adenomatous polyposis (FAP) and its variants, Cowden syndrome, Werner syndrome, Carney complex, and DICER1 syndrome (Table 65–1). The association between these syndromes and developing thyroid cancer is strong, especially in patients with pathogenic germline mutations.[1]

In this chapter, we review the current approaches to the diagnosis and management of patients with syndromic FNMTC.

FAMILIAL ADENOMATOUS POLYPOSIS (FAP)

FAP is an autosomal dominant disease caused by an inactivating mutation of the *APC* tumor suppressor gene located on chromosome 5q21.[1] The frequency of this mutation ranges from 1 in 6,850 to 29,000 people, with 10%-30% of cases being *de novo* without any family history. FAP is clinically characterized by the development of multiple (more than 100) adenomatous polyps with malignant potential and an almost 100% lifetime risk of colorectal cancer (CRC). While the development of multiple colonic polyps is the hallmark of FAP, patients with FAP are also at high risk of developing extracolonic disease, including osteomas, desmoid tumors, epidermal cysts, hepatoblastomas, and thyroid tumors.[2]

Thyroid nodules are found in up to 38% of patients with FAP; however, the risk of developing thyroid cancer is approximately 2%.[3] In this patient population, follicular thyroid cancer (FTC) and papillary thyroid cancer (PTC) are the most common histologic subtypes[4] with nearly 90% of these cases seen in women.[3] Recent research suggests an increased prevalence of thyroid cancer (up to 12%) among patients with FAP who are screened with a thyroid ultrasound.[3] The risk of thyroid cancer is greatest during the second and third decades of life. Compared to those with no history of FAP, thyroid cancer occurs at about a 10-fold greater frequency among patients with FAP, with the thyroid cancer diagnosis preceding the diagnosis of FAP in one-third of patients.[4]

Clinical Findings

The hallmark of FAP is the development of multiple gastrointestinal tract polyps, which often leads to a diagnosis

Table 65–1. Summary and characteristics of syndromic familial nonmedullary thyroid cancer.

Syndrome	Susceptibility Gene(s)	Type of Thyroid Cancer	Associated Tumors and Clinical Manifestations
Familial adenomatous polyposis, Gardner syndrome, Turcot syndrome	*APC*	CMV-PTC and PTC	Adenomatous polyps or malignant tumors in GI tract, desmoid tumors, hepatoblastomas, and osteomas
Cowden syndrome	*PTEN*	PTC and FTC	Hamartomatous changes and epithelial tumors of breast, thyroid, kidney, colon, and endometrium
Werner syndrome	*WRN*	PTC, FTC, and ATC	Premature aging, scleroderma-like skin changes, cataracts, and age-related diseases (type 2 diabetes mellitus and osteoporosis)
Carney complex	*PRKAR1A*	PTC and FTC	Spotty skin pigmentation, myxomas, endocrine tumors, and schwannomas
DICER1 syndrome	*DICER1*	DTC	Pleuropulmonary blastomas, Sertoli-Leydig cell tumors, and cystic nephromas

ATC, anaplastic thyroid cancer; CMV-PTC, cribriform molecular variant papillary thyroid cancer; DTC, differentiated thyroid cancer; FTC, follicular thyroid cancer; PTC, papillary thyroid cancer.

of CRC by the fourth decade of life. Patients with thyroid involvement may present with a neck mass or local obstructive symptoms if the tumor is large or infiltrating surrounding structures.[4]

Essentials of Diagnosis

FAP is typically diagnosed using a combination of clinical findings and genetic testing for the *APC* gene (Table 65–2). FTC and PTC are the most common diagnoses among these patients; however, 0.1%-0.2% of FAP-related thyroid cancers can have a rare variant of PTC called the "cribriform-morular variant of papillary thyroid cancer" (CMV-PTC). Development of CMV-PTC among patients with FAP is associated with a better prognosis compared to other variants. Because of the high risk of developing thyroid cancer in the second and third decades of life, it is recommended that a thorough neck exam to identify any thyroid nodules and/or screening ultrasound be performed annually beginning in the teenage years for all patients diagnosed with FAP.[4]

Table 65–2. Diagnostic criteria for familial adenomatous polyposis.

Syndrome	Diagnostic Criteria
Familial adenomatous polyposis (FAP)	• ≥100 colorectal adenomatous polyps • <100 polyps but with a family history of FAP • Extracolonic manifestations, including desmoid tumors, thyroid tumors, and brain tumors

Treatment

A total or near-total thyroidectomy and therapeutic lymph node dissection is the best surgical treatment for patients with FAP-related thyroid cancer given their high risk of developing multifocal and bilateral thyroid cancers. Adjunct treatment (radioactive iodine therapy or TSH suppression with thyroxine) in patients with FAP-associated thyroid cancer is similar to that in patients with sporadic thyroid cancer.[3]

Prognosis

If left untreated, patients with FAP typically have a poor prognosis, with most not surviving past the fourth decade of life. With a near 100% risk of developing CRC, colorectal malignancy remains the leading cause of death in patients with FAP, followed by duodenal/periampullary carcinoma.[4]

GARDNER SYNDROME

Gardner syndrome, caused by a mutation in the *APC* gene, is a variant of FAP characterized by the development of extracolonic disease. As such these patients can develop both intestinal and colorectal polyps. While its key manifestations include intestinal polyps and CRC, it is also linked with a 2% risk of developing thyroid cancer. Screening, treatment, and management are similar to that of patients with FAP, as discussed in the FAP section above.[4]

TURCOT SYNDROME

Also considered to be a variant of FAP, Turcot syndrome is characterized by the presence of brain tumors in a patient diagnosed with hereditary nonpolyposis colorectal cancer

(HNPCC) or FAP. Type 1 Turcot syndrome (TS1) arises from a mutation in two DNA mismatch repair (MMR) genes associated with HNPCC (*MLH1* and *PMS2*), while type 2 Turcot syndrome (TS2, otherwise known as Crail syndrome) is caused by a mutation of the *APC* gene, which is implicated in FAP. Compared to the single allele or heterozygous mutations seen in HNPCC and FAP, the mutations in the *MLH1*, *PMS2*, and *APC* genes in Turcot syndrome are typically biallelic. Research has shown that 12% of patients with an HNPCC/FAP diagnosis are eventually diagnosed with thyroid cancer. Due to the rarity of the disease, epidemiologic information on Turcot syndrome is lacking.

Clinical Findings

Along with the typical symptoms and signs seen in FAP, patients with Turcot syndrome have an approximately 40% risk of developing medulloblastomas. Patients with TS1 may present with hematologic malignancies, cafe-au-lait spots, and glioblastoma multiforme. Most patients with a diagnosis of TS1 have fewer but larger colonic polyps that have a greater chance of becoming malignant, while TS2 is characterized by smaller but more numerous colonic polyps. Patients with Turcot syndrome may also present with a neck mass or local obstructive symptoms if the tumor is large or infiltrating surrounding structures.

Essentials of Diagnosis

Guidelines for the diagnosis of Turcot syndrome are lacking, but family history is an extremely important consideration in the workup, management, and surveillance of the disease. Because the cost-effectiveness of genetic testing remains in question, clinicians generally prefer to follow screening guidelines similar to those for FAP. It is of utmost importance to recognize the presence of inherited CRC within the family and to be aware of the presence of other disease-related manifestations, such as brain tumors.

Treatment

Patients with Turcot syndrome who develop thyroid cancer should undergo total thyroidectomy and therapeutic lymph node dissection for definitive treatment.

Prognosis

Poor prognostic indicators include the development of metastatic disease, as well as glioblastoma multiforme, which is associated with an average overall survival of 27 months.

COWDEN SYNDROME

Cowden syndrome (CS) is an autosomal dominant disease that occurs due to a mutation in the *PTEN* tumor suppressor gene located on chromosome 10q23.[5] Patients with CS develop hamartomatous changes and epithelial tumors of the breast, thyroid, kidney, colon, and endometrium. The incidence of CS is approximately 1 in 200,000 people, with the majority of patients being Caucasian and female.[6] Over two-thirds of patients with CS develop CS-related thyroid tumors, and at least 10% of these patients develop thyroid cancer. CS is part of a wider classification of syndromes called PTEN-hamartoma tumor syndrome (PHTS), with most of the variants sharing similar clinical presentations despite being due to different germline mutations. Combined with the Cleveland Clinic score, which can be used as a CS risk predictor, genetic testing for germline *PTEN* gene mutations provides a definitive diagnosis.[5]

Due to the increased risk of developing both benign and malignant thyroid tumors at an early age, screening for thyroid masses by ultrasound is recommended to begin by the age of 7 years and continued every 2 years throughout childhood.[7]

Clinical Findings

The hallmark feature of CS is macrocephaly, which first presents in childhood and progresses into adulthood, along with several neurodevelopmental disorders. Many patients present with developmental delays, intellectual disability, and autism. Other associated diagnoses may include gastrointestinal polyps, vascular malformations, and lipomas. Patients have a lifetime risk of developing malignancies, including thyroid cancer, renal cell carcinoma, melanoma, and CRC.[7] Specific facial and skin features such as trichilemmomas, acral keratoses, and tongue papillomas may also be present (Table 65–3).[5]

Differentiated thyroid cancer (DTC) is one of the most common diagnoses among children diagnosed with CS. The risk of DTC is much greater in patients with CS than that of the general population, with more recent studies reporting a risk of up to 35%-38%. Thyroid nodules, multinodular goiters, and adenomas are common in adults with PHTS, and can be detected early in childhood. Rates of metastatic disease and mortality from thyroid cancer are, however, low because of appropriate screening, which allows for early detection and treatment.[6]

Table 65–3. Diagnostic criteria for Cowden syndrome.

Cowden Syndrome Diagnostic Criteria	
• Pathognomonic mucocutaneous lesions, two or more major criteria, one major and three minor, or four or more minor criteria	
Major Criteria	**Minor Criteria**
• Breast cancer	• Multiple GI hamartomas
• Differentiated thyroid cancer (FTC and PTC)	• Colon cancer
• Macrocephaly	• Neurodevelopmental disorders
• Endometrial cancer	• Intellectual disability
	• Autism
	• Lipomas

Essentials of Diagnosis

Genetic testing for germline mutation in the *PTEN* gene should be performed. If genetic testing is unavailable or negative but a high clinical suspicion remains, the Cleveland Clinic score is a clinical scoring system based on case studies and prospective data that provides an approximate risk-prediction of the presence of a *PTEN* mutation or variant. Due to the potential development of thyroid cancer, screening neck ultrasound should be performed beginning in childhood, although the overall impact of early screening is still up for debate.[8]

Treatment

Although thyroid cancer among patients with CS is not as aggressive as sporadic thyroid cancer, most patients elect to undergo total thyroidectomy for definitive treatment. Prophylactic total thyroidectomy may also be considered in select patients, especially those with developmental disorders and a significant family history.[8]

Prognosis

The prognosis of CS is fair, and if cancers are detected and treated at an early stage, patients may live close to a normal life expectancy.[7]

WERNER SYNDROME

Werner syndrome (WS) is a rare autosomal recessive mutation of the *WRN* gene on chromosome 8p11-21. The *WRN* gene mutation impairs the function of telomere maintenance, which leads to many of the distinct WS phenotypes. Approximately 17% of patients with WS develop thyroid tumors, including follicular, papillary, and anaplastic thyroid carcinomas, as well as thyroid adenomas.[1] The relative risk of developing thyroid cancer in Japanese populations appears to be significantly higher, with an observed incidence ratio of 14 compared to the standardized proportionate incidence ratio of 9.6. WS is characterized by premature aging, scleroderma-like skin changes, short stature, cataracts, and common age-related diseases (such as type 2 diabetes mellitus, osteoporosis, and malignancies).[9,10] Clinical criteria for diagnosing WS are based on the International Registry of WS, with the most common manifestations being bilateral cataracts, premature aging, and short stature (Table 65–4).[9]

Table 65–4. Diagnostic criteria for Werner syndrome.

Werner Syndrome Diagnostic Criteria	
• Four cardinal signs and two additional signs or three cardinal signs and two additional signs	
Cardinal Signs	Additional Signs
• Bilateral cataracts • Premature aging • Short stature • Accelerated skin atrophy and graying of hair	• Hypogonadism • Diabetes mellitus • Atherosclerosis • Osteoporosis • Neoplasms, including but not limited to thyroid carcinomas, malignant melanomas, and meningiomas • Thyroid carcinoma, PTC, FTC, and ATC

Clinical Findings

The spectrum of clinical presentations seen in patients with WS are all consistent with premature aging, which generally begins in early adolescence. Short stature and lack of a growth spurt are characteristic in these patients, who by the third decade of life show signs of aging (including skin atrophy and gray hair). Due to their premature aging, patients may also develop medical complications common among the elderly, including type 2 diabetes mellitus, malignancies, osteoporosis, atherosclerosis, early loss of fertility, and hypogonadism, even at a young biological age. Interestingly, Alzheimer-related dementias are not common in patients with WS, despite their prevalence in normal aging populations.[9] The most common neoplasms that develop in patients with WS include malignant melanomas, meningiomas, soft tissue sarcomas, leukemia and preleukemic conditions of the bone marrow, primary bone neoplasms, and thyroid cancers.[10]

Essentials of Diagnosis

Genetic testing for the *WRN* mutation is required to confirm a diagnosis of WS, in addition to clinical criteria for the four cardinal signs: bilateral cataracts, premature aging and thinning of scalp hair, dermatologic changes, and short stature. The high prevalence of thyroid cancer in patients with WS warrants routine screening for early detection and treatment, especially among patients of Japanese descent.[9]

Treatment

Total thyroidectomy and therapeutic lymph node dissection should be performed in those with thyroid cancer or thyroid nodules concerning for thyroid cancer.

Prognosis

The prognosis is poor in patients with WS, with a median life expectancy of 54 years. The most common causes of death in patients with WS are myocardial infarction and cancers, including thyroid cancer and nonepithelial cancer.[10]

CARNEY COMPLEX

Carney complex (CC) is an autosomal dominant disease caused by a mutation in the *PRKAR1A* gene on chromosome 17q22-24.[11] The most common clinical characteristics of CC include spotty skin pigmentation, myxomas, and endocrine tumors. Thyroid lesions are common in patients with CC, with nearly 60% of patients having thyroid cysts or multinodular thyroids on ultrasound. Approximately 25% of patients have thyroid tumors, and 2.5% of patients develop thyroid cancer. FTC is more common than PTC; a finding that is contrary to what is seen among the general population (where PTC is the most common type).[11] Additionally, while FTCs are typically solitary and slow-growing tumors with a low risk for lymph node metastasis, FTCs seen among patients with CC were found in some cases to be multifocal with lymph node metastasis present, suggesting more aggressive disease. Fortunately, thyroid disorders among patients with CC are uncommon and generally develop later in life. As such, appropriate screening with thyroid ultrasound can help in early detection and treatment. Primary pigmented nodular adrenocortical disease (PPNAD) may also be seen in patients with CC, which can result in Cushing syndrome. Growth-hormone-secreting pituitary adenoma or pituitary somatotropic hyperplasia, both of which can manifest clinically as acromegaly, also occur in patients with CC.[12]

Clinical Findings

As discussed above, CC is characterized by spotty skin pigmentation; myxomas of the heart, skin, and breast; and PPNAD, leading to ACTH-independent Cushing syndrome and acromegaly (Table 65–5). Compared to those seen in patients without CC, the myxomas in patients with CC are more aggressive, and cardiac myxomas account for more than 50% of patient mortality. PPNAD is the most common endocrine lesion, presenting as normal-sized or enlarged adrenal glands with bilateral adrenocortical nodules that are pigmented and surrounded by atrophic adrenocortical tissue. While only 12% of patients with CC develop acromegaly, the vast majority have elevated levels of growth hormone and insulin-like growth factor 1 (IGF-1).[11]

Essentials of Diagnosis

A diagnosis of CC is made if two or more clinical manifestations are present and confirmed by histologic evaluation, biochemical testing, and imaging. Genetic testing for the *PRKAR1A* mutation is not recommended, except for individuals with a known family history of CC.[12]

Table 65–5. Diagnostic criteria for Carney complex.

Carney Complex Diagnostic Criteria
• Two or more manifestations or single manifestation with a germline *PRKAR1A* mutation and/or first-degree relative with Carney complex
• Spotty skin pigmentation • Myxomas • PPNAD • Acromegaly • Thyroid carcinoma, PTC, and FTC • Pituitary adenomas and pituitary somatotropic hyperplasia

Treatment

Total thyroidectomy and therapeutic lymph node dissection should be performed in those with thyroid cancer or thyroid nodules suspicious for thyroid cancer.[13]

Prognosis

The life expectancy of patients with CC is 50-55 years, even with proper surveillance and treatment.[11]

DICER1 SYNDROME

DICER1 syndrome is an autosomal dominant disorder caused by mutations in the *DICER1* gene on chromosome 14q32.13. Patients with this mutation commonly develop pleuropulmonary blastomas (PPBs), macrocephaly, pulmonary cysts, cystic nephromas, thyroid gland neoplasia, Sertoli-Leydig cell tumors (SLCTs), and Wilms tumor.[7] Patients have an increased risk of developing thyroid cancer and multinodular goiter. Approximately 1 in 2529 to 1 in 10,600 individuals carry a pathogenic mutation in the *DICER1* gene.[14]

Clinical Findings

Most commonly, patients with *DICER1* syndrome present with PPBs, macrocephaly, and multinodular goiter. Rarer tumor predispositions include but are not limited to cystic nephromas, ovarian sex cord-stromal tumors, ciliary body medullo-epitheliomas, and nasal chondromesenchymal hamartomas (Table 65–6). The majority of patients diagnosed with *DICER1* syndrome develop PPBs as early as infancy and can present with weight loss, fever, respiratory distress, and chest pain. Patients also have a higher risk of developing thyroid nodules, multinodular goiters, and thyroid cancer.[14] In the United States, the likelihood of

Table 65–6. Diagnostic criteria for DICER1 syndrome.

DICER1 Syndrome Diagnostic Criteria Consider diagnostic testing in individuals with one major or two minor criteria	
Major Criteria	Minor Criteria
• Pleuropulmonary blastomas	• Pulmonary cysts
• Cystic nephromas	• Wilms tumor
• Thoracic embryonal rhabdomyosarcomas	• Multinodular goiter
• Thyroid gland neoplasia with family history of *DICER1* syndrome	• Childhood onset DTC
• Sertoli-Leydig cell tumors	• Macrocephaly
• Medullo-epitheliomas	

developing a multinodular goiter or undergoing thyroidectomy by the age of 20 years in a patient with *DICER1* syndrome was 32% in women and 13% in men. Over a patient's lifetime, there is a 16- to 24-fold increased risk for DTC. PTC is the most common type of thyroid cancer among patients with *DICER1*.[14]

Essentials of Diagnosis

The diagnosis of *DICER1* syndrome is established by genetic testing which detects a heterozygous germline mutation in the *DICER1* gene. Screening ultrasound has been recommended to begin as early as the age of 8 years, with follow-up ultrasounds every 3 years, due to the increased risk of thyroid cancer.[15]

Treatment

Total thyroidectomy and therapeutic lymph node dissection should be performed in those with thyroid cancer or thyroid nodules suspicious for thyroid cancer.[15]

Prognosis

Most patients with DICER1 syndrome have a good prognosis when surveillance imaging and appropriate screening are performed to allow early detection and treatment.[15]

REFERENCES

1. Nosé V. Familial thyroid cancer: a review. *Mod Pathol.* 2011; 24:S19-S33.
2. Waller A, Findels S, Lee MJ. Familial adenomatous polyposis. *J Pediatr Genet.* 2016;5(2):78-83.
3. Jarrar AM, Milas M, Mitchell J, et al. Screening for thyroid cancer in patients with familial adenomatous polyposis. *Ann Surg.* 2011;253(3):515-521.
4. Dinarvand P, Davaro EP, Doan JV, et al. Familial adenomatous polyposis syndrome: an update and review of extraintestinal manifestations. *Arch Path Lab Med.* 2019;143(11):1382-1398.
5. Macken WL, Tischkowitz M, Lachlan KL. PTEN hamartoma tumor syndrome in childhood: a review of the clinical literature. *Am J Med Genet. C Semin Med Genet.* 2019;181(4):591-610.
6. Szabo Yamashita T, Baky FJ, McKenzie TJ, et al. Occurrence and natural history of thyroid cancer in patients with Cowden syndrome. *Eur Thyroid J.* 2020;9(5):243-246.
7. Schultz KAP, Rednam SP, Kamihara J, et al. *PTEN, DICER1, FH*, and their associated tumor susceptibility syndromes: clinical features, genetics, and surveillance recommendations in childhood. *Clin Cancer Res.* 2017;23(12):e76-e82.
8. Milas M, Mester J, Metzger R, et al. Should patients with Cowden syndrome undergo prophylactic thyroidectomy? *Surgery.* 2012;152(6):1201-1210.
9. Oshima J, Sidorova JM, Monnat RJ Jr. Werner syndrome: Clinical features, pathogenesis and potential therapeutic interventions. *Ageing Res Rev.* 2017;33:105-114.
10. Lauper JM, Krause A, Vaughan TL, Monnat RJ Jr. Spectrum and risk of neoplasia in Werner syndrome: a systematic review. *PLoS One.* 2013;8(4):e59709.
11. Kamilaris CDC, Faucz FR, Voutetakis A, Stratakis CA. Carney complex. *Exp Clin Endocrinol Diabetes.* 2019;127(2-03):156-164.
12. Stratakis CA. Carney complex: a familial lentiginosis predisposing to a variety of tumors. *Reviews in Endocrine & Metabolic Disorders.* 2016;17(3):367-371.
13. Carney JA, Lyssikatos C, Seethala RR, et al. The spectrum of thyroid gland pathology in Carney complex: the importance of follicular carcinoma. *Am J Surg Pathol.* 2018;42(5):587-594.
14. Schultz KAP, Williams GM, Kamihara J, et al. *DICER1* and associated conditions: identification of at-risk individuals and recommended surveillance strategies. *Clin Cancer Res.* 2018;24(10):2251-2261.
15. Schultz KAP, Stewart D, Kamihara J, et al. *DICER1* tumor predisposition. In: Adam MP, Ardinger HH, Pagon RA, Wallace SE, Bean LJH, Mirzaa G, et al. eds. *GeneReviews.* Seattle (WA): University of Washington; 1993.

66 Familial Primary Hyperparathyroidism

Robert Grant, MD
William F. Simonds, MD
Naris Nilubol, MD

INTRODUCTION

Primary hyperparathyroidism (PHPT) is characterized by excess production of parathormone, also called parathyroid hormone (PTH), by one or more parathyroid glands. With the advent of modern molecular analysis and routine laboratory testing, the number of people diagnosed with PHPT has risen over the past several decades worldwide, with a current incidence between 0.1% and 0.7% of the world population.[1] Ninety-five percent of these cases are from what is termed sporadic disease—a case that occurs randomly with no apparent inciting environmental or genetic risk factors. Of these sporadic cases, the most common form of PHPT presents as excess PTH from a solitary parathyroid adenoma approximately 80% of the time. The other 20% of patients have multiple gland disease characterized by generalized hyperplasia rather than a discrete adenomatous lesion. In 2% to 5% of patients, PHPT is a phenotype associated with a familial syndrome or inherited genotype. The most well-known familial syndrome associated with PHPT is multiple endocrine neoplasia (MEN) type 1 (MEN1). Specifically, in MEN1 PHPT is the predominant phenotype in conjunction with pituitary and pancreatic lesions. In MEN type 2A (MEN2A), PHPT is a less common feature compared to medullary thyroid cancer and pheochromocytoma. In MEN type 4 (MEN4), PHPT is the predominant phenotype with pituitary and other lesions. Another rare syndromic disease is the hyperparathyroidism-jaw tumor syndrome (HPT-JT) which, as its name suggests, comprises PHPT from benign and/or malignant parathyroid tumors, bony lesions of the upper or lower jaw, and renal cysts or tumors. PHPT can also be associated with nonsyndromic isolated familial forms. Familial isolated primary hyperparathyroidism (FIHP), familial hypocalciuric hypercalcemia (FHH), and neonatal severe primary hyperparathyroidism (NSHPT) are discussed here. In patients with a new diagnosis of PHPT, physicians should maintain a high level of clinical suspicion for the familial and syndromic forms, and, when diagnosed, these patients should be referred to centers with specific expertise in treating them. In this chapter, we discuss PHPT in all its forms, with a specific focus on the familial types, both syndromic and isolated.

Clinical Pathophysiology

Calcium is vital for the normal functioning of many cellular processes in vertebrates including mammals. Such processes include the excitability of nerves and muscles, the rhythmicity of cardiac pacemaker cells, the release of neurotransmitters and neuromodulators, muscular contraction, the actions of multiple calcium-dependent enzymes, membrane permeability, and second-messenger signaling within cells. To ensure the proper function of several vital cellular processes that depend on calcium, a system of calcium homeostasis has evolved to rely on bone tissue as a reservoir for calcium.

The principal endocrine factor that governs calcium balance and ensures proper circulating levels of calcium is PTH. PTH is a peptide hormone secreted from parathyroid glands that serves to maintain ambient serum calcium concentration close to a defined physiologic "set-point." Many of the common genes associated with inherited PHPT, which will be discussed in detail later, play important roles in calcium homeostasis by regulating the growth and function of cells of the parathyroid gland. These genes include *GCM2, CASR, GNA11, AP2S1, MEN1, CDC73, CDKN1B,* and *RET* (Table 66–1).

The release of PTH from parathyroid glands is principally controlled by changes in the ambient ionized calcium level in a classic negative feedback loop. Calcium sensing by parathyroid cells is mediated by the calcium-sensing receptor (CASR), a G protein-coupled receptor (GPCR) positioned on the plasma membrane of parathyroid chief cells and an essential regulator of PTH secretion.[2,3] After its release into the circulation, PTH targets the bones by binding to specific

Table 66–1. Familial primary hyperparathyroidism

Disorder	Gene	Chromosomal Locus	Molecular Mechanism	Typical Clinical Features
Syndromic PHPT				
Multiple Endocrine Neoplasia (MEN)				
MEN Type 1	*MEN1*	11q13	TS; LoF	Multigland PHPT, enteropancreatic NET, and anterior pituitary adenomas. Associated features: foregut (including bronchial and thymic) NET, cutaneous lipomas, collagenomas, facial angiofibromas; leiomyomas (eg, of esophagus and uterus)
MEN Type 2A	*RET*	10q11.21	PO; GoF	Medullary thyroid carcinoma, bilateral pheochromocytoma; PHPT due to benign parathyroid disease
MEN Type 4	*CDKN1B*	12p13.1	TS; LoF	Multigland PHPT; pituitary adenoma; reproductive organ tumors (eg, testicular cancer, neuroendocrine cervical carcinoma); adrenal and renal
Hyperparathyroidism-Jaw Tumor Syndrome (HPT-JT)	*CDC73 (formerly called HRPT2)*	1q31.2	TS; LoF	Single- or multigland PHPT with an increased incidence of parathyroid cancer; cemento-ossifying fibromas of the maxilla or mandible; Wilms tumor, renal MEST; uterine pathology (eg, adenomyosis and leiomyoma)
Isolated PHPT				
Familial Hypocalciuric Hypercalcemia (FHH)				
FHH Type 1	*CASR*	3q13.3-q21.1	ICSST; LoF	Lifelong elevation of serum calcium with low urinary calcium excretion (FeCa < 1%) in association with normal or mildly elevated PTH
FHH Type 2	*GNA11*	19p13.3	ICSST; LoF	
FHH Type 3	*AP2S1*	19q13.32	ICSST; LoF	
Neonatal Severe Primary Hyperparathyroidism (NSHPT)	*CASR*	3q13.3-q21.1	ICSST; LoF	Severe neonatal hypercalcemia with bone demineralization and failure to thrive (associated with bi-allelic LoF of *CASR*)
Familial Isolated Hyperparathyroidism (FIHP)				Multigland PHPT
GCM2	*GCM2*	6p24.2	PO; GoF	Multigland PHPT (enriched among those of Ashkanazi Jewish ethnicity)

PHPT, primary hyperparathyroidism; TS, tumor supressor gene, LoF, loss of function; NET, neuroendocrine tumor; PO, proto-oncogene; GoF, gain of function; MEST, mixed epithelial and stromal tumor [of the kidney]; ICSST, impaired calcium sensing or signal transduction.

receptors present on the surface of osteoblasts, parathyroid hormone 1 receptor (PTH1R). Activation of PTH1R on osteoblasts stimulates the synthesis and release of the cytokine RANKL (receptor activator of nuclear factor-kappa-B ligand), which binds to RANK receptors present on nascent and mature osteoclasts promoting their proliferation, differentiation, and activation. Activated osteoclasts resorb bone and mobilize calcium thus increasing the circulation ionized calcium concentration,[4] a metabolic change that can be sensed by parathyroid cell CASRs and may lead to diminished PTH release once the calcium "set-point" is reached. In a parallel homeostatic negative feedback loop, 1,25-dihydroxy vitamin D, the bioactive form of cholecalciferol whose 1α-hydroxylation in the proximal renal tubule is stimulated by PTH, feeds back to cells of the parathyroid gland, inhibiting the synthesis and release of PTH.[5-8] PHPT has been defined as the demonstration of hypercalcemia concurrently with an elevated or inappropriately normal serum PTH.[9] PHPT is asymptomatic in 70% to 80% of cases and is often diagnosed during an evaluation triggered by the incidental discovery of hypercalcemia on a routine blood chemistry panel. When symptomatic, common manifestations include osteoporosis, nephrolithiasis, polyuria, anorexia, constipation, fatigue, weakness, and neurocognitive changes.[9-11] A syndrome of advanced skeletal demineralization characterized by *osteitis fibrosa cystica* classically accompanies advanced disease.[12,13] The overwhelming majority of sporadic parathyroid tumors are benign neoplasms (ie, adenomas), with parathyroid carcinoma comprising <1% of cases of PHPT in most published series.

Hypophosphatemia is frequently observed in PHPT. While PHPT is only one consideration in the differential diagnosis of hypophosphatemia, the simultaneous demonstration of hypercalcemia and hypophosphatemia strongly suggests PHPT.[14] The mechanism of hypophosphatemia in PHPT involves PTH1R present in cells of the proximal renal tubule. Activation of PTH1R by PTH decreases the expression of type II sodium phosphate cotransporters present on the proximal renal tubule apical cell membranes resulting in PTH-dependent phosphaturia and often renal phosphate wasting.[15,16]

Etiology

The vast majority of cases of PHPT are sporadic, a small fraction of which have been associated with prior radiation exposure, especially when such exposure occurs in childhood.[17]

Familial PHPT comprises some 2% to 5% of total cases. As shown in Table 66–1, the study of the molecular genetics of this small subcategory of PHPT has nevertheless yielded critical insights into the genes and dysregulated molecular pathways that contribute to both sporadic and familial parathyroid neoplasia. The most frequently encountered inherited disorders that predispose to PHPT are MEN1, HPT-JT, FIHP, and MEN2A.[18-22] A related condition, FHH (known also as familial benign hypercalcemia), is an autosomal dominant disorder characterized by lifelong hypercalcemia that is largely asymptomatic but often misdiagnosed as PHPT. FHH results from diminished calcium-sensing or impaired downstream signal transduction. The attempted treatment of FHH by partial or even subtotal parathyroid resection does not remedy hypercalcemia.[23] The relevance of these rare familial PHPT syndromes to the underlying etiology of parathyroid neoplasia will be discussed later.

The transformation of a normal cell into a neoplasm, or the process of tumorigenesis, typically involves dysregulation of genes encoding proteins that control cell growth and proliferation. Tumorigenesis can be initiated by the loss of the normal balance between cell growth and inhibition, as genes that negatively regulate cell growth (tumor suppressor genes) or promote cell growth (proto-oncogenes) are either mutationally inactivated or activated, respectively.

A. Multiple Endocrine Neoplasia Type 1

The recognition of an autosomal dominantly inherited constellation of parathyroid hyperplasia, anterior pituitary tumors, and pancreatic islet cell tumors was reported in 1954,[24] a syndrome now known as MEN1. Additional manifestations of the syndrome have been subsequently recognized to create our current concept of a disorder involving neoplasms affecting multiple (including nonendocrine) organs (Table 66–1). The MEN1 trait in affected families linked to a putative tumor suppressor gene on chromosome 11q13[25] that was ultimately identified by positional cloning in 1997 as the *MEN1* gene.[26] Many of the functions of the 67 kDa tumor suppressor protein encoded by the *MEN1* gene, menin, remain elusive. Thus, an accurate genotype-phenotype correlation does not exist. While highly conserved across animal species, the amino acid sequence of menin does not contain recognized functional domains or modules nor does it share sequence homology with other known proteins. Menin is targeted to the cell nucleus by intrinsic nuclear localization signals.[27,28] The 3-dimensional structures of invertebrate and human menin have been solved.[29,30] Menin is a multifunctional protein that can act as a transcriptional co-repressor or co-activator, and also function in DNA repair in response to DNA damage, cell division, cell signaling, cytoskeletal structure, cell adhesion, and cell motility.[31] Because menin connects several transcription factors to histone-modifying proteins to regulate chromatin accessibility and gene transcription,[32] *MEN1* mutations can alter the expression of other tumor suppressor genes and oncogenes resulting in tumor initiation and progression.

B. Multiple Endocrine Neoplasia Type 2A

MEN2A is a familial endocrine tumor syndrome in which PHPT is but one endocrine feature. Apart from PHPT, patients with MEN2A are predisposed to develop medullary thyroid cancer (MTC) and pheochromocytoma which is typically benign and often bilateral.[33] MEN2A is inherited as an autosomal dominant trait and is caused by an activating missense mutation in the *RET* proto-oncogene on chromosome 10 (Figure 66–1). The *RET* gene encodes a receptor tyrosine kinase that binds members of the GDNF (glial cell line-derived neurotrophic factor) family of neurotrophic ligands. The RET receptor functions together with co-receptor glycosylphosphatidylinositol-anchored protein Gfra1.[34]

Germline activating mutations of *RET* are associated with three separate familial endocrine neoplasia syndromes. The three syndromes are all associated with MTC: MEN2A, MEN type 2B (MEN2B), and familial medullary thyroid cancer (FMTC) (Figure 66–1). Usually, PHPT and parathyroid tumors are not part of the spectrum of disease in MEN2B or FMTC. Particular RET mutations give rise to distinct patterns of disease establishing an apparent genotype-phenotype correlation. Approximately 95% of MEN2A cases result from codon substitutions affecting the cysteine-rich region present in RET's large extracellular domain, namely germline missense mutations of *RET* codons 609, 611, 618, 620, or 634.[35] In fact, germline missense mutation of RET residue cysteine-634 accounts for approximately 85% of cases of MEN2A.[33,36]

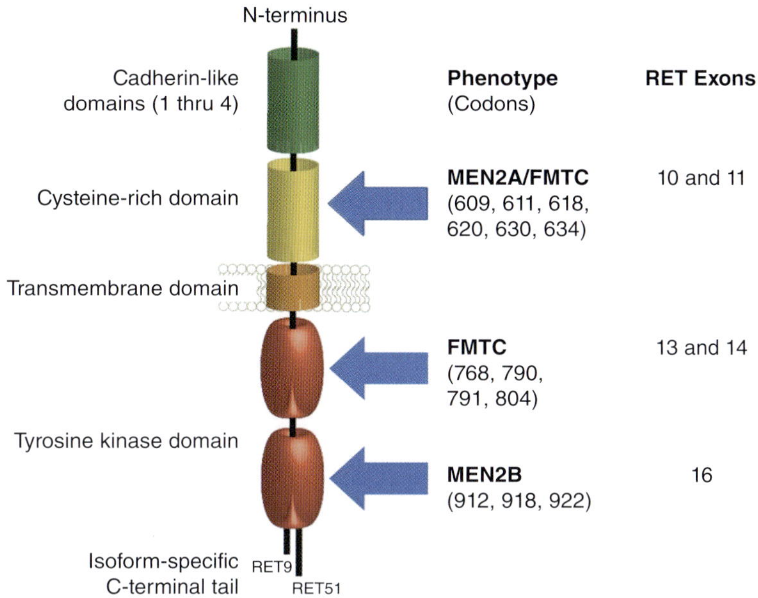

Figure 66–1. Correlations of germline mutations in the *RET* proto-oncogene with multiple endocrine neoplasia type 2A and other disease phenotypes. Graphic illustration of the protein domains encoded by the RET proto-oncogene. The extracellular cadherin-like domains (1-4) contain a calcium-binding site required for RET protein function and for its ability to interact with ligand. The cysteine-rich domain (CRD), also a component of RET's large extracellular domain, is followed by a transmembrane-spanning domain. The intracellular region of RET contains a tyrosine kinase domain split by a short linker region into two subdomains. There are two types of C-terminal tail because of alternative mRNA splicing: a "short" RET isoform contains nine unique C-terminal residues (RET9), whereas the "long" RET isoform contains 51 unique C-terminal residues (RET51). Germline activating mutations of RET are associated with three separate familial endocrine neoplasia syndromes. The three syndromes are all associated with medullary thyroid cancer: multiple endocrine neoplasia type 2A (MEN2A), multiple endocrine neoplasia type 2B (MEN2B), and familial medullary thyroid cancer (FMTC). Usually, primary hyperparathyroidism and parathyroid tumors are not part of the spectrum of disease in MEN2B or FMTC. Different RET mutations give rise to distinct patterns of disease establishing an apparent genotype-phenotype correlation, as illustrated. Approximately 95% of MEN2A cases result from codon substitutions affecting the CRD, namely germline missense mutations of RET codons 609, 611, 618, 620 (in exon 10), or 634 (in exon 11). Indeed, germline missense mutation of RET residue cysteine-634 accounts for approximately 85% of cases of MEN2A. Germline missense mutation in one of the RET tyrosine kinase subdomains typically gives rise only to FMTC or MEN2B (exons 13 -16).

C. Multiple Endocrine Neoplasia Type 4

Approximately 5% to 10% of patients with clinical phenotypes of MEN1 do not have mutations of *MEN1*.[37] MEN4 was first described in multigenerational kindred with features overlapping those of MEN1 but not associated with germline *MEN1* mutation.[38,39] In the study by Pellegata et al., the proband had PHPT and acromegaly and harbored a germline heterozygous truncation mutation in *CDKN1B* which encodes the cyclin dependent-kinase inhibitor p27 (Kip1), a mutation shared with several other members of this kindred who lacked PHPT.[38] Subsequently, a large multigenerational MEN4 kindred from Denmark was reported in which a germline frameshift *CDKN1B* mutation was identified in 13 family members with PHPT.[40] The tumors associated with MEN4 include parathyroid adenomas, pituitary tumors, pancreatic NET, adrenal tumors, lipomas, and meningiomas.[40]

D. The Hyperparathyroidism-Jaw Tumor Syndrome

HPT-JT is an autosomal dominant inherited syndrome with variable penetrance and expressivity that was recognized as a genetically distinct form of familial PHPT in 1990 by Gene Jackson and co-workers.[41] Key to this recognition was the follow-up of a previously reported kindred with familial PHPT,[42] in which multiple members developed ossifying fibromas of the maxilla and mandible, histologically distinct from the "brown tumors" of PHPT. The jaw tumors in HPT-JT have subsequently been classified as cemento-ossifying fibromas.[43]

PHPT is the most penetrant expression of HPT-JT and most often brings affected members to medical attention.

Apart from PHPT, the main features of HPT-JT include cemento-ossifying fibromas of the upper or lower jaw, renal cysts or tumors, and uterine pathology of several types frequently causing menorrhagia and requiring early hysterectomy.[41,44-46] In contrast to other forms of familial and even sporadic HPT, parathyroid cancer in the context of HPT-JT is relatively frequent, affecting some 20% of those with PHPT.[41,44,45,47,48]

A germline inactivating mutation of the *CDC73* putative tumor suppressor gene (formerly called *HRPT2*) can be identified in most HPT-JT kindreds.[20,49] The *CDC73* gene encodes a protein of 531 residues called parafibromin and is considered a tumor suppressor because its loss-of-function predisposes to the neoplastic features of HPT-JT.[49] Parafibromin is a component of the RNA polymerase II and chromatin-associated human Paf1 complex. Parafibromin and the associated cleavage and polyadenylation specific factor and cleavage stimulation factor play a critical role in mRNA maturation.[50] The inhibition of parafibromin resulted in increased cell proliferation and increased the *c-Myc* proto-oncogene product.[51] Most HPT-JT-associated germline *CDC73* gene variants are predicted to inactivate gene function via truncation or frameshift mutation, with only a minority encoding missense mutations.[48,52] Deletion of the *CDC73* gene has also been reported in the context of HPT-JT.[53-56] A genotype-phenotype correlation has been reported among *CDC73*-mutation carriers. Those harboring frameshift, nonsense, or deletion *CDC73* mutations are some sevenfold more likely to develop parathyroid carcinoma than those harboring missense mutations.[48]

E. Familial Isolated Hyperparathyroidism

Familial isolated hyperparathyroidism (FIHP) describes a category of familial PHPT in which families that contain two or more individuals with HPT also lack obvious features characteristic of one of the syndromic forms of familial PHPT: MEN1, MEN2A, HPT-JT, or FHH.[57] As such, FIHP is a diagnosis of exclusion. Following the initial clinical evaluation of potential FIHP kindreds, gene testing may uncover a germline mutation of *MEN1*, *CDC73*, *CDKN1B*, or *CASR*. Thus, a fraction of the FIHP kindreds under investigation in fact have previously unrecognized MEN1, HPT-JT, MEN4, or FHH.[21,58-61] Nevertheless, the majority of FIHP kindreds have been shown to lack a germline mutation in the established PHPT-susceptibility genes.[21,58,62]

Missense mutations in GCM2, which is a nuclear transcription factor required for parathyroid gland organogenesis, have been reported in the germline DNA of eight different FIHP kindreds.[22] Two germline *GCM2* mutant variants associated with FIHP act as gain-of-function mutations.[22] The missense mutations in GCM2 associated with FIHP map to its C-terminal conserved inhibitory domain (CCID) and result in increased transcriptional activity when studied *in vitro* suggesting that *GCM2* is a parathyroid proto-oncogene in the context of FIHP. Among FIHP kindreds and sporadic PHPT patients with Ashkenazi Jewish ethnicity, specific germline mutations affecting the CCID of *GCM2* are enriched.[63] Approximately 18% of FIHP kindreds harbor activating germline GCM2 mutations,[22] with the inference that some 80% of well-studied FIHP families currently lack a defined genetic basis.

F. Familial Hypocalciuric Hypercalcemia

Familial hypocalciuric hypercalcemia (FHH) is a typically benign condition of PTH-dependent hypercalcemia, resembling, and in the differential diagnosis of, PHPT (Table 66–1).[23,64] FHH is inherited in an autosomal dominant fashion and is genetically heterogeneous. The disorder results from germline mutations that cause parathyroid gland insensitivity to extracellular calcium. This insensitivity to ambient calcium levels results in a rightward shift of the usual physiologic set-point for suppression of PTH secretion by calcium. As a consequence of this insensitivity of the parathyroids to suppression by extracellular calcium, trait carriers from FHH kindreds nearly always demonstrate persistent hypercalcemia following partial or even subtotal parathyroid gland resection. The typical phenotype of FHH includes mild hypercalcemia, relative hypocalciuria, and nonsuppressed or mildly elevated PTH. In FHH, hypercalcemia is highly penetrant across all ages, including in infants.[23,65] Most cases of FHH result from germline loss-of-function mutation of the calcium-sensing receptor, encoded by the *CASR* gene.[2,66] FHH due to an inactivating mutation in the *CASR* gene is the most common type and is categorized as type 1 FHH (FHH1).[67] NSHPT is a rare autosomal recessive disorder typically presenting as severe hypercalcemia occurring in the first 6 months of life. NSHPT is usually a consequence of the compound heterozygous or homozygous inheritance of two mutant *CASR* alleles.[68] Type 2 FHH (FHH2) is caused by inactivating mutation in the *GNA11* gene encoding the G protein α11 subunit that signals downstream of the CASR.[69-71] Type 3 FHH (FHH3) is caused by a loss-of-function mutation in AP2S1 (adaptor-related protein complex 2 subunit sigma 1), an adaptor protein involved in clathrin-mediated endocytosis.[72-75] In FHH3 the majority of cases result from missense substitutions of codon Arg-15 in AP2S1.[76] Such mutant forms of AP2S1 may exert dominant-negative effects on CASR signaling.[74]

Epidemiology

PHPT is the most common cause of hypercalcemia worldwide. It is almost three times more common in women with an incidence of 66 per 100,000 person-years compared to men with an incidence of 25 per 100,000 person-years and peaks in the sixth decade.[1] It is more common in black patients, followed by white patients, Asians, and Hispanics, in descending order.[1] In China, Europe, and the United States, the incidence has been increasing over the past decades, likely due to the increase in biochemical testing and the incorporation of a serum calcium determination in many health-care screening systems. Symptomatic cases are declining worldwide as well, and the incidence of asymptomatic hypercalcemia is increasing. However, this finding is not uniform. A study published in the year 2000 comparing the PHPT population of Beijing to New York found that during the last 15 years of the twentieth century that 97% of Chinese patients studied had target organ damage in the form of skeletal lesions or nephrolithiasis while only 20% of New York patients were symptomatic.[77] A follow-up study comparing the United States and Chinese patients in 2013 found that while patients in China still more commonly present with symptoms of nephrolithiasis and fracture than do the US patients, asymptomatic Chinese patients took up a significantly greater proportion of the overall PHPT population.[78] This phenomenon is also likely due to testing; as more patients are diagnosed earlier more patients receive treatment.[78,79] These descriptive statistics capture all patients with sporadic and familial forms of PHPT. The incidences of each of the syndromic and isolated forms of familial PHPT account for approximately 2% to 5% of cases. Syndromic cases have variable phenotypes and PHPT is not always present at the same rate in all families with MEN1, for instance. The isolated familial forms, FHH, NSHPT, and FIHP, are defined by the presence of PHPT.

Clinical Presentation

Clinical presentations of PHPT are caused by excess plasma levels of calcium as well as effects of PTH on target tissues and generally vary based on the severity of the disease. Most commonly, PHPT is asymptomatic. Patients present with one of three phenotypes: asymptomatic with mild hypercalcemia, asymptomatic with high PTH levels and normal serum ionized calcium levels, or symptomatic with target organ complications or injury specifically with renal and bone manifestations. When patients are symptomatic, they can experience hypertension, neurocognitive changes, fatigue, weakness, gastrointestinal symptoms, polyuria, nephrolithiasis, or osteoporosis.[9-11] The severity of symptoms is usually directly related to the severity of hypercalcemia, but rapid shifts and older age can cause a patient to be more sensitive to smaller total calcium levels. The hypophosphatemia associated with renal phosphate loss adds to fatigue and weakness. Severe symptomatic PHPT, or "classic PHPT" as it was the most common presentation before the advent of routine laboratory testing, is characterized by nephrolithiasis and fractures or osteitis fibrosa cystica, which is severe bone demineralization with fractures, long-bone deformities such as bowing, and cyst-like bone lesions.

In patients with MEN1, PHPT is present and is the only manifestation of the syndrome in 90% of diagnoses by early in the third decade of life. Increased serum calcium can worsen symptoms from the gastrinomas associated with MEN1 by causing increased gastrin and therefore acid production, and parathyroidectomy has been shown to decrease the severity of Zollinger-Ellison syndrome in these patients.[80]

Parathyroid disease is present in about 20% to 30% of patients with MEN2A and usually presents in the late 30s in a milder form than in MEN1. Unlike MEN1-associated PHPT, MEN2-associated PHPT commonly presents as a single-gland disease. Before parathyroidectomy, all patients with MEN2A must be screened biochemically and with imaging for pheochromocytoma. Patients who receive general anesthesia and experience stress from surgery can have potentially fatal blood pressure fluctuations if an unrecognized pheochromocytoma is present.

MEN4 is similar to MEN1 in that PHPT is a primary manifestation along with pituitary tumors, although the gene mutation is different (Table 66–1). In patients with MEN4, PHPT is present in 80% to 90% and is the most common presentation.

Ossifying fibromas causing tooth displacement or jaw deformities can be a presentation of HPT-JT. However, patients can also first present with symptoms of severe hypercalcemia due to PHPT as they are at increased risk of both parathyroid adenoma and parathyroid carcinoma. This presentation contrasts with MEN1 and MEN4 where multiple gland hyperplasia is the characteristic parathyroid abnormality.

Familial hypocalciuric hypercalcemia is rarely symptomatic. Patients can experience the neurocognitive manifestations of hypercalcemia, fatigue, or mild gastrointestinal or genitourinary symptoms such as constipation, polyuria, or polydipsia.

Diagnosis, Laboratory Studies, & Imaging

The diagnosis of PHPT is made by measuring the serum concentrations of both albumin-corrected serum calcium and ionized calcium, and intact PTH. When a patient has PHPT, PTH levels can either be high with normal or elevated calcium, or inappropriately normal when the calcium level is high. High levels of calcium that are not caused by PTH overproduction will suppress PTH secretion from normally functioning parathyroid glands. Pathologies such as renal disease, malabsorptive syndromes like Crohn disease, and vitamin D deficiency cause poor absorption of calcium or calcium wasting and may be associated with elevated serum PTH. Drugs such as thiazide and loop diuretics, lithium, or bisphosphonates have various effects on calcium homeostasis. Ultimately, these are examples of diseases and medications that cause elevated PTH levels—secondary hyperparathyroidism—which must be ruled out before a diagnosis of PHPT is confirmed. In contrast to inappropriately normal or elevated PTH in the presence of hypercalcemia in PHPT, secondary HPT is defined as an appropriate physiologic elevation of PTH in response to conditions described above that cause hypocalcemia. In approximately 70% to 80% of cases, the diagnosis of PHPT is an asymptomatic, incidental finding on routine laboratory testing panels.[81] To distinguish PHPT from FHH, both calcium and creatinine are measured from a 24-hour urine collection sample. Patients with FHH will excrete less than 100 mg of calcium in 24 hours and have a calcium to creatine renal clearance ratio of less than 0.01.

After the diagnosis is confirmed and FHH as well as the causes of both secondary HPT and nonparathyroid-related hypercalcemia are ruled out, the patient must be assessed for the sequela of hypercalcemia and elevated PTH on target tissues. This includes workup for renal dysfunction (serum/urine creatinine and creatinine clearance, GFR), osteoporosis by DEXA (dual-energy X-ray absorptiometry) scan to measure bone density, and a serum phosphate level. High levels of PTH release both calcium and phosphorous from the bone via indirect activation of osteoclasts and stimulation of bone resorption, but the hormone also causes increased renal excretion of phosphate leading to an overall depleted state of this essential mineral.

After the biochemical workup is complete imaging is obtained to localize the lesion(s), which can prove challenging due to their small size and not infrequently variable location. Imaging is not done to confirm the diagnosis as PHPT is diagnosed by biochemical workup. Nor is the goal of imaging to determine if a patient needs an operation as patients with PHPT and nonlocalizing imaging studies for enlarged parathyroid glands are still operative candidates. The goal of anatomical imaging studies such as neck ultrasound or CT scan is to localize the enlarged parathyroid gland(s) and assess whether the patient is a candidate for focused parathyroidectomy. A normal-sized parathyroid gland is approximately 6 × 3-4 mm, and is relatively flat and disk shaped. The two superior parathyroid glands are almost always found at the posterior aspect of the bilateral superior poles of the thyroid gland, an infrequently variable location. The superior parathyroid glands can reside in the retroesophageal space which is not easily visible during surgical exploration and can lead to persistent PHPT if a gland is missed. They develop from the fourth pharyngeal pouch and have a shorter distance to travel than the inferior parathyroids during embryogenesis. The inferior glands develop from the third pharyngeal pouch with the thymus gland and must travel farther during development in a caudal direction than do the superior glands. As such, the inferior glands are more frequently found in ectopic locations anywhere from the mandible to the mediastinum. Thirteen percent of patients have supernumerary glands, which are most commonly found within the thymus.[82] An echogenic capsule can be seen separating the parathyroid from the thyroid tissue, and an adenoma is frequently seen as homogenously hypoechoic. Parathyroid scintigraphy, in which technetium Tc99m sestamibi is usually coupled with either single-photon emission computed tomography or dual-phase modality, is used to detect an overactive and enlarged parathyroid gland. This radiotracer is taken up by both the thyroid and parathyroid glands, but washes out more quickly from the thyroid, while an enlarged parathyroid gland commonly retains the radioisotope for a longer duration. Early and late images are taken, and enlarged overactive parathyroid glands, as well as ectopic glands, are able to be identified. The limitation of Tc99m sestamibi scan in patients with inherited PHPT such as MEN1 is the failure to identify multiple other enlarged parathyroid glands in the presence of one that is dominantly enlarged. Because multiple synchronous enlarged parathyroid glands are common in most patients with inherited PHPT, the extent of initial parathyroidectomy should include bilateral neck exploration with the identification of all four glands. The greatest benefit of preoperative Tc99m sestamibi is in patients who need reoperative parathyroidectomy or in highly selected patients who are the candidates for initial unilateral parathyroidectomy.

The role of other imaging studies recently used in patients with PHPT such as multiphase CT scan or 4-D CT scan and 18F-fluorocholine PET/CT in patients with inherited PHPT is largely limited to the reoperative setting with unclear benefit in patients undergoing initial parathyroidectomy.[83]

For all patients with a new diagnosis of PHPT, thorough family history is required. The diagnosis of each familial form is made by identifying the gene mutations listed in Table 66–1, but strong family history also meets the criteria. For instance, MEN1 is diagnosed by the presence of involvement of two endocrine tumors associated with its usual constellation or a *MEN1* germline mutation with one organ involved ex. PHPT. MEN2A is diagnosed if a patient or the patient and a close relative have involvement of two organs or if a *RET* proto-oncogene pathologic variant is identified. MEN4, HPT-JT, NSHPT, and FIHP are diagnosed by family history and identification of their specific associated germline mutations. FHH can be diagnosed by low calcium excretion on 24-hour urine collection and urine calcium to creatinine clearance ratio in conjunction with hypercalcemia and family history.

Medical Management & Treatment

Since PHPT is frequently asymptomatic, guidelines have been established based on expert opinion as to when intervention is indicated in patients lacking obvious symptoms.[84,85] For symptomatic cases, surgery remains the sole definitive therapy (see the following section). Medical therapy for hypercalcemia prior to definitive surgery may be required, however, for patients with serum calcium levels greater than ~12 mg/dL associated with neurocognitive changes, and in patients with total calcium levels greater than 14 mg/dL, regardless of symptoms.

In contrast to patients with inherited PHPT associated with benign parathyroid tumors, patients with persistent or recurrent parathyroid cancer with or without *CDC73* germline mutations frequently require medical treatments as hypercalcemia can be severe and symptomatic. Treatment of acute and/or severe hypercalcemia most often requires inpatient therapy and is typically established with intravenous normal saline infusion. Such saline hydration can be initiated at a rate of 250 to 300 mL/h in the absence of heart failure, or other cardiac or renal contraindications. Severe hypercalcemia is dehydrating due to impaired free water reabsorption, and the goal of saline hydration is to restore intravascular volume, improve glomerular filtration, and increase renal calcium excretion. Saline hydration is usually titrated to maintain a urine output of 100 to 150 mL/h. Routine treatment with furosemide or other loop diuretics is no longer recommended because of the risk of unintentional volume depletion but can be considered in cases of congestive heart failure or obvious volume overload.

In addition to normal saline hydration, treatment with calcitonin is a useful adjunct for the initial treatment of acute hypercalcemia. Salmon calcitonin, usually administered at a dose of 4 IU/kg subcutaneously or intramuscularly every 12 hours, acts pharmacologically to inhibit bone resorption following binding to calcitonin receptors present on the surface of mature osteoclasts. Although useful in the initial treatment of hypercalcemia, the efficacy of calcitonin is limited by the early development of tachyphylaxis, and is, therefore, typically used only during the first 24 to 48 hours of treatment.[86]

Treatment with intravenous bisphosphonates is a mainstay in the treatment of acute hypercalcemia, even though maximal calcium-lowering effects of IV bisphosphonates are not seen for 2 to 4 days. Bisphosphonates are stable analogs of inorganic pyrophosphate which bind to the surface of mineralized bone and interfere with bone resorption, likely by inducing osteoclast apoptosis.[87] Among available intravenous bisphosphonates, zoledronic acid, at a dose of 4 mg IV given over 15 minutes, is commonly used as the first-line agent, with pamidronate an alternative option if zoledronic acid is not available. Pamidronate is less potent than zoledronic acid and is given at a dosage of 60 to 90 mg IV over 2 hours. Intravenous bisphosphonates are usually well tolerated, but side effects can include fever, arthralgias, myalgias, hypocalcemia, osteonecrosis of the jaw, and atypical femoral fractures of the femur.[88,89] Bisphosphonates have potential renal toxicity and should be used cautiously in patients with impaired renal function. Denosumab, a monoclonal antibody targeting RANKL given subcutaneously and approved for the treatment of osteoporosis, is an alternative antihypercalcemic therapeutic option in patients for whom bisphosphonates are contraindicated because of renal impairment. As with bisphosphonates, osteonecrosis of the jaw and atypical femur fractures have been reported in patients receiving denosumab.[89]

The calcimimetic agent cinacalcet has been used to treat PTH-dependent hypercalcemia, including patients with inoperable PHPT, those with parathyroid cancer, and patients with chronic renal disease and severe secondary HPT. Initial dosing for patients with PHPT due to parathyroid cancer or benign parathyroid disease who are not operative candidates is 30 mg by mouth every 12 hours. The dose can be increased at 2 to 4 weeks intervals as needed to normalize serum calcium up to a maximum of 90 mg every 6 hours. Calcimimetics work by increasing the sensitivity of the CASR in parathyroid tissue to activation by extracellular calcium, resulting in decreased PTH release.

In select cases, hemodialysis may be indicated for the treatment of hypercalcemia.[90] These may include hypercalcemic and symptomatic patients in whom saline hydration is not possible because of anuria or severe impairment of renal function or hemodynamically stable patients with acute hypercalcemia in a range above ~18 mg/dL associated with neurocognitive changes for whom rapid and aggressive therapy is clinically warranted.

Surgical Treatment

Surgical management in the form of parathyroidectomy is the only definitive treatment for PHPT. Unless the patient is not a surgical candidate due to severe comorbidities which would preclude them from receiving general anesthesia, parathyroidectomy is indicated in all symptomatic cases. Other indications according to current American Association of Endocrine Surgeons (AAES) Guidelines include serum calcium more than 1 mg/dL above the normal institutional range, any evidence of bone loss or renal involvement including hypercalciuria, and age below 50 years, among others (Table 66–2).[91]

Sporadic cases are most commonly caused by an adenoma of a single parathyroid gland, which is localized with preoperative imaging and removed for cure. Both isolated and syndromic cases of familial PHTP are usually caused by hyperplasia of multiple glands. For this type of disease, parathyroidectomy is performed in which the goal is to remove all enlarged parathyroid glands, leaving behind one to two normal parathyroid gland equivalents (~50-80 mg of parathyroid tissue), which could be an intact normal-appearing gland or a portion of a hyperplastic gland. An inferior parathyroid gland is a preferred parathyroid remnant as the anatomical location is anterior to the recurrent laryngeal nerve and more superficial compared to a superior parathyroid gland, which facilitates identification and may reduce the risk of nerve injury during reoperation. The parathyroid remnant is either left in its normal anatomic location in a procedure termed subtotal parathyroidectomy, or morcellated and implanted into the sternocleidomastoid or brachioradialis muscle—total parathyroidectomy with autotransplantation. The purpose of reimplanting the remaining parathyroid tissue in a nonanatomic location is to facilitate reoperation with no risk for recurrent laryngeal nerve injury and without a need for general anesthesia. Reoperative parathyroidectomy is more difficult because of scar tissue which forms after the index procedure and increases the risk of the most dreaded complication, recurrent laryngeal nerve injury,

Table 66–2. Indications for parathyroidectomy after diagnosis of primary hyperparathyroidism

Indication	Qualifications
Symptomatic PHPT	—
Serum Calcium >1 mg/dL above institutional normal	Regardless of symptoms
Renal involvement	Asymptomatic nephrolithiasis, nephrocalcinosis, hypercalciuria, or GFR <60 mL/min
Bone involvement	Osteoperosis, fragility fractures, or asymptomatic spinal compression fractures
Less than 50 years of age	—
Concern for parathyroid cancer	—
High risk for loss of follow-up	—
Neurocognitive or psychiatric symptoms	—
Cardiovascular disease	Cardiovascular risk mitigation for high-risk candidates
Nontraditional symptoms	Weakness, fatigue, abnormal sleep, decreased daily functioning, GERD, fibromyalgia

PHPT, primary hyperparathyroidism; GFR, glomerular filtration rate; GERD, gastroesophageal reflux disease.

and resulting vocal cord paralysis. The use of intraoperative laryngeal nerve monitoring can aid the identification of the recurrent laryngeal nerve and can assess its conductivity to confirm functional integrity. Although nonconclusive, recent studies suggest that intraoperative laryngeal nerve monitoring reduces transient and permanent recurrent laryngeal nerve injury.[92] Recurrent PHTP from continuing hyperplastic changes in syndromic cases is expected since the underlying germline mutation is untreatable with modern therapy. These nonanatomic locations, such as brachioradialis or sternocleidomastoid muscles, specifically are chosen because they are easily accessible and give the reimplanted parathyroid access to the formidable blood supply inherent in muscle tissue. When recurrence occurs, for instance in MEN1, the incision in the arm or in the neck over the sternocleidomastoid is opened and the parathyroid tissue is debulked. Cryopreservation of a patient's parathyroid tissue is done at high-volume centers and can be reimplanted if the immediate autograft or the parathyroid remnant at the time of the index procedure does not provide sufficient parathyroid hormone to maintain serum calcium in the normal range.

Parathyroid tumors can be small and are often difficult to identify even with preoperative localization imaging. Intraoperative PTH monitoring is done to functionally confirm the adequacy of the resection and reduce the rate of persistent PHPT. However, the benefit of intraoperative PTH monitoring in patients with inherited PHPT, such as MEN1, undergoing initial parathyroidectomy remains unproven[93] because the PTH values and dynamics do not change the extent of the initial operation nor predict or improve the outcomes. However, the use of intraoperative PTH monitoring can be helpful in reoperative parathyroidectomy to determine the adequacy of the operation. A baseline level measured from peripheral blood is drawn prior to the start of surgery. Intraoperatively a PTH level is measured at time zero (pre-excision up to the moment the blood supply to the gland is ligated) followed by additional levels in 5, 10, and (optional) 20 minutes after resection. The half-life of PTH is approximately 3 to 5 minutes, and if the hyperfunctioning glands are appropriately removed, the surgeon will observe a precipitous drop. In patients with *sporadic* PHPT, a 50% decrease in PTH from the highest PTH level (preincision or pre-excision) predicts operative success and postoperative eucalcemia more than 92% of the time.[94] The cutoff of intraoperative PTH drop ≥75% from the baseline was associated with 87% resolution of hypercalcemia in patients with MEN1 undergoing initial parathyroidectomy. The biochemical resolution of hypocalcemia in patients who had three or more parathyroid glands identified was also 87%.[93]

Eucalcemia and normal PTH levels postoperatively indicate surgical success. Persistent or recurrent disease (hypercalcemia within or after 6 months, respectively) is diagnosed

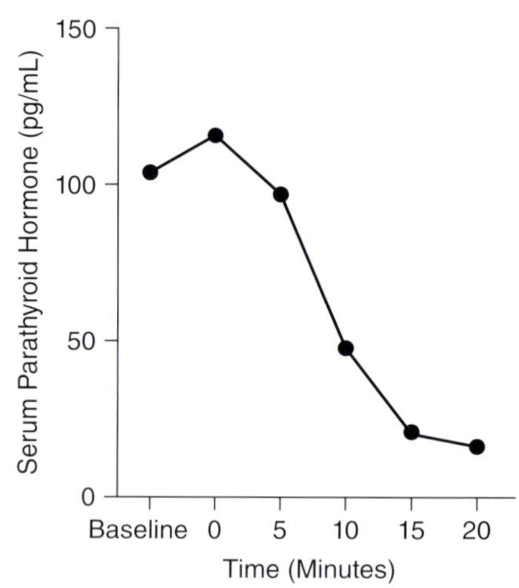

Figure 66–2. Serum dynamics of parathyroid hormone intraoperatively. Graph of serum PTH level taken prior to surgery (baseline), at excision (time 0 minutes), and at 5-minute intervals. The kinetics of intraoperative PTH during an initial parathyroidectomy for MEN1-related primary hyperparathyroidism after excision predict the resolution of hypercalcemia postoperatively.

in approximately 2.5% to 5% of patients after surgery.[95] Conversely, transient or persistent hypoparathyroidism resulting in hypocalcemia and the need for calcium replacement therapy occur from inadequate PTH production to maintain eucalcemia. Patients who had multiple parathyroid glands removed are at high risk for hypoparathyroidism and immediate parathyroid autotransplantation should be considered if the offending gland is believed to be the last gland. A hungry bone syndrome is a serious complication characterized by severe hypocalcemia, hypophosphatemia, and hypomagnesemia which occurs rarely but more often in patients with preoperative evidence of bone loss from severe PHPT.

Prognosis

Patients with syndromic disorders do frequently have a shorter life expectancy than the general population but this shortening is most often not due to PHPT. For instance, a diagnosis of MEN1 carries decreased survival probability compared to the general population; however, this is due to metastatic duodenopancreatic neuroendocrine tumors and not the manifestations of PHPT.[96] Patients with MEN2A currently die most commonly from metastatic medullary thyroid cancer, whereas in the past before the ubiquity of biochemical testing the culprit was usually pheochromocytoma.[97] After successful surgery for PHPT, calcium and PTH levels rapidly normalize. Data on long-term follow-up after definitive treatment for PHPT in sporadic cases show excellent results in bone mineral density, with patients seeing improvement in the spine, hip, and radius on DEXA scan, as well as a decrease in the incidence of fractures in preoperatively symptomatic patients.[9] Also in patients with sporadic disease, renal symptoms improve as well, with consistent decreases in the rate of hypercalciuria and nephrolithiasis. However, other data are more mixed. Among all patients with treated PHPT, improvement in neurocognitive symptoms such as confusion, fogginess, and fatigue is not consistent. Also, PHPT imparts an increased risk of cardiovascular disease, specifically in the form of hypertension, atherosclerosis, and ventricular remodeling, as well as cardiovascular mortality.[98] Data, however, is mixed on the reduction of this risk after parathyroidectomy with seemingly the most benefit imparted to those patients with sporadic PHPT with severely elevated serum calcium. Additional studies are needed to definitively answer this question.

REFERENCES

1. Yeh MW, Ituarte PHG, Zhou HC, et al. Incidence and prevalence of primary hyperparathyroidism in a racially mixed population. *J Clin Endocrinol Metab*. 2013;98(3):1122-1129.
2. Brown EM. Role of the calcium-sensing receptor in extracellular calcium homeostasis. *Best Pract Res Clin Endocrinol Metab*. 2013;27(3):333-343.
3. Zhang C, Miller CL, Gorkhali R, et al. Molecular basis of the extracellular ligands mediated signaling by the calcium sensing receptor. *Front Physiol*. 2016;7:441.
4. Silva BC, Bilezikian JP. Parathyroid hormone: anabolic and catabolic actions on the skeleton. *Curr Opin Pharmacol*. 2015;22:41-50.
5. Cantley LK, Russell J, Lettieri D, Sherwood LM. 1,25-Dihydroxyvitamin D3 suppresses parathyroid hormone secretion from bovine parathyroid cells in tissue culture. *Endocrinology*. 1985;117(5):2114-2119.
6. Russell J, Lettieri D, Sherwood LM. Suppression by 1,25(OH)2D3 of transcription of the pre-proparathyroid hormone gene. *Endocrinology*. 1986;119(6):2864-2866.
7. Silver J, Yalcindag C, Sela-Brown A, Kilav R, Naveh-Many T. Regulation by vitamin D metabolites of parathyroid hormone gene transcription in vivo in the rat. *J Clin Invest*. 1986;78(5):1296-1301.
8. Silver J, Russell J, Sherwood LM. Regulation by vitamin D metabolites of messenger ribonucleic acid for preproparathyroid hormone in isolated bovine parathyroid cells. *Proc Natl Acad Sci USA*. 1985;82(12):4270-4273.
9. Bilezikian JP. Primary hyperparathyroidism. *J Clin Endocrinol Metab*. 2018;103(11):3993-4004.
10. Fraser WD. Hyperparathyroidism. *Lancet*. 2009;374(9684):145-158.
11. Walker MD, Bilezikian JP. Primary hyperparathyroidism, in K.R. Feingold et al., eds. *Endotext*. South Dartmouth (MA); 2000.
12. Minisola S, Gianotti L, Bhadada S, Silverberg SJ. Classical complications of primary hyperparathyroidism. *Best Pract Res Clin Endocrinol Metab*. 2018;32(6):791-803.
13. Naji Rad S, Deluxe L. Osteitis Fibrosa Cystica, in *StatPearls*. Treasure Island (FL); 2021.
14. Weber TJ, Quarles LD. Molecular control of phosphorus homeostasis and precision treatment of hypophosphatemic disorders. *Curr Mol Biol Rep*. 2019;5(2):75-85.
15. Jacquillet G, Unwin RJ. Physiological regulation of phosphate by vitamin D, parathyroid hormone (PTH) and phosphate (Pi). *Pflugers Arch*. 2019;471(1):83-98.
16. Farrow EG, White KE. Recent advances in renal phosphate handling. *Nat Rev Nephrol*. 2010;6(4):207-217.
17. Schneider AB, Gierlowski TC, Shore-Freedman E, Stovall M, Ron E, Lubin J. Dose-response relationships for radiation-induced hyperparathyroidism. *J Clin Endocrinol Metab*. 1995;80(1):254-257.
18. Insogna KL. Primary hyperparathyroidism. *N Engl J Med*. 2018;379(11):1050-1059.
19. Marx SJ. Molecular genetics of multiple endocrine neoplasia types 1 and 2. *Nat Rev Cancer*. 2005;5(5):367-375.
20. Hyde SM, et al. CDC73-Related Disorders. 2008 Dec 31 [Updated 2018 Apr 26]. Seattle (WA): University of Washington, Seattle; 1993-2019. GeneReviews® [Internet].
21. Simonds WF, James-Newton LA, Agarwal SK, et al. Familial isolated hyperparathyroidism: clinical and genetic characteristics of thirty-six kindreds. *Medicine*. 2002;81:1-26.
22. Guan B, Welch JM, Sapp JC, et al. GCM2-activating mutations in familial isolated hyperparathyroidism. *Am J Hum Genet*. 2016;99(5):1034-1044.
23. Marx SJ, Attie MF, Levine MA, Spiegel AM, Downs RW Jr, Lasker RD. The hypocalciuric or benign variant of familial hypercalcemia: clinical and biochemical features in fifteen kindreds. *Medicine*. 1981;60(6):397-412.
24. Wermer P. Genetic aspects of adenomatosis of endocrine glands. *Am J Med*. 1954;16(3):363-371.
25. Larsson C, Skogseid B, Oberg K, Nakamura Y, Nordenskjöld M. Multiple endocrine neoplasia type 1 gene maps to chromosome 11 and is lost in insulinoma. *Nature*. 1988;332(6159):85-87.

26. Chandrasekharappa SC, Guru SC, Manickam P, et al. Positional cloning of the gene for multiple endocrine neoplasia-type 1. *Science*. 1997;276(5311):404-407.
27. Guru SC, Goldsmith PK, Burns AL, et al. Menin, the product of the MEN1 gene, is a nuclear protein. *Proc Natl Acad Sci USA*. 1998;95(4):1630-1634.
28. La P, Desmond A, Hou Z, Silva AC, Schnepp RW, Hua X. Tumor suppressor menin: the essential role of nuclear localization signal domains in coordinating gene expression. *Oncogene*. 2006;25(25):3537-3546.
29. Huang J, Gurung B, Wan B, Wan K, Hua X, Lei M. The same pocket in menin binds both MLL and JUND but has opposite effects on transcription. *Nature*. 2012;482(7386):542-546.
30. Murai MJ, Chruszcz M, Reddy G, Grembecka J, Cierpicki T. Crystal structure of menin reveals binding site for mixed lineage leukemia (MLL) protein. *J Biol Chem*. 2011;286(36): 31742-31748.
31. Agarwal SK. The future: genetics advances in MEN1 therapeutic approaches and management strategies. *Endocr Relat Cancer*. 2017;24(10):T119-T134.
32. Dreijerink KMA, Timmers HTM, Brown M. Twenty years of menin: emerging opportunities for restoration of transcriptional regulation in MEN1. *Endocr Relat Cancer*. 2017;24(10): T135-T145.
33. Eng C. Multiple endocrine neoplasia type 2. 1999 Sep 27 [updated 2019 Aug 15], in Adam MP, et al. eds. *GeneReviews [Internet]*. Seattle, WA: University of Washington, Seattle; 1993-2020.
34. Wells SA Jr, Santoro M. Targeting the RET pathway in thyroid cancer. *Clin Cancer Res*. 2009;15(23):7119-7123.
35. Frank-Raue K, Raue F. Hereditary medullary thyroid cancer genotype-phenotype correlation. *Recent Results Cancer Res*. 2015;204:139-156.
36. Eng C, Clayton D, Schuffenecker I, et al. The relationship between specific RET proto-oncogene mutations and disease phenotype in multiple endocrine neoplasia type 2. International RET mutation consortium analysis. *JAMA*. 1996;276(19):1575-1579.
37. Lemos MC, Thakker RV. Multiple endocrine neoplasia type 1 (MEN1): analysis of 1336 mutations reported in the first decade following identification of the gene. *Hum Mutat*. 2008; 29(1):22-32.
38. Pellegata NS, Quintanilla-Martinez L, Siggelkow H, et al. Germ-line mutations in p27Kip1 cause a multiple endocrine neoplasia syndrome in rats and humans. *Proc Natl Acad Sci USA*. 2006;103(42):15558-15563.
39. Alrezk R, Hannah-Shmouni F, Stratakis CA. MEN4 and CDKN1B mutations: the latest of the MEN syndromes. *Endocr Relat Cancer*. 2017;24(10):T195-T208.
40. Frederiksen A, Rossing M, Hermann P, Ejersted C, Thakker RV, Frost M, et al. Clinical features of multiple endocrine neoplasia type 4: novel pathogenic variant and review of published cases. *J Clin Endocrinol Metab*. 2019;104(9):3637-3646.
41. Jackson CE, Norum RA, Boyd SB, et al. Hereditary hyperparathyroidism and multiple ossifying jaw fibromas: a clinically and genetically distinct syndrome. *Surgery*, 1990;108(6):1006-1012; discussion 1012-1013.
42. Jackson CE. Hereditary hyperparathyroidism associated with recurrent pancreatitis. *Ann Intern Med*. 1958;49(4):829-836.
43. Kramer IR, Pindborg JJ, Shear M. The WHO histological typing of odontogenic tumours. A commentary on the Second Edition. *Cancer*. 1992;70(12):2988-2994.
44. Bradley KJ, Hobbs MR, Buley ID, et al. Uterine tumours are a phenotypic manifestation of the hyperparathyroidism-jaw tumour syndrome. *J Intern Med*. 2005;257(1):18-26.
45. Chen JD, Morrison C, Zhang C, Kahnoski K, Carpten JD, Teh BT. Hyperparathyroidism-jaw tumour syndrome. *J Intern Med*. 2003;253(6):634-642.
46. Torresan F, Iacobone M. Clinical features, treatment, and surveillance of hyperparathyroidism-jaw tumor syndrome: an up-to-date and review of the literature. *Int J Endocrinol*. 2019;2019:1761030.
47. Mehta A, Patel D, Rosenberg A, et al. Hyperparathyroidism-jaw tumor syndrome: results of operative management. *Surgery*. 2014;156(6):1315-1324; discussion 1324-1325.
48. Li Y, Zhang J, Adikaram PR, et al. Genotype of CDC73 germline mutation determines risk of parathyroid cancer. *Endocr Relat Cancer*. 2020;27(9):483-494.
49. Carpten JD, Robbins CM, Villablanca A, et al. HRPT2, encoding parafibromin, is mutated in hyperparathyroidism-jaw tumor syndrome. *Nat Genet*. 2002; 32(4): 676-680.
50. Rozenblatt-Rosen O, Nagaike T, Francis JM, et al. The tumor suppressor Cdc73 functionally associates with CPSF and CstF 3' mRNA processing factors. *Proc Natl Acad Sci USA*. 2009;106(3):755-760.
51. Lin L, Zhang J-H, Panicker LM, Simonds WF. The parafibromin tumor suppressor protein inhibits cell proliferation by repression of the c-myc proto-oncogene. *Proc Natl Acad Sci USA*. 2008;105(45):17420-17425.
52. Newey PJ, Bowl MR, Thakker RV. Parafibromin–functional insights. *J Intern Med*. 2009;266(1):84-98.
53. Domingues R, Tomaz RA, Martins C, Nunes C, Bugalho MJ, Cavaco BM. Identification of the first germline HRPT2 whole-gene deletion in a patient with primary hyperparathyroidism. *Clin Endocrinol*. 2012;76(1):33-38.
54. Cascón A, Huarte-Mendicoa CV, Leandro-García LJ, et al. Detection of the first gross CDC73 germline deletion in an HPT-JT syndrome family. *Genes Chromosomes Cancer*. 2011;50(11):922-929.
55. Bricaire L, Odou M-F, Cardot-Bauters C, et al. Frequent large germline HRPT2 deletions in a French National cohort of patients with primary hyperparathyroidism. *J Clin Endocrinol Metab*. 2013;98(2):E403-E408.
56. Guarnieri V, Seaberg RM, Kelly C, et al. Large intragenic deletion of CDC73 (exons 4-10) in a three-generation hyperparathyroidism-jaw tumor (HPT-JT) syndrome family. *BMC Med Genet*. 2017;18(1):83.
57. Marx SJ. New concepts about familial isolated hyperparathyroidism. *J Clin Endocrinol Metab*. 2019;104:4058-4066.
58. Simonds WF, Robbins CM, Agarwal SK, et al. Familial isolated hyperparathyroidism is rarely caused by germline mutation in HRPT2, the gene for the hyperparathyroidism-jaw tumor syndrome. *J Clin Endocrinol Metab*. 2004;89(1):96-102.
59. Warner J, Epstein M, Sweet A, et al. Genetic testing in familial isolated hyperparathyroidism: unexpected results and their implications. *J Med Genet*. 2004;41(3):155-160.
60. Cetani F, Pardi E, Ambrogini E, et al. Genetic analyses in familial isolated hyperparathyroidism: implication for clinical assessment and surgical management. *Clin Endocrinol*. 2006;64(2):146-152.
61. Vierimaa O, Villablanca A, Alimov A, et al. Mutation analysis of MEN1, HRPT2, CASR, CDKN1B, and AIP genes in primary hyperparathyroidism patients with features of genetic predisposition. *J Endocrinol Invest*. 2009;32(6):512-518.
62. Pontikides N, Karras S, Kaprara A, et al. Genetic basis of familial isolated hyperparathyroidism: a case series and a narrative review of the literature. *J Bone Miner Metab*. 2014;32(4):351-366.
63. Guan B, Welch JM, Vemulapalli M, et al. Ethnicity of patients with germline GCM2-activating variants and primary hyperparathyroidism. *J Endocr Soc*. 2017;1(5):488-499.

64. Lee JY, Shoback DM. Familial hypocalciuric hypercalcemia and related disorders. *Best Pract Res Clin Endocrinol Metab.* 2018;32(5):609-619.
65. Papadopoulou A, Gole E, Melachroinou K, et al. Identification and functional characterization of a calcium-sensing receptor mutation in an infant with familial hypocalciuric hypercalcemia. *J Clin Res Pediatr Endocrinol.* 2016;8(3):341-346.
66. Brown EM. Familial hypocalciuric hypercalcemia and other disorders with resistance to extracellular calcium. *Endocrinol Metab Clin North Am.* 2000;29(3):503-522.
67. Mariathasan S, Andrews KA, Thompson E, et al. Genetic testing for hereditary hyperparathyroidism and familial hypocalciuric hypercalcaemia in a large UK cohort. *Clin Endocrinol.* 2020;93:409-418.
68. Brown EM. Mutations in the calcium-sensing receptor and their clinical implications. *Horm Res.* 1997;48(5):199-208.
69. Nesbit MA, Hannan FM, Howles SA, et al. Mutations affecting G-protein subunit alpha11 in hypercalcemia and hypocalcemia. *N Engl J Med.* 2013;368(26):2476-2486.
70. Gorvin CM, Cranston T, Hannan FM, et al. A G-protein subunit-alpha11 loss-of-function mutation, Thr54Met, causes familial hypocalciuric hypercalcemia type 2 (FHH2). *J Bone Miner Res.* 2016;31(6):1200-1206.
71. Hannan FM, Babinsky VN, Thakker RV. Disorders of the calcium-sensing receptor and partner proteins: insights into the molecular basis of calcium homeostasis. *J Mol Endocrinol.* 2016;57(3):R127-R142.
72. Nesbit MA, Hannan FM, Howles SA, et al. Mutations in AP2S1 cause familial hypocalciuric hypercalcemia type 3. *Nat Genet.* 2013;45(1):93-97.
73. Hendy GN, Canaff L, Newfield RS, et al. Codon Arg15 mutations of the AP2S1 gene: common occurrence in familial hypocalciuric hypercalcemia cases negative for calcium-sensing receptor (CASR) mutations. *J Clin Endocrinol Metab.* 2014;99(7): E1311-E1315.
74. Hannan FM, Howles SA, Rogers A, et al. Adaptor protein-2 sigma subunit mutations causing familial hypocalciuric hypercalcaemia type 3 (FHH3) demonstrate genotype-phenotype correlations, codon bias and dominant-negative effects. *Hum Mol Genet.* 2015;24(18):5079-5092.
75. Vargas-Poussou R, Mansour-Hendili L, Baron S, et al. Familial hypocalciuric hypercalcemia types 1 and 3 and primary hyperparathyroidism: similarities and differences. *J Clin Endocrinol Metab.* 2016;101(5):2185-2195.
76. Gorvin CM, Metpally R, Stokes VJ, et al. Large-scale exome datasets reveal a new class of adaptor-related protein complex 2 sigma subunit (AP2sigma) mutations, located at the interface with the AP2 alpha subunit, that impair calcium-sensing receptor signalling. *Hum Mol Genet.* 2018;27(5):901-911.
77. Bilezikian JP, Meng X, Shi Y, Silverberg SJ. Primary hyperparathyroidism in women: a tale of two cities—New York and Beijing. *Int J Fertil Womens Med.* 2000;45(2):158-165.
78. Liu JM, Cusano NE, Silva BC, et al. Primary hyperparathyroidism: A tale of two cities revisited—New York and Shanghai. *Bone Res.* 2013;1(2):162-169.
79. Sun B, Guo B, Wu B, et al. Characteristics, management, and outcome of primary hyperparathyroidism at a single clinical center from 2005 to 2016. *Osteoporos Int.* 2018; 29(3):635-642.
80. Norton JA, Venzon DJ, Berna MJ, et al. Prospective study of surgery for primary hyperparathyroidism (HPT) in multiple endocrine neoplasia-type 1 and Zollinger-Ellison syndrome: long-term outcome of a more virulent form of HPT. *Ann Surg.* 2008;247(3):501-510.
81. Blau JE, Simonds WF. Familial hyperparathyroidism. *Front Endocrinol (Lausanne).* 2021;12:623667.
82. Sung JY. Parathyroid ultrasonography: the evolving role of the radiologist. *Ultrasonography.* 2015;34(4):268-274.
83. Gauthé M, Dierick-Gallet A, Delbot T, et al. (18)F-fluorocholine PET/CT in MEN1 patients with primary hyperparathyroidism. *World J Surg.* 2020;44(11):3761-3769.
84. Bilezikian JP, Brandi ML, Eastell R, et al. Guidelines for the management of asymptomatic primary hyperparathyroidism: summary statement from the Fourth International Workshop. *J Clin Endocrinol Metab.* 2014;99(10):3561-3569.
85. Silva BC, Cusano NE, Bilezikian JP. Primary hyperparathyroidism. *Best Pract Res Clin Endocrinol Metab.* 2018:101247.
86. McLaughlin MB, Jialal I. Calcitonin, in *StatPearls.* Treasure Island (FL); 2021.
87. Hughes DE, Wright KR, Uy HL, et al. Bisphosphonates promote apoptosis in murine osteoclasts in vitro and in vivo. *J Bone Miner Res.* 1995;10(10):1478-1487.
88. Reyes C, Hitz M, Prieto-Alhambra D, Abrahamsen B. Risks and benefits of bisphosphonate therapies. *J Cell Biochem.* 2016;117(1):20-28.
89. Jara MA, Varghese J, Hu MI. Adverse events associated with bone-directed therapies in patients with cancer. *Bone.* 2022;128:115901.
90. Trabulus S, Oruc M, Ozgun E, Altiparmak MR, Seyahi N. The use of low-calcium hemodialysis in the treatment of hypercalcemic crisis. *Nephron.* 2018;139(4):319-331.
91. Wilhelm SM, Wang TS, Ruan DT, et al. The American Association of Endocrine Surgeons guidelines for definitive management of primary hyperparathyroidism. *JAMA Surg.* 2016;151(10):959-968.
92. Bai B, Chen W. Protective effects of intraoperative nerve monitoring (IONM) for recurrent laryngeal nerve injury in thyroidectomy: meta-analysis. *Sci Rep.* 2018;8(1):7761.
93. Nilubol N, Weisbrod AB, Weinstein LS, et al. Utility of intraoperative parathyroid hormone monitoring in patients with multiple endocrine neoplasia type 1-associated primary hyperparathyroidism undergoing initial parathyroidectomy. *World J Surg.* 2013;37(8):1966-1972.
94. Irvin GL 3rd, Solorzano CC, Carneiro DM. Quick intraoperative parathyroid hormone assay: surgical adjunct to allow limited parathyroidectomy, improve success rate, and predict outcome. *World J Surg.* 2004;28(12):1287-1292.
95. Guerin C, Paladino NC, Lowery A, et al. Persistent and recurrent hyperparathyroidism. *Updates Surg.* 2017;69(2):161-169.
96. Conemans EB, Nell S, Pieterman CRC, et al. Prognostic factors for survival of MEN1 patients with duodenopancreatic tumors metastatic to the liver: results from the DMSG. *Endocr Pract.* 2017;23(6):641-648.
97. Wells SA Jr, Pacini F, Robinson BG, Santoro M. Multiple endocrine neoplasia type 2 and familial medullary thyroid carcinoma: an update. *J Clin Endocrinol Metab.* 2013;98(8):3149-3164.
98. Walker MD, Silverberg SJ. Cardiovascular aspects of primary hyperparathyroidism. *J Endocrinol Invest.* 2008;31(10):925-931.

67 Familial Hypocalciuric Hypercalcemia Syndrome

Francesca Giusti, MD, PhD
Francesca Marini, PhD
Maria Luisa Brandi, MD, PhD

GENERAL CONSIDERATIONS

Familial hypocalciuric hypercalcemia (FHH) (ORPHA 405), also known as familial benign hypercalcemia, comprises a genetically heterogenous group of rare heritable disorders of calcium homeostasis, characterized by lifelong mild to moderate elevation of serum calcium levels (hypercalcemia), associated with an inappropriately low urinary excretion of calcium (hypocalciuria) and with normal or mildly elevated circulating level of intact parathyroid hormone (PTH). Three genetic forms (phenocopies) are described, based on the causative gene defect: Type 1 (FHH1; OMIM #145980) caused by mutations of the *CASR* gene, type 2 (FHH2; OMIM #145981) caused by mutations of the *GNA11* gene, and type 3 (FHH3; OMIM #600740) caused by mutations of *AP2S1* gene.[1]

All three genetic forms are transmitted as a monogenic autosomal dominant trait, with a very high degree of penetrance and an equal distribution among genders. No ethnic or geographical prevalence has been reported.

An extremely rare and severe form of autosomal recessive FHH, the neonatal severe primary hyperparathyroidism (NSHPT), has been reported.[2]

Exact FHH prevalence is unknown and difficult to calculate, given the subclinical nature of the disease in many cases. FHH1 is estimated to account for about 65% of cases. According to a recent study, the estimated frequency of FHH1 would be about 74.1/100,000.[3]

PATHOGENESIS

FHHs are Mendelian-inherited monogenic diseases presenting with an autosomal dominant pattern of inheritance. The genetic defect is inherited by the affected parent, who has a 50% probability of transmitting the mutation to their offspring independent of sex. Hypercalcemia penetrance is almost 100% at birth in mutation carriers.

FHH1 is caused by germline heterozygote loss-of-function mutations of the calcium-sensing receptor (*CASR*) gene on chromosome 3q13-q21, encoding a homodimeric G-protein transmembrane receptor (CaSR protein),[1] widely expressed in the cells of parathyroid glands and kidney tubules and responsible for the maintenance of physiological levels of ionized calcium in the blood. Inactivating mutations make the receptor less sensitive to serum calcium ion variations, leading, at the parathyroid level, to continuous release of PTH even when serum calcium is high, resulting in constant hypercalcemia, while at the kidney level the decreased sensitivity accounts for the inappropriately low urinary calcium excretion in the presence of hypercalcemia. Biochemical signatures in FHH1 are suspected to be *CASR* mutation dependent. Truncating mutations, presumably not exerting a dominant-negative effect on the homodimeric conformation of CaSR, are associated with less severe hypercalcemia and a minor increase of PTH levels (but not with urinary calcium excretion, calcium/creatinine clearance or symptoms), than *CaSR* missense mutations which are responsible for a dominant-negative effect on the receptor function.

NSHPT is caused by germline homozygote loss-of-function mutations of the *CASR* gene, inherited by both FHH1-affected parents.

FHH2 is caused by heterozygote inactivating mutations of the G-protein alpha 11 (*GNA11*) gene on chromosome 19p13, encoding the alpha subunit of an intracellular G protein coupled with CaSR (G11), acting as transducer of CaSR-mediated signaling, to block the production and release of PTH in the parathyroids, and the reabsorption of calcium from the filtered fluids in the renal tubules.[1] To date, only three *GNA11* gene mutations have been reported in FHH2—p.Thr54Met, p.Leu135Gln, and p.Ile200del.

FHH3 is caused by heterozygote loss-of-function mutations of the Adaptor Protein 2 Sigma 1 (*AP2S1*) gene on chromosome 19q13, encoding the 17-kD component of the AP2 clathrin-associated protein complex (AP17), which is necessary for the correct membrane trafficking of CaSR.[1] All the identified *AP2S1* mutations affect the arginine residue at codon 15 of the AP17 protein (p.Arg15Cys, p.Arg15His, or p.Arg15Leu). Individuals bearing the p.Arg15Leu mutation showed the most severe hypercalcemia among FHH3 patients, with mild hypophosphatemia and elevated PTH concentrations.

In extremely rare cases an acquired, nongenetic, form of FHH is caused by autoantibodies against the CaSR protein.

PREVENTION

In first-degree relatives of an FHH patient, it is recommended to perform serum calcium screening; if hypercalcemia is identified, it is advisable to perform the measurement of PTH and the assessment of the relationship between clearance of calcium and creatinine.

Genetic testing, starting with the *CASR* gene, can be performed in a suspected case of FHH to confirm the clinical diagnosis, or for a differential diagnosis with primary hyperparathyroidism (PHPT). A positive genetic testing enables the possibility to genetically screen first-degree relatives for the family-specific mutation.

Given the fact that FHHs are benign diseases, prenatal genetic testing is not commonly recommended. However, prenatal genetic testing or a genetic test at birth for the *CASR* gene are strongly recommended when both parents have been found to be carriers of *CASR* mutations and/or present clinical signs of FHH, as the inheritance of both maternal and paternal *CASR* mutated alleles leads to the development of NSHPT.

Pregnant women with FHH should be constantly monitored during pregnancy, since during fetal development marked maternal hypercalcemia leads to the inhibition of endogenous secretion of PTH with a consequent high risk of developing severe hypocalcemia during the first days of life.

CLINICAL FINDINGS

Symptoms & Signs

Biochemically, FHH patients show mild to moderate and nonprogressive hypercalcemia, hypocalciuria featured by low calcium-to-creatinine clearance ratio, and normal (80% of cases) or slightly elevated (20% of cases) serum PTH levels.[4]

Clinically, the majority of FHH patients are asymptomatic, though some with moderate-to-severe hypercalcemia may present with classical hypercalcemic symptoms such as fatigue, weakness, excessive thirst, concentration problems, gallstones, polyuria, and polydipsia. Some adult patients can also manifest chondrocalcinosis, relapsing pancreatitis, and premature vascular calcification.

In the FHH2 form marked hypocalciuria is noted. FHH3 patients usually have a relatively higher hypercalcemia and hypermagnesemia, and a more marked hypocalciuria, compared to those with FHH1. Low bone mineral density (BMD) and cognitive disorders have also been reported in FHH3.[1]

In contrast to the three autosomal dominant forms of FHH, NSHPT is a symptomatic severe form of neonatal-onset FHH, characterized by PHPT occurring at birth or within the first 6 months of life and causing life-threatening severe hypercalcemia (>3.5 mmol/L), hypotonia, bone demineralization, fragility fractures, and respiratory distress.

Laboratory Findings

1. Mild to moderate hypercalcemia.
2. Normal or slightly elevated serum intact PTH.
3. Inappropriate hypocalciuria in the presence of hypercalcemia (in presence of normal value of vitamin D and correct calcium intake, a urinary calcium <100 mg/day and fractional excretion of calcium <0.01 are suggestive of FHH).
4. Low calcium-to-creatinine clearance ratio (<0.01).[4]
5. Values of active form of vitamin D (calcitriol) are usually normal or slightly elevated.
6. Serum levels of magnesium are usually elevated.
7. Unaltered BMD (only rare FHH3 cases may have low BMD values).[1]
8. No increased incidence of fragility fracture.

Imaging Studies

Imaging of the parathyroids in patients with FHH by ultrasound is typically unrevealing, since in FHH the parathyroid glands can be normal in size. Surgically excised parathyroids from FHH patients can range from normal size and histology to clearly enlarged glands consistent with an adenoma.

Genetic Testing

Genetic testing is useful for differentiating FHH from PHPT, mostly in those cases in which biochemical findings do not support a clear FHH diagnosis. Discriminating FHH from PHPT is fundamental for the therapeutic management, since, in FHH patients, parathyroid surgery is not curative, and should be avoided.

Genetic testing should start by the analysis of the *CASR* gene (since FHH1 accounts for about 65% of cases). Target genetic testing of the *GNA11* gene is recommended for FHH phenotypes in whom mutational analysis of the *CASR* gene was negative. Screening of exon 2 of the *AP2S1* gene (estimated to cause over 20% of *CASR*-negative FHH cases) is indicated in FHH phenotypes showing a marked hypermagnesemia, cognitive impairment, or low BMD and in FHH cases negative for both *CASR* and *GNA11* mutations.

Prenatal genetic testing for FHH1, FHH2, and FHH3 is not recommended, while *CASR* prenatal or at-birth genetic testing is strongly indicated if both parents are carriers of *CASR* mutations of present clinical signs of FHH1.

DIFFERENTIAL DIAGNOSIS

FHH should be differentiated from mild forms of PHPT prior to parathyroid surgery, as parathyroidectomy, normally indicated for PHPT patients, does not improve hypercalcemia in FHH patients. Usually, FHH is easily distinguished from PHPT, as the former usually has mildly elevated calcium levels and a normal PTH level, while the latter is typically characterized by elevated PTH levels. However, this differentiation can be difficult in the case of FHH presenting a mildly elevated PTH, and of PHPT patients showing mild hypercalcemia and normal PTH (10%-20% of cases). A recent study[5] confirmed the heterogeneity in FHH biochemical phenotypes with possible overlap with PHPT that could lead to inappropriate management.

Clinical signatures characterizing FHH that are valuable in the differential diagnosis between FHH and PHPT are:

1. A reduced urinary excretion of calcium
2. Absence of nephrolithiasis and/or nephrocalcinosis
3. Unaltered BMD

Genetic testing provides a clear path to resolve a differential diagnosis of FHH with PHPT and other diseases (acute or chronic renal failure, adrenal insufficiency, osteolytic metastases, humoral malignant hypercalcemia, and sarcoidosis).

COMPLICATIONS

Chondrocalcinosis, recurrent pancreatitis, and premature vascular calcification can manifest in some rare cases of adults with FHH.

NSHPT presents a spectrum of severe complications, including respiratory distress due to hypotonia and rib cage deformities, bone under mineralization, and multiple fragility fractures.

MANAGEMENT & TREATMENT

FHH is usually a benign disorder and the majority of FHH patients do not develop complications from the disease, with calcium and PTH levels remaining usually stable over the years. Therefore, it is important to reassure patients about the benign nature of their disease and about the fact that therapy is not usually necessary.

FHH-related hypercalcemia does not respond to diuretics or bisphosphonates.

Subtotal parathyroidectomy does not cure hypercalcemia in FHH patients, and it should be avoided. Total parathyroidectomy can be indicated in rare FHH cases with constant severe hypercalcemia (>14 mg/dL), or in some patients with atypical clinical features, such as recurrent pancreatitis, to reduce the risk of further pancreatitis relapse.

In contrast to FHH, NSHPT requires an aggressive therapeutic approach, starting at birth, to control PHPT and severe hypercalcemia. The primary line of hypercalcemia treatment can consist of progressive use of bisphosphonates, dialysis, or calcimimetics. If these approaches are unsuccessful, total parathyroidectomy, followed by a life-long supplementation with calcidiol is required.

Calcimimetics (CaSR agonists) are positive allosteric modulators of the CaSR protein that increase the sensitivity of the CaSR to extracellular calcium ion. Studies on cell models showed that calcimimetics lower PTH secretion, decrease the proliferation of parathyroid chief cells, and correct signaling and/or trafficking defects caused by mutant CaSR, G11, or AP17 proteins. Cinacalcet showed to ameliorate symptomatic hypercalcemia in all the three genetic forms of FHH.[6,7] However, the requirement of a long-term use of cinacalcet in FHH patients associated with the high cost of this drug may be limiting factors to this therapy.

PROGNOSIS

FHH1, FHH2, and FHH3 do not lower life expectancy and have a benign, stable course.

Patients with NSHPT can die from complications of dramatic hypercalcemia or respiratory distress during the neonatal period.

REFERENCES

1. Tőke J, Czirják G, Enyedi P, Tóth M. Rare diseases caused by abnormal calcium sensing and signalling. *Endocrine.* 2021;71(3):611-617.
2. Marx SJ, Sinaii N. Neonatal severe hyperparathyroidism: novel insights from calcium, PTH, and the CASR gene. *J Clin Endocrinol Metab.* 2020;105(4):1061-1078.
3. Dershem R, Gorvin CM, Metpally RPR, et al. Familial hypocalciuric hypercalcemia type 1 and autosomal-dominant hypocalcemia type 1: prevalence in a large healthcare population. *Am J Hum Genet.* 2020;106(6):734-747.
4. Lee JY, Shoback DM. Familial hypocalciuric hypercalcemia and related disorders. *Best Pract Res Clin Endocrinol Metab.* 2018;32:609-619.
5. Lasbleiz A, Paladino NC, Romanet P, et al. Familial hypocalciuric hypercalcemia: the challenge of diagnosis. *Endocrine.* 2022;75(2):646-649.
6. Marx SJ. Calcimimetic use in familial hypocalciuric hypercalcemia-a perspective in endocrinology. *J Clin Endocrinol Metab.* 2017;102(11):3933-3936.
7. Hannan FM, Olesen MK, Thakker RV. Calcimimetic and calcilytic therapies for inherited disorders of the calcium-sensing receptor signalling pathway. *Br J Pharmacol.* 2018;175(21):4083-4094.

SUGGESTED READING

Bertocchio JP, Tafflet M, Koumakis E, et al. Pro-FHH: a risk equation to facilitate the diagnosis of parathyroid-related hypercalcemia. *J Clin Endocrinol Metab.* 2018;103(7):2534-2542.

Mariathasan S, Andrews KA, Thompson E, et al. Genetic testing for hereditary hyperparathyroidism and familial hypocalciuric hypercalcaemia in a large UK cohort. *Clin Endocrinol (Oxf).* 2020;93(4):409-418.

Parathyroid Cancer & the Hyperparathyroidism-Jaw Tumor Syndrome

68

William F. Simonds, MD
Electron Kebebew, MD, FACS

GENERAL CONSIDERATIONS

Calcium is required for diverse cellular processes ranging from neuromuscular excitability, muscular contraction, and neurotransmitter release to the functioning of calcium-dependent enzymes and cardiac pacemaker cells. A system of physiologic calcium homeostasis ensures the continued normal functioning of the many intracellular processes that depend on calcium. To maintain the ambient calcium concentration within a physiologic range, PTH secretion from the parathyroid glands is normally tightly regulated in response to changes in circulating ionized calcium. In parathyroid cancer (PC), the inappropriate release of PTH from malignant parathyroid tissue drives serum calcium levels upward into the pathologic range, producing the metabolic syndrome known as PHPT.[1]

PC is an extraordinarily rare endocrine malignancy, with an annual incidence in Western nations ranging from 2 to 11 new cases per 10 million person-years.[2-5] PC accounts for <1% of all cases of PHPT. Most parathyroid carcinomas secrete PTH and cause marked hypercalcemia, though a small fraction can be nonfunctional. The malignant character of parathyroid tumors can be challenging to diagnose preoperatively. Most of the histopathological features of PC are not specific, such as the presence of fibrous bands, elevated mitotic index, and nuclear atypia, so that the tissue diagnosis may depend on the demonstration of tumoral invasion of the capsule, adjacent tissues, nerves, blood vessels, or the lymphatic vasculature. Sometimes PC is only recognized months to years after initial parathyroid surgery when PHPT recurs and is found to be the result of locally invasive or metastatic disease. PC is usually associated with higher serum calcium and PTH levels than PHPT due to benign parathyroid adenoma and patients with PC are more likely to be symptomatic at the time of presentation (Table 68–1). There is no known racial or ethnic predilection for PC. The prevalence of PC is higher in kindreds with Hyperparathyroidism-Jaw Tumor syndrome (HPT-JT), associated with germline inactivating mutation of the *CDC73* tumor suppressor gene (formerly called *HRPT2*).[6] Germline mutation of *CDC73* can also be demonstrated in about a quarter of patients with apparently sporadic PC.

Since the best opportunity for cure of PC is complete surgical resection at the initial exploration, the possibility of surgical cure depends on both preoperative suspicion and the experience of the surgeon. PC usually follows an indolent but progressive clinical course, characterized initially by local recurrence and later by distant metastases, usually to lung, bone, or liver. The major morbidity of PC is due to severe PHPT and the complications of intractable hypercalcemia, such as neurocognitive impairment (altered mental status, confusion, lethargy, and coma), progressive dehydration and renal failure, and pathologic skeletal fractures.

PATHOGENESIS OF PARATHYROID CANCER & THE HYPERPARATHYROIDISM-JAW TUMOR SYNDROME

The etiology of PC likely involves the interplay of multiple environmental and genetic factors.[3,4] Exposure to radiation, especially during childhood, increases the risk of both thyroid and parathyroid neoplasia but whether such exposure plays a causative factor in PC remains unclear. Cases of PC developing in patients with secondary or tertiary HPT due to chronic kidney disease or other conditions have been reported but represent only a tiny fraction of all PC.

Our current understanding of the pathogenesis of PC derives largely from the clinical and molecular genetic characterization of HPT-JT, a rare autosomal dominant familial cancer syndrome associated with a high frequency of PC.[7,8] In HPT-JT, affected individuals may develop PHPT due to benign or malignant parathyroid tumors, benign

Table 68–1. Clinical features typical of parathyroid cancer versus benign parathyroid disease.

	Parathyroid Cancer	Benign PHPT
Gender ratio (M:F)	1:1	1:3
Age at presentation	40s to 50s	50s to 70s
Symptomatic at time of diagnosis (%)	>90	<20
Serum calcium (mg/dL)	≥14	≤12
PTH level	3 to 10× ULN	<2× ULN
Concurrent skeletal and renal disease	Common	Rare
Palpable neck mass	Common	Rare

PHPT, primary hyperparathyroidism; PTH, parathyroid hormone; ULN, upper limit of the normal range.

cemento-ossifying fibrous jaw tumors, as well as renal cysts or tumors and/or uterine abnormalities (Figure 68–1). The vast majority of kindreds with HPT-JT harbor germline mutation or deletion of the *CDC73* gene, at chromosomal locus 1q31. The high frequency of PC is a hallmark of HPT-JT, unique among the familial forms of PHPT (Table 68–2). A subset of kindreds with familial isolated PHPT (FIHP) also harbor germline *CDC73* mutation, suggesting that such patients may represent *formes frustes* of HPT-JT.

The *CDC73* gene encodes parafibromin, a protein of 531 residues, considered to be a tumor suppressor.[6] Tumor suppressors are proteins that normally restrain cell growth and proliferation.

Tumors can develop when the balance between cell growth and inhibition is lost such as when tumor suppressor genes, encoding proteins that normally inhibit cell growth, are constitutively inactivated by mutation or deletion. The majority of germline *CDC73* mutations in HPT-JT kindreds are predicted to disrupt gene function via frameshift or truncation mutation, with only a minority encoding missense mutations. Partial or complete deletion of the *CDC73* gene has also been described in patients and kindreds with HPT-JT. A genotype-phenotype correlation has been described in *CDC73*-mutation carriers such that those with frameshift, truncation, or deletion mutations are much more likely to develop PC than patients harboring *CDC73* missense mutations.[9] Dysregulation of several microRNAs may contribute to the pathogenesis of PC harboring *CDC73* mutation. In apparently sporadic PC, somatic mutations of *CDC73* in tumor DNA have been identified in 60% to 100% of cases. In addition, germline loss-of-function mutation in *CDC73* may be found in some 25% of patients with apparently sporadic PC. This suggests that some cases of apparently sporadic PC may harbor *de novo* mutations of *CDC73* or, like a subset of FIHP kindreds, may represent an incomplete expression of HPT-JT (Figure 68–2). Because of the potential benefit for offspring and other family members, germline DNA analysis for *CDC73* mutation is recommended in all patients with apparently sporadic PC.

Apart from *CDC73*, several other gene changes have been implicated in parathyroid cancer, based on analysis of tumor DNA by gene profiling or by whole genome or whole exome next-generation sequencing. These include overexpression of *CCND1*, alterations of genes in the *PI3KCA/MTOR* pathway, *ADCK1*, *AKAP9*, *PRUNE2*, and *ZEB1*, as well as evidence of the *APOBEC* mutational signature.[10-13]

Clinical Findings

A. Symptoms & Signs

The clinical presentation of PC usually reflects symptoms caused by the effects of markedly elevated serum PTH and hypercalcemia, rather than mass effects from local tumor infiltration or distant metastatic disease. There can therefore be a broad spectrum of clinical presentations, reflecting the multiple actions of PTH on target tissues as well as the myriad potential signs and symptoms of hypercalcemia.[2,14] Patients with PHPT due to PC tend to be more symptomatic than those with PHPT due to benign parathyroid disease (Table 68–1). Common symptoms of hypercalcemia include fatigue, generalized weakness, neurocognitive changes such as impaired memory and difficulty concentrating, gastrointestinal symptoms including anorexia, constipation and bloating, polyuria, renal colic from nephrolithiasis, and bone pain and fractures from osteoporosis. The severity of symptoms is usually proportional to the degree of hypercalcemia. Older patients tend to be more sensitive to the neurocognitive and neuromuscular manifestations of hypercalcemia.

Hypophosphatemia resulting from renal phosphate wasting associated with metabolically severe PHPT as is seen in PC may worsen patients' fatigue and weakness. Advanced PHPT in PC is often accompanied by *osteitis fibrosa cystica*, a syndrome of skeletal demineralization associated with radiolucent cyst-like "brown tumors," bone pain, fractures, and bone deformities including bowing of the weight-bearing bones.[15,16] Although uncommon in patients with PHPT due to benign parathyroid adenomas, patients with PC may present with concurrent nephrolithiasis and skeletal disease. Other clinical findings highly suggestive of PC a include a palpable neck mass and hoarseness (which may indicate vocal cord paralysis and laryngeal nerve damage) (Table 68–1).

B. Laboratory Findings

Hypercalcemia, often with serum calcium levels of 14 mg/dL or greater, and intact PTH values greater than 3 to 10 times the upper limit of the normal range are typically

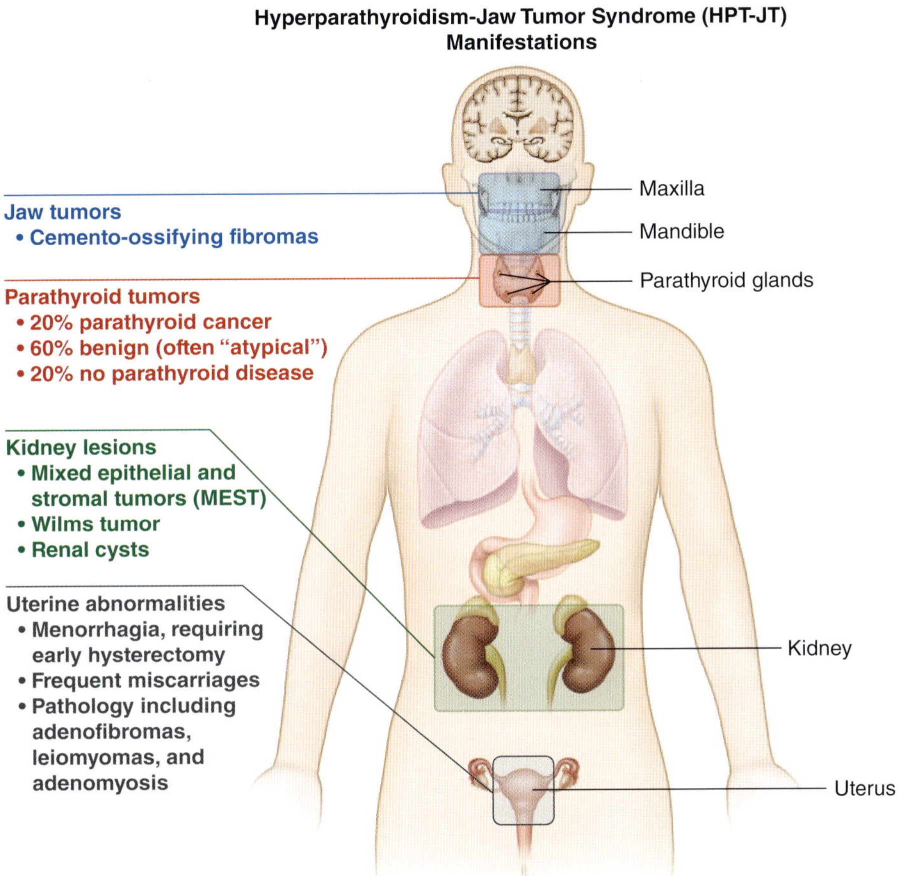

Figure 68–1. Manifestations of the hyperparathyroidism-jaw tumor syndrome (HPT-JT). Manifestations of HPT-JT may include cemento-ossifying tumors of the maxilla or mandible; parathyroid disease (~20% with parathyroid cancer, 60% with benign adenomas that often include "atypical parathyroid adenomas," ~20% with no parathyroid disease); kidney lesions including mixed epithelial and stromal tumors (MEST), Wilms tumor, or renal cysts; and uterine abnormalities that frequently manifest as menorrhagia requiring early hysterectomy, a high incidence of miscarriages, and uterine lesions such as adenofibromas, leiomyomas, and adenomyosis. Because of the incomplete penetrance associated with germline *CDC73* loss-of-function mutation, the manifestations of HPT-JT in any individual patient or within affected kindreds can be quite variable.

Table 68–2. Frequency of parathyroid cancer in sporadic and familial parathyroid disease.

Context of PHPT	Frequency of PC (%)
Sporadic parathyroid disease	<1
Multiple endocrine neoplasia type 1 (MEN1)	<1
Multiple endocrine neoplasia type 2A (MEN2A)	<1
Hyperparathyroidism-jaw tumor syndrome (HPT-JT)	~20

PC, parathyroid cancer; PHPT, primary hyperparathyroidism.

seen in PC. A subset of PC demonstrates normal serum calcium despite PTH elevation at the time of diagnosis but no threshold level for malignancy has been defined. Alkaline phosphatase, a sensitive marker of bone turnover, is usually elevated in PC. Low-normal or overtly low serum phosphate caused by PTH-mediated phosphaturia, and renal phosphate wasting can be seen in PC. Severe PHPT associated with benign parathyroid disease is uncommon, but it can be difficult to distinguish on clinical grounds from PC. There are no accepted specific circulating biomarkers that can reliably distinguish PC from PHPT due to benign parathyroid adenomas, but this is an area of active research.

Spectrum of clinical phenotypes associated with germline *CDC73* mutation

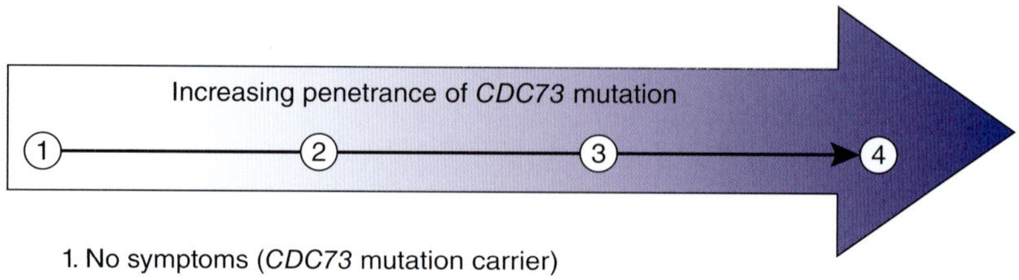

1. No symptoms (*CDC73* mutation carrier)
2. Parathyroid cancer ("sporadic")
3. Familial isolated hyperparathyroidism (+/– parathyroid cancer)
4. Hyperparathyroidism-jaw tumor syndrome (+/– parathyroid cancer)

▲ **Figure 68–2.** The variable and incomplete penetrance of germline *CDC73* mutation results in a spectrum of different clinical phenotypes. Some ~20% of known or obligate *CDC73* mutation carriers may be asymptomatic, while 25% of patients with apparently sporadic parathyroid cancer harbor germline mutation of *CDC73*. Other manifestations of germline *CDC73* mutation include familial isolated hyperparathyroidism, with or without individuals in the kindred with parathyroid cancer, and the hyperparathyroidism-jaw tumor syndrome with primary hyperparathyroidism due to benign adenomas or parathyroid cancer, cemento-ossifying tumors of the maxilla or mandible, renal cysts or tumors, and uterine tumors.

C. Tumor Localization and Other Imaging Studies

Parathyroid malignancies arise from parathyroid glands present in the neck or anterior mediastinum. Preoperative imaging employing such noninvasive modalities as computed tomography scanning (CT), magnetic resonance imaging, ultrasound, and technetium Tc-99m sestamibi is frequently helpful for tumor localization.[17,18] Positron emission tomography employing 18F-fluorocholine (fluoromethylcholine) is a more recently available nuclear medicine modality for parathyroid localization that may have superior sensitivity compared to ultrasound or sestamibi.[19-21] With respect to the evaluation of primary parathyroid tumors such noninvasive studies cannot reliably distinguish PC from parathyroid adenomas; however, even though the former tend to be larger, with an average diameter of ~3 cm. Certain ultrasonographic features of parathyroid tumors often correlate with malignancy, including hypoechogenicity, tumor inhomogeneity, and irregularity of borders, but their absence does not exclude PC.

The manifestations of PC and/or HPT-JT may be evident in other imaging studies. The cemento-ossifying fibromas of HPT-JT can be seen on CT scan or by panoramic dental X-ray and are usually well circumscribed and either radiolucent (when smaller) or mixed radiolucent-radiopaque (when more mature). Whereas the radiolucent "brown tumors" seen in association with the severe bone disease of PC can occur anywhere in the axial or appendicular skeleton, the jaw tumors found in HPT-JT are restricted to the maxilla and mandible. Plain radiographs may reveal subperiosteal bone resorption, "salt and pepper" skull, absence of the lamina dura, and diffuse osteopenia or osteoporosis. Generalized osteoporosis from metabolically severe PHPT can be quantitated by the estimation of bone mineral density using dual-energy X-ray absorptiometry (DEXA). The presence of nephrocalcinosis or nephrolithiasis may be documented by plain radiographs, CT, or ultrasound.

In patients with suspected PC, parathyroid biopsy by percutaneous fine-needle aspiration of cervical masses should be avoided due to the possibility of tumor rupture and the documented risk of seeding malignant cells along the needle track. Furthermore, it is difficult to differentiate benign from malignant tumor based on cytologic features alone using the small specimen obtained through fine-needle biopsy. However, in patients with suspected metastatic PC, when iatrogenic seeding is of lesser concern, biopsy of the metastatic lesions may help establish the diagnosis by histopathological examination and determination of PTH levels in the aspirated sample.

Differential Diagnosis

Apart from PHPT, the differential diagnosis of hypercalcemia includes nonparathyroid etiologies such as sarcoidosis and other granulomatous diseases, the humor hypercalcemia of malignancy, the milk-alkali syndrome, and vitamin D intoxication.[22,23] The differential diagnosis of PHPT includes both sporadic (95%) and familial disorders (5%) such as multiple endocrine neoplasia type 1, multiple endocrine neoplasia type 2A, HPT-JT, FIHP, and familial hypocalciuric hypercalcemia, justifying the ascertainment of a thorough family medical and dental history. Table 68–1 lists clinical features that may help distinguish PHPT caused by benign parathyroid disease from PC; however, severe PHPT caused by benign parathyroid adenomas, though uncommon, can be difficult to distinguish from PC. Certainly, PHPT or suspected PC in association with a personal or family history of cemento-ossifying fibromas of the maxilla or mandible, or other features typical of HPT-JT (Figure 68–1) support that syndromic diagnosis. As noted earlier, there are no specific circulating biomarkers or radiographic tumor characteristics that can reliably distinguish PC from PHPT due to benign parathyroid disease.

Hypophosphatemia is a frequent concomitant of PHPT due to PC. PHPT figures prominently in the differential diagnosis of hypophosphatemia, which also includes vitamin D deficiency, malnutrition, and diuretic use. The coincidence of hypercalcemia and hypophosphatemia is highly suggestive of PHPT.

The differential diagnosis of jaw tumors in patients under consideration for HPT-JT include, besides cemento-ossifying fibromas and "brown tumors" from metabolically severe PHPT, fibrous dysplasia, ameloblastic fibroodontoma, odontogenic cyst, cementoblastoma, osteochondroma, and osteosarcoma.

The differential diagnosis of a palpable anterior neck mass includes nonfunctional PC, an extremely rare phenomenon. Patients are normocalcemic at diagnosis and may have normal intact PTH. The vast majority present with an anterior neck mass, with other common findings that include dysphagia, and hoarseness or vocal cord paralysis. Grossly, tumors are similar in appearance to functional PC, and they may also appear similar histologically (see following discussion).

Histopathology of Parathyroid Cancer & Atypical Parathyroid Adenomas

The tissue diagnosis of PC is very challenging for surgical pathologists. Often the malignant nature of parathyroid tumors is only recognized retrospectively, long after the initial parathyroid surgery when recurrent PHPT is found to result from locally invasive or distant metastatic disease. The World Health Organization has identified histopathological features associated with PC and formalized criteria to facilitate its diagnosis.[24] These features such as the presence of fibrous bands forming trabecular architecture, elevated mitotic index, aneuploidy, and nuclear atypia are not specific so that the tissue diagnosis may depend on the demonstration of tumoral invasion of the capsule, adjacent tissues, nerves, blood vessels, or the lymphatic vasculature. Tumors lacking clear evidence of such invasion, yet with unusual features suggestive of PC such as fibrous bands, high mitotic index, and nuclear atypia, can be classified as atypical parathyroid adenomas and represent a class of tumors with indeterminate malignant potential to be distinguished from PC. There is a high frequency of atypical parathyroid adenomas in patients and families with PHPT associated with germline *CDC73* mutation (Figure 68–3).

In PC, as in benign parathyroid tumors, immunohistochemical staining is positive for chromogranin A and PTH, and negative for calcitonin, thyroglobulin, and thyroid transcription factor 1 (TTF1). Immunostaining for parafibromin, the protein product of *CDC73*, has shown promise in the differential diagnosis of benign from malignant parathyroid neoplasms.[25-27] Parafibromin is normally expressed in the cell nucleus, and absent or diminished nuclear staining for parafibromin has been reported in a high proportion of PC specimens, but not in benign parathyroid tumors, studied in several centers. Immunohistochemical studies of atypical parathyroid adenomas frequently show an overlap with parathyroid carcinoma in parafibromin staining patterns that is distinct from benign parathyroid adenomas.[28-30] Aberrant parafibromin staining patterns in atypical parathyroid adenomas like those in PC may portend more malignant behavior. The utility of parafibromin staining to distinguish PC from benign parathyroid tumors has not been confirmed by all investigators; however, possibly due to differences in primary antibodies, immunohistochemical techniques, and the algorithms and controls used to define positive and negative (or reduced) parafibromin nuclear staining. When used in conjunction with classical histopathology, the employment of an immunohistochemical panel against multiple tissue markers may be superior to the use of any single marker in the diagnosis of PC. Immunohistochemical panels that can detect overexpression of PGP9.5, MKI67 (marker of proliferation Ki-67), and galectin-3, and screen for negative or diminished nuclear staining for parafibromin (as described above), as well as reduced or absent staining for the tumor suppressor adenomatosis polyposis coli (APC), have been used by surgical pathologists to enhance the ability to distinguish PC from parathyroid adenomas.

Complications

The complications of untreated PC include the metabolic, renal, and skeletal consequences of PHPT as well as the effects of local tumor invasion. The signs and symptoms of hypercalcemia and the renal and skeletal complications of PHPT have been described above. Potential complications of untreated cervical or mediastinal PC include tumoral compression or invasion of the esophagus, trachea, or recurrent laryngeal nerves that can result in dysphagia, dyspnea, and hoarseness or vocal cord paralysis.

A complication that may follow surgery for PC in patients with significant hyperparathyroid bone disease is prolonged postoperative hypocalcemia and hypophosphatemia resulting from the so-called hungry bone syndrome. Patients with elevated preoperative total or bone-specific serum alkaline phosphatase, a marker of bone turnover, are at increased risk. The pathophysiology involves the net shift of calcium and phosphate from the extracellular fluid into bone because of

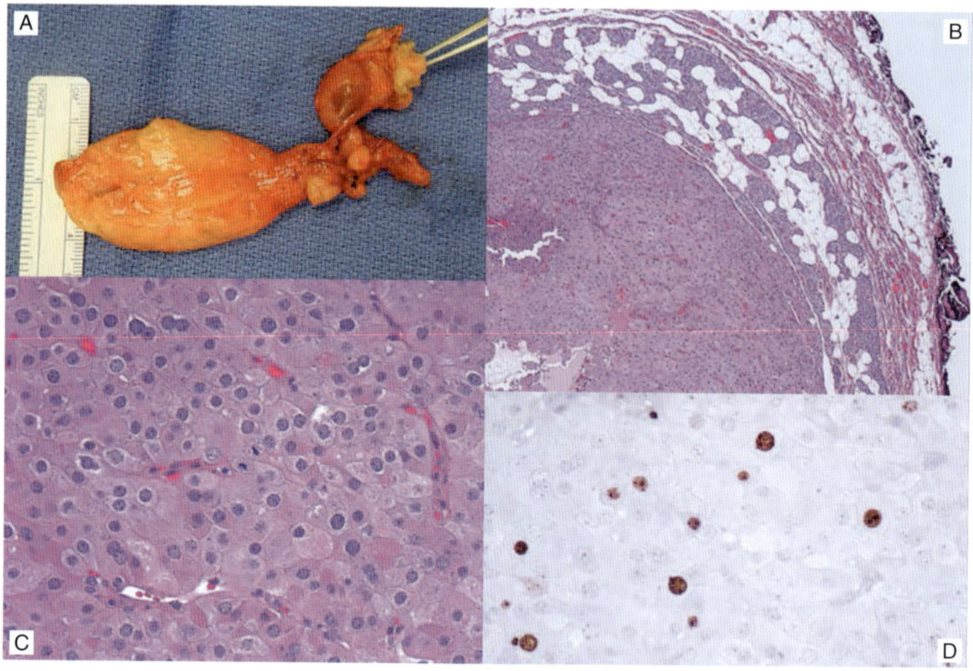

▲ **Figure 68–3.** Atypical parathyroid adenoma from a patient with germline *CDC73* mutation. **(A)** Gross surgical pathology of an intrathymic parathyroid adenoma following its excision. **(B)** Hematoxylin and eosin-stained section at low power demonstrates sheets of predominantly oxyphilic tumor cells with pleiomorphic nuclei compressing a rim of normal parathyroid tissue (upper right; with abundant adipocytes), but with no clear evidence of capsular or lymphovascular invasion by the tumor cells. **(C)** High-power view demonstrates frequent mitotic figures, nuclear atypia, and prominent nucleoli. **(D)** Section of same tumor shows numerous cell nuclei with strong staining by MIB-1 monoclonal antibody to MKI67 (marker of proliferation Ki-67) (brown coloration).

the sudden drop in serum PTH level following a prolonged period of elevation. The sudden postoperative reduction in PTH results in a rapid deceleration of osteoclast activity and the unopposed anabolic action of osteoblasts with influx of calcium and phosphorus into bone. Hungry bone syndrome can usually be satisfactorily treated with high-dose oral calcium and calcitriol supplementation.

Surgical Treatment of Parathyroid Cancer

Patients with or suspected to have PC (based on tumor size, calcium >14 mg/dL, and or PTH >10 upper limit normal, a white-hard tumor adherent to surrounding structures at the time of exploration) should have *en bloc* resection with ipsilateral hemithyroidectomy to ensure negative tumor margins. An ipsilateral central and lateral therapeutic neck dissection should be performed if lymph node involvement is suspected based on preoperative imaging studies or is documented at the time of the operation, based on frozen section analysis. In patients with vocal cord paralysis and tumor involvement of the recurrent laryngeal nerve, the nerve should be resected along with the tumor as these patients have a high rate of local recurrence. Nerve reconstruction can be performed primarily if a short segment, or via the ansa cervicalis.

The evidence for selecting focused parathyroidectomy or bilateral neck exploration with four gland identification and removal of enlarged parathyroid gland(s) in patients with HPT-JT syndrome is based on limited retrospective data. Based on the high rates of synchronous multigland disease, higher rate of PC at initial presentation or at the time of recurrent disease, and the overall higher rate of recurrence, we recommend a bilateral neck exploration with four gland identification and removal of enlarged parathyroid gland(s) with cervical thymectomy. In selected patients with HPT-JT syndrome, a focused approach may be considered if (1) multiple localizing studies suggest single-gland disease, (2) the biochemical profile and imaging studies are not suspicious for PC, (3) intraoperative PTH monitoring will be used as an adjunct to confirm biochemical cure, (4) the patient is young with no family members who had PC, and (5) prefers a focused approach, or has had a previous thyroid or parathyroid operation and presents with persistent/recurrent disease. In our opinion, the morbidity of PC and the high rate of synchronous multigland disease outweigh the morbidity of bilateral neck exploration, especially when done by specialized endocrine surgeons.

Nonsurgical Treatments

PC is generally believed to be insensitive to irradiation. There have been some reports suggesting that adjuvant radiation treatment following surgical treatment may reduce the chance of local recurrence, however. The efficacy of such adjuvant external beam radiotherapy is difficult to assess since some patients with PC may have prolonged disease-free intervals following parathyroidectomy alone and therefore adjuvant radiotherapy is not routinely recommended.

Inoperable PC due to diffuse metastases can be palliated by selective metastasectomy, by treatment with radiofrequency ablation (RFA) or by a combination of RFA and transcatheter arterial embolization, depending on the location of the metastases. Recurrent PC in the neck has been treated with ultrasound-guided percutaneous injection of ethanol.

In general, cytotoxic chemotherapy has not been demonstrated to be beneficial in PC. Short-term responses have been demonstrated with single-agent dacarbazine, and combination chemotherapy regimens of fluorouracil, cyclophosphamide, and dacarbazine or methotrexate, lomustine, doxorubicin, and cyclophosphamide in patients with metastatic PC, but a survival benefit has not been demonstrated. In contrast, therapy with the multitarget tyrosine kinase inhibitors (TKIs) sorafenib and cabozantinib that potentially inhibit both tumor cell proliferation and angiogenesis have shown some efficacy in treating PC, but prospective large-scale clinical trials using TKIs for the treatment of PC are lacking.

Because the major morbidity and ultimate cause of death in most patients with PC is severe hypercalcemia, medical management has focused on ameliorating high serum calcium levels in patients with persistent disease (Table 68–3). Acute hypercalcemia can be treated with standard therapies

Table 68–3. Medical treatments for parathyroid cancer-associated hypercalcemia.

Treatment	Dosage (or Rate)	Mechanism	Comments
Intravenous normal saline infusion	250-300 mL/h, adjusted to maintain a urine output at 100-150 mL/h	Volume expansion improves renal function and clearance of calcium; forced natriuresis promotes urinary excretion of calcium	May be contraindicated in heart failure, other cardiac or renal disease. Although no longer routinely recommended, auxiliary treatment with loop diuretics such as furosemide can be considered in cases of congestive heart failure or obvious fluid overload.
Calcitonin (salmon)	4 IU/kg SC or IM every 12 hours	Direct inhibition of osteoclast-mediated bone resorption	Useful in initial 24-48 hours only, since tachyphylaxis rapidly develops
Intravenous bisphosphonates	Zoledronic acid, 4 mg IV, infused over >15 minutes Pamidronate, 60-90 mg IV, infused over 2-24 hours	Indirect inhibition of osteoclast-mediated bone resorption	Initial calcium-lowering effects seen in 1-2 days, maximal effects in 4-7 days. Side effects can include fever, arthralgias, myalgias, hypocalcemia, osteonecrosis of the jaw, and atypical subtrochanteric and diaphyseal femoral fractures. Should be used cautiously in patients with impaired renal function.
Denosumab	(Xgeva) 120 mg SC every 4 weeks; give additional 120 mg doses on days 8 and 15 during first month of therapy	Monoclonal antibody that targets the receptor activator of nuclear factor kappa-B ligand (RANKL)	For patients refractory to bisphosphonates, or for whom bisphosphonates are contraindicated because of renal impairment. As with bisphosphonates, side effects can include osteonecrosis of the jaw and atypical femur fractures. To prevent or treat hypocalcemia, administer calcium and vitamin D as necessary.
Cinacalcet	Initial: 30 mg PO every 12 hours; can increase sequentially as needed, at 2 to 4-week intervals, up to 90 mg every 6 hours	Calcimimetic; increases the sensitivity of the CASR to activation by extracellular calcium, decreasing PTH release	Major intolerance due to gastrointestinal side effects such as nausea and vomiting

CASR, calcium sensing receptor; IM, intramuscularly; IV, intravenous; PO, by mouth; PTH, parathyroid hormone; RANKL, receptor activator of nuclear factor kappa-B ligand; SC, subcutaneously.

and may require inpatient management. Treatment is typically established with intravenous normal saline infusion at a rate of 250 to 300 mL/h in the absence of heart failure, or other cardiac or renal contraindications. Hydration with normal saline is critical in patients with severe hypercalcemia to correct volume depletion that typically results from nausea, vomiting, and hypercalcemia-mediated nephrogenic diabetes insipidus. Routine treatment with loop diuretics such as furosemide is no longer recommended because of the risk of excessive volume depletion but can be considered in cases of congestive heart failure or obvious fluid overload. Treatment with calcitonin is a useful adjunct for the initial treatment of acute hypercalcemia. Salmon calcitonin is usually given at a dose of 4 IU/kg SC or IM every 12 hours. Although useful in the initial treatment of hypercalcemia, calcitonin's efficacy is limited by the rapid development of tachyphylaxis so is typically used only during the first 24 to 48 hours.

Following rehydration with normal saline, treatment with intravenous bisphosphonates can be very effective for the treatment of acute hypercalcemia, even though maximal calcium-lowering effects are not seen for 4 to 7 days. Among available bisphosphonates for parenteral use, zoledronic acid, at a dose of 4 mg IV given over 15 minutes, is commonly the first-line agent, with pamidronate an alternative option if zoledronic acid is not available. Side effects of intravenous bisphosphonates can include fever, arthralgias, myalgias, hypocalcemia, osteonecrosis of the jaw, and atypical subtrochanteric and diaphyseal femoral fractures. Bisphosphonates should be used cautiously in patients with impaired renal function.

Denosumab, a monoclonal antibody targeting RANKL (receptor activator of nuclear factor kappa-B ligand), is an alternative antihypercalcemic therapeutic option given subcutaneously for patients who are refractory to bisphosphonates or for whom treatment with the latter is contraindicated because of renal impairment. As with bisphosphonates, osteonecrosis of the jaw and atypical femur fractures have been reported in patients receiving denosumab. Denosumab-associated hypocalcemia can be prevented or treated with calcium and vitamin D supplementation as necessary.

The calcimimetic agent cinacalcet has been used to treat patients with PC. Initial dosing is 30 mg by mouth every 12 hours. The dose can be increased at 2 to 4 weeks intervals as needed to normalize serum calcium up to a maximum of 90 mg every 6 hours. Calcimimetics work by increasing the sensitivity of the CASR in parathyroid tissue to activation by extracellular calcium, resulting in decreased PTH release.

In select cases, hemodialysis may be indicated for the treatment of hypercalcemia. This might include hypercalcemic patients in whom saline hydration is not possible because of anuria or severely impaired renal function, or hemodynamically stable patients with acute hypercalcemia in a range above ~18 mg/dL associated with neurocognitive changes for whom rapid therapy is clinically warranted.

Prognosis

The overall survival of patients with PC is 82% and 66% at 5 and 10 years, respectively.[31] There is no American Joint Committee on Cancer or Union for International Cancer Control TNM (tumor, node, metastasis) staging system widely accepted and utilized for PC given its rarity. However, the overall survival is highest for patients with localized disease followed by those with regional disease (locally invasive, lymph node metastasis) and distant metastases. Prognostic factors associated with worse overall survival, in addition to extent of disease at diagnosis, found in most studies include tumor size (>3 cm), older age (>57-65 years old), male sex, and positive tumor margins.[2,32,33]

REFERENCES

1. Bilezikian JP. Primary hyperparathyroidism. *J Clin Endocrinol Metab*. 2018;103(11):3993-4004.
2. Lenschow C, Schragle S, Kircher S, et al. Clinical presentation, treatment, and outcome of parathyroid carcinoma: results of the NEKAR retrospective international multicenter study. *Ann Surg*. 2022;275(2):e479-e487.
3. Salcuni AS, Cetani F, Guarnieri V, et al. Parathyroid carcinoma. *Best Pract Res Clin Endocrinol Metab*. 2018;32(6):877-889.
4. Machado NN, Wilhelm SM. Parathyroid cancer: a review. *Cancers (Basel)*. 2019;11(11):1676.
5. Perrier ND, Arnold A, Costa-Guda J, et al. Hereditary endocrine tumours: current state-of-the-art and research opportunities: new and future perspectives for parathyroid carcinoma. *Endocr Relat Cancer*. 2020;27(8):T53-T63.
6. Carpten JD, Robbins CM, Villablanca A, et al. HRPT2, encoding parafibromin, is mutated in hyperparathyroidism-jaw tumor syndrome. *Nat Genet*. 2002;32(4):676-680.
7. Skefos CM, Waguespack SG, Perrier ND, Hu MI. CDC73-related disorders. In: Adam MP, Feldman J, Mirzaa GM, et al., eds. *GeneReviews®* [Internet]. Seattle (WA): University of Washington, Seattle; 1993-2021. 2008 Dec 31 [updated 2023 Sep 21].
8. Tora R, Welch J, Sun J, et al. Phenotypic profiling and molecular mechanisms in hyperparathyroidism-jaw tumor syndrome. *J Clin Endocrinol Metab*. 2023;108(12):3165-3177.
9. Li Y, Zhang J, Adikaram PR, et al. Genotype of CDC73 germline mutation determines risk of parathyroid cancer. *Endocr Relat Cancer*. 2020;27(9):483-494.
10. Brewer K, Costa-Guda J, Arnold A. Molecular genetic insights into sporadic primary hyperparathyroidism. *Endocr Relat Cancer*. 2019;26(2):R53-R72.
11. Clarke CN, Katsonis P, Hsu TK, et al. Comprehensive genomic characterization of parathyroid cancer identifies novel candidate driver mutations and core pathways. *J Endocr Soc*. 2019;3(3):544-559.
12. Pandya C, Uzilov AV, Bellizzi J, et al. Genomic profiling reveals mutational landscape in parathyroid carcinomas. *JCI Insight*. 2017;2(6):e92061.
13. Kutahyalioglu M, Nguyen HT, Kwatampora L, et al. Genetic profiling as a clinical tool in advanced parathyroid carcinoma. *J Cancer Res Clin Oncol*. 2019;145(8):1977-1986.
14. Cetani F, Pardi E, Marcocci C. Parathyroid carcinoma. *Front Horm Res*. 2019;51:63-76.

15. Misiorowski W, Czajka-Oraniec I, Kochman M, Zgliczynski W, Bilezikian JP. Osteitis fibrosa cystica—a forgotten radiological feature of primary hyperparathyroidism. *Endocrine.* 2017;58(2):380-385.
16. Naji Rad S, Deluxe L. Osteitis fibrosa cystica. In: *StatPearls.* Treasure Island (FL): StatPearls Publishing; 2024.
17. Itani M, Middleton WD. Parathyroid imaging. *Radiol Clin North Am.* 2020;58(6):1071-1083.
18. Shirali AS, Clemente-Gutierrez U, Perrier ND. Parathyroid surgery: what radiologists need to know. *Neuroimaging Clin N Am.* 2021;31(3):397-408.
19. Thanseer N, Bhadada SK, Sood A, et al. Comparative effectiveness of ultrasonography, 99mTc-sestamibi, and 18F-fluorocholine PET/CT in detecting parathyroid adenomas in patients with primary hyperparathyroidism. *Clin Nucl Med.* 2017;42(12):e491-e497.
20. Whitman J, Allen IE, Bergsland EK, Suh I, Hope TA. Assessment and comparison of (18)F- fluorocholine PET and (99m) Tc-sestamibi scans in identifying parathyroid adenomas: a metaanalysis. *J Nucl Med.* 2021;62(9):1285-1291.
21. Graves CE, Hope TA, Kim J, et al. Superior sensitivity of (18) F-fluorocholine: PET localization in primary hyperparathyroidism. *Surgery.* 2022, Jan;171(1):47-54.
22. Goltzman D. Nonparathyroid hypercalcemia. *Front Horm Res.* 2019;51:77-90.
23. Bollerslev J, Pretorius M, Heck A. Parathyroid hormone independent hypercalcemia in adults. *Best Pract Res Clin Endocrinol Metab.* 2018;32(5):621-638.
24. DeLellis RA, Larsson C, Arnold A, et al. Tumors of the parathyroid glands. In: Lloyd R, Osamura R, Kloppel G, Rosai J, eds. *WHO Classification of Tumors of Endocrine Organs.* 4th ed. Lyon, France: IARC Press; 2017:145-159.
25. Kruijff S, Sidhu SB, Sywak MS, Gill AJ, Delbridge LW. Negative parafibromin staining predicts malignant behavior in atypical parathyroid adenomas. *Ann Surg Oncol.* 2014;21(2):426-433.
26. Erickson LA, Mete O. Immunohistochemistry in diagnostic parathyroid pathology. *Endocr Pathol.* 2018;29(2):113-129.
27. Juhlin CC, Nilsson IL, Lagerstedt-Robinson K, et al. Parafibromin immunostainings of parathyroid tumors in clinical routine: a near-decade experience from a tertiary center. *Mod Pathol.* 2019;32(8):1082-1094.
28. Cetani F, Marcocci C, Torregrossa L, Pardi E. Atypical parathyroid adenomas: challenging lesions in the differential diagnosis of endocrine tumors. *Endocr Relat Cancer.* 2019;26(7):R441-R464.
29. Silva-Figueroa AM, Bassett R Jr, Christakis I, et al. Using a novel diagnostic nomogram to differentiate malignant from benign parathyroid neoplasms. *Endocr Pathol.* 2019;30(4):285-296.
30. Gill AJ, Lim G, Cheung VKY, et al. Parafibromin-deficient (HPT-JT Type, CDC73 Mutated) parathyroid tumors demonstrate distinctive morphologic features. *Am J Surg Pathol.* 2019;43(1):35-46.
31. Sadler C, Gow KW, Beierle EA, et al. Parathyroid carcinoma in more than 1,000 patients: a population-level analysis. *Surgery.* 2014;156(6):1622-1629; discussion 1629-1630.
32. Asare EA, Sturgeon C, Winchester DJ, et al. Parathyroid carcinoma: an update on treatment outcomes and prognostic factors from the national cancer data base (NCDB). *Ann Surg Oncol.* 2015;22(12):3990-3995.
33. Rodrigo JP, Hernandez-Prera JC, Randolph GW, et al. Parathyroid cancer: an update. *Cancer Treat Rev.* 2020; 86:102012.

69 Multiple Endocrine Neoplasia Type 1 (MEN1)

Crystal D. C. Kamilaris, MD
Constantine A. Stratakis, MD, D(Med)Sc

INTRODUCTION

Multiple endocrine neoplasia type 1 (MEN1) is a rare autosomal dominant hereditary tumor syndrome with a high degree of penetrance that is caused by inactivating mutations of the tumor suppressor gene MEN1 and is characterized by a predisposition to a multitude of endocrine and nonendocrine tumors. MEN1 was first described as early as 1903 by Erdheim and was defined by Underdahl and Werner approximately five decades later. The syndrome is classically comprised of hyperplasia and/or tumors of parathyroid, enteropancreatic, and/or anterior pituitary origin that develop in 90%, 30% to 70%, and 30% to 40% of patients, respectively, by age 40. Other endocrine tumors noted with increased frequency in MEN1 include foregut carcinoid tumors, such as thymic and bronchial carcinoid, and gastric enterochromaffin-like tumors, which each have a penetrance of 2%, 2%, and 10%, respectively by 40 years of age. Adrenocortical tumors develop in 40% of affected individuals by this age, whereas pheochromocytomas are rare (<1%). Nonendocrine manifestations are predominantly comprised of neoplasms of the central nervous system, including meningiomas, ependymomas, and schwannomas; cutaneous lesions such as lipomas, angiofibromas, and collagenomas, and smooth muscle tumors such as leiomyomas. Women with MEN1 may also have an increased risk of breast cancer. MEN1 can affect all age groups, with an estimated prevalence of 2 per 100,000 and no apparent gender predilection. Though extensive data is lacking regarding MEN1 in young individuals, in a cohort of 924 patients with MEN1, 160 patients, or 17%, developed MEN1-associated tumors before 21 years of age. In these young patients, primary hyperparathyroidism (PHPT) was diagnosed in 75% by age 21, followed by pituitary adenomas in 34%, pancreatic neuroendocrine tumors (pNETs) in 34% (14% nonfunctional pNETs [NF-pNETs], 12% insulinomas, 2% gastrinomas), adrenal tumors in 1% (two patients), and thymic neuroendocrine tumor (th-NET) in 1% (one patient). MEN1-associated neoplasms were diagnosed as early as within the first 5 years of life, though the majority were diagnosed after the age of 10 with increasing disease penetrance with age.

Despite advances in the diagnosis and treatment of MEN1-associated tumors, patients with this syndrome continue to have a decreased life expectancy compared to the rest of the population, with a mean age of death of 55 to 60 years. Furthermore, delayed MEN1 diagnosis has been associated with potential harm to patients, as demonstrated in a recent study where family members of MEN1 index cases developed metastatic NETs before or during the lag time (median lag time 3.5 years) between the diagnosis of MEN1 in the index case and genetic testing of family members for the disease. The cause of death in 50% to 70% of patients with MEN1 is related to the disease itself. Through the advent of new treatments, the most common cause of death has shifted from the complications of hormone-excess states, primarily due to gastrinomas, to malignant NETs, most notably pNETs and th-NETs. The most recent Endocrine Society clinical practice guidelines for MEN1 published in 2012 recommend an intensive surveillance approach for patients with MEN1 and asymptomatic carriers starting at the age of 5 years, based on the assumption that early detection and management of MEN1-associated neoplasms may lead to decreased morbidity and mortality.

Genetics & Molecular Pathogenesis

MEN1 may be inherited in an autosomal dominant manner, with 90% of individuals diagnosed with this disease having an affected parent and only 10% having a *de novo MEN1* germline mutation. The *MEN1* gene, located on chromosome 11 (11q13), was first identified in 1997 and spans approximately 9000 base pairs of genomic DNA containing 10 exons. This gene encodes the protein *menin*. Germline heterozygous mutations in *MEN1* are identified in 70% to

90% of familial MEN1 cases, with the frequency of finding a *de novo* mutation being significantly lower in sporadic MEN1 cases. More than 1200 germline mutations in the *MEN1* gene have been identified, which are scattered over the entire coding region of the gene without any significant hot spots or genotype-phenotype correlations. The majority of *MEN1* germline mutations (69%) predict pathologic consequences due to either premature truncation of menin due to frameshift mutations (42%) and nonsense mutations (14%), or exon region deletions that are attributed to splicing defects (10.5%) and large deletions (2.5%). Other *MEN1* germline mutations include missense mutations (25.5%) and single or few amino acid in-frame deletions or insertions (5.5%), which require further investigation to determine their pathogenicity.

Approximately 5% to 25% of patients with MEN1 may not have mutations in the *MEN1* coding region, and may have whole or partial gene deletions, or mutations in the promoter or untranslated regions. In addition, the occurrence of phenocopies, or patients that develop disease manifestations typically associated with mutations in the *MEN1* gene but instead are due to another etiology, has been described in 5% to 10% of MEN1 kindreds. These phenocopies may occur in individuals with a family history of MEN1 and one MEN1-associated tumor or in patients with two MEN1-associated tumors with other gene involvement.

MEN1 phenocopies can be attributed to multiple endocrine neoplasia type 4 (MEN4) in 1% to 2% of cases. This syndrome results from inactivating mutations of the tumor suppressor gene *CDKN1B,* which encodes the $p27^{kip1}$ inhibitor of cyclin-dependent kinase 2, with manifestations such as parathyroid and pituitary adenomas, neuroendocrine tumors, and various benign and malignant tumors. Less common germline mutations that may be identified in another 1% to 2% of phenocopies include those attributed to mutations in genes encoding additional members of the cyclin-dependent kinase inhibitor (CDKN) family, such as *CDKN1A* ($P21^{cip1}$), *CDKN2B* ($p15^{Ink4b}$), or *CDKN2C* ($p18^{Ink4c}$). These CDKN genetic defects should be evaluated in patients that present as MEN1-like (phenocopies).

Additional genes to be considered for screening in phenocopies include *CDC73* (also known as *HRPT2*) which is a tumor suppressor gene that encodes the protein parafibromin (mutations implicated in hyperparathyroid-jaw tumor syndrome), *CaSR* which encodes the calcium-sensing receptor (mutations associated with familial benign hypocalciuric hypercalcemias), *GNA11* which encodes the G-protein alpha 11, and *AP2S1* which encodes the adaptor-related protein complex 2, sigma 1 subunit, particularly in patients with familial hyperparathyroidism. Defects in *AIP,* which encodes the aryl hydrocarbon receptor-interacting protein and is associated with familial isolated pituitary adenomas, should also be evaluated in children and adolescents with prolactinoma or somatotropinoma. Germline *MEN1* mutations have also been noted in families with a parathyroid-only disorder, familial isolated primary hyperparathyroidism, where there is a higher frequency of missense mutations compared to patients with the MEN1 syndrome. Similarly, germline *MEN1* mutations have been reported in five cases of "sporadic" pNETs.

MEN1 acts as a tumor-suppressor gene. Patients with germline inactivating mutations in *MEN1* demonstrate loss of heterozygosity (LOH) in more than 90% of their tumors, though LOH involving chromosome 11q13 has also been observed in 5% to 50% of sporadic endocrine tumors. Neoplasms develop as described in Knudson's two-hit hypothesis when a second somatic inactivating mutation occurs in one *MEN1* allele in the setting of the preexisting germline inactivating mutation in the alternate allele. The protein product of *MEN1,* menin, is implicated in the regulation of transcription, genome stability, cell division, and cell proliferation, though the exact role of menin in tumorigenesis is yet to be elucidated. Menin is composed of 610 amino acids and is a highly conserved, ubiquitously expressed, predominantly nuclear protein that does not show homology to any other protein. Two main nuclear localization signals (NLS), NLS1 and NLS2, as well as a third accessory NLS, NLSa, are harbored within the amino acid sequence of menin. Mutations in *MEN1* that lead to premature protein truncation may lead to functional inactivation of menin through the loss of one or both main NLSs. Menin has not been demonstrated to have intrinsic enzymatic activity, but studies of protein-protein interaction by multiple groups have identified more than 50 proteins that could partner with menin. Furthermore, the crystal structure of menin demonstrates a deep pocket that can serve as a binding site for interacting proteins. Menin is predicted to be a multifunctional protein that plays a role in epigenetic regulation and gene transcription through interaction with proteins in chromatin-associated protein complexes and transcription factors, with regulation of gene expression of target genes such as those that control cell proliferation. Similarly, through its protein partners, menin has also been implicated in playing a possible role in DNA repair associated with response to DNA damage, cell signaling, cytoskeletal structure, cell division, cell adhesion, and/or cell motility. In genetically engineered mouse models, germline targeted deletion of both copies of the *MEN1* gene leads to death in utero, whereas germline targeted deletion of one copy of the *MEN1* gene results in live mice that develop endocrine tumors similar to those in humans.

Screening for *MEN1* mutations in the appropriate setting has several benefits, including confirmation of the clinical diagnosis of MEN1, identification of family members that are carriers of *MEN1* mutations so that appropriate screening and/or treatment can be implemented, and identification of the 50% of family members that do not harbor a pathogenic mutation in *MEN1* and thus do not require screening. Genetic testing for defects in the

MEN1 gene currently includes PCR-based screening for mutations in the coding region and splice junctions. If a mutation is not identified by the aforementioned method, then multiplex ligation probe amplification (MLPA)-based screening is performed to detect large deletions of the *MEN1* gene. This testing should be performed in a clinical genetics laboratory that is accredited to perform *MEN1* mutational analysis. Twenty-four different polymorphisms of the *MEN1* gene have been described and should be distinguished from mutations. According to the most recent clinical practice guidelines published in 2012 by Thakker et al. *MEN1* mutational analysis should be performed in index cases with two or more MEN1-associated endocrine tumors (parathyroid, pancreatic, or pituitary tumors), asymptomatic first-degree relatives of a known *MEN1* mutation carrier, first-degree relatives of a *MEN1* mutation carrier expressing familial MEN1 (to exclude phenocopies), and in patients with suspicious or atypical MEN1 (individuals with parathyroid adenomas occurring prior to 30 years of age or multigland parathyroid disease, gastrinoma, or multiple pNET at any age, or those who have at least two MEN1-associated tumors not part of the classical triad of parathyroid, entero-pancreatic, and anterior pituitary tumors) (Table 69–1). When possible, this testing should be undertaken in the first decade of life and as early as before the age of 5 to detect and prevent significant morbidity and even mortality. All individuals should be provided genetic counseling prior to and following testing.

Table 69–1. Indications for MEN1 mutational analysis.*

1. Index case with two or more MEN1-associated endocrine tumors (ie, parathyroid adenoma, enteropancreatic tumor, and pituitary adenoma).
2. Patients with suspicious or atypical MEN1, which includes individuals with parathyroid adenomas occurring before the age of 30 years; or multigland parathyroid disease, gastrinoma, or multiple pancreatic neuroendocrine tumors at any age; or individuals who have two or more MEN1-associated tumors that are not part of the classical triad of parathyroid, pancreatic islet, and anterior pituitary tumors.
3. Asymptomatic first-degree relatives of a known *MEN1* mutation carrier.
4. First-degree relative of an *MEN1* mutation carrier expressing familial MEN1 (ie, having symptoms, signs, biochemical, or radiological evidence for one or more MEN1-associated tumors).

MEN1: multiple endocrine neoplasia type 1

*MEN1 mutational analysis should be undertaken as early as possible (eg, before the age of 5 for asymptomatic individuals); however, there is no clear genotype-phenotype correlation and surveillance should follow guidelines for all patients with documented MEN1.
Source: Thakker RV, Newey PJ, Walls GV, et al. Clinical Practice Guidelines for Multiple Endocrine Neoplasia Type 1 (MEN1). *J Clin Endocrinol Metabol*. 2012;97:2990-3011.

Table 69–2. Diagnostic criteria for MEN1.*

1. Occurrence of two or more primary MEN1-associated endocrine tumors (ie, parathyroid adenoma, enteropancreatic tumor, and pituitary adenoma).
2. Occurrence of one of the MEN1-associated tumors in a first-degree relative of a patient with a clinical diagnosis of MEN.
3. Identification of a germline *MEN1* mutation in an individual who may be asymptomatic and has not yet developed serum biochemical or radiological abnormities indicative of tumor development.

*To make a diagnosis of MEN1, a patient must fulfill at least one of three criteria.
MEN1: multiple endocrine neoplasia type 1.
Source: Thakker RV, Newey PJ, Walls GV, et al. Clinical Practice Guidelines for Multiple Endocrine Neoplasia Type 1 (MEN1). *J Clin Endocrinol Metabol*. 2012;97:2990-3011.

Clinical Manifestations & Diagnosis

The diagnosis of MEN1 can be made based on clinical, familial, or genetic criteria (Table 69–2). Per the most recent clinical practice guidelines, a patient can be diagnosed with MEN1 by meeting any one of the following three conditions: the occurrence of at least two primary MEN1-associated endocrine tumors (ie, parathyroid adenoma, enteropancreatic tumor, and pituitary adenoma); the development of one MEN1-associated tumor in a first-degree relative of a patient with a clinical diagnosis of MEN1; and the identification of a germline *MEN1* mutation in an individual, who may be asymptomatic without biochemical or radiological evidence of MEN1. Genetic evaluation in family members of patients with MEN1 was recently shown to result in the diagnosis of MEN1, 10 years earlier than clinical or biochemical diagnosis.

A. Parathyroid Tumors

Primary hyperparathyroidism (PHPT), which is due to parathyroid hyperplasia and/or adenoma, and is the most common and often earliest endocrine manifestation in MEN1 and occurs primarily in the third decade of life with 100% penetrance by the age of 50. Though PHPT in children is predominantly diagnosed after the age of 10, asymptomatic PHPT has been described in patients with MEN1 as young as 4 years old, with symptomatic disease diagnosed as early as 8 years of age. Furthermore, it is estimated that 1% to 18% of patients diagnosed with PHPT will have MEN1. The degree of hypercalcemia in these individuals is usually mild, and patients may be asymptomatic or present with polydipsia, polyuria, constipation, malaise, altered mentation, nephrolithiasis, decreased bone mineral density with increased fracture risk, hypertension, shortened QT interval, or peptic ulcer disease. Severe hypercalcemia or parathyroid cancer is rare.

Compared to sporadic PHPT, parathyroid disease in MEN1 occurs at an earlier age (20-25 years of age vs 55 years) with an equal male-to-female ratio (1:1 vs 1:3), and typically has multiple gland involvement, with ultimate involvement of all four glands (as compared to 80%-85% patients with sporadic PHPT that have single-gland disease). MEN1-associated PHPT has a high recurrence rate after apparently successful subtotal parathyroidectomy that reaches up to 50% 12 years postoperatively (compared to 4%-16% recurrence in sporadic PHPT). In addition, a greater decline in bone mineral density is noted in patients with PHPT due to MEN1 when compared to patients with sporadic PHPT, with decreased bone mineral density recovery 1 year postoperatively compared to sporadic cases. Parathyroid tumors in patients with multigland disease are asynchronous and vary in size, with each tumor likely representing a different clonal adenoma. In addition, a "negative feedback loop" between miR-24-1 and menin has recently been suggested in MEN1-associated parathyroid tumorigenesis. This "negative feedback loop" mimics the second hit in the Knudson hypothesis by silencing the expression of the second *MEN1* wild-type allele through a post-transcriptional, reversible, epigenetic effect, which may precede the permanent genetic deletion or inactivation of the second wild-type allele.

PHPT is often diagnosed incidentally by biochemical testing that demonstrates hypercalcemia in association with inappropriately increased parathyroid hormone (PTH) levels. Given the multiglandular nature of parathyroid involvement in MEN1, preoperative imaging to localize the parathyroid tumors, such as ultrasound of the neck or Tc99m-sestamibi parathyroid scintigraphy or chest computed tomography (CT), is of limited value. Bilateral neck exploration during surgery should be planned in an attempt to identify all pathological parathyroid glands. Preoperative localization may be of benefit in recurrent or persistent PHPT.

Surgery is the treatment of choice for PHPT though the optimal timing, type, and extent of parathyroid surgery are unclear and should be decided on a case-by-case basis. Whether early parathyroid surgery reduces morbidity and mortality in patients with MEN1 is yet to be elucidated. Some clinicians favor early intervention to reduce the years a patient is at risk of developing bone disease, while others prefer delaying surgery as much as possible with the goal of avoiding the risk of postsurgical hypoparathyroidism and limiting the number of surgeries a patient may need to undergo for management of recurrent PHPT. Indications for parathyroidectomy in patients with MEN1 are similar to those for individuals with sporadic PHPT and include symptomatic or marked hypercalcemia/hypercalciuria, nephrolithiasis, and/or evidence of bone disease. Furthermore, parathyroidectomy may be required in the treatment of patients with severe peptic ulcer disease or other symptoms caused by gastrinoma (the Zollinger-Ellison syndrome [ZES]) that are poorly controlled with medical management, as hypercalcemia typically worsens hypergastrinemia. The recommended surgical approach for the treatment of MEN1-associated PHPT is subtotal parathyroidectomy with the removal of 3.5 parathyroid glands. Total parathyroidectomy with heterotopic autotransplantation of fresh or cryopreserved normal parathyroid tissue into the forearm or neck may also be an option for certain patients, particularly those that have extensive disease either at initial or repeat surgery. Previous observational studies have noted that the total parathyroidectomy approach has been associated with lower rates of persistent hyperparathyroidism but higher rates of hypoparathyroidism. This was demonstrated in a review of 18 reports that included 2 to 73 patients with MEN1 followed for 4 to 12 years after subtotal parathyroidectomy with or without cervical thymectomy, where persistent hyperparathyroidism was noted in 0% to 33%, recurrent hyperparathyroidism in 0% to 6%, and persistent hypoparathyroidism in 0% to 35% of patients. The same review analyzed 10 reports that included 4 to 36 patients with MEN1 who underwent total parathyroidectomy with cervical thymectomy and heterotopic autotransplantation of a small parathyroid graft, where after a mean follow up of 6 to 10 years, patients were noted to have persistent hyperparathyroidism in 0% to 3%, recurrent hyperparathyroidism in 0% to 55%, and hypoparathyroidism in 0% to 46%. Furthermore, in prior observational studies, patients who underwent less than subtotal parathyroidectomy more commonly had persistent disease, with 42% of patients who underwent less than three gland parathyroidectomy having persistent disease compared to 0% to 12% of those who had three or more parathyroid glands resected. However, a recent retrospective study from a single institution that compared eight patients with MEN1 that underwent "unilateral clearance" (preoperative localization of a single enlarged parathyroid gland with resection of that parathyroid gland, the remaining ipsilateral parathyroid gland, as well as ipsilateral transcervical thymectomy) to 16 patients with MEN1 who underwent subtotal parathyroidectomy, showed that one patient from each group had persistent disease (12.5% and 6.25%, respectively), 13% of patients with unilateral clearance and 31% of patients with subtotal parathyroidectomy had recurrent PHPT after a mean follow-up of 47 (2-112) and 68 (1-223) months, whereas no unilateral clearance patients and 2 (12.5%) patients who underwent subtotal parathyroidectomy had permanent hypoparathyroidism. During parathyroidectomy, intraoperative monitoring of PTH is suggested to monitor the correct excision of all adenomatous and/or hyperplastic parathyroid glands. Furthermore, transcervical thymectomy is recommended in all patients with MEN1 during initial parathyroid surgery, as supernumerary glands are identified in 6% to 20% of MEN1 patients, and intrathymic parathyroid tissue may be a source of PTH excess. Calcimimetics, such as cinacalcet, have been used to treat patients with hyperparathyroidism in whom surgery has failed or who were poor surgical candidates. Though data are limited in patients with MEN1, cinacalcet has been shown to have calcium-lowering effects, but current evidence does not show an improvement in bone mineral density in the spine or femur or in hypercalciuria.

B. Enteropancreatic Neuroendocrine Tumors

Pancreatic neuroendocrine tumors (pNETs) are estimated to occur in 30% to 80% of patients with MEN1 and up to 80% to 100% of patients in postmortem studies. MEN1 is the most common hereditary syndrome associated with pNETs, with approximately 10% of all pNETs being associated with MEN1. In addition, somatic *MEN1* mutations can be observed in greater than 40% of sporadic pNETs. These tumors may secrete excessive quantities of hormones such as gastrin, insulin, vasoactive intestinal polypeptide (VIP), glucagon, or somatostatin and may be associated with distinct clinical syndromes, with approximately one-third of these neoplasms becoming clinically apparent. Also, these tumors may be nonfunctional (NF-pNET), either nonsecretory, or releasing hormonally inactive peptides such as pancreatic polypeptide, chromogranin A, neurotensin, neuron-specific enolase, or ghrelin. By the age of 40, the prevalence of gastrinoma is 30% to 40%, that of insulinoma is 10%, and that of other pNETs such as glucagonoma, VIPoma, somatostatinoma, etc. is 2%, whereas the prevalence of nonfunctioning enteropancreatic tumors including those that secrete pancreatic polypeptide is 20% to 55%. Pancreatic neuroendocrine tumors have an earlier age of onset in patients with MEN1 when compared to sporadic cases (10-50 years of age vs 50-80 years), and tend to be multiple (as opposed to single in sporadic pNETs), most commonly leading to diffuse microadenomatosis (tumors <0.5 cm), with less than 13% of patients developing larger tumors (>2 cm) which are often nonfunctional. As previously mentioned, given the effective treatment of PHPT, pituitary disease, and Zollinger-Ellison syndrome (ZES), the malignant potential of enteropancreatic NETs, particularly NF-pNETs, is now the primary cause of death in patients with MEN1. Several MEN1 genotype-phenotype correlations associated pNET growth and/or malignant potential have been identified (mutations in JunD, CHES1, truncating mutations in the N- or C-terminal regions of the menin gene [exons 2,8,9] and the *CDKN1B* V109G polymorphism), and particular pathological characteristics such as high mitotic count in large NF-pNETs, may characterize more aggressive tumors; however, these have not been studied prospectively and are not broadly used.

Gastrinoma is the most common functional enteropancreatic tumor in MEN1 and may lead to ZES (hypergastrinemia with recurrent peptic ulcerations), with ZES being the initial clinical manifestation in up to 40% of patients with MEN1. Up to 60% of patients with MEN1 have either ZES or asymptomatic elevation in serum gastrin concentration. Furthermore, 20% to 60% of patients with ZES have underlying MEN1. ZES may present with gastroesophageal reflux disease (GERD) and peptic ulcer disease (PUD), which are often refractory, with or without diarrhea. In a study of 160 patients with MEN1 below the age of 21, 6 patients (or 2%) developed ZES before the age of 21, with the youngest patient to develop the disease being 6 years of age. Gastrinomas in MEN1 are typically diagnosed by the age of 40 (on average 10 years earlier than sporadic gastrinomas) and are most commonly microadenomas that occur primarily in the duodenum (>80%), and less frequently in the pancreas. They may be complicated by lymph node metastases in 34% to 85% of cases, and hepatic metastases in 6% to 16% of cases at the time of diagnosis. The diagnosis of gastrinoma is indicated by elevated fasting serum gastrin concentration (gastrin levels 10 times greater than the upper limit of normal) in the presence of hyperchloridria or gastric pH <2. If fasting gastrin levels are below this threshold (1000 pg/mL), then gastrin stimulation (either by secretin or calcium infusion) may be necessary for diagnosis. Localization, which should include evaluation for metastases, may be comprised of gastroscopy and endoscopic ultrasound (EUS), particularly for duodenal gastrinomas, as well as other imaging procedures (ultrasound [US], CT, magnetic resonance imaging [MRI], selective abdominal angiography, somatostatin receptor scintigraphy [with In-DPTA-octreotide or octreoscan], ^{68}Ga-DOTATATE-PET [positron emission tomography]/CT), with combined EUS and MRI being the most sensitive for pancreatic disease. The combined use of intra-arterial calcium injections with hepatic venous gastrin sampling may also be used for diagnosis. Though they typically grow slowly, gastrinomas can frequently metastasize to the peripancreatic lymph nodes and less commonly to the liver, with a higher mortality rate than insulinomas but not to other pNETs. Lymph node metastases do not inevitably result in a poor prognosis or a high probability that clinically significant metastases will occur, and the risk of death from lymph node metastases due to MEN1-associated gastrinoma is less than that for sporadic cases. The prognosis of patients with MEN1-associated gastrinomas is associated with tumor size and the presence of hepatic metastases, with an increased risk of hepatic metastases with increasing tumor size. Treatment of MEN1-associated gastrinomas is primarily comprised of medical therapy which aims to decrease gastric acid secretion through the use of histamine 2 receptor antagonists, proton pump inhibitors, and/or somatostatin analogs (SSAs). These medications have shown long-term effectiveness and safety in controlling hypergastrinemia and the complications of ZES. Furthermore, SSAs have been demonstrated to have an antineoplastic effect, though data is lacking regarding their effectiveness in malignant and/or metastatic gastrinoma. Surgical treatment of gastrinomas/ZES in patients with MEN1 is controversial given the multiplicity and small size of these tumors that leads to rare surgical cure without aggressive resections. Surgery is suggested when concomitant NF-NETs double in size over 6 months or exceed 2 cm in diameter, with possible surgical approaches including Thompson's procedure (excision of the duodenal gastrinoma through a longitudinal excision), duodenopancreatectomy, or pancreas-preserving surgery. The use of surgical resection is also limited in advanced metastatic disease, with treatment involving several approaches that may include medical therapy (with everolimus or tyrosine kinase inhibitors such as sunitinib or chemotherapy), peptide radioreceptor therapy with lutetium-177-labeled somatostatin analog, chemotherapy, or liver-directed therapies (such as embolization, chemoembolization, or radioembolization). As aforementioned, hypercalcemia from concomitant PHPT may worsen the symptoms of ZES, with parathyroidectomy leading to decreased fasting and secretin-simulated gastrin levels and basal acid secretion. Another special consideration in patients with ZES is the increased incidence of Cushing's syndrome that has been described in these patients, which is due to a corticotroph pituitary adenoma causing Cushing's disease, as opposed to ectopic ACTH secretion from an islet cell tumor which is more commonly seen in conjunction with sporadic gastrinomas.

Insulinomas are the second most common type of functional enteropancreatic neoplasm in patients with MEN1, representing 10% to 30% of pNETs in this group. They are the most frequent cause of endogenous hyperinsulinemic hypoglycemia in adult patients, with approximately 4% of insulinomas occurring in patients with MEN1. These tumors comprise the first MEN1-associated manifestation in 10% of patients with the syndrome. In contrast to sporadic insulinomas, which tend to occur after the age of 40, MEN1-associated insulinomas occur primarily in patients younger than 40 years old, with many of these tumors arising in patients younger than 20 years of age. In the aforementioned cohort of 160 patients with MEN1 below the age of 21, insulinoma occurred in 10% of patients and as early as 5 years of age. These tumors are solitary in 85% and multiple in 6% to 13% of cases, and are associated with other pNETs at the time of diagnosis in 10% of patients. They are scattered across the pancreas and tend to be small, with 82% of these neoplasms measuring less than 2 cm and 47% measuring less than 1 cm, which may make them difficult to localize. Diagnosis is established with a 72-hour fast through documentation of hypoglycemia with characteristic symptoms that are rapidly reversed by glucose administration and with demonstration of inappropriately increased plasma insulin, c-peptide, and/or proinsulin, in the setting of hypoglycemia. Localization is pursued with ultrasound, CT, and/or MRI, with EUS demonstrating a sensitivity of 94%. If these studies fail to localize the insulinoma(s), more invasive techniques such as selective angiography with intra-arterial calcium stimulation and hepatic venous sampling for insulin levels may localize more than 80% of these neoplasms. In addition, more novel somatostatin receptor-targeting PET modalities such as ^{68}Ga-DOTATATE-PET/CT may aid in localization, with PET imaging with labeled glucagon-like peptide 1 (GLP1) analogs being a promising possible future modality. Medical therapy is often unsuccessful in patients with MEN1-associated insulinomas, with surgery being the treatment of choice. Unlike patients with MEN1-associated gastrinoma/ZES that are rarely cured with pNET enucleation or local gastrinoma excision, and often require more extensive resections, those with other functional pNETs including insulinomas are often cured without extensive surgical resections, but may have recurrent disease. There is no consensus on the optimal extent of surgical resection in patients with insulinoma, which can range from enucleation of a single tumor, to distal pancreatectomy or partial pancreatectomy, to excision of all the macroscopic pancreatic neoplasms and enucleation of nodules in the remaining pancreas. Monitoring the insulin/glucose ratio during surgery may be helpful in assessing successful insulinoma excision. Many experts suggest distal pancreatic resection associated with enucleation of any additional pancreatic head tumors as the treatment of choice. Metastatic insulinoma is rare, occurring in 4% to 14% of cases, with the goal of treatment, as in other malignant functioning pNETs, being symptom control and tumor volume reduction with possible resection of lesions that are amenable to surgery. In cases with unresectable disease or in patients that need further symptom control, adjuvant therapy may vary from diazoxide and SSAs to everolimus and chemotherapy, as well as local therapies (radiofrequency ablation [RFA], chemoembolization, or radiotherapy) or peptide receptor radionuclide therapy (PRRT).

Glucagonomas occur in less than 3% of MEN1 patients, though NF-pNETs may have positive immunostaining for glucagon. These tumors most frequently occur in the tail of the pancreas, and 50% to 80% of patients have metastases at the time of diagnosis. Patients may present with characteristic symptoms such as skin rash (necrolytic migratory erythema), weight loss, anemia, and stomatitis. Asymptomatic patients may be detected incidentally through findings on imaging and/or biochemical evidence of glucose intolerance or hyperglucagonemia. VIP-secreting tumors or VIPomas are rare in MEN1 and present with watery diarrhea, hypokalemia, and achlorhydria (WDHA). Like glucagonomas, these neoplasms are primarily located in the pancreatic tail. The diagnosis of a VIPoma is made through evidence of a fasting stool volume greater than 1 to 2 L per day and a significantly increased plasma VIP concentration, in the absence of laxative or diuretic use. The treatment approach for both glucagonomas and VIPomas is similar to that for insulinomas as described above.

Nonfunctioning pNETs are among the most common enteropancreatic tumors in MEN1. Detection of NF-pNETs has significantly increased in the setting of standardized biochemical and imaging protocols in patients with MEN1.

Furthermore, pathology from pancreatic resections in patients with MEN1 has revealed numerous microtumors that were not shown preoperatively on imaging. NF-pNETs have been detected in patients with MEN1 as early as 12 to 14 years of age, and patients between the ages of 10 and 20 years old have been reported as developing large tumors. EUS is the most sensitive modality for detecting NF-pNETs, with a combined strategy of EUS and MRI being the most useful. ^{68}Ga-DOTATATE-PET/CT has been reported to have high sensitivity for detecting NETs in MEN1, at times leading to change in management. This study may be added to identify metastases in patients with NF-pNETs. In addition, ^{18}F-fluorodeoxyglucose (FDG) PET/CT imaging can be valuable in predicting the malignant potential of pNETs. There is lack of agreement regarding the optimal indications for surgery in patients with NF-pNETs, with major considerations including the size of the neoplasm and other considerations being the growth rate, presence of metastases, and tumor histology. Previous studies have shown an increased rate of metastases in patients with larger tumors. However, there is controversy among experts regarding the tumor size cutoff for offering surgery, with suggested cutoff ranging between 1 and 3 cm. There is a consensus that withholding surgery for tumors that reach or exceed 3 cm in size leads to a negative prognosis; however, the indication for surgical intervention in smaller-sized tumors is unclear. The Endocrine Society clinical practice guidelines for MEN1 suggest surgical resection for NF-pNETs greater than 1 cm in size, or tumors less than 1 cm in size with significant growth, such as doubling of tumor size over 3 to 6 months and exceeding 1 cm in size. The 1-cm cutoff for surgical NF-pNET resection has also been suggested by several other groups of experts including the Uppsala group, the Marburg group, and the MEN consortium in Japan. However, the European Neuroendocrine Tumor Society and the Groupe d'Etude des Tumeurs Endocrines (GTE) suggest conservative management for tumors less than 2 cm in size that do not demonstrate characteristics of aggressive behavior such as rapid growth. Furthermore, two recent studies advocate conservative management for NF-pNETs that are 2 cm or less in size, with low disease-specific mortality and without loss of oncologic safety at this threshold. In terms of surgical approach, the least invasive procedure is typically considered best, with lymph node dissection in addition to pancreatic resection according to the type and location of the tumors. Treatment options for unresectable pNETs or advanced metastatic disease may include biotherapies such as SSAs, interferon alpha, mechanistic target of rapamycin (mTOR) inhibitors, receptor tyrosine kinase (RTK) inhibitors, including platelet-derived growth factor receptor (PDGFR) and vascular endothelial growth factor receptor (VEGFR) inhibitors, and vascular endothelial growth factor A (VEGFA) antibodies. Chemotherapy may be appropriate for patients with metastatic pNETs with a high tumor burden, high proliferative index, rapid tumor progression, and/or symptoms not controlled with biotherapy. Radiological therapies such as PRRT, or localized interventional radiological treatment using RFA, transarterial embolization (TAE), transarterial chemoembolization (TACE), and selective internal radiation therapy (SIRT) may also be considered in select cases.

C. Anterior Pituitary Tumors

The prevalence of anterior pituitary tumors in patients with MEN1 varies widely among series between 10% and 60% and was noted to be 42% and 38.1% in two large cohorts. Pituitary tumors (PITs) have been reported as early as the age of 5 years and can occur as late as the ninth decade of life, with onset primarily in the fourth decade. Furthermore, these tumors were noted in 35% of patients in a large cohort of pediatric patients, comprising the second most common MEN1-associated neoplasm in this group, and the first lesion identified in 21% of cases. Overall, PITs may be the first MEN1-associated lesion to develop in at least 10% to 15% of cases, and up to 3% of patients with the diagnosis of a PIT will have MEN1. Approximately 60% of these tumors secrete prolactin (PRL), 25% release growth hormone (GH), 5% secrete ACTH, and the remaining are primarily nonfunctional (NFTs). This profile is similar to that of sporadic PITs but differs from that of other hereditary pituitary tumors (due to *GNAS, AIP,* or *PRKAR1A* defects) that secrete primarily GH. In a study that included 324 patients, MEN1-associated PITs were described as being larger (macroadenomas in 85% vs 42% in sporadic cases), with more aggressive behavior (one-third of MEN1-associated cases were observed to have invasive features), and reduced response to medical therapy (42% vs 90% in sporadic cases), without increased prevalence of pituitary carcinoma. However, in a subsequent study that included 323 patients with MEN1, two-thirds of PITs were microadenomas. Tumors detected by screening were predominantly nonfunctional microadenomas that did not require treatment and were stable in size over time. Symptom development that required treatment was rare during long-term follow-up (median 6 years). Furthermore, the response rate to medical therapy for prolactinomas was more than 90%. MEN1-associated PITs have been shown to demonstrate plurihormonal expression more frequently than sporadic tumors. However, in contrast with other MEN1-associated neoplasms, multiple pituitary tumors are rare. Clinical manifestations of PITs in MEN1 are similar to those with sporadic PITs, and include those that are due to hormone excess, and those that are related to the size of the tumor. Patients with prolactinomas may present with amenorrhea, galactorrhea, and infertility in women, or erectile dysfunction and infertility in men. Those with excess GH or ACTH secretion may present with signs or symptoms of gigantism or acromegaly, or Cushing syndrome, respectively. Individuals with enlarging PITs may experience headaches and signs of compression of adjacent structures such as visual field disturbances in the setting of optic chiasm compression, and/or hypopituitarism. Biochemical evaluation can lead to the diagnosis of hormone excess syndromes, whereas MRI of the pituitary gland is the imaging study of choice to diagnose PITs. Treatment of PITs in patients with MEN1 is similar to treatment of sporadic disease. Medical therapy with dopamine agonists is first line for prolactinomas, whereas transsphenoidal surgery (TSS) and radiotherapy are reserved for drug-resistant tumors. For GH- and ACTH-secreting tumors the initial treatment of choice is often TSS. When surgery is indicated, TSS is also the primary treatment for nonfunctioning PITs, particularly in macroadenomas associated with visual signs and symptoms or that are in close proximity to the optic chiasm and/or those that demonstrate rapid growth.

D. Other Tumors

Several other neoplasms occur with increased frequency in MEN1 including foregut carcinoid tumors, adrenocortical tumors, cutaneous tumors, meningiomas and ependymomas, tumors of smooth muscle, and very rarely pheochromocytoma.

MEN1-associated carcinoid tumors include thymic, bronchial, and gastric enterochromaffin-like cell NETs. Thymic NETs (th-NETs) occur in 2% to 8% of patients with MEN1 and are associated with strong heritability and a poor prognosis with frequent recurrence and increased risk of death. They occur mostly in men, whereas carcinoids in women are primarily bronchial. Heavy smoking may be a risk factor. Th-NETs have been identified as early as 16 years of age and may be fatal even in young patients. These tumors are primarily nonfunctional and are the most common cause of anterior mediastinal masses in MEN1. Most individuals may be asymptomatic at diagnosis; however, liver, bone, and lung metastases may be identified. Biochemical evaluation is not useful diagnostically in these patients with the diagnostic studies of choice being CT or MRI of the chest. MEN1-associated th-NETs comprise the second most common MEN1-related cause of death and have a high mortality rate, with the 10-year survival rate in several larger studies ranging between 25% and 45%. Treatment is primarily surgical and complete resection of thymic tumors is recommended. Adjuvant radiotherapy may be used for incomplete resection and/or positive surgical margins. Medical treatments that can be considered for unresectable/metastatic disease, include those that are implemented in sporadic th-NETs such as SSAs, chemotherapy, mTOR inhibitors, and PRRT. Prophylactic transcervical thymectomy is typically performed at the time of parathyroidectomy for PHPT; however, this does not eliminate the risk of development of th-NETs, due to residual thymic tissue. The frequency of bronchial NETs (br-NETs) in MEN1 has been reported from 3% to 13%, and may even reach 31%, depending on the mode of diagnosis (imaging and/or pathology), with the frequency of histologically proven br-NETs ranging from 4.6% to 6.6%. Br-NETs have not been described in patients younger than 20 years old, with increasing penetrance with age which reaches 8.1% at 60 years. Presenting symptoms may include dyspnea, hemoptysis, cough, and/or flushing; however, most patients are asymptomatic. Several cases of br-NETs have been described in the same families. Most br-NETs are typical or atypical carcinoids, though small- and large-cell neuroendocrine carcinomas were identified in 10% of cases in a cohort of 51 patients. Although br-NETs do not decrease overall survival in patients with MEN1, poorly differentiated and aggressive br-NETs can lead to death. Chest CT or MRI may be used to detect these tumors. Management is similar to that for sporadic br-NETs, with surgical resection being the recommended treatment modality, though it is possible that small noncentral lesions can be followed without affecting mortality. Gastric carcinoids (type II gastric enterochromaffin-like cell [ECL] carcinoids) and ECL proliferation (a precursor to gastric carcinoid) have been described in patients with MEN1 and ZES. In a cohort of 57 patients with MEN1 and ZES ECL, proliferative changes were universally present, whereas advanced changes were noted in 53% and carcinoids were diagnosed in 23%. Recent studies have demonstrated that these type II gastric carcinoids may be aggressive and metastasize to the liver. However, the disease is localized in at least 70% to 90% of cases and these tumors can often be excised endoscopically after assessment of the extent of invasion by EUS. In certain patients, tumors are present in excessive numbers or are large and may be invasive. In these patients, more aggressive resection and additional therapy with SSAs or CCK-B receptor antagonists may be considered. Annual surveillance with endoscopy is recommended.

Asymptomatic adrenocortical tumors (ACTs) may be detected in 20% to 73% of patients with MEN1 depending on the imaging modality used for screening. These lesions are primarily nonfunctioning and may include cortical adenomas that may be multiple, hyperplasia, cysts, or carcinomas. Less than 10% of MEN1-associated ACTs demonstrate hormone hypersecretion, which can lead most commonly to primary hyperaldosteronism and/or ACTH-independent Cushing syndrome. Hyperandrogenemia may occasionally be detected, particularly in the setting of an adrenocortical carcinoma (ACC). ACC has been described in 1% of patients, manifesting as early as 3 years of age. In the previously described group of 160 young patients under 21 years of age, 2 patients were diagnosed with ACC. Pheochromocytoma is rare with a prevalence of less than 1% by age 40. Patients with signs or symptoms concerning a functional ACT or pheochromocytoma, and those with tumors greater than 1 cm on imaging should be evaluated biochemically for hormone excess. The incidence of ACC in tumors greater than 1 cm in size rises to 13%. Patients with MEN1 and adrenal tumors should receive annual imaging, with consideration for surgical tumor resection if tumors are larger than 4 cm, display atypical radiological features and are 1 to 4 cm in size, or show significant growth over 6 months. Treatment of functional adrenal tumors in MEN1 is similar to that of sporadic neoplasms.

Cutaneous manifestations are common in MEN1 and may include lipomas, angiofibromas, and collagenomas, with the penetrance of these lesions by age 40 being 30%, 85%, and 70%, respectively. Angiofibromas and collagenomas tend to be multiple and are more common in patients with MEN1 than in the general population (64% vs 8% and 62% vs 5%, respectively). The presence of angiofibromas and/or collagenomas may be a strong indicator of the diagnosis of MEN1. In one study that included 110 patients with gastrinoma, including 48 individuals with MEN1 and 62 without MEN1, the presence of angiofibromas or collagenomas (single or multiple) had a sensitivity of 50% to 65% for MEN1 and a specificity of 92% to 100%. The combined finding of at least three angiofibromas and any collagneoma had a sensitivity of 75% and a specificity of 95%.

Surveillance

As outlined in Table 69–3, the diagnostic criteria include those stated in the text, the most recent Endocrine Society clinical practice guidelines for MEN1 recommend a comprehensive surveillance scheme commencing at the age of 5, with the goal of early detection and management of MEN1-associated manifestations and tumors. Unfortunately, there is no clear genotype-phenotype correlation and individual mutation-dependent surveillance is not possible at this time.

Screening for hyperparathyroidism with annual biochemical evaluation of calcium and PTH is recommended starting at the age of 8, which is the age at which the earliest symptomatic patient with PHPT has been described (asymptomatic hyperparathyroidism has been observed as early as age 4). Biochemical evaluation for gastrinoma is recommended beginning at the age of 20, though 2% of cases have been detected in patients younger than 21 years old. Screening for gastrinoma is performed through an annual evaluation of gastrin (+/− gastric pH). Evaluation for insulinoma should commence at age 5, which is the age at which the earliest symptomatic case has been reported, and should include annual insulin and glucose measurement. For other pNETs, the annual measurement of chromogranin-A, pancreatic polypeptide, glucagon, and VIP is recommended beginning before the age of 10. However, the sensitivity of these measurements to detect foregut NETs is unclear, as two retrospective analyses of the use of chromogranin-A, pancreatic polypeptide, and glucagon to screen for the emergence of MEN1-associated neoplasms found that these tests were not effective in early tumor diagnosis, either singly or in combination. Imaging with MRI, CT, or EUS is also recommended annually to evaluate for pNETs beginning before the age of 10 years, as large pancreatic tumors may develop between 10 and 20 years of age. Surveillance for anterior PITs is recommended starting at age 5, which is consistent with the age of the earliest case of MEN1-associated PIT that has been reported and includes

Table 69–3. Recommended biochemical and radiological surveillance for MEN1-associated tumors in patients with MEN1 and MEN1 mutation carriers.*

Tumor	Age to Begin Screening (years)	Biochemical Test (Serum or Plasma) Annually	Imaging Test (Time Interval)
Parathyroid	8	Calcium, PTH	None
Gastrinoma	20	Gastrin (+/− gastric pH)	None
Insulinoma	5	Fasting glucose, insulin	None
Other pNETs	<10	CgA; PPP; glucagon; VIP	MRI, CT, or EUS (annually)
Anterior pituitary	5	Prolactin, IGF-1	MRI (every 3 years)
Adrenal	<10	None unless symptoms or signs of functioning tumor and/or tumor >1 cm identified on imaging	MRI or CT (annually with pancreatic imaging)
Thymic and bronchial carcinoid	15	None	CT or MRI (every 1-2 years)

*To make a diagnosis of MEN1, a patient must fulfill at least one of three criteria.

CgA, chromogranin-A; CT, computed tomography; EUS, endoscopic ultrasound; IGF-1, insulin like growth factor-1; MEN1, multiple endocrine neoplasia type 1; MRI, magnetic resonance imaging; pNET, pancreatic neuroendocrine tumor; PPP, pancreatic polypeptide; PTH, parathyroid hormone; VIP, vasoactive intestinal peptide.

Source: Thakker RV, Newey PJ, Walls GV, et al. Clinical practice guidelines for multiple endocrine neoplasia type 1 (MEN1). *J Clin Endocrinol Metabol.* 2012;97:2990-3011.

annual measurement of serum PRL and insulin-like growth factor 1 (IGF-1) and MRI of the pituitary every 3 years. Evaluation for MEN1-associated adrenal tumors is primarily based on imaging either with CT or MRI that can be performed in conjunction with pancreatic imaging, with biochemical testing indicated only in the setting of symptoms or signs of a functional tumor or the presence of a tumor greater than 1 cm. Screening for adrenal neoplasms is recommended beginning before the age of 10 years, as ACC has been identified in a child as young as 3 years of age. Lastly, screening for thymic and bronchial NETs is recommended starting at the age of 15, with CT or MRI recommended every 1-2 years. This is consistent with the diagnosis of fatal cases of th-NETs in patients as young as 16 years old, though br-NETs have not been reported in patients younger than 20 years old.

Acknowledgments

This work was supported by the research project Z01-HD008920 (Principal Investigator: Dr. Constantine A. Stratakis) of the Intramural Research Program of the *Eunice Kennedy Shriver* National Institute of Child Health & Human Development (NICHD), National Institutes of Health (NIH), Bethesda, MD, USA.

SUGGESTED READING

Agarwal SK. Exploring the tumors of multiple endocrine neoplasia type 1 in mouse models for basic and preclinical studies. *Int J Endocr Oncol*. 2014;1:153-161.

Agarwal SK. The future: genetics advances in MEN1 therapeutic approaches and management strategies. *Endocr Relat Cancer*. 2017;24:T119-T34.

Agarwa SK, Mateo CM, Marx SJ. Rare germline mutations in cyclin-dependent kinase inhibitor genes in multiple endocrine neoplasia type 1 and related states. *J Clin Endocrinol Metab*. 2009;94:1826-1834.

Agarwal SK, Ozawa A, Mateo CM, Marx SJ. The MEN1 gene and pituitary tumours. *Horm Res*. 2009;71(Suppl 2):131-138.

Akerstrom G, Hellman P. Surgery on neuroendocrine tumours. *Best Pract Res Clin Endocrinol Metab*. 2007;21:87-109.

Akerstrom G, Stalberg P, Hellman P. Surgical management of pancreatico-duodenal tumors in multiple endocrine neoplasia syndrome type 1. *Clinics (Sao Paulo)*. 2012;67(Suppl 1):173-178.

Anlauf M, Schlenger R, Perren A, et al. Microadenomatosis of the endocrine pancreas in patients with and without the multiple endocrine neoplasia type 1 syndrome. *Am J Surg Pathol*. 2006;30:560-574.

Antwi K, Fani M, Nicolas G, et al. Localization of hidden insulinomas with (6)(8)Ga-DOTA-Exendin-4 PET/CT: a pilot study. *J Nucl Med*. 2015;56:1075-1078.

Asgharian B, Turner ML, Gibril F, Entsuah LK, Serrano J, Jensen RT. Cutaneous tumors in patients with multiple endocrine neoplasm type 1 (MEN1) and gastrinomas: prospective study of frequency and development of criteria with high sensitivity and specificity for MEN1. *J Clin Endocrinol Metab*. 2004;89:5328-5336.

Balogh K, Patocs A, Hunyady L, Racz K. Menin dynamics and functional insight: take your partners. *Mol Cell Endocrinol*. 2010;326:80-84.

Barbe C, Murat A, Dupas B, et al. Magnetic resonance imaging versus endoscopic ultrasonography for the detection of pancreatic tumours in multiple endocrine neoplasia type 1. *Dig Liver Dis*. 2012;44:228-234.

Bartsch DK, Albers MB, Lopez CL, et al. Bronchopulmonary neuroendocrine neoplasms and their precursor lesions in multiple endocrine neoplasia type 1. *Neuroendocrinology*. 2016;103:240-247.

Bartsch DK, Fendrich V, Langer P, Celik I, Kann PH, Rothmund M. Outcome of duodenopancreatic resections in patients with multiple endocrine neoplasia type 1. *Annals of Surgery*. 2005;242:757-764, discussion 64-6.

Bartsch DK, Langer P, Wild A, et al. Pancreaticoduodenal endocrine tumors in multiple endocrine neoplasia type 1: surgery or surveillance? *Surgery*. 2000;128:958-966.

Bartsch DK, Slater EP, Albers M, et al. Higher risk of aggressive pancreatic neuroendocrine tumors in MEN1 patients with MEN1 mutations affecting the CHES1 interacting MENIN domain. *J Clin Endocrinol Metab*. 2014;99:E2387-E2391.

Baudin E, Caron P, Lombard-Bohas C, et al. [Malignant insulinoma: recommendations for workup and treatment]. *Presse Med*. 2014; 43:645-659.

Beckers A, Betea D, Valdes Socin H, Stevenaert A. The treatment of sporadic versus MEN1-related pituitary adenomas. *J Intern Med*. 2003;253:599-605.

Berna MJ, Annibale B, Marignani M, et al. A prospective study of gastric carcinoids and enterochromaffin-like cell changes in multiple endocrine neoplasia type 1 and Zollinger-Ellison syndrome: identification of risk factors. *J Clin Endocrinol Metab*. 2008;93:1582-1591.

Brandi ML, Gagel RF, Angeli A, et al. Guidelines for diagnosis and therapy of MEN type 1 and type 2. *J Clin Endocrinol Metab*. 2001; 86:5658-5671.

Brown CK, Bartlett DL, Doppman JL, et al. Intraarterial calcium stimulation and intraoperative ultrasonography in the localization and resection of insulinomas. *Surgery*. 1997;122:1189-1193; discussion 93-4.

Burgess JR, Nord B, David R, et al. Phenotype and phenocopy: the relationship between genotype and clinical phenotype in a single large family with multiple endocrine neoplasia type 1 (MEN 1). *Clin Endocrinol*. 2000;53:205-211.

Chandrasekharappa SC, Guru SC, Manickam P, et al. Positional cloning of the gene for multiple endocrine neoplasia-type 1. *Science*. 1997;276:404-407.

Christakis I, Qiu W, Hyde SM, et al. Genotype-phenotype pancreatic neuroendocrine tumor relationship in multiple endocrine neoplasia type 1 patients: a 23-year experience at a single institution. *Surgery*. 2018;163:212-217.

Christakis I, Qiu W, Silva Figueroa AM, et al. Clinical features, treatments, and outcomes of patients with thymic carcinoids and multiple endocrine neoplasia type 1 syndrome at MD anderson cancer center. *Horm Cancer*. 2016;7:279-287.

Circelli L, Ramundo V, Marotta V, et al. Prognostic role of the CDNK1B V109G polymorphism in multiple endocrine neoplasia type 1. *J Cell Mol Med*. 2015;19:1735-1741.

Concolino P, Costella A, Capoluongo E. Multiple endocrine neoplasia type 1 (MEN1): an update of 208 new germline variants reported in the last nine years. *Cancer Genetics*. 2016;209: 36-41.

Conemans EB, Brosens LAA, Raicu-Ionita GM, et al. Prognostic value of WHO grade in pancreatic neuro-endocrine tumors in multiple endocrine neoplasia type 1: results from the Dutch-MEN1 study group. *Pancreatology*. 2017;17:766-772.

Cougard P, Goudet P, Peix JL, et al. [Insulinomas in multiple endocrine neoplasia type 1. Report of a series of 44 cases by the multiple endocrine neoplasia study group]. *Ann Chir.* 2000;125:118-123.

de Laat JM, Dekkers OM, Pieterman CR, et al. Long-term natural course of pituitary tumors in patients with MEN1: results from the DutchMEN1 study group (DMSG). *J Clin Endocrinol Metab.* 2015;100:3288-3296.

de Laat JM, Pieterman CR, van den Broek MF, et al. Natural course and survival of neuroendocrine tumors of thymus and lung in MEN1 patients. *J Clin Endocrinol Metab.* 2014; 99:3325-3333.

de Laat JM, Pieterman CR, Weijmans M, et al. Low accuracy of tumor markers for diagnosing pancreatic neuroendocrine tumors in multiple endocrine neoplasia type 1 patients. *J Clin Endocrinol Metab.* 2013;98:4143-4151.

de Laat JM, van der Luijt RB, Pieterman CR, et al. MEN1 redefined, a clinical comparison of mutation-positive and mutation-negative patients. *BMC Med.* 2016;14:182.

Dean PG, van Heerden JA, Farley DR, et al. Are patients with multiple endocrine neoplasia type I prone to premature death? *World J Surg.* 2000;24:1437-1441.

Di Meo G, Sgaramella LI, Ferraro V, Prete FP, Gurrado A, Testini M. Parathyroid carcinoma in multiple endocrine neoplasm type 1 syndrome: case report and systematic literature review. *Clin Exp Med.* 2018;18(4):585-593.

Doherty GM. Multiple endocrine neoplasia type 1. *J Surg Oncol.* 2005;89:143-150.

Doherty GM, Olson JA, Frisella MM, Lairmore TC, Wells SA, Norton JA. Lethality of multiple endocrine neoplasia type I. *World J Surg.* 1998;22:581-587.

Dralle H, Krohn SL, Karges W, Boehm BO, Brauckhoff M, Gimm O. Surgery of resectable nonfunctioning neuroendocrine pancreatic tumors. *World J Surg.* 2004;28:1248-1260.

Dwight T, Nelson AE, Theodosopoulos G, et al. Independent genetic events associated with the development of multiple parathyroid tumors in patients with primary hyperparathyroidism. *Am J Pathol.* 2002;161:1299-1306.

Eller-Vainicher C, Chiodini I, Battista C, et al. Sporadic and MEN1-related primary hyperparathyroidism: differences in clinical expression and severity. *J Bone Miner Res.* 2009;24:1404-1410.

Elston MS, McDonald KL, Clifton-Bligh RJ, Robinson BG. Familial pituitary tumor syndromes. *Nat Rev Endocrinol.* 2009;5:453-461.

Erdheim J. Normal and pathological histology of the glandula thyroidea, parathyroidea and hypophysis. *Beitrage Zur Pathologischen Anatomie Und Zur Allgemeinen Pathologie.* 1903;33:158-236.

Falchetti A, Marini F, Luzi E, et al. Multiple endocrine neoplasia type 1 (MEN1): not only inherited endocrine tumors. *Genet Med.* 2009;11:825-835.

Falconi M, Eriksson B, Kaltsas G, et al. ENETS Consensus Guidelines update for the management of patients with functional pancreatic neuroendocrine tumors and non-functional pancreatic neuroendocrine tumors. *Neuroendocrinology.* 2016;103:153-171.

Ferolla P, Falchetti A, Filosso P, et al. Thymic neuroendocrine carcinoma (carcinoid) in multiple endocrine neoplasia type 1 syndrome: the Italian series. *J Clin Endocrinol Metab.* 2005;90:2603-2609.

Fink G, Krelbaum T, Yellin A, et al. Pulmonary carcinoid: presentation, diagnosis, and outcome in 142 cases in Israel and review of 640 cases from the literature. *Chest.* 2001;119:1647-1651.

Frost M, Lines KE, Thakker RV. Current and emerging therapies for PNETs in patients with or without MEN1. *Nat Rev Endocrinol.* 2018;14:216-227.

Gatta-Cherifi B, Chabre O, Murat A, et al. Adrenal involvement in MEN1. Analysis of 715 cases from the Groupe d'etude des Tumeurs Endocrines database. *Eur J Endocrinol.* 2012;166: 269-279.

Geerdink EA, Van der Luijt RB, Lips CJM. Do patients with multiple endocrine neoplasia syndrome type 1 benefit from periodical screening? *Eur J Endocrinol.* 2003;149:577-582.

Gibril F, Chen YJ, Schrump DS, et al. Prospective study of thymic carcinoids in patients with multiple endocrine neoplasia type 1. *J Clin Endocrinol Metab.* 2003;88:1066-1081.

Gibril F, Jensen RT. Advances in evaluation and management of gastrinoma in patients with Zollinger-Ellison syndrome. *Curr Gastroenterol Rep.* 2005;7:114-121.

Gibril F, Schumann M, Pace A, Jensen RT. Multiple endocrine neoplasia type 1 and Zollinger-Ellison syndrome: a prospective study of 107 cases and comparison with 1009 cases from the literature. *Medicine (Baltimore).* 2004;83:43-83.

Giudici F, Nesi G, Brandi ML, Tonelli F. Surgical management of insulinomas in multiple endocrine neoplasia type 1. *Pancreas.* 2012;41:547-553.

Giusti F, Cianferotti L, Boaretto F, et al. Multiple endocrine neoplasia syndrome type 1: institution, management, and data analysis of a nationwide multicenter patient database. *Endocrine.* 2017;58:349-359.

Giusti F, Cianferotti L, Gronchi G, et al. Cinacalcet therapy in patients affected by primary hyperparathyroidism associated to multiple endocrine neoplasia syndrome type 1 (MEN1). *Endocrine.* 2016;52:495-506.

Goncalves TD, Toledo RA, Sekiya T, et al. Penetrance of functioning and nonfunctioning pancreatic neuroendocrine tumors in multiple endocrine neoplasia type 1 in the second decade of life. *J Clin Endocrinol Metab.* 2014;99:E89-E96.

Goudet P, Bonithon-Kopp C, Murat A, et al. Gender-related differences in MEN1 lesion occurrence and diagnosis: a cohort study of 734 cases from the Groupe d'etude des Tumeurs Endocrines. *Eur J Endocrinol.* 2011;165:97-105.

Goudet P, Dalac A, Le Bras M, et al. MEN1 disease occurring before 21 years old: a 160-patient cohort study from the Groupe d'etude des Tumeurs Endocrines. *J Clin Endocrinol Metab.* 2015;100:1568-1577.

Goudet P, Murat A, Binquet C, et al. Risk factors and causes of death in MEN1 disease. A GTE (Groupe d'Etude des Tumeurs Endocrines) cohort study among 758 patients. *World J Surg.* 2010;34:249-255.

Goudet P, Murat A, Cardot-Bauters C, et al. Thymic neuroendocrine tumors in multiple endocrine neoplasia type 1: a comparative study on 21 cases among a series of 761 MEN1 from the GTE (Groupe des Tumeurs Endocrines). *World J Surg.* 2009;33:1197-1207.

Guettier JM, Kam A, Chang R, et al. Localization of insulinomas to regions of the pancreas by intraarterial calcium stimulation: the NIH experience. *J Clin Endocrinol Metab.* 2009;94:1074-1080.

Guru SC, Goldsmith PK, Burns AL, et al. Menin, the product of the MEN1 gene, is a nuclear protein. *Proc Natl Acad Sci USA.* 1998;95:1630-1634.

Hanazaki K, Sakurai A, Munekage M, et al. Surgery for a gastroenteropancreatic neuroendocrine tumor (GEPNET) in multiple endocrine neoplasia type 1. *Surg Today.* 2013;43:229-236.

Hannan FM, Nesbit MA, Christie PT, et al. Familial isolated primary hyperparathyroidism caused by mutations of the MEN1 gene. *Nat Clin Pract Endocrinol Metab.* 2008;4:53-58.

Hellman P, Goretzki P, Simon D, Dotzenrath C, Roher HD. Therapeutic experience of 65 cases with organic hyperinsulinism. *Langenbecks Arch Surg*. 2000;385:329-336.

Hendy GN, Kaji H, Canaff L. Cellular functions of menin. *Adv Exp Med Biol*. 2009;668:37-50.

Huang J, Gurung B, Wan B, et al. The same pocket in menin binds both MLL and JUND but has opposite effects on transcription. *Nature*. 2012;482:542-546.

Imamura M, Komoto I, Ota S, et al. Biochemically curative surgery for gastrinoma in multiple endocrine neoplasia type 1 patients. *World J Gastroenterol*. 2011;17:1343-1353.

Ito T, Igarashi H, Uehara H, Berna MJ, Jensen RT. Causes of death and prognostic factors in multiple endocrine neoplasia type 1: a prospective study: comparison of 106 MEN1/Zollinger-Ellison syndrome patients with 1613 literature MEN1 patients with or without pancreatic endocrine tumors. *Medicine (Baltimore)*. 2013;92:135-181.

Jensen RT, Berna MJ, Bingham DB, Norton JA. Inherited pancreatic endocrine tumor syndromes: advances in molecular pathogenesis, diagnosis, management, and controversies. *Cancer*. 2008;113:1807-1843.

Jiao YC, Shi CJ, Edil BH, et al. DAXX/ATRX, MEN1, and mTOR pathway genes are frequently altered in pancreatic neuroendocrine tumors. *Science*. 2011;331:1199-1203.

Kluijfhout WP, Beninato T, Drake FT, et al. Unilateral clearance for primary hyperparathyroidism in selected patients with multiple endocrine neoplasia type 1. *World J Surg*. 2016;40:2964-2969.

Knudson AG. Mutation and cancer—statistical study of retinoblastoma. *Proc Natl Acad Sci USA*. 1971;68:820-823.

Kornaczewski Jackson ER, Pointon OP, Bohmer R, Burgess JR. Utility of FDG-PET imaging for risk stratification of pancreatic neuroendocrine tumors in MEN1. *J Clin Endocrinol Metab*. 2017;102:1926-1933.

Kouvaraki MA, Shapiro SE, Cote GJ, et al. Management of pancreatic endocrine tumors in multiple endocrine neoplasia type 1. *World J Surg*. 2006;30:643-653.

La P, Desmond A, Hou Z, Silva AC, Schepp RW, Hua X. Tumor suppressor menin: the essential role of nuclear localization signal domains in coordinating gene expression. *Oncogene*. 2006;25:3537-3546.

Lairmore TC, Piersall LD, DeBenedetti MK, et al. Clinical genetic testing and early surgical intervention in patients with multiple endocrine neoplasia type 1 (MEN 1). *Ann Surg*. 2004;239:637-645; discussion 45-7.

Langer P, Cupisti K, Bartsch DK, et al. Adrenal involvement in multiple endocrine neoplasia type 1. *World J Surg*. 2002;26: 891-896.

Langer P, Kann PH, Fendrich V, et al. Prospective evaluation of imaging procedures for the detection of pancreaticoduodenal endocrine tumors in patients with multiple endocrine neoplasia type 1. *World J Surg*. 2004;28:1317-1322.

Lecomte P, Binquet C, Le Bras M, et al. Histologically proven bronchial neuroendocrine tumors in MEN1: a GTE 51-case cohort study. *World J Surg*. 2018;42:143-152.

Lemmens I, VandeVen WJM, Kas K, et al. Identification of the multiple endocrine neoplasia type 1 (MEN1) gene. *Hum Mol Genet*. 1997;6:1177-1183.

Lemos MC, Thakker RV. Multiple endocrine neoplaslia type 1 (MEN 1): analysis of 1336 mutations reported in the first decade following identification of the gene. *Hum Mutat*. 2008;29:22-32.

Luzi E, Marini F, Giusti F, Galli G, Cavalli L, Brandi ML. The negative feedback-loop between the Oncomir Mir-24-1 and Menin modulates the MEN1 tumorigenesis by mimicking the "Knudson's Second Hit." *PLoS One*. 2012;7(6):e39767.

Machens A, Schaaf L, Karges W, et al. Age-related penetrance of endocrine tumours in multiple endocrine neoplasia type 1 (MEN1): a multicentre study of 258 gene carriers. *Clin Endocrinol*. 2007;67:613-622.

Mai HD, Sanowski RA. Regression of duodenal gastrinomas in a patient with multiple endocrine neoplasia type I after parathyroidectomy. *Gastrointest Endosc*. 1992;38:706-708.

Manoharan J, Albers MB, Bartsch DK. The future: diagnostic and imaging advances in MEN1 therapeutic approaches and management strategies. *Endocr Relat Cancer*. 2017;24:T209-T225.

Marini F, Giusti F, Tonelli F, Brandi ML. Management impact: effects on quality of life and prognosis in MEN1. *Endocr Relat Cancer*. 2017;24:T227-T242.

Marx SJ, Simonds WF. Hereditary hormone excess: genes, molecular pathways, and syndromes. *Endocr Rev*. 2005;26:615-661.

Matkar S, Thiel A, Hua XX. Menin: a scaffold protein that controls gene expression and cell signaling. *Trends Biochem Sci*. 2013;38:394-402.

Maton PN, Gardner JD, Jensen RT. Cushing's syndrome in patients with the Zollinger-Ellison syndrome. *N Engl J Med*. 1986;315:1-5.

McLean AM, Fairclough PD. Endoscopic ultrasound in the localisation of pancreatic islet cell tumours. *Best Pract Res Clin Endocrinol Metab*. 2005;19:177-193.

Melmed S. Pathogenesis of pituitary tumors. *Nat Rev Endocrinol*. 2011;7:257-266.

Moyes VJ, Monson JP, Chew SL, Akker SA. Clinical use of cinacalcet in MEN1 hyperparathyroidism. *Int J Endocrinol*. 2010; 2010:906163.

Murai MJ, Chruszcz M, Reddy G, Grembecka J, Cierpicki T. Crystal structure of menin reveals binding site for mixed lineage leukemia (MLL) protein. *J Biol Chem*. 2011;286:31742-31748.

Nell S, Borel Rinkes IHM, Verkooijen HM, et al. Early and late complications after surgery for MEN1-related nonfunctioning pancreatic neuroendocrine tumors. *Ann Surg*. 2018;267:352-356.

Nell S, Verkooijen HM, Pieterman CRC, et al. Management of MEN1 related nonfunctioning pancreatic NETs: a shifting paradigm: results from the DutchMEN1 study group. *Ann Surg*. 2018;267:1155-1160.

Newey PJ, Jeyabalan J, Walls GV, et al. Asymptomatic children with multiple endocrine neoplasia type 1 mutations may harbor nonfunctioning pancreatic neuroendocrine tumors. *J Clin Endocrinol Metab*. 2009;94:3640-3646.

Newey PJ, Thakker RV. Role of multiple endocrine neoplasia type 1 mutational analysis in clinical practice. *Endocrine Practice*. 2011;17:8-17.

Nilubol N, Weisbrod AB, Weinstein LS, et al. Utility of intraoperative parathyroid hormone monitoring in patients with multiple endocrine neoplasia type 1-associated primary hyperparathyroidism undergoing initial parathyroidectomy. *World J Surg*. 2013;37:1966-1972.

Nockel P, Babic B, Millo C, et al. Localization of insulinoma using 68Ga-DOTATATE PET/CT scan. *J Clin Endocrinol Metab*. 2017;102:195-199.

Norton JA, Foster DS, Ito T, Jensen RT. Gastrinomas: medical or surgical treatment. *Endocrinol Metab Clin North Am*. 2018;47:577-601.

Norton JA, Fraker DL, Alexander HR, et al. Surgery to cure the Zollinger-Ellison syndrome. *N Engl J Med*. 1999;341:635-644.

Norton JA, Krampitz G, Jensen RT. Multiple endocrine neoplasia: genetics and clinical management. *Surg Oncol Clin N Am*. 2015;24:795-832.

Norton JA, Krampitz G, Zemek A, Longacre T, Jensen RT. Better survival but changing causes of death in patients with multiple endocrine neoplasia type 1. *Ann Surg.* 2015;261:e147-e148.

Norton JA, Venzon DJ, Berna MJ, et al. Prospective study of surgery for primary hyperparathyroidism (HPT) in multiple endocrine neoplasia-type 1 and Zollinger-Ellison syndrome: long-term outcome of a more virulent form of HPT. *Ann Surg.* 2008;247:501-510.

Pavel M, Baudin E, Couvelard A, et al. ENETS Consensus Guidelines for the management of patients with liver and other distant metastases from neuroendocrine neoplasms of foregut, midgut, hindgut, and unknown primary. *Neuroendocrinology.* 2012;95:157-176.

Pellegata NS. MENX and MEN4. *Clinics (Sao Paulo).* 2012;67(Suppl 1):13-18.

Pellegata NS, Quintanilla-Martinez L, Siggelkow H, et al. Germline mutations in p27Kip1 cause a multiple endocrine neoplasia syndrome in rats and humans. *Proc Natl Acad Sci USA.* 2006;103:15558-15563.

Pieterman CR, Conemans EB, Dreijerink KM, et al. Thoracic and duodenopancreatic neuroendocrine tumors in multiple endocrine neoplasia type 1: natural history and function of menin in tumorigenesis. *Endocr Relat Cancer.* 2014;21:R121-R142.

Pipeleers-Marichal M, Somers G, Willems G, et al. Gastrinomas in the duodenums of patients with multiple endocrine neoplasia type 1 and the Zollinger-Ellison syndrome. *N Engl J Med.* 1990; 322:723-727.

Plockinger U. Diagnosis and treatment of gastrinomas in multiple endocrine neoplasia type 1 (MEN-1). *Cancers (Basel).* 2012; 4:39-54.

Powell AC, Alexander HR, Pingpank JR, et al. The utility of routine transcervical thymectomy for multiple endocrine neoplasia 1-related hyperparathyroidism. *Surgery.* 2008;144:878-883; discussion 83-4.

Qiu W, Christakis I, Silva A, et al. Utility of chromogranin A, pancreatic polypeptide, glucagon and gastrin in the diagnosis and follow-up of pancreatic neuroendocrine tumours in multiple endocrine neoplasia type 1 patients. *Clin Endocrinol (Oxf).* 2016;85:400-407.

Rizzoli R, Green J 3rd, Marx SJ. Primary hyperparathyroidism in familial multiple endocrine neoplasia type I. Long-term follow-up of serum calcium levels after parathyroidectomy. *Am J Med.* 1985;78:467-474.

Sachithanandan N, Harle A, Burgess JR. Bronchopulmonary carcinoid in multiple endocrine neoplasia type 1. *Cancer.* 2005; 103:509-515.

Sadowski SM, Cadiot G, Dansin E, Goudet P, Triponez F. The future: surgical advances in MEN1 therapeutic approaches and management strategies. *Endocr Relat Cancer.* 2017;24:T243-T260.

Sadowski SM, Millo C, Cottle-Delisle C, et al. Results of (68) Gallium-DOTATATE PET/CT scanning in patients with multiple endocrine neoplasia type 1. *J Am Coll Surg.* 2015; 221:509-517.

Sadowski SM, Neychev V, Millo C, et al. Prospective study of 68Ga-DOTATATE positron emission tomography/computed tomography for detecting gastro-entero-pancreatic neuroendocrine tumors and unknown primary sites. *J Clin Oncol.* 2016;34:588-596.

Sakurai A, Suzuki S, Kosugi S, et al. Multiple endocrine neoplasia type 1 in Japan: establishment and analysis of a multicentre database. *Clin Endocrinol.* 2012;76:533-539.

Scarpa A, Chang DK, Nones K, et al. Whole-genome landscape of pancreatic neuroendocrine tumours. *Nature.* 2017;543:65-71.

Scarsbrook AF, Thakker RV, Wass JA, Gleeson FV, Phillips RR. Multiple endocrine neoplasia: spectrum of radiologic appearances and discussion of a multitechnique imaging approach. *Radiographics.* 2006;26:433-451.

Schaefer S, Shipotko M, Meyer S, et al. Natural course of small adrenal lesions in multiple endocrine neoplasia type 1: an endoscopic ultrasound imaging study. *Eur J Endocrinol.* 2008; 158:699-704.

Schreinemakers JMJ, Pieterman CRC, Scholten A, Vriens MR, Valk GD, Rinkes IHMB. The optimal surgical treatment for primary hyperparathyroidism in MEN1 patients: a systematic review. *World J Surg.* 2011;35:1993-2005.

Service FJ, McMahon MM, O'Brien PC, Ballard DJ. Functioning insulinoma—incidence, recurrence, and long-term survival of patients: a 60-year study. *Mayo Clin Proc.* 1991;66: 711-719.

Silva AM, Vodopivec D, Christakis I, et al. Operative intervention for primary hyperparathyroidism offers greater bone recovery in patients with sporadic disease than in those with multiple endocrine neoplasia type 1-related hyperparathyroidism. *Surgery.* 2017;161:107-115.

Simonds WF, James-Newton LA, Agarwal SK, et al. Familial isolated hyperparathyroidism: clinical and genetic characteristics of 36 kindreds. *Medicine (Baltimore).* 2002;81:1-26.

Singh MH, Fraker DL, Metz DC. Importance of surveillance for multiple endocrine neoplasia-1 and surgery in patients with sporadic Zollinger-Ellison syndrome. *Clin Gastroenterol Hepatol.* 2012;10:1262-1269.

Singh Ospina N, Thompson GB, Nichols FC 3rd, Cassivi SD, Young WF Jr. Thymic and bronchial carcinoid tumors in multiple endocrine neoplasia type 1: the Mayo Clinic experience from 1977 to 2013. *Horm Cancer.* 2015;6:247-253.

Stalberg P, Carling T. Familial parathyroid tumors: diagnosis and management. *World J Surg.* 2009;33:2234-2243.

Stratakis CA, Schussheim DH, Freedman SM, et al. Pituitary macroadenoma in a 5-year-old: an early expression of multiple endocrine neoplasia type 1. *J Clin Endocrinol Metab.* 2000;85: 4776-4780.

Syro LV, Scheithauer BW, Kovacs K, et al. Pituitary tumors in patients with MEN1 syndrome. *Clinics (Sao Paulo).* 2012;67(Suppl 1): 43-48.

Teh BT, McArdle J, Chan SP, et al. Clinicopathologic studies of thymic carcinoids in multiple endocrine neoplasia type 1. *Medicine (Baltimore).* 1997;76:21-29.

Thakker, RV. Multiple endocrine neoplasia type 1 (MEN1). *Best Pract Res Clin Endocrinol Metab.* 2010;24:355-370.

Thakker RV. Multiple endocrine neoplasia type 1 (MEN1) and type 4 (MEN4). *Mol Cell Endocrinol.* 2014;386:2-15.

Thakker RV, Newey PJ, Walls GV, et al. Clinical Practice Guidelines for multiple endocrine neoplasia type 1 (MEN1). *J Clin Endocrinol Metab.* 2012;97:2990-3011.

Tham E, Grandell U, Lindgren E, Toss G, Skogseid B, Nordenskjold M. Clinical testing for mutations in the MEN1 gene in Sweden: a report on 200 unrelated cases. *J Clin Endocrinol Metab.* 2007; 92:3389-3395.

Thevenon J, Bourredjem A, Faivre L, et al. Unraveling the intrafamilial correlations and heritability of tumor types in MEN1: a Groupe d'etude des Tumeurs Endocrines study. *Eur J Endocrinol.* 2015;173:819-826.

Thevenon J, Bourredjem A, Faivre L, et al. Higher risk of death among MEN1 patients with mutations in the JunD interacting domain: a Groupe d'etude des Tumeurs Endocrines (GTE) cohort study. *Hum Mol Genet.* 2013;22:1940-1948.

Thomas-Marques L, Murat A, Delemer B, et al. Prospective endoscopic ultrasonographic evaluation of the frequency of nonfunctioning pancreaticoduodenal endocrine tumors in patients with multiple endocrine neoplasia type 1. *Am J Gastroenterol.* 2006;101:266-273.

Tonelli F, Marcucci T, Giudici F, Falchetti A, Brandi ML. Surgical approach in hereditary hyperparathyroidism. *Endocr J.* 2009;56:827-841.

Triponez F, Dosseh D, Goudet P, et al. Epidemiology data on 108 MEN 1 patients from the GTE with isolated nonfunctioning tumors of the pancreas. *Ann Surg.* 2006;243:265-272.

Triponez F, Goudet P, Dosseh D, et al. Is surgery beneficial for MEN1 patients with small (< or = 2 cm), nonfunctioning pancreaticoduodenal endocrine tumor? An analysis of 65 patients from the GTE. *World J Surg.* 2006;30:654-662; discussion 63-4.

Triponez F, Sadowski SM, Pattou F, et al. Long-term follow-up of MEN1 patients who do not have initial surgery for small ≤2 cm nonfunctioning pancreatic neuroendocrine tumors, an AFCE and GTE Study: Association Francophone de Chirurgie Endocrinienne & Groupe d'Etude des Tumeurs Endocrines. *Ann Surg.* 2018;268:158-164.

Trouillas J, Labat-Moleur F, Sturm N, et al. Calender, and Endocrines Groupe d'etudes des Tumeurs. Pituitary tumors and hyperplasia in multiple endocrine neoplasia type 1 syndrome (MEN1): a case-control study in a series of 77 patients versus 2509 non-MEN1 patients. *Am J Surg Pathol.* 2008;32:534-543.

Trump D, Farren B, Wooding C, et al. Clinical studies of multiple endocrine neoplasia type 1 (MEN1). *QJM.* 1996;89:957-958.

Turner JJO, Christie PT, Pearce SHS, Turnpenny PD, Thakker RV. Diagnostic challenges due to phenocopies: lessons from multiple endocrine neoplasia type 1 (MEN1). *Hum Mutat.* 2010; 31:E1089-E1101.

Turner JJ, Wren AM, Jackson JE, Thakker RV, Meeran K. Localization of gastrinomas by selective intra-arterial calcium injection. *Clin Endocrinol (Oxf).* 2002;57:821-825.

Underdahl LO, Woolner LB, Black BM. Multiple endocrine adenomas; report of 8 cases in which the parathyroids, pituitary and pancreatic islets were involved. *J Clin Endocrinol Metab.* 1953;13:20-47.

van Leeuwaarde RS, Dreijerink KM, Ausems MG, et al. MEN1-dependent breast cancer: indication for early screening? Results from the Dutch MEN1 Study Group. *J Clin Endocrinol Metab.* 2017;102:2083-2090.

van Leeuwaarde RS, van Nesselrooij BPM, Hermus AR, et al. Impact of delay in diagnosis in outcomes in MEN1: results from the dutch MEN1 study group. *J Clin Endocrinol Metab.* 2016;101:1159-1165.

van Treijen MJC, van Beek DJ, van Leeuwaarde RS, Vriens MR, Valk GD. Diagnosing nonfunctional pancreatic NETs in MEN1: the evidence base. *J Endocr Soc.* 2018;2:1067-1088.

Verges B, Boureille F, Goudet P, et al. Pituitary disease in MEN type 1 (MEN1): data from the France-Belgium MEN1 multicenter study. *J Clin Endocrinol Metab.* 2002;87:457-465.

Wamsteker EJ, Gauger PG, NW Thompson, Scheiman JM. EUS detection of pancreatic endocrine tumors in asymptomatic patients with type 1 multiple endocrine neoplasia. *Gastrointest Endosc.* 2003;58:531-535.

Welch K, McHenry CR. The role of transcervical thymectomy in patients with hyperparathyroidism. *Am J Surg.* 2012;203:292-295; discussion 95-6.

Wermer P. Genetic aspects of adenomatosis of endocrine glands. *Am J Med.* 1954;16:363-371.

Wolin EM. The expanding role of somatostatin analogs in the management of neuroendocrine tumors. *Gastrointest Cancer Res.* 2012;5:161-168.

Yates CJ, Newey PJ, Thakker RV. Challenges and controversies in management of pancreatic neuroendocrine tumours in patients with MEN1. *Lancet Diabetes Endocrinol.* 2015;3:895-905.

70 Multiple Endocrine Neoplasia Type 2 Syndrome (MEN2)

Andreas Machens, MD
Henning Dralle, MD

GENERAL CONSIDERATIONS

Multiple endocrine neoplasia type 2 (MEN2) is characterized by strong genotype-phenotype correlations (Figure 70–1), which are extremely useful for clinical diagnosis and risk assessment.[1,2]

The neuroendocrine components of MEN2 (Figure 70–1, left panel) include

- medullary thyroid cancer (MTC) in ~100% (MEN2A and MEN2B);
- pheochromocytoma (epinephrine phenotype) in ~10%-50% (MEN2A and MEN2B); and
- primary hyperparathyroidism (pseudonodular parathyroid hyperplasia) in ≤20% (MEN2A).

The nonendocrine components of MEN type 2 (Figure 70–1, right panel) include

- congenital megacolon (Hirschsprung's disease) in <10% (MEN2A, limited to mutations in codon 609, 611, 618, and 620)[3];
- renal agenesis, ureteropelvicalyceal dilatation, or polycystic kidney disease in <10% (MEN2A, limited to mutations in codon 609, 611, 618, and 620);[3]
- cutaneous lichen amyloidosis affecting the interscapular region (dermatomes C4-T5) in ~10%-20% (MEN2A, limited to mutations in codon 634);
- intestinal ganglioneuromatosis ("pseudo-Hirschsprung's disease") in ~10%-20% (MEN2B);
- multiple ocular, buccal, lingual and lip neuromas, neurofibromas and thickened nerve sheaths (Figure 70–2) in ~100% (MEN2B);
- skeletal malformations in ~100% (MEN2B).

The treatment paradigm for MEN2 has moved away from a "one-size-fits-all" approach based on genetic risk alone toward precision medicine.[4,5] Barring sample mix-up or laboratory errors, there are no false-positive genomic test results.

Remarkably, many national health-care systems do not reimburse genomic testing for sporadic-appearing medullary thyroid cancer or pheochromocytoma so that less penetrant mutations are missed. Indeed, some 6.5% to 9.5% of patients with seemingly sporadic MTC harbor germline mutations causing MEN2A. These gene carriers cannot be recognized unless all relevant exons of the susceptibility gene have been screened.

Large pedigree analyses found that RET mutations can be inherited over centuries,[6] for instance:

- p.Cys618Ser in Sweden, dating back to 1896 or earlier.
- p.Cys611Phe in Germany, dating back to 1876 or earlier.
- p.Cys634Trp in Germany, dating back to 1865 or earlier.
- p.Ser891Ala in Italy, dating back to 1493 or earlier.

By way of contrast, p.Met918Thr is passed on to offspring only in < 5% by an affected MEN2B parent.[7]

For an age-dependent hereditary disease, DNA-based screening yields more definitive results earlier than biochemical screening that hinges on the presence of syndromic components. Of note, gene carriers may die of unrelated causes before developing syndromic components of MEN2.

One of the most reliable population-based estimates of age-standardized incidence (0.06 per 100,000 per year) and prevalence (1.3 per 100,000) for hereditary MTC are based on a cohort of Danish gene carriers constructed with the support of the Danish Civil Registration System and the Danish National Archives, the Danish Thyroid Cancer Database, the Danish Cancer Registry, and the Danish Pathology Register.[8]

Comprehensive genomic data also have been reported from France, Italy, and Germany[6] where genomic screening is supported by the national health-care systems. These

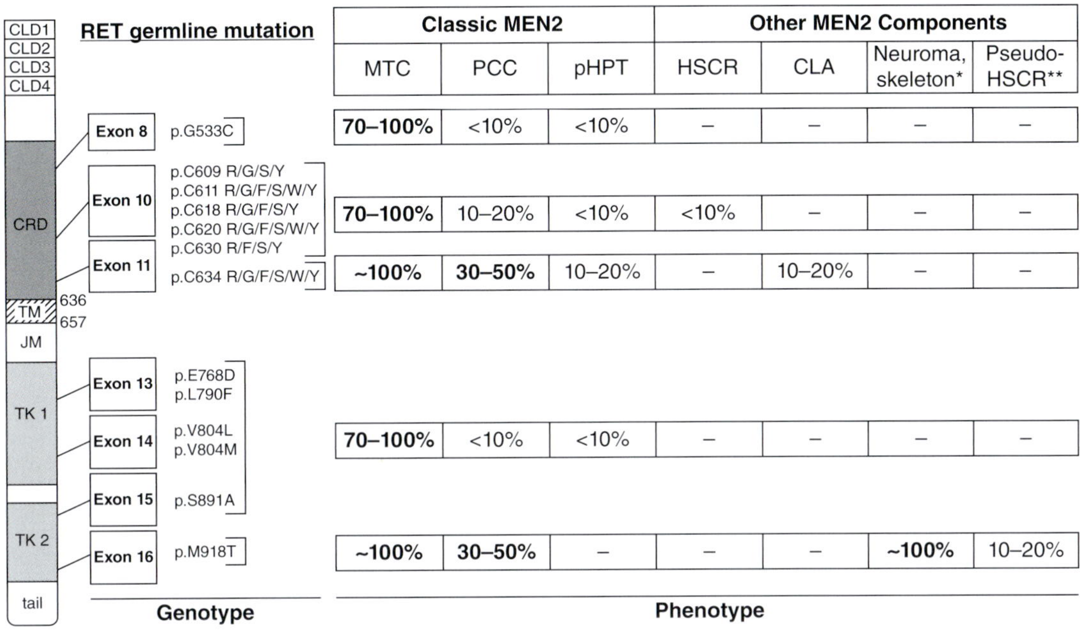

Figure 70–1. RET receptor mutations and clinical penetrance of MEN2.*

Bolded percents denote most common MEN2 characteristics. CLA, cutaneous lichen amyloidosis; CLD, cadherin-like domain; CRD, cysteine-rich domain; HSCR, Hirschsprung disease (aganglionic megacolon); JM, juxtamembrane domain; MTC, medullary thyroid carcinoma; PCC, pheochromocytoma; pHPT, primary hyperparathyroidism; TK, tyrosine kinase; TM, transmembrane domain.

*Multiple ocular, buccal, lingual, and lip neuromas and skeletal Malfarnoid malformations.

**Intestinal gangioneuromatosis.

Western European data showed broadly comparable distributions of clinically relevant mutational categories across countries[6,9-12] (Figure 70–3).

However, p.Cys634Arg is more prevalent than p.Cys634Tyr in the French, Italian, and German data, whereas the converse holds true for the data in the Spanish Online National Database and from the Brazilian Bras-MEN study.

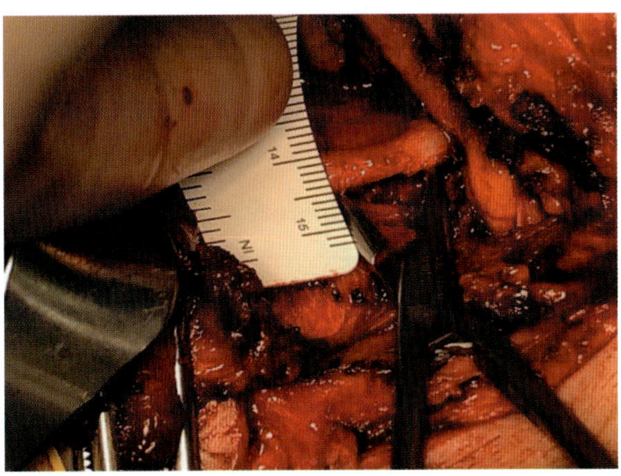

Figure 70–2. Thickened recurrent laryngeal nerve in a 33-year-old male p.Met918Thr carrier.

Founder mutations, although rare, have been described:[6]

- p.Gly533Cys, clustering in the southern part of central Greece (Fokis and around Lake Trichonis; 10 families) and in the Peleponnese (Laconia, mount Parnon region, and Arcadia; 11 families).
- p.Gly533Cys, which migrated from Spain (Catalunia region) to Southeastern Brazil in the late 1800s and may have originated from Greece.
- p.Cys611Tyr, clustering in Denmark.
- p.Cys618Arg, clustering in Cyprus (5 of the 9 families were from the same village in the Northwestern part of the Limassol province).
- p.Ser891Ala, clustering in Northern Italy (28 genetically related families), namely in Castione della Presolana in the mountainous Seriana valley, province of Bergamo, and the plain of Breccia.
- p.Met918Val, which migrated from Portugal (city of Braga) to the state of Ceará in Northeastern Brazil (currently 9 families) in the 1600s.

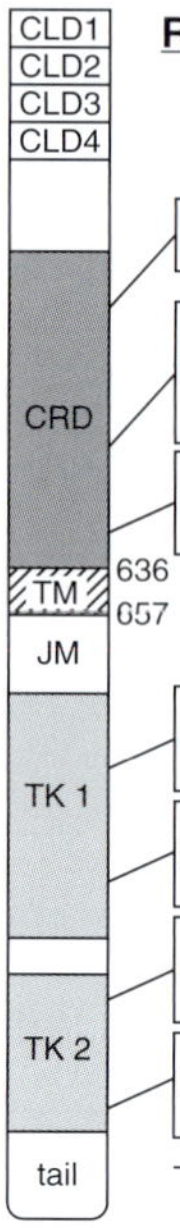

Exon	RET germline mutation	UK (103)	Germany (530)	France (420)	Italy (234)	Greece (119)	Brazil* (533)	China* (214)
Exon 8	p.G533C	1.0%	–	0.7%	–	28.6%	11.0%	–
Exon 10, Exon 11	p.C609 R/G/S/Y; p.C611 R/G/F/S/W/Y; p.C618 R/G/F/S/Y; p.C620 R/G/F/S/W/Y; p.C630 R/F/S/Y	25.2%	27.2%	18.6%	15.3%	27.7%	17.4%	33.2%
Exon 11	p.C634 R/G/F/S/W/Y	31.1%	34.7%	34.3%	37.1%	36.1%	49.2%	45.8%
Exon 13, Exon 14, Exon 15	p.E768D; p.L790F; p.V804L; p.V804M; p.S891A	31.1%	30.8%	39.3%	40.2%	3.4%	16.3%	18.7%
Exon 16	p.M918T	14.6%	7.4%	7.1%	7.4%	4.2%	6.0%	2.3%

Genotype (Exon, RET germline mutation); Phenotype (Country)

Figure 70–3. Geographic prevalence of RET receptor mutations.

*Limited to RET carriers with medullary thyroid cancer.

Column percents denote proportions of the respective RET mutations among all RET mutations per country, the numbers of which are given in parentheses in the column headers. CLD, cadherin-like domain; CRD, cysteine-rich domain; JM, juxtamembrane domain; TK, tyrosine kinase; TM, transmembrane domain.

Compared to the general population, gene carriers diagnosed at an older age have decreased life expectancies owing to pheochromocytoma-associated hypertensive crisis and metastatic medullary thyroid cancer.

PATHOGENESIS

RET Proto-oncogene & RET Tyrosine Kinase Receptor

The *RET* (*RE*arranged during *T*ransfection) proto-oncogene, located on chromosome 10q11.2, encodes for a transmembrane RET receptor tyrosine kinase. The RET receptor comprises an extracellular domain, a transmembrane domain, and an intracellular tyrosine kinase domain (Figure 70–1).

This RET receptor tyrosine kinase plays an important role in

- the proliferation and differentiation of neuroendocrine thyroid, adrenal, and parathyroid cells, producing a *"gain of function"* phenotype when mutated (Figure 70–1, left panel); and
- the craniocaudal migration of enteric neurons during the 5th to 12th week of gestation and in interactions critical for renal tubule formation between the epithelium at the tips of the ureteric bud and the metanephric mesenchyme, giving rise to "*loss of function*" phenotype when mutated (Figure 70–1, right panel).

RET mutations, clustering in "hot spot" regions and referred to as the "*primary hit*," are potent oncogenic drivers causing MEN2A and MEN2B. They typically are heterozygous (one mutated allele inherited from one parent), predominantly missense mutations, substituting one amino acid for another. Conceptually, homozygous patients who carry two mutated RET alleles inherited from consanguineous parents develop tumors earlier and MEN2A phenotypes more frequently.[13,14]

Gain of Function Phenotype

RET mutations set a genetic frame inside which MEN2A and MEN2B evolve (Figure 70–4).[1,2,15,16] Ligand-independent activation of the RET receptor (*gain of function*) drives the time-dependent development of MEN2A in a tissue-specific manner (parafollicular C cell hyperplasia > adrenal medullary hyperplasia > parathyroid chief cell hyperplasia).

The time when these neuroendocrine cells acquire somatic mutations in RET or other genes ("*second hits*") is difficult to predict, and may differ even within the same

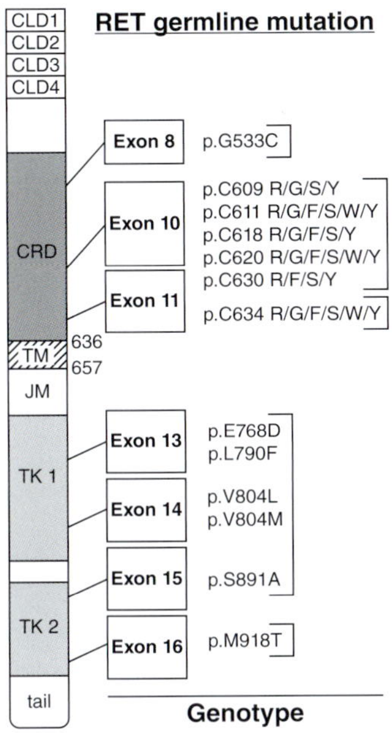

RET germline mutation	Age at diagnosis, yr, mean (range)					Mutational risk	
	MTC		PCC		pHPT	ATA[1]	MTC
	NO	N1	first	second*		(modif.)[2]	onset[15]
p.G533C	45 (23-72)	51 (21-72)	51 (34-65)	54 (45-66)	56	MOD (L-MOD)	D
p.C609/C611/C618/C620/C630	33 (1-67)	42 (15-75)	41 (22-57)	38 (36-38)	39 (32-45)	MOD–H	E
p.C634	19 (1-69)	31 (9-63)	35 (14-67)	36 (19-64)	40 (22-57)	H	EE
p.E768D, p.L790F, p.V804L, p.V804M, p.S891A	44 (12-75)	55 (10-81)	57 (39-72)	51 (44-55)	55 (54-55)	MOD (L-MOD)	D
p.M918T	6 (0.5-31)	16 (5-31)	26 (19-31)	29 (23-37)	–	HST	EEE

Phenotype

Figure 70–4. RET receptor mutations and development of MEN2.[2,16]

*Numbers indicate mean age (range) at surgery for the respective condition contralateral adrenal.

ATA, American Thyroid Association; CLD, cadherin-like domain; CRD, cysteine-rich domain; D, delayed; E, early; H, high; HST, highest; JM, juxtamembrane domain; L, low; MOD, moderate; MTC, medullary thyroid carcinoma; N0/1, node-negative/ node-positive; PCC, pheochromocytoma; pHPT, primary hyperparathyroidism; TK, tyrosine kinase; TM, transmembrane domain.

RET family, because these somatic events are subject to the play of chance.

As depicted in Figure 70–4, RET mutations are grouped into highest-risk (p.Met918Thr, always associated with MEN2B), high-risk (p.Cys634, associated with classic MEN2A), and moderate-risk mutations.[1] Moderate-risk mutations can be subdivided further into moderate-high (p.Cys609/611/618/620/630, occasionally associated with MEN2A) and low-moderate risk mutations (p.Glu768Asp, p.Leu790Phe, p.Val804Leu/Met, and p.Ser891Ala, infrequently associated with MEN2A).[2]

The greater the mutational strength, the faster the age-dependent progression from neoplastic C cell hyperplasia to node-negative, and ultimately to node-positive medullary thyroid cancer when not surgically treated; and the earlier and more frequent the development of pheochromocytoma and primary hyperparathyroidism. In carriers of strongly activating RET mutations, tumors typically are multifocal and involve both thyroid lobes and both adrenals. For high and moderate-high RET mutations, which are situated in the extracellular domain of the RET receptor, the transforming activity is the weaker the farther these mutations are positioned away from the cell membrane.

Loss of Function Phenotype

The *loss of function* phenotype, including Hirschsprung disease and renal malformations, likely is due to trapping of precursor RET receptors in the endoplasmatic reticulum, interfering with the transport of these proteins to the cell membrane, which decreases cell surface concentrations of the RET receptor.[3]

In patients exhibiting a *loss of function* phenotype, surgical intervention is more directed at the avoidance and correction of intestinal complications, which are fraught with significant morbidity.

These strong genotype-phenotype relationships (Figure 70–4) lay the groundwork for precision medicine in gene carriers harboring the trait.

PREVENTION

Appreciation of an individual's genetic predisposition to MEN2A or MEN2B is important to treat at an earlier stage, screen for other syndromic components, and initiate family cascade testing, moving from symptom-based to preventative medicine.[17]

Genomic screening is able to disclose a RET carrier's genetic susceptibility to medullary thyroid cancer, even before neoplastic C cell disease comes into being. The tight genotype-phenotype relationships in MEN2 provide a genetic framework within which unfolds the malignant transformation into early medullary thyroid cancer. Molecular information alone cannot predict this point in time precisely.

Prevention of tumor formation is the more feasible the earlier the person at risk is identified; the more adverse the consequences of tumor progression and metastasis; and the more expendable the affected organ. The thyroid is the organ that meets these requirements best, enabling prophylactic thyroidectomy in RET carriers.[18]

Biochemical screening, being more sensitive than high-resolution ultrasonography, is extremely useful to fill this void. When basal calcitonin serum levels start rising beyond the upper reference limit of the assay, typically <10 pg/mL for children aged 2 years and older,[19] transformation to medullary thyroid cancer is impending or just may have occurred. This biochemical threshold marks the last opportunity for prophylactic thyroidectomy without need for concomitant central node dissection.

The slow growth of medullary thyroid cancer provides some latitude for carriers of weakly transforming RET mutations whose basal calcitonin levels remain within normal limits. As long as basal calcitonin serum levels are ≤30 pg/mL, node metastases are absent.

This allows one, navigating between these biochemical landmarks, to delay, but not avoid, prophylactic thyroidectomy for some time.[18]

CLINICAL FINDINGS

Technological improvements in imaging, such as high-resolution ultrasonography, and in laboratory technology, notably the advent of sensitive hormone assays and gene tests, have been instrumental in capturing MEN2-associated tumors while they are still in their infancy and asymptomatic.[17]

- Recognition of the *signs and symptoms* produced by tumor growth and/or secretion of hormones by tumor cells used to be the backbone of MEN2A and MEN2B management.
- Starting in the 1980s, *laboratory findings* obtained routinely by systematic measurement of calcitonin, metanephrines, and normetanephrines, and intact parathyroid hormone started to dominate the scene because these biomarkers spot small tumors better than imaging.
- The laboratory finding of raised tissue-specific biomarkers, in turn, triggered *imaging studies* targeted at the putative source(s) of hormone production.
- If necessary, the clinical workup is complemented by *special tests and special examinations* to confirm the diagnosis and/or locate occult neuroendocrine tumor(s).

These advances have augmented tumor lead time in MEN2, which is defined as the length of time between tumor detection by screening and the usual clinical manifestations of the disease, and provide clinicians and patients with unprecedented "*windows of opportunity*."[17]

DIFFERENTIAL DIAGNOSIS

The differential diagnosis of the various neuroendocrine and nonendocrine features of MEN2A and MEN2B is basically the same as for each corresponding condition that occurs sporadically.

Nonetheless, there are important clinical clues pointing to MEN2A and MEN2B:

- Very early tumor development (eg, medullary thyroid cancer by age ≤20 years)
- Multiple tumor growth, especially when bilateral, within the same organ system
- Concurrence of rare tumors in one patient or within a patient's family (eg, medullary thyroid cancer and pheochromocytoma)
- Unusual combinations of signs and symptoms preceding tumor formation (eg, tearless crying and severe constipation in MEN2B; cutaneous lichen amyloidosis in MEN2A)

The more that these conditions coincide, the greater is the likelihood of a diagnosis of MEN2.

Severe constipation and bowel obstruction in early infancy call for a targeted clinical workup, which includes rectal suction biopsy and acetylcholine immunochemistry, to discriminate between congenital megacolon and intestinal ganglioneuromatosis.

Congenital megacolon (Hirschsprung disease), which may be connected to MEN2A, is characterized by colonic dilatation and lack of ganglionic nerve cells, and increased acetylcholinesterase activity in the aganglionic segment.

Intestinal ganglioneuromatosis (pseudo-Hirschsprung disease), indicative of MEN2B, in contrast is defined by ganglion cell hyperplasia of the submucosal and myenteric plexus.

As a rule, all thyroid tumors should be immunostained for calcitonin and CEA in order not to miss medullary thyroid cancer, which frequently is the first manifestation of MEN2A.

Upon diagnosis, all newly diagnosed patients with medullary thyroid cancer should be offered RET testing, regardless of family history, to rule out hereditary disease definitively.

DETERMING THE BEST COURSE OF ACTION

Before embarking on any treatment, the benefits to be expected from the intervention need to be weighed against the risks of that treatment and the natural course of the disease if left untreated.

Surgery is the most effective treatment for neuroendocrine tumors and usually the first choice in MEN2.

The benefit of total thyroidectomy (with vs without lymph node dissection), adrenalectomy (tissue-sparing vs total), and parathyroidectomy (of one vs more glands) is a continuous function of

- the risk of morbidity if left untreated (high for pheochromocytoma and medullary thyroid cancer; lower for primary hyperparathyroidism)
- the relative risk reduction achievable by the intervention (surgical cure, high in experienced hands)
- the risk of harm by the intervention (operative morbidity, low in experienced hands)

An important point in the trade-off between harms and benefits of surgical interventions is that many of the harms are front-loaded and occur much earlier than the benefits, in particular in asymptomatic patients.

All these considerations support the notion that RET carriers should ideally be treated at specialist centers experienced in the management of MEN2A and MEN2B.

TREATMENT

The concept of precision medicine entails that the intervention must be commensurate with the disease or risk at hand, with minimum ill consequences and maximum efficacy.

For MEN2A and MEN2B, surgery is the mainstay of therapy because it alone offers prevention of medullary thyroid cancer and cure of the neuroendocrine components of MEN2A and MEN2B.

Total Thyroidectomy

The objective of prophylactic thyroidectomy is not so much to prevent malignancy from occurring in the first place but to take out the thyroid gland before the disease has spread beyond the thyroid capsule. Involvement of neck lymph nodes makes it much more challenging to clear the tumor completely.

Before embarking on neck surgery for MEN2A or MEN2B, it is critical to rule out coexistent pheochromocytoma, which, if present, needs to be tackled first.

Total thyroidectomy is the procedure of choice in MEN2A and MEN2B because it removes the risk of malignant transformation inherent in each parafollicular C cell.

The optimal point in time for early total thyroidectomy is when a normal calcitonin test becomes abnormal by exceeding the upper normal reference limit of the calcitonin assay.

This biochemical conversion from normal to abnormal typically occurs:

- within the first year of life in carriers of highest-risk mutations (MEN2B)[7,18,20,21]
- before or around the age of 5 years in carriers of high-risk mutations (classic MEN2A)[18]
- after the age of 5 years in carriers of moderate-risk mutations[18]

Timing of early thyroidectomy, triggered by abnormal basal calcitonin test results which are more sensitive, has largely replaced timing of early thyroidectomy based on mutation-specific age thresholds.

To keep surgical morbidity to a minimum, the inferior parathyroid glands and recurrent laryngeal nerves are identified and preserved in situ before dissecting the thyroid gland off its bed, keeping the line of dissection as closely as possible to the thyroid capsule. Very useful for this purpose are optical magnification and bipolar forceps coagulation, nerve monitoring equipment, and in situ preservation of parathyroid glands or autografting of parathyroid glands that have become completely devascularized.

Space for maneuvering is more limited in infants and young children whose parathyroid glands are small, translucent, and hard to distinguish from soft tissues, thymus, and neck nodes.[18] In pediatric gene carriers, the thymus can take the size of a normal thyroid gland, compromising surgical exposure further. In experienced hands, infants aged ≤3 years have no greater operative morbidity than older children.[18]

Carriers who have normal basal calcitonin levels may safely forgo lymph node dissection, sparing them excess surgical morbidity inherent in the procedure, specifically postoperative hypoparathyroidism.

Compartment-Oriented Neck Dissection

In conjunction with total thyroidectomy, compartment-oriented microdissection[22] is the mainstay of therapy for hereditary MTC.

The authors' surgical concept, which is delineated in Figure 70–5, is centered on the presence of

- RET p.Met918Thr, substratified by diagnosis ≤4 versus >4 years of age, versus
- RET mutations other than p.Met918Thr, substratified by calcitonin status (normal vs increased)

For non-p.Met918Thr RET carriers whose basal serum calcitonin is raised, the clinical nodal status helps to calibrate the extent of microdissection (central versus central plus bilateral microdissection).

Adrenalectomy

Laparoscopic or retroperitoneoscopic adrenalectomy is the procedure of choice for the treatment of unilateral or bilateral pheochromocytoma.

Unless the tumor occupies most or all of the adrenal gland, subtotal (also referred to as "*tissue-sparing*") adrenalectomy is the preferred option, even for unilateral pheochromocytoma.[17]

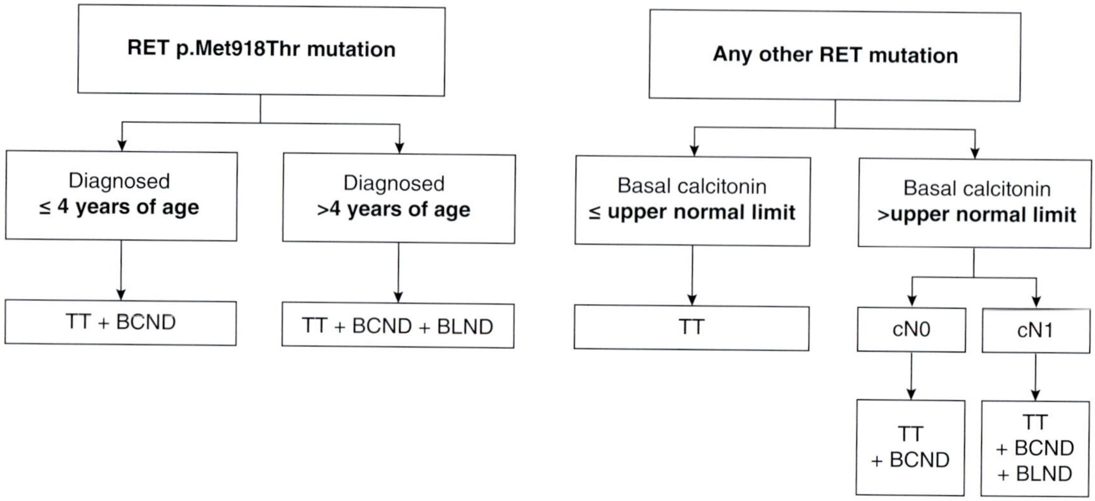

Figure 70–5. Authors' surgical concept for hereditary medullary thyroid cancer.
BCND, bilateral central node dissection; BLND, bilateral lateral node dissection; cN0/cN1, clinically (pre-/intraoperatively) node-negative/node-positive; TT, total thyroidectomy.

Although some subclinical postoperative compromise is common, adrenal remnants can usually compensate for the loss of 70% to 85% of adrenal tissue.[17]

The goal of subtotal adrenalectomy is to minimize the risk of postoperative adrenal insufficiency and Addisonian crisis, which used to be the most frequent life-limiting event.

Parathyroidectomy

Extirpation of grossly enlarged parathyroids alone usually is sufficient because primary hyperparathyroidism is almost always mild in MEN2A.[17] Wherever feasible, normal parathyroids should be preserved in situ. Total parathyroidectomy with autografting of parathyroid slivers has been abandoned because it carries a 6% risk of permanent hypoparathyroidism.

Parathyroidectomy for primary hyperparathyroidism is curative when the intraoperative quick test shows a ≥50% fall of the intact parathyroid hormone serum level relative to the upper normal reference limit of the PTH assay after parathyroid resection.

PROGNOSIS

The clinical outcome of surgery for MEN2A and MEN2B hinges on "*what has been left behind.*" In general, interventions for MEN2 are deemed successful when raised tumor markers normalize or become unmeasurable after the operation.

When *the organ is more expendable* such as the thyroid, the one-time cost of achieving definitive cure and the cost of daily thyroxine supplementation may be smaller from a societal perspective than the need for continual biochemical follow-up and imaging studies, which may prompt further operations at additional cost.

When *the organ is less expendable* such as adrenals and parathyroids, preservation of organ function (subtotal adrenalectomy and parathyroidectomy of single glands) becomes the primary objective. The benefit of intact organ function must be balanced against the risk of *de novo* tumors arising from the residual adrenal or parathyroid tissue.

Postoperatively, gene carriers need regular follow-up investigations, not just for recurrence but also for adequate hormone substitution. The risk of subsequent tumor formation, which would require another operation, is more relevant to carriers of highest and high-risk mutations (Figure 70–4) and ordinarily low.

Earlier surgical intervention at specialist centers experienced in the management of MEN2A and MEN2B has resulted in superior clinical outcome: biochemical cure rates approximating 100%; absence of residual structural disease or recurrence; and rarely any permanent operative morbidity.

These achievements hold the hope that death and major morbidity from MEN2A and MEN2B can be eliminated in our lifetime.

REFERENCES

1. Wells SA Jr, Asa SL, Dralle H, et al. Revised American Thyroid Association guidelines for the management of medullary thyroid carcinoma. *Thyroid.* 2015;25(6):567-610.
2. Machens A, Lorenz K, Weber F, Dralle H. Genotype-specific progression of hereditary medullary thyroid cancer. *Hum Mutat.* 2018;39(6):860-869.

3. Machens A, Lorenz K, Dralle H. Kidney malformations and Hirschsprung's disease in carriers of cysteine mutations in exon 10 of the RET proto-oncogene. *Endocrine.* 2021;73(1):217-222.
4. Machens A, Elwerr M, Lorenz K, Weber F, Dralle H. 100-year evolution of precision medicine and surgery for multiple endocrine neoplasia type 2A. *Endocrine.* 2020;68(2):368-376.
5. Machens A, Lorenz K, Weber F, Dralle H. Recurrent ipsilateral pheochromocytoma in carriers of RET p.Cys634 missense mutations. *Endocrine.* 2022;77(1):160-167.
6. Machens A, Dralle H. Long-term outcome after DNA-based prophylactic neck surgery in children at risk of hereditary medullary thyroid cancer. *Best Pract Res Clin Endocrinol Metab.* 2019;33(4):101274.
7. Machens A, Lorenz K, Weber F, Dralle H. Prophylactic neck surgery for second-generation multiple endocrine neoplasia type 2B. *Eur J Surg Oncol.* 2021;47(4):924-927.
8. Mathiesen JS, Kroustrup JP, Vestergaard P, et al. Incidence and prevalence of sporadic and hereditary MTC in Denmark 1960-2014: a nationwide study. *Endocr Connect.* 2018;7(6): 829-839.
9. Fussey JM, Smith JA, Cleaver R, et al. Diagnostic RET genetic testing in 1,058 index patients: a UK centre perspective. *Clin Endocrinol.* 2021;95(2):295-302.
10. Sarika HL, Papathoma A, Garofalaki M, et al. Genetic screening of patients with medullary thyroid cancer in a referral center in Greece during the past two decades. *Eur J Endocrinol.* 2015;172(4):501-509.
11. Maciel RMB, Camacho CP, Assumpção LVM, et al. Genotype and phenotype landscape of MEN2 in 554 medullary thyroid cancer patients: the BrasMEN study. *Endocr Connect.* 2019;8(3):289-298.
12. Qi XP, Zhao JQ, Fang XD, et al. Spectrum of germline RET variants identified by targeted sequencing and associated Multiple Endocrine Neoplasia type 2 susceptibility in China. *BMC Cancer.* 2021;21(1):369.
13. Schirwani S, Frazer S, Mushtaq T, et al. Homozygosity for the pathogenic RET hotspot variant p.Cys634Trp: a consanguineous family with MEN2A. *Eur J Med Genet.* 2021;64(2):104141.
14. Machens A, Dralle H. Accelerated MEN2A in homozygous RET carriers in the context of consanguinity. *Eur J Endocrinol* 2024;190(3):K43-K46.
15. Machens A, Lorenz K, Weber F, Dralle H. Exceptionality of distant metastasis in node-negative hereditary and sporadic medullary thyroid cancer: lessons learned. *J Clin Endocrinol Metab.* 2021;13;106(8):e2968-e2979.
16. Machens A, Lorenz K; Dralle H. Peak incidence of pheochromocytoma and primary hyperparathyroidism in multiple endocrine neoplasia 2: need for age-adjusted biochemical screening. *J Clin Endocrinol Metab.* 2013;98(2):E336-E345.
17. Machens A, Lorenz K, Brandenburg T, Führer-Sakel D, Weber F, Dralle H. The changing face of multiple endocrine neoplasia 2A: from symptom-based to preventative medicine. *J Clin Endocrinol Metab.* 2023;108(9):e734-e742.
18. Machens A, Ellwerr M, Lorenz K, Weber F, Dralle H. Long-term outcome of prophylactic thyroidectomy in children carrying RET germline mutations. *Br J Surg.* 2018;105(2):e150-e157.
19. Castagna MG, Fugazzola L, Maino F, et al. Reference range of serum calcitonin in pediatric population. *J Clin Endocrinol Metab.* 2015;100(5):1780-1784.
20. Raue F, Dralle H, Machens A, Bruckner T, Frank-Raue K. Long-term survivorship in multiple endocrine neoplasia type 2B diagnosed before and in the new millennium. *J Clin Endocrinol Metab.* 2018;103(1):235-243.
21. Castinetti F, Waguespack SG, Machens A, et al. Natural history, treatment, and long-term follow up of patients with multiple endocrine neoplasia type 2B: an international, multicentre, retrospective study. *Lancet Diabetes Endocrinol.* 2019;7(3):213-220.
22. Dralle H, Damm I, Scheumann GF, et al. Compartment-oriented microdissection of regional lymph nodes in medullary thyroid carcinoma. *Surg Today.* 1994;24(2):112-121.

71 Multiple Endocrine Neoplasia Type 4 (MEN 4)

Oliver Gimm, MD
Natalia S. Pellegata, PhD

GENERAL CONSIDERATIONS (INCLUDES EPIDEMIOLOGY & CLINICALLY HELPFUL BACKGROUND STATEMENTS)

Various multiple endocrine neoplasia (MEN) syndromes are known. Patients with multiple endocrine neoplasia type 1 (MEN 1) which is caused by mutations in the *MEN1* gene[1] have mainly an increased risk of developing primary hyperparathyroidism (pHPT), adenomas of the anterior pituitary gland, and neuroendocrine neoplasms (NEN) in the foregut (pancreas, duodenum, stomach).

Multiple endocrine neoplasia type 2 (MEN 2) is subdivided into MEN 2A and MEN 2B. Patients with MEN 2A mainly have an increased risk of developing medullary thyroid carcinoma (MTC), pheochromocytoma (PCC), and pHPT. Patients with MEN 2B also have an increased risk of developing MTC and PCC, whereas pHPT is not part of the MEN 2B phenotype. Instead, patients with MEN 2B develop mucosal neuromas, thickened corneal nerves, and present with a marfanoid habitus. The term multiple endocrine neoplasia type 3 (MEN 3) was initially used for patients with MEN 2B since the phenotype of these patients differed from those having MEN 2A, which at that time was named simply MEN 2. However, when it was recognized that germline mutations in the same gene are responsible for both the MEN 2A and MEN 2B variants.[2,3] MEN 2 was subdivided into MEN 2A and MEN 2B and the term MEN 3 was abandoned.

A "fourth" multiple endocrine neoplasia syndrome (MEN 4) was identified in humans during the first decade of the second millennium.[4] The syndrome was initially reported in rats, where it was named MENX.[5] In humans, MEN 4 mostly resembles MEN 1, while in rats MENX shares phenotypic features with both MEN 1 and MEN 2.[6]

PATHOGENESIS

Inactivating germline mutations in the *CDKN1B* gene, which encodes the cyclin-dependent kinase (CDK) inhibitor P27KIP1, cause MEN 4. A summary of the germline *CDKN1B* mutations so far identified in humans is shown in Table 71–1. Under normal conditions, P27KIP1 binds to and inhibits cyclin E,A/CDK2 complexes in the nucleus. By doing so, P27KIP1 inhibits cell cycle progression.[7] *CDKN1B* mutations identified in MEN 4 were mostly found to be inactivating[8] leading to reduced or absent expression of P27KIP1, to impaired interaction with protein partners, to protein mislocalization, or enhanced degradation.

P27KIP1 is a pleiotropic protein with functions that go beyond cell cycle regulation, including cell motility, and transcriptional regulation.[9] The precise molecular mechanisms linking reduced/absent P27KIP1 expression to the formation of various diseases including (neuro)endocrine tumors are not fully understood but are likely not limited to deregulated cell cycle progression.

PREVENTION

In humans, the inheritance of MEN 4 is autosomal dominant. If one inherits an MEN 4-specific germline mutation in *CDKN1B*, nothing can be done to prevent the development of tumors/diseases associated with MEN 4. Thus, the aim must be to identify reasonable surveillance guidelines that are lacking as of today. It should be kept in mind that the penetrance of a *CDKN1B* mutation (the probability that the mutation carrier develops a neoplasm) is not necessarily 100% (see following discussion).

CLINICAL FINDINGS

Due to the limited number of patients identified as of today, the phenotype of MEN 4 is still not well defined (Table 71–1). Currently, also due to the lack of any known genotype-phenotype correlation, it is unknown how mutation carriers should be screened for the development of potential tumors/diseases. Of note, more than 75% of the patients identified so far are women.

Table 71–1. Genotype-phenotype correlation in MEN 4.

CDKN1B/P27KIP2 Sequence Variant	Reported Phenotype/ Clinical Findings
5′ UTR	
-456_-453delCCTT	fPA (GH), pancreatic NEN
-80C>T	Sporadic pHPT
-73G>A	Gigantism, neurodevelopmental defects
-32_-29delGAGA	pHPT, gastric NEN
-29_-26delAGAG	Sporadic pHPT, gigantism, Cushing disease
-7G->C	pHPT, bilateral nonfunctioning adrenal tumors
Exon 1	
G9R	Sporadic pHPT
K25fs	pHPT, fPA (ACTH), NEN
L41fs	pHPT, fPA, nfPA, NEN
A55T	pHPT, NEN (gastrinoma)
Q65H	Colorectla cancer
P69L	pHPT, nfPA, lung NEN, papillary thyroid carcinoma
W76X	pHPT, fPA (GH)
F80Q	Hairy cell leukemia
P94L	Hairy cell leukemia
P95S	pHPT, pancreatic NEN (gastrinoma)
K96Q	fPA (prolactin)
V109G	nfPA
I119T	fPA (ACTH)
S125X	pHPT, gastric NEN
E126D	pHPT
P133T	pHPT, papillary thyroid carcinoma, goiter, meningioma

fPA = functioning pituitary adenoma; fs = frameshift; NEN = neuroendocrine neoplasm; nfPA = nonfunctioning pituitary adenoma; pHPT = primary hyperparathyroidism.

(Neuro)endocrine Tumors

A. Primary Hyperparathyroidism

The commonest phenotypic feature of patients with MEN 4 is pHPT. Overall, the penetrance of pHPT seems to be very high (>85%)[10] which is very similar to MEN 1-associated pHPT. However, in contrast to MEN 1, only one gland has been reported to be affected in about 50% of MEN 4 patients.[11]

B. Pituitary Gland Adenomas

The second most common manifestation of the MEN 4 syndrome is adenomas of the anterior pituitary gland.[11] Looking at all the published cases, these tumors seem to develop in 30% to 40% of the patients. In a large family, they have been reported in about 30% of all mutation carriers.[10] Both nonfunctioning and functioning (ACTH-, GH-, prolactin-, somatotropin-secreting) pituitary adenomas have been reported. One polymorphism in *CDKN1B* (rs2066827, V109G) has been reported to be associated with ACTH-secreting pituitary adenomas.[12]

C. Neuroendocrine Neoplasms

The third most common endocrine manifestation in MEN 4 is neuroendocrine neoplasms (NEN). They have been reported in about 25% of all available mutation carriers but may be less common in some families.[10] As in MEN 1, NENs in MEN 4 develop in the foregut (lungs, stomach, duodenum, and pancreas). Both functioning (gastrin-secreting) and nonfunctioning NENs have been reported.

D. Other (Neuro)endocrine Tumors

Apart from these (neuro)endocrine tumors, patients with MEN 4 have reported to develop various types of thyroid tumors including thyroid cancers, in particular the follicular variant of papillary thyroid cancer.[13] In addition, bilateral adrenal tumors have been reported.[14]

Non-(Neuro)endocrine Tumors

Non-(neuro)endocrine tumors reported in patients with germline mutation in *CDKN1B* include colorectal carcinoma,[15] prostate cancer,[16] and testicular cancer[5] as well as meningiomas.[11]

DIFFERENTIAL DIAGNOSIS

MEN 4 may clinically appear as MEN 1 (Table 71–2). Thus, MEN 1 is the main differential diagnosis. Due to the rarity of MEN 4, patients should first be screened for mutations in the *MEN1* gene. Based on published studies, up to 10% of patients with clinically typical signs of MEN 1 do not harbor a germline mutation or a large genomic alteration in the *MEN1* gene.[8] If no mutation in the *MEN1* gene is found, patients may be candidates for mutation screening in the *CDKN1B* gene. When analyzing these patients for inactivating alterations in *CDKN1B*, mutations have only

Table 71–2. (Neuro)endocrine findings in patients with MEN 4.

Clinical Finding	Frequency
Primary hyperparathyroidism	85%-95%
Pituitary adenomas (both functioning and nonfunctioning)	30%-40%
Neuroendocrine neoplasms	25%
Goiter, thyroid cancer, adrenal tumors	Few case reports

been found in about 2% of cases[11,14,18] or slightly more often.[19,20] Of note, about 2% of patients undergoing surgery for apparently sporadic parathyroid adenomas harbor a germline mutation in *CDKN1B*.[21,22] The same applies to patients with familial isolated pituitary adenomas (FIPA), where germline mutations in *CDKN1B* have been found in less than 3% of cases.[23]

It is of interest that most of the clinical manifestations in female patients seem to arise around the age of menopause, which is later in comparison to MEN 1,[11] but exceptions exist.[8]

COMPLICATIONS

While the phenotype of MEN 4 is still not well defined (Table 71–1), it appears that the syndrome is mainly associated with the development of a variety of endocrine tumors. Due to the overall very low number of patients, no MEN 4-specific complications are known. However, the complications that can be expected are probably very similar to those associated to the sporadic counterpart of MEN 4-associated tumors, for example, osteoporosis, kidney stones, and cardiovascular disease for pHPT.

TREATMENT

In general, (neuro)endocrine tumors are mainly treated surgically. As the number of patients diagnosed with germline *CDKN1B* mutations is still very low, recommendations on the treatment of tumors that are associated with MEN 4 have to be given cautiously. So far, treatments to be performed have been recommended on a case-by-case basis, following existing guidelines for other MEN syndromes.[8]

Primary Hyperparathyroidism

As in MEN 1, multiglandular parathyroid gland involvement has been reported in patients with MEN 4. Nevertheless, it seems that many MEN 4 patients do not develop multiglandular disease. Thus, bilateral neck exploration with removal of only enlarged parathyroid glands seems to be a justified approach.[8,24] Even a more limited approach including the use of intraoperative PTH measurement may be reasonable since about 50% of the patients only seem to develop uniglandular disease.

Pituitary Gland Adenoma

In comparison to patients with MEN 1, pituitary adenomas appear to be smaller and less aggressive in patients with MEN 4.[8] Theoretically, this could imply that the surgical treatment of pituitary adenomas in patients with MEN 4 is associated with a higher rate of cure and a lower rate of side effects but this awaits further confirmation once additional patients are available.

Neuroendocrine Neoplasms

As in MEN 1, neuroendocrine neoplasms associated with MEN 4 have been found in the foregut (Table 71–1). Since the number of patients is very low, no MEN 4-specific recommendation can be given with regard to the surgical treatment of these tumors.

PROGNOSIS

Due to the very low number of published cases, little is known regarding the prognosis of patients with MEN 4. Since some diseases (eg, pHPT, pituitary gland adenomas) seem to be milder as compared to MEN 1, the prognosis of patients with MEN 4 may therefore be better.

WHEN TO REFER/WHEN TO ADMIT

Patients that clinically fulfill the criteria of having MEN 1, but are negative for mutations in the *MEN1* gene, are potential candidates for mutation analysis of the *CDKN1B* gene in these patients, something which has been recommended.[8] However, since germline mutations in the *CDKN1B* gene are found in only 2% to 3% of potential candidate patients, *CDKN1B* mutation screening has not become routine in clinical practice. Nevertheless, if every patient suspected of having MEN 1[25] but without a mutation in the *MEN1* gene would be screened for mutations in *CDKN1B*, more MEN 4 patients should be rapidly identified. This would enable more precise determination of the natural course of the various tumors/diseases associated with MEN 4, as well as the ability to confirm whether any genotype-phenotype correlations exist. Subsequently, more informed recommendations regarding surveillance and treatment could be given to *CDKN1B* mutation-positive patients.

REFERENCES

1. Chandrasekharappa SC, Guru SC, Manickam P, et al. Positional cloning of the gene for multiple endocrine neoplasia-type 1. *Science*. 1997;276:404-407.
2. Carlson KM, Dou S, Chi D, et al. Single missense mutation in the tyrosine kinase catalytic domain of the RET protooncogene is associated with multiple endocrine neoplasia type 2B. *Proc Natl Acad Sci USA*. 1994;91:1579-1583.
3. Mulligan LM, Kwok JB, Healey CS, et al. Germ-line mutations of the RET proto-oncogene in multiple endocrine neoplasia type 2A. *Nature*. 1993;363:458-460.
4. Georgitsi M. MEN-4 and other multiple endocrine neoplasias due to cyclin-dependent kinase inhibitors (p27(Kip1) and p18(INK4C)) mutations. *Best Pract Res Clin Endocrinol Metab*. 2010;24:425-437.
5. Pellegata NS, Quintanilla-Martinez L, Siggelkow H, et al. Germ-line mutations in p27Kip1 cause a multiple endocrine neoplasia syndrome in rats and humans. *Proc Natl Acad Sci USA*. 2006;103:15558-15563.
6. Pellegata NS. MENX and MEN4. *Clinics (Sao Paulo)*. 2012;67 Suppl 1:13-18.

7. Lee M, Pellegata NS. Multiple endocrine neoplasia syndromes associated with mutation of p27. *J Endocrinol Invest.* 2013;36:781-787.
8. Alrezk R, Hannah-Shmouni F, Stratakis CA. MEN4 and *CDKN1B* mutations: the latest of the MEN syndromes. *Endocr Relat Cancer.* 2017;24:T195-T208.
9. Razavipour SF, Harikumar KB, Slingerland JM. p27 as a transcriptional regulator: new roles in development and cancer. *Cancer Res.* 2020;80:3451-3458.
10. Frederiksen A, Rossing M, Hermann P, Ejersted C, Thakker RV, Frost M. Clinical features of multiple endocrine neoplasia type 4: novel pathogenic variant and review of published cases. *J Clin Endocrinol Metab.* 2019;104:3637-3646.
11. Tonelli F, Giudici F, Giusti F, et al. A heterozygous frameshift mutation in exon 1 of CDKN1B gene in a patient affected by MEN4 syndrome. *Eur J Endocrinol.* 2014;171:K7-K17.
12. Sekiya T, Bronstein MD, Benfini K, et al. p27 variant and corticotropinoma susceptibility: a genetic and in vitro study. *Endocr Relat Cancer.* 2014;21:395-404.
13. Landa I, Montero-Conde C, Malanga D, et al. Allelic variant at −79 (C>T) in *CDKN1B* (p27Kip1) confers an increased risk of thyroid cancer and alters mRNA levels. *Endocr Relat Cancer.* 2010;17:317-328.
14. Agarwal SK, Mateo CM, Marx SJ. Rare germline mutations in cyclin-dependent kinase inhibitor genes in multiple endocrine neoplasia type 1 and related states. *J Clin Endocrinol Metab.* 2009;94:1826-1834.
15. Esteban-Jurado C, Vila-Casadesus M, Garre P, et al. Whole-exome sequencing identifies rare pathogenic variants in new predisposition genes for familial colorectal cancer. *Genet Med.* 2015;17:131-142.
16. Chang BL, Zheng SL, Isaacs SD, et al. A polymorphism in the CDKN1B gene is associated with increased risk of hereditary prostate cancer. *Cancer Res.* 2004;64:1997-1999.
17. Bugalho MJ, Domingues R. Uncommon association of cerebral meningioma, parathyroid adenoma and papillary thyroid carcinoma in a patient harbouring a rare germline variant in the CDKN1B gene. *BMJ Case Rep.* 2016;2016.
18. Occhi G, Regazzo D, Trivellin G, et al. A novel mutation in the upstream open reading frame of the CDKN1B gene causes a MEN4 phenotype. *PLoS Genet.* 2013;9:e1003350.
19. Molatore S, Marinoni I, Lee M, et al. A novel germline CDKN1B mutation causing multiple endocrine tumors: clinical, genetic and functional characterization. *Hum Mutat.* 2010;31:E1825-E1835.
20. Borsari S, Pardi E, Pellegata NS, et al. Loss of p27 expression is associated with MEN1 gene mutations in sporadic parathyroid adenomas. *Endocrine.* 2017;55:386-397.
21. Costa-Guda J, Marinoni I, Molatore S, Pellegata NS, Arnold A. Somatic mutation and germline sequence abnormalities in CDKN1B, encoding p27Kip1, in sporadic parathyroid adenomas. *J Clin Endocrinol Metab.* 2011;96:E701-E706.
22. Georgitsi M, Raitila A, Karhu A, et al. Germline CDKN1B/p27Kip1 mutation in multiple endocrine neoplasia. *J Clin Endocrinol Metab.* 2007;92:3321-5.
23. Tichomirowa MA, Lee M, Barlier A, et al. Cyclin-dependent kinase inhibitor 1B (CDKN1B) gene variants in AIP mutation-negative familial isolated pituitary adenoma kindreds. *Endocr Relat Cancer.* 2012;19:233-241.
24. Marini F, Cianferotti L, Giusti F, Brandi ML. Molecular genetics in primary hyperparathyroidism: the role of genetic tests in differential diagnosis, disease prevention strategy, and therapeutic planning. A 2017 update. *Clin Cases Miner Bone Metab.* 2017;14:60-70.
25. Kamilaris CDC, Stratakis CA. Multiple endocrine neoplasia Type 1 (MEN1): an update and the significance of early genetic and clinical diagnosis. *Front Endocrinol (Lausanne).* 2019;10:339.

72 Familial Endocrine Syndromes Associated With Adrenomedullary Tumors (Recklinghausen Disease, von Hippel Lindau Syndrome, Pheochromocytoma-Paraganglioma Syndrome)

Tobias Åkerström, MD, PhD Per Hellman, MD, PhD

INTRODUCTION

Pheochromocytomas/paragangliomas (PPGL) are endocrine tumors derived from neural crest cells—pheochromocytomas from the adrenal medulla and paragangliomas from the sympathetic/parasympathetic paraganglia. PPGLs have the highest likelihood of being driven by germline mutations, with 40% being caused by inherited constitutional mutations in susceptibility genes. The genetic background of hereditary PPGL has been elucidated in great detail in recent years. Mutations in different genes are associated with different phenotypes. Knowledge of this genotype-phenotype correlation is clinically important in guiding biochemical analyses, imaging, and treatment modalities, including the type of surgery as well as appropriate follow-up. Therefore, genetic testing is recommended for all patients with PPGL. Malignancy is rare, and difficult to diagnose based on histopathology alone. Certain genetic mutations indicate an increased risk for malignancy, which should be taken into consideration when following the patient. For example, the most concerning mutations are SDHB gene mutations which present clinically with larger tumor size (>5 cm), and high Ki67 index.

CLUSTERS

Global gene analyses on tumor tissue have shown that PPGL may be divided into three distinct clusters.[1] Cluster 1 tumors are characterized by a pseudohypoxic response (~100% germline), with a risk of malignancy of about 25%. Cluster 2 tumors are characterized by mutations in genes involved in kinase signaling (25% germline, 4% malignant), and Cluster 3 with mutations associated with derangement in the Wnt signaling pathways (0% germline, 11% malignant).[1,2] This three-cluster taxonomy is useful in predicting the tumor behavior and can guide physicians in clinical decision-making. Hence, we will use this as a framework in our further discussion for describing the different susceptibility genes and their clinical consequences. The RET gene belonging to Cluster 2 and causing MEN2 syndrome will be discussed in a separate chapter.

CLUSTER 1

For Cluster 1 tumors there is a defect in the hypoxia response pathway.[3] In normal cells and in normoxic conditions, hypoxia-inducible factors (HIFs) are rapidly degraded due to hydroxylation on prolyl residues, which leads to recognition by a complex with the VHL protein, subsequent ubiquination, and degradation by the proteasome.[4] Genetic alterations that cause a constitutively active hypoxic response may lead to familial PPGL disease with tumors showing Cluster 1 properties. The Cluster 1 is further divided into those that alter components of the TCA cycle (Cluster C1A) and those that alter the hypoxia signaling pathway (Cluster C1B).[5] The susceptibility genes for Cluster C1A include succinate dehydrogenase subunits (*SDHA, SDHB, SDHC, SDHD*), succinate dehydrogenase complex assembly factor-2 (*SDHAF2*), fumarate hydrogenase (*FH*), mitochondrial glutamic-oxaloacetic transaminase (*GOT2*), 2-oxoglutarate-malate-carrier (*SLC25A11*), malate dehydrogenase (*MDH2*).

Dihydrolipoamide S-succinyltransferase (*DLST*) and those for Cluster C1B include von-Hippel Lindau (*VHL*), hypoxia-inducible factor 2α (*HIF2A/EPAS1*), and Egl-9 prolyl hydroxylase-1 and -2 (*EGLN1/2*).[6] Those with a C1A phenotype are associated with oncometabolite accumulation (succinate, fumarate, and 2-hydroxyglutarate) which ultimately affect the HIF pathway. Those with a C1B phenotype instead directly alter the HIF pathway.[6]

CLUSTER 1–C1A

Pathophysiology

Constitutional mutations in the succinate dehydrogenase complex subunits (*SDHA*, *SDHB*, *SDHC,* and *SDHD*) are the most common inherited forms of PPGL.[7] Mutations in *SDHAF2*, *FH*, *GOT2*, *SLC25A11*, and *MDH2* are much rarer. Cluster C1A mutations are inherited in an autosomal dominant fashion. For *SDHD* and *SDHAF2*, only inheritance of the paternal allele carries risk of disease due to maternal allele imprinting.[7,8] Characteristic of these genes is a tumor suppressor role, where inactivation leads to accumulation of oncometabolites, succinate for SDHx, and fumarate for FH patients. This accumulation stabilizes HIFs which in turn creates a pseudohypoxic state leading to increased angiogenesis and cell proliferation.[9,10] Further, activation of alpha-ketoglutarate-dependent dioxygenases leads to alterations in histone and DNA methylation, creating a hypermethylator phenotype, known as CpG island methylator phenotype (CIMP).[10,11] High CIMP is mainly related to SDHx mutations and especially SDHB.[11] CIMP leads to silencing of genes involved in chromaffin differentiation, an epithelial to mesenchymal transition, and are linked to malignant behavior. Finally, in SDHx tumors, inhibition of lysine demethylases causes suppressed homologous repair.[12] This is a process necessary for DNA strand repair, which provides another mechanistic basis for oncogenic potential, but also for treatment with poly (ADP)-ribose polymerase (PARP) inhibitors.[12,13]

Biochemical

Because of tumor expression profiles of key enzymes in catecholamine synthesis, patients with C1A tumors have a distinct secretory profile. Most are noradrenergic due to low expression of the enzyme dopamine-β-hydroxylase and phenyl-ethanolamine-N-methyltransferase responsible for the conversion to epinephrine.[1,14] Some only produce dopamine or its metabolite methoxytyramine, which is associated with a more aggressive phenotype.[11,15,16] Some may lack expression of tyrosine hydroxylase, the rate-limiting enzyme in catecholamine synthesis, leading to nonfunctioning tumors.[17,18] These cases pose a diagnostic problem and biochemical screening should not be restricted to metanephrines/normetanephrines/metoxythyramines. Instead, chromogranin A has been suggested as a complementary diagnostic laboratory test, and imaging tests become more important.[19]

Imaging

PPGL have variable expression of proteins on their cell surface that are dependent on genotype and differentiation.[20] These may be used for different imaging and treatment modalities. MIBG is a guanidine analogue structurally comparable to norepinephrine; it concentrates in cells expressing catecholamine transporters. For SDHx tumors there is relatively low expression of these transporters.[21] Therefore, MIBG imaging shows less sensitivity/specificity especially in malignant disease in the background of SDHx mutations.[22] Due to their defects in the electron transport chain and the TCA (Krebs) cycle they display increased anaerobic metabolism, which in turn increases glycolysis and expression of glucose transporters on the cell surface, a phenomenon called the Warburg effect.[23] Therefore, 18FDG PET shows high sensitivity and specificity.[20] Importantly, SDHx tumors have high expression of somatostatin receptors (SSTR), especially type 2 (SSTR2), even in dedifferentiated malignant tumors, making them detectable with somatostatin receptor-based imaging and theranostic treatment.[24,25] Currently, ^{68}Gallium-DOTATATE PET/CT scanning has shown the highest sensitivity/specificity in C1A tumors and is considered the gold standard for detection when available. If unavailable, 18FDG PET is the preferred modality.[20,26] For patients with FH mutations data are scarce but their tumors may be better visualized with ^{18}F-FDOPA.[27]

Clinical/Treatment Considerations for Cluster C1A

Tumors with C1A mutations present in younger patients with extra-adrenal disease, and there is an increased risk of malignancy, especially in *SDHB*-mutated patients.[2] There is high expression of somatostatin receptors and usually, there is a distinct expression pattern of enzymes involved in the synthesis of catecholamines.[28] Patients with germline SDHx mutations may also develop renal cell carcinomas, pituitary tumors, pulmonary chondromas, and gastrointestinal stromal tumors (GIST).[17] Germline mutations in *FH* cause hereditary leiomyomatosis renal cell carcinoma syndrome.[29]

Surgery is the first line of treatment for extra-adrenal PGLs and PCCs in most patients with C1A tumors. In *SDHB*-mutated patients' special considerations include the higher risk of malignancy. Therefore, a more aggressive surgical approach should be considered.[30] In heritable adrenal disease in general, there is an increased risk of bilateral adrenal disease and multifocal tumors. Therefore, adrenal-sparing surgery is usually considered.[31] However, it is usually not recommended for SDHx tumors and especially not in *SDHB*-mutated tumors.[32]

HEAD & NECK PARAGANGLIOMAS

Another common presentation in SDHx tumors are head and neck tumors that may arise in the carotid body, near the vagal nerve and the jugular foramen, usually arising from parasympathetic tissue, and therefore rarely hormone producing. They usually have an indolent course even in localized metastatic disease with 5-year survival rates of 60% to 82%, though it drops to 12% to 41% with systemic disease.[33] They are associated with germline mutations (especially *SDHD* and *SDHB*) and frequently affect young people. Unfortunately, there is considerable morbidity associated with these tumors when performing surgery as they may grow in close proximity to nerves, muscles, and large blood vessels. Hence, it is of importance to choose patients who may benefit from a more watchful wait approach (more often *SDHD* mutated patients), and those needing more aggressive surgery. In general, young patients with small tumors, growing tumors, those invading vital nerve or cranial structures, the rare ones which secrete hormones and those with risk of malignancy should be considered for surgery.

In *SDHB* patients with HNPGL, the malignancy risk seems lower than other PPGL. Hence an active surveillance may be advocated; however, in growing tumors or in those that are small and do not risk major neurological deficits, surgery may be appropriate.[30] Importantly, for both *SDHB* and *SDHD* mutations there is usually slow growth over time which can make surgery more difficult and associated with higher morbidity.[30,34] Tumor-shrinking methods like embolization may be used to lower complications.[35] *SDHD* carriers have a lower risk of metastasis but often have multiple tumors that may require several interventions with increased risk of complications. Hence, multidisciplinary discussions regarding surgery, stereotactic surgery, radiation, and embolization treatments are necessary.[35] Debulking in metastatic disease may be used to alleviate symptoms and could possibly aid in delivery of guided therapy but will likely not affect overall survival.[36]

NONSURGICAL TREATMENT

There are today low-grade evidence for systemic treatment in metastatic PPGL. In rapidly growing metastatic PPGL, CVD (cyclophosphamide, vincristine, and dacarbazine) is usually considered, with a partial response seen in 37% and complete response in 4% of all PPGL patients.[37] There are some data that *SDHB*-mutated tumors may respond better.[38] For head and neck paragangliomas (HNPGL) with localized metastatic disease radiation treatment, specifically stereotactic radiosurgery may be used.[33,35] I-131-MIBG, where MIBG is labeled with a high-energy beta-emitting particle, is used in metastatic disease with reported clinical response rates of 24% to 45%.[39] However, because of the low expression of catecholamine transporters in SDHx patients the response rate is lower.[39] Due to higher expression of somatostatin receptors in SDHx patients, there is a rationale for peptide receptor radionuclide therapy (PRRT). This uses a radioactive isotope, in most cases ^{177}Lutetium, bound to a somatostatin analogue to deliver beta radiation and subsequently cause cell death in somatostatin receptor (SSR) expressing tissues. Multiple retrospective reports have shown a clinical utility in metastatic PPGL. It is usually considered in more slow growing metastatic disease. Only a few case series have investigated PRRT in patients with SDHx mutations (reviewed in Mak et al.[39]). There seems to be a good response in these patients and future trials will hopefully shed more light on this topic. It is currently recommended to enroll patients in PRRT clinical trials if the tumors show expressions of SSR.[33] Finally, the tyrosine kinase inhibitor Sunitinib has shown promise in metastatic PPGL.

THE DIFFERENT SUSCEPTIBILITY GENES IN CLUSTER 1 TUMORS (C1A)

SDHA Mutations

SDH is a mitochondrial enzyme involved in the respiratory chain and the TCA cycle where it catalyzes the oxidation of succinate to fumarate. SDHA encodes a subunit of the complex. Mutations in *SDHA* cause pheochromocytoma/paraganglioma syndrome 5 (PPGL5) and are relatively rare events in familial PPGL cases with an estimated frequency of 1% to 3% in PPGL cases.[40,41] These patients may also develop GIST tumors and rarely pituitary adenomas. Most of mutation carriers develop solitary PGL and often nonfunctioning head and neck PGL.[41,42] Some PGL produce methoxytyramines, and most PCC and extra-adrenal PGL produce normetanephrines. There seems to be a relatively high degree of metastatic PPGL[41] (12%) associated with SDHA mutations. Compared to other SDHx mutations, patients with SDHA mutations have a lower disease penetrance, 10% by age 70 years for non-index carriers.[42] Most of these patients have no family history of PPGL.[40] This makes it difficult to correctly diagnose the syndrome and to decide appropriate clinical follow up. The current expert recommendation suggests to start the first tumor screening in asymptomatic patients between 10 and 15 years of age and then continue annual follow-up.[43] In a single institution series, a 100% detection rate was shown for ^{68}Ga-DOTATATE PET/CT in metastatic cases.[44]

SDHB Mutations

In patients with PPGL the frequency of germline *SDHB* mutations are ~10% and cause PPGL4.[1,45] These tumors become metastatic in about 25%.[2] Those with concomitant somatic alterations in *ATRX* or *TERT* have a higher risk of metastasis.[46] This is caused by cellular immortalization, an event common in other malignant neoplasms. Most *SDHB* patients present as a solitary PGL. The tumor location is most often along the sympathetic chain (68%), head and neck (17%), and (14%) in the adrenal gland.[47] Other manifestations include a 4% risk of developing renal tumors and rarely thyroid tumors.[48] Compared to sporadic PPGL these patients usually present at a younger age (~30 years).[49] Some children are affected at a very young age and biochemical screening has been proposed to commence at age 6 to 10.[43] The disease penetrance is reported to be 21% at age 50 and 42% at age 70.[50] Interestingly, male patients have a higher disease penetrance.[48] Because of the high rate of metastasis, surgical treatment is usually more aggressive and adrenal-sparing techniques should seldomly be utilized.

Like other SDHx mutated PPGL these tumors express high amounts of somatostatin receptors and are therefore avidly visualized by ^{68}Ga-DOTATATE PET/CT and may respond to PRRT. Immunohistochemistry for SDHB may be used and loss is associated with a more aggressive phenotype.

Chemotherapy using CVD seems to be effective in patients with *SDHB* mutation.[38] In a retrospective case series of temozolamide monotherapy given to 10 patients with germline *SDHB* mutations, a partial response was seen in five patients.[51] These all showed deficient MGMT expression which previously was linked to response to temozolamide in glioblastoma patients.[52] The tyrosine kinase inhibitor Sunitinib has also shown response in *SDHB*-mutated PPGL and a randomized placebo-controlled trial is running (FIRSTMAPPP, NCT01371201).[53] Finally, in SDHB-mutated PPGL there seems to be an increased dependence on the PARP DNA repair system. In an SDHB-mutated mouse model the PARP inhibitor Olaparib potentiated the effect of temozolamide leading to increased survival.[13] Therefore, a phase II trial using temozolamide and Olaparib is also under way (NCT04394858).

SDHC Mutations

Mutations in *SDHC* cause PPGL3 and is responsible for <2% of PPGL patients.[48] The main presentation seems to be head and neck paraganglioma with occasional thoracic PGL, other PGL and PCC.[54,55] The malignant potential seems low, however cases of malignancy have been described.[48,56] A clinical workup similar to *SDHD* mutated patients has been suggested with initial screening in kindred aged 10 to 15 years.[43]

SDHD Mutations

Like other *SDH* mutations, *SDHD* mutations are inherited in an autosomal dominant pattern and cause PPGL1. However, because of imprinting of the maternal allele only affected alleles inherited from the father will give a clinical phenotype. Mutations in *SDHD* may be found in around 4% to 9% of PPGL.[45,57] The disease penetrance is high with 90% being diagnosed with tumors. Multifocal disease is observed in 75%.[58] Most often the patient presents at a relatively young age with parasympathetic HNPGL (71% at 60 years of age) with other forms of PPGL occurring as well.[49,58] The risk of malignancy has been estimated to be around 5%-8%.[59] In those with HNPGL there is rarely catecholamine excretion and patients usually present with a neck mass.[60] Some HNPGL (both *SDHB* and *SDHD*) are detected by increased plasma 3-methoxytyramine, which is associated with malignancy. MRI and CT provide a sensitive method for detecting primary tumors. Functional imaging using 68Ga-radiolabelled somatostatin analogues are usually positive. HNPGL may invade adjacent organs like cranial nerves, vessels, and brainstem causing significant morbidity with attempted surgical resection. Hence, an initial observational period or minimally invasive methods for surgery should be considered. Due to the often multicentric disease, low malignancy rate and varied catecholamine secretion, a multimodal treatment strategy with surgery, radiotherapy, and theranostics may be needed.[61] Close follow up in these patients for new tumors or recurrences is advocated.

SDHAF2 Mutations

The protein SDHAF2 is involved in the flavination of SDHA and loss of expression leads to destabilization of the SDH complex. Germline mutation of SDHAF2 is a rare cause of FPPGL. Similar to *SDHD* mutations only paternally inherited variants will cause disease. In a Dutch family with 57 screened individuals, 12/16 carrying the mutation (75%) developed disease. The median age of onset was 33, and there was usually multiple tumors. Only HNPGL was observed, and none developed malignant tumors.[8]

FH Mutations

Fumarate hydratase acts one step over SDH in the TCA cycle where it converts fumarate to malate. Inactivating mutations leads to accumulation of fumarate that inhibits prolyl hydroxylases, thereby stabilizing HIF and creates a pseudohypoxic signal like other cluster 1 tumors. Also, there is an increase in methylation similar to SDHx tumors.[62] Germline *FH* mutations occur in hereditary leiomyomatosis renal cell carcinoma syndrome.[29] Rarely, patients with germline *FH* mutations develop PPGL. In patients without mutations in PCC/PGL susceptibility genes, the frequency of germline *FH* mutations was 1%.[62] In the same series of five patients, multiple tumors were seen in 3/5, metastases in 3/5 and there were both PCCs and PGLs diagnosed.[62] Like in metastatic *SDHB* patients, *ATRX* and *TERT* may immortalize tumors in *FH* patients, an event linked to metastatic behavior.[46] There seems to be a better detection rate with 18F-DOPA than ^{68}Ga-DOTATATE PET/CT compared with the other Cluster C1A tumors.

Other Rare Forms of Cluster C1A Mutations

A. *SLC25A11*

SLC25A11 encodes the mitochondrial 2-oxoglutarate/malate carrier that reconstitutes the NADH pool, necessary for normal function of mitochondrial complex 1. One explanation for the link to FPPGL susceptibility is increased levels of glutamate and aspartate that may inhibit HIF enzymes.[63] Germline *SLC25A11* mutations were found in 1% of screened PPGL patients and were associated with a malignant phenotype.[63]

B. *DLST*

Dihydrolipoamide S-succinyltransferase (DLST) is a protein involved in the TCA cycle. It is involved in a subunit of mitochondrial α-ketoglutarate dehydrogenase (OGDH) complex which facilitates conversion of α-ketoglutarate to succinyl-CoA. Recurrent germline mutations in *DSLT* have been found in apparently sporadic cases.[64,65] Mutations were shown to increase the ratio of α-ketoglutarate to fumarate and increase the level of the oncometabolite 2-hydroxyglutarate.[65]

C. *MDH2*

Malate dehydrogenase 2 (*MDH2*) mutations cause a rare form of FPPGL accounting for <1% in patients not carrying a mutation in another susceptibility gene. Due to its rarity, clinical data are hard to determine. There are both benign and malignant cases described.[66,67]

D. *GOT2*

GOT2 mutations have been reported in a few familial cases.[68] GOT2 converts oxaloacetate into aspartate by transamination, with the subsequent conversion of glutamate to α-ketoglutarate. The tumors had a high succinate to fumarate ratio, a "CIMP" high phenotype.

CLUSTER 1 C1B—*VHL, EPAS1, EGLN1/2, MDH2* MUTATIONS

Pathophysiology

The cluster C1B tumors are found in both somatic and heritable disease (25% are heritable). Most patients in this cluster have a VHL mutation with the other mutations being much rarer. The affected genes are involved in the hypoxia pathway, leading to these tumors displaying a pseudohypoxic signal, similar to that seen in Cluster C1A. VHL belongs to the degradation complex targeting HIF proteins, such as EPAS1/HIF2alfa which encodes one of the members of the HIF family that regulate the hypoxic response.[69] Mutations disrupt the normal prolyl hydroxylation leading to less degradation. EGLN1/2/PHD1/2 encodes one of the prolyl hydroxylases. These proteins, under normoxic conditions, hydroxylate HIF proteins leading to their ultimate degradation.

Biochemistry

Like the Cluster 1A tumors the C1B tumors usually overproduce norepinephrine.[70] *VHL* patients with PPGL, which constitutes the major part of this cluster, have a low expression of the *PNMT* gene leading to less conversion of noradrenaline to adrenaline, and subsequent high noradrenaline secretion.[71] Patients with germline *VHL* mutations and PPGL may have nonfunctional and asymptomatic tumors in up to 70% in some studies.[71,72]

Compared to SDHx-related tumors, VHL-mutated tumors more rarely secrete dopamine.[73]

Imaging

Patients with Cluster C1B often present with PCC.[71,72,74] Tumors in the adrenal seen with CT/MRI with concomitant elevation of noradrenaline are usually sufficient for diagnosis of PCC. When considering metastatic disease these modalities may be insufficient. Functional imaging in C1B differs somewhat from C1A. C1B tumors tend to be harder to diagnose with SSTR imaging because of the lower SSTR expression and background uptake in the surrounding adrenal. Also, there seems to be higher expression of L-type amino transporters as these tumors display high sensitivity/specificity with ^{18}F-DOPA; hence this modality is recommended.[26,75] There is some evidence showing reduced uptake of 123-MIBG in these tumors and imaging should not rely solely on this method.[76]

Clinical/Treatment Considerations

Because *VHL* patients with PPGL tumors constitute the majority of patients with hereditary C1B tumors, the usual presentation of C1B tumors is a solitary PCC and when functional, there is commonly overproduction of noradrenaline.[71,74] Importantly, age at onset may be very young; hence screening in *VHL* kindred is recommended from 5 years of age.[77] Only rarely do patients with *VHL* succumb to metastatic PCC and the estimated frequency of malignancy is around 5%.[78] For tumors arising outside of the adrenal, estimating the rate of malignancy is harder due to their rarity. However, bilateral disease occurs in up to 50% in *VHL* patients and there is a 10% risk of recurrence after adrenalectomy.[74]

To avoid lifelong adrenal insufficiency, surgical treatment with adrenal-sparing techniques is an option.[79-81] This method allows minimizing the risk of Addisonian crisis and avoiding lifelong cortisol supplementation, which carries a risk of osteoporosis, diabetes, and hypertension. Today, adrenal-sparing surgery using minimally invasive retroperitoneal/transperitoneal surgery is a safe method and has been validated in many different types of adrenal tumors.[82] It is recommended to leave no less than one-third of one adrenal (>15% of both).[83] The risk with this method is development of malignant disease in the remnant adrenal[81] and recurrent tumors (up to 20%[81,84]). In a multicenter study involving 191 *VHL* patients undergoing adrenal-sparing surgery, the success rate was 87%, 12% had an ipsilateral recurrence and 2% developed metastatic disease.[81] Most recurrences develop approximately 10 years following surgery or later, and early recurrences likely represent missed synchronous tumors. When performing bilateral adrenal sparing surgery, one should take into consideration that the patient will have benefit from the remnant tissue and likely avoid cortisol supplementation for a prolonged period, even if there is a recurrence. It is also feasible to try to preserve remnant tissue at reoperation for a recurrence, although the risk of adrenal insufficiency is higher in this instance. Both retroperitoneal and transperitoneal approaches may be used and have their pros and cons. Relative contraindications for a retroperitoneal approach are large tumors (>8 cm) and severe obesity[31] while previous abdominal surgery and cardiac disease are relative contraindications for the transperitoneal approach.[85]

THE DIFFERENT SUSCEPTIBILITY GENES IN CLUSTER 1B TUMORS

Von Hippel Lindau (*VHL*)

In total about 3/100,000 children per year are born carrying a disease-causing mutation in *VHL*. *VHL* encodes the tumor suppressor von Hippel Lindau protein, which is part of a complex that is required for the degradation of HIFs. Mutations cause an abnormal hypoxic response leading to risk of tumor formation.[86] The disease is inherited in an autosomal dominant fashion. Patients develop vascularized tumors like retinal angiomas, CNS hemangioblastomas, clear cell renal carcinomas, and PCCs. Depending on the type of mutation, the presentation of disease can vary considerably, and in particular, some missense mutations (Type IIB, IIC - syndrome) are at risk for PPGL development.[77,87]

Pheochromocytomas are the usual manifestation and occur in 10% to 20% of patients, which accounts for about 5% to 7% of all PPGL.[45,88] Pheochromocytomas are usually functional with overproduction of noradrenaline.[71,74] First age of presentation may be as early as 5 years and screening is recommended from this age.[74] Patients often develop bilateral and recurrent disease.[89] Hence, there is a rationale for using adrenal-sparing techniques. For imaging, ^{18}F-DOPA PET/CT is the most sensitive in identifying tumors.[90]

Other Rare Forms of Cluster C1B Tumors

HIF2alfa or *EPAS1* encodes one of the members of the HIF family that regulate the hypoxic response.[69] Mutations disrupt the normal prolyl hydroxylation leading to less degradation. Mutations have been described in patients with congenital polycythemia with concurrent somatostatinoma and PGL.[91] Interestingly, no germline mutation was detected, although the same somatic mutation was observed in multiple tumors.[91] This suggests a postzygotic mutation as a cause of the clinical phenotype.[91] Further reports have found somatic *EPAS1* mutations in additional patients. These patients have PPGLs that may develop in early childhood, both single/multiple PPGLs and in those with and without congenital polycythemia.[92,93] Another rare form of hereditary PPGL with a pseudohypoxic expression profile is *EGLN1/2/PHD1/2* mutation, which encodes a prolyl hydroxylase. It accounts for <1% of all PPGL.[1] Prolyl hydroxylase proteins, as mentioned earlier, under normoxic conditions hydroxylate HIF proteins causing their ultimate degradation. Loss of function of *EGLN1/2* has been described in hereditary erythrocytosis and in some cases of hereditary PPGL.[94,95]

FAMILIAL PPGL DUE TO CLUSTER 2 TUMORS

Pathophysiology

The Cluster 2 group includes the susceptibility genes *RET*, *TMEM127*, *MAX* and *NF1*, and about 20% are germline mutations. The most frequent alteration in this group is *RET* mutations and will be further discussed in a separate chapter. Hereditary PPGL tumors caused by *NF1*, *TMEM127*, and *MAX* mutations constitute about 5% to 10% of all PPGL. These mutations are associated with activation in kinase signaling pathways like PI3 kinase/AKT, RAS/RAF/ERK, and mTORC1.[96-99] *NF1* encodes Neurofibromin, a GTPase-activating protein that negatively regulates RAS. Other signaling pathways affected are mTOR and MAPK pathways.[100] *TMEM127* mutations lead to increased mTOR association with lysosomes, and induced mTOR signaling[97,101,102] while MAX is a component of the MYC-MAX-MXD1 network, a commonly deregulated pathway in other cancers.

Biochemistry

Cluster 2 tumors display an adrenergic phenotype, characterized by a more differentiated and mature expression of secretory genes with retained expression of PNMT. Hence, they mainly secrete epinephrine and seldomly dopamine.[1,14] MAX-mutated tumors are an exception and have an intermediate phenotype with excretion of noradrenaline. Cluster C2 tumors have a high tumor catecholamine content[28] but seem to have lower secretory activity and are more responsive to stimuli with large variations in their catecholamine secretion.[28] They display a more paroxysmal clinical presentation than functional C1 tumors with typically episodic attacks of hypertension, palpitations, and tachycardia.[103]

Imaging

Like with C1B tumors, the intra-adrenal location together with usually functional tumors makes diagnosis with metanephrines and CT/MRI sufficient. In metastatic disease, multifocality, or in the rare instance of extra-adrenal disease, functional imaging should be considered. Compared to C1 tumors these have a more differentiated phenotype with higher expression of catecholamine transporters compared to SSTRs making the detection rate with ^{18}F-DOPA better than ^{68}Ga-DOTATATE PET/CT imaging.[104] Also, the background expression of SSTR in the adrenal may hide smaller tumors in SSTR imaging.[105]

Clinical Considerations

Cluster 2 tumors almost invariably originate from the adrenal glands.[28] Importantly, the risk of malignancy is much lower than C1 tumors and only about 2% to 4% are metastatic.[2] For *TMEM127* and *MAX*-mutated patients the risk of malignancy is higher and special clinical considerations apply for them. Cluster C2 tumors are often multifocal and recurrence after surgery is not uncommon. Like in *VHL*-mutated patients, adrenal-sparing surgery can be considered, especially for MEN2 patients but also *NF1* patients. In three studies of 24 *NF1* patients there were no metachronous malignancies.[81,106,107] The data are more scarce on *TMEM127* and *MAX*; however, there seems to be a higher risk of malignancy in these patients and adrenal sparing surgery is therefore debated and a case by case approach with multidisciplinary discussion is advocated.[108] In metastatic disease, CVD should be considered, and depending on receptor uptake, PRRT or MIBG treatment may be indicated. Because of the alteration in kinase signaling pathways there is hope that kinase inhibitors may work in these tumors. There are now multiple trials ongoing with different kinase inhibitors (discussed in Crona et al.,[17] Wachtel and Fishbein,[88] Nölting and Grossman,[99] and De Filpo et al.[109]).

THE DIFFERENT SUSCEPTIBILITY GENES IN CLUSTER 2 TUMORS

NF1

Neurofibromatosis type 1 (also known as von Recklinghausen disease) is a syndrome with an autosomal dominant mode of inheritance and frequently childhood onset. Patients develop neurofibromas, lisch nodules, café au lait spots, optic gliomas, skeletal dysplasias, and PPGLs. The prevalence is about 1/3000 births. Of all PPGLs 3.3% have a germline *NF1* mutation but *NF1* mutations can occur sporadically as well.[45] Systematic screening of *NF1* will likely increase the prevalence of PPGLs due to asymptomatic cases.[110] First presentation is usually similar as with sporadic cases and most patients develop PCCs, which occasionally are bilateral.[110,111] Metastasis has been described in 5% to 11% of patients.[112] Most patients will have increased metanephrines and many have symptoms of catecholamine excess.[112] Like in the other Cluster 2 tumors the current recommendation is ^{18}F-DOPA PET/CT imaging.[104] Adrenal sparing surgery can be considered in *NF1* patients, especially in those with bilateral disease.[108,112]

TMEM127

TMEM127 is a highly conserved 3-spanner transmembrane protein that is associated with different cellular organelles and is a susceptibility gene for hereditary PPGL.[97] Mutations are inherited in an autosomal dominant fashion. The prevalence of *TMEM127*-associated disease seems to be around 1%-2% of all PPGL.[41,113] Most patients develop disease around 40 years of age and there is rarely a family history. In one family with 47 individuals carrying a mutation, 11/47 (32%) eventually developed disease.[114] The main presentation is PCC; however, PGL may be found in all locations. All tumors are catecholamine producing (both epinephrine and norepinephrine). The majority of patients have benign disease, and about 10% are malignant. There is often multifocal disease.[113,114] There are currently conflicting recommendations for adrenal sparing surgery.[108,115] For best imaging results it is suggested to start with ^{18}F-DOPA PET/CT.[104]

MAX

MAX is a component of the MYC-MAX-MXD1 network, a commonly deregulated pathway in cancers. When MAX interacts with MYC family proteins it increases transcription while it represses it when interacting with other proteins. It acts as a tumor suppressor in PPGL with inherited mutations in one allele and loss of the other, by either large CNVs or uniparental disomy.[116] In a large screening study of *MAX* mutations for both germline and somatic mutations, germline mutations were observed in about 1% and somatic mutations in 1.5%.[117] There was a familial history in about one-third of patients and a paternal inheritance. All developed PCCs, but 15% recurred with a PGL. In addition there was a high risk of multifocal disease and 10% developed malignant tumors. Most had a noradrenergic phenotype.[117] Due to a relatively high metastatic rate adrenal sparing surgery is usually not recommended.[108]

CONCLUSION

Today the genetic background of PPGL can guide the clinician in all parts of the medical workup, from diagnosis to prognosis, systemic treatment, surgery, imaging, and follow-up after treatment. The genetic information makes it possible to group the tumors into larger, more phenotypically similar groups which has paved the way for a more comprehensive understanding and confident treatment strategies. Cluster C1 and C2 tumors have distinct genetic alterations with their own expressional, metabolomic, and methylomic alterations. Surgical considerations affected by these underlying genetic differences include how aggressive the surgeon should be during the operation, when to operate and what technique to use. Adrenal sparing surgery is a safe and effective method that is important to consider in heritable disease and especially in those with cluster C1B and C2 tumors. Also, patients with mutations in *SDHB* should suggest more aggressive and early surgery, while other family kindreds (eg, *SDHD* carriers) should be monitored more closely for development of multiple tumors. Without genetic testing on these patients, opportunity to devise the optimal treatment strategy is likely missed. Hopefully current understanding of the genetic background can pave the way for better systemic treatment in patients with metastatic disease.

REFERENCES

1. Fishbein L, Leshchiner I, Walter V, et al. Comprehensive molecular characterization of pheochromocytoma and paraganglioma. *Cancer Cell.* 2017;31:181-193.
2. Crona J, Lamarca A, Ghosal S, Welin S, Skogseid B, Pacak K. Genotype-phenotype correlations in pheochromocytoma and paraganglioma: a systematic review and individual patient meta-analysis. *Endocr Relat Cancer.* 2019;26:539-550.
3. Jochmanová I, Yang C, Zhuang Z, Pacak K. Hypoxia-inducible factor signaling in pheochromocytoma: turning the rudder in the right direction. *J Nat Cancer Inst.* 2013;105:1270-1283.
4. Hon WC, Wilson MI, Harlos K, et al. Structural basis for the recognition of hydroxyproline in HIF-1 alpha by pVHL. *Nature.* 2002;417:975-978.
5. Castro-Vega LJ, Letouzé E, Burnichon N, et al. Multi-omics analysis defines core genomic alterations in pheochromocytomas and paragangliomas. *Nat Commun.* 2015;6:6044.
6. Nölting S, Bechmann N, Taieb D, et al. Personalized management of pheochromocytoma and paraganglioma. *Endocr Rev.* 2021.
7. Baysal Bora E, Ferrell RE, Willett-Brozick JE, et al. Mutations in SDHD, a mitochondrial complex II gene, in hereditary paraganglioma. *Science.* 2000;287:848-851.
8. Kunst HP, Rutten MH, de Mönnink JP, et al. SDHAF2 (PGL2-SDH5) and hereditary head and neck paraganglioma. *Clin Cancer Res.* 2011;17:247-254.
9. Selak MA, Armour SM, MacKenzie ED, et al. Succinate links TCA cycle dysfunction to oncogenesis by inhibiting HIF-α prolyl hydroxylase. *Cancer Cell.* 2005;7:77-85.
10. Xiao M, Yang H, Xu W, et al. Inhibition of α-KG-dependent histone and DNA demethylases by fumarate and succinate that are accumulated in mutations of FH and SDH tumor suppressors. *Genes Dev.* 2012;26:1326-1338.
11. Letouzé E, Martinelli C, Loriot C, et al. SDH mutations establish a hypermethylator phenotype in paraganglioma. *Cancer Cell.* 2013;23:739-752.
12. Sulkowski PL, Sundaram RK, Oeck S, et al. Krebs-cycle-deficient hereditary cancer syndromes are defined by defects in homologous-recombination DNA repair. *Nat Genet.* 2018;50:1086-1092.
13. Pang Y, Lu Y, Caisova V, et al. Targeting NAD(+)/PARP DNA repair pathway as a novel therapeutic approach to *SDHB*-mutated cluster I pheochromocytoma and paraganglioma. *Clin Cancer Res.* 2018;24:3423-3432.
14. Huynh TT, Pacak K, Wong DL, et al. Transcriptional regulation of phenylethanolamine N-methyltransferase in pheochromocytomas from patients with von Hippel-Lindau syndrome and multiple endocrine neoplasia type 2. *Ann N Y Acad Sci.* 2006;1073:241-252.
15. Eisenhofer G, Lenders JW, Timmers H, et al. Measurements of plasma methoxytyramine, normetanephrine, and metanephrine as discriminators of different hereditary forms of pheochromocytoma. *Clin Chem.* 2011;57:411-420.
16. Gimenez-Roqueplo AP, Caumont-Prim A, Houzard C, et al. Imaging work-up for screening of paraganglioma and pheochromocytoma in SDHx mutation carriers: a multicenter prospective study from the PGL.EVA investigators. *J Clin Endocrinol Metab.* 2013;98:E162-E173.
17. Crona J, Taïeb D. Pacak K. New perspectives on pheochromocytoma and paraganglioma: toward a molecular classification. *Endocr Rev.* 2017;38: 489-515.
18. Timmers HJLM, Pacak K, Huynh TT, et al. Biochemically silent abdominal paragangliomas in patients with mutations in the succinate dehydrogenase subunit B gene. *J Clin Endocrinol Metab.* 2008;93:4826-4832.
19. Zuber S, Wesley R, Prodanov T, Eisenhofer G, Pacak K, Kantorovich V. Clinical utility of chromogranin A in SDHx-related paragangliomas. *Eur J Clin Invest.* 2014;44: 365-371.
20. Kan Y, Zhang S, Wang W, Liu J, Yang J, Wang Z. ^{68}Ga-somatostatin receptor analogs and ^{18}F-FDG PET/CT in the localization of metastatic pheochromocytomas and paragangliomas with germline mutations: a meta-analysis. *Acta Radiol.* 2018;59:1466-1474.
21. Elston MS, Meyer-Rochow GY, Conaglen HM, et al. Increased SSTR2A and SSTR3 expression in succinate dehydrogenase-deficient pheochromocytomas and paragangliomas. *Hum Pathol.* 2015;46:390-396.
22. Timmers HJ, Chen CC, Carrasquillo JA, et al. Staging and functional characterization of pheochromocytoma and paraganglioma by 18F-fluorodeoxyglucose (18F-FDG) positron emission tomography. *J Natl Cancer Inst.* 2012;104:700-708.
23. Favier J, Brière JJ, Burnichon N, et al. The Warburg effect is genetically determined in inherited pheochromocytomas. *PLoS One.* 2009;4:e7094.
24. Janssen I, Blanchet EM, Adams K, et al. Superiority of [68Ga]-DOTATATE PET/CT to other functional imaging modalities in the localization of SDHB-associated metastatic pheochromocytoma and paraganglioma. *Clin Cancer Res.* 2015;21:3888-3895.
25. Janssen I, Chen CC, Taieb D, et al. 68Ga-DOTATATE PET/CT in the localization of head and neck paragangliomas compared with other functional imaging modalities and CT/MRI. *J Nucl Med.* 2016;57:186-191.
26. Taïeb D, Hicks RJ, Hindié E, et al. European Association of Nuclear Medicine Practice Guideline/Society of Nuclear Medicine and Molecular Imaging Procedure Standard 2019 for radionuclide imaging of phaeochromocytoma and paraganglioma. *Eur J Nucl Med Mol Imaging.* 2019;46:2112-2137.
27. Nambuba J, Därr R, Janssen I, et al. Functional imaging experience in a germline fumarate hydratase mutation–positive patient with pheochromocytoma and paraganglioma. *AACE Clinical Case Reports.* 2016;2:e176-e181.
28. Eisenhofer G, Klink B, Richter S, Lenders JW, Robledo M. Metabologenomics of phaeochromocytoma and paraganglioma: an integrated approach for personalised biochemical and genetic testing. *Clin Biochem Rev.* 2017;38:69-100.
29. Tomlinson IP, Alam NA, Rowan AJ, et al. Germline mutations in FH predispose to dominantly inherited uterine fibroids, skin leiomyomata and papillary renal cell cancer. *Nat Genet.* 2002;30:406-410.
30. Ellis RJ, Patel D, Prodanov T, Nilubol N, Pacak K, Kebebew E. The presence of SDHB mutations should modify surgical indications for carotid body paragangliomas. *Ann Surg.* 2014;260:158-162.
31. Castinetti F, Taieb D, Henry JF, et al. Management of endocrine disease: outcome of adrenal sparing surgery in heritable pheochromocytoma. *Eur J Endocrinol.* 2016;174:R9-R18.
32. Iacobone M, Belluzzi A, Torresan F. Surgical approaches and results of treatment for hereditary paragangliomas. *Best Pract Res Clin Endocrinol Metab.* 2019;33:101298.

33. Fishbein L, Del Rivero J, Else T, et al. The North American Neuroendocrine Tumor Society Consensus Guidelines for Surveillance and Management of Metastatic and/or Unresectable Pheochromocytoma and Paraganglioma. *Pancreas.* 2021;50(4):469-493.
34. Assadipour Y, Sadowski SM, Alimchandani M, et al. SDHB mutation status and tumor size but not tumor grade are important predictors of clinical outcome in pheochromocytoma and abdominal paraganglioma. *Surgery.* 2017;161:230-239.
35. Moore MG, Netterville JL, Mendenhall WM, Isaacson B, Nussenbaum B. Head and neck paragangliomas: an update on evaluation and management. *Otolaryngol Head Neck Surg.* 2016;154:597-605.
36. Ellis RJ, Patel D, Prodanov T, et al. Response after surgical resection of metastatic pheochromocytoma and paraganglioma: can postoperative biochemical remission be predicted? *J Am Coll Surg.* 2013;217:489-496.
37. Niemeijer ND, Alblas G, van Hulsteijn LT, Dekkers OM, Corssmit EP. Chemotherapy with cyclophosphamide, vincristine and dacarbazine for malignant paraganglioma and pheochromocytoma: systematic review and meta-analysis. *Clin Endocrinol (Oxf).* 2014;81:642-651.
38. Fishbein L, Ben-Maimon S, Keefe S, et al. *SDHB* mutation carriers with malignant pheochromocytoma respond better to CVD. *Endocr Relat Cancer.* 2017;24:L51-L55.
39. Mak IYF, Hayes AR, Khoo B, Grossman A. Peptide receptor radionuclide therapy as a novel treatment for metastatic and invasive phaeochromocytoma and paraganglioma. *Neuroendocrinology.* 2019;109:287-298.
40. Maniam P, Zhou K, Lonergan M, Berg JN, Goudie DR, Newey PJ. Pathogenicity and penetrance of germline SDHA variants in pheochromocytoma and paraganglioma (PPGL). *J Endocr Soc.* 2018;2:806-816.
41. Bausch B, Schiavi F, Ni Y, et al. Clinical characterization of the pheochromocytoma and paraganglioma susceptibility genes SDHA, TMEM127, MAX, and SDHAF2 for gene-informed prevention. *JAMA Oncology.* 2017;3:1204-1212.
42. van der Tuin K, Mensenkamp AR, Tops CMJ, et al. Clinical aspects of SDHA-related pheochromocytoma and paraganglioma: a nationwide study. *J Clin Endocrinol Metab.* 2018;103:438-445.
43. Amar, L, Pacak K, Steichen O, et al. International consensus on initial screening and follow-up of asymptomatic SDHx mutation carriers. *Nat Rev Endocrinol.* 2021;17:435-444.
44. Jha A, de Luna K, Balili CA, et al. Clinical, diagnostic, and treatment characteristics of SDHA-related metastatic pheochromocytoma and paraganglioma. *Front Oncol.* 2019; 9:53.
45. Lenders JWM, Duh QY, Eisenhofer G, et al. Pheochromocytoma and paraganglioma: an endocrine society clinical practice guideline. *J Clin Endocrinol Metab.* 2014;99:1915-1942.
46. Job S, Draskovic I, Burnichon N, et al. Telomerase activation and ATRX mutations are independent risk factors for metastatic pheochromocytoma and paraganglioma. *Clin Cancer Res.* 2019;25:760-770.
47. Jochmanova I, Wolf KI, King KS, et al. SDHB-related pheochromocytoma and paraganglioma penetrance and genotype-phenotype correlations. *J Cancer Res Clin Oncol.* 2017;143:1421-1435.
48. Andrews KA, Ascher DB, Pires DEV, et al. Tumour risks and genotype-phenotype correlations associated with germline variants in succinate dehydrogenase subunit genes SDHB, SDHC and SDHD. *J Med Genet.* 2018;55:384-394.
49. Ricketts CJ, Forman JR, Rattenberry E, et al. Tumor risks and genotype-phenotype-proteotype analysis in 358 patients with germline mutations in SDHB and SDHD. *Hum Mutat.* 2010;31:41-51.
50. Rijken JA, Niemeijer ND, Jonker MA, et al. The penetrance of paraganglioma and pheochromocytoma in SDHB germline mutation carriers. *Clin Genet.* 2018;93:60-66.
51. Hadoux J, Favier J, Scoazec JY, et al. SDHB mutations are associated with response to temozolomide in patients with metastatic pheochromocytoma or paraganglioma. *Int J Cancer.* 2014;135:2711-2720.
52. Hegi ME, Diserens AC, Gorlia T, et al. MGMT gene silencing and benefit from temozolomide in glioblastoma. *N Engl J Med.* 2005;352:997-1003.
53. Ayala-Ramirez M, Chougnet CN, Habra MA, et al. Treatment with sunitinib for patients with progressive metastatic pheochromocytomas and sympathetic paragangliomas. *J Clin Endocrinol Metab.* 2012;97:4040-4050.
54. Vandy FC, Sisk G, Berguer R. Synchronous carotid body and thoracic paraganglioma associated with a germline SDHC mutation. *J Vasc Surg.* 2011;53:805-807.
55. Schiavi F, Boedeker CC, Bausch B, et al. Predictors and prevalence of paraganglioma syndrome associated with mutations of the SDHC gene. *JAMA.* 2005;294:2057-2063.
56. Bickmann JK, Sollfrank S, Schad A, et al. Phenotypic variability and risk of malignancy in SDHC-linked paragangliomas: lessons from three unrelated cases with an identical germline mutation (p.Arg133*). *J Clin Endocrinol Metab.* 2014;99:E489-E496.
57. Neumann HPH, Pawlu C, Peczkowska M, et al. Distinct clinical features of paraganglioma syndromes associated with SDHB and SDHD gene mutations. *JAMA.* 2004;292:943-951.
58. Benn DE, Gimenez-Roqueplo AP, Reilly JR, et al. Clinical presentation and penetrance of pheochromocytoma/paraganglioma syndromes. *J Clin Endocrinol Metab.* 2006;91:827-836.
59. van Hulsteijn LT, Dekkers OM, Hes FJ, Smit JW, Corssmit EP. Risk of malignant paraganglioma in SDHB-mutation and SDHD-mutation carriers: a systematic review and meta-analysis. *J Med Genet.* 2012;49:768-776.
60. Davila VJ, Chang JM, Stone WM, et al. Current surgical management of carotid body tumors. *J Vasc Surg.* 2016;64:1703-1710.
61. Elenkova A, Robeva R, Gimenez-Roqueplo AP, Zacharieva S. A 40-year follow-up of a patient with multiple paragangliomas and a SDHD mutation. *Acta Endocrinol (Buchar).* 2019;15:254-260.
62. Castro-Vega LJ, Buffet A, De Cubas AA, et al. Germline mutations in FH confer predisposition to malignant pheochromocytomas and paragangliomas. *Hum Mol Genet.* 2014;23:2440-2446.
63. Buffet A, Morin A, Castro-Vega LJ, et al. Germline mutations in the mitochondrial 2-oxoglutarate/malate carrier *SLC25A11* gene confer a predisposition to metastatic paragangliomas. *Cancer Res.* 2018;78:1914-1922.
64. Buffet A, Zhang J, Rebel H, et al. Germline DLST variants promote epigenetic modifications in pheochromocytoma-paraganglioma. *J Clin Endocrinol Metab.* 2020;106:459-471.
65. Remacha L, Pirman D, Mahoney CE, et al. Recurrent germline DLST mutations in individuals with multiple pheochromocytomas and paragangliomas. *Am J Hum Genet.* 2019;104: 651-664.
66. Cascón A, Comino-Méndez I, Currás-Freixes M, et al. Whole-exome sequencing identifies MDH2 as a new familial paraganglioma gene. *J Natl Cancer Inst.* 2015;107:djv053.

67. Calsina B, Currás-Freixes M, Buffet A, et al. Role of MDH2 pathogenic variant in pheochromocytoma and paraganglioma patients. *Genet Med*. 2018;20:1652-1662.
68. Remacha L, Comino-Méndez I, Richter S, et al. Targeted exome sequencing of Krebs cycle genes reveals candidate cancer–predisposing mutations in pheochromocytomas and paragangliomas. *Clin Cancer Res*. 2017;23:6315-6324.
69. Tian H, McKnight SL, Russell DW. Endothelial PAS domain protein 1 (EPAS1), a transcription factor selectively expressed in endothelial cells. *Genes Dev*. 1997;11:72-82.
70. Eisenhofer G, Lenders JW, Linehan WM, Walther MM, Goldstein DS, Keiser HR. Plasma normetanephrine and metanephrine for detecting pheochromocytoma in von Hippel-Lindau disease and multiple endocrine neoplasia type 2. *N Engl J Med*. 1999;340:1872-1879.
71. Eisenhofer G, Walther MM, Huynh TT, et al. Pheochromocytomas in von Hippel-Lindau syndrome and multiple endocrine neoplasia type 2 display distinct biochemical and clinical phenotypes. *J Clin Endocrinol Metab*. 2001;86:1999-2008.
72. Li SR, Nicholson KJ, McCoy KL, Carty, S.E, Yip L. Clinical and biochemical features of pheochromocytoma characteristic of von Hippel–Lindau syndrome. *World J Surg*. 2020;44:570-577.
73. Eisenhofer G, Pacak K, Huynh TT, et al. Catecholamine metabolomic and secretory phenotypes in phaeochromocytoma. *Endocr Relat Cancer*. 2011;18:97-111.
74. Aufforth RD, Ramakant P, Sadowski SM, et al. Pheochromocytoma screening initiation and frequency in von Hippel-Lindau syndrome. *J Clin Endocrinol Metab*. 2015;100:4498-4504.
75. Janssen I, Chen CC, Zhuang Z, et al. Functional imaging signature of patients presenting with polycythemia/paraganglioma syndromes. *J Nucl Med*. 2017;58:1236-1242.
76. Kaji P, Carrasquillo JA, Linehan WM, et al. The role of 6-[18F] fluorodopamine positron emission tomography in the localization of adrenal pheochromocytoma associated with von Hippel-Lindau syndrome. *Eur J Endocrinol*. 2007;156:483-487.
77. Rednam SP, Erez A, Druker H, et al. von Hippel–Lindau and hereditary pheochromocytoma/paraganglioma syndromes: clinical features, genetics, and surveillance recommendations in childhood. *Clin Cancer Res*. 2017;23:e68-e75.
78. Maher ER, Neumann HPH, Richard S. von Hippel–Lindau disease: a clinical and scientific review. *Eur J Hum Genet*. 2011;19:617-623.
79. Volkin D, Yerram N, Ahmed F, et al. Partial adrenalectomy minimizes the need for long-term hormone replacement in pediatric patients with pheochromocytoma and von Hippel-Lindau syndrome. *J Pediatr Surg*. 2012;47:2077-2082.
80. Benhammou JN, Boris RS, Pacak K, Pinto PA, Linehan WM, Bratslavsky G. Functional and oncologic outcomes of partial adrenalectomy for pheochromocytoma in patients with von Hippel-Lindau syndrome after at least 5 years of followup. *J Urol*. 2010;184:1855-1859.
81. Neumann HPH, Tsoy U, Bancos I, et al. Comparison of pheochromocytoma-specific morbidity and mortality among adults with bilateral pheochromocytomas undergoing total adrenalectomy vs cortical-sparing adrenalectomy. *JAMA Netw Open*. 2019;2:e198898.
82. Nagaraja V, Eslick GD, Edirimanne S. Recurrence and functional outcomes of partial adrenalectomy: a systematic review and meta-analysis. Int J Surg. 2015;16:7-13.
83. Alesina PF, Hinrichs J, Meier B, Schmid KW, Neumann HP, Walz MK. Minimally invasive cortical-sparing surgery for bilateral pheochromocytomas. *Langenbecks Arch Surg*. 2012;397:233-238.
84. Castinetti F, Qi XP, Walz MK, et al. Outcomes of adrenal-sparing surgery or total adrenalectomy in phaeochromocytoma associated with multiple endocrine neoplasia type 2: an international retrospective population-based study. *Lancet Oncol*. 2014;15:648-655.
85. Ip JCY, Lee JC, Sidhu SB. Laparoscopic adrenalectomy: the transperitoneal approach. *Curr Surg Rep*. 2013;1:26-33.
86. Hes FJ, Hoppener JW, Lips CJ. Clinical review 155: pheochromocytoma in von Hippel-Lindau disease. *J Clin Endocrinol Metab*. 2003;88:969-974.
87. McNeill A, Rattenberry E, Barber R, Killick P, MacDonald F, Maher ER. Genotype-phenotype correlations in VHL exon deletions. *Am J Med Genet A*. 2009;149a:2147-2151.
88. Wachtel H, Fishbein L. Genetics of pheochromocytoma and paraganglioma. *Curr Opin Endocrinol Diabetes Obes*. 2021;28:283-290.
89. Walther MM, Keiser HR, Choyke PL, Rayford W, Lyne JC, Linehan WM. Management of hereditary pheochromocytoma in von Hippel-Lindau kindreds with partial adrenalectomy. *J Urol*. 1999;161:395-398.
90. Weisbrod AB, Kitano M, Gesuwan K, et al. Clinical utility of functional imaging with ^{18}F-FDOPA in von Hippel-Lindau syndrome. *J Clin Endocrinol Metab*. 2012;97:E613-E617.
91. Zhuang Z, Yang C, Lorenzo F, et al. Somatic HIF2A gain-of-function mutations in paraganglioma with polycythemia. *N Engl J Med*. 2012;367:922-930.
92. Comino-Méndez I, de Cubas AA, Bernal C, et al. Tumoral EPAS1 (HIF2A) mutations explain sporadic pheochromocytoma and paraganglioma in the absence of erythrocytosis. *Hum Mol Genet*. 2013;22:2169-2176.
93. Därr R, Nambuba J, Del Rivero J, et al. Novel insights into the polycythemia-paraganglioma-somatostatinoma syndrome. *Endocr Relat Cancer*. 2016;23:899-908.
94. Ladroue C, Carcenac R, Leporrier M, et al. PHD2 mutation and congenital erythrocytosis with paraganglioma. *N Engl J Med*. 2008;359:2685-2692.
95. Yang C, Zhuang Z, Fliedner SM, et al. Germ-line PHD1 and PHD2 mutations detected in patients with pheochromocytoma/paraganglioma-polycythemia. *J Mol Med (Berl)*. 2015;93:93-104.
96. Johannessen CM, Johnson BW, Williams SM, et al. TORC1 is essential for NF1-associated malignancies. *Curr Biol*. 2008;18:56-62.
97. Qin Y, Yao L, King EE, et al. Germline mutations in TMEM127 confer susceptibility to pheochromocytoma. *Nat Genet*. 2010;42:229-233.
98. Segouffin-Cariou C, Billaud M. Transforming ability of MEN2A-RET requires activation of the phosphatidylinositol 3-kinase/AKT signaling pathway. *J Biol Chem*. 2000;275:3568-3576.
99. Nölting S, Grossman AB. Signaling pathways in pheochromocytomas and paragangliomas: prospects for future therapies. *Endocr Pathol*. 2012;23:21-33.
100. Gottfried ON, Viskochil DH, Couldwell WT. Neurofibromatosis type 1 and tumorigenesis: molecular mechanisms and therapeutic implications. *Neurosurg Focus*. 2010;28:E8.
101. Qin Y, Deng Y, Ricketts CJ, et al. The tumor susceptibility gene TMEM127 is mutated in renal cell carcinomas and modulates endolysosomal function. *Hum Mol Genet*. 2014;23:2428-2439.
102. Deng Y, Qin Y, Srikantan S, et al. The TMEM127 human tumor suppressor is a component of the mTORC1 lysosomal nutrient-sensing complex. *Hum Mol Genet*. 2018;27:1794-1808.

103. Eisenhofer G, Huynh TT, Elkahloun A, et al. Differential expression of the regulated catecholamine secretory pathway in different hereditary forms of pheochromocytoma. *Am J Physiol Endocrinol Metab*. 2008;295:E1223-E1233.
104. Taïeb D, Jha A, Treglia G, Pacak K. Molecular imaging and radionuclide therapy of pheochromocytoma and paraganglioma in the era of genomic characterization of disease subgroups. *Endocr Relat Cancer*. 2019;26:R627-R652.
105. Taïeb D, Pacak K. New insights into the nuclear imaging phenotypes of cluster 1 pheochromocytoma and paraganglioma. *Trends Endocrinol Metab*. 2017;28:807-817.
106. Grubbs EG, Rich TA, Ng C, et al. Long-term outcomes of surgical treatment for hereditary pheochromocytoma. *J Am Coll Surg*. 2013;216:280-289.
107. Yip L, Lee JE, Shapiro SE, et al. Surgical management of hereditary pheochromocytoma. *J Am Coll Surg*. 2004;198:525-534.
108. Rossitti HM, Söderkvist P, Gimm O. Extent of surgery for phaeochromocytomas in the genomic era. *Br J Surg*. 2018;105:e84-e98.
109. De Filpo G, Maggi M, Mannelli M, Canu L. Management and outcome of metastatic pheochromocytomas/paragangliomas: an overview. *J Endocrinol Invest*. 2021;44:15-25.
110. Moramarco J, El Ghorayeb N, Dumas N, et al. Pheochromocytomas are diagnosed incidentally and at older age in neurofibromatosis type 1. *Clin Endocrinol (Oxf)*. 2017;86:332-339.
111. Gimenez-Roqueplo AP, Dahia PL, Robledo M. An update on the genetics of paraganglioma, pheochromocytoma, and associated hereditary syndromes. *Horm Metab Res*. 2012;44:328-333.
112. Gruber LM, Erickson D, Babovic-Vuksanovic D, Thompson GB, Young WF Jr, Bancos I. Pheochromocytoma and paraganglioma in patients with neurofibromatosis type 1. *Clin Endocrinol (Oxf)*. 2017;86:141-149.
113. Yao L, Schiavi F, Cascon A, et al. Spectrum and prevalence of FP/TMEM127 gene mutations in pheochromocytomas and paragangliomas. *JAMA*. 2010;304:2611-2619.
114. Toledo SP, Lourenço DM Jr, Sekiya T, et al. Penetrance and clinical features of pheochromocytoma in a six-generation family carrying a germline TMEM127 mutation. *J Clin Endocrinol Metab*. 2015;100:E308-E318.
115. Paredes SCS, Lopes SGC, Torres IMBF, Alves MLF. Pheochromocytoma due to *TMEM127* mutation: the importance of genetic testing for clinical decision. *Eur Endocrinol*. 2020;16:72-74.
116. Comino-Méndez I, Gracia-Aznárez FJ, Schiavi F, et al. Exome sequencing identifies MAX mutations as a cause of hereditary pheochromocytoma. *Nat Genet*. 2011;43:663-667.
117. Burnichon N, Cascón A, Schiavi F, et al. MAX mutations cause hereditary and sporadic pheochromocytoma and paraganglioma. *Clin Cancer Res*. 2012;18:2828-2837.

Thyroid Storm

73

Rajam Raghunathan, MD, PhD
Jesse D. Pasternak, MD, MPH

INTRODUCTION

Thyroid storm is a severe and exaggerated clinical manifestation of hyperthyroidism. It is characterized by fever, hemodynamic instability, cardiovascular dysregulation, gastrointestinal dysfunction, and altered mental status.[1] Precipitating factors and events include longstanding untreated hyperthyroidism, trauma, surgery, infection, iodine load—commonly from contrast or amiodarone use, and erratic use or abrupt discontinuation of antithyroid medication.[2] The exact pathophysiology of thyroid storm remains unknown.[2] Without a universally validated scoring system or pathognomonic diagnostic criteria, thyroid storm remains a clinical diagnosis in the presence of confirmatory thyroid function tests, suppressed TSH, and elevated T4 and/or T3 that establish hyperthyroidism.[2,3] Mortality in thyroid storm remains significant; some series estimate it at between 10% and 25%, with the highest mortality rates seen among patients requiring ICU admission.[1,2] Early identification of its manifesting symptoms, treatment of precipitating factors, and aggressive supportive therapy in an intensive care setting form the cornerstone of therapy.[4] Medical management is the first line in addressing thyroid storm. Radioiodine ablative (RAI) therapy and thyroidectomy are definitive therapies for hyperthyroidism and the prevention of recurrence in thyrotoxic patients recalcitrant to maximal medical intervention.[4,5]

CLINICAL PATHOPHYSIOLOGY

It is unclear what factors contribute to inciting thyroid storm.[2,5] A rapid increase in serum thyroid hormone levels, increased catecholamine responsiveness and heightened responses to thyroid hormone at the cellular level are among the hypotheses proposed to account for its development.[3,4] The quantity of thyroid hormone (T4 and T3) excess and TSH suppression is not reflective of risk when patients who have uncomplicated thyrotoxicosis are compared to those progressing to thyroid storm.[3]

ETIOLOGY

Thyroid storm can develop in patients with known or undiagnosed hyperthyroidism which can be secondary to Graves' disease (most common), toxic multinodular goiter, or solitary toxic adenoma. The risk factors for its development, however, are unclear.[2] It can be precipitated by an acute stress event such as surgery (thyroidectomy or non-thyroid surgery), trauma, infection, childbirth, or a load of iodine-containing medication (amiodarone or iodinated contrast).[5,6] Erratic or irregular use of antithyroid medication, or its abrupt discontinuation, are reported to be more common precipitants.[7,8] In oncology patients, the use of checkpoint inhibitor therapy leading to a destructive thyroiditis can be associated with thyroid storm.[9,10] A rare but important cause occurs when patients with hyperthyroidism may be prescribed SSKI or Lugol's solution in anticipation of thyroidectomy.[7] While it can help thyroid surgery outcomes in these patients, extended use of this preoperative treatment can lead to the Wolff-Chaikoff effect and thus, thyroid storm can ensue.[7]

EPIDEMIOLOGY

Recent estimates of the incidence of thyroid storm in the United States are 0.57 to 0.7 cases per 100,000 persons per year in the overall population and 4.8 to 5.6 cases per 100,000 persons per year among hospitalized patients.[11] A nationwide survey in Japan showed the incidence of thyroid storm in Japan to be about 0.22% of all thyrotoxic patients and 5.4% of all admitted thyrotoxic patients.[6,12] The average age found in the Japanese study was between 42 and 44 years, which was similar to those with thyrotoxicosis without thyroid storm.[6,12] The male to female ratio for thyroid storm incidence was 1:3, similar to the gender ratio of the group of patients who had thyrotoxicosis without storm.[6,12]

CLINICAL PRESENTATION

Clinical manifestations of storm are multisystem in nature and characterized by an amplification of typical symptoms of hyperthyroidism. These include hyperpyrexia (with temperatures greater than 40°C), cardiovascular dysfunction (tachycardia greater than 130-140 beats/minute, atrial fibrillation, congestive heart failure, cardiovascular collapse), gastrointestinal symptoms (nausea, vomiting, diarrhea, abdominal cramps, hepatic failure, jaundice), and altered mentation (agitation, delirium, obtundation, or coma).[12,13] The use of antithyroid drug therapy in the context of hyperthyroidism, recent thyroidal or nonthyroidal surgery, and recent exposure to iodinated contrast materials are also important details to note in history. When thyroid storm occurs in the operating room, it is usually recognized by the anesthesiologist on induction into general anesthesia and may result in an acute hemodynamic collapse.[14]

DIAGNOSIS, LABORATORY, & IMAGING STUDIES

In the absence of precise criteria or a universally accepted clinical score, thyroid storm is diagnosed based on the presence of life-threatening symptoms in a patient with biochemical hyperthyroidism.[15] Burch and Wartofsky introduced a clinical scoring system for the identification of thyroid storm (Table 73–1).[4] A score of 45 or more is highly suggestive of the diagnosis, less than 25 is highly unlikely, and scores between 25 and 44 are suggestive of an impending thyroid storm. This scoring system has not gained universal acceptance given the tool's performance. Although the specificity is quite high, the sensitivity is seen to be low.[12] Another set of clinical criteria has been introduced by the Japanese Thyroid Association (Table 73–2) based on the manifestations of thyroid storm and severe hyperthyroidism.[15] Subsequent literature, however, has highlighted that it also has a low sensitivity for diagnosis.[12,15]

Along with a detailed history and physical exam, patients in whom there is suspicion for thyroid storm risk should have biochemical workup of hyperthyroidism. While suppressed TSH and elevated free T4 and/or T3 may signal that a patient is at increased risk to develop storm,[16] it is important to note that the degree of biochemical hyperthyroidism is not diagnostic of thyroid storm: the level of TSH suppression and T4 and/or T3 elevation in thyroid storm is comparable to that seen in hyperthyroid patients without thyroid storm.[3,16]

Given the mortality associated with thyroid storm, the priority for the clinician is aggressive, supportive therapy.[17] Once stabilized, investigation of etiology, whether through radioactive iodine uptake scan (Plummer disease) or further

Table 73–1. Burch Wartofsky point scale for thyroid storm diagnosis (1993).

Thermoregulatory dysfunction		
Temperature °F (°C)		
99-99.5 (37.2-37.7)	0	
100-100.9 (37.8-38.2)	10	
101-101.9 (38.3-38.8)	15	
102-102.9 (38.9-39.2)	20	
103-103.9 (39.3-39.9)	25	
≥104 (≥40)	30	
Cardiovascular		
Tachyardia (beats/min)		
100-109	5	
110-119	10	
120-129	15	
130-139	20	
≥140	25	
Atrial fibrillation		
Absent	0	
Present	10	
Congestive heart failure		
Absent	0	
Mild	5	Pedal edema
Moderate	10	Bibasilar rales
Severe	20	Pulmonary edema
Gastrointestinal–hepatic dysfunction		
Absent	0	
Moderate	10	Diarrhea, abdominal pain, nausea/vomiting
Severe	20	Unexplained jaundice
CNS effects		
Absent	0	
Mild	10	Agitation
Moderate	20	Delirium, psychosis, extreme lethargy
Severe	30	Seizure, coma
Precipitant history		
Status		
Positive	0	
Negative	10	
Score–Total		
≥45	Highly suggestive of thyroid storm	
25-44	Suggestive of impending thyroid storm	
<25	Unlikely to represent thyroid storm	

Source: Modified with permission from Burch HB, Wartofsky L. Life-threatening Thyrotoxicosis. Thyrotoxic storm. *Endocrinol Metab Clin North Am*. 1993; 22(2):263-277.

Table 73–2. Japanese Thyroid Association criteria for thyroid storm (2016).

Prerequisite = Thyrotoxicosis (elevated FT3 and/or FT4) **Plus** • Altered mentation (delirium, psychosis, lethargy, somnolence coma) • Fever (38 Celsius/100.4 Fahrenheit or greater) • Tachycardia (130 beats per minute or higher) • CHF (pulmonary edema, rales, cardiogenic shock, or NYHA class IV) • GI symptoms (nausea, vomiting, diarrhea, total Bilirubin 3 mg/dL or greater)
Definite thyroid storm Thyrotoxicosis (elevated FT3 and/or FT4) **Plus** At least one CNS manifestation **Plus** One or more other symptom: fever, tachycardia, CHF, GI/hepatic manifestations) **or** A combination of ≥ three features among: fever, GI symptoms, CHF, or tachycardia
Suggested thyroid storm A combination of at least two features: tachycardia, CHF, GI/hepatic, fever **or** History of thyroid disease, presence of goiter and exophthalmos Meets criteria for TS1; TFTs not available

Source: Adapted from Satoh T, Isozaki O, Suzuki A, et al. 2016 Guidelines for the Management of Thyroid Storm from The Japan Thyroid Association and Japan Endocrine Society (1st ed). *Endocr J.* 2016;63(12):1025-1064.

biochemical workup with thyrotropin receptor antibody (Graves' disease) testing, should ensue.[15,17,18]

MEDICAL MANAGEMENT & TREATMENT

Early identification, immediate initiation of medical treatment, and supportive management in an intensive care setting are essential to survival in thyroid storm. The therapeutic regimen for thyroid storm is multifactorial (Table 73–3). From a cardiovascular standpoint, heart rate control with a beta-blocker or calcium channel blocker is central to address the signs and symptoms of increased adrenergic tone.[4] Propranolol is the first line, at a dose of 60 to 80 mg every 4 to 6 hours, with appropriate titration for heart rate and blood pressure control.[4,19] Propranolol is chosen as initial therapy as it inhibits type 1 deiodinase in high doses, which further helps to reduce serum T3 levels.[19] It can also be given intravenously in a monitored setting at an initial dose of 0.5 to 1 mg over 10 minutes followed by 1 to 2 mg over 10 minutes every 2 to 3 hours.[20]

A thionamide should be initiated to block *de novo* thyroid hormone synthesis and iodine given to block thyroid

Table 73–3. Medical management of thyroid storm.

Intervention	Effect
ICU admission and management • IV fluid support +/− diuretics • IV antibiotics (as required) • Acetaminophen for fever (avoid ASA)	• Aggressive supportive management • Identification and treatment of precipitating factors (ie, infection) • Control of hyperpyrexia
Beta blocker • Propranolol 60-80 mg PO q 4-6h **or** • Propranolol 0.5-1 mg IV over 10 min followed by 1-2 mg IV over 10 min q2-3h	• Heart rate and BP control • Inhibits type 1 deiodinase in high doses, further helps to reduce serum T3 levels
Thionamide • Propylthiouracil (PTU) 200 mg PO q4h **or** • Methimazole 20 mg PO q4-6h	• Blocks *de novo* thyroid hormone synthesis
Iodine • Saturated solution of potassium iodide (5 drops PO q6h) **or** • Lugol's solution (10 drops PO q8h)	• Blocks thyroid hormone release • Administer at least one hour after the administration of thionamide to prevent iodine being used as substrate in *de novo* hormone synthesis
Glucocorticoids • Hydrocortisone 100 mg IV q8h	• Inhibit peripheral conversion of T4 to T3 • May treat the autoimmune process in Graves' disease • May address any associated relative adrenal insufficiency
Bile acid sequestrants • Cholestyramine 4 g PO QID	• Use in severe thyrotoxicosis and thyroid storm • Decreases enterohepatic recycling of thyroid hormones

hormone release.[21,22] Thionamides include either Propylthiouracil (PTU) 200 mg orally every 4 hours or Methimazole 20 mg orally every 4 to 6 hours.[22] While they have no effect on preformed hormones from the thyroid itself, they begin blocking *de novo* synthesis of thyroid hormone within 1 to 2 hours of administration.[16,18] Propylthiouracil is favored due to its capacity to block T4-to-T3 conversion; as a result, T3 levels can drop by approximately 45% within the first 24 hours of PTU administration, compared to only 10% to 15% after methimazole administration.[16,18] Given altered GI absorption of medications during storm, higher doses of thionamide are used than those necessary to completely block thyroid hormone synthesis.[16] Both drugs can be administered orally via nasogastric tube or rectally via enema.[23,24] PTU can also be prepared for intravenous administration at a dose of 576 mg/24 hours.[25] Patients initiated on PTU in the ICU or in hospital should be transitioned to Methimazole prior to discharge.[22]

One hour after the administration of the first dose of thionamide, iodine is given, in the form of saturated solution of potassium iodide (5 drops orally every 6 hours) or Lugol's solution (10 drops orally every 8 hours).[22] It is essential to delay iodine administration for at least an hour after dosing of the Thionamide to prevent the iodine from being taken up and used as a substrate for new hormone synthesis in instances where the patient has a toxic adenoma or toxic multinodular goiter. Further, prolonged use of Lugol's solution can itself elicit thyroid storm due to the Wolf-Chaikoff effect.[7]

Glucocorticoids (Hydrocortisone IV 100 mg every 8 hours) are given to inhibit the peripheral conversion of T4 to T3; they also treat the autoimmune process in Graves' disease.[22] Though uncommon, relative adrenal insufficiency associated with Graves' disease is addressed by glucocorticoids as well.[26,27] Bile acid sequestrants (Cholestyramine 4 g orally, four times daily) can be used in severe cases of thyroid storm to decrease the enterohepatic recycling of thyroid hormones.[22] Supportive management should also include the recognition and treatment of any inciting factors such as infection. Intravenous fluids should be administered judiciously; some patients may require significant fluid support, while others may need diuresis due to the symptoms of congestive heart failure.[22] Hyperpyrexia (temperatures greater than 104°F or 41°C) should be aggressively addressed and corrected with acetaminophen; ASA should be avoided as it can increase serum-free T4 and T3 concentrations by inhibiting the binding of triiodothyronine (T3) and free thyroxine (T4) to thyroxine-binding globulin and thyroxine-binding prealbumin.[28]

If clinical improvement is seen with medical therapy—evidenced by defervescence, hemodynamic stability, and the resolution of any CNS manifestations—glucocorticoids can be tapered and discontinued and iodine can be stopped.[22] Beta blockers or calcium channel blockers should only be withdrawn once thyroid function tests normalize and thionamides should be dose-titrated to euthyroidism, with propylthiouracil (PTU) switched to methimazole prior to patient discharge.[22]

Definitive treatment in Graves' patients consists of radioactive iodine (RAI) therapy or thyroidectomy.[22] RAI is the classic first-line definitive therapy in the absence of orbitopathy or contraindication to radioactive treatment given evidence of lower cost and low complication rates. Surgical management, however, has become more commonly used given its comparable patient quality of life after treatment.[22,29]

SURGICAL TREATMENT

Surgical treatment via total thyroidectomy is recommended for definitive management of thyrotoxicosis in certain patients and newer evidence has shown it to be preferred in many scenarios.[29] These include in patients:

- unable to take a thionamide
- recalcitrant to maximal medical management
- with coexisting primary hyperparathyroidism requiring surgery
- with confirmed thyroid malignancy
- in whom radioactive iodine treatment is contraindicated

Patients who require surgery and are at high risk of thyroid storm should be considered for preoperative treatment of thyrotoxicosis with beta blockade or calcium channel blockade to achieve adequate rate control, glucocorticoids to inhibit T4 to T3 conversion, bile acid sequestrants to reduce enterohepatic circulation of thyroid hormone, and SSKI or iodine in patients with Graves' disease.[21,22] Treatment with SSKI/Lugol's solution can be initiated up to 5 to 7 days prior to surgery, which should not be extended beyond 8 to 10 days due to the phenomenon of the escape from the Wolff-Chaikoff effect.[7,21] The Wolff-Chaikoff effect refers to the capacity of exogenous iodine in large doses to inhibit the organification of iodine in the thyroid gland. This effect, however, is transient in nature as the iodide transport system can adapt to higher concentrations of iodine, which permits thyroid hormone synthesis to resume, potentially worsening and intensifying thyrotoxicosis.[7] This highlights the importance of expeditious surgical intervention once thyrotoxic symptoms are controlled preoperatively. If traditional preoperative therapy to control thyrotoxicosis in patients awaiting thyroid surgery is unsuccessful, plasmapheresis may be tried as an alternative.[30,31] Plasmapheresis removes thyroid hormones, cytokines, and antibodies from plasma; case reports demonstrate clinical improvement in thyrotoxicosis. There is no current consensus regarding its role, safety, or efficacy at producing any mortality benefit.[30,31]

PROGNOSIS

Given the rarity of thyroid storm, predictive features associated with increased morbidity and mortality have not been clearly identified. A nationwide database in Japan showed the overall in-hospital mortality rate of thyroid storm to be 10.1%, with older age (60 years or more), central nervous system dysfunction, need for mechanical ventilation and/or hemodialysis, and nonuse of antithyroid drugs and beta blockers associated with higher mortality.[2,6] Both the Japanese study and an American retrospective cohort study highlighted CNS dysfunction as an important feature distinguishing in-hospital morbidity and mortality in patients with thyroid storm, suggesting that the identification of thyrotoxic patients developing altered mentation and early initiation of aggressive supportive measures in these patients are essential to survival.[2,6,13]

CONCLUSION

While thyroid storm is extremely rare, its consequences are often fatal. Good control of thyrotoxicosis and sharp clinical suspicion, especially during times of stress, should be a priority for thyroidologists. Aggressive supportive care and subsequent definitive management of thyrotoxicosis should be the main tenets of treatment.

REFERENCES

1. Bourcier S, Coutrot M, Kimmoun A, et al. Thyroid storm in the ICU: a retrospective multicenter study. *Crit Care Med.* 2020;48:83-90.
2. Ono Y, Ono S, Yasunaga H, Matsui H, Fushimi K, Tanaka Y. Factors associated with mortality of thyroid storm: analysis using a national inpatient database in Japan. *Medicine (Baltimore).* 2016;95(7):e2848.
3. Brooks MH, Waldstein SS. Free thyroxine concentrations in thyroid storm. *Ann Intern Med.* 1980;93:694-697.
4. Burch HB, Wartofsky L. Life-threatening thyrotoxicosis. Thyroid storm. *Endocrinol Metab Clin North Am.* 1993;22(2):263-277.
5. Sarlis NJ, Gourgiotis L. Thyroid emergencies. *Rev Endocr Metab Disord.* 2003;4:129-136.
6. Akamizu T, Satoh T, Isozaki O, et al. Diagnostic criteria, clinical features and incidence of thyroid storm based on nationwide surveys. *Thyroid.* 2012;22(7):661-679.
7. Eng PHK, Cardona GR, Fang S-L, et al. Escape from the acute Wolff-Chaikoff effect is associated with a decrease in thyroid sodium/iodide symporter messenger ribonucleic acid and protein. *Endocrinology.* 1999;140(8):3404-3410.
8. Rivas AM, Larumbe E, Thavaraputta S, Juarez E, Adiga A, Lado-Abeal J. Unfavorable socioeconomic factors underlie high rates of hospitalization for complicated thyrotoxicosis in some regions of the United States. *Thyroid.* 2019;29(1):27-35.
9. Ferrari SM, Fallahi P, Galetta F, Citi E, Benvenga S, Antonelli A. Thyroid disorders induced by checkpoint inhibitors. *Rev Endocr Metab Disord.* 2018;19(4):325-333.
10. Swee du S, Chang CL, Lim A. Clinical characteristics and outcome of thyroid storm: a case series and review of neuropsychiatric derangements in thyrotoxicosis. *Endocr Pract.* 2015;21(2):182-189.
11. Galindo RJ, Hurtado CR, Pasquel FJ, García Tome R, Peng L, Umpierrez GE. National trends in incidence, mortality and clinical outcomes of patients hospitalized for thyrotoxicosis with and without thyroid storm in the United States, 2004-2013. *Thyroid.* 2019;29(1):36-43.
12. Akamizu T. Thyroid storm: a Japanese perspective. *Thyroid.* 2018;28(1):32-40.
13. Angell TE, Lechner MG, Nguyen CT, Salvato VL, Nicoloff JT, LoPresti JS. Clinical features and hospital outcomes in thyroid storm: a retrospective cohort study. *J Clin Endocrinol Metab.* 2015(2);100:451-459.
14. Grimes CM, Muniz H, Montgomery WH. Intraoperative thyroid storm: a case report. *AANA Journal.* 2004;72(1):53-55.
15. Satoh T, Isozaki O, Suzuki A, et al. 2016 Guidelines for the management of thyroid storm from The Japan Thyroid Association and Japan Endocrine Society (First Edition). *Endocr J.* 2016;63(12):1025-1064.
16. Abuid J, Larsen PR. Triiodothyronine and thyroxine in hyperthyroidism. Comparison of the acute changes during therapy with antithyroid agents. *J Clin Invest.* 1974;54(1):201-208.
17. Chiha M, Samarasinghe S, Kabaker AS. Thyroid storm: an updated review. *J Intensive Care Med.* 2015;30(3):131-140.
18. Cooper DS, Saxe VC, Meskell M, Maloof F, Ridgway EC. Acute effects of propylthiouracil (PTU) on thyroidal iodide organification and peripheral iodothyronine deiodination: correlation with serum PTU levels measured by radioimmunoassay. *J Clin Endocrinol Metab.* 1982;54(1):101-107.
19. Cooper DS, Daniels GH, Ladenson PW, Ridgway EC. Hyperthyroxinemia in patients treated with high-dose propranolol. *Am J Med.* 1982;73(6):867-871.
20. Das G, Krieger M. Treatment of thyrotoxic storm with intravenous administration of propranolol. *Ann Intern Med.* 1969;70(5):985-988.
21. Langley RW, Burch HB. Perioperative management of the thyrotoxic patient. *Endocrinol Metab Clin North Am.* 2003;32(2):519-534.
22. Ross DS, Burch HB, Cooper DS, et al. 2016 American Thyroid Association Guidelines for Diagnosis and Management of Hyperthyroidism and Other Causes of Thyrotoxicosis. *Thyroid.* 2016;26(10):1343-1421.
23. Yeung SC, Go R, Balasubramanyam A. Rectal administration of iodide and propylthiouracil in the treatment of thyroid storm. *Thyroid.* 1995 Oct;5(5):403-5.
24. Jongjaroenprasert W, Akarawut W, Chantasart D, et al. Rectal administration of propylthiouracil in hyperthyroid patients: comparison of suspension enema and suppository form. *Thyroid.* 2002 Jul;12.
25. Alfadhli E, Gianoukakis AG. Management of severe thyrotoxicosis when the gastrointestinal tract is compromised. *Thyroid.* 2011 Mar;21(3):215-220.
26. Naik D, Jebasignh KF, Thomas N. Delayed diagnosis of Graves' thyrotoxicosis presenting as recurrent adrenal crisis in primary adrenal insufficiency. *J Clin Diagn Res.* 2016;10(4):OD20-OD22.
27. Tsatsoulis A, Johnson EO, Kalogera CH, Seferiadis K, Tsolas O. The effect of thyrotoxicosis on adrenocortical reserve. *Eur J Endocrinol.* 2000;142(3):231-235.
28. Larsen PR. Salicylate-induced increases in free triiodothyronine in human serum. Evidence of inhibition of triiodothyronine binding to thyroxine-binding globulin and thyroxine-binding prealbumin. *J Clin Invest.* 1972;51(5):1125-1134.
29. Liu X, Wong CKH, Chan WWL, et al. Outcomes of Graves' disease patients following antithyroid drugs, radioactive iodine, or thyroidectomy as the first-line treatment. *Ann Surg.* 2021;273(6):1197-1206.
30. Vinan-Vega M, Mantillia B, Jahan N, et al. Usefulness of plasmapheresis in patients with severe complicated thyrotoxicosis. *Proc (Bayl Univ Med Cent).* 2021;34(2):279-282.
31. Vyas AA, Vyas P, Fillipon NL, Vijayakrishnan R, Trivedi N. Successful treatment of thyroid storm with plasmapheresis in a patient with methimazole-induced agranulocytosis. *Endocr Pract.* 2010;16(4):673-676.

74 Myxedema Coma

Radwa Osman, MD
Ahmed Ahmed, MD
David Lieb, MD, FACE

GENERAL CONSIDERATIONS

Myxedema coma (MC), also called decompensated hypothyroidism or myxedema crisis, is a life-threatening condition requiring emergent, intensive care. While rare, it carries a high mortality—ranging between 30% and 60% depending on available medical resources.[1] The incidence of MC, estimated to be 0.22 to 1.08 cases per million patients per year worldwide, is likely underreported in the literature, especially given that its predecessor, hypothyroidism, is quite common.[1] That said, it's important for clinicians such as surgeons, endocrinologists, emergency medicine physicians, and intensivists to be able to recognize MC, and to identify those individuals at highest risk for morbidity and mortality, especially older individuals, and those who present in colder winter months.

While many patients presenting with MC will have a clear history of hypothyroidism—either autoimmune or postsurgical—this will not always be clear on presentation. Given their altered mental status patients will typically not be able to provide their relevant medical history. MC tends to be more common in women and older adults, as these populations are at higher risk for developing autoimmune thyroiditis.[2] It has been rarely reported in children and adolescents, though prognosis in this population may be better than in adults.[3] MC may be medication-related, as can be seen with amiodarone therapy (in treatment of cardiac arrhythmias), with thionamide therapy (ie, methimazole, propylthiouracil, carbimazole) in treatment of hyperthyroidism and with tyrosine kinase inhibitors and immune checkpoint inhibitors used for the treatment of a variety of cancers.[4-6] The latter two are associated with the development of thyroiditis (Table 74–1). There have also been cases of MC described in patients with coronavirus disease 2019 (COVID-19), which has been associated with the development of autoimmune thyroiditis and hypothyroidism.[7,8]

Those at particularly high risk for death include older patients (those >65 years of age), and those that present with hemodynamic instability, sepsis, or require mechanical ventilation.[1] Any systemic stressor in a predisposed patient can trigger a myxedema crisis (Table 74–2). Infections are the most frequently reported precipitating factor, but MC can occur following surgery, burn, trauma, cerebrovascular accidents, heart failure or myocardial injury, gastrointestinal bleeding, and pulmonary embolism.[1] These events will disrupt normal homeostatic responses that hypothyroid patients mount to prevent organ damage, that is, significant volume loss or respiratory compromise. Of note, up to half of individuals with MC will not have a clear precipitating factor.[1]

Special attention should be given to the medically disadvantaged. Those without medical insurance and regular access to routine health care are more likely to have hypothyroidism that may be undiagnosed and may present late in the course of their disease process. They may develop symptoms of significant hypothyroidism over time due to lack of access to thyroid hormone, or unwillingness or inability (eg, due to distance or cost) to seek hospital care. Further, individuals living in more remote or rural locations may not have ready access to advanced and intensive care. Preventive measures, such as the use of mobile-free clinics and health insurance sign-up assistance, should be carried out when possible for these communities.

Pathogenesis of Myxedema Coma

Thyroid hormone production and its regulation are controlled by the hypothalamic-pituitary-thyroid (HPT) axis. This axis operates under continuous feedback to maintain normal thyroid hormone concentrations. Approximately 80% of thyroid hormone release by the thyroid gland is thyroxine or T4.[9] The remaining thyroid hormone released is triiodothyronine or T3. T3 is the active hormone, with T4 serving as a prohormone. T4 and T3 are released by the thyroid gland in response to stimulation of the thyroid by thyroid stimulating hormone (TSH), produced by

Table 74–1. Medications associated with the development of hypothyroidism/myxedema coma.

- Amiodarone
- Thionamides (methimazole, propylthiouracil, carbimazole)
- Lithium
- Tyrosine kinase inhibitors
  - Sunitinib
  - Sorafenib
- Immune checkpoint inhibitors
  - Anti-CTLA4 monoclonal antibodies (ipilimumab)
  - Anti-PD-1 monoclonal antibodies (nivolumab, pembrolizumab)
  - Anti-PD-L1 monoclonal antibodies (atezolizumab)

thyrotrophs in the anterior pituitary under control from the hypothalamus. T4 in the circulation is then deiodinated to T3, which then enters cell nuclei of target tissues where it binds to the thyroid hormone receptor (TR) that leads to gene transcription.[9]

Any insult to this axis can lead to the development of hypothyroidism, which, if left untreated, may lead to MC. This may include abnormalities involving the hypothalamus which produces thyrotropin-releasing hormone (TRH), the pituitary which is responsible for the production of TSH, or the thyroid gland itself.[9] Individuals may also have abnormalities involving the production of thyroid hormone (including iodine deficiency), its transport in blood, or its action at target tissues via the thyroid hormone receptor. Those with treated hypothyroidism may have a condition that affects adequate absorption of thyroid hormone, such as inflammatory bowel disease, celiac disease, or previous bariatric surgery.[2]

Thyroid hormone is necessary for life. Thyroid hormone regulates gene expression involved in metabolism of fats, carbohydrates, and proteins, determines the basal metabolic rate, and amplifies the effect of catecholamines.[9] While individuals may tolerate periods of hypothyroidism with mild symptoms, eventually the end-organ effects of lack of thyroid hormone on the cardiovascular and central nervous systems will be overwhelming, especially in the setting of additional stressors such as infection, ischemia, and infarction.

Prevention of Myxedema Coma

A number of strategies can help to reduce the likelihood of an individual developing MC. Patient education is very critical. All individuals with preexisting hypothyroidism, especially those who are older and may be a risk for developing MC, should be made aware of its existence and precipitating factors. It is important that families also be involved in this education, so that they may recognize symptoms and signs of less severe hypothyroidism that require evaluation. Patients should understand the consequences of missing thyroid hormone doses and should be encouraged to ask for assistance if they are having difficulty with paying for or otherwise obtaining their medication. Those taking medications that may interfere with thyroid hormone absorption (ie, calcium, lithium, iron) should be educated on how best to take their thyroid medication (on an empty stomach, with water at least 30 minutes prior to eating or drinking anything else each day or separate from all other medications and food for approximately 4 hours). Individuals should have their thyroid function assessed at least annually, with adjustments in thyroid hormone as indicated.

Provider education is equally important. Those who work in the emergency room should be able to identify serious and severe symptoms of hypothyroidism, as should those who work in the intensive care unit. Primary care providers should feel comfortable screening for and initiating treatment in individuals with hypothyroidism and should also have access to endocrinology consultative care when needed.

Clinical Findings in Myxedema Coma

A. Symptoms and Signs

Patients with MC can present with a variety of symptoms and signs reflecting multiorgan dysfunction, as a result of their slower metabolic state and changes in catecholamine action (Table 74-3). Diagnosis should be suspected in a patient presenting with altered mental status with a thyroidectomy scar, a history of radioactive iodine therapy, or hypothyroidism. History of preceding events from family members is often helpful. Providers should remember that not all patients

Table 74–2. Precipitating factors associated with the development of myxedema coma.

- Infections (including sepsis)
- Surgery
- Burns
- Trauma
- Cerebrovascular accidents
- Heart failure
- Myocardial injury/infarction
- Gastrointestinal bleeding
- Pulmonary embolism

Table 74–3. Clinical findings in patients with myxedema coma.

- Altered mental status (ranging from confusion to obtundation)
- Hypothermia
- Myxedema (nonpitting edema of lower extremities)
- Dry skin
- Brittle hair
- Delayed relaxation phase of deep tendon reflexes
- Pleural and pericardial effusions
- Bradycardia
- Hypotension

will have a history of hypothyroidism, and that their initial presentation may come in the form of severe, decompensated hypothyroidism.

Many patients with MC will present with significantly altered mental status with obtundation and may require intubation with mechanical ventilation. Thus, not all patients will be able to provide their symptoms. Patients or their families may be able to describe a history of cold intolerance, weight gain, fluid retention, fatigue, constipation, dry skin, brittle hair, hoarse voice, and forgetfulness. Older patients may be more likely to present with apathetic symptoms, including decreased appetite, weight loss, and depressed mood. Those with more severe hypothyroidism may note a recent history of muscular discomfort due to hypothyroidism-related myopathy. On examination, patients will have delayed relaxation phase of deep tendon reflexes.

Patients with severe, long-standing hypothyroidism may develop myxedematous changes. Typically described as a nonpitting edema of the lower extremities ("pretibial myxedema"), myxedema develops when individuals cannot clear glycosaminoglycans and hyaluronic acids from the dermis. Though it may begin in the legs, it can become more generalized causing hoarse voice (due to laryngeal myxedema) and cardiovascular disease.[10] There may be evidence of the "myxedematous facies"—with periorbital puffiness and swelling, and an enlarged tongue. Patients with MC may present with significant pleural and pericardial effusions causing dyspnea and chest discomfort. Rarely a pericardial effusion may become larger enough to cause cardiac tamponade, a cardiovascular emergency involving impaired venous return to the heart with hypotension and shock that requires immediate treatment.[11]

Patients with MC, given their severe decompensated hypothyroidism, may present with hypothermia and significant bradycardia, with reduced cardiac output and hypotension. The hypoventilation seen in patients with decompensated hypothyroidism is multifactorial, with altered mental status and weakened respiratory musculature each playing a significant role. Each of these requires supportive care that typically requires intensive care evaluation and management.

B. Laboratory Findings, Imaging Studies, and Special Tests

Patients presenting with MC will typically have an elevated thyroid stimulation hormone (TSH) level, in association with low thyroxine (T4) and triiodothyronine (T3) levels.[12] Patients with a history of hypothalamic or pituitary disease or surgery may have an inappropriately normal TSH level in the setting of low thyroid hormone levels. If the individual has autoimmune thyroiditis, antithyroid peroxidase (TPO) and/or antithyroglobulin antibodies may be elevated.[12]

A number of additional laboratory findings can be seen in patients with severe hypothyroidism. These include electrolyte abnormalities such as hyponatremia (due to increased free water retention), a reduced glomerular filtration rate (GFR) due to poor renal perfusion, hypoglycemia, and anemia (which can be micro-, normo-, or macrocytic). Individuals may also have elevated muscle-derived creatinine kinase and hyperlipidemia.[12] Those with respiratory failure will have an associated respiratory acidosis.

Evaluation for a concomitant infection is mandatory and may include imaging (chest X-ray to evaluate for pneumonia), urinalysis, and blood cultures. Viral etiologies including SARS-CoV-2 (the pathogenic agent in COVID-19) and influenza should be considered, as should viral and bacterial meningitis.

In addition to a chest film to evaluate for pneumonia, an electrocardiogram (EKG) should be done to evaluate for any cardiac arrhythmias, and an echocardiogram may be considered to identify evidence of heart failure or pericardial effusion.[12] A plain film of the abdomen should be performed to evaluate for ileus and bowel obstruction. Thyroid ultrasound can be considered in a stable patient to evaluate for goiter, or ultrasonographic evidence of autoimmune thyroid disease.

Differential Diagnosis

The differential diagnosis for myxedema coma is broad, and there are many causes of altered mental status that may have additional symptoms and signs that overlap. Therefore, clinicians must be actively looking to make a diagnosis of MC, otherwise it may be easily missed. Further, as patients often present with comorbid diagnoses that precipitate MC, such as sepsis, much attention may be paid to that condition rather than the MC itself. MC may also come to attention with atypical presentations. Hepatic encephalopathy (HE) is a particular diagnosis that can lead clinicians toward an incorrect diagnosis, as hyperammonemia can be seen in both HE and MC. There are reports in the literature of patients presenting with significant psychiatric manifestations of MC, including psychosis and mania.[13] There are also reports of stroke-like presentations, with patients having altered mental status, slurred speech, and weakness without clear evidence of stroke on brain imaging.[14]

Nonthyroidal illness (NTI), formerly called sick euthyroid syndrome, presents a particularly vexing situation for the clinician, as many of the conditions that may precipitate MC can be associated with NTI.[15] In early NTI the TSH will be low or suppressed, differentiating this condition from severe primary hypothyroidism (ie, related to thyroid gland dysfunction). However, it may be difficult to differentiate NTI from central hypothyroidism (ie, related to hypothalamic or pituitary dysfunction) as both will present with a low TSH. Some have suggested the use of reverse T3 measurements in this setting (as those with central hypothyroidism should have a low reverse T3 while it will be elevated in those with NTI), though this is not consistently reliable. While both NTI and MC will require treatment of the underlying condition leading to the abnormal thyroid function tests, only MC will necessitate treatment with thyroid hormone.

Popveniuc et al. developed a scoring system that can help to predict the presence of myxedema coma.[16] This scoring system includes abnormalities in body temperature, cardiovascular dysfunction, gastrointestinal findings, metabolic disturbances, and central nervous system effects of hypothyroidism, and accounts for whether a precipitating factor is present or not. A score >60 is considered highly suggestive or diagnostic of MC, while a score between 25 and 59 is suggestive. Those with a score <25 are not considered to have MC.

Complications

Hypothyroidism affects every organ system, and patients with MC are very ill. Patients need to be monitored for respiratory failure and many will require ventilatory assistance. Patients need to be monitored for the development of cardiac abnormalities including bradyarrhythmias, and thus should be placed on telemetry. Arrhythmias may also be precipitated by treatment with thyroid hormone (see following discussion). Bladder dysfunction should be managed with urethral catheterization. Patients may require hemodialysis for acute renal failure. An aggressive bowel regimen including laxatives may be needed to reduce fecal impaction and bowel obstruction. Hypothermia should be managed with passive warming (ie, warm blankets) rather than active warming to reduce cutaneous vasodilation which may worsen hypotension. Those with cardiogenic shock will require vasopressor agents to restore normotension.

Treatment

Myxedema coma is an emergency and when considered as a diagnosis, supportive care and therapy should begin immediately (Table 74–4). MC is a rare entity, and data guiding its management is sparse. As above, patients should be monitored for cardiac arrhythmias via telemetry, and most likely will require intensive care unit admission.[17] Many patients will require mechanical ventilation, intravenous fluids, and vasopressor agents. If there are concerns for infection, appropriate antibiotic therapy should be initiated. Given the potential for concomitant adrenal insufficiency, all patients with MC should receive stress-dose glucocorticoid therapy (typically provided as 100 mg of hydrocortisone intravenously every 8 hours).[18] If the patient is stable, a serum cortisol and ACTH can be drawn prior to initiating glucocorticoid therapy to confirm that diagnosis, and if normal, the steroid therapy can be discontinued. All patients require treatment with levothyroxine (T4), typically as a bolus of 200 to 400 μg followed by a daily dose of 50 to 100 μg. Many experts also recommend treatment with liothyronine (T3), though this may not be available at all medical centers.[18] This dose is 5 to 20 μg initially, followed by 2.5 to 10 μg every 8 hours. While liothyronine has a faster onset of action and stronger potency compared with levothyroxine, it can also increase oxygenation demands on the body. For this reason, the lowest dose necessary should be used in older individuals and in those with cardiac complications or comorbidities.

Table 74–4. Supportive care and therapeutic interventions in patients with myxedema coma.

Supportive care
- Respiratory assistance, potentially including mechanical ventilation
- Monitoring for cardiac arrhythmias with telemetry
- Urethral catheterization for bladder dysfunction
- Aggressive bowel regimen to prevent bowel obstruction
- Passive warming to treat hypothermia
- Intravenous fluids and vasopressor agents in those with hypotension

Therapeutic interventions
- Antibiotic therapy to treat any coexisting infections
- Stress-dose glucocorticoid therapy (hydrocortisone 100 mg IV every 8 hours)
- Levothyroxine (T4)—single IV bolus (200-400 μg) followed by daily dose of 50 to 100 μg
- Liothyronine (T3)—single IV bolus (5-20 μg) followed by 2.5-10 μg every 8 hours (Use caution in older patients and in those with cardiac complications/comorbidities)

Thyroid hormone—both levothyroxine and liothyronine—is typically provided intravenously. There are very few anecdotal reports of patients with MC succeeding with oral thyroid hormone replacement, and this is not recommended.[19] Once the patient is stable, the liothyronine can be discontinued and a daily oral dose of levothyroxine can be continued. In patients receiving enteral feeding, the tube feed will need to be held for at least 1 hour prior to and after thyroid hormone dosing to avoid malabsorption. For most patients with MC, endocrine consultation should be obtained if available. The endocrine consultant can assist with hospital management, and also ensure that the patient has appropriate outpatient follow-up care.

Prognosis

Myxedema coma carries a high mortality rate, up to 60%, though this may improve with better recognition and initiation of more immediate treatment.[1] As previously noted, there are particular risk factors that increase morbidity and mortality in patients presenting with MC, including older age (>65 years), and those presenting with hypotension, sepsis, and/or the need for mechanical ventilation.[1]

Given the high mortality associated with this condition, health-care providers must be able to diagnose and treat it quickly and ensure that all patients with MC receive appropriate supportive and therapeutic care.

When to Refer/When to Admit

Myxedema coma is an emergency requiring urgent, immediate care and management. All patients should be admitted to the intensive care unit with appropriate treatment and observant care as outlined in this chapter.

REFERENCES

1. Bridwell RE, Willis GC, Gottlieb M, Koyfman A, Long B. Decompensated hypothyroidism: a review for the emergency clinician. *Am J Emerg Med.* 2021;39:207-212.
2. Acharya R, Cheng C, Bourgeois M, Masoud J, McCray E. Myxedema coma: a forgotten medical emergency with a precipitous onset. *Cureus.* 2020;12(9):e10478.
3. De Sanctis V, Soliman A, Daar S, et al. The myxedema coma in children and adolescents: a rare endocrine emergency—personal experience and review of literature. *Acta Biomed.* 2021;92(5):e2021481.
4. Alaie M, Tramutola A, Mukamal D. A case report on methimazole-induced severe hypothyroidism. *Curerus.* 2022; 14(1):e21339.
5. Gummalla S, Manjunath M, Phillips B. Myedema coma: a life-threatening condition in patients using pembrolizumab. *Case Re Endocrinol.* 2020;2020:8855943.
6. Zagrski E, Jayatilaka S, Hirani F, et al. Amiodarone-associated myxedema coma. *Am J Case Rep.* 2020;21:e926757.
7. Dixit NM, Truong KP, Rabadia SV, et al. Sudden cardiac arrest in a patient with myxedema coma and COVID-19. *J Endocr Soc.* 2020;4(10):bvaa130.
8. Tutal E, Ozaras R, Leblebicioglu H. Systematic revie of COVID-19 and autoimmune thyroiditis. *Travel Med Infect Dis.* 2022;47:102314.
9. Shahid M, Ashraf M, Sharma S. Physiology, thyroid hormone. *StatPearls.* 2022.
10. Iftikhar M, Raziq F, Coll P, Dar AY. Laryngeal myxoedema: a literature review of an uncommon complication of hypothyroidism. *BMJ Case Reports.* 2021;14(4):e241313.
11. Baldwin C, Newman J, Vallejo F, Peck V, Greene LW, Goldberg IJ. Myxedema heart and pseudotamponade. *J Endocr Soc.* 2021 Jan 1;5(1):bvaa125.
12. McDermott M. Hypothyroidism. *Ann Intern Med.* 2020; 173(1):ITC1-ITC16.
13. Kaplan J, Castro-Revoredo I. Severe hypothyroidism manifested as acute mania with psychotic features: a case report and review of the literature. *J Psychiatr Pract.* 2020;26(5):417-422.
14. Butter C, Rashid N, Banatwalla R, FitzGerald T. Myxoedema coma masquerading as acute stroke. *Eur J Case Rep Intern Med.* 2020;7(7):001563.
15. Lies L, Jacobs A, Van den Berghe G. Nonthyroidal illness syndrome across the ages. *J Endocr Soc.* 2019;3(12):2313-2325.
16. Ylli D, Klubo-Gwiezdzinska J, Wartofsky L. Thyroid emergencies. *Pol Arch Intern Med.* 2019;129(7-8):526-534.
17. Elkattawy S, Dhanoa P, Kotys J, Fichadiya H, Eckman A. Myxedema coma: case report and literature review. *Cureus.* 2021; 13(5):e15277.
18. Wilson SA, Stem LA, Bruehlman RD. Hypothyroidism: diagnosis and treatment. *Am Fam Physician.* 2021;103(10):605-613.
19. Gadaen RJ, Tummers-de Lind van Wiingaarden RF. Hypothyroid crisis: oral or intravenous treatment? A report of two cases. *Eur J Case Rep Intern Med.* 2021;8(9):002752.

Acute Hyperparathyroidism

Marcella Donovan Walker, MD, MS
Ananya V. Kondapalli, MD
Shonni J. Silverberg, MD

75

INTRODUCTION

Parathyroid crisis refers to an episode of life-threatening hypercalcemia of abrupt onset in a patient with primary hyperparathyroidism (PHPT). There is no accepted definition or calcium threshold that defines parathyroid crisis, though numerous reports suggest a serum calcium concentration of 14 mg/dL or higher is consistent with the diagnosis. The first description, albeit incompletely recognized, was in 1923. At that time, Dawson and Struthers described a 49-year-old man with history of a humerus fracture months before who presented with an acute myocardial infarction and sudden death.[1,2] Postmortem exam indicated *osteitis fibrosa cystica* and a one-inch tumor near the left lower pole of the thyroid.

The first laboratory demonstration of parathyroid crisis dates to 1926 when James Collip, a Canadian biochemist, known for his work on purifying insulin, repeatedly administered large quantities of parathyroid extract to dogs, resulting in marked hypercalcemia associated with soft tissue calcium deposition, renal failure, and rapid demise.[3,4] Subsequently, Hanes is credited with reporting the first recognized human case of death from spontaneous parathyroid intoxication in his 1939 paper "Parathyroid Adenoma with Death, Due to Parathormone Intoxication."[1] This manuscript described a 49-year-old woman with history of pyelitis and hydronephrosis, admitted with fatigue and found to have a peak calcium of 22 mg/dL. Radiographs demonstrated calcium deposits in her kidneys and demineralized bones and ultimately she succumbed to her condition. Autopsy demonstrated a cystic and partially necrotic parathyroid tumor and widespread calcification and injury to the connective tissue, organs, and arteries. In addition, extensive myocardial injury and chronic tubular and glomerular nephritis with extensive medullary calcium deposits were present. Since that time, several hundred cases of the rare phenomenon of parathyroid crisis have been reported in the literature with varying features. Initially described as uniformly fatal, recognition of the surgical urgency of the condition and improvement in medical management has led to better outcomes in most cases.[5-7] While most of the information regarding acute hyperparathyroidism is limited to case reports and surgical case series, this chapter summarizes the available data on the condition.

EPIDEMIOLOGY

The incidence of acute PHPT is unknown, but it appears to be a relatively rare phenomenon today and less common since it was initially described.[7,8] Prevalence rates are variable and range from approximately 1.6% to 6.7% of patients with PHPT.[6,7] In one series of 152 patients with PHPT from the 1970s, acute hyperparathyroid crisis occurred in eight patients or 5.3%.[9] A review of 1310 consecutive patients with PHPT who underwent parathyroidectomy at a single institution from April 1970 through July 2009 indicated a similar prevalence of 6.7%.[10] Other surgical series that included similar time periods noted prevalence rates ranging from 2% to 4%.[11,12] A more recent study of patients from 1990 to 2007 indicated a similar prevalence with 2.7% presenting in crisis.[7] Such prevalence rates are almost exclusively derived from surgical series in patients undergoing parathyroidectomy. Thus, the true prevalence among all patients with PHPT is likely lower. PHPT is seen more commonly in women than in men. In parathyroid crisis, a few reports have demonstrated increased prevalence in women while other studies have shown a ratio closer to 1:1.[10,13,14] There does not appear to be an age predilection.[7,8,11] A small percentage of women present during pregnancy.[7,8]

ETIOLOGY & PATHOPHYSIOLOGY

Parathyroid storm is thought to be due to an external precipitant in many cases. Such precipitants may increase bone resorption or reduce calcium clearance. Case reports have documented parathyroid storm incited by dehydration, intercurrent illness, thiazide initiation, hyperemesis gravidarum, thyrotoxicosis, childbirth, or immobilization among others.[7] One case precipitated by vitamin D supplementation has been reported.[15] On the other hand, parathyroid storm has been hypothesized, in some cases, to be the result of a sudden outpouring of parathyroid hormone (PTH) into the bloodstream, leading to catastrophic hypercalcemia. Typically, parathyroid storm is due to a parathyroid adenoma, rather than parathyroid hyperplasia or carcinoma, though these have both been reported.[7,16] Parathyroid carcinoma may be more frequent in those with crisis. In a review of 252 cases of hyperparathyroid crisis reported from 1978 to 2007, parathyroid carcinoma was present in 5%, which contrasts with a prevalence of <1% reported in the literature for sporadic PHPT.[7] Figures 75–1A and B show pathological images from a patient presenting at our institution with parathyroid crisis found to have parathyroid carcinoma.

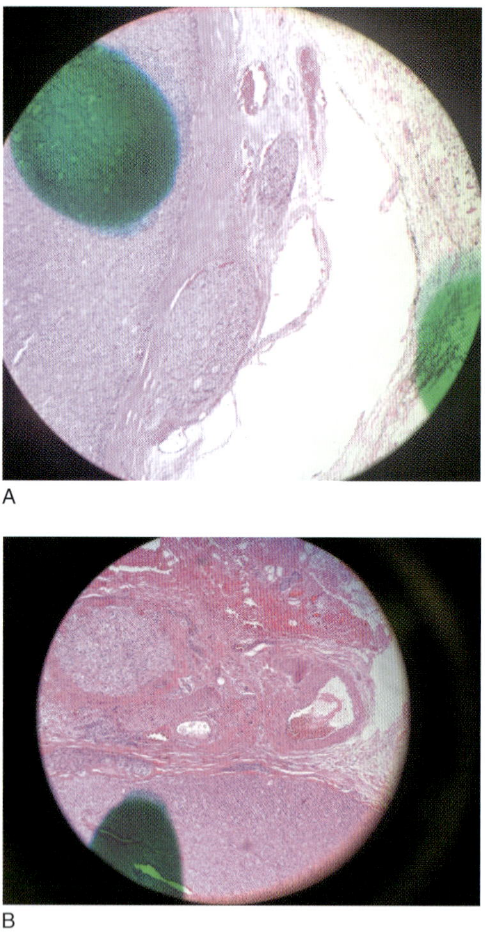

▲ **Figure 75–1.** Parathyroid carcinoma in a patient with primary hyperparathyroidism. **(A)** Parathyroid carcinoma can be seen extending into the capsule. **(B)** Invasion into neurovascular bundle.

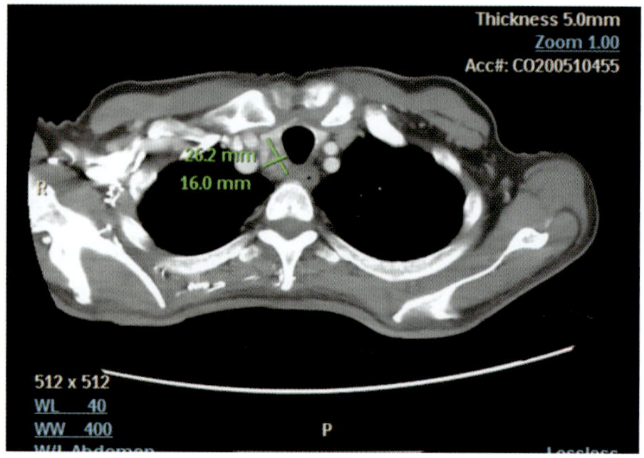

▲ **Figure 75–2.** Neck CT indicating a "thyroid nodule" measuring 2.6 × 1.6 cm, consistent with an intrathyroidal parathyroid.

Numerous cases describe associations with parathyroid hemorrhage, cysts, and/or infarction and necrosis, suggesting that some cases are, indeed, likely attributable to an acute parathyroid event that provokes presentation.[17-19] Some data indicate those presenting with crisis have larger and more "abnormal glands" than those presenting without crisis, potentially signifying that large glands may be vulnerable.[7,10] Another study, however, provides contradictory data to this hypothesis. It found no difference in gland size between those with and without crisis and reported that most tumors were <2 cm;[17] Figure 75–2 shows representative images from a neck computed tomography (CT) in a patient presenting with parathyroid crisis. The image indicates an enlarged parathyroid measuring 2.6 × 1.6 cm. The parathyroid was initially thought to be a thyroid nodule due to its intrathyroidal location.

One study assessed postparathyroidectomy histopathological characteristics between those with and without parathyroid crisis. It found no differences in histopathological characteristics except mitotic activity, which was greater in those with crisis.[17] Figure 75–3 demonstrates the parathyroid cytological findings from the patient corresponding to imaging in Figure 75–2. While parathyroid biopsy is not recommended in those with crisis or for diagnosis, the specimen was originally obtained by endocrine surgery to further evaluate the "thyroid nodule" seen on CT. The cytology indicates pleomorphic cells in syncytial and solid cellular arrangements, focally linked by traversing capillaries. The cells have rather monotonous hyperchromatic nuclei with very occasional pseudoinclusions and conspicuous nucleoli. The cytoplasm is somewhat abundant with clear cell features. Immunohistochemical staining was positive for PTH.

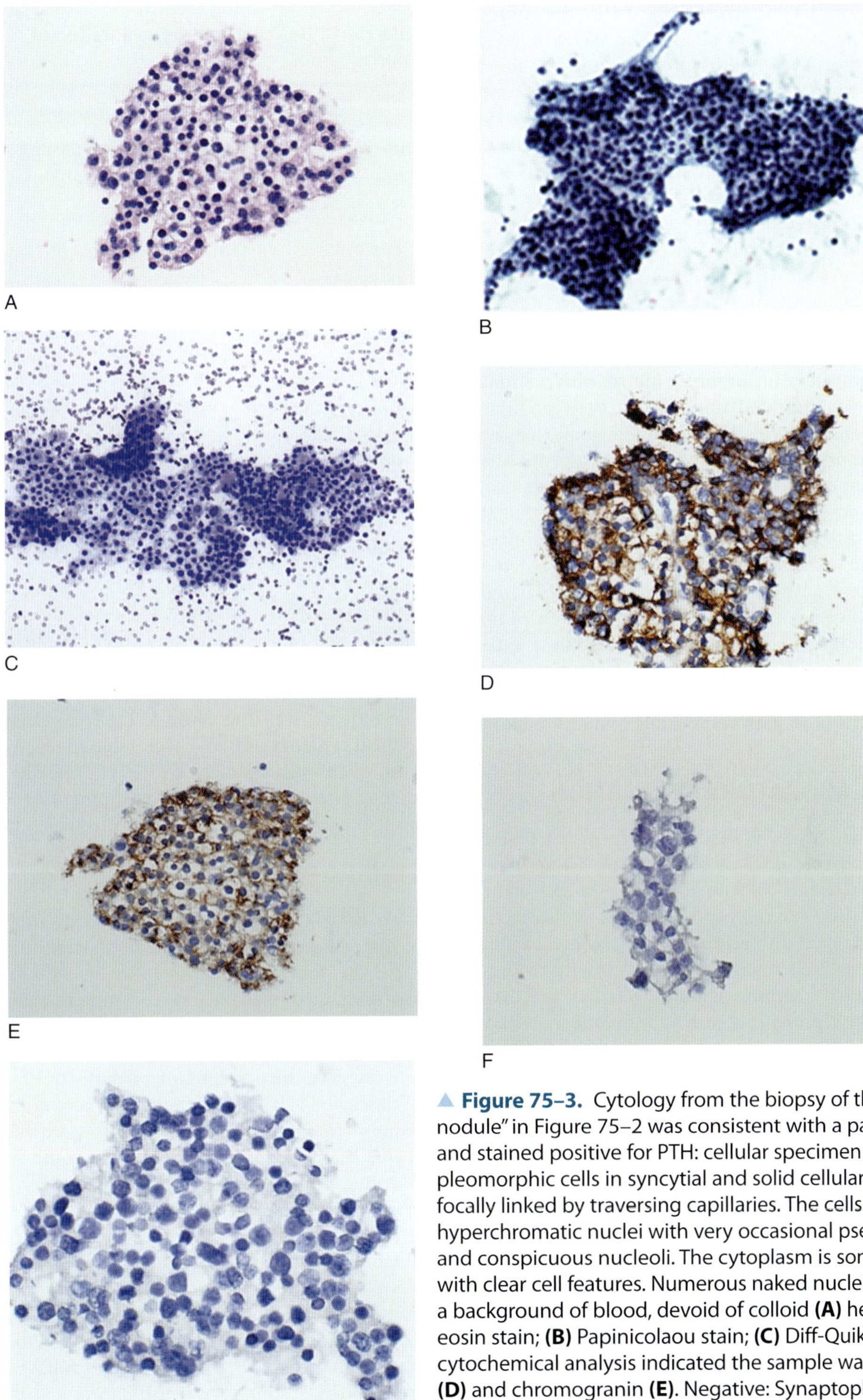

▲ **Figure 75–3.** Cytology from the biopsy of the "thyroid nodule" in Figure 75–2 was consistent with a parathyroid lesion and stained positive for PTH: cellular specimen composed of pleomorphic cells in syncytial and solid cellular arrangements, focally linked by traversing capillaries. The cells had monotonous hyperchromatic nuclei with very occasional pseudoinclusions and conspicuous nucleoli. The cytoplasm is somewhat abundant with clear cell features. Numerous naked nuclei are present in a background of blood, devoid of colloid **(A)** hematoxylin and eosin stain; **(B)** Papinicolaou stain; **(C)** Diff-Quik stain. Immunocytochemical analysis indicated the sample was positive for PTH **(D)** and chromogranin **(E)**. Negative: Synaptophysin, Calcitonin, Thyroglobulin **(F)**, TTF1 **(G)**; Ki-67 (proliferative rate) is 0%.

In the 1980s, Cundy et al. hypothesized that the source of the calcium in parathyroid crisis was the skeleton.[20] He suggested those who have "rapidly growing tumors, short clinical histories, and more marked bone involvement are at greatest risk of developing parathyroid crisis."[20,21] He based this on his observations that the majority of patients with parathyroid crisis had no radiologically apparent evidence of parathyroid bone disease. This is, however, not uniformly true as numerous case reports indicate *osteitis fibrosa cystica*, lytic lesions, and osteoporosis.[1,2,7] Cundy et al. suggested that those with a more prolonged course and chronic hyperparathyroid bone disease were protected due to a secondary increase in bone formation rate which offsets parathyroid hormone's hypercalcemic action on bone. His postmortem histomorphometric observations in a patient with crisis indicated an imbalance between bone resorption and formation, which he suggested supported the notion that bone resorption in parathyroid crisis was of acute onset;[20,21] he documented a "low level of bone formation despite a massive increase in osteoclastic activity. The extent of the trabecular osteoid surface was at the lower limit of normal (57% of the total trabecular surface) and the osteoid consisted of only one lamella, when viewed under polarized light. No plump 'active' osteoblasts were seen. There was no woven bone visible under polarized light and only a little patchy marrow fibrosis was present. The trabecular bone volume was slightly reduced."[20] Whether the mechanism proposed by Cundy et al. is, in part, responsible remains unclear.

DIAGNOSIS & LABORATORY EVALUATION

As with all presentations of PHPT, the diagnosis of PHPT in those with parathyroid crisis is biochemical. There is no uniformly accepted serum calcium level that defines acute parathyroid crisis, but several papers suggest a threshold of 14 mg/dL or greater.[8] In various series, serum calcium has been as high as 24.5 mg/dL and many of those presenting with crisis have serum calcium levels that are over 16 mg/dL.[7,9,16] Patients presenting with parathyroid crisis may or may not have been previously recognized to have PHPT.[22] The most common presentation, however, is more severe and symptomatic hypercalcemia in a patient with long-standing, mild, asymptomatic hypercalcemia.[8] PTH levels may be 10 to 20 times the upper limit of normal or higher.[7,15,18] Thus, the biochemical profile is similar to that often seen in parathyroid carcinoma. As with serum calcium, there is no PTH threshold that defines the diagnosis. A nonsuppressed PTH (>20 pg/dL) or frankly high PTH is consistent with the diagnosis of PHPT. Because an antecedent history of hypercalcemia is not always obvious from the patient's history, initially the hypercalcemia associated with parathyroid crisis may be mistaken for hypercalcemia of malignancy due to its severity. The PTH level, however, usually quickly clarifies the diagnosis. Hypercalcemia of malignancy, the other main cause of hypercalcemia, is characterized by a suppressed PTH. Similarly, hypercalcemia caused by less common conditions such as vitamin D intoxication and granulomatous disease is associated with suppressed serum PTH. It may, in some cases, be prudent to exclude a coexisting cause of hypercalcemia, despite biochemical evidence of PHPT (see Table 75–1). An acute rise in serum calcium in a patient with PHPT may be due to crisis, but may also be due to the development of a second concomitant cause of hypercalcemia with stable PHPT.

Table 75–1. Basic laboratory evaluation of hypercalcemia.

Test	Rationale for Test
PTH	Primary hyperparathyroidism*
PTHrP	Humoral hypercalcemia of malignancy
25-hydroxyvitamin D	Vitamin D intoxication
1,25-dihydroxyvitamin D	Granulomatous disease, lymphoma
Adjunctive tests: phosphate, creatinine, alkaline phosphatase	Low phosphate is often seen in PTH-mediated causes; hypercalcemia often causes AKI. Alkaline phosphatase may provide helpful information regarding bone turnover
Other: SPEP, UPEP, TSH, cortisol, CXR, other scan, etc.	Myeloma, hyperthyroidism, adrenal insufficiency, osteolytic metastases

PTH, parathyroid hormone; PTHrP, PTH-related peptide; *and other less common causes of PTH-mediated hypercalcemia such as familial FHH, lithium-induced PHPT, thiazide-induced hypercalcemia, etc.

CLINICAL PRESENTATION

Today, PHPT is usually characterized by mild, asymptomatic hypercalcemia and it generally has an indolent, benign course. In contrast, the rare phenomenon of parathyroid crisis is characterized by severe, symptomatic hypercalcemia associated with multisystemic effects that impact neurological, cardiovascular, gastrointestinal, and renal function.[16] In some respects, the presentation of acute PHPT can be similar to "classical PHPT" or parathyroid carcinoma. Presenting symptoms are typically related to the sequelae of marked hypercalcemia itself. Table 75–2 shows the major possible presenting symptoms of parathyroid crisis by system as reported in case series. In one surgical series of 43 patients, the most common presenting symptoms were musculoskeletal complaints, fatigue, mental status changes, anorexia, constipation, and polyuria.[17] The prevalence of pancreatitis is variable, ranging from 7% to 25%, but it appears to be much more common in those with crisis compared to those without parathyroid crisis.[9,11,12] Other case reports have described status epilepticus, respiratory arrest/failure, a positive bone scan, osteolytic lesions, soft tissue calcification, electrocardiogram

Table 75–2. Possible presenting symptoms in patients with parathyroid crisis.

Constitutional	Fatigue, weakness, malaise, lethargy, weight loss
Gastrointestinal	Anorexia, nausea, vomiting, constipation, pancreatitis, abdominal pain, dyspepsia
Renal	Nephrocalcinosis, nephrolithiasis, renal dysfunction, polyuria, polydipsia
Skeletal	Fracture, bone pain, osteitis fibrosa cystica, osteoporosis/demineralization
Neurological	Mental status changes, confusion, status epilepticus, coma, depression
Cardiovascular	Myocardial infarction, cardiovascular arrest, death, PVC's, EKG changes
Other	Respiratory arrest, ectopic tissue calcification, neck mass

changes, confusion, coma, depression, conversion disorder, weakness, abdominal pain, dyspepsia, lethargy, renal insufficiency, nephrocalcinosis, and urolithiasis.[6,7,9,16,18,23-25] Figure 75–4 shows abdominal CT images from a 76-year-old patient presenting with mental status changes, polyuria, polydipsia, and decreased appetite found to be in parathyroid crisis with calcium 15.5 mg/dL and PTH level 299.5 pg/mL. A bladder stone can be seen. The imaging did not show evidence of any gross bone disease or pathologic fractures.

ANATOMIC LOCATION & PATHOLOGY

Most often parathyroid crisis is due to a single adenoma.[7] One large surgical series, indicated rates of multi-glandular disease in those with parathyroid crisis were similar to those with PHPT without crisis.[10] Distinctly unusual in mild asymptomatic PHPT, neck masses have been reported in case series with a relatively high prevalence, ranging from 5% to 50% in patients with parathyroid crisis.[6,7,11] Some analyses suggest that ectopic glands are more common in those with parathyroid crisis compared to those without crisis.[7,10,26] The intrathyroidal location of a parathyroid from a patient in crisis can be seen in Figure 75–2. While imaging should not delay surgery, imaging prior to surgery in patients with crisis is suggested by some for this reason.[7] Because patients with parathyroid crisis often have renal insufficiency, some imaging modalities, such as CT with contrast, may not be feasible. The use of sestamibi and neck ultrasound has been reported in patients with PHPT crisis.[9,16,27] In one series of 88 patients with crisis, sestamibi correctly localized the culprit gland in 78% of cases.[10] Local expertise and diagnostic accuracy should guide selection of imaging modality.

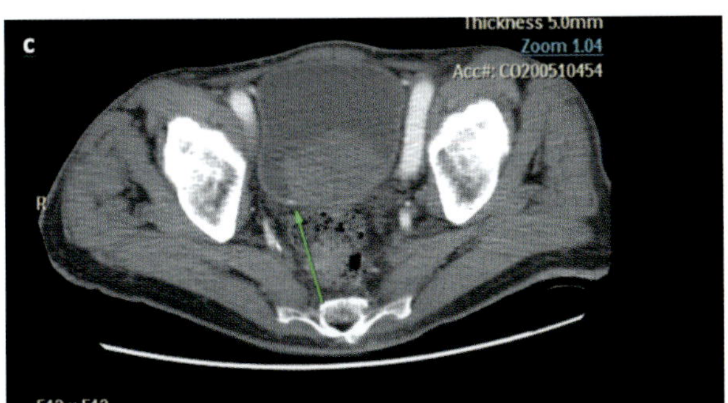

▲ **Figure 75–4.** Abdominal CT indicates a small bladder stone (green arrow) but absence of gross skeletal disease.

MEDICAL MANAGEMENT

Initial Measures

Medical management to decrease serum calcium prior to definitive cure with parathyroidectomy is routinely initiated on the patient's presentation. As with the treatment of marked hypercalcemia due to any etiology, lowering serum calcium initially predominantly relies on increasing renal excretion of calcium with intravascular volume expansion. Agents that decrease bone resorption and reduce the gastrointestinal absorption of calcium may also subsequently be necessary. Medical therapies that may be utilized in the treatment of hypercalcemia are shown in Table 75–3. Patients presenting in crisis are usually profoundly volume depleted. Aggressive hydration usually utilizing normal saline at an initial rate of 200 to 300 mL per hour and then adjusted to maintain urine output at 100 to 150 mL per hour is recommended. Rates should be adjusted depending on the patient's underlying medical comorbidities such as congestive heart and renal failure. Hydration with saline increases glomerular filtration and the filtered load of calcium. In one series, patients with parathyroid crisis received an average of 16 L of saline to achieve euvolemia.[7]

Calcitonin, which is both a calciuretic and weak skeletal antiresorptive agent, administered at a dose of 4 IU/kg intramuscularly or subcutaneously every 12 hours is effective at reducing serum calcium by 1 to 2 mg/dL over 4 to 6 hours in hypercalcemia of many etiologies.[6,16] Therefore, it may be a helpful adjunct to hydration that enables the rapid lowering of serum calcium. It is FDA-approved for the treatment of hypercalcemia.[28] Tachiphylaxis soon develops, however, and it becomes ineffective.[28] We therefore recommend discontinuation after four doses. Loop diuretics were once a mainstay of the treatment of hypercalcemia. However, they are no longer routinely recommended. They may be helpful in patients who are becoming volume overloaded with aggressive hydration and may increase renal excretion of serum calcium further. Care must be taken to avoid initiation of diuretics until the patient is euvolemic, as administration in the setting of hypovolemia will worsen hypercalcemia.[29] Figure 75–5 indicates serum calcium levels and response to intravenous saline hydration, calcitonin, and furosemide in a patient presenting with parathyroid crisis.

Table 75–3. Medical treatment of hypercalcemia.

Treatment	Usual Agent/Dose*	Mechanism	Major Potential Side Effects
Hydration	Normal saline 200-300 mL/h	Increase renal excretion of calcium	Volume overload
Calcitonin	4 IU/kg q 12 hours × 4 doses	Increase renal excretion of calcium and decrease bone resorption	Allergic reaction, flushing, tachyphylaxis
Loop diuretics	Furosemide 20-40 mg IV	Increase renal calcium excretion	Dehydration, worsening renal function, hypokalemia
Bisphosphonates	Zoledronic acid 4 mg IV over 15 min or longer Pamidronate 30-90 mg IV over 2 hours or more	Anti-resorptives/decrease bone resorption	Acute phase reaction, joint/bone pain, hypocalcemia, renal dysfunction
Denosumab	60-120 mg SQ once	RANKL inhibitor/decrease bone resorption	Hypocalcemia, rash,
Cinacalcet	30-90 mg bid to qid	Calcimimetic/decreased PTH secretion	Nausea, vomiting
Glucocorticoids	Prednisone 20-60 mg daily	Decrease calcium absorption and increase renal excretion	Hyperglycemia, hypertension, immunosuppression
Dialysis	No or low calcium dialysate	Removes calcium from intravascular space	Hypotension

*Rates and doses may need adjustment based on individual patient factors including but not limited to volume status, renal and cardiac function, serum calcium level; patients may have contraindications.

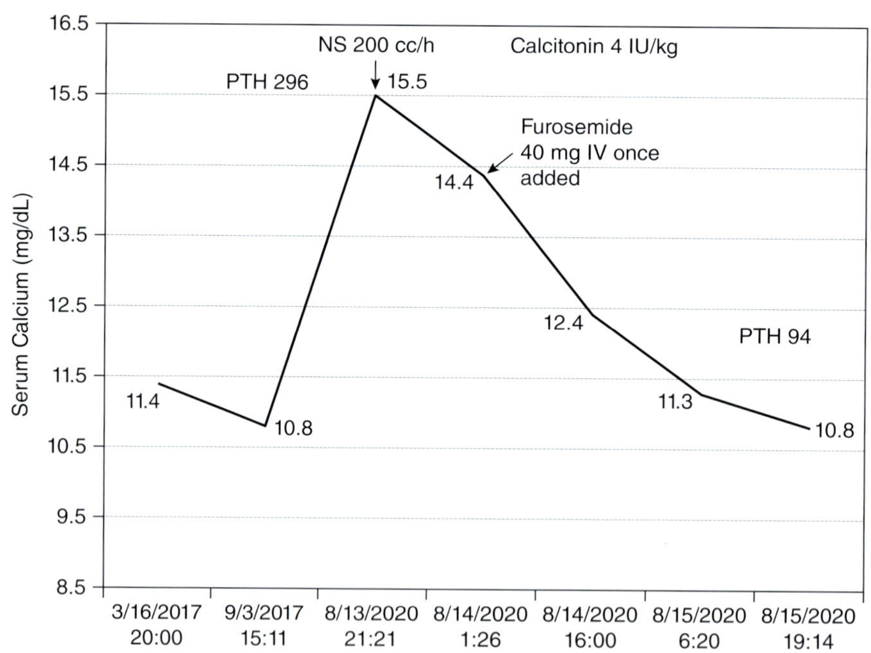

▲ **Figure 75–5.** The patient's serum calcium decreased with initiation of normal saline administered intravenously at 200 cc/h. Calcitonin was added to further decrease serum calcium along with hydration. Furosemide was initiated due to volume overload. Zometa was subsequently administered as patient refused parathyroidectomy.

Bisphosphonates

Administration of bisphosphonates including pamidronate or zoledronic acid can be considered depending on the patient's clinical presentation, degree of hypercalcemia, response to other measures, renal function, and timing of surgery. These agents act as skeletal antiresorptives and decrease the entry of calcium into the serum from the skeleton by interfering with the action of osteoclasts. They are more potent and effective than calcitonin and are the preferred agents for other types of hypercalcemia, such as hypercalcemia of malignancy. Both pamidronate and zoledronic acid are FDA-approved for the treatment of hypercalcemia of malignancy. There are no data comparing pamidronate with zoledronic acid in parathyroid crisis. Temporary normalization of serum calcium preoperatively with both agents has been reported in the setting of parathyroid crisis.[7,30] In a head-to-head trial in patients with hypercalcemia of malignancy, zoledronic acid 4 mg intravenously was more effective at normalizing calcium than pamidronate 90 mg intravenously.[31] In trials evaluating both drugs for the chronic treatment of metastatic bone disease, there were more renal events in those allocated to zoledronic acid compared to those receiving pamidronate. While patients with creatinine levels up to 4.5 mg/dL were included in this trial, pamidronate is sometimes preferentially used in those with renal insufficiency for this reason.[31] However, pamidronate requires a much longer infusion time compared to zoledronic acid (2 hours compared with 15 minutes). Dose adjustment and slower infusion rates with both agents are recommended in patients with renal insufficiency to reduce risk of further renal impairment. The peak effect of bisphosphonates is approximately 2 days after infusion, but the duration of their effects on bone metabolism and serum calcium is longer. The reduction in serum calcium achieved with intravenous bisphosphonates is, however, transient. Thus, bisphosphonates are not usually an effective long-term primary treatment approach to managing patients with parathyroid crisis. On the other hand, hypocalcemia may occur after treatment with intravenous bisphosphonates in some patients, particularly in those with vitamin D deficiency and renal insufficiency. Use of intravenous bisphosphonates prior to parathyroidectomy may further predispose to hypocalcemia that can develop postoperatively. Patients with parathyroid crisis are already at high risk for "hungry bone syndrome."[7]

Other Agents

A. Denosumab

Denosumab is a skeletal antiresorptive agent approved for the treatment of hypercalcemia of malignancy refractory to treatment with bisphosphonates. It is a human monoclonal antibody against receptor activator of nuclear factor-kB ligand (RANKL). RANKL is a protein secreted by osteoblasts that binds to its receptor on osteoclasts and stimulates bone resorption. There are two reports of the use of denosumab in the treatment of parathyroid crisis with successful reduction in serum calcium. Hypocalcemia remains a risk after parathyroidectomy and may be greater in those treated with denosumab than intravenous bisphosphonates.[32,33] Denosumab may be used in those with renal insufficiency and does not cause kidney injury but risk of hypocalcemia is heightened in this setting.

B. Cinacalcet

Cinacalcet is a calcimimetic that binds to the calcium-sensing receptor (CaSR). It increases the sensitivity of the CaSR to extracellular calcium, resulting in a reduction in PTH and serum calcium. Cinacalcet has been shown to reduce and normalize serum calcium in patients with mild PHPT.[34,35] It also has efficacy in patients with a similar biochemical picture to patients in crisis, namely parathyroid cancer.[36] In an open-label study, titration of cinacalcet from 30 mg twice daily to 90 mg four times daily over 16 weeks, reduced serum calcium by 1 mg/dL in 62% of patients. In the responders, serum calcium fell from a mean of 15 mg/dL to 11.2 mg/dL. Cinacalcet is FDA-approved for the treatment of hypercalcemia in patients with parathyroid cancer and in those with PHPT with severe hypercalcemia who are unable to undergo parathyroidectomy. There is no systematic investigation of cinacalcet in parathyroid crisis. However, it has been studied in patients with moderate to severe inoperable PHPT.[37] In 17 patients with serum calcium greater than 12.5 mg/dL, cinacalcet was titrated using the same approach described above. Eighty-eight percent of patients achieved a 1 mg/dL or greater reduction in serum calcium. Adverse events with cinacalcet include nausea, vomiting, and paresthesias. Since a rapid reduction in serum calcium is required in parathyroid crisis and the maximal effect of cinacalcet often requires dose titration, its use is limited in the acute setting.

C. Glucocorticoids

While glucocorticoids have traditionally been used to treat hypercalcemia related to vitamin D intoxication and 1,25-dihydroxyvitamin D mediated hypercalcemia, they can be considered as needed in patients with parathyroid crisis depending on the degree of hypercalcemia, presentation, and responsiveness to other treatments. Glucocorticoids reduce the absorption of calcium from the gastrointestinal tract and increase renal excretion. In PHPT, bone resorption is the major mechanism leading to hypercalcemia. However, there is a component of gastrointestinal hyperabsorption due to PTH's effect to increase transcription of the 1-alpha-hydroxylase responsible for the conversion of 25-hydroxyvitamin D to 1,25-dihydroxyvitamin D. Thus, they may be a helpful adjunctive treatment. Their use has been reported in a case series of patients with hyperparathyroid crisis.[6]

D. Dialysis

Dialysis with a no calcium or low calcium bath may be considered in patients with crisis depending on their calcium level, presentation, and response to other treatments. Dialysis is an important therapy, particularly in those with acute kidney injury with oliguria, refractory hypercalcemia despite above therapies, and those in whom fluids cannot be administered safely. There are reports of using dialysis in patients with parathyroid crisis, though most case reports predate the availability of potent bisphosphonates.[6,16]

SURGICAL TREATMENT

Traditionally, emergency surgery had been recommended within 72 hours of presentation with parathyroid crisis.[5-7] There is little data regarding the optimal timing of surgery. Early surgery after medical stabilization is currently favored rather than emergent surgery to optimize the patient's stability.[8,38] A retrospective single-center study reported no difference in long-term survival in a series of 43 patients who underwent parathyroidectomy within 72 hours, compared to those medically treated for >72 hours before surgery.[11] Both gland exploration and minimally invasive surgery have been used as surgical approaches in patients with parathyroid crisis.[10] Overall, lower operative success has been reported in patients with crisis compared to those without crisis in one series.[10] Failures were due to missed glands, misdiagnosis, and parathyroid carcinoma.[10] Mortality rates in PHPT patients who underwent parathyroidectomy with hypercalcemic crisis were higher compared to those without crisis.[39] In one surgical series of 43 patients, 98% were eucalcemic/cured by parathyroidectomy.[11]

A. Postsurgical Hypocalcemia

Hypocalcemia is a potentially life-threatening complication that has been reported after parathyroidectomy in patients presenting with crisis, but the prevalence rate varies widely from 0% to 100%.[7,11,15] A paper summarizing the data available up until 2008 indicated hypocalcemia had occurred in 42.8% (57/133) of patients reported in the literature.[7] Hypocalcemia may be related to "bone hunger" as well as the use of bisphosphonates prior to surgery. Hungry bone syndrome refers to hypocalcemia precipitated by the sudden shift from bone resorption to bone formation after cure of the hyperparathyroid condition. Patients with concomitant renal dysfunction or vitamin D deficiency may be particularly at risk due to the independent hypocalcemic effects of these conditions.

There are no systematic investigations regarding the optimal management or prevention of postoperative hypocalcemia. There are only anecdotal reports regarding the use of oral calcium supplementation for the prevention or treatment of postoperative hypocalcemia in the setting of crisis. High-dose oral calcium supplementation (1 g four times per day) with or without calcitriol is used as a prophylactic regimen in some centers. Oral and intravenous calcium may be necessary to treat hypocalcemia after its development along with cholecalciferol or ergocalciferol and calcitriol. Intravenous calcium is recommended in those with symptoms of hypocalcemia (paresthesias, muscle spasm/tetany, etc.), a prolonged QT interval on electrocardiogram or those with a decline in calcium to ≤7.5 mg/dL.[40] Intravenous calcium should be administered as an infusion. Calcium gluconate is preferred to calcium chloride due to the greater risk of tissue necrosis with the latter if extravasation occurs. Typically 1 to 2 amps (90-180 mg elemental calcium) of 10% calcium gluconate is given in 50 to 100 mL of D5 and infused over 15 minutes. This is followed by a subsequent slower infusion containing 1 mg/mL of elemental calcium (11 g of calcium gluconate, which is equivalent to ~1000 mg of elemental calcium) in 1000 ml of D5 at a rate of 0.5-1.5 mg/kg elemental calcium per hour.[40]

MORTALITY & PROGNOSIS

Initially, the parathyroid crisis was uniformly fatal. In reviews from the 1970s and 1980s, the condition was reported to be lethal if not operated upon.[16] Over the last half century mortality has declined.[7] Mortality was reported to be 93% in 1956 and 60% in 1967.[7,14,41] The mortality rate was 52.5% in a series published in 1976.[9] A more recent case series of patients operated on from 1990 to 2007 indicated a mortality rate of 0%.[7] Since the 1980s, most case series report low mortality rates ranging from 0% to 4%, though there are isolated case reports of patients succumbing to their condition.[11,39] In most such cases, death occurred in patients with parathyroid carcinoma or pancreatitis.[7,42,43] Little information is available about recurrence or long-term outcomes. In one surgical series of 43 patients who underwent parathyroidectomy, the recurrence rate of PHPT was 7%.[11] Median survival after parathyroidectomy was 11.7 years in this series.[11] Younger age was associated with better survival.[11] On the other hand, preoperative calcium and number of preoperative symptoms did not affect long-term survival.[11]

SUMMARY & CONCLUSIONS

Parathyroid crisis is a rare condition with a historically high mortality rate. Recognition of the urgency of parathyroid crisis, improved medical management, and early parathyroidectomy have improved the care and prognosis of patients with crisis over the last century. The precise precipitants are unclear in some cases, but may include parathyroid hemorrhage or necrosis, dehydration, inter-current illnesses, and immobility. The clinical presentation usually involves multisystemic neurological, gastrointestinal, renal, and other symptoms that accompany marked and rapidly developing hypercalcemia. Diagnosis is based on an elevated or nonsuppressed PTH level that accompanies marked elevations in serum calcium. While early parathyroidectomy is the definitive treatment, aggressive medical therapy with hydration and other agents that lower calcium provides an effective bridge to parathyroidectomy.

ACKNOWLEDGMENTS

We are grateful to the patients whose images are documented within this report. All patients provided consent for their images to be utilized.

REFERENCES

1. Hanes FM. Parathyroid adenoma with death, due to parathormone intoxication. *Trans Am Clin Climatol Assoc.* 1938;54:152-162.
2. Dawson JW, Struthers JW. Generalised osteitis fibrosa. *Edinb Med J.* 1923;30(10):421-564.
3. Collip JB. The production of some of the phenomena peculiar to parathyroid overdosage in dogs by means of certain inorganic salts. *Am J Physiol.* 1926;76:472-476.
4. Collip JB, Clark EP, Scott JW. The effects of parathyroid hormone on normal animals. *JBC.* 1925(2):439-460.
5. Nelson AR, Cantrell JR. Acute parathormone poisoning complicating parathyroid adenoma. *Arch Surg.* 1961;83:1-10.
6. Wang CA, Guyton SW. Hyperparathyroid crisis: clinical and pathologic studies of 14 patients. *Ann Surg.* 1979;190(6):782-790.
7. Phitayakorn R, McHenry CR. Hyperparathyroid crisis: use of bisphosphonates as a bridge to parathyroidectomy. *J Am Coll Surg.* 2008;206(6):1106-1115.
8. Ahmad S, Kuraganti G, Steenkamp D. Hypercalcemic crisis: a clinical review. *Am J Med.* 2015;128(3):239-245.
9. Kistler H. [Primary hyperparathyroidism. An analysis of 152 patients with special references to acute life threatening complications (acute hyperparathyroidism)]. *Schweiz Med Wochenschr.* 1976;106(suppl 3):1-61.
10. Cannon J, Lew JI, Solorzano CC. Parathyroidectomy for hypercalcemic crisis: 40 years' experience and long-term outcomes. *Surgery.* 2010;148(4):807-812; discussion 12-13.
11. Lew JI, Solorzano CC, Irvin GL, 3rd. Long-term results of parathyroidectomy for hypercalcemic crisis. *Arch Surg.* 2006;141(7):696-699; discussion 700.
12. Kelly TR. Primary hyperparathyroidism. A personal experience with 242 cases. *Am J Surg.* 1980;140(5):632-635.
13. Payne RL, Jr., Fitchett CW. Hyperparathyroid crisis: survey of the literature and a report of two additional cases. *Ann Surg.* 1965;161:737-747.
14. MacLeod WA, Holloway CK. Hyperparathyroid crisis. A collective review. *Ann Surg.* 1967;166(6):1012-1015.
15. Asghar A, Ikram M, Islam N. A case report: giant cystic parathyroid adenoma presenting with parathyroid crisis after Vitamin D replacement. *BMC Endocr Disord.* 2012;12:14.
16. Bayat-Mokhtari F, Palmieri GM, Moinuddin M, Pourmand R. Parathyroid storm. *Arch Intern Med.* 1980;140(8):1092-1095.
17. Bondeson AG, Bondeson L, Thompson NW. Clinicopathological peculiarities in parathyroid disease with hypercalcaemic crisis. *Eur J Surg.* 1993;159(11-12):613-617.
18. Minisola S, Romagnoli E, Scarnecchia L, Pacitti MT, Rosso R, Carnevale V, et al. Parathyroid storm: immediate recognition and pathophysiological considerations. *Bone.* 1993;14(5):703-706.
19. Ma SK, Oh TR, Choi YD, Kim SW. Parathyroid crisis caused by a large parathyroid adenoma. *Intern Med.* 2014;53(2):165-166.
20. Cundy T, Darby AJ, Berry HE, Parsons V. Bone metabolism in acute parathyroid crisis. *Clin Endocrinol (Oxf).* 1985;22(6):787-793.
21. Parfitt AM. Equilibrium and disequilibrium hypercalcaemia: new light on an old subject. *Metabolic Bone Disease.* 1979;1:279-293.
22. Ntaios G, Savopoulos C, Chatzinikolaou A, Kaiafa G, Hatzitolios A, Karamitsos D. Parathyroid crisis as first manifestation of primary hyperparathyroidism. *Eur J Intern Med.* 2007;18(7):551-552.
23. Ikegaki S, Otoshi T, Hirai T, Hirabayashi M. A rare case of parathyroid crisis with respiratory failure successfully treated using extracorporeal membrane oxygenation. *Respir Med Case Rep.* 2020;30:101088.
24. Nora EH, Wermers RA. Visual vignette. Acute parathyroid crisis due to primary hyperparathyroidism. *Endocr Pract.* 2004;10(1):88.
25. Maselly MJ, Lawrence AM, Brooks M, et al. Hyperparathyroid crisis. Successful treatment of ten comatose patients. *Surgery.* 1981;90(4):741-746.
26. Zhou W, Chen M. A case report of mediastinal ectopic parathyroid adenoma presented as parathyroid crisis localized by SPECT/CT. *Medicine (Baltimore).* 2016;95(41):e5157.
27. Chacon A, Vilar A, Arroyo D, et al. Acute kidney injury secondary to very severe hypercalcaemic crisis caused by primary hyperparathyroidism. *Nefrologia.* 2015;35(2):224-226.
28. Calcitonin Prescribing information [Available from: https://www.accessdata.fda.gov/drugsatfda_docs/label/2014/017808s035lbl.pdf.]
29. LeGrand SB, Leskuski D, Zama I. Narrative review: furosemide for hypercalcemia: an unproven yet common practice. *Ann Intern Med.* 2008;149(4):259-263.
30. Jansson S, Tisell LE, Lindstedt G, Lundberg PA. Disodium pamidronate in the preoperative treatment of hypercalcemia in patients with primary hyperparathyroidism. *Surgery.* 1991;110(3):480-486.
31. Major P, Lortholary A, Hon J, et al. Zoledronic acid is superior to pamidronate in the treatment of hypercalcemia of malignancy: a pooled analysis of two randomized, controlled clinical trials. *J Clin Oncol.* 2001;19(2):558-567.
32. Eremkina A, Krupinova J, Dobreva E, et al. Denosumab for management of severe hypercalcemia in primary hyperparathyroidism. *Endocr Connect.* 2020;9(10):1019-1027.
33. Mamedova E, Kolodkina A, Vasilyev EV, Petrov V, Belaya Z, Tiulpakov A. Successful use of denosumab for life-threatening hypercalcemia in a pediatric patient with primary hyperparathyroidism. *Horm Res Paediatr.* 2020;93(4):272-278.
34. Shoback DM, Bilezikian JP, Turner SA, McCary LC, Guo MD, Peacock M. The calcimimetic cinacalcet normalizes serum calcium in subjects with primary hyperparathyroidism. *J Clin Endocrinol Metab.* 2003;88(12):5644-5649.
35. Peacock M, Bilezikian JP, Klassen PS, Guo MD, Turner SA, Shoback D. Cinacalcet hydrochloride maintains long-term normocalcemia in patients with primary hyperparathyroidism. *J Clin Endocrinol Metab.* 2005;90(1):135-141.

36. Silverberg SJ, Rubin MR, Faiman C, et al. Cinacalcet hydrochloride reduces the serum calcium concentration in inoperable parathyroid carcinoma. *J Clin Endocrinol Metab*. 2007;92(10):3803-3808.
37. Marcocci C, Chanson P, Shoback D, et al. Cinacalcet reduces serum calcium concentrations in patients with intractable primary hyperparathyroidism. *J Clin Endocrinol Metab*. 2009;94(8):2766-2772.
38. Basok AB, Rogachev B, Haviv YS, Vorobiov M. Treatment of extreme hypercalcaemia: the role of haemodialysis. *BMJ Case Rep*. 2018;2018:bcr2017223772.
39. Gasparri G, Camandona M, Mullineris B, Raggio E, Vigna S, Dei Poli M. Acute hyperparathyroidism: our experience with 36 cases. *Ann Ital Chir*. 2004;75(3):321-324.
40. Tohme JF, Bilezikian JP. Hypocalcemic emergencies. *Endocrinol Metab Clin North Am*. 1993;22(2):363-375.
41. James PR, Richards PG. Parathyroid crisis: treatment by emergency parathyroidectomy. *AMA Arch Surg*. 1956;72(4):553-556.
42. Love GL, Samuels M. Fatal acute hyperparathyroidism and parathyroid carcinoma. *South Med J*. 1983;76(3):407-408.
43. Matthias GS, Helliwell TR, Williams A. Postpartum hyperparathyroid crisis. Case report. *Br J Obstet Gynaecol*. 1987;94(8):807-810.

Endocrine Hypertensive Emergencies

76

Nicole Lunardi, MD
Sarah C. Oltmann, MD, FACS

INTRODUCTION

Hypertension is a common medical condition affecting nearly half of the adult population in the United States.[1] While the vast majority have essential hypertension, approximately 15% to 30% have a secondary cause of hypertension. Secondary hypertension is more prevalent among children and young adults, with estimates ranging from 30% to 50% of hypertensive youth.[2,3] The prevalence of endocrine hypertension is not well established, but is estimated to account for 5% to 10% of all hypertensive patients.[4] Patients with hypertension may already be under treatment; however, not all obtain or have access to regular medical care, and/or additional underlying causes of episodic endocrine hypertension may be undiagnosed. These patients may interact with the health-care system under urgent or emergent scenarios when a hypertensive emergency may occur. Additional patient symptomology may prompt elective workup which uncovers an underlying endocrine driver of their hypertension.[4,5] We discuss both scenarios herein.

PHEOCHROMOCYTOMA & PARAGANGLIOMA

General Considerations

Pheochromocytoma (PHEO) and paraganglioma (PGL) are catecholamine-secreting tumors arising from neural crest-derived chromaffin cells from the adrenal gland or sympathetic/parasympathetic chain, respectively. PHEO/PGLs are rare with an incidence of 1 in 300,000 people annually. They affect men and women equally, most commonly detected between the third and fifth decade of life. PHEO is more common than PGL (incidence of 2-8 per million vs 0.5 per million, respectively).[6] PHEO and PGL are the underlying cause of secondary hypertension in 0.2% to 0.6% adults and 1.7% of children.[6,7]

Pathophysiology

The basics of catecholamine synthesis, stimulation of adrenergic receptors, and catecholamine metabolism are helpful in understanding the diagnosis and treatment of PHEO/PGL hypertensive emergency. Norepinephrine and epinephrine are broken down to normetanephrine, metanephrine, or vanillylmandelic acid (VMA) depending on the metabolic pathway. Only PHEO patients can have elevation of epinephrine and metanephrine because of an enzyme (phenylethanolamine N-methyltransferase) unique to the adrenal medulla.[6,8] Catecholamines act on adrenergic receptors throughout the body as summarized in Figure 76–1 resulting in hypertension.[8]

Clinical Findings

Symptomatic patients may have brief paroxysms of palpitations, pallor, tremor, headache, and diaphoresis. These episodes can be spontaneous or triggered by postural changes, exercise, or increased intraabdominal pressure. Blood pressure in these patients can be labile, due to the combination of catecholamine surges and volume depletion, paroxysmal or sustained hypertension. Patients may present with less common symptoms or even be asymptomatic, clinical scenarios are discussed in separate chapters. Evaluation for catecholamine-secreting tumors should be considered in patients with hyperadrenergic paroxysms, resistant hypertension, hypertensive emergency triggered by prior procedures, incidentaloma, or family history.[6,7] The differential diagnosis is broad and summarized in Table 76–1.

Laboratory Findings

Biochemical confirmation is the first step in diagnosis. The 24-hour urine collection measures catecholamines, metanephrines, and creatinine. It has a 98% sensitivity and specificity, but is a cumbersome and inconvenient test for

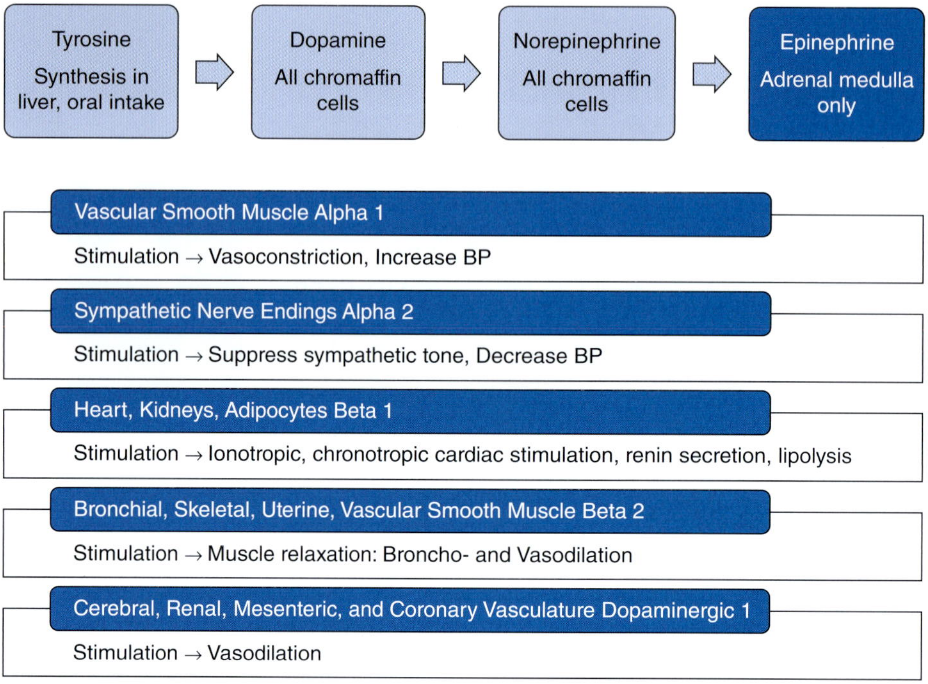

▲ **Figure 76–1.** Catecholamine synthesis and adrenergic receptors.

Table 76–1. Additional diagnoses to consider during workup of pheochromocytoma and/or paraganglioma.

Endocrine
Thyrotoxicosis
Pancreatic endocrine tumors
Hypoglycemia
Cardiovascular
Essential hypertension
Renovascular disease
Arrhythmias
Vasovagal syncope
Psychological
Anxiety
Withdrawal
Factitious
Neurological
Migraine
Postural orthostatic tachycardia syndrome
Autonomic seizures
Pharmacological
Cocaine, phencyclidine
Sympathomimetics
Polypharmacy
Other
Carcinoid
Anaphylaxis

the patient. Plasma metanephrines, with 96% to 100% sensitivity and 77% to 89% specificity, should be selectively used in circumstances with high index of suspicion—resistant hypertension, known familial syndromes, known mass, or previous pheochromocytoma. Medications that have been shown to reduce the efficacy of biochemical testing include tricyclic antidepressants, levodopa, adrenergic receptor agonists, amphetamines, buspirone, antipsychotics, and ethanol.[6,7,9]

Imaging Studies

The next step in diagnosis is localization. CT of the chest, abdomen, and pelvis will identify a chromaffin-secreting tumor with 95% sensitivity and 65% specificity. Extra-adrenal tumors can be superior para-aortic (46%), inferior para-aortic (29%), bladder (10%), mediastinum (10%), head and neck (3%), and pelvis (2%). MRI may be more appropriate for patients with metastatic disease, contrast allergy, children, and pregnant patients. PHEOs and PGLs are round, smooth masses that are nonhomogeneous and hyperenhancing with delayed washout.[9,10]

Additional imaging modalities may include ^{123}I-metaiodobenzylguanidine (MIBG) single photon emission-computed tomograph or PET scan. Tagged ^{123}I-MIGB scan can be performed for multifocal or extra-adrenal disease as the tracer is preferentially taken up by catecholamine tumors. PET scans are useful in patients with metastatic disease.[9,10]

Genetic Testing

Patients who are found to have PHEO/PGL should be referred to genetic counseling. Based on family history and associated symptoms, a host of genetic tests may be suggested. Syndromes include multiple endocrine neoplasia 1, 2A, and 2B (RET, MEN), von Hipple Lindau (VHL), neurofibromatosis type 1 (NF1), succinate dehydrogenase mutations (SDH), ataxia telangiectasia, tuberous sclerosis, Sturge Webber, and Carney Triad.[9,11]

Treatment

While surgical resection is ultimately curative, patients must first be appropriately medically blocked prior to proceeding with surgery. The mass can be resected laparoscopically or open, depending on size, solitary versus bilateral, difficulty of the dissection (adhesions, invasions), and surgeon experience. Careful preoperative and intraoperative treatment of hypertension is essential in preventing and promptly treating hypertensive crisis. If the Endocrine, Surgical, and or Anesthesia teams do not feel comfortable managing such a patient, transfer to higher level of care should be initiated.[6,7,9]

The first step in management is alpha blockade to allow for vasodilation, coupled with increased salt and fluid intake for volume repletion/expansion. The agent typically used is phenoxybenzamine, which is a nonspecific, irreversible, long-acting alpha blocker. It is started at 10 mg twice daily and up-titrated to achieve a goal blood pressure of 120/80; however, this medication can be expensive and hard to come by. Alternatively, selective alpha-1 blockade with agents like terazosin, doxazosin, and prazosin can be used; however, patients will not generally develop reflex tachycardia (Table 76–2).[6,7,9]

Only once adequate alpha blockade has been established, may beta blockers be initiated to assist with tachycardia

Table 76–2. Pharmacological treatment of pheochromocytoma and/or paraganglioma.

Drug	Indication	Dose	Side Effects
Alpha Blocker			
Phenoxybenzamine	Preoperative preparation	20-100 mg/day	Postural hypotension, tachycardia, miosis, nasal congestion, diarrhea, fatigue
Phentolamine	Hypertensive crisis	30-120 mg/day 2-5 mg/h IV	Orthostatic hypotension, nausea, vomiting diarrhea, abdominal pain
Prazosin, terazosin, doxazosin	Alternative preoperative preparation	1-32 mg/day	Dizziness, fatigue, headache, palpitations, nausea
Beta Blocker			
Esmolol	Hypertensive crisis, intraoperative management	50 μg/kg/min to 300 μg/kg/min	Dizziness, fatigue, peripheral edema, asthma exacerbation
Propranolol	After adequate alpha blockade, if tachycardia present	30-120 mg/day	Dizziness, fatigue, impotence
Atenolol	After adequate alpha blockade, if tachycardia present	25-50 mg/day	Dizziness, fatigue
Metoprolol	After adequate alpha blockade, if tachycardia present	40 mg/day	Dizziness, fatigue, nausea, impotence
Calcium Channel Blocker			
Nicardipine	Refractory hypertension, alternative to alpha/beta blocker, crisis	30-60 mg/day 5-12 mg/h drip	Edema, dizziness, headache, flushing, nausea, dyspnea
Amlodipine	Refractory hypertension, alternative to alpha/beta blocker, crisis	5-10 mg/day	Peripheral edema, dizziness, fatigue, gastrointestinal distress
Nitrous Oxide Releasing Agent			
Nitroprusside	Hypertensive crisis	2 μg/kg/min	Chest pain, palpitations, dizziness, bradycardia
Catecholamine Synthesis Inhibitor			
Metyrosine	Used in conjunction with alpha blockers in short term, tumor manipulation/ablation	500-4000 mg/day	Sedation, diarrhea, anxiety, nightmare, extrapyramidal symptoms

control. Metoprolol should be started 10 mg every 6 hours. If this is well tolerated, the patient can be transitioned to a longer-acting agent. Patients with a history of cardiomyopathy or asthma should be monitored for symptoms of pulmonary edema and bronchospasm, respectively.[6,7,9]

If a patient continues to have uncontrolled hypertension, or cannot tolerate alpha and beta blockade, a calcium channel blocker is indicated. Nicardipine can be used as an oral agent or as a drip. Catecholamine synthesis inhibitors are another alternative to alpha and beta blockade and may be particularly useful in patients with tumor manipulation or ablation. Metyrosine can be started at 250 mg every 6 hours and up-titrated over 3 days. It is, unfortunately, poorly tolerated with side effects including diarrhea, urolithiasis, galactorrhea, extrapyramidal symptoms, depression, anxiety, and nightmares.[6,7,9]

Complications

Operative management requires close hemodynamic monitoring with arterial line and, in some cardiac patients, a swan-ganz catheter may be indicated. Fentanyl, morphine, ketamine, and parasympathetic blockade should all be avoided as they can trigger catecholamine release. Propofol, etomidate, and barbiturates are preferred agents. As many of these agents may cause significant vasodilation, additional preoperative volume repletion can be beneficial. Intraoperatively, the patient can be treated with combinations of esmolol, nitroprusside, nitroglycerine, and/or phentolamine, all of which have a rapid onset of action and short half-lives. Nicardipine may also be considered. A summary of blood pressure treatments is available in Table 76–3. There should be an ongoing dialogue between the surgeon and anesthesiologist as manipulation of the tumor can induce hypertensive crisis. This dialogue can ensure the surgeon pauses to minimize ongoing spikes of catecholamines and allow the anesthesiologist time to catch up.[6,7,9]

Once the venous drainage has been controlled, hypotension may be immediate due to sudden catecholamine withdrawal. Robust preoperative alpha blockade coupled with volume expansion may minimize this risk. Initial management should be aggressive fluid resuscitation, but additional use of vasopressors may be necessary for a short period of time. Adrenocortical insufficiency and hypoglycemia may also occur, and patients should be appropriately monitored in the immediate postoperative period. Alpha blockade can be immediately discontinued postoperatively, and beta blockade weaned as appropriate.[6,7,9]

Postoperative hypertension is possible for 5 to 8 weeks. The surgeon must also consider incomplete resection, metastatic disease, renal artery injury, and concomitant essential hypertension. The residual disease would be evident on postoperative plasma or 24-hour urine metanephrines in 1 to 2 weeks.[6,7,9]

Prognosis

Patients who are found to have benign disease and who have been properly treated will ultimately succumb to other ailments. However, patients with malignant disease can be characterized as fast or slow growing. If left untreated, life expectancy is 1 to 3 years. Metastatic disease can spread locally to adjacent nodes and omentum and have distant metastasis including lung and bone.[12] Blood pressure control is an ongoing challenge in these patients and should be achieved with pharmacological blockade of alpha, beta, and catecholamine synthesis.[6,7,9]

PRIMARY HYPERALDOSTERONISM

General Considerations

Primary hyperaldosteronism (PA) typically presents between the third and sixth decade of life with moderate to severe hypertension, poorly controlled on multiple agents. It accounts for 5% to 15% of hypertensive patients, much higher than previously thought, thanks to increased screening in hypertensive patients.[13,14]

Table 76–3. Pharmacological treatment of hyperaldosteronism and Cushing's syndrome hypertension.

Drug	Indication	Dose	Side Effects
Mineralocorticoid Receptor Antagonist			
Spironolactone	First line antihypertensive	12.5-25 mg/day, max 400 mg/day	Gynecomastia, erectile dysfunction, decreased libido and menstrual activity
Eplerenone	First-line antihypertensive, unable to tolerate spironolactone	25 mg BID, max 100 mg/day	Dizziness, headache, fatigue, diarrhea, hypertriglyceridemia, and elevated liver enzymes
Thiazide Diuretics			
Hydrochlorothiazide or chlorthalidone	Second-line antihypertensive	12.5-25 mg/day	Hypokalemia, dizziness, photosensitivity, gastrointestinal distress, paresthesias

Pathophysiology

Normally, decreased circulating volume is detected by the kidney's macula densa, triggering the renin-angiotensin pathway, and stimulating release of aldosterone. Aldosterone acts to increase resorption of sodium (bringing with it water) at the expense of hydrogen and potassium. There are many subtypes of hyperaldosteronism, but they are all unified in that they produce aldosterone independent of renin. This results in hypertension, atrial fibrillation, diabetes, kidney disease, and cardiac disease. Subtypes of PA include aldosterone-producing adenoma (30%), bilateral idiopathic hyperaldosteronism (60%), familial hyperaldosteronism (1%), unilateral hyperplasia (1%-2%), pure aldosterone-producing adrenocortical carcinomas (1%), and ectopic aldosterone-producing tumors (1%).[13-15]

Clinical Findings

Initial laboratory findings may include an upper limit of normal sodium, metabolic alkalosis, and/or hypokalemia. Only 9% to 36% of patients will have hypokalemia. This may be exacerbated by a potassium-wasting diuretic, like furosemide. In severe cases of hypokalemia, the patient may experience muscle weakness, cramping, headaches, palpitations, polydipsia, and polyuria.[13,14] The following patients should be considered for evaluation of PA:

- Three or more visits with BP >150/100
- BP >140/90 despite three or more antihypertensives
- Hypertension with any of the following: hypokalemia, adrenal incidentaloma on cross-sectional imaging, sleep apnea, family history of early onset hypertension, stroke, or known primary hyperaldosteronism

Laboratory Tests

There are three components of diagnosis and treating PA: detection, confirmation, and subtype identification. They will be briefly reviewed here with more thorough discussion available elsewhere in this text.

Initial laboratory tests suggest renin-independent aldosterone production with the following findings: plasma renin below the level of detection, high plasma aldosterone (>20 ηg/dL), and high aldosterone/renin ratio (institution dependent). The combination of the plasma aldosterone to renin ratio and plasma aldosterone concentration is 90% sensitive and 91% specific for PA. Potassium-sparing diuretics, spironolactone, and eplerenone can affect these tests and should be held for at least 2 weeks prior to laboratory analysis. Confirmation tests using oral or intravenous sodium chloride or, less commonly, fludrocortisone will fail to suppress aldosterone production in the patient with PA as it is autonomously produced.[13,14]

Once the patient is determined to have PA, the next step is to identify the subtype with imaging, adrenal vein sampling (AVS), and, when appropriate, genetic testing. CT scans may be helpful in identifying large unilateral lesions; however, the majority of aldosterone-producing adenomas are 1.5 cm or smaller. Nonspecific CT findings may include unilateral adrenal limb thickening, unilateral microadenomas, or bilateral adenomas. Several studies have demonstrated that imaging alone is not always sufficient to determine subtype and appropriate treatment.[13,14]

AVS is recommended in most patients to help determine which gland is the source of aldosterone overproduction. This testing may be less useful in a small minority of patients with hypertensive hypokalemic hyperaldosteronism, who are less than 35 years old with a unilateral adrenal adenoma and a normal-appearing contralateral gland on appropriate imaging, as adrenal incidentalomas in this patient population are very rare. A dominant gland with AVS will have three- to fourfold higher aldosterone than the nondominant gland. Failure to demonstrate a clear dominant gland indicates that the patient has bilateral hypersecretion and will likely not benefit from surgical intervention. Sixty percent of patients with hyperaldosteronism have bilateral disease.[13,14]

Genetic testing maybe considered for young patients (<20 years old), patients with early-onset stroke (<40 years old) or known family history of PA.[13,14]

Treatment

Initial treatment of all PA patients should include a sodium-restricted diet (<100 mEq/day). They should be encouraged to maintain an ideal body weight, exercise daily, and quit smoking. Medical management of PA hypertension should include a mineralocorticoid receptor antagonist, spironolactone, or eplerenone. Spironolactone can be started 12.5 to 25 mg/day and be up-titrated as needed to max 400 mg/day. The side effects can be unbearable to some, as they include gynecomastia, erectile dysfunction, decreased libido, and menstrual activity. Eplerenone is a more selective antagonist and therefore has less affinity for androgen and progesterone receptors. This medication can be started with 25 mg twice daily and up-titrated to maximum of 100 mg daily. Side effects are more tolerable and can include dizziness, headache, fatigue, diarrhea, hypertriglyceridemia, and elevated liver enzymes. Eplerenone has the added benefit of having a substantially reduced pharmacologic half-life, which is useful if AVS is anticipated. Potassium and creatinine should be monitored with either drug. If blood pressure is still poorly controlled, additional agents may include low-dose thiazide diuretics and sulfonamide diuretics. Glucocorticoids have a limited role for those with familial disease. Isolated medical management is appropriate for patients with bilateral adrenal disease, those with prohibitive surgical risk, and those not interested in surgical treatment.[13,14]

Patients with unilateral disease should be offered a laparoscopic adrenalectomy. Surgical management may be curative of hypertension in up to 40% of patients. Another 50% will have a partial clinical response to surgery, resulting in improved control of blood pressure with fewer medications and/or lower doses. Patients with family history of hypertension, kidney disease, and those requiring more than two antihypertensive agents preoperatively are less likely to achieve complete resolution of their hypertension postoperatively. Patients should be started on spironolactone or eplerenone preoperatively.[16-18]

Complications

PA patients have a chronically suppressed renin-angiotensin axis. Postoperatively, these patients can experience hyperkalemia and hypoaldosteronism. Clinically significant hyperkalemia is experienced by 5% of patients. Fludrocortisone may be considered in these patients for treatment. It is more likely that these patients will experience persistent hypertension postoperatively.[13,14,16-18]

Prognosis

Patients with PA have higher rates of cardiovascular events, stroke, and renal failure even when compared to those with the same degree of hypertension due to essential hypertension. These rates are decreased with appropriate biochemical control via medical management or surgical resection. For unilateral disease, surgery may be curative, decrease pill burden, and increase quality of life.[14,16-18]

CUSHING DISEASE/SYNDROME

General Considerations

Cushing syndrome represents a constellation of disease processes, all joined by hypercortisolism. Eighty percent of Cushing syndrome patients have an ACTH-dependent process, the majority of which are Cushing disease from the pituitary and the minority are ectopic (small-cell lung cancer, pulmonary neuroendocrine tumors, etc). Cushing disease is 3 to 8 times more common in women and presents in the third to fourth decade of life. Ectopic Cushing syndrome, once a majority male disease, is now equalizing between men and women as the incidence of lung cancer in women has increased. These patients tend to present later in life, over the age of 50.[19,20]

Twenty percent of patients with Cushing syndrome have an ACTH-independent process, adrenal adenoma (10%), carcinoma (8%), or hyperplasia (<1%). These processes are more common among women. There is a bimodal age distribution in the first and fourth to fifth decades of life.[19,20]

Pathophysiology

Eighty percent of all Cushing syndrome patients have hypertension. The increased cortisol levels result in increased peripheral vascular sensitivity to epinephrine and angiotensin II. Cortisol itself can also act on renal tubule receptors and have direct cardiotoxic effects. It is through these mechanisms that hypercortisolism increases blood pressure.[19,21,22]

Clinical Findings

Cushing syndrome may present with a constellation of symptoms. Common symptoms include decreased libido, menstrual changes, hirsutism, weight gain, round facies, lethargy, depression, elevated glucose levels, and hypertension. Other, less common symptoms include atherosclerosis, striae, proximal muscle weakness, acne, balding, and recurrent infections. Clinicians should have a high index of suspicion for not only the presence of these symptoms, but increasing severity of the symptoms over time.[19,20] The following patients should be considered for evaluation of Cushing syndrome:

- Chronic diseases presenting at an early age, osteoporosis and hypertension
- Unexplained resistant hypertension and osteoporosis at any age
- Multiple and progressive Cushing syndrome symptoms
- Adrenal incidentalomas

A thorough review of a patient's medications, prescribed and over-the-counter supplements to rule out exogenous Cushing syndrome. The differential diagnosis for Cushing syndrome includes severe obesity, polycystic ovarian syndrome, psychological or physical stress, chronic alcohol abuse, obstructive sleep apnea, and glucocorticoid resistance.[19,20]

Laboratory Findings

The first step in diagnosing Cushing syndrome is to evaluate hypercortisolism. This is typically done with three separate midnight salivary cortisol levels (greater than 1.5 times normal). Other tests include 24-hour urinary-free cortisol or 1 mg dexamethasone suppression test. The next step is to determine if it is an ACTH-dependent or -independent process. ACTH levels greater than 20 ρg/mL are ACTH dependent and levels less than 5 ρg/mL are ACTH independent. Pituitary versus ectopic ACTH-dependent processes can be distinguished by CRH/desmopressin stimulation and/or dexamethasone suppression tests. ACTH levels between 5 to 10 pg/mL are indeterminant. Serum dehydroepiandrosterone sulfate (DHEAS) or CRH stimulation test can be used to distinguish between ACTH-independent and -dependent hypercortisolism. ACTH-dependent hypercortisolism will have decreased DHEAS and will respond appropriately to CRH stimulation.[19,20,22]

Imaging Studies

ACTH-independent processes, like adrenal carcinomas, adenomas (unilateral, bilateral, micro, or macronodular), and hyperplasia, should be first delineated on an adrenal protocol CT. Adrenal adenomas tend to be small with low Hounsfield units (<10 HU). Carcinomas, on the other hand, tend to be larger and have necrosis, hemorrhage, or calcifications, higher Hounsfield units (>10 HU). Concern for carcinoma should be followed with MRI and/or PET. Bilateral hyperplasia could be macro or micronodular. Adrenal tissue outside of the nodule may be atrophic.[19,20,22]

Treatment

The goal in treating hypertension secondary to Cushing syndrome is to reduce hypercortisolism, excise hypersecreting tumors, and minimize hormone deficiency. In Cushing disease, the size of the pituitary tumor, desire for fertility, and degree of hypercortisolism determine treatment. A small pituitary tumor can be excised with trans-sphenoidal total or subtotal micro-adenectomy. There is a 70% to 90% cure rate and 5% to 20% recurrence rate. For recurrent or residual disease, the patient may undergo re-resection, radiation, or medical therapy. In patients with ectopic Cushing syndrome, resection of the ectopic source of ACTH is preferred when possible. In nonresectable diseases, options may include cryoablation, transplantation (liver), chemotherapy, and radiation, depending on the source of the disease. In primary adrenal disease, the patient may undergo unilateral or bilateral adrenalectomy. Patients with bilateral disease who undergo subtotal or unilateral resection will recur. Bilateral adrenalectomy for pituitary or ectopic sources is reserved for patients who have failed medical management.[21,23]

Preoperatively patients can be given metyrapone or ketoconazole to reduce cortisol secretion and prevent surge during the stress of surgery. Hypertension should be controlled preoperatively on mineralocorticoid receptor antagonists, like spironolactone. If a second-line agent is needed, a thiazide diuretic should be considered. Communication with anesthesia should be constant during tumor manipulation and resection.[23]

Complications

Hypercortisolism is associated with an increased risk for thromboembolism. Cortisol acts to activate the coagulation cascade and impair fibrinolysis. Patients should be kept on prophylactic anticoagulation. Regardless of the etiology of the Cushing syndrome, patients are prone to adrenal insufficiency postoperatively either due to the suppressed pituitary-adrenal axis, atrophic adrenal parenchyma, or bilateral adrenalectomy. Patients will need glucocorticoids postoperatively, and most will require long-term therapy.[23]

Prognosis

Cushing syndrome, left untreated, is fatal. Leading causes of death include cardiovascular (myocardial infarction, hypertensive complications), thromboembolic disease (pulmonary embolism), or recurrent bacterial or fungal infections. In this scenario, mortality is 50% in 5 years after symptom onset. The prognosis for malignant Cushing syndrome (adrenal carcinoma or ectopic ACTH from small-cell lung cancer, gastrinoma, medullary thyroid cancer, etc.) depends on the stage of disease and degree of hypercortisolism. Indolent disease is survivable for many years, whereas patients with metastatic disease life expectancy can be on the order of months. Patients with treated pituitary or benign adrenal disease typically have symptom improvement within 2 to 12 months. Many patients will continue to have residual problems with hypertension, glucose tolerance and weight control, cholesterol, and bone density. These patients should be under close management with a primary care or endocrinologist postoperatively.[21,23]

THYROTOXICOSIS/THYROID STORM

General Considerations

Thyroid storm is rare, accounting for only 0.57 to 0.76 cases per 100,000 persons per year. It is more common among hospitalized patients at a rate of 4.8 to 5.7 per 100,000 hospitalized persons per year. This translates to 16% of inpatients with thyrotoxicosis develop thyroid storm.[24–26]

Pathophysiology

The increased thyroid hormone levels in thyrotoxicosis increases the propensity for cellular response to thyroid hormone as well as thyroid hormone receptor sensitivity to catecholamines. Importantly, total thyroxine (T4) and triiodothyronine (T3) levels in thyroid storm are similar to those with uncomplicated thyrotoxicosis. The free T4 and T3 levels, however, are significantly higher. The increase in free thyroid hormone interacting with thyroid hormone receptors increases systemic sensitivity and responsiveness to catecholamines. As previously discussed, catecholamine action on adrenergic receptors increases vasoconstriction and renin secretion, thereby increasing blood pressure.[25,26]

Clinical Findings

Patients at risk for thyroid storm typically have longstanding untreated or poorly controlled hyperthyroidism due to Graves' disease, toxic multinodular goiter, solitary toxic adenoma, or destructive thyroiditis. Storm may be brought on by an acute event like surgery (thyroid and nonthyroidal alike), trauma, infection, or acute iodine load, usually an iodine-containing contrast. Amiodarone can cause either increased thyroid hormone synthesis or thyroid tissue destruction, resulting in thyrotoxicosis. However, these patients are more likely to present with arrhythmia and heart failure and less likely to have the adrenergic symptoms of thyrotoxicosis because of the beta-blocking effect of amiodarone.[25,26]

Patients present with hyperpyrexia, altered mental status (agitation, anxiety, mania, delirium, psychosis), gastrointestinal distress (nausea, vomiting, diarrhea, pain), and cardiovascular changes (tachycardia, tachyarrhythmias, high cardiac output, decreased peripheral vascular resistance, and increased systolic blood pressure). On exam, patients may have a palpable or visible goiter, palpable thrill or audible bruit over the thyroid, ophthalmopathy, lid lag, tremor, pressured speech, and warm/moist skin.[25,26]

Laboratory Findings

Patients in thyroid storm will have low TSH, and elevated free T3 and T4. They may also present with hyperglycemia from increased glycogenolysis and inhibition of insulin release, hypercalcemia from hemoconcentration, elevated liver enzymes, and leukocytosis or leukopenia.

Laboratory findings, along with the life-threatening symptoms of hyperpyrexia, cardiovascular dysfunction, and altered mental status, are diagnostic for thyroid storm. Clinical identification of the triggering event is helpful in treatment. If the underlying hyperthyroid disease is not known, thyroid ultrasound and radioiodine uptake studies may play a role. Imaging, however, is not essential in diagnosing thyroid storm. Antibody studies may also help solidify the diagnosis; evaluation of thyrotropin receptor antibody or thyroid-stimulating immunoglobulin can be done in lieu of radioiodine uptake scan.[25,26]

Treatment

Thyroid storm can be prevented with adequate medical treatment of hyperthyroid patients, particularly prior to surgery (thyroidal or nonthyroidal). If a patient develops thyroid storm, they should immediately be transferred to the intensive care unit. Treatment should include thyroid-targeted therapy, supportive therapy, and reversal of any precipitating factors.[25,26]

Thyroid-targeted therapy includes beta blockade, thioamide blockade, iodine solution, glucocorticoids, and cholestyramine (Table 76–4). Nonselective beta blockers help treat increased adrenergic tone and reduce peripheral conversion of thyroid hormone. Patients should be started on 60 to 80 mg of oral propranolol every 4 to 6 hours, or in patients with acute heart failure an esmolol drip can also be initiated and titrated to heart rate and blood pressure. Metoprolol and atenolol are safer in patients with reactive airway disease as these agents are cardioselective; however, they will not help with blockage of peripheral thyroid hormone conversion. Calcium channel blockers are an alternative antihypertensive for patients who cannot tolerate a beta blocker.[25,26]

Thioamide blockade inhibits new hormone synthesis within 2 hours. Propylthiouracil (PTU) is preferred to methimazole (MMI) as it decreases thyroid hormone conversion peripherally, as well as blockade of synthesis. T3 levels drop 45% within 24 hours when PTU is used. They are only reduced by 10% to 15% when methimazole is used. PTU is dosed at 200 mg every 4 hours, and MMI is 20 mg every 4 to 6 hours. Patients should be monitored for agranulocytosis and hepatoxicity. If the patient has a severe reaction, thyroidectomy should be considered.[25,26]

After PTU or MMI is administered, iodine solutions (saturated solution of potassium iodide [SSKI] or Lugol's solution) block the release of synthesized thyroid hormone. If this medication is administered prior to thioamide blockade, the iodine will be used as a substrate for hormone synthesis. Patients are at risk for esophageal and duodenal mucosal injury; to avoid this, drops of the solution are diluted in an 8 oz glass of water or juice, and taken with food.[25,26]

Glucocorticoids may be used to reduce thyroid hormone conversion, stabilize cardiovascular symptoms, particularly if there is underlying adrenal insufficiency, and reduce autoimmune processes, that is, Graves'. Patients can be started on 100 mg IV every 8 hours. Studies have shown there is no mortality benefit in the use of glucocorticoids in thyroid storm. In patients who are difficult to control with conventional methods, bile acid sequestrants can be used to decrease enterohepatic recycling of thyroid hormones with cholestyramine 4 g four times daily.[25,26]

Critical care supportive therapy is an essential cornerstone in surviving thyroid storm. Volume status should be measured continuously; crystalloid resuscitation and diuretics should be administered as appropriate. Hyperpyrexia should be aggressively controlled. Acetaminophen is the preferred medical therapy as aspirin can increase free T4 and T3 concentration. Other supportive therapy includes antiemetics, pain control, and delirium precautions.[25,26]

The underlying precipitating factors for thyroid storm must be addressed. This may include physiologic stress (trauma, surgery), infection, or untreated Graves' disease. Definitive treatment of Graves' disease is recommended in patients who have a history of thyroid storm with either radioactive iodine or thyroidectomy. Radioactive iodine is contraindicated in patients with ocular involvement or active thyroid storm. Thyroidectomy is particularly recommended if the patient has a large goiter and/or compressive symptoms.[25-27]

Thyroidectomy has a role not only in Graves' disease, but also in patients with thyroid storm who do not tolerate

Table 76–4. Pharmacologic treatment of thyroid storm.

Drug	Indication	Dose	Side Effects
Beta Blocker			
Propranolol	Blocks peripheral conversion of thyroid hormone	60-80 mg/4-6 h	Dizziness, fatigue, impotence, insomnia
Esmolol	Blocks peripheral conversion of thyroid hormone in patients with acute heart failure	50-100 μg/kg/min	Dizziness, fatigue, peripheral edema, asthma exacerbation
Atenolol	Antihypertensive, does not block peripheral conversion of thyroid hormone	25-50 mg/day	Dizziness, fatigue, gastrointestinal distress
Metoprolol	Antihypertensive, does not block peripheral conversion of thyroid hormone	40 mg/day	Dizziness, fatigue, nausea, impotence, gastrointestinal distress
Calcium Channel Blocker			
Nicardipine	Refractory hypertension	30-60 mg/day 5-12 mg/h drip	Peripheral edema, dizziness, headache, flushing, dyspnea
Amlodipine	Refractory hypertension	5-10 mg/day	Peripheral edema, dizziness, fatigue, gastrointestinal distress
Thioamide Blockade			
Propylthiouracil	Decreases synthesis and blocks peripheral conversion of thyroid hormone	200 mg/4 h	Gastrointestinal distress, neuropathy, headache, hair loss
Methimazole	Decreases synthesis of thyroid hormone	20 mg/6 h	Agranulocytosis, hepatotoxicity, gastrointestinal distress, neuropathy
Iodine Solution			
Potassium iodide—SSKI or Lugol's solution	Blocks the release of thyroid hormone, after thioamide blockade initiated	1 mL/8 h	Esophageal and duodenal mucosal injury
Glucocorticoids			
Hydrocortisone	Reduces thyroid hormone conversion, stabilizes cardiovascular symptoms	5 mg/kg (up to 100 mg) IV/8 h	Insomnia, mood changes, muscle weakness, headache, fragile skin, delayed wound healing
Bile Acid Sequestrants			
Cholestyramine	Decreases enterohepatic recycling of thyroid hormones	4 g/6 h	Constipation, bloating, poor appetite

thioamide blockade. Surgical intervention should not be considered unless the patient has been initiated on medical therapy. Delay for more than 10 days while on iodine is associated with escape from the Wolff-Chaikoff effect whereby the body starts to utilize iodine for thyroid hormone synthesis once again which can exacerbate thyrotoxicosis. If the patient is not medically optimized prior to surgical intervention, plasmapheresis can be considered to remove cytokines, antibodies, and thyroid hormone from circulation.[25-27]

Complications and Prognosis

Patients are at high risk of coma, arrhythmia, and cardiovascular collapse. Thyroid storm has a mortality rate of 10% to 30%. Treatment should occur in a facility with a multidisciplinary critical care, endocrine, surgery, and anesthesia team as these patients are at increased risk of morbidity and mortality. With clinical improvement, iodine therapy can be discontinued. Glucocorticoids should be tapered. Beta blockers should be stopped with normal thyroid function tests. A euthyroid state should be targeted with thioamides. If undergoing thyroidectomy, patients can stop thioamides, iodine, and cholestyramine immediately. Beta blockers and glucocorticoids should be tapered in the postoperative period. Thyroid hormone replacement should not be initiated until the patient has reached normal free T4/T3 levels. The time required to achieve this will vary from patient to patient based on how well controlled they became prior to surgery.[25-27]

Patients who undergo thyroidectomy for the management of acute thyrotoxicosis and/or storm are at much higher risk of having issues with hypocalcemia post-op. Aggressive replacement of calcium, as well as vitamin D 25-OH is critical.[25-27]

OTHER HYPERTENSIVE ENDOCRINOPATHIES

While not typically associated with hypertensive emergencies, the following endocrinopathies can cause hypertension if not managed appropriately: congenital adrenal hyperplasia, hypothyroidism, hyperparathyroidism, and acromegaly.[28]

Congenital Adrenal Hyperplasia

Congenital deficiency of either 11-beta-hydroxylase or 17-alpha-hydroxylase results in the inability to produce cortisol. Both result in the increased production of mineralocorticoids including aldosterone. High aldosterone levels result in retention of sodium-causing hypertension. Patients with 11-beta hydroxylase deficiency will also have increased androgen production, resulting in hirsutism, acne, pseudoprecocious puberty in males, and virilization in females. To the contrary, patients with 17-alpha hydroxylase deficiency present low androgens resulting in hermaphroditism in genetic males (XY) and amenorrhea in females (XX). Treatment in both requires glucocorticoid replacement which will decrease aberrant mineralocorticoid production.[29]

Hypothyroidism

Patients with severe, untreated hypothyroidism develop decreased cardiac output, narrowed pulse pressure, and increased systemic vascular resistance, resulting in diastolic hypertension. Appropriate treatment with thyroid replacement hormone will treat corresponding hypertension.[28,30]

Primary Hyperparathyroidism

Patients with primary hyperparathyroidism will have hypertension related to hypercalcemia, 10% to 60% of the time. The exact mechanism is unclear. Symptomatic patients can present with polydipsia, polyuria, constipation, osteoporosis, renal lithiasis, peptic ulcer disease, and hypertension. The hypertension may or may not resolve with parathyroidectomy, and frequently does not; however, it may become easier to control.[28,30]

Acromegaly

Acromegaly is the aberrant production of growth hormone. Patients present with soft tissue overgrowth, arthritis, voice changes, perineural expansion, cardiac dysfunction, and/or hypertension. About 20% to 40% of the hypertension is due to sodium retention resulting in high circulating volume. This is best treated with diuretics. Surgical resection and/or radiation of the primary tumor can be curative.[28,31]

REFERENCES

1. Facts About Hypertension. Centers for Disease Control and Prevention. https://www.cdc.gov/bloodpressure/facts.htm. Published September 27, 2021. Accessed November 5, 2021.
2. Charles L, Triscott J, Dobbs B. Secondary hypertension: discovering the underlying cause. *Am Fam Physician.* 2017;96(7):453-461.
3. Gupta-Malhotra M, Banker A, Shete S, et al. Essential hypertension vs. secondary hypertension among children. *Am J Hypertens.* 2015;28(1):73-80.
4. Young WF, Calhoun DA, Lenders JWM, Stowasser M, Textor SC. Screening for endocrine hypertension: an endocrine society scientific statement. *Endocrine Reviews.* 2017;38(2):103-122.
5. Koch C, Papadopoulou-Marketou N, Chrousos GP. Overview of Endocrine Hypertension. In: Feingold KR, Anawalt B, Boyce A, et al., eds. *Endotext.* South Dartmouth (MA): MDText.com, Inc.; February 4, 2020.
6. Lenders JWM, Kerstens MN, Amar L, et al. Genetics, diagnosis, management and future directions of research of phaeochromocytoma and paraganglioma: a position statement and consensus of the Working Group on Endocrine Hypertension of the European Society of Hypertension. *J Hypertens.* 2020;38(8):1443-1456.
7. Jain A, Baracco R, Kapur G. Pheochromocytoma and paraganglioma—an update on diagnosis, evaluation, and management. *Pediatr Nephrol.* 2020;35(4):581-594.
8. Motiejunaite J, Amar L, Vidal-Petiot E. Adrenergic receptors and cardiovascular effects of catecholamines. *Annales d'endocrinologie.* 2021;82(3-4):193-197.
9. Lenders JW, Duh QY, Eisenhofer G, et al. Pheochromocytoma and paraganglioma: an endocrine society clinical practice guideline. *J Clin Endocrinol Metab.* 2014;99(6):1915-1942.
10. Baez JC, Jagannathan JP, Krajewski K, et al. Pheochromocytoma and paraganglioma: imaging characteristics. *Cancer Imaging.* 2012;12(1):153-162.
11. Currás-Freixes M, Piñeiro-Yañez E, Montero-Conde C, et al. PheoSeq: a targeted next-generation sequencing assay for pheochromocytoma and paraganglioma diagnostics. *J Mol Diagn.* 2017;19(4):575-588.
12. Hescot S, Curras-Freixes M, Deutschbein T, et al. Prognosis of malignant pheochromocytoma and paraganglioma (MAPP-PronO study): a European network for the study of adrenal tumors retrospective study. *J Clin Endocrinol Metab.* 2019;104(6):2367-2374.
13. Funder JW, Carey RM, Mantero F, et al. The management of primary aldosteronism: case detection, diagnosis, and treatment: an Endocrine Society Clinical Practice Guideline. *J Clin Endocrinol Metab.* 2016;101(5):1889-1916.
14. Brown JM, Siddiqui M, Calhoun DA, et al. The unrecognized prevalence of primary aldosteronism: a cross-sectional study. *Ann Intern Med.* 2020;173(1):10-20.
15. Rossi GP, Bernini G, Caliumi C, et al. A prospective study of the prevalence of primary aldosteronism in 1,125 hypertensive patients. *J Am Coll Cardiol.* 2006;48(11):2293-2300.
16. Monticone S, D'Ascenzo F, Moretti C, et al. Cardiovascular events and target organ damage in primary aldosteronism compared with essential hypertension: a systematic review and meta-analysis. *Lancet Diabetes Endocrinol.* 2018;6(1):41-50.
17. Puar TH, Loh LM, Loh WJ, et al. Outcomes in unilateral primary aldosteronism after surgical or medical therapy. *Clin Endocrinol (Oxf).* 2021;94(2):158-167.

18. Williams TA, Lenders JWM, Mulatero P, et al. Outcomes after adrenalectomy for unilateral primary aldosteronism: an international consensus on outcome measures and analysis of remission rates in an international cohort. *Lancet Diabetes Endocrinol.* 2017;5(9):689-699.
19. Barbot M, Zilio M, Scaroni C. Cushing's syndrome: overview of clinical presentation, diagnostic tools and complications. *Best Pract Res Clin Endocrinol Metab.* 2020;34(2):101380.
20. Pivonello R, De Martino MC, De Leo M, Simeoli C, Colao A. Cushing's disease: the burden of illness. *Endocrine.* 2017;56(1): 10-18.
21. Nieman LK. Hypertension and cardiovascular mortality in patients with Cushing syndrome. *Endocrinol Metab Clin North Am.* 2019;48(4):717-725.
22. Nieman LK. Diagnosis of Cushing's syndrome in the modern era. *Endocrinol Metab Clin North Am.* 2018;47(2):259-273.
23. Di Dalmazi G, Reincke M. Adrenal surgery for Cushing's syndrome: an update. *Endocrinol Metab Clin North Am.* 2018;47(2):385-394.
24. Bourcier S, Coutrot M, Kimmoun A, et al. Thyroid storm in the ICU: a retrospective multicenter study. *Crit Care Med.* 2020;48(1):83-90.
25. Doubleday AR, Sippel RS. Hyperthyroidism. *Gland Surg.* 2020;9(1):124-135.
26. Radhi MA, Natesh B, Stimpson P, Hughes J, Vaz F, Dwivedi RC. Thyroid storm in head and neck emergency patients. *J Clin Med.* 2020;9(11):3548.
27. Koh H, Kaushik M, Loh JK, Chng CL. Plasma exchange and early thyroidectomy in thyroid storm requiring extracorporeal membrane oxygenation. *Endocrinol Diabetes Metab Case Rep.* 2019;2019(1):1-6.
28. Charles L, Triscott J, Dobbs B. Secondary hypertension: discovering the underlying cause. *Am Fam Physician.* 2017;96(7):453-461.
29. El-Maouche D, Arlt W, Merke DP. Congenital adrenal hyperplasia [published correction appears in *Lancet.* 2017;390(10108):2142]. *Lancet.* 2017;390(10108):2194-2210.
30. Fisher SB, Perrier ND. Primary hyperparathyroidism and hypertension. *Gland Surg.* 2020;9(1):142-149.
31. Berg C, Petersenn S, Lahner H, et al. Cardiovascular risk factors in patients with uncontrolled and long-term acromegaly: comparison with matched data from the general population and the effect of disease control. *J Clin Endocrinol Metab.* 2010;95:3648-3656.

77 Carcinoid Crisis

Rodney F. Pommier, MD

INTRODUCTION

Operating on patients with neuroendocrine tumors can be more challenging and stressful than operations on patients with other diagnoses because the patient may have an intraoperative event known as carcinoid crisis. Carcinoid crisis has no strict, or even agreed upon, definition, but is characterized by sudden, marked hemodynamic instability which may or may not be accompanied by characteristics of carcinoid syndrome, such as flushing or bronchospasm. Carcinoid crisis has been reported to occur spontaneously, during abdominal examinations, during procedures including transesophageal echocardiography, colonoscopy, and mammography, during biopsy of tumors, during liver embolization, and during operations, including at induction of anesthesia.[1-7]

The hemodynamic instability may be characterized by hypertension or hypotension, but intraoperative crises usually manifest as profound hypotension. This presents a difficult and dangerous problem. The profound hypotension results in hypoperfusion of vital organs that, in turn, may lead to acute kidney injury, liver damage, stroke, or myocardial infarction. It can lead to complete circulatory collapse and death.

Not surprisingly, the occurrence of intraoperative carcinoid crisis has been associated with increased risk of both minor and major postoperative complications.

Neuroendocrine tumors synthesize and release a variety of vasoactive compounds including serotonin, histamine, bradykinin, tachykinin, kallikrein, and many others.

These compounds have been implicated in causing the symptoms of carcinoid syndrome.

Early reports of carcinoid crisis involved patients with carcinoid syndrome and their authors assumed crisis is a severe manifestation of carcinoid syndrome.

They hypothesized that the etiology of carcinoid crisis is a sudden, massive release of those hormones. This theory is still prevalent today. However, this theory had never been proven.

Based largely on this theory, various efforts have been made over the years to reduce the incidence of intraoperative carcinoid crisis through administration of specific pharmacologic agents, such as anxiolytics and antihistamines, while avoiding the administration of others, particularly catecholamines which are believed to provoke release of carcinoid hormones.

Over time, however, management of carcinoid crisis has shifted almost entirely to prophylactic administration of the somatostatin analog octreotide.

Recommendations for prophylactic use of octreotide abound. They also vary widely with respect to patient selection, dose, route of administration, timing of administration, and duration of administration.

However, data supporting the use of any of these regimens are scant. Much of it has been in the form of single case reports which, with an N of one, do not allow any reasonable conclusions to be drawn. Other literature on intraoperative carcinoid crisis has been in the form of case series, which have provided some valuable information on incidence, clinical risk factors, and outcomes. To date, seven single institution retrospective case series[8-10,18-22] and two single institution prospective case series have been published.[10,23]

Many statements about carcinoid crisis have been made within the body of literature, some of which have become dogmatic.[1-43] The list of dogmas includes: crisis is caused by massive release of carcinoid hormones, particularly serotonin, crisis occurs only in patients with carcinoid syndrome, prophylactic administration of octreotide prevents (or reduces the incidence of) crisis, octreotide is the best treatment for crisis, antihistamines (both histamine 1 and histamine 2 receptor blockers) should be used to prevent and treat crisis, and beta-adrenergic agonists, especially catecholamines, should not be given to patients with neuroendocrine tumors because they will provoke a crisis or worsen an ongoing crisis. This chapter will review the literature on carcinoid crisis and examine these issues in detail. In the course of review, it will analyze whether these statements are supported or refuted by more recent findings and data.

THE HISTORY OF CARCINOID SYNDROME & CARCINOID CRISIS

Carcinoid syndrome was first described in 1954 among 16 patients with a diverse constellation of diarrhea, abdominal pain, bronchial asthma, patchy peculiar flushing, malar telangiectasia, right-sided heart failure, and edema.[20]

The authors implicated serotonin as the hormone responsible for many of these findings. It was subsequently established that patients with carcinoid syndrome had a high prevalence of elevated levels of 5-hydroxyindolacetic acid (5-HIAA), the breakdown product of serotonin, in 24-hour collections of their urine and some patients also had elevated levels of urinary histamine.

However, reports soon followed which questioned the role of serotonin in flushing. Almost no patients demonstrated elevation of serum serotonin or its metabolites in serum or urine after spontaneous flushing episodes.[11]

Some patients with severe flushing had normal urinary 5-HIAA levels.[21]

Intravenous injection of serotonin into normal subjects and patients with carcinoid syndrome did not induce flushing.[22,23]

The serotonin antagonists cyproheptadine and methysergide were ineffective at controlling flushing.[11]

Rather, it had been shown that patients with carcinoid flushing had elevated levels of bradykinin and kallikrein in their hepatic venous blood and such elevations could be provoked with intravenous injections of epinephrine. These elevations were accompanied by episodes of flushing. Thus, it was far from clear which hormones were responsible for causing flushing. But contrary to what is still a popular belief today, data actually supported bradykinin and kallikrein as the cause of flushing rather than serotonin.[11-14]

The first report of "carcinoid crisis" was published in 1964.[24] A 41-year-old woman was admitted to the hospital with liver metastases and carcinoid syndrome, including carcinoid heart disease, years after resection of an ileal primary tumor. On her 13th hospital day, she left to visit her family but, 15 minutes after returning to the ward, she had abrupt onset of apprehension, oppressive chest pain, excruciating abdominal cramps, frequent diarrhea, facial flushing, pale cold extremities, and cyanotic nail beds. Although her apical cardiac impulse was strong and rapid, her peripheral pulses were absent and her blood pressure could not be recorded. She was not responsive to doses of metaraminol, an alpha-adrenergic agonist with some beta effect, nor the beta-adrenergic agonist norepinephrine. Over the next hour, her symptoms of apprehension, flushing, and burning and itching skin worsened. She was given a single intravenous dose of cyproheptadine, which gave her dramatic relief of her chest and abdominal pain. A few minutes later, her femoral pulse became transiently palpable. Thirty minutes later, she had a normal blood pressure and peripheral pulses. Her symptoms, but not hypotension, returned 12 hours later and were again relieved with cyproheptadine. A norepinephrine infusion was continued for the next 15 hours, during which her blood pressure remained stable. The patient had been having daily measurement of her 24-hour urinary 5-HIAA levels and the level on the day of the crisis was higher than on any previous day.

While this may have been the first report of carcinoid crisis by that name, the authors immediately point out in the background of their manuscript that profound hypotension in patients with carcinoid syndrome had been noted during anesthesia and palpation of the tumor at operation. These are clear references to intraoperative carcinoid crises.

The authors point out that the mechanism of hypotension in those cases was not clear, but an excessive amount of circulating serotonin was assumed to be a major causative factor. Neither did they know what triggered the crisis in their patient, but reported the patient's consumption of tryptophan, a precursor to serotonin, had been changed from 300 to 1200 mg/day on the day of the crisis. They also thought it is possible she had a surge of serotonin from tumor necrosis, but actually cited the literature described above reporting that rises in patients' serum serotonin levels during flushing episodes were infrequent as an argument against that conclusion. They doubted histamine played a role. They found it interesting the patient had relief of symptoms with the serotonin antagonist cyproheptadine, but her blood pressure responded neither to it nor to adrenergic vasopressors. They cited literature that patients with carcinoid syndrome had been reported to experience transient flushing and significant reductions in blood pressure when receiving intravenous norepinephrine and epinephrine.

Therefore, they stated that when the need for vasopressor therapy arises in a patient with carcinoid syndrome, the use of norepinephrine and epinephrine should be avoided. This statement likely began, or at least contributed to, the dogma that patients in crisis do not respond to beta-adrenergic agonists like norepinephrine and epinephrine, that beta-adrenergic agonists worsen crises, and that they should not be administered to patients with carcinoid syndrome, a dogma that persists to the present day. It is difficult to justify this statement given the fact that they administered a continuous intravenous infusion of norepinephrine to their patient for 15 hours with the result being stable blood pressure and that no additional hypotensive crises were triggered. Although they reported that her symptoms of apprehension and flushing, burning, and itching skin increased after norepinephrine, they did not report worsening of her hypotension.

What is often overlooked is that this patient had carcinoid heart disease, which could have significantly altered the interpretations of events and responses to treatment. Patients with carcinoid heart disease are very sensitive to loss of cardiac preload and can be extremely difficult to resuscitate from any hypotensive event, regardless of the etiology. Carcinoid heart disease typically consists of marked tricuspid insufficiency with the pulmonic valve exhibiting a combination of stenosis and regurgitation.

This results in reflux of blood back out of the right heart into the venous circulation with each heartbeat. There is also fibrosis of the endocardium with decreased contractility. As a result, the delivery of intravenous drugs to the systemic circulation can be significantly delayed. Therefore, apparent lack of responses and timing of responses to intravenous drugs administered in this case are all questionable. Although it appears the patient did have timely relief of symptoms and a transient return of pulses with the intravenous administration of the cyproheptadine, it should be noted that her pulses and blood pressure did not return to normal for another 30 minutes. So, it is difficult to know whether to ascribe their return to cyproheptadine, the norepinephrine given prior to it, or simply spontaneous recovery from the crisis.

The elevated 24-hour urinary 5-HIAA level on the day of the crisis certainly seems to lend credence to the theory of massive release of hormones as the pathophysiologic cause of her crisis. However, examination of the graph published in the manuscript shows that while the level was about 550 mg/24 h on the day of the crisis, it had typically been above 400 mg/24 h and as high as 480 mg/24 h during the 12 preceding days without any crises. Does that degree of rise support the theory of massive release? Also, if one believes catecholamines trigger release of hormones like serotonin, then wouldn't one expect the urinary 5-HIAA level to be higher on a day when they received a continuous intravenous infusion of norepinephrine for 15 hours?

In 1976, Mason and Steane published a comprehensive review of the literature on patients with carcinoid syndrome undergoing anesthesia. They found a total of 40 operations reported within nine papers. The incidence of intraoperative complications, including hypotension, hypertension, or bronchospasm, was very high, occurring in 27 (54%) of cases; more clear references to intraoperative crises.

OCTREOTIDE AS TREATMENT FOR CARCINOID CRISIS

The first report of octreotide treating a carcinoid crisis was published in 1985 by Kvols et al. from the Mayo Clinic, initially as a letter to the editor of the *New England Journal of Medicine* and subsequently published by his group as a manuscript in an anesthesiology journal.[16]

Dr. Kvols has personally told me the story many times. He was investigating octreotide for treatment of carcinoid syndrome[34] and had given lectures on its effects at the Mayo Clinic. A patient with small bowel neuroendocrine tumor causing stenosis of the ileum with liver metastases and carcinoid syndrome was taken to the operating for primary tumor resection to relieve obstructive symptoms and ligation of the hepatic artery to induce necrosis of metastases to improve carcinoid syndrome symptoms. Following induction of anesthesia, as the abdominal skin was being prepared with povidone-iodine solution, the patient experienced flushing of the abdominal skin followed by profound, life-threatening hypotension. No blood pressure could be obtained and only the carotid pulse was palpable. The authors report the patient did not respond to intravenous fluids, intravenous calcium, nor intravenous conventional vasopressors, including neosynephrine and, eventually, epinephrine. The surgeon knew of the work Dr. Kvols was doing with octreotide and had him paged. When Dr. Kvols responded, he was told of the life-threatening situation and asked if he could bring some octreotide to the operating room. Dr. Kvols rushed to the investigational pharmacy, procured some octreotide despite the protests of the pharmacist, and took it to the operating room. Several minutes after the onset of the crisis, the patient was given an intravenous dose of 50 μg of octreotide. The dose was repeated 15 seconds later. Thirty to 40 seconds later, the patient had bounding pulses and blood pressure returned to normal. About five minutes later, the flushing resolved. The authors state that the response to octreotide was dramatic and life-saving and recommended octreotide be kept available in operating rooms during operations on patients with carcinoid syndrome.

Interpretation of timing of administration of pharmacologic agents and their corresponding responses should also be questioned in this case. If one looks at the graph of blood pressure versus time published in the manuscript,[7] one can see a V-shaped dip of blood pressure, down to zero at the vertex, followed by rapid recovery to normal. The graph indicates octreotide was administered at the nadir of the blood pressure and then the blood pressure immediately begins to rise. However, it also indicates epinephrine was administered 3.5 minutes before that nadir and the octreotide administration. So, is the rise in blood pressure really an almost instantaneous effect of the octreotide administration in a patient who concurrently had almost no blood pressure? Or had the epinephrine delivered earlier finally been distributed to the systemic circulation and began taking effect? Or was it a combination of the two? In any event, this report had an effect of further strengthening the belief that patients with neuroendocrine tumors do not respond to beta-adrenergic agonists during hypotensive crises.

Treating crises with octreotide raises a very important question that has never been answered to the author's satisfaction. How would octreotide work to reverse an ongoing crisis? This is particularly difficult to explain if one subscribes to the predominant theory that crisis is due to the sudden massive release of carcinoid hormones from tumors. Octreotide is known to inhibit both synthesis and release of vasoactive hormones from neuroendocrine tumor cells. But if a crisis is ongoing then, according to that theory, the hormones must have already been released. Octreotide is not a hormone receptor blocker. It is incapable of blocking the effects of hormones already released. One could argue that an ongoing crisis requires continued massive release of hormones to be sustained. Therefore, octreotide could inhibit the release of additional hormones and, ultimately, relieve the crisis. But that doesn't adequately explain the rapid reversal of crises that have been reported.[16,35-37]

It would still take time for those hormones that have already been released to be metabolized before the crisis would abate, let alone for the vascular system to reset itself to normal from whatever massive perturbation had occurred. Octreotide therapy rapidly reversing a crisis doesn't make sense physiologically, and it certainly requires massive release of hormones by the tumor to be the pathophysiology behind crisis.

The first publication of a large series of operations suggesting that octreotide administration might reduce the incidence of intraoperative carcinoid crisis also came from the Mayo Clinic in 2001. Kinney et al. reported their experience with 119 patients with metastatic carcinoid tumors undergoing abdominal operations between 1983 and 1996.[18]

Octreotide became available after Food and Drug Administration approval in 1988 and they began administering it both preoperatively and intraoperatively to some patients, likely spurred by their case report described above. Accordingly, some received no octreotide, some received a preoperative dose, and some received an intraoperative dose, either with or without a preoperative dose. Seventy percent of the patients had preoperative diarrhea and 64% had preoperative flushing.

They reviewed patients' records for what they termed as intraoperative complications, including flushing, urticaria, ventricular dysrhythmias, bronchospasm, acidosis, hypoxemia, hypotension, systolic blood pressure (SBP) less than 80 mmHg for >10 minutes, and total duration of sustained tachycardia. They also recorded perioperative complications and deaths. They found that 15 patients experienced a perioperative complication, including death in three. Among those 15 patients, eight had one or more intraoperative complications including flushing in four, sustained hypotension in two, and bronchospasm, acidosis, and ventricular tachycardia in one patient each. They found that eight of 73 patients (11%) who did not receive any octreotide and one of six patients (17%) who received only preoperative octreotide had an intraoperative complication. However, none of the 45 patients who received intraoperative octreotide had an intraoperative complication. The difference in intraoperative complications between the 45 patients who received intraoperative octreotide and the 73 who received none was statistically significant. They concluded that the administration of intraoperative octreotide was associated with a decreased incidence of those intraoperative complications.

Octreotide for Prophylaxis Against Carcinoid Crisis

Two years after the report by Kinney et al., two surgeons from the Mayo Clinic published a monograph on hepatic surgery for neuroendocrine tumor metastases in which they claimed that preoperative preparation of patients with a dose of 150 to 500 μg of octreotide decreases the chance of carcinoid crisis.[38]

However, no data supporting this claim were provided. Soon, numerous recommendations for prophylactic octreotide regimens also emerged within the literature. They varied widely in terms of dose, route of administration, timing, and duration. A textbook of endocrine surgery stated that preoperative administration of octreotide LAR alone essentially eliminates the risk of crisis.[32]

Others recommended a preoperative dose of 250 to 500 μg. Still, others recommended subcutaneous administration of 100 μg of octreotide three times per day for 2 weeks prior to operation and then 100 μg administered intravenously at the induction of anesthesia. The North American Neuroendocrine Tumor Society recommended continuous intravenous infusion at doses of 50 to 500 μg per hour.[33] Guidelines from the United Kingdom recommended beginning a continuous infusion of intravenous octreotide at a dose of 50 μg per hour for 12 hours prior to and continued at least 48 hours after operation.[36] Many authors recommended having additional vials of octreotide available for intravenous administration if crises still arise during the operation despite the prophylactic measures taken. Generally, these recommendations were made only for patients with carcinoid syndrome. However, data supporting any of these diverse regimens were lacking. For example, the references supporting the NANETS guidelines of continuous infusion of octreotide were two single case reports in which infusions were given and no events occurred during those cases.

Given that the claim about prophylactic octreotide reducing the incidence of carcinoid crisis came from the Mayo Clinic, it is logical to conclude that the concept might have arisen from and been supported by the earlier report by Kinney et al. from the same institution. Indeed, it is quite common to see the report by Kinney et al. referenced as evidence for prophylactic octreotide on slides at conferences and in some literature. However, one cannot actually interpret that report as providing any supportive evidence for efficacy of prophylactic octreotide. An intraoperative complication still occurred in one of the six patients given only a preoperative dose, yielding a rate of intraoperative complications similar to that seen among the 73 who received none. Crises can occur with induction, yet no recommendation was made to administer it prior to induction. The doses of intraoperative octreotide given in their series ranged from 30 to 4000 μg. So, how much octreotide must be given to prevent a crisis? The timing of intraoperative doses was not specified, so when should it be given to prevent crisis? In fact, the authors specifically state in the discussion that their study was not able to evaluate the efficacy of intraoperative octreotide to prevent intraoperative carcinoid crises. So, other than an occasional case report where preoperative octreotide was given and nothing occurred during that particular case, there were as yet no published data supporting the concept of octreotide prophylaxis.

CARCINOID CRISIS RESEARCH AT OREGON HEALTH & SCIENCE UNIVERSITY

Recognizing the lack of data on outcomes of various octreotide prophylaxis protocol being recommended, the author decided to implement octreotide protocols in a systematic fashion, progressing through preoperative octreotide LAR, preoperative prophylactic doses, intraoperative doses, and eventually the use of continuous intravenous infusion, if necessary. The plan was to periodically analyze the outcomes of these various approaches and modify them accordingly. Based on recommendations in a consensus report in 2004, our initial prophylactic octreotide protocol was to prescribe octreotide LAR preoperatively and administer an additional preoperative dose of 250 to 500 μg of octreotide either subcutaneously or intravenously prior to induction of anesthesia.[45] Additional vials of octreotide would be available for intraoperative intravenous administration as boluses of 250 to 500 μg for treatment of bronchospasm, flushing, or changes in blood pressure or heart rate not attributable to other causes such as blood loss or hypovolemia. At first, this was done only for syndromic patients, but it was soon discovered that asyndromic patients could also have carcinoid crises and the protocol was soon extended to include all patients.[8]

In 2011, we reviewed our results with the first 97 patients. Seventy-five patients (77%) had hepatic metastases and 57 (59%) carried a diagnosis of carcinoid syndrome. Seventy patients (72%) had received preoperative octreotide LAR and 87 (90%) received a preoperative bolus of octreotide, with a median dose of 500 μg. The principal procedure was hepatic resection in 50% of cases. Twenty-three patients (24%) had an intraoperative complication. This is a rate over three times higher than the overall rate of 7% reported by Kinney et al. The most common intraoperative complication was SBP <80 mmHg for 10 or more minutes not attributable to any other cause, such as blood loss or hypovolemia, by either the attending surgeon or attending anesthesiologist, which occurred in 18 patients (19%). Marked hemodynamic instability was reported to be a severe carcinoid crisis by either the attending anesthesiologist in the anesthesia record and/or by the attending surgeon in the operative report in an additional five cases (5%). Crises were statistically just as likely to occur in patients without carcinoid syndrome as in patients with syndrome. The only independent predictor of carcinoid crisis was the presence of hepatic metastases, as all crises occurred in patients with them.

Analyses showed neither preoperative octreotide LAR administration nor a preoperative bolus of octreotide was associated with a statistically significant lower incidence of crises compared to no administration. Furthermore, 54 patients (55%) received intraoperative boluses of octreotide to treat intraoperative hypotension. Despite previous reports of rapid, dramatic improvement in hypotension, 37 of those patients did not respond adequately and also required administration of intravenous vasopressors, including seven who required continuous intravenous infusion of vasopressors. Twenty-six percent of the patients who received intraoperative octreotide experienced yet another hypotensive event during their operation. Patients who had intraoperative complications were statistically significantly more likely to have postoperative complications. Moreover, they were statistically more likely to have major complications. The overall 30-day postoperative complication rate for patients having an intraoperative event was 60.8%, with 39.1% having major complications.

The conclusions derived from this series were that the rate of intraoperative complications is substantial at 23%, that a major risk factor is the presence of liver metastases, that they also occur in patients without carcinoid syndrome, and patients who have them are at markedly increased risk for both minor and major postoperative complications. The most important findings were that neither preoperative octreotide LAR nor preoperative bolus administration of octreotide showed any significant reduction in their occurrence compared to no octreotide therapy. Furthermore, intraoperative administration of octreotide often failed to resolve a crisis.

Following the publication of this series, Woltering et al. hypothesized that a preoperative bolus of octreotide, with a half-life of 90 to 120 minutes, might not last long enough for protection against carcinoid crises during long operations and that this could be remedied by continuous intravenous infusion. Their practice was to give a preoperative 500 μg bolus followed by continuous infusion at 500 μg/h. They reviewed their experience with 179 operations, which had an average duration of 6.3 hours. Based on our report, they reviewed their records specifically for instances of SBP <80 mmHg for ≥10 minutes, hemodynamic instability, or either the attending surgeon or anesthesiologist having declared that a crisis occurred in the operative and anesthesia reports. They found an incidence of only 3.6%. Thus, this series showed a possible beneficial effect of a continuous octreotide infusion for reducing the incidence of intraoperative carcinoid crisis.[40]

In the meantime, because of high rates of crisis and associated complications with our original regimen, we modified it by adding a continuous intravenous infusion of octreotide at 500 μg/h. We also realized that we had to modify our criteria for declaring crises and initiating treatment of hypotension. Previously, it had been our practice to observe an SBP <80 mmHg for several minutes, to see if it spontaneously resolved, before declaring it to be a crisis and initiating therapy. However, our data showed that the mean time between initiating therapy and having SBP recover to >80 mmHg was about 9 minutes. Importantly, patients who were hypotensive for ≥10 minutes were significantly more likely to have postoperative complications. Therefore, we considered it unethical to observe hypotension for more than a minute without initiating therapy to try to keep crises <10 minutes in duration.

Our definition of carcinoid crisis was changed to be hemodynamic instability, such as SBP <80 or >180 mmHg, heart rate >120 beats/minute, or display of any physiology that, if sustained, would be expected to lead to end-organ dysfunction, such as ventricular arrhythmias, or bronchospasm. It had to be unattributable to any other cause, such as being behind on fluid resuscitation, hemorrhage, or compression of the vena cava. Both attending surgeon and attending anesthesiologist had to agree there was no other plausible cause before declaring a crisis. On declaration, therapy was begun immediately. These changes were applied prospectively to the next 150 operations, after which we again reviewed and published our results.

We found that the incidence of intraoperative events with continuous octreotide infusion was no lower, at 30%, than it had been without it. Crises again correlated with presence of liver metastases, but also, with this larger sample, older age, carcinoid syndrome, and duration of anesthesia. They did not correlate with serum chromogranin A or 24-hour urinary 5-HIAA levels. Again, the predominant type of event was intraoperative hypotension, occurring in 23% of patients. An encouraging finding was immediate treatment had shortened the mean duration of crisis from 19 minutes in our previous study to 8.9 minutes. Crises no longer correlated with major postoperative complications, except among the 8% of patients where hypotension still persisted ≥10 minutes. Three operations were aborted due to medically refractory intraoperative carcinoid crises.[41]

Superficially, the results of our study using continuous infusion do not appear to agree with those of Woltering et al.[19] But, perhaps they actually do. Woltering et al. reviewed records only for episodes of hypotension lasting ≥10 minutes. Treatments for hypotension were not reported and events lasting <10 minutes with treatment would not have been captured by their methodology. In our series, hypotensive events lasting ≥10 minutes despite treatment occurred at a rate of 8%, which is similar to the 3.6% rate they reported. Although continuous infusion of octreotide was not the panacea we had hoped for, this study did identify additional risk factors for crises and did show that prompt, aggressive treatment of hypotensive crises can shorten their duration. At this point, it also appeared that shortening the duration of crises to <10 minutes reduced the rate of subsequent major postoperative complications.

Kinney et al. from the Mayo Clinic subsequently published a series in which they did use prophylactic preoperative doses of octreotide for some patients with liver metastases undergoing partial hepatic resection.[42] Patients with liver metastases were then known to be high risk for crisis based on our previous reports. The authors clearly took issue with the evolving definition of carcinoid crisis to include hemodynamic instability not attributable to other causes, particularly hypotension, given that there could be multiple other causes for intraoperative hypotension during major operations. Accordingly, they changed their definition of crisis to be sudden or abrupt onset of at least two of the following: flushing or urticaria that is not explained by an allergic reaction, bronchospasm or bronchodilator administration, hypotension (SBP <80 mmHg for >10 minutes and treated with vasopressors) not explained by volume status or hemorrhage, tachycardia ≥120 beats/minute. Among the 169 cases reviewed, 130 (77%) received a preoperative subcutaneous injection of 500 μg of octreotide and 39 did not, regardless of octreotide LAR use.

Using their new definition, they reported their incidence of intraoperative carcinoid crisis was 0%. It should be noted, however, that sustained hypotension occurred in 5.3% and sustained tachycardia occurred in another 8.9% of patients, but because none of those patients exhibited any other of their criteria, none of those events were declared to be crises. The authors do once again state in the discussion section that their review is not able to evaluate the efficacy of octreotide to prevent or ameliorate intraoperative carcinoid crisis. Indeed, within their data set and using their new definition, no treatment with octreotide was statistically just as effective as giving octreotide. However, based on their clinical experience, the authors did recommend preoperative treatment with octreotide LAR, a preoperative dose of short-acting octreotide to reduce hormone release during induction of anesthesia, and having additional octreotide available in the operating room to treat events for patients undergoing hepatic resection.

Another report on the outcomes of prophylactic octreotide was made by the group at the University of California, San Francisco.[9] They reported on 75 patients, 38 of whom underwent operation and 37 of whom received embolotherapy. They found the incidence of carcinoid crisis or hemodynamic instability among all patients was 32%, but it was 42% among patients undergoing operation. Neither long-acting somatostatin analog therapy, preprocedure octreotide, intraprocedural octreotide, nor any combination thereof was associated with a lower incidence of crisis or hemodynamic instability. Treatments of hypotension included additional octreotide and vasopressors, but norepinephrine and epinephrine were only rarely given in their series. Patients who had events had a significantly higher incidence of postprocedure complications.

DETERMINING THE PATHOPHYSIOLOGY OF CARCINOID CRISIS

Having been disappointed by the lack of reduction of the incidence of carcinoid crisis by continuous infusion of octreotide, we concluded that determining proper pharmacologic intervention, let alone prevention, for carcinoid crisis was severely hampered by lack of understanding of the actual pathophysiology and identifications of the responsible hormones. Again, it didn't make sense that sudden massive release of serotonin, the most potent vasoconstrictor known to science, would cause profound hypotension. However, we could imagine three potential mechanisms by which it, or other hormones, might. Hormones could cause pulmonary artery vasoconstriction, severely impeding cardiac output. Alternatively, they could constrict coronary vessels or directly affect heart muscle contractility resulting in cardiac failure or cardiogenic shock. Lastly, they could cause peripheral vasodilation.

To obtain data about what is actually occurring physiologically and hormonally during carcinoid crisis, we prospectively studied hemodynamic parameters and serum hormone levels during elective major operations on patients with carcinoid tumors. To increase our odds of collecting data during crises, we intentionally selected patients at higher risk for crises based on our previously identified risk factors. They included requiring liver metastases, an anticipated long anesthesia time, and older age. To avoid introducing any new variables, all patients received the same octreotide prophylaxis protocol of preoperative octreotide LAR, a preoperative 500 μg bolus of octreotide, and continuous intravenous infusion of octreotide at 500 μg/h, as used in our prior study.[19]

Forty-six patients were enrolled and had pulmonary artery catheters inserted to obtain measurements of pulmonary artery pressure, cardiac output, and systemic vascular resistance. They also had transesophageal echocardiography probes inserted to monitor cardiac function. Patients had serial measurement of serum levels of the "usual suspect" carcinoid hormones serotonin, histamine, bradykinin, and kallikrein. Complete data sets were collected prior to incision, prior to closing, and during any crises declared. We used the same criteria for declaring crises as in the previous study. The strategy of selecting patients with risk factors appeared to have worked as 16 patients experienced intraoperative hypotensive crises for a rate of 34%. During crises, pulmonary artery pressures exhibited a statistically significant reduction, ruling out pulmonary vascular vasoconstriction as the mechanism. Echocardiography during crises was normal and unchanged from pre-incision parameters, ruling out coronary vasoconstriction or cardiac failure as the mechanism. However, cardiac hypovolemia was consistently observed. Systemic vascular resistance had a statistically significant reduction during crises. Thus, the pathophysiology of hypotensive intraoperative carcinoid crisis was consistent with distributive shock.

Serum hormone levels obtained prior to incision exhibited strikingly diverse profiles; no two patient profiles were alike. Many patients had remarkably high serum hormone levels despite octreotide LAR and a preoperative octreotide bolus. Furthermore, they did not change significantly as a result of continuous high-dose intravenous octreotide infusions. The most significant finding was the mean pre-incision serum serotonin level in patients who had crises was significantly higher at 1064 ng/mL than the mean value of 453 ng/mL in patients who did not. Contrary to expectations, there were no significant changes in the mean values of any of the four hormone levels during crises. Actually, all mean values were lower than pre-incision values, but not significantly lower. We found highly significant negative linear correlations between individual pre-incision serotonin levels and the individual systemic vascular resistance values during the crisis. Because serum serotonin levels did not change significantly during crises, similar significantly negative linear correlations between individual mid-crisis serotonin levels and systemic vascular resistance during crisis were also found. Thus, the higher a patient's pre-existing serum serotonin level was, the lower their systemic vascular resistance was during a hypotensive crisis.

Conclusions drawn from this study were that there is no typical hormone profile for a carcinoid patient, and that an elevated serum serotonin level is a marker for increased risk of carcinoid crisis occurring and for the severity of the crisis when it occurs. The most important conclusion was that, contrary to long-standing popular theory, indeed dogma, there was no evidence of any sudden massive release of hormones during a crisis. We also took the strong correlations we derived between serum serotonin levels and occurrence of crisis, as well as with reductions in systemic vascular resistance, to be strong evidence that the events we were calling as hypotensive crises with our new definition were in fact crises and were not due to other possible causes of intraoperative hypotension. If they had been due to blood loss or hypovolemia, we would not have expected these correlations to be so statistically significant. Furthermore, given the diversity of hormone profiles seen among patients in this study, given that no surge of any hormones was seen, and given that we don't yet know which hormones cause flushing and urticarial and bronchospasm in carcinoid patients, it now seems unreasonable to require another manifestation of carcinoid syndrome, such as flushing, urticarial or bronchospasm to declare a crisis.

The results of this study greatly weakened the argument for efficacy of prophylactic octreotide. It also weakened the argument for octreotide as a treatment for crisis. The correct treatment for distributive shock is intravenous fluids and vasopressors, not octreotide. Given what we now know about the actual pathophysiology of crisis, it seems very unlikely that the intravenous octreotide administered to the patient in the report by Kvols et al. resulted in the immediate rise in SBP. While the patient was in distributive shock, with very little blood returning to the heart, it is likely that the intravenous octreotide if it was administered peripherally (the site was not reported, but it seems unlikely the patient would have had a central venous catheter placed for the intended procedures) would have lingered peripherally and not make it to the heart for systemic distribution for some time. By the same token, it is also now more conceivable that the epinephrine administered 3.5 minutes earlier was finally being distributed systemically and could have been responsible for the observed recovery.

We were still curious about the published reports of dramatic recovery from carcinoid crisis following administration of intravenous octreotide. Accordingly, we have made invasive physiologic observations in a few patients treated with intravenous octreotide via a central venous catheter during crises. We observed some minor increase in systemic vascular resistance and a return of some blood to the hypovolemic heart seen on echocardiography. We suspect these findings were due to the vasoconstrictor effect of octreotide on splanchnic vasculature, which is well known and why it is specifically used to treat gastrointestinal hemorrhage. Thus, it is plausible that if octreotide was given via a central venous catheter, it could have improved blood pressure in some reports simply because it is another vasopressor, but not because it blocks hormone release. However, because the correct treatment of distributive shock is intravenous fluids and vasopressors, it makes more sense to use a vasopressor with wider systemic, not just splanchnic, effects.

This presents a conundrum. Beta-adrenergic catecholamines are vasopressors with wide systemic effects that would normally be used to treat distributive shock. But it has become dogma that these agents be avoided in patients with neuroendocrine tumors because they might trigger hormone release, provoking yet another crisis, known as a secondary crisis. Instead, alpha-adrenergic vasopressors and vasopressin are recommended. The arsenal of available drugs is somewhat limited, particularly for patients in crisis not responding to vasopressin or alpha-adrenergic pressors. Accordingly, we have also examined the effects of beta-adrenergic agonists among our patients. Many doses of vasopressors have been given to treat hypotensive crises at our institution, and in some instances, we had been forced to give beta-adrenergic agonists such as ephedrine, norepinephrine, and epinephrine when patients failed to respond to other agents, such as vasopressin and phenylephrine.[43] Reviewing our data, we analyzed the hemodynamic parameters for the 15-minute period after administration of over 800 doses of pressor agents.[46] We found that patients responded just as well to beta-adrenergic agonists as to other pressors. Blood pressure recovered quickly with their administration, usually under our 10-minute time limit, which is remarkable given that they are usually withheld until 8 or 9 minutes into a crisis. Furthermore, no worsening of crisis or secondary crises were ever observed after administration of beta-adrenergic agonists. Therefore, we believe that beta-adrenergic agents should be administered when standard measures fail.

Based on our research, we modified our protocol yet again, this time to eliminate use of perioperative octreotide due to inefficacy and lack of scientific grounds. If patients experienced intraoperative crises, they would be treated for distributive shock with intravenous fluids and vasopressors, including beta-adrenergic agonists, if necessary, but no octreotide. Before recommending this to others, we thought it prudent to report data from a large prospective series using this protocol. We would need to show that neither the crisis rate nor the rate of major postoperative complications associated with them increased compared to previous studies using octreotide. Because in our previous study crises correlated only with crises lasting >10 minutes, we believed we would also need to show there was no increase in mean crisis duration compared to previous studies using octreotide. Being the mean crisis duration in the previous study was 8.9 minutes, increased duration of crisis of about a minute would lengthen them to >10 minutes and possibly increase the incidence of complications.

We reported on 195 consecutive operations with no perioperative octreotide. The incidence of crisis was 25%, which is not demonstrably increased compared to previous series using octreotide. There was no difference in the use of long-acting somatostatin analog use between patients who did and did not have crises. Crises are again correlated with clinical factors such as carcinoid syndrome, anesthesia time, and older age. In this series, they also correlated with higher blood loss and need for transfusion. Accordingly, we are willing to consider that, in this series, some hypotensive events might have been overcalled as crises when they were due to hypovolemia. However, this only means that the actual rate of crisis was lower than the 25% reported. Mean duration of crisis was dramatically shorter at 3 minutes and no crises lasted more than 10 minutes and no operations were aborted due to refractory crisis. Despite no crises lasting more than 10 minutes, their occurrence again correlated with major complications. Thus, it now appears that crisis of any duration increases risk of major postoperative complications. However, the incidence of postoperative major complications at 29% was no higher than in previous series using octreotide. Based on the results of this study, we conclude that use of perioperative octreotide may be safely discontinued due to lack of efficacy without concern it would result in increases in crisis rates, crisis duration, or incidence of major postoperative complications associated with crisis. However, because crisis of any duration is associated with increased rates of major postoperative complications, the search for an effective prophylactic agent should continue.

CONCLUSION

Here is what we currently know about carcinoid crisis. It can occur in patients spontaneously, during procedures, and especially during operations. The incidence during operations is about 25%, typically manifested by profound hypotension. It may or may not exhibit other manifestations of carcinoid syndrome, such as flushing, bronchospasm, or urticaria. Identified risk factors for crisis include liver metastases, small bowel primary tumors, carcinoid syndrome, older age, and longer anesthesia times. However, it can occur in patients without carcinoid syndrome. Intraoperative crises are associated with higher rates of major postoperative complications. Contrary to long-held belief, it is not due to sudden massive release of carcinoid hormones. However, patients who have higher serum serotonin levels are at higher risk of having crises. Also contrary to popular belief, the data are not convincing that its incidence is reduced or that it can be prevented by perioperative administration of octreotide.

Pathophysiology studies have shown that crisis is actually a form of distributive shock for which the proper treatment is intravenous fluids and vasopressors. Eliminating perioperative octreotide does not increase the incidence of crisis or the postoperative complications associated with it and results in a shorter duration of crisis. Contrary to long-held belief, beta-adrenergic pressors may be used in patients with carcinoid tumors and will not provoke a secondary crisis.

Because crisis of any duration is associated with increased risk of complications, the search for an effective prophylactic agent should be continued, but that search should be based on the available science. The only scientific clue we have is that patients who have crises have higher serum serotonin levels than patients who do not. It appears that we need a new model to explain crisis, one other than the old, unproven model that is due to sudden massive release of carcinoid hormones. Perhaps a new model might be that chronic exposure of the vascular system to high serum levels of serotonin makes it sensitive to certain perturbations that result in sudden vasodilatation and/or sudden vasospasm. It will be interesting to see if future research endeavors can find evidence that this is the case and whether medical science can develop ways to ameliorate those effects.

REFERENCES

1. Kahil ME, Brown H, Fred HL. The carcinoid crisis. *Arch Intern Med.* 1964;114:26-28.
2. Morrisroe K, Sim IW, MacLachlan K, Inder WJ. Carcinoid crisis induced by repeated abdominal examinations. *Intern Med J.* 2012;42(3):432-434.
3. Manssen M, Salm EF, Breburda CS, et al. Carcinoid crisis during transesophageal echocardiography. *Intensive Care Med.* 2000; 26(2):254.
4. Ozgen A, Demirkazik FB, Arat A, Arat AR. Carcinoid crisis provoked by mammographic compression of metastatic carcinoid tumour of the breast. *Clin Radiol.* 2001;56(3):250-251.
5. Magabe PC, Bloom AL. Sudden death from carcinoid crisis during image-guided biopsy of a lung mass. *J Vasc Interv Radiol.* 2014;25(3):484-487.
6. Fujie S, Zhou W, Fann P, Yen Y. Carcinoid crisis 24 hours after bland embolizations: a case report. *Bisoci Treds.* 2010; 4(3):143-144.
7. Kvols LK, Marin JK, Marsh HM, Moertel CG. Rapid reversal of carcinoid crisis with a somatostatin analogue. *N Engl J Med.* 1985;313(19):1229-1230.
8. Massimino K, Harrskog O, Pommier S, Pommier R. Octreotide LA and bolus octreotide are insufficient for preventing intraoperative complications in carcinoid patients. *J Surg Oncol.* 2013;107(8):842-846.
9. Kwon DH, Paciorek A, Mulvey CK, et al. Periprocedural management of patients undergoing liver resection or embolotherapy for neuroendocrine tumor metastases. *Pancreas.* 2019;48(4):496-503.
10. Wonn SM, Ratzlaff AN, Pommier SJ, McCully BH, Pommier RF. A prospective study of carcinoid crisis with no perioperative octreotide. *Surgery.* 2021;S0039-6060(21):00452-9.
11. Mason DT, Melmon KL. New understanding of the mechanism of the carcinoid flush. *Ann Intern Med.* 1966;65(6):1334-1339.
12. Oates JA, Melmon K, Sjoerdsma A, Gillespie L, Mason DT. Release of a kinin peptide in the carcinoid syndrome. *Lancet.* 1964;1(7332):514-517.
13. Goedert M, Otten U, Suda K, et al. Dopamine, norepinephrine and serotonin production by an intestinal carcinoid tumor. *Cancer.* 198;45(1):104-107.
14. Oates JA, Pettinger WA, Doctor RB. Evidence of release of bradykinin in carcinoid syndrome. *J Clin Invest.* 1966;45(2):173-178.
15. Miller R, Patel Au, Warner RR, Parnes IH. Anaesthesia for the carcinoid syndrome: a report of nine cases. *Can Anaesth Soc J.* 1978;25(3):240-244.
16. Marsh HM, Martin JK Jr, Kvols LK, et al. Carcinoid crisis during anesthesia: successful treatment with a somatostatin analogue. *Anesthesiology.* 1987;66(1):89-91.
17. Parris WC, Oates JA, Kambam J, Shmerling R, Sawyers JF. Pre-treatment with somatostatin in the anaesthetic management of a patient with carcinoid syndrome. *Can J Anaesth.* 1988;3594):413-416.
18. Kinney MA, Wanter ME, Nagorney DM, et al. Perianaesthetic risks and outcomes of abdominal surgery for metastatic carcinoid tumours. *Br J Anaesth.* 2001;87(3):447-452.
19. Condron ME, Jameson NE, Limbach KE, et al. A prospective study of the pathophysiology of carcinoid crisis. *Surgery.* 2019;165(1):158-165.
20. Thorson A, Bioreck G, Bjokman G, Waldenstrom J. Malignant carcinoid of the small intestine with metastases to the liver, valvular disease of the right heart (pulmonary stenosis and tricuspid regurgitation without septal defects), peripheral vasomotor symptoms, bronchoconstriction, and an unusual type of cyanosis: a clinical and pathologic syndrome. *Am Heart J.* 1954;47(5):795-817.
21. Pernow B, Waldenstrom J. Determination of 5-hydroxytryptamine, 5-hydroxyindole acetic acid and histamine in thirty-three cases of carcinoid tumor (argentaffinoma). *Am J Med.* 1957;23(1):16-25.
22. Robertson JI, Peart WS, Andrews TM. The mechanism of facial flushes in the carcinoid syndrome. *Q J Med.* 1962;31.
23. Levine RJ, Sjoerdsma A. Pressor amines and the carcinoid flush. *Ann Intern Med.* 1963;58:818-828.
24. Sjoerdsma A, Melmon KL. The carcinoid spectrum. *Gastroenterology.* 1964;47:104-107.

25. Jones WP. Serotonin release from carcinoid tumours. *Can Anaesth Soc J*. 1962;9:42-50.
26. Snow PJ, Lennard-Jones JE, Curzon G, Stacey RS. Humoral effects of metastasizing carcinoid tumours. *Lancet*. 1955;269(6898):1004-1009.
27. Bean WB, Funk D. The vasculo-cardiac syndrome of metastatic carcinoid. *AMA Arch Intern Med*. 1959;103(2):189-199.
28. Daugherty GW, Manger WM, Roth GM, Flock EV, Childs DS Jr., Waugh JM. Malignant carcinoid with hyperserotoninemia occurring spontaneously or induced by palpation of the tumor or by intravenous histamine: report of a case. *Proc Staff Meet Mayo Clin*. 1955;30(25):595-601.
29. Veall GR, Peacock JE, Bax ND, Reilly CS. Review of the anaesthetic management of 21 patients undergoing laparotomy for carcinoid syndrome. *Br J Anaesth*. 1994;72(3):335-341.
30. Warner RR, Mani S, Profeta J, Grunstein E. Octreotide treatment of carcinoid hypertensive crisis. *Mt Sinai J Med*. 1994;61(4):349-355.
31. Sarmiento JM, Que FG. Hepatic surgery for metastases from neuroendocrine tumors. *Surg Oncol Clin N Am*. 2003;12(1):231-242.
32. Thompson GB. *Textbook of Endocrine Surgery*. Mayo Clin Proc.
33. Phan AT, Oberg K, Choi J, et al. NANETS consensus guidelines for the diagnosis and management of neuroendocrine tumors: well differentiated neuroendocrine tumors of the thorax (includes lung and thymus). *Pancreas*. 2010;39(6):784-798.
34. Vaughan DIJ, Brunner MD. Anesthesia for patients with carcinoid syndrome. *Int Anesthesiol Clin*. 1997;35(4):129-142.
35. Boudreaux JP, Klimstra DS, Hassan MM, et al. The NANETS consensus guidelines for the diagnosis and management of neuroendocrine tumors: well differentiated neuroendocrine tumors of the jejunum, ileum, appendix, and cecum. *Pancreas*. 2010;39(6):753-766.
36. Ramage JK, Davies AH, Ardill J, et al. Guidelines for the management of gastroenteropancreatic neuroendocrine (including carcinoid) tumours. *Gut*. 2005;54(Suppl 4):iv1-v16.
37. Dierdorf SF. Carcinoid tumor and carcinoid syndrome. *Curr Opin Anaesthsiol*. 2003;16(3):343-347.
38. Quinlivan JK, Roberts WA. Intraoperative octreotide for refractory carcinoid-induced bronchospasm. *Anesth Analg*. 1994;78(2):400-402.
39. Oberg K, Kvols L, Caplin M, et al. Consensus report on the use of somatostatin analogs for the management of neuroendocrine tumors of the gastroenteropancreatic system. *Ann Oncol*. 2004;14(6):966-973.
40. Woltering EA, Wright AE, Stevens MA, et al. Development of effective prophylaxis against intraoperative carcinoid crisis. *J Clin Anesth*. 2016;32:189-193.
41. Condron ME, Pommier SJ, Pommier RF. Continuous infusion of octreotide combined with perioperative octreotide bolus does not prevent intraoperative carcinoid crisis. *Surgery*. 2016;159(1):358-365.
42. Kinney MAO, Nagorney DM, Clark DF, et al. Partial hepatic resections for metastatic neuroendocrine tumors: perioperative outcomes. *J Clin Anesth*. 2018;51:93-96.
43. Limbach KE, Condron ME, Bingham AE, Pommie SJ, Pommier RF. B-adrenergic agonist administration is not associated with secondary carcinoid crisis in patients with carcinoid tumor. *Am J Surg*. 2019;217(5):932-936.

78 Approach to the Pregnant Patient With Endocrine Disease

Jessica E. Gosnell, MD
Terrance Peng, MPH

INTRODUCTION

Pregnancy creates a state of physiologic dynamism with which the endocrine system is inexorably linked. As dramatic changes in maternal anatomy and metabolism occur, the endocrine system engages in continuous and complex recalibration to support the body's new demands. While such changes are typically nonpathological and instead representative of the natural course of pregnancy, endocrine derangements in pregnant women can be life-threatening without prompt recognition and appropriate treatment. Diseases and disorders of the endocrine system are common during pregnancy but rarely necessitate surgical intervention. It is nonetheless critical to recognize those clinical scenarios during pregnancy for which endocrine surgery is indicated and employ a multidisciplinary approach to facilitate appropriate surgical evaluation and treatment. The American College of Obstetricians and Gynecologists recently released a Committee Opinion on nonobstetric surgery during pregnancy, stating: "A pregnant woman should never be denied medically necessary surgery or have that surgery delayed regardless of trimester because this can adversely affect the pregnant woman and her fetus."[1] Thus, the objective of this chapter is to discuss common endocrine disorders that may warrant surgical intervention during pregnancy and provide an overview of the literature that guides treatment recommendations in this arena.

THYROID

MATERNAL HYPERTHYROIDISM

Essentials of Diagnosis

- Reductions in maternal serum thyroid stimulating hormone (TSH) can be normal in pregnancy, particularly in the first trimester, but concomitant inappropriately elevated total/free thyroxine (T_4) and/or triiodothyronine (T_3) are indicative of hyperthyroidism.
- Uncontrolled maternal hyperthyroidism is associated with adverse effects for both mother and fetus, including thyroid storm, maternal congestive heart failure, intrauterine growth restriction, and pregnancy loss.
- In the setting of classic signs such as diffusely enlarged goiter and proptosis, thyroid receptor antibodies (TRAb) are typically confirmatory for Graves' disease.

General Considerations

Graves' disease, an autoimmune disorder characterized by TRAb-mediated stimulation of TSH receptors, is the most common cause of hyperthyroidism in women of childbearing age and occurs in approximately 0.2% of pregnancies.[2] Left uncontrolled, thyrotoxicosis in pregnancy can have significant consequences for both maternal and fetal health.[3] The clinical presentation of hyperthyroidism in pregnancy is similar to that of nonpregnant patients, but changes to the normal reference ranges for thyroid function tests may present challenges for biochemical diagnosis. Treatment of Graves' disease in pregnancy must be approached judiciously, given the consequences of uncontrolled hyperthyroidism and risks associated with each therapeutic modality.

Prevention

All women diagnosed with Graves' disease who are of childbearing age and wish to become pregnant should receive preconception counseling. Current American Thyroid Association (ATA) guidelines indicate that patients with Graves' disease should seek to postpone pregnancy until a stable euthyroid state is achieved; this can be defined as two consecutive sets of thyroid function test results within reference ranges, provided that the tests are performed ≥1 month apart with no interim adjustments in therapy.[4] Patients with Graves' disease who are not currently pregnant but desire future pregnancy may be treated with radioactive iodine, anti-thyroid drug therapy (ADT) therapy, or thyroidectomy. If electing to receive radioactive iodine ablation, patients should undergo a pregnancy test 48 hours prior to treatment and delay conception for 6 months after treatment and until reaching a stable euthyroid state on levothyroxine.[4] If ATD therapy is chosen, patients should be counseled on the increased risk of birth defects with propylthiouracil and methimazole in early pregnancy.[4] However, patients with no prior history of Graves' disease still face a theoretical 0.05% risk of developing hyperthyroidism during pregnancy.[2] For these patients, a thorough history and physical with appropriate thyroid function testing are critical for accurate diagnosis and treatment selection. Currently, universal screening for thyroid dysfunction in pregnancy is not recommended due to a lack of proven benefit.[5]

Clinical Findings

A. Symptoms and Signs

The clinical presentation of maternal hyperthyroidism mirrors that of thyrotoxicosis in nonpregnant patients. Typical signs and symptoms include but are not limited to weight loss, hyperactivity, anxiety, tremulousness, palpitations, diarrhea, polyuria, polydipsia, excessive sweating, and heat intolerance. Stigmata of Graves' disease include diffusely enlarged goiter and ophthalmic manifestations such as proptosis, dry eyes, excessive tearing, and blurred vision. The severity of Graves' disease varies throughout pregnancy, with thyrotoxicosis typically at its worst in the first trimester.[6,7] In pregnant patients, clinical suspicion for Graves' disease should be higher in individuals who have a history of hyperthyroidism, were experiencing hyperthyroid symptoms before pregnancy, or have previously given birth to an infant with thyroid dysfunction.[6]

B. Laboratory Findings

During pregnancy, serum TSH and total T_4 concentrations vary in response to normal physiological changes such as increased thyroxine binding protein and β-hCG stimulation of thyroid receptors.[4,8,9] To aid in interpretation, current ATA guidelines recommend using trimester-specific reference ranges when available.[4] As a general estimate, upper and lower reference ranges for serum TSH concentration in weeks 7 to 12 of the first trimester can be reduced by 0.5 mU/L and 0.4 mU/L, respectively.[4] In the second and third trimesters, these thresholds gradually return to the standard reference range used for nonpregnant patients. Clinicians should also be aware of geographic and ethnic diversity in serum TSH concentrations, but population-based data to account for these variations are inconsistently available.[4] Low but detectable maternal TSH is unlikely to be clinically significant, and subclinical hyperthyroidism has not been associated with adverse outcomes in pregnancy.[10] In combination with elevated total/free T_4 and/or T_3, however, a low or undetectable TSH indicates overt hyperthyroidism. Testing for TRAbs can be useful for identifying Graves' disease as the underlying cause of thyrotoxicosis.[11]

C. Imaging Studies

Ultrasound is the mainstay imaging modality in the evaluation of Graves' disease for pregnant patients with hyperthyroidism. Findings consistent with Graves' disease include a diffusely enlarged thyroid, evidence of hypervascularity, and/or heterogeneous echotexture. For pregnant patients with hyperthyroidism, the ATA recommends that an ultrasound be performed to evaluate nodularity in those who have negative TRAb testing or suspicion for nodules on clinical exam.[4] Ultrasonography to evaluate fetal thyroid function is not routinely recommended but can be performed in select cases, such as in pregnant patients who have poorly controlled hyperthyroidism, have TRAb concentrations >3 times the upper limit of normal, exhibit persistent fetal tachycardia, or have had a previous fetus or neonate with thyroid dysfunction.[5,6] While radionuclide scintigraphy and radioiodine uptake scans are useful diagnostic tools in the evaluation of nonpregnant patients with hyperthyroidism, these methods are contraindicated in pregnancy.[4]

Differential Diagnosis

In early pregnancy, it is particularly critical to differentiate Graves' disease from gestational transient thyrotoxicosis. While both present with typical symptoms of hyperthyroidism, gestational transient thyrotoxicosis is the more likely diagnosis in the absence of a prior history of thyroid disease or hallmark signs of Graves' disease, such as diffusely enlarged goiter or orbitopathy. Ultrasound has not been shown to be useful in differentiating the two conditions.[4] Gestational transient thyrotoxicosis is diagnosed in 1% to 5% of pregnancies and typically resolves by weeks 14 to 18 of gestation; it occurs secondary to elevated β-hCG and has a strong association with hyperemesis gravidarum.[12] ATD therapy should not be used in gestational transient thyrotoxicosis, given the absence of proven therapeutic benefits and increased risk of birth defects.[4] Instead, treatment of this self-limited condition consists of supportive therapy and short-term use of β-adrenergic blocking agents, if required for symptomatic management. Thus, exclusion of gestational transient thyrotoxicosis in a pregnant patient with hyperthyroidism is imperative to avoid inappropriate use of ATDs.

Additional considerations in the differential diagnosis for maternal hyperthyroidism during pregnancy include toxic adenoma, toxic multinodular goiter, and factitious intake of thyroid hormone.[4] Thyroiditis during pregnancy may also cause a thyrotoxic state secondary to the release of preformed thyroid hormone. Other rare causes of maternal hyperthyroidism include TSH-secreting pituitary adenoma and struma ovarii, a rare ovarian tumor composed of thyroid tissue.[13,14]

Complications

Poorly controlled hyperthyroidism can lead to severe maternal and fetal adverse outcomes, including thyroid storm, maternal congestive heart failure, intrauterine growth restriction, and pregnancy loss.[3,6] Pregnant women with uncontrolled Graves' disease face a significantly greater risk of developing severe preeclampsia, undergoing preterm delivery, and having a neonate with low birth weight.[3,6] The risk of low birth weight decreases when maternal Graves' disease is controlled but nonetheless remains elevated compared to pregnant patients without Graves' disease.[6] Maternal thyroid hormone and TRAbs cross the placental barrier and increase the risk of fetal and neonatal hyperthyroidism if persistently elevated.[4,15,16] In addition, fetal exposure to excessive maternal thyroid hormone increases the risk for developing epilepsy and attention-deficit/hyperactivity disorder during childhood.[17]

Treatment

Although radioactive iodine ablation can be used for Graves' disease in nonpregnant patients, this modality is strictly contraindicated in pregnancy. ATDs (including propylthiouracil, methimazole, and carbimazole) are the standard treatment for Graves' disease during pregnancy but should be used with caution, given the increased risk for birth defects and liver failure.[4,6] In general, pregnant women should seek to avoid ATD therapy in the first trimester; if necessary during this period, propylthiouracil is preferred over methimazole as it is associated with a less severe teratogenic profile.[4] After the first trimester, however, methimazole should be favored to avoid the greater risk of maternal hepatotoxicity with propylthiouracil. These differences are summarized in Table 78–1. Transient leukopenia is observed in 10% of pregnant patients receiving ATDs and requires no change in therapy, but providers should be aware of agranulocytosis as an additional severe, albeit rare, side effect.[5,18] Pregnant patients previously diagnosed with Graves' disease who appears to be in remission may choose to withdraw ATD therapy and undergo serial thyroid function testing during the first trimester, but certain risk factors (eg, <6 months of ATD therapy, elevated TRAb, orbitopathy) are associated with an increased likelihood of rapid relapse.[4,19]

Current ATA guidelines outline the following ranges for initial ATD dosing and recommend adjustments based on the severity of thyrotoxicosis and associated symptoms: propylthiouracil, 100 to 600 mg/day; methimazole, 5 to 30 mg/day; carbimazole, 10 to 40 mg/day.[4] As a general principle, the lowest dosages of ATDs should be used whenever feasible. ATDs exert a stronger effect on the fetal thyroid than

Table 78–1. Comparison of propylthiouracil and methimazole for treatment of maternal hyperthyroidism.

	Propylthiouracil	Methimazole
Initial Dosing	• 100-600 mg/day	• 5-30 mg/day
Considerations	• Greater risk of maternal hepatotoxicity • Less severe teratogenic profile	• Lower risk of maternal hepatotoxicity • More severe teratogenic profile
Timing	• Favored over MMI during first trimester	• Favored over PTU after first trimester

MMI, methimazole; PTU, propylthiouracil.
Source: Recommendations summarized from the 2017 Guidelines of the American Thyroid Association for the Diagnosis and Management of Thyroid Disease During Pregnancy and the Postpartum.[4]

the maternal thyroid and can lead to fetal goiter, fetal hypothyroidism, and elevated neonatal serum TSH; thus, overtreatment carries significant risks.[20,21] During pregnancy, maternal total/free T_4 and TSH should be measured every 2 to 4 weeks after initiation of ATD therapy.[8,20,21] Testing frequency can be liberalized to every 4 to 6 weeks after serum total/free T_4 and TSH reach target ranges. Symptomatic control with β-adrenergic blocking agents may be helpful for patients who have not achieved a euthyroid state but should not be used for long-term therapy in pregnancy.[4,22]

Thyroidectomy should be considered for pregnant patients with Graves' disease in the context of refractory disease on high doses of ATDs; allergies and/or contraindications to ATDs; noncompliance with ATD therapy; or very large goiter.[4,6] If surgical intervention is chosen, thyroidectomy is optimally performed in the second trimester. Preoperative potassium iodide solution and β-adrenergic blocking agents are recommended for patients with poor response to ATDs.[4,23] After thyroidectomy, treatment with levothyroxine should be initiated on postoperative day 1 using a weight-based dosing estimate (0.8 μg/lb or 1.7 μg/kg). Many patients with Graves' disease have at least temporary hypocalcemia after thyroidectomy, given their hyperthyroidism, high bone turnover, and intraoperative trauma to parathyroid glands.[24] Elevated maternal TRAb concentrations remain prognostic for fetal hyperthyroidism even postthyroidectomy and, therefore, warrant continued monitoring of fetal thyroid function throughout pregnancy.[25] The major risks and benefits of ATD and thyroidectomy are summarized in Figure 78–1.

Prognosis

Approximately 9% of pregnant women with uncontrolled hyperthyroidism are diagnosed with heart failure and pulmonary hypertension secondary to thyrotoxicosis.[26] While

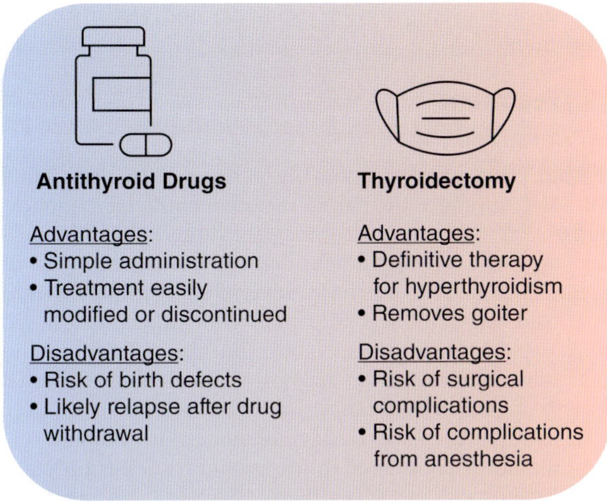

▲ **Figure 78–1.** Associated advantages and disadvantages of antithyroid drug and thyroidectomy.

its incidence in pregnancy is not well defined, thyroid storm is a life-threatening complication of uncontrolled Graves' disease associated with a significantly increased risk for maternal congestive heart failure.[6,26] Fetal and/or neonatal hyperthyroidism occurs in 1% to 5% of pregnancies in women with active Graves' disease or prior diagnosis of Graves' disease.[6,27]

When to Refer or Admit

Endocrine surgery referral for thyroidectomy is warranted for pregnant patients with refractory thyrotoxicosis despite high doses of ATDs, allergies, and/or contraindications to ATDs or large goiter with compression. Inpatient admission is required for thyroid storm, a life-threatening medical emergency characterized by severe thyrotoxicosis with decompensation of organ function. Without treatment, preferably in the ICU setting, thyroid storm can rapidly progress to multiorgan failure.[6] Specific treatment strategies vary based on the affected organ systems but generally include ATD therapy, β-adrenergic blocking agents, and supportive measures.

THYROID NODULES & CANCER

Essentials of Diagnosis

- Thyroid nodules are very common, typically benign, and often discovered incidentally without associated symptoms.
- Thyroid nodules with concerning ultrasonographic features may require fine needle aspiration biopsy to evaluate for malignancy.
- In the setting of low serum TSH and symptoms of hyperthyroidism, a thyroid nodule may be a toxic adenoma.

General Considerations

Among pregnant women, thyroid nodules have a prevalence of 3% to 21% and are more common with older age and higher gravidity.[28,29] Pregnancy has been associated both with the formation of new thyroid nodules and with the growth of preexisting nodules.[28] The estimated prevalence of thyroid cancer in pregnancy per California Cancer Registry data (1991-1999) is 14.4 cases per 100,000, with 3.3 cases per 100,000 being diagnosed before delivery and 10.8 cases per 100,000 being diagnosed within 1 year postpartum.[30] Similar to the general population, papillary thyroid cancer is the most common pathological type diagnosed in pregnant women.[30]

Prevention

The risk of thyroid cancer increases with older age, family history of thyroid cancer, and history of exposure to ionizing radiation.[31,32] There are no specific recommendations for reducing the risk of thyroid cancer in pregnant women. While radiation exposure is a modifiable factor for which avoidance can reduce the risk of thyroid cancer, this may be impossible in patients who require radiotherapy for head and neck or breast cancer. Special screening for patients with familial follicular cell-derived differentiated thyroid cancer may lead to earlier detection but is not recommended under current ATA guidelines.[32] Additionally, there is no data to characterize the impact of pregnancy on the progression of residual or metastatic medullary thyroid cancer.[4]

Clinical Findings

A. Symptoms and Signs

Most thyroid nodules cause no symptoms and are generally found incidentally on physical exam or ultrasonography. However, nodules may grow large enough to cause compressive symptoms, including dysphagia, dyspnea, voice changes, or a sense of neck fullness. In the case of a hyperfunctioning thyroid nodule, the patient may report symptoms of hyperthyroidism, such as weight loss, tremulousness, or tachycardia. Thyroid nodules can be palpable and/or grossly visible on physical exam but may be detected only on ultrasound, depending on size and location.

B. Laboratory Findings

Serum TSH should be measured in all women presenting with a thyroid nodule, regardless of pregnancy status.[4] Thyroid cancer is typically associated with normal thyroid function tests, whereas a thyroid nodule in the setting of suppressed TSH is more suggestive of a toxic adenoma.[4] Interpretation of thyroid function tests may be challenging due to normal fluctuations in serum TSH throughout pregnancy. At present, routine measurements of calcitonin and thyroglobulin are not recommended in the evaluation of pregnant patients presenting with a thyroid nodule.[4]

C. Imaging Studies

As in the nonpregnant patient, ultrasound is the recommended imaging modality during pregnancy for the detection and evaluation of thyroid nodules and assessment of cervical lymph nodes.[4,32] Sonographic features associated with malignancy include solid composition, hypoechogenicity, irregular margins or extrathyroidal extension, microcalcifications, and taller than wide shape.[32,33] In estimating the risk of malignancy, these features should be interpreted in combination rather than in isolation.[34,35] The risk profile associated with the sonographic appearance of the thyroid nodule can be used to inform decisions regarding biopsy, as discussed later.

D. Special Tests

Fine-needle aspiration biopsy with or without molecular testing may be indicated for evaluation of thyroid nodules that demonstrate sonographic features concerning malignancy. Decision-making regarding fine-needle aspiration biopsies should be informed using the 2015 ATA guidelines and/or the 2017 American College of Radiology (ACR) Thyroid Imaging, Reporting, and Data System (TI-RADS), which have demonstrated similar accuracy with respect to predicting malignancy.[32,33,36] Radionuclide scintigraphy may be helpful for identifying toxic adenomas in non-pregnant patients but is contraindicated during pregnancy.[4] Genetic counseling with discussion of preimplantation or prenatal testing should be considered for pregnant women with a known *RET* mutation.[4]

Differential Diagnosis

In pregnant and nonpregnant patients, the overwhelming majority of solitary thyroid nodules are benign lesions.[31] However, it is critical to differentiate benign nodules from thyroid cancers and toxic adenomas. Ultrasonography and fine-needle aspiration biopsy are used to evaluate the risk for malignancy.[32-34] Low serum TSH alongside signs and symptoms of hyperthyroidism would be more suggestive of a hyperfunctioning thyroid nodule.

Complications

Thyroid nodules typically pose low risk to both pregnant and nonpregnant patients, and many thyroid cancers can be treated effectively with minimal adverse impact on survival.[4,32] However, a rapidly enlarging thyroid nodule may cause significant compressive symptoms, such as dysphagia, dyspnea, or voice change. Although differentiated thyroid cancer generally progresses slowly, anaplastic thyroid cancer and medullary thyroid cancer behave more aggressively with greater propensity for metastasis and worse survival outcomes.[37,38]

Treatment

Surgery remains the standard treatment for differentiated thyroid cancer and is optimally performed in the second trimester to reduce the risk of maternal and fetal complications.[4,5,32,39,40] However, deferment of surgery for differentiated thyroid cancer until after delivery has not been found to influence survival outcomes adversely.[41-43] Surgery should be considered in the second trimester for women diagnosed with papillary thyroid carcinoma during pregnancy who have advanced disease at diagnosis, experience substantial growth of their thyroid cancer by 24 weeks gestation, or have metastatic disease to cervical lymph nodes.[4] In addition, surgery should be considered in the second trimester for pregnant patients with medullary thyroid carcinoma or anaplastic carcinoma.[4] Although tyrosine kinase inhibitor agents have been FDA-approved for the treatment of metastatic differentiated thyroid cancer and medullary thyroid cancer, these have shown teratogenicity and embryotoxicity in animal studies.[4] Pregnant patients with cytologically proven benign thyroid nodules can defer surgery until after delivery and do not require pregnancy-specific surveillance.[4,32]

Prognosis

Large database studies have identified no differences in overall and disease-free survival between pregnant patients and nonpregnant patients with differentiated thyroid cancer.[41-43] However, other studies have suggested that patients diagnosed with differentiated thyroid cancer during pregnancy or within 1 to 2 years postpartum may face higher rates of disease persistence or recurrence after definitive therapy.[44,45] It is unknown whether survival outcomes differ between pregnant and nonpregnant patients with medullary thyroid carcinoma or anaplastic thyroid carcinoma.[4]

When to Refer or Admit

A referral to endocrine surgery is warranted for the pregnant patient presenting with a thyroid nodule causing compressive symptoms, thyroid cancer, or a toxic adenoma in the context of hyperthyroidism refractory to medical management. In general, thyroid nodules are highly unlikely to warrant inpatient admission.

PARATHYROID

Essentials of Diagnosis

- Primary hyperparathyroidism (PHPT) is characterized by hypercalcemia with an inappropriately normal or elevated serum parathyroid hormone (PTH) level.

- Physiologic elevations in PTH-related protein (PTHrP) during pregnancy can partially suppress serum PTH levels, which may cloud the diagnosis of PHPT in pregnant patients.
- PHPT is typically the result of a solitary parathyroid adenoma, but localization of such a lesion is not required for diagnosis.

General Considerations

The prevalence of PHPT is an estimated 0.05% among women of reproductive age.[46] This condition is characterized by hypercalcemia alongside an inappropriately normal or elevated serum PTH and most commonly occurs due to a solitary parathyroid adenoma. With pregnant patients representing a generally younger age group, an underlying genetic mutation may be present in >10% of cases of PHPT in this population.[47]

Prevention

Given that PHPT typically occurs secondary to a sporadic parathyroid adenoma, there are no specific measures that should be taken to prevent this condition in the pregnant patient. However, early recognition of PHPT is critical for reducing the risk of adverse maternal and fetal/neonatal health outcomes.[48] Careful monitoring of serum calcium levels should be considered for patients who are pregnant or wish to become pregnant and who have a strong family history of PHPT or confirmed genetic mutation associated with PHPT.

Clinical Findings

A. Symptoms and Signs

Classic signs and symptoms of hypercalcemia in PHPT include nephrolithiasis, osteoporosis, abdominal or epigastric pain, hypertension, depression, and memory problems. Other manifestations of PHPT, such as lethargy, polyuria, and hyperemesis gravidarum, may be conflated with common changes in pregnancy. Pregnant patients with PHPT occurring as part of a syndrome may also present with relevant stigmata, including lesions of the pituitary gland, pancreas, adrenal gland, or mandible. However, approximately 80% of pregnant patients with a biochemical diagnosis of PHPT are asymptomatic at presentation.[47]

B. Laboratory Findings

The diagnosis of PHPT is made on a biochemical basis and is characterized by an elevated serum ionized calcium or serum calcium corrected for albumin in the setting of an inappropriately normal or elevated serum PTH. A 24-hour urine collection for calcium and creatinine should be performed for the purposes of distinguishing PHPT from familial hypocalciuric hypercalcemia (FHH); the calcium to creatinine clearance ratio (CCCR) is expected to be >0.02 in PHPT and <0.01 in FHH.[49] It should also be noted that pregnancy is associated with absorptive hypercalciuria, which would ostensibly lend greater diagnostic value to a low CCCR.[50] When evaluating pregnant patients with hypercalcemia, it is also critical to consider that physiologic elevations in PTHrP during pregnancy can partially suppress serum PTH levels.[51,52] Thus, pregnant patients with PHPT may be more likely to present with hypercalcemia alongside a nonsuppressed, rather than overtly elevated, serum PTH. Table 78–2 lists special considerations in the laboratory evaluation of PHPT during pregnancy.

C. Imaging Studies

Ultrasound imaging is the mainstay modality for localization of a parathyroid adenoma in the pregnant patient with PHPT. While X-ray and computed tomography (CT) with 99mTc Sestamibi and four-dimensional CT are useful in the nonpregnant population, these modalities should be avoided in pregnancy to reduce the risk of adverse fetal outcomes associated with radiation exposure.[53] Magnetic resonance imaging (MRI) without gadolinium can be considered as an adjunct imaging technique for localization, though this technique demonstrates limited sensitivity.[54] Special considerations for imaging in pregnant patients with PHPT are listed in Table 78–2.

D. Special Tests

Genetic mutation testing should be considered in pregnant patients with PHPT who present with or have relatives exhibiting stigmata of syndromes such as MEN1, MEN2A, MEN4, or hyperparathyroidism-jaw tumor syndrome. While

Table 78–2. Considerations in the evaluation of primary hyperparathyroidism during pregnancy.

	Measurement/ Modality	Considerations
Laboratory	Serum PTH	PTH suppressed due to elevations in PTHrP
	CCCR	Absorptive hypercalciuria
Imaging	99mTc Sestamibi X-ray SPECT 4D CT DEXA scan	Not recommended due to radiation exposure

4D CT, four-dimensional computed tomography; 99mTc, Technetium 99m; CCCR, calcium to creatinine clearance ratio; DEXA, dual-energy X-ray absorptiometry; PTH, parathyroid hormone; PTHrP, parathyroid hormone-related protein; SPECT, single proton emission computed tomography.

dual-energy X-ray absorptiometry (DEXA) scans are often performed in the assessment of PHPT in the general population, this modality should be avoided in pregnant patients.[53]

Differential Diagnosis

In evaluating pregnant patients presenting with hypercalcemia and nonsuppressed PTH, it is critical to first exclude FHH via calculation of the CCCR. Other potential causes of hypercalcemia, such as malignancy, granulomatous disease, or adrenal insufficiency, would likely present with a suppressed PTH but can be considered in the differential diagnosis.[55] PHPT due to a solitary adenoma should also be distinguished from parathyroid hyperplasia and parathyroid carcinoma, both of which occur far less frequently.[47]

Complications

PHPT during pregnancy poses significant risks to maternal and fetal health. Maternal complications of PHPT may include nephrolithiasis, acute pancreatitis, preeclampsia, and hyperemesis gravidarum, whereas fetal and neonatal consequences include intrauterine growth restriction, fetal demise, as well as neonatal hypocalcemia, seizure, and tetany.[56-60] Postpartum maternal hypercalcemic crisis has also been reported and postulated as occurring secondary to the cessation of transplacental transfer of calcium after delivery.[61]

Treatment

Treatment planning for PHPT during pregnancy should be individualized and consider the patient's full clinical picture, including symptom severity, degree of hypercalcemia, and gestational age at diagnosis. Parathyroidectomy with intraoperative PTH monitoring remains the definitive treatment for PHPT and is optimally pursued in the second trimester.[1,62,63] Nonsurgical options such as cinacalcet and calcitonin have limited data to demonstrate efficacy or safety in pregnancy.[47,64] Furthermore, medical management of PHPT in pregnancy has been associated with an increased risk of pregnancy loss and preeclampsia.[59,60] Bisphosphonates and denosumab are not recommended during pregnancy due to increased risk of fetal skeletal defects.[65,66]

Prognosis

Outcomes are typically favorable for pregnant patients with PHPT who are treated with parathyroidectomy.[47,58] In contrast, fetal mortality rates appear to be substantially higher in pregnant patients with PHPT who are managed medically (16%) relative to those treated surgically (3%).[67] It should be further noted that the comparatively poorer outcomes of PHPT in pregnancy reported in older literature are thought to be partially attributable to previously limited awareness and, consequently, delayed diagnoses.[47]

When to Refer or Admit

An endocrine surgery referral is warranted for all pregnant patients with PHPT, as parathyroidectomy remains the definitive treatment for this condition. Critically, pregnant patients with PHPT should still be referred to endocrine surgery even when imaging studies are nonlocalizing for a parathyroid adenoma. Ultimately, however, deferral of surgical intervention until after delivery may be considered for patients who are asymptomatic and have only mild hypercalcemia. Pregnant patients with PHPT who develop complications such as acute pancreatitis and severe preeclampsia may require inpatient admission. Similarly, inpatient management is warranted for patients who experience hypercalcemic crisis in the postpartum period.

ADRENAL

Essentials of Diagnosis

- Pheochromocytomas are catecholamine-releasing tumors with potentially life-threatening consequences.
- Patients with pheochromocytoma present with paroxysmal symptoms of catecholamine excess, including hypertension, diaphoresis, headache, and arrhythmias.
- A biochemical diagnosis of pheochromocytoma can be made by measuring plasma fractionated metanephrines and 24-hour urinary fractionated metanephrines and catecholamines.

General Considerations

While exceptionally rare among pregnant patients, pheochromocytomas may have life-threatening consequences and necessitate early detection and appropriate treatment. Pheochromocytomas and paragangliomas have a combined estimated prevalence during pregnancy between 1/15,000 and 1/54,000, with the majority being diagnosed during the third trimester or after delivery.[68-72] Nearly 50% of pheochromocytomas and paragangliomas occur in the setting of an inherited pathogenic variant.[73,74]

Prevention

Women with a family history of pheochromocytoma or a known inherited pathogenic mutation associated with pheochromocytoma who wish to become pregnant should undergo preconception biochemical evaluation and cross-sectional imaging. If a pheochromocytoma is discovered, surgical resection should be performed prior to attempting conception. However, patients with metastatic pheochromocytoma, which is associated with an indolent course and comparatively low levels of catecholamines, can conceive with the expectation of favorable pregnancy outcomes.[72]

Clinical Findings

A. Symptoms and Signs

Pregnant patients with pheochromocytomas present with paroxysmal symptoms of catecholamine excess, including hypertension, diaphoresis, arrhythmias, and headaches. Relative to preeclampsia, pheochromocytoma is less commonly associated with signs of end-organ damage.[75]

B. Laboratory Findings

Biochemical testing for pheochromocytoma includes measurement of plasma fractionated metanephrines and/or 24-hour urine fractionated metanephrines and catecholamines.[76] It should be noted that a normal, transient physiologic elevation may occur in urinary epinephrine and norepinephrine levels at the time of delivery, persisting for multiple days.[77]

C. Imaging Studies

During the first trimester, ultrasound may be a feasible imaging modality for identifying pheochromocytoma.[75] MRI without gadolinium is likely to provide greater visualization and should be preferred in the second and third trimester. Due to the risk to fetal health, other methods commonly used in the evaluation of pheochromocytoma, such as CT and metaiodobenzylguanidine scintigraphy, should be avoided.[53,75]

D. Special Tests

Genetic testing may be considered in pregnant patients with a family history of MEN2A, MEN2B, Von-Hippel-Lindau syndrome, or other inherited syndromes associated with pheochromocytoma. Similarly, pregnant patients who are diagnosed with pheochromocytoma without a known inherited pathogenic variant should be offered genetic testing. Mutations associated with pheochromocytoma include *RET*, *VHL*, *MAX*, and various mutations in succinate dehydrogenase subunits (SDH).[75,78]

Differential Diagnosis

Hypertension secondary to pheochromocytoma during pregnancy should be differentiated from gestational hypertension, which typically presents after 20-weeks' gestation.[75,79] Pheochromocytomas should also be distinguished from other lesions of the adrenal gland (eg, cortisol-secreting adrenal adenoma, aldosteronoma, adrenal carcinoma) and paragangliomas, which also secrete catecholamines but arise from sympathetic paraganglia.

Complications

Catecholamine release from pheochromocytomas can lead to significant adverse maternal and fetal health outcomes. These include maternal cardiac arrest, acute heart failure, and stroke, as well as fetal hypoxia or demise.[72] Other severe complications include hypertensive crisis and flash pulmonary edema. Providers should be aware that pregnant patients with pheochromocytoma are also at increased risk for acute catecholamine surge during delivery.[80]

Treatment

Medical therapy with α-adrenergic blockade (eg, doxazosin, phenoxybenzamine) is the mainstay intervention for pheochromocytoma during pregnancy, and treatment initiation at the time of diagnosis is preferred.[72,75] When administered for at least 2 weeks, α-adrenergic blockade reduces the risk of adverse maternal and fetal health outcomes.[72] The β-adrenergic blockade, preferably with cardioselective β-1 blockers (eg, metoprolol succinate), should not be initiated until the patient has received α-adrenergic blockade for ≥7 days.[75] Of note, atenolol, propranolol, and labetalol are not recommended for the treatment of pheochromocytoma during pregnancy.[75,81,82] Dihydropyridine calcium channel blockers (eg, nifedipine, amlodipine) do not directly address catecholamine excess but may be considered for pheochromocytoma during pregnancy in patients who have refractory hypertension despite α-adrenergic and β-adrenergic blockade.[75] Specific medication and dosing recommendations are summarized in Table 78–3.[75]

Table 78–3. Medical therapy for pheochromocytoma during pregnancy.

	Doxazosin	Phenoxybenzamine	Metoprolol Succinate
Class	• Selective α-1 adrenergic blocker	• Irreversible, nonselective α-adrenergic blocker	• Selective β-1 adrenergic blocker
Initial Dosing	• 1 mg QHS	• 10 mg QDay	• 25 mg QDay
Adjustments	• Advance to 1 mg QDay vs BID • Advance by 1 mg each day to goal blood pressure	• Advance by 10 mg every 1-2 days to goal blood pressure	• Advance by 25 mg every 1-2 days to goal heart rate

Source: Recommendations summarized from Gruber and colleagues.[75]

Patients who undergo surgery for pheochromocytoma during pregnancy do not experience improved outcomes compared to those who defer surgery until after delivery.[72] However, surgery should be considered during pregnancy for patients unable to adhere to medical therapy or those with refractory hypertension on maximal doses of α-adrenergic blockade.[75] If surgical intervention is ultimately pursued during pregnancy, it is optimally performed in the second trimester.[1,83]

Prognosis

Pregnant patients with untreated pheochromocytoma or paraganglioma experience a 27-fold increased risk of adverse maternal or fetal health outcomes.[72] In addition, there is a 42-fold increased risk of maternal mortality and 2.6-fold increased risk of fetal/neonatal mortality among pregnant patients who are diagnosed with pheochromocytoma or paraganglioma after delivery or at autopsy relative to those diagnosed before delivery.[84] Compared to sporadic cases, inherited pheochromocytomas are associated with fewer adverse outcomes during pregnancy.[72] Metastatic pheochromocytoma is typically associated with a more indolent course and does not appear to confer worse outcomes during pregnancy for maternal or fetal health.[72,85]

When to Refer or Admit

Although medical therapy with α-adrenergic blockage is the mainstay treatment for pheochromocytoma during pregnancy, an endocrine surgery referral is warranted for all patients at diagnosis for the purposes of surgical planning. A pregnant patient with pheochromocytoma may require inpatient management for severe complications such as flash pulmonary edema, acute myocardial infarction, or hypertensive crisis.

REFERENCES

1. ACOG Committee Opinion No. 775 Summary: Nonobstetric Surgery During Pregnancy. *Obstet Gynecol.* 2019;133(4): 844-845.
2. Cooper DS, Laurberg P. Hyperthyroidism in pregnancy. *Lancet Diabetes Endocrinol.* 2013;1(3):238-249.
3. Millar LK, Wing DA, Leung AS, Koonings PP, Montoro MN, Mestman JH. Low birth weight and preeclampsia in pregnancies complicated by hyperthyroidism. *Obstet Gynecol.* 1994;84(6):946-949.
4. Alexander EK, Pearce EN, Brent GA, et al. 2017 Guidelines of the American Thyroid Association for the Diagnosis and Management of Thyroid Disease During Pregnancy and the Postpartum. *Thyroid.* 2017;27(3):315-389.
5. Thyroid Disease in Pregnancy: ACOG Practice Bulletin, Number 223. *Obstetrics & Gynecology.* 2020;135(6).
6. Nguyen CT, Sasso EB, Barton L, Mestman JH. Graves' hyperthyroidism in pregnancy: a clinical review. *Clin Diabetes Endocrinol.* 2018;4(1):4.
7. Andersen SL, Olsen J, Carlé A, Laurberg P. Hyperthyroidism incidence fluctuates widely in and around pregnancy and is at variance with some other autoimmune diseases: a Danish population-based study. *J Clin Endocrinol Metab.* 2015;100(3):1164-1171.
8. Glinoer D, Spencer CA. Serum TSH determinations in pregnancy: how, when and why? *Nat Rev Endocrinol.* 2010;9: 526-529.
9. Lambert-Messerlian G, McClain M, Haddow JE, et al. First- and second-trimester thyroid hormone reference data in pregnant women: a FaSTER (First- and Second-Trimester Evaluation of Risk for aneuploidy) Research Consortium study. *Am J Obstet Gynecol.* 2008;199(1):62. e1-6.
10. Casey BM, Dashe JS, Wells CE, McIntire DD, Leveno KJ, Cunningham FG. Subclinical hyperthyroidism and pregnancy outcomes. *Obstet Gynecol.* 2006;107(2 Pt 1):337-341.
11. Bell L, Hunter AL, Kyriacou A, Mukherjee A, Syed AA. Clinical diagnosis of Graves' or non-Graves' hyperthyroidism compared to TSH receptor antibody test. *Endocrine Connections.* 2018;7(4):504-510.
12. Goldman AM, Mestman JH. Transient non-autoimmune hyperthyroidism of early pregnancy. *J Thyroid Res.* 2011; 2011:142413.
13. Merza Z, White D, Khanem N. Struma ovarii in pregnancy: an uncommon cause of hyperthyroidism. *Clin Nucl Med.* 2015; 40(8):687-688.
14. Bolz M, Körber S, Schober HC. [TSH secreting adenoma of pituitary gland (TSHom) - rare cause of hyperthyroidism in pregnancy]. TSH-sezernierendes Hypophysenadenom (TSHom) - seltene Ursache einer Hyperthyreose in der Schwangerschaft. *Dtsch Med Wochenschr.* 2013;138(8):362-366.
15. Abeillon-du Payrat J, Chikh K, Bossard N, et al. Predictive value of maternal second-generation thyroid-binding inhibitory immunoglobulin assay for neonatal autoimmune hyperthyroidism. *Eur J Endocrinol.* 2014;171(4):451-460.
16. Donnelly MA, Wood C, Casey B, Hobbins J, Barbour LA. Early severe fetal Graves disease in a mother after thyroid ablation and thyroidectomy. *Obstet Gynecol.* 2015;125(5):1059-1062.
17. Andersen SL, Olsen J, Laurberg P. Foetal programming by maternal thyroid disease. *Clin Endocrinol (Oxf).* 2015;83(6):751-758.
18. Watanabe N, Narimatsu H, Noh JY, et al. Antithyroid drug-induced hematopoietic damage: a retrospective cohort study of agranulocytosis and pancytopenia involving 50,385 patients with Graves' disease. *J Clin Endocrinol Metab.* 2012;97(1): E49-E53.
19. Laurberg P, Krejbjerg A, Andersen SL. Relapse following antithyroid drug therapy for Graves' hyperthyroidism. *Curr Opin Endocrinol Diabetes Obes.* 2014;21(5):415-421.
20. Momotani N, Noh J, Oyanagi H, Ishikawa N, Ito K. Antithyroid drug therapy for Graves' disease during pregnancy. Optimal regimen for fetal thyroid status. *N Engl J Med.* 1986; 315(1):24-28.
21. Patil-Sisodia K, Mestman JH. Graves hyperthyroidism and pregnancy: a clinical update. *Endocr Pract.* 2010;16(1):118-129.
22. Rubin PC. Current concepts: beta-blockers in pregnancy. *N Engl J Med.* 1981;305(22):1323-1326.
23. Momotani N, Hisaoka T, Noh J, Ishikawa N, Ito K. Effects of iodine on thyroid status of fetus versus mother in treatment of Graves' disease complicated by pregnancy. *J Clin Endocrinol Metab.* 1992;75(3):738-744.
24. Lebrun B, De Block C, Jacquemyn Y. Hypocalcemia after thyroidectomy and parathyroidectomy in a pregnant woman. *Endocrinol.* 2020;161(7).

25. Laurberg P, Bournaud C, Karmisholt J, Orgiazzi J. Management of Graves' hyperthyroidism in pregnancy: focus on both maternal and foetal thyroid function, and caution against surgical thyroidectomy in pregnancy. *Eur J Endocrinol*. 2009;160(1):1-8.
26. Sheffield JS, Cunningham FG. Thyrotoxicosis and heart failure that complicate pregnancy. *Am J Obstet Gynecol*. 2004;190(1):211-217.
27. Zimmerman D. Fetal and neonatal hyperthyroidism. *Thyroid*. 1999;9(7):727-733.
28. Kung AW, Chau MT, Lao TT, Tam SC, Low LC. The effect of pregnancy on thyroid nodule formation. *J Clin Endocrinol Metab*. 2002;87(3):1010-1014.
29. Struve CW, Haupt S, Ohlen S. Influence of frequency of previous pregnancies on the prevalence of thyroid nodules in women without clinical evidence of thyroid disease. *Thyroid*. 1993;3(1):7-9.
30. Smith LH, Danielsen B, Allen ME, Cress R. Cancer associated with obstetric delivery: results of linkage with the California cancer registry. *Am J Obstet Gynecol*. 2003;189(4):1128-1135.
31. Hegedüs L. Clinical practice. The thyroid nodule. *N Engl J Med*. 2004;351(17):1764-1771.
32. Haugen BR, Alexander EK, Bible KC, et al. 2015 American Thyroid Association Management Guidelines for Adult Patients with Thyroid Nodules and Differentiated Thyroid Cancer: The American Thyroid Association Guidelines Task Force on Thyroid Nodules and Differentiated Thyroid Cancer. *Thyroid*. 2016;26(1):1-133.
33. Tessler FN, Middleton WD, Grant EG, et al. ACR Thyroid Imaging, Reporting and Data System (TI-RADS): White Paper of the ACR TI-RADS Committee. *J Am Coll Radiol*. 2017;14(5):587-595.
34. Horvath E, Majlis S, Rossi R, et al. An ultrasonogram reporting system for thyroid nodules stratifying cancer risk for clinical management. *J Clin Endocrinol Metab*. 2009;94(5):1748-1751.
35. Russ G, Royer B, Bigorgne C, Rouxel A, Bienvenu-Perrard M, Leenhardt L. Prospective evaluation of thyroid imaging reporting and data system on 4550 nodules with and without elastography. *Eur J Endocrinol*. 2013;168(5):649-655.
36. Liu J, Guo Y, Xiao J, Chen L, Liang Z. Comparison of the Efficacy and Safety of the American Thyroid Association Guidelines and American College of Radiology TI-RADS. *Endocr Pract*. 2021;27(7):661-667.
37. Bible KC, Kebebew E, Brierley J, et al. 2021 American Thyroid Association Guidelines for Management of Patients with Anaplastic Thyroid Cancer. *Thyroid*. 2021;31(3):337-386.
38. Wells SA Jr, Asa SL, Dralle H, et al. Revised American Thyroid Association guidelines for the management of medullary thyroid carcinoma. *Thyroid*. 2015;25(6):567-610.
39. Mestman JH, Goodwin TM, Montoro MM. Thyroid disorders of pregnancy. *Endocrinol Metab Clin North Am*. 1995;24(1):41-71.
40. Uruno T, Shibuya H, Kitagawa W, Nagahama M, Sugino K, Ito K. Optimal timing of surgery for differentiated thyroid cancer in pregnant women. *World J Surg*. 2014;38(3):704-708.
41. Herzon FS, Morris DM, Segal MN, Rauch G, Parnell T. Coexistent thyroid cancer and pregnancy. *Arch Otolaryngol Head Neck Surg*. 1994;120(11):1191-1193.
42. Moosa M, Mazzaferri EL. Outcome of differentiated thyroid cancer diagnosed in pregnant women. *J Clin Endocrinol Metab*. 1997;82(9):2862-2866.
43. Yasmeen S, Cress R, Romano PS, et al. Thyroid cancer in pregnancy. *Int J Gynaecol Obstet*. 2005;91(1):15-20.
44. Vannucchi G, Perrino M, Rossi S, et al. Clinical and molecular features of differentiated thyroid cancer diagnosed during pregnancy. *Eur J Endocrinol*. 2010;162(1):145-151.
45. Messuti I, Corvisieri S, Bardesono F, et al. Impact of pregnancy on prognosis of differentiated thyroid cancer: clinical and molecular features. *Eur J Endocrinol*. 2014;170(5):659-666.
46. Hirsch D, Kopel V, Nadler V, Levy S, Toledano Y, Tsvetov G. Pregnancy outcomes in women with primary hyperparathyroidism. *J Clin Endocrinol Metab*. 2015;100(5):2115-2122.
47. Ali DS, Dandurand K, Khan AA. Primary hyperparathyroidism in pregnancy: literature review of the diagnosis and management. *J Clin Med*. 2021;10(13).
48. Abood A, Vestergaard P. Pregnancy outcomes in women with primary hyperparathyroidism. *Eur J Endocrinol*. 2014;171(1):69-76.
49. Gunn IR, Gaffney D. Clinical and laboratory features of calcium-sensing receptor disorders: a systematic review. *Ann Clin Biochem*. Nov 2004;41(Pt 6):441-458.
50. Kovacs CS. Maternal mineral and bone metabolism during pregnancy, lactation, and post-weaning recovery. *Physiol Rev*. Apr 2016;96(2):449-547.
51. Bertelloni S, Baroncelli GI, Pelletti A, Battini R, Saggese G. Parathyroid hormone-related protein in healthy pregnant women. *Calcif Tissue Int*. Mar 1994;54(3):195-197.
52. Yadav S, Yadav YS, Goel MM, Singh U, Natu SM, Negi MP. Calcitonin gene- and parathyroid hormone-related peptides in normotensive and preeclamptic pregnancies: a nested case-control study. *Arch Gynecol Obstet*. 2014;290(5):897-903.
53. Committee Opinion No. 656 Summary: Guidelines for Diagnostic Imaging During Pregnancy and Lactation. *Obstet Gynecol*. 2016;127(2):418.
54. Gotway MB, Reddy GP, Webb WR, Morita ET, Clark OH, Higgins CB. Comparison between MR imaging and 99mTc MIBI scintigraphy in the evaluation of recurrent of persistent hyperparathyroidism. *Radiology*. 2001;218(3):783-790.
55. Dandurand K, Ali DS, Khan AA. Primary hyperparathyroidism: a narrative review of diagnosis and medical management. *J Clin Med*. 2021;10(8).
56. Davis C, Nippita T. Hyperparathyroidism in pregnancy. *BMJ Case Rep*. 2020;13(2).
57. Dale AG, Holbrook BD, Sobel L, Rappaport VJ. Hyperparathyroidism in pregnancy leading to pancreatitis and preeclampsia with severe features. *Case Rep Obstet Gynecol*. 2017;2017:6061313.
58. DiMarco AN, Meeran K, Christakis I, et al. Seventeen cases of primary hyperparathyroidism in pregnancy: a call for management guidelines. *J Endocr Soc*. 2019;3(5):1009-1021.
59. Norman J, Politz D, Politz L. Hyperparathyroidism during pregnancy and the effect of rising calcium on pregnancy loss: a call for earlier intervention. *Clin Endocrinol (Oxf)*. 2009;71(1):104-109.
60. Rigg J, Gilbertson E, Barrett HL, Britten FL, Lust K. Primary hyperparathyroidism in pregnancy: maternofetal outcomes at a quaternary referral obstetric hospital, 2000 through 2015. *J Clin Endocrinol Metab*. 2019;104(3):721-729.
61. Nilsson IL, Adner N, Reihnér E, Palme-Kilander C, Edstrom G, Degerblad M. Primary hyperparathyroidism in pregnancy: a diagnostic and therapeutic challenge. *J Womens Health (Larchmt)*. 2010;19(6):1117-1121.
62. Pothiwala P, Levine SN. Parathyroid surgery in pregnancy: review of the literature and localization by aspiration for parathyroid hormone levels. *J Perinatol*. 2009;29(12):779-784.

63. Khan AA, Hanley DA, Rizzoli R, et al. Primary hyperparathyroidism: review and recommendations on evaluation, diagnosis, and management. A Canadian and international consensus. *Osteoporos Int.* 2017;28(1):1-19.
64. Horjus C, Groot I, Telting D, et al. Cinacalcet for hyperparathyroidism in pregnancy and puerperium. *J Pediatr Endocrinol Metab.* 2009;22(8):741-749.
65. Djokanovic N, Klieger-Grossmann C, Koren G. Does treatment with bisphosphonates endanger the human pregnancy? *J Obstet Gynaecol Can.* 2008;30(12):1146-1148.
66. Boyce RW, Varela A, Chouinard L, et al. Infant cynomolgus monkeys exposed to denosumab in utero exhibit an osteoclast-poor osteopetrotic-like skeletal phenotype at birth and in the early postnatal period. *Bone.* 2014;64:314-325.
67. Kelly TR. Primary hyperparathyroidism during pregnancy. *Surgery.* Dec 1991;110(6):1028-1033; discussion 1033-4.
68. Harper MA, Murnaghan GA, Kennedy L, Hadden DR, Atkinson AB. Phaeochromocytoma in pregnancy. Five cases and a review of the literature. *Br J Obstet Gynaecol.* 1989;96(5):594-606.
69. Antonelli NM, Dotters DJ, Katz VL, Kuller JA. Cancer in pregnancy: a review of the literature. Part I. *Obstet Gynecol Surv.* 1996;51(2):125-134.
70. Antonelli NM, Dotters DJ, Katz VL, Kuller JA. Cancer in pregnancy: a review of the literature. Part II. *Obstet Gynecol Surv.* 1996;51(2):135-142.
71. Harrington JL, Farley DR, van Heerden JA, Ramin KD. Adrenal tumors and pregnancy. *World J Surg.* 1999;23(2):182-186.
72. Bancos I, Atkinson E, Eng C, Young WF Jr, Neumann HPH. Maternal and fetal outcomes in phaeochromocytoma and pregnancy: a multicentre retrospective cohort study and systematic review of literature. *Lancet Diabetes Endocrinol.* 2021; 9(1):13-21.
73. Fishbein L, Merrill S, Fraker DL, Cohen DL, Nathanson KL. Inherited mutations in pheochromocytoma and paraganglioma: why all patients should be offered genetic testing. *Ann Surg Oncol.* 2013;20(5):1444-1450.
74. Gimenez-Roqueplo AP, Dahia PL, Robledo M. An update on the genetics of paraganglioma, pheochromocytoma, and associated hereditary syndromes. *Horm Metab Res.* 2012;44(5):328-333.
75. Gruber LM, Young WF Jr, Bancos I. Pheochromocytoma and paraganglioma in pregnancy: a new era. *Curr Cardiol Rep.* 2021;23(6):60.
76. Lenders JW, Pacak K, Walther MM, et al. Biochemical diagnosis of pheochromocytoma: which test is best? *JAMA.* 20 2002;287(11):1427-1434.
77. Zuspan FP. Urinary excretion of epinephrine and norepinephrine during pregnancy. *J Clin Endocrinol Metab.* 1970;30(3): 357-360.
78. Bausch B, Schiavi F, Ni Y, et al. Clinical characterization of the pheochromocytoma and paraganglioma susceptibility genes SDHA, TMEM127, MAX, and SDHAF2 for gene-informed prevention. *JAMA Oncol.* 2017;3(9):1204-1212.
79. Leavitt K, Običan S, Yankowitz J. Treatment and prevention of hypertensive disorders during pregnancy. *Clin Perinatol.* 2019;46(2):173-185.
80. Oishi S, Sato T. Pheochromocytoma in pregnancy: a review of the Japanese literature. *Endocr J.* 1994;41(3):219-225.
81. Bellos I, Pergialiotis V, Papapanagiotou A, Loutradis D, Daskalakis G. Comparative efficacy and safety of oral antihypertensive agents in pregnant women with chronic hypertension: a network metaanalysis. *Am J Obstet Gynecol.* 2020;223(4):525-537.
82. MacCarthy EP, Bloomfield SS. Labetalol: a review of its pharmacology, pharmacokinetics, clinical uses and adverse effects. *Pharmacotherapy.* 1983;3(4):193-219.
83. Pacak K, Taieb D. Phaeochromocytoma and pregnancy: looking towards better outcomes, less fear, and valuable recommendations. *Lancet Diabetes Endocrinol.* 2021;9(1):2-3.
84. Langton K, Tufton N, Akker S, et al. Pregnancy and phaeochromocytoma/paraganglioma: clinical clues affecting diagnosis and outcome—a systematic review. *BJOG.* 2021;128(8):1264-1272.
85. Hamidi O, Young WF Jr, Iñiguez-Ariza NM, et al. Malignant pheochromocytoma and paraganglioma: 272 patients over 55 years. *J Clin Endocrinol Metab.* 2017;102(9):3296-3305.

Adrenal Insufficiency

79

Sharon T. Mackin, MRCP (UK), MD
Gemma Currie, MRCP (UK), PhD
David Carty, FRCP (UK), PhD

ADRENAL INSUFFICIENCY

Adrenal insufficiency is the inability of the adrenal glands to produce vital steroid hormones, primarily glucocorticoids, although can also involve mineralocorticoid and androgen deficiencies depending on the pathology involved. In this chapter, we will discuss the presentation of adrenal insufficiency, the common aetiologies and how to differentiate between them, and treatment in acute and chronic settings.

A BRIEF HISTORY

Adrenal insufficiency was one of the first endocrine disorders to be recognized. The adrenal glands were discovered by renowned anatomist Eustachius in 1563, but it wasn't until three centuries later in 1855 that Thomas Addison (Figure 79–1) first recognized the typically fatal clinical syndrome of adrenal insufficiency. He described a case series of preterminal patients with peculiar sickly "anemia," irritability, GI disturbance, and flexural pigmentation. Crucially, he observed an association with diseased "suprarenal capsules" at autopsy in these patients. Shortly after this observation, Brown-Séquard showed that adrenalectomized animals suffered a similar rapidly terminal event, and that injection of adrenal extract could temporize such mortality. At the turn of the twentieth century, Sir William Osler administered oral adrenal extracts to human subjects with the described Addison syndrome and found similar temporary mortality benefit. Over the next 50 years, recognition and extraction of the individual adrenal hormones took place. Most notably two chemists, Edward Kendall (Mayo Clinic) and Tadeusz Reichstein (University of Basle), won the Nobel Prize in Medicine and Physiology for their isolation of the adrenocortical hormones (11-dehydrocorticosterone, corticosterone, cortisone, and cortisol). Furthermore, they were able to demonstrate that some of these compounds had differential effects on enhanced gluconeogenesis (glucocorticoid effects of cortisone and cortisol), whilst others altered electrolyte balance, which we now know as mineralocorticoid effects (11-dehydrocorticosterone). Progress has continued over the years, such that we better understand the complex steroidogenesis pathway (Figure 79–2), are able to reliably measure these hormones, and can offer effective steroid replacement therapies.

ADRENAL STEROIDOGENESIS & PHYSIOLOGICAL EFFECTS

Steroids are grouped into three categories, depending on their main target receptor and downstream biological effects (Table 79–1).

All steroid hormones originate from a cholesterol precursor. Within the adrenal mitochondria, the cholesterol molecule undergoes side-chain cleavage by CYP11A1 to form the steroid precursor Pregnenolone. This is the main rate-limiting step in adrenal steroidogenesis. Pregnenolone is then released from the adrenal mitochondria, and via a series of oxidation and hydroxylation reactions within individual zones of the adrenal cortex is converted to the various steroid hormones. Figure 79–2 shows the enzymatic reactions that occur within each layer of the adrenal cortex. The outermost zona glomerulosa is where mineralocorticoids are produced and are highlighted in the blue box. Aldosterone is the key final product in this pathway and is largely under the control of the renin-angiotensin-aldosterone system (RAAS). The middle zona fasciculata is where glucocorticoids are produced (highlighted by the green box), and adrenal androgens are formed in the innermost zona reticularis (highlighted by the yellow box). These latter two regions are regulated by the hypothalamic-pituitary-adrenal axis (Figure 79–2). To summarize, corticotropin-releasing hormone (CRH) is produced from the hypothalamus and stimulates the pituitary gland to produce the peptide precursor, proopiomelanocortin (POMC). POMC is a 241 amino acid peptide that is cleaved under various enzymatic reactions to form other peptides, such as melanocortin and adrenocorticotrophic hormone (ACTH).

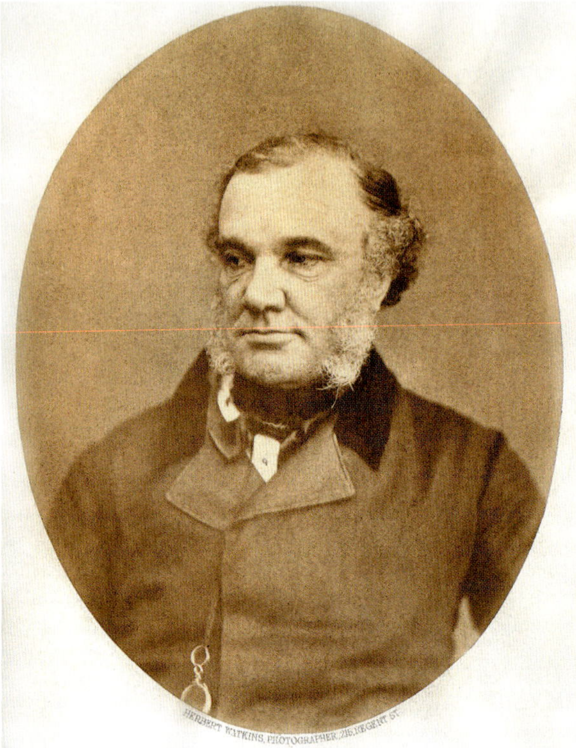

▲ **Figure 79–1.** Portrait of Thomas Addison. (Used with permission from ARCHIVIO GBB/Alamy Stock Photo.)

ACTH then binds to receptors on the adrenal cortex, and through cAMP pathways activates gene transcription of the enzymes 3β-hydroxysteroid dehydrogenase, 21-hydroxylase, and 11-β2 hydroxylase, thereby increasing glucocorticoid and androgen production. In the presence of optimal glucocorticoid levels, negative feedback to reduce CRH and ACTH production should occur.

CLASSIFICATION

To understand classification of adrenal insufficiency, an understanding of the hypothalamic-pituitary-adrenal negative feedback system is important (Figure 79–3).

Primary adrenal insufficiency refers to intrinsic failure of the adrenal cortex to produce glucocorticoids despite the presence of appropriate ACTH stimulation from the pituitary gland, as a result of destruction or dysfunction of the adrenal cortex. Glucocorticoid production is universally affected, and because it can involve the whole adrenal cortex, it often encompasses failure of mineralocorticoid and androgen production also. Alternatively, secondary and tertiary adrenal insufficiency refers to glucocorticoid deficiency that occurs as a result of absolute or relative ACTH deficiency (Table 79–2). Secondary adrenal insufficiency refers to ACTH deficiency as a result of pituitary disease, while tertiary insufficiency can be iatrogenic as a result of long-term administration of corticosteroids, or due to hypothalamic disease. Unlike primary adrenal insufficiency, in these cases, mineralocorticoid function is usually preserved since this is not predominantly under ACTH control. This is also useful to consider when thinking about presentation of disease. For example, dilutional hyponatremia is common to all subgroups of adrenal insufficiency as free water excretion is

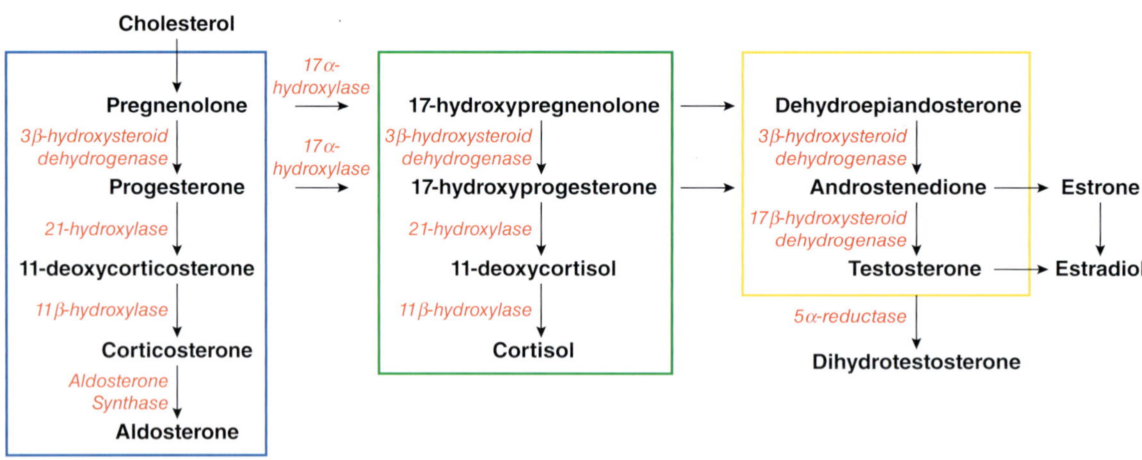

▲ **Figure 79–2.** Adrenal steroid pathway. Following side-chain cleavage of cholesterol to form pregnenolone, a series of enzymatic steps take place within the adrenal cortex to form mineralocorticoids (blue box), glucocorticoids (green box), and adrenal androgens (yellow box). The enzyme catalyst at each step of adrenal steroid metabolism is highlighted in red.

Table 79–1. Physiological effects of steroid hormones.

Mineralocorticoid	Aldosterone	• Binds to mineralocorticoid receptors • ↑ Na^+ and H_2O reabsorption at proximal tubule leading to increased plasma Na^+, expanded plasma volume, and increased blood pressure • ↑ K^+ and H^+ urinary excretion
Glucocorticoid	Cortisol	• Binds to glucocorticoid receptors • ↑ gluconeogenesis • "stress" response inducing alert state and catabolism for energy • Immunomodulatory and anti-inflammatory effects • Regulates free water excretion via ↓ADH/↓CRH (an ADH secretagogue) • In high concentrations, endogenous cortisol and some exogenous glucocorticoids have affinity for mineralocorticoid receptors. One such disorder that demonstrates this is Apparent Mineralocorticoid Excess due to 11β-hydroxysteroid-dehydrogenase 2 deficiency. This enzyme converts cortisol to inactive cortisone, and so deficiency leads to increased cortisol concentrations, which subsequently activate the mineralocorticoid receptor causing hypertension.
Androgens	Dehydroepiandrosterone (adrenal-specific precursor) Testosterone	• Sexual function • Hirsutism • Lesser role than androgens of testicular/ovarian origin but can have virilizing effects if produced in excess

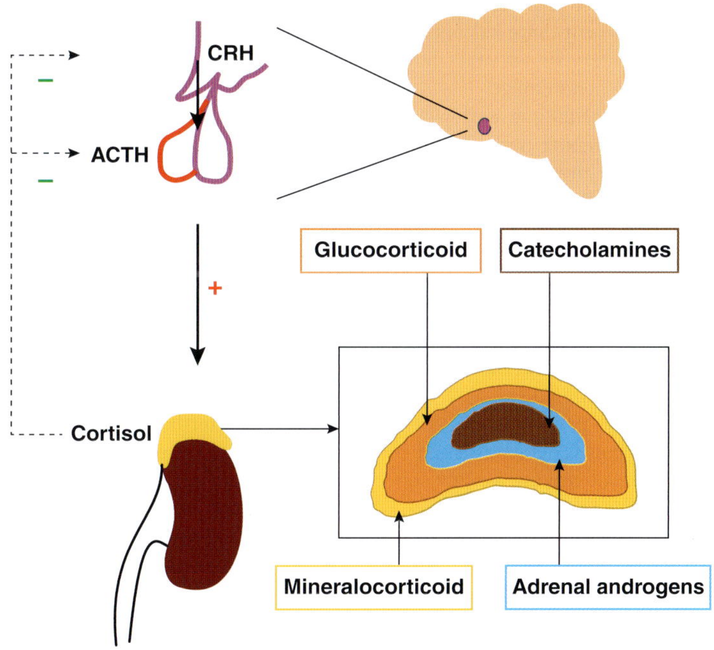

▲ **Figure 79–3.** Hypothalamic pituitary adrenal axis negative feedback. CRH is released from the hypothalamus (shown in purple connected to the posterior pituitary gland) in response to low circulating levels of cortisol. CRH binds to G-protein-coupled receptors in the anterior pituitary (shown in red) where it stimulates production of the ACTH precursor proopiomelanocortin (POMC). Upregulation of this leads to increased ACTH release from the anterior pituitary, with subsequent activation of glucocorticoid, and a modest activation of adrenal androgen production from the adrenal gland. The mineralocorticoids produced by the zona glomerulosa are under RAAS control, and catecholamine production from the inner adrenal medulla under sympathetic nervous system control.

Table 79–2. Typical hormone patterns in primary, secondary, and tertiary adrenal insufficiency.

	Primary	Secondary	Tertiary
CRH	↑	↑	↓
ACTH	↑	↓	↓
Cortisol	↓	↓	↓
Aldosterone	Often ↓	↔	↔

reduced in the absence of adequate cortisol; however, hypotension and hyperkalemia are less likely to be associated with secondary or tertiary adrenal insufficiency as mineralocorticoid function should be intact.

SYMPTOMS & SIGNS

Most cases of adrenal insufficiency have an indolent presentation in the initial stages. Adrenal crisis as first presentation is thankfully less common and tends to occur in those with a longer history of classical symptoms that have yet to be diagnosed, in those with abrupt cessation of prolonged courses of supraphysiological glucocorticoids or if there has been an acute catastrophic insult to the pituitary or adrenal glands such as pituitary apoplexy or adrenal hemorrhage.

In the more indolent presentation, fatigue and weight loss are common. Patients may also report nausea, vomiting, abdominal pain, diarrhea, and myalgia, and oligo-amenorrhoea can occur in female patients. Hypoglycemia can occur due to glucocorticoid deficiency, and an assessment of glucocorticoid production should therefore be undertaken in any patient presenting with unexplained hypoglycemia. These symptoms are common to both primary and secondary causes of hypoadrenalism and are reflective of hypocortisolaemia, but some signs can help us differentiate clinically between primary and secondary hypoadrenalism.

In primary adrenal insufficiency, patients may notice additional effects of mineralocorticoid deficiency such as postural dizziness, hypotension, or salt craving as they subconsciously look to regulate electrolyte levels in the absence of aldosterone. The classic pattern of electrolyte disturbance seen is hyponatremia and hyperkalemia, but electrolytes can be normal in patients with adrenal insufficiency and so should not be solely relied on to pursue diagnosis in patients. Hyperkalaemia reflects aldosterone deficiency. The astute clinician may also notice increased skin pigmentation in patients presenting with primary adrenal insufficiency, which can be generalized, or more sparse with darker patches of pigmentation evident on the buccal mucosa, around the gum line, on flexural surfaces, in palmar creases, and knuckle folds (Figure 79–4). In the low cortisol state, CRH production is upregulated, which in turn stimulates the ACTH precursor POMC. POMC is cleaved to smaller peptides, including ACTH and melanocyte-stimulating hormone (MSH), resulting in coincident activation of melanocytes in the skin.

Alternatively, in secondary and tertiary adrenal insufficiency, patients usually do not exhibit the low mineralocorticoid effects or POMC-stimulated hyperpigmentation symptoms. If ACTH deficiency is because of hypothalamic-pituitary disease, the clinician may notice symptoms or signs associated with other pituitary hormone deficits, for example, hypothyroidism from low TSH production, symptoms of hypogonadism if LH/FSH is low, or diabetes insipidus if posterior pituitary function is affected. In the case of pituitary apoplexy or pituitary mass, symptoms of headache, visual disturbance with bitemporal hemianopia, or ophthalmoplegia may also be evident.

Acute Adrenal Crisis

Acute adrenal crisis is a life-threatening emergency and occurs as a result of acute cortisol deficiency that leads to severe physiological disturbance. Patients can rapidly progress from symptoms of nausea, vomiting, abdominal pain, and diarrhea to being obtunded with hypotension, hypoglycemia, and coma within hours. Epidemiological data from Europe suggest a prevalence of 6 to 8 per 100 patient-years in those with known adrenal insufficiency, with mortality from a crisis as high as 6% in prospective studies. Prompt recognition and treatment with parenteral glucocorticoids and intravenous fluids are lifesaving in these patients. Treatment is discussed later in the chapter.

EPIDEMIOLOGY

Epidemiological data are difficult to fully capture internationally, but European and US registry studies suggest a prevalence of 40 to 140 cases per 1,000,000 population of primary adrenal insufficiency, with some suggesting that prevalence is increasing in recent decades. Incidence is approximately 6 new cases per 1,000,000 population in Western societies. Secondary and tertiary adrenal insufficiency are often grouped collectively as "secondary" adrenal insufficiency in studies. Unsurprisingly, with the burden of supraphysiological steroid prescriptions in Western population, the prevalence of secondary/tertiary adrenal insufficiency is much higher than that of primary adrenal disease at 150 to 280 cases per 1,000,000 population, although this may reflect a gross underestimate of iatrogenic adrenal insufficiency secondary to long-term steroid or opiate use. A UK review of prescribing practice suggested that 1% of the adult population is prescribed corticosteroids at any one time, with this increasing to 2.5% in older adults. Of those on steroids, approximately one-fifth of them were prescribed for >6 months duration suggesting a group at high risk of adrenal suppression.

Table 79–3 outlines the demographic associations with each subgroup of adrenal insufficiency.

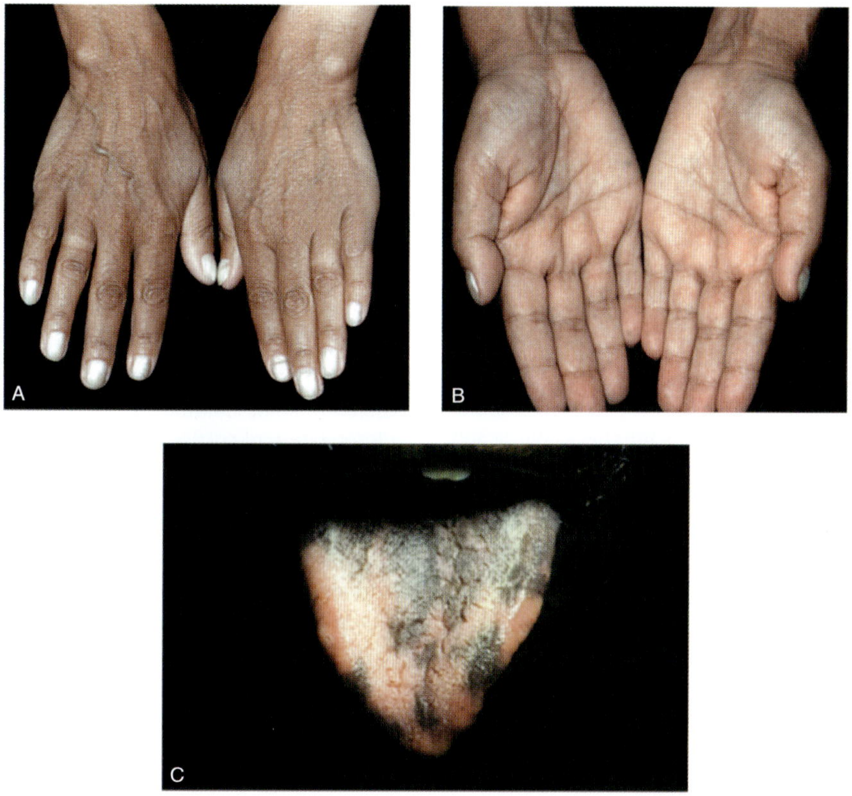

▲ **Figure 79–4.** Arms of a girl who had Addison disease. (Reproduced with the permission from Saavedra AP, Roh EK, Mikailov A. *Fitzpatrick's Color Atlas and Synopsis of Clinical Dermatology*, 9 ed. McGraw Hill LLC Copyright © 2023.)

DIAGNOSIS

Any patient who has potential symptoms of adrenal insufficiency should be considered for diagnostic testing. Furthermore, it should be considered in hemodynamically unstable patients whereby the cause of illness is unclear, or they are failing to respond as expected to supportive treatment. In the acute scenario, testing should not delay prompt administration of potentially lifesaving glucocorticoid treatment. If suspected in the more stable patient, testing should still be done with urgency. If there is ever doubt about the diagnosis, safe practice would be to treat with glucocorticoids and consider subsequent testing once stabilized.

Table 79–3. Demographics associated with adrenal insufficiency subtypes.

Primary Adrenal Insufficiency	Secondary/Tertiary Adrenal Insufficiency
Affects 40-140 individuals per 1,000,000 population	Affects 150-280 individuals per 1,000,000 population but may be underestimated
2-4 fold higher in women	Females more commonly affected
Peak incidence age 30-40 years	Peak incidence age 50-60 years
Associated with other autoimmune diseases	

An ACTH stimulation test, also known as a cosyntropin or short Synacthen™ test, is the gold standard for diagnosing primary adrenal insufficiency. This requires a baseline blood sample for cortisol to be taken, followed by intravenous or intramuscular administration of 250 μg tetracoside (Synacthen™) and subsequent measurement of serum cortisol at 30- and 60-minute postinjection. ACTH should be measured concurrently at baseline. For those patients already taking hydrocortisone, it is recommended to perform the test at least 18 hours following their previous dose of glucocorticoid. Since hydrocortisone is short-acting, this should allow an accurate interpretation of endogenous cortisol production.

Current guidelines recommend that a postcosyntropin cortisol of >500 nmol/L (>18 μg/dL) is sufficient to exclude primary adrenal insufficiency. Those who have a normal baseline cortisol, and who increment by >200 nmol/L (7 μg/dL) are also likely to have adequate adrenal function. However, guidelines also acknowledge that normal values are based on older generation assays, and more modern cortisol assays have improved. Modern lab techniques are less likely to use polyclonal antibodies prone to interference and cross-reactivity with other steroid hormones, and may show more specific cortisol values that read up to 20% lower than some of the older tests. For this reason, each lab should have its own normalized reference range for cortisol, and this should be consulted when interpreting any cortisol test.

A cosyntropin test can be performed at any time of day if wishing to exclude primary adrenal insufficiency; however, it is less reliable in excluding secondary adrenal insufficiency in the context of acute or subacute insult to ACTH production. In these cases, the adrenal gland is still capable of generating an appropriate physiological response to ACTH, and so the postcosyntropin cortisol may exceed the normal threshold. A low baseline cortisol, provided it is measured early in the morning (between 8 and 9 am), is often used to identify glucocorticoid deficiency in such scenarios. This is a cost-effective means of screening for secondary adrenal insufficiency but requires consideration of the pretest clinical probability to interpret. Furthermore, there are similar caveats to normal thresholds given the lack of standardization between cortisol assays. The Endocrine Society guidelines suggest an early morning cortisol <83 nmol/L (<3 μg/dL) confirms adrenal insufficiency, and levels >413 nmol/L (>15 μg/dL) exclude adrenal insufficiency. Early morning cortisol values between these are indeterminate, and should be considered against the pretest clinical probability and followed up with confirmatory testing using a cosyntropin test, or the insulin tolerance test. If high suspicion of adrenal insufficiency and indeterminate early morning cortisol values, it would be clinically reasonable to treat whilst awaiting confirmatory testing or with serial testing several weeks apart.

An insulin tolerance test (ITT) involves administering insulin intravenously at a dose of 0.05-0.15 U/kg, to cause hypoglycemia (blood glucose <2.2 mmol/L or <40 mg/dL) and a resultant stimulation of ACTH and cortisol in response to this physiological stress. Blood sampling for glucose and cortisol occurs at 30-minute intervals from before insulin administration, until 2 hours after. Peak cortisol should exceed 500 nmol/L (18.1 μg/dL) if HPA function is intact, and is reliable even in the acute ACTH-deficiency setting. For these reasons, guidelines may refer to it as the gold standard. However, it is rarely practical, and important safety considerations significantly limit its use. Not only is it more time-consuming than the cosyntropin test, but the test has to be performed in a setting with close physician supervision and access to resuscitation facilities. Hypoglycaemia can be unpleasant for patients at best, and be associated with increased risks of adverse outcomes including seizures. ITTs are contraindicated in patients with known seizures or at risk of them such as in frail patients and in those with established cerebrovascular disease. Patients at risk of cardiac arrhythmia should also be considered for alternative testing to ITT. It is more commonly used in pediatric populations where simultaneous assessment of growth hormone deficiency can occur.

Table 79–4 outlines other useful tests that may be considered to help establish the cause of adrenal insufficiency, or to detect other associated endocrinopathy once the initial diagnosis is confirmed.

Common Caveats to Consider With Cortisol Testing

There are some common clinical scenarios that can make interpretation of cortisol tests challenging.

- Critical illness: In the severely unwell patient with normal adrenal function, random cortisol levels can be extremely high in response to extreme physiological stress. Acute phase response can also attenuate production of binding proteins such as cortisol binding globulin (CBG) and albumin. In such patients, total cortisol secretion may increase, and simultaneously have lower protein binding meaning more active free cortisol in plasma whilst cortisol metabolism and clearance is decreased. Referenced normal cortisol levels, measured in the well patient, are therefore unlikely to be applicable or "normal" in the critically unwell patient. There is ongoing debate without consensus on what is a normal cortisol range in such patients. A taskforce statement from the American College of Critical Care Medicine has suggested a failure of cortisol to increment by >250 nmol/L (9 μg/dL) following a cosyntropin test, or a random cortisol <275 nmol/L (10 μg/dL) can be used to diagnose adrenal insufficiency. With such patients, repeat testing when well would be good practice to confirm longer-term need for steroid replacement.
- Pregnancy: Cortisol and binding globulins are increased in pregnancy. Cortisol-binding globulin can be two- to threefold higher in the context of high estrogen, as demonstrated in both pregnancy and in those taking estrogen-containing contraceptives. Physiological adaptations also occur which may aid the mother in coping with the increased physiological stress in pregnancy. Women who are on glucocorticoid replacement therapy often need higher doses, particularly in the third trimester of pregnancy when metabolic demands are increased.
- Beware of the endocrinopathy mimics related to adrenal insufficiency. For example, TSH can be elevated in the context of cortisol deficiency and will be remedied with glucocorticoid replacement. If suspicious of adrenal insufficiency, assess adrenal function prior to thyroid replacement. Correction of hypothyroidism in patients with cortisol deficiency may precipitate an adrenal crisis.

Table 79–4. Additional tests to consider when investigating the cause of adrenal insufficiency.

Primary Adrenal Insufficiency		
Renin and aldosterone	↓ Aldosterone, ↑ Renin in mineralocorticoid deficiency	Affected by medications such as antihypertensives, salt intake, and posture. Can also be difficult to interpret in the context of acute illness where fluid resuscitation may cloud the picture.
Adrenal antibodies	Positive in Addison disease/autoimmune adrenalitis	
CT adrenals	To look for masses (benign or malignant), infiltrative disease such as TB, granuloma	Dedicated CT adrenals can provide superior radiological phenotyping of adrenal lesions than CT abdomen.
Short synacthen test with 17-hydroxyprogesterone (17-OHP) measurement	If suspected Congenital Adrenal Hyperplasia due to 21-hydroxylase deficiency and early morning 17-OHP >6 nmol/L, a confirmatory rise to >30 nmol/L after cosyntropin 250 mg IV/IM is diagnostic.	24-hour urinary steroid profiles (when not on steroids) can also be used to help diagnose CAH from 21-hydroxylase as well as other enzyme deficiencies.
Secondary Adrenal Insufficiency		
Full pituitary functions tests	Prolactin, insulin-like growth factor-1, prolactin, luteinizing hormone, follicular stimulating hormone, estradiol/testosterone, thyroid function tests	May have deficits or excess of various hormones in context of pituitary disease.
MRI pituitary	To look for pituitary masses (most commonly benign adenomas), hypophysitis, empty sella syndrome, etc.	10% risk of identifying incidentalomas.

CAUSES

Primary Adrenal Insufficiency

In developed nations, the commonest cause of primary adrenal insufficiency is autoimmune adrenalitis, accounting for >80% of presentations. In countries where tuberculosis infection is prevalent, TB of adrenals is more common. Bilateral adrenalectomy and adrenal hemorrhage are other common causes of adrenal insufficiency. These and other aetiologies are discussed below.

- **Autoimmune adrenalitis:** Progressive antibody-mediated destruction of the adrenal cortex leads to glucocorticoid, mineralocorticoid, and androgen deficiencies. At the time of presentation, a sizeable proportion of the adrenal cortex has been damaged, with some studies estimating that as much as 90% of cortical destruction occurs prior to clinically evident sequelae. Susceptible individuals may have a genetic predisposition, with HLA-B8, HLA-DR3, and HLA-DR4 conferring increased risk. The pathogenesis is not fully understood, but like many autoimmune conditions, an environmental trigger such as a viral stimulus, is thought to be an important trigger. In susceptible individuals, such triggers activate a pathological T-cell immune response and the production of antibodies that direct a cytotoxic response to the adrenal cortex. 25-Hydroxylase antibodies are found in approximately 90% of recent-onset autoimmune adrenalitis. Autoimmune adrenalitis can occur as an isolated presentation, or as part of an autoimmune polyglandular syndrome (APS).
- **APS type 1 (APS-1), also known as autoimmune polyendocrinopathy candidiasis ectodermal dystrophy (APECED):** A rare, autosomal recessively inherited condition associated with multiple autoimmune-mediated endocrinopathy, which occurs in the context of defects in the *AIRE* autoimmune-regulator gene located on the short arm of chromosome 21. The AIRE protein is produced by medullary cells in the thymus and has a key role in immune tolerance. An APS-1, a classic triad of chronic mucocutaneous candidiasis, hypoparathyroidism, and Addison disease, is well recognized, but other autoimmune pathologies are also identified. These include hypothyroidism, type 1 diabetes mellitus, primary and secondary hypogonadism, vitiligo, alopecia, pernicious anemia, and hepatitis. Affected children also require screening for dental hypoplasia and keratitis. It typically presents in childhood and has a prevalence that ranges from 1 in 10,000 to 100,000 population. However, cases have also been diagnosed in early adulthood depending on the clinical phenotype and onset of endocrinopathy. Candidiasis in early childhood is the most prevalent manifestation of APS-1. Hypoparathyroidism is one of the earliest endocrine presentations of disease, and 90% of APS-1 individuals will be affected. Addison disease typically develops after hypoparathyroidism, and will

affect approximately two-thirds of patients with APS-1. Diagnosis can be confirmed if two of the three classical triad conditions are present, or one of these with a known APS-1 affected sibling, or if defects in the *AIRE* gene are identified. Other antibodies linked with APS-1 include interferon, aromatic L-amino acid decarboxylase, tryptophan-hydroxylase, and tyrosine hydroxylase antibodies. Whilst these latter antibodies are not confirmatory for APS-1, their presence in an affected individual should alert the clinician to a possible diagnosis, and appropriate autoimmune screening offered.

- **APS-2, also known as Schmidt syndrome:** Multiple endocrinopathies can occur due to lymphocytic infiltration and destruction of endocrine glands. APS-2 is most classically associated with the triad of autoimmune thyroid disease, type 1 diabetes, and Addison disease, and is more common than APS-1. Other manifestations include hypogonadism, hypophysitis, pernicious anemia, myasthenia gravis, coeliac disease, IgA deficiency, rheumatoid arthritis, and stiff-man syndrome. In contrast to APS-1, where presentation is typically in childhood, APS-2 is more often associated with a diagnosis in adulthood. Peak incidence occurs between 20 and 40 years of age and affects females more commonly than males. There are genetic associations with certain HLA haplotypes (DR-3, DR-4, DQ-2, and DQ-8) and other gene polymorphisms linked to T-lymphocyte function, but no single gene is diagnostic. Diagnosis is instead dependent on the presence of two or more of the classic thyroid, type 1 diabetes, and Addison disease cluster.
- **Congenital Adrenal Hyperplasia (CAH):** CAH is a group of congenital autosomal recessive disorders associated with enzyme deficiencies important to steroidogenesis, and is the commonest cause of adrenal insufficiency presenting in childhood. 21-Hydroxylase deficiency is the commonest CAH disorder with mutations in the *CYP21A2* gene accounting for 95% of cases. It affects 1 in 14,000 births and has a varied phenotype depending on severity of genetic deletions and enzyme deficiency. Deficiency of 21-hydroxylase prevents the conversion of 17-hydroxyprogesterone to the cortisol precursor 11-deoxycortisol, and progesterone to the aldosterone precursor deoxycorticosterone (Figure 79–2). Glucocorticoid and mineralocorticoid deficiency therefore occurs, which stimulates ACTH release from the pituitary and subsequent adrenal gland hypertrophy. Furthermore, the excess progesterone and 17-hydroxyprogesterone are shared precursors for adrenal androgens, leading to increased androgen production and virilization. Classic-type CAH is the most severe phenotype and presents in the neonatal period. It can be classified as either "salt wasting" or "non-salt wasting" depending on the severity of mineralocorticoid loss. In the severe salt-wasting type, both cortisol and aldosterone levels are very low due to absent 21-hydroxylase, whilst in the non-salt-wasting type aldosterone levels are more typically normal or mildly deficient in comparison. Both phenotypes are associated with glucocorticoid deficiency and significant virilization. This may be more apparent in female infants who are born with ambiguous genitalia. If not promptly recognized, infants can develop life-threatening adrenal and salt-wasting crises. Current guidelines recommend that 17-hydroxyprogesterone testing be offered as part of routine neonatal screening in the United States to detect potential cases. If suspected, a cosyntropin stimulation test with simultaneous measurement of 17-hydroxyprogesterone should be performed to diagnose the condition, with a rise in 17-hydroxyprogesterone to >30 nmol/L considered confirmatory (Table 79–4).

  Late-onset nonclassical CAH due to 21-hydroxylase deficiency is much milder and is often not detected until the teenage years or adulthood. In these cases, enzyme deficiency is only mildly affected and often has sufficient glucocorticoid and mineralocorticoid production. These patients may present with precocious puberty, menstrual irregularities, and features of hyperandrogenism. In females, it may be confused for polycystic ovarian syndrome. An elevated 17-hydroxyprogesterone in these individuals should trigger diagnostic testing with a cosyntropin-stimulation test. Other steroid pathway enzymes can be involved in other CAH phenotypes, but this is not in the scope of this chapter.
- **Adrenoleukodystrophy:** This is a rare X-linked recessive disorder associated with mutations in the *ABCD1* gene, which is responsible for producing adrenoleukodystrophy protein. This protein helps transport very long-chain fatty acids into peroxisomes for subsequent metabolism. As such, mutations in this gene lead to accumulation of these fatty acids in tissues, leading to inflammatory damage of the myelin sheath in the central nervous system, destruction of the adrenal cortex, and disruption of Leydig cell function in the gonads. There is significant variation in severity of genotype-phenotype and not all patients will manifest symptoms in all these areas. Males are typically affected and can present with progressive neurological disorders, bladder and bowel dysfunction, hypogonadism, and adrenal insufficiency of varying degrees.
- **Infective adrenalitis:** Tuberculosis (TB) is the most common cause of infective adrenalitis, but is uncommon in nonendemic areas. Due to clinician unfamiliarity and the inherent challenges of low-yield diagnostic tests in non-pulmonary TB, it can go undiagnosed. It should be considered in the nonspecifically unwell patient with adrenal masses (typically bilateral) and a previous history or risk factors for TB. Adrenal biopsy with staining for acid-fast bacilli may help with diagnosis. An important safety

point prior to biopsy of any adrenal mass is to ensure that phaeochromocytoma is excluded. Other infective causes of adrenalitis include HIV, fungal infections such as cryptococcus and aspergillus, and syphilis.

- **Bilateral adrenal hemorrhage:** Adrenal hemorrhage is an uncommon presentation, but if severe and bilateral can lead to adrenal insufficiency. Despite their small size, the adrenal glands are very vascular being supplied by three suprarenal arteries—the superior adrenal artery branching off the inferior phrenic artery, the middle adrenal artery from the aorta, and the inferior adrenal artery from the renal arteries. Many cases of adrenal hemorrhage are spontaneous with unknown etiology, but risk factors include large adrenal masses (phaeochromocytomas, adrenocortical carcinomas, and tumors >5 cm at greatest risk), pregnancy especially if complicated by preeclampsia, severe sepsis, trauma, and concomitant risk factors with anticoagulation. If adrenal insufficiency occurs due to adrenal hemorrhage, recovery of the adrenal axis may occur with resolution of the hemorrhage and thus repeat testing is warranted.
- **Bilateral adrenal malignancy:** Primary adrenal lymphoma can present with abdominal pain, classic B-symptoms of weight loss, fever and night sweats, and bilateral adrenal masses. Adrenal insufficiency is common in this group. Bilateral secondary malignancies can also occur in the adrenal glands with common primary sites including breast, colon, lung, and stomach.
- **Bilateral infiltrative adrenal disease:** Infiltrative disease from sarcoidosis, amyloidosis, and hemochromatosis rarely manifest with adrenal insufficiency.
- **Drugs:** Many commonly used drugs inhibit enzymes involved in steroidogenesis or induce cytochrome P450 enzymes that upregulate cortisol metabolism, and can lead to adrenal insufficiency. Separately to this, some newer immune checkpoint inhibitors used in oncology have revolutionized cancer treatments and their prognosis, but have also been linked to a variety of endocrinopathies. Although uncommon, they can induce immune-mediated adrenalitis sufficient to disrupt adrenal function. Table 79–5 lists some of the drugs known to cause adrenal insufficiency and their mechanisms.

Table 79–5. Drugs with potential to affect adrenal cortical function and proposed mechanisms.

Drug	Effects That Lead to Reduced Cortisol
Antifungals, eg, ketoconazole, fluconazole	Inhibit cytochrome P450 enzymes responsible for steroidogenesis, eg, inhibit CYP11A1 which converts cholesterol to pregnenolone, the first step in steroid hormone production (Figure 79–2).
Antiepileptics, eg, phenytoin, phenobarbital	Enzyme inducers of CYP2B1, CYP2B2, and CYP3A4 which upregulate steroid hydroxylase activity and increase cortisol metabolism.
Rifampicin	Strong enzyme inducer of CYP3A4 leading to increased cortisol clearance.
Etomidate, metyrapone	Inhibits 11β-hydroxylase thereby preventing production of corticosterone and cortisol (Figure 79–2).
Mitotane	Used in treatment of adrenocortical cancer. Multiple effects including inhibition of CYP11A1 in steroidogenesis, but also direct toxic effects on the adrenal cortex resulting in cell death.
Immune checkpoint inhibitors, eg, nivolumab, pembrolizumab, ipilimumab	Exact mechanism unclear but mechanisms similar to autoimmune adrenalitis, with dysregulated immune response. Can also induce a secondary adrenal insufficiency secondary to hypophysitis.

Secondary and Tertiary Adrenal Insufficiency

Secondary adrenal insufficiency is typically due to a direct pathology or insult to the pituitary and may coexist with other anterior and posterior pituitary hormone dysfunction.

The commonest cause of tertiary adrenal insufficiency is iatrogenic secondary to chronic glucocorticoid use, with rarer causes involving hypothalamic disease that has a negative effect on CRH release. There is a common misconception that only those administered glucocorticoids systemically via oral or injectable routes are at risk of adrenal insufficiency. Typically, those administered a steroid equivalence of >5 mg/day oral prednisolone for three or more weeks are deemed at risk. Whilst patients on systemic corticosteroids are at the highest risk, those with recurrent use of potent inhaled, intra-articular, and topical glucocorticoid may also develop adrenal axis suppression. A retrospective UK study suggested as many as one-fifth of patients prescribed inhaled glucocorticoid showed suppression of their adrenal axis. Meta-analysis has suggested that the lowest risk route of steroid administration is seen with topical and nasal preparations, but there is still some risk.

Table 79–6 outlines common causes of secondary and tertiary adrenal insufficiency.

TREATMENT

Treatment of adrenal insufficiency involves replacement of the glucocorticoid, and if appropriate mineralocorticoid. Treatment with glucocorticoid should take priority over any other hormone replacement including thyroid and sex hormones, since replacement of others first can precipitate

Table 79–6. Common causes of secondary and tertiary adrenal insufficiency.

Pituitary and hypothalamic tumors, eg, adenomas (functioning and nonfunctioning), craniopharyngioma, meningioma	Look for coexisting pituitary endocrinopathy. More common to have secondary adrenal insufficiency associated with craniopharyngiomas than adenomas.
Pituitary or other head and neck irradiation	Late effects from pituitary and head and neck irradiation have shown prevalence of secondary adrenal insufficiency ranging from 12% to 68%, with a dose- and time-dependent effect seen. Other anterior pituitary hormones can also be affected.
Pituitary surgery	Prevalence of ACTH deficiency postpituitary surgery varies widely in studies (<10%-50%) and will be affected by extent of initial surgery, preexisting pathology, and the experience of the pituitary surgeon. Early ACTH deficiency postsurgery may recover, and so repeat testing of adrenal function should occur 6-12 weeks postsurgery.
Pituitary apoplexy	Life-threatening acute infarction and/or hemorrhage of pituitary gland. Has a prevalence of 6 per 100,000 population and complicates between 2% and 12% of pituitary adenomas. Risk factors include recent dopamine agonist therapy, anticoagulation, hypertension, major surgery, or dynamic pituitary function testing. Classic presentation of acute severe headache, visual disturbance, ophthalmoplegia, and potential for acute ACTH deficiency. In cases where early cortisol testing is normal, repeat assessment should take place 4-6 weeks following the event or earlier if clinically suspicious. Should be managed in a specialist center with neurosurgical and endocrine expertise.
Sheehan's syndrome	Acute pituitary necrosis secondary to large volume blood loss in the peripartum period. Rare with a prevalence of 5 per 100,000 women.
Hypophysitis—most commonly lymphocytic, but can be associated with granulomatous disease or other inflammatory disease	Autoimmune-mediated lymphocytic infiltration of the pituitary gland, resulting in anterior and pituitary function. Converse to adenomas where ACTH is one of the last hormonal axes to be lost, in hypophysitis, ACTH deficiency typically occurs earlier than other pituitary hormone deficiencies. Associations with IgG4 disease. Typical symptoms are of acute headache, vomiting, cranial nerve defects and may include symptoms of diabetes insipidus. MRI pituitary demonstrates a homogenously enhancing, potentially enlarged gland with absence of the posterior pituitary bright spot. Diagnosis often made clinically, since can only be confirmed by biopsy.
Infiltrative disease	Very rare but pituitary infiltration from TB and sarcoid can occur.
Pituitary metastases	Very rare. Most common primary is lung in men and breast in women.
Drugs	Glucocorticoids largest group of medications implicated in suppression of hypothalamic-pituitary-adrenal axis. Others include opiate medications and GABA receptor agonists such as benzodiazepines and some antipsychotics. Immune checkpoint inhibitors can activate an immune-mediated hypophysitis.

an adrenal crisis. Treatment of adrenal crisis is discussed separately in the following discussion.

Glucocorticoid Replacement

In an ideal situation, glucocorticoid treatment would mimic cortisol circadian rhythm, but the currently available preparations are imperfect in this regard. Individuals with an intact cortisol axis and typical wake-sleep cycle will have a surge in cortisol in the early morning hours, with a gradual decline over the day to very low levels by evening and overnight (Figure 79–5). For this reason, shorter-acting glucocorticoids are preferred over longer-acting preparations for cortisol replacement as their rapid absorption and short half-life allow us to attempt to replicate this diurnal rhythm with multiple daily dosing. Total daily cortisol production increases with body mass and surface area, with studies approximating daily secretion of 6 mg/m^2.

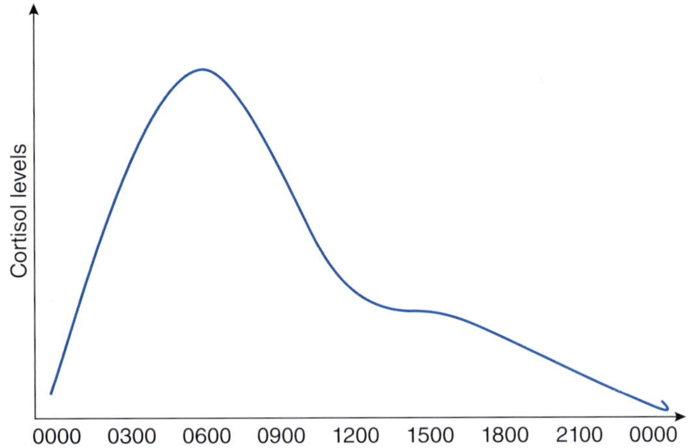

Figure 79–5. Circadian rhythm of endogenous cortisol production in an individual with typical wake-sleep cycle.

The current preferred glucocorticoid replacement is hydrocortisone 15 to 25 mg/day in the adult patients given over 2 to 3 divided doses. The highest dose should be given first thing in the morning with a smaller dose mid-afternoon. An example would be 15 mg hydrocortisone on wakening, followed by 5 mg hydrocortisone 2 hours after lunch. Some individuals may feel effects wear off between morning and afternoon doses, and so a trial of three divided doses may be helpful in such cases. For example, 10 mg is taken on wakening, 5 mg at lunch, and 5 mg later afternoon. Thrice daily dosing may also be preferred in the pediatric population, with a total daily dose of 8 mg/m^2 hydrocortisone. Hydrocortisone is also preferred in pregnancy since placental 11β-hydroxylase enzymes metabolize it effectively, thereby reducing placental passage of high cortisol levels to the fetus.

In some countries, clinicians are more familiar with cortisone, which is an acceptable short-acting glucocorticoid replacement therapy and should be given similar to hydrocortisone but at higher total daily doses (25 to 35 mg/day in adult populations).

Prednisolone is an intermediate-acting glucocorticoid and for this reason, is less preferred. Situations where it may be useful are in those patients who have iatrogenic adrenal insufficiency who intermittently require frequent doses of supraphysiological steroids, or in those where compliance with twice-daily regimes is challenging. For example, an individual with difficult chronic airways disease who requires acute monthly prescriptions of higher dose prednisolone despite optimized treatment for their lung condition may find it easier to maintain on prednisolone 5 mg/day for adrenal replacement than to switch between steroid preparations regularly. Very long-acting glucocorticoids are not recommended for routine steroid replacement.

Modified-release preparations of hydrocortisone have been developed (Chronocort™ in the United States and Efmody™ in Europe). Currently, they are approved by the European Medicine Agency and the UK Medicine and Health Regulation Authority for use in CAH and are undergoing special protocol assessment by the FDA for the same indication. Chronocort™ is not currently approved for use for adrenal insufficiency. In CAH, the dose of glucocorticoid required to switch off excess androgen production and control CAH symptoms can be higher than that used to control adrenal insufficiency. Studies exploring the modified-release preparations have shown that they are safe and biochemical control may be achieved with potentially lower dose of glucocorticoid than when using immediate-release preparations in CAH patients, thereby potential for reducing long-term effects of high glucocorticoid exposure.

Table 79–7 details glucocorticoid dose equivalence, and approximate half-lives.

Mineralocorticoid Replacement

Should only be required in primary adrenal insufficiency. Fludrocortisone at a starting dose of 50 to 100 μg is recommended in adults and can be titrated up according to response and blood pressure. It is rare that significantly higher doses are required in primary adrenal insufficiency. Suboptimal mineralocorticoid replacement may result in hyperkalemia, postural hypotension, and salt craving. Whilst not routinely required, plasma renin levels can sometimes be useful as will be very high in suboptimally treated mineralocorticoid deficiency. In addition, these patients should not be salt restricted.

Overreplacement with mineralocorticoid may present with hypokalaemia, edema, and hypertension. The presence

Table 79–7. Oral glucocorticoid steroid dose equivalence and biological half-life.*

Glucocorticoid	Oral Steroid Dose Equivalence	Mineralocorticoid Effect	Biological Half-Life
Hydrocortisone	20 mg	High—approx. equivalent to 125 μg fludrocortisone	Short-acting
Prednisolone	5 mg	High—approx. equivalent to 100 μg fludrocortisone	Intermediate-acting
Dexamethasone	0.75 mg	Negligible	Long-acting
Methylprednisolone	4 mg	Negligible	Intermediate-acting
Betamethasone	0.6 mg	Negligible	Long-acting

*Short-acting 8-12 hours, intermediate-acting 12-36 hours, long-acting >36 hours.

of these factors should prompt assessment to see if dose reduction is necessary.

TREATMENT OF ADRENAL CRISIS

Prompt treatment of adrenal crisis is essential to reduce serious morbidity and mortality. In the unwell adult with suspected or confirmed adrenal crisis, 100 mg hydrocortisone should be administered as an intravenous bolus immediately, and rapid fluid resuscitation should be undertaken. They should then be administered hydrocortisone 200 mg/day as a continuous intravenous infusion or as 50 mg administered 6 hourly via intramuscular boluses. Intravenous boluses are not mentioned in some guidelines as can get peaks and troughs in cortisol concentrations, but in practice are often used. In the pediatric population, hydrocortisone doses are

Table 79–8. Example of sick day rules for steroid-dependent adults.

Type and Severity of Physiological Stress	Stress Dosing Example
Mild to moderate acute illness, eg, fever, infections requiring antibiotics	Double usual dose of hydrocortisone for a few days until feeling better. Maintain hydration with isotonic fluids.
Acute gastrointestinal disturbance	If vomiting and unable to keep steroids down, adults should administer intramuscular hydrocortisone 100 mg and seek urgent medical review. In children, the recommended emergency intramuscular dose of hydrocortisone is 50 mg/m^2. Likely to need parenteral hydrocortisone, and intravenous fluid rehydration if ongoing symptoms.
Severe acute illness, eg, sepsis, critical illness	Administer 100 mg intravenously followed by 200 mg/day continuous intravenous infusions or 50 mg intramuscular/intravenous every 6 hours.
Minor procedures under local anesthetic and of short duration, eg, tooth extraction	Double dose of hydrocortisone before and after the procedure, before returning to usual maintenance treatment.
Surgery involving anesthesia, or major surgeries	Administer 100 mg intravenously at induction followed by 200 mg/day continuous intravenous infusions or 50 mg intramuscular/intravenous every 6 hours until eating and drinking, and no post-op vomiting. If well at this stage, consider stepdown to double usual dose of oral hydrocortisone for a few days until well.
Endoscopy requiring bowel preparation	Admit for bowel preparation and list patient for earliest slot. During preparation, intravenous fluids, and parenteral hydrocortisone 50 mg every 6 hours should be considered. Consider 100 mg intravenous hydrocortisone at the start of the procedure. If well after the procedure, revert to double usual hydrocortisone for 24-48 hours.
Labor and cesarean section delivery	Administer 100 mg hydrocortisone intravenous or intramuscular at onset of labor or at start of cesarean, followed by 200 mg/day continuous intravenous infusions or 50 mg intramuscular/intravenous every 6 hours. After delivery, revert to double dose hydrocortisone for 24-48 hours.

50 mg/m^2 for the initial bolus, followed by 50 to 100 mg/m^2 over 24 hours. Additional fludrocortisone is not usually required in the acute phase since hydrocortisone at high doses exhibits good mineralocorticoid cross activity.

This treatment is usually continued until improving and stable, after which a weaning regime can be individualized. One such example would be to reduce the patient to 100 mg/day intravenous hydrocortisone after 24 hours, and then if well reduce further to double their usual hydrocortisone doses for a period, followed by further reduction to usual maintenance doses when well.

PREVENTION OF ADRENAL CRISIS

"Sick Day" Rules

All patients on long-term steroids, regardless of indication, should have advice on steroid management during acute illness or in the event of medical procedures. They should be advised never to omit steroids unless advised safe to do by a medical professional and should carry a steroid card or bracelet alerting medical personnel to their steroid dependency. All steroid-dependent patients should also be educated on the requirement and use of intramuscular hydrocortisone, for situations where symptoms of an impending adrenal crisis are evident or in situations where vomiting prevents them from taking their usual oral medications.

In the patient with normal adrenal function, physiological stress caused by acute illness, medical procedures, or extreme emotional stress would ordinarily trigger a rise in endogenous cortisol. In those with adrenal insufficiency, this response will be blunted and so need increased "stress-dosing" of glucocorticoid during such periods. It should be noted that patients with mineralocorticoid deficiency are at greater risk of fluid and electrolyte disturbance during procedures.

Table 79–8 details common sick day rules that can be used to guide patients.

SUGGESTED READING

Arlt W, Allolio B. Adrenal insufficiency. *Lancet*. 2003;361(9372): 1881-1893.

Betterle C, Lazzarotto F, Presotto F. Autoimmune polyglandular syndrome type 2: the tip of an iceberg. *Clin Exp Immunol*. 2004;137(2):225-233.

Bornstein SR, Allolio B, Arlt W, et al. Diagnosis and treatment of primary adrenal insufficiency: an endocrine society clinical practice guideline. *J Clin Endocrinol Metab*. 2016:101(2): 364-389.

Briet C, Salenave S, Bonneville JF, Laws ER, Chanson P. Pituitary apoplexy. *Endoc Rev*. 2015;36(6):622-645.

Broerson LHA, Pereira AM, Jørgenson JOL, Dekkers OM. Adrenal insufficiency in corticosteroid use: systematic review and meta-analysis. *J Clin Endocrinol Metab*. 2015;100(6):2171-2180.

Ceccato F, Scaroni C. Central adrenal insufficiency: open issues regarding diagnosis and glucocorticoid treatment. *Clin Chem Lab Med*. 2019;57(8):1125-1135.

Chabre O, Goichot B, Zenaty D, Bertherat J. Group 1: epidemiology of primary and secondary adrenal insufficiency: prevalence and incidence, acute adrenal insufficiency. *Ann Endocrinol (Paris)*. 2017;78(6):490-494.

Charmandari E, Nicolaides NC, Chrousos GP. Adrenal insufficiency. *Lancet*. 2014:383(9935):2152-2167.

Erichsen MM, Løvås K, Skinningsrud B, et al. Clinical, immunological, and genetic features of autoimmune primary adrenal insufficiency: observations from a Norwegian registry. *J Clin Endocrinol Metab*. 2009;94(12):4882-4890.

Esteban NV, Loughlin T, Yergey AL, et al. Daily cortisol production rate in man determined by stable isotope dilution/mass spectrometry. *J Clin Endocrinol Metab*. 1991;72(1):39-45.

Fleseriu M, Hashim IA, Karavitaki N, et al. Hormonal replacement in hypopituitarism in adults: an endocrine society clinical practice guideline. *J Clin Endocrinol Metab*. 2016;101(11): 3888-3921.

Freda PU. Pituitary incidentaloma: an endocrine society clinical practice guideline. *J Clin Endocrinol Metab*. 2011;96(4): 894-904.

Grouthier V, Lebrun-Vignes B, Moey M, et al. Immune-checkpoint inhibitor associated primary adrenal insufficiency: WHO VigiBase report analysis. *Oncologist*. 2020;25(8):696-701.

Gruber LM, Bancos I. Secondary adrenal insufficiency: recent updates and new directions for diagnosis and management. *Endocrine Practice*. 2022;28(1):110-117.

Husebye ES, Perheentupa J, Rauetemaa R, Kämpe O. Clinical manifestations, and management of patients with autoimmune polyendocrine syndrome type 1. *J Int Med*. 2009;265: 514-529.

Joshi MN, Whitelaw BC, Carroll PV. Mechanisms in endocrinology: hypophysitis: diagnosis and treatment. *Eur J Endocrinol*. 2018;179(3):R151-R163.

Karwacka IM, Obołończyk L, Sworczak K. Adrenal haemorrhage: a single centre experience and literature review. *Adv Clin Exp Med*. 2018;27(5):681-687.

Kristjansdottir HL, Bodvarsdottir SP, Sigurjonsdottir HA. Sheehan's syndrome in modern times: a nationwide retrospective study in Iceland. *Eur J Endocrinol*. 2011;164:349-354.

Leoutsakos B, Leoutsakos A. The adrenal glands: a brief historical perspective. *Hormones*. 2008;7(4):334-336.

Li X, Li Y, Cao Y, et al. Safety and efficacy of fractionated stereotactic radiotherapy and stereotactic radiosurgery for treatment of pituitary adenomas: a systematic review and meta-analysis. *J Neurol Sci*. 2017;372(15):110-116.

Lousada LM, Mendonca BB, Bachega TASS. Adrenal crisis and mortality rate in adrenal insufficiency and congenital adrenal hyperplasia. *Arch Endocrinol Metab*. 2021;65(4):488-494.

Marik PE, Pastores SM, Annane D, et al. Recommendations for the diagnosis and management of corticosteroid insufficiency in critically unwell adult patients: consensus statements from an international task force by the American College of Critical Care Medicine. *Crit Care Med*. 2008;36(6):1937-1948.

Merke DP, Mallappa A, Arlt W, et al. Modified-release hydrocortisone in congenital adrenal hyperplasia. *J Clin Endocrinol Metab*. 2021;106(5):e2063-e2077.

Simpson H, Tomlinson J, Wass J, Dean J, Arlt W. Guidance for the prevention and emergency management of adult patients with adrenal insufficiency. *Clin Med*. 2020;20(4):371-378.

Speiser PW, Arlt W, Auchus RJ, et al. Congenital adrenal hyperplasia due to steroid 21-hydroxylase deficiency: an endocrine society clinical practice guideline. *J Clin Endocrinol Metab*. 2018;103(11):4043-4088.

Timmermans S, Souffriau J, Libert C. A general introduction to glucocorticoid biology. *Front Immunol.* 2019;10:1545.

Van Staa TP, Leufkens HG, Abenhaim L, Begaud B, Zhang B, Cooper C. Use of oral corticosteroids in the United Kingdom. *QJM*. 2000;93:105-111.

Woods CP, Argese N, Chapman M, et al. Adrenal suppression in patients taking inhaled glucocorticoids is highly prevalent and management can be guided by morning cortisol. *Eur J Endocrinol.* 2015;173(5):633-642.

Yedinak C, Hameed N, Gassner M, Brzana J, McCartney S, Fleseriu M. Recovery rate of adrenal function after surgery in patients with acromegaly is higher than in those with non-functioning pituitary tumours: a large single centre study. *Pituitary*. 2015;18:701-709.

Index

Note: Page numbers by an "*f*" indicate figures; page numbers followed by a "*t*" indicate tables.